CYCLOSPORINE
Biological Activity and Clinical Applications

A Transplantation Proceedings Reprint
of Supplement 1, Volume XV, 1983

CYCLOSPORINE

VOLUME I

Biological Activity and Clinical Applications

Edited by

BARRY D. KAHAN, PH.D., M.D.
University of Texas Medical School
Houston, Texas

GRUNE & STRATTON, INC.
(Harcourt Brace Jovanovich, Publishers)
Orlando San Diego San Francisco New York London
Toronto Montreal Sydney Tokyo São Paulo

Cyclosporine: Biological Activity and Clinical Applications is the hardcover edition of Supplement 1 of the December 1983 issue (Volume XV, Number 4) of the bimonthly journal *Transplantation Proceedings*, an official publication of the Transplantation Society.

Grune & Stratton, Inc.
Orlando, FL 32887

Distributed in the United Kingdom by
Grune & Stratton, Ltd.
24/28 Oval Road, London NW 1

Library of Congress Catalog Number 84-47553
International Standard Book Number 0-8089-1651-3
Printed in the United States of America

84 85 86 87 10 9 8 7 6 5 4 3 2 1

THE FIRST INTERNATIONAL CONGRESS ON CYCLOSPORINE

President and Guest Editor

B.D. KAHAN, Ph.D., M.D.
Houston, Texas, USA

Honorary President

J.F. BOREL, Ph.D.
Basel, Switzerland

May 16–19, 1983
Houston, Texas

ACKNOWLEDGMENT

The Congress organizers acknowledge with gratitude the support of

SANDOZ PRODUCTS LTD.

for a very substantial contribution to the organization of the Congress, the publication costs of the *Proceedings,* and for a number of other services rendered to the Congress.

CONTENTS

Foreword .... *F. G. Moody* xxi

PREFACE

Cosmas and Damian Revisited .... *B. D. Kahan* xxv

MECHANISMS OF ACTION

Cyclosporine: Historical Perspectives .... *J. F. Borel* 3

Synthesis of Cyclosporine and Analogues: Structure, Activity, Relationships of New Cyclosporine Derivatives .... *R. Wenger* 14

Cyclosporine-A (CsA): Models for the Mechanism of Action .... *K. J. Lafferty, J. F. Borel, and P. Hodgkin* 26

Effect of Cyclosporine on the Induction of Cytotoxic T Lymphocytes: Role of Interleukin-1 and Interleukin-2 .... *A. D. Hess, P. J. Tutschka, and G. W. Santos* 32

Lack of Evidence for a Cyclosporine Receptor on Human Lymphocyte Membranes *S. J. LeGrue, A. W. Friedman, and B. D. Kahan* 43

Cyclosporine Binding Component in BW5147 Lymphoblasts and Normal Lymphoid Tissue .... *M. Merker, J. Rice, B. Schweitzer, and R. E. Handschumacher* 49

Effects of Cyclosporine on Experimental Infections .... *G. A. Cole, S. P. Nickell, F. Mokhtarian, and L. W. Scheibel* 55

Potential for Tolerance Induction With Cyclosporine ... *D. J. G. White, H. ff. S. Davies, N. Kamada, and T. Nagao* 62

CONTENTS

(continued)

IMMUNOSUPPRESSIVE PROPERTIES

CELL-MEDIATED IMMUNITY

The Effect of Cyclosporine A on Lymphocytes in Animal Models of Tissue Transplantation .... *P. J. Morris, D. W. Mason, and I. V. Hutchinson* 71

Cyclosporine Effects on Immunoregulatory Cells in Man .... *C. T. Van Buren, R. Kerman, S. Flechner, and B. D. Kahan* 77

Analysis of Lymphocytes Concerned in Spontaneous Blastogenesis During Acute Rejection.............. *T. Oka, N. Yoshimura, Y. Ohmori, I. Aikawa, T. Matsumura, T. Usui, K. Arakawa, and I. Hashimoto* 82

Immunologic Monitoring of Renal Allograft Recipients Treated with Cyclosporine *R. H. Kerman, S. M. Flechner, C. T. Van Buren, W. Payne, and B. D. Kahan* 86

Cyclosporine Effects on Mitogen-Induced T- and B-Cell Proliferation *H. G. A. Bouwer and D. J. Hinrichs* 90

Cyclosporine Selectively Inhibits Certain Mitotic Responses to Thymocytes *I. Gery, W. R. Benjamin, S. Jones, and R. B. Nussenblatt* 95

Cyclosporine Modulates the Human In Vitro T-Dependent Antigen-Induced Synthesis of Specific Antibody .... *J. B. Harley and A. S. Fauci* 99

Dissociation of T Helper-Cell Function and Helper-Cell Priming by Cyclosporine *G. G. B. Klaus and A. Kunkl* 105

Differential Effect of Cyclosporine on the Generation of Allogeneic Versus Syngeneic Cytotoxic T Lymphocytes .... *Z. K. Ballas and W. E. Schulte* 107

Differential In Vitro Action of Cyclosporine on Non-T-Cell and T-Cell Responses to Non-HLA Alloantigens: Significance for MHC-Independent Graft-Versus-Host Disease.. *L. Delmonte* 112

Induction of Suppressor T Lymphocytes in Mice Treated with Cyclosporine *N. Yoshimura, T. Oka, Y. Ohmori, I. Aikawa, M. Fukuda, Y. Kondoh, and I. Hashimoto* 118

Suppressor Cells in Cyclosporine-Induced Long-Term Graft Acceptance in the Rat *K. Sakamoto, T. Ochiai, N. Shinohara, T. Asano, and H. Sato* 124

Suppressor-Cell Amplification Circuitry in Cyclosporine-Treated MLR Cultures *A. D. Hess, A. D. Donnenberg, P. Engel, P. J. Tutschka, and G. W. Santos* 127

The Immunosuppressive Action of Cyclosporine in Man........................ *R. M. Ferguson and R. Fidelus-Gort* 134

Population of Cyclosphosphamide-Sensitive T Suppressor Cells Maintain Cyclosporine-Induced Allograft Survival .... *J. W. Kupiec-Weglinski, P. A. Lear, T. B. Strom, and N. L. Tilney* 141

Effects of Cyclosporine on the Efferent Limb of the Immune Response *M. Mochizuki, R. B. Nussenblatt, T. Kuwabara, and I. Gery* 148

CONTENTS
(continued)

Pulmonary Macrophage and Polymorphonuclear Leukocyte Function in Response to Immunosuppressive Therapy .... *D. B. Drath and B. D. Kahan* 151

Effect of Cyclosporine Alone or Combined with Prednisolone or Azathioprine on Macrophage Phagocytosis .... *A. Rios, L. H. Toledo-Pereyra, and S. Buscetta* 157

Inhibitory Effect of Cyclosporine on Adherent Cells in Oxidation-Induced Lymphocyte Proliferation .... *K. Uyemura, J. F. P. Dixon, and J. W. Parker* 160

HUMORAL MEDIATORS

Effect of Cyclosporine on Human Leukocyte Interferon Production: Selective Inhibition of IFN-Gamma Synthesis .... *J. Abb and H. Abb* 164

Effects of Cyclosporine on the Production of Various Interferons *V. K. Kalman and G. R. Klimpel* 167

Cyclosporine Inhibits Interleukin-2 and Interferon Gamma Synthesis by Human Thymocytes .... *G. H. Reem, L. A. Cook, and M. A. Palladino* 171

Cyclosporine and Lymphokines Affecting Macrophage Behavior *A. W. Thomson, D. K. Moon, C. L. Geczy, and D. S. Nelson* 174

Relationship Between IL-2 Receptors and Cyclosporine-Induced Suppression of T Leukemia and T Helper Cells .... *C. C.-Y. Shih, R. L. Truitt, P. Abramoff, and M. M. Bortin* 178

Effect of Cyclosporine on Prostacyclin Synthesis by Vascular Tissue in Rabbits *G. H. Neild, G. Rocchi, L. Imberti, F. Fumagalli, Z. Brown, G. Remuzzi, and D. G. Williams* 182

PHARMACOKINETICS

Methods to Measure Cyclosporine Levels—High Pressure Liquid Chromatography, Radioimmunoassay, and Correlation .... *W. T. Robinson, H. F. Schran, and E. P. Barry* 187

Cyclosporine: Pharmacokinetics, Metabolism, and Drug Interactions .... *A. J. Wood, G. Maurer, W. Niederberger, and T. Beveridge* 193

Cyclosporine Pharmacokinetics in Man .... *J. Newburger and B. D. Kahan* 197

Pharmacokinetics and Toxicity of Cyclosporine in Marrow Transplant Patients *M. S. Kennedy, G. C. Yee, H. J. Deeg, R. Storb, and E. D. Thomas* 200

Distribution and Binding of Cyclosporine in Blood and Tissues .... *W. Niederberger, M. Lemaire, G. Maurer, K. Nussbaumer, and O. Wagner* 203

In Vitro Stability and Storage of Cyclosporine in Human Serum and Plasma *J. Smith, J. Hows, and E. C. Gordon-Smith* 206

Distribution and Transfer of Cyclosporine Among the Various Human Lipoprotein Classes .... *W. Mraz, R. A. Zink, A. Graf, D. Preis, W. D. Illner, W. Land, W. Siebert, and H. Zöttlein* 210

CONTENTS

(continued)

Blood and Tissue Distribution of Cyclosporine in Humans and Mice .... *K. Atkinson, J. Boland, K. Britton, and J. Biggs* 214

Cyclosporine Levels in Human Tissues of Patients Treated for One Week to One Year *M. Ried, S. Gibbons, D. Kwok, C. T. Van Buren, S. Flechner, and B. D. Kahan* 218

The Clinical Relevance of Cyclosporine Blood Levels As Measured by Radioimmunoassay .... *P. A. Keown, C. R. Stiller, N. R. Sinclair, G. Carruthers, W. Howson, M. Stawecki, J. McMichael, J. Koegler, N. McKenzie, and W. Wall* 222

Pharmacologic Monitoring in the Clinical Use of Cyclosporine *F. Lokiec, A. Devergie, O. Poirier, and E. Gluckman* 226

Detrimental Effect of Intestinal Disease on Absorption of Orally Administered Cyclosporine .... *K. Atkinson, K. Britton, P. Paull, C. Farrell, A. Concannon, A. Dodds, and J. Biggs* 230

Variable Tempo of Cyclosporine Peaks and Troughs in a Lung Transplant Recipient: Importance of Frequent Monitoring .... *S. L. Nehlsen-Cannarella, F. J. Veith, S. L. Kamholz, C. M. Montefusco, F. P. Mollenkopf, J. Goldsmith, and R. Kaleya* 234

CLINICAL TRANSPLANTATION

KIDNEY TRANSPLANTATION

The Colorado-Pittsburgh Cadaveric Renal Transplantation Study with Cyclosporine *T. E. Starzl, T. R. Hakala, J. T. Rosenthal, S. Iwatsuki, and B. W. Shaw, Jr.* 243

Comparison of Cyclosporine Versus Azathioprine-Antilymphocyte Globulin in Renal Transplantation .... *J. S. Najarian, M. Strand, D. S. Fryd, R. M. Ferguson, R. L. Simmons, N. L. Ascher, and D. E. R. Sutherland* 247

Cyclosporine Immunosuppression Mitigates Immunologic Risk Factors in Renal Allotransplantation .... *B. D. Kahan, C. T. Van Buren, S. M. Flechner, W. D. Payne, M. Boileau, and R. H. Kerman* 253

The Canadian Trial of Cyclosporine: Cyclosporine Therapy Compared to Standard Immunosuppression in Renal Transplants: An Exploration of Nephrotoxicity *C. Stiller, London, Canada, for The Canadian Transplant Study Group* 263

Australian Trial of Cyclosporine (Csa) in Cadaveric Donor Renal Transplantation *A. G. R. Sheil, B. M. Hall, D. J. Tiller, M. S. Stephen, J. P. Harris, G. G. Duggin, J. S. Horvath, J. R. Johnson, J. R. Rogers, and J. Boulas* 269

The Requirements for Maintenance Steroids in Cyclosporine-Treated Renal Transplant Recipients .... *C. Stiller, London, Canada, for The Canadian Transplant Study Group* 274

A Prospective Randomized Substitutive Trial of Cyclosporine as a Prophylactic Agent in Human Renal Transplant Rejection .... *R. A. Sells* 279

CONTENTS

(continued)

Living Related Kidney Transplants Treated with Cyclosporine....... *T. Oka, Y. Ohmori, I. Aikawa, J. Ioka, Y. Kadotani, H. Nomura, S. Suzuki, and I. Hashimoto* 285

Improved Outcome in Renal Transplant Recipients Above 55 Years of Age Treated with Cyclosporine and Low Doses of Steroids ....*O. Ringdén, L. Öst, G. Klintmalm, A. Tillegård, I. Fehrman, H. Wilczek, and C. G. Groth* 291

Randomized Comparison Between Cyclosporine and Conventional Therapy Plus Minnesota Antilymphocyte Globulin in Cadaveric Renal Transplantation *P. Halloran, D. Ludwin, M. Aprile, J. Lien, N. White, and the Canadian Transplant Study Group* 297

Cadaveric Renal Transplantation with Cyclosporine: Experiences in 148 Patients at a Single Institution .... *W. Land, L. A. Castro, K. Günther, C. Hammer, C. Hillebrand, W. -D. Illner, N. Schmeller, B. Schneider, W. Siebert, R. A. Zink, and H. Zöttlein* 301

Cyclosporine in Cadaveric Renal Transplantation: A Prospective Randomized Trial *P. McMaster, I. G. Haynes, J. Michael, D. Adu, T. Vlassis, S. Roger, J. Turney, S. Stock, J. Buckels, P. Mackintosh, and M. Ezzibdeh* 307

Renal Transplantation Using Cyclosporine in Pediatric Patients 3 to 17 Years Old *S. B. Conley, E. D. Brewer, S. M. Flechner, C. T. Van Buren, and B. D. Kahan* 312

Cyclosporine and Steroids: Effects on the Clinical Course After Renal Allotransplantation ....*H. Bunzendahl, K. Wonigeit, J. Klempnauer, C. Brölsch, and R. Pichlmayr* 315

Cyclosporine for Steroid-Resistant Rejection in Azathioprine-Treated Renal Graft Recipients .... *A. S. MacDonald, P. Belitsky, A. Cohen, J. Crocker, R. Gupta, S. G. Lannon, and J. White* 319

A Critical Look at Renal Allografts That Failed in Patients Receiving Cyclosporine *T. Kovithavongs, W. H. Lakey, R. Boake, K. B. Bettcher, P. McCormick, and J. B. Dossetor* 322

HEART AND LUNG TRANSPLANTATION

Cyclosporine in Cardiac Transplantation: A 2½ Year Follow-Up.................. *P. E. Oyer, E. B. Stinson, S. W. Jamieson, S. A. Hunt, M. Perlroth, M. Billingham, and N. E. Shumway* 330

Experience with Cyclosporine in Cardiac Transplantation..................... *R. L. Hardesty, B. P. Griffith, R. F. Debski, and H. T. Bahnson* 337

Cyclosporine for Cardiac Transplantation: U. K. Trial ....*J. Wallwork, R. Cory-Pearce, and T. A. H. English* 343

Cardiac and Cardiopulmonary Transplantation Using Cyclosporine For Immunosuppression: Recent Texas Heart Institute Experience *D. A. Cooley, O. H. Frazier, G. A. Painvin, L. Boldt, and B. D. Kahan* 351

CONTENTS
(continued)

New Onset of Hypertension Following Cardiac Transplantation: A Preliminary Report and Analysis .... *M. E. Thompson, A. P. Shapiro, A. M. Johnsen, R. Reeves, J. Itzkoff, E. Ginchereau, R. L. Hardesty, B. L. Griffith, H. T. Bahnson, and R. McDonald, Jr.* 357

Single Lung Transplantation with Cyclosporine Immunosuppression *S. L. Kamholz, F. J. Veith, C. M. Montefusco, K. L. Pinsker, F. P. Mollenkopf, R. Kaleya, J. Goldsmith, A. J. Norin, E. E. Emeson, S. N. Cannarella, and M. L. Gliedman* 362

LIVER AND PANCREAS TRANSPLANTATION

Report of Colorado-Pittsburgh Liver Transplantation Studies .... *T. E. Starzl, S. Iwatsuki, D. H. Van Thiel, J. C. Gartner, B. J. Zitelli, J. J. Malatack, R. R. Schade, B. W. Shaw, Jr., T. R. Hakala, and J. T. Rosenthal* 366

Special Aspects of Immunosuppression with Cyclosporine in Liver Transplantation *K. Wonigeit, C. Brölsch, P. Neuhaus, M. Burdelski, E. Schmidt, W. Lang, and R. Pichlmayr* 370

Hepatic Homograft Survival in Pediatric Orthotopic Liver Transplantation with Cyclosporine and Steroids .... *B. J. Zitelli, J. C. Gartner, Jr., J. J. Malatack, B. W. Shaw, Jr., S. Iwatsuki, and T. E. Starzl* 376

Pancreas Transplantation: Overview and Current Status of Cases Reported to the Registry Through 1982 .... *D. E. R. Sutherland* 381

Cyclosporine in Clinical Pancreatic Transplantation.........*J. Traeger, J. M. Dubernard, E. Bosi, A. Gelet, S. El Yafi, A. Secchi, G. Pozza, and J. L. Touraine* 386

Experience with Cyclosporine Versus Azathioprine for Pancreas Transplantation *D. E. R. Sutherland, P. L. Chinn, F. C. Goetz, B. A. Elick, and J. S. Najarian* 390

BONE MARROW TRANSPLANTATION

Cyclosporine in Clinical Marrow Transplantation: The Baltimore Experience *P. J. Tutschka, A. D. Hess, W. E. Beschorner, E. R. Farmer, R. Saral, R. Brookmeyer, and G. W. Santos* 397

Allogeneic Bone Marrow Transplantation: The Basel Trial with Cyclosporine *B. Speck, A. Gratwohl, B. Osterwalder, E. Signer, C. Nissen, M. Corneo, and M. Jeannet* 401

Preliminary Results of Prospective Randomized Trials Comparing Methotrexate and Cyclosporine for Prophylaxis of Graft-vs.-Host-Disease After HLA-Identical Marrow Transplantations ......*R. Storb, H. J. Deeg, E. D. Thomas, C. D. Buckner, R. A. Clift, N. Flournoy, M. S. Kennedy, K. Doney, F. R. Appelbaum, J. E. Sanders, P. Stewart, H. Shulman, K. M. Sullivan, and R. P. Witherspoon* 404

CONTENTS

(continued)

Cyclosporine for the Prevention of Graft-vs.-Host Disease in 72 Patients with Acute Myeloblastic Leukemia in First Remission Receiving Matched Sibling Bone Marrow Transplants
R. L. Powles, B. Evans, C. Poole, A. Pedrazzini, M. Crofts, C. Pollard, and G. Hughes 408

Use of Cyclosporine as Prophylaxis of Graft-vs.-Host Disease After Human Allogeneic Bone Marrow Transplantation: Report of 38 Patients
E. Gluckman, A. Devergie, O. Poirier, and F. Lokiec 412

Postgraft Immunosuppression with Cyclosporine in Allogeneic Bone Marrow Transplantation for Severe Aplastic Anemia
J. M. Hows, J. L. Yin, P. M. Chipping, S. M. Fairhead, S. Palmer, and E. C. Gordon-Smith 418

CLINICAL CASE PRESENTATIONS

The Management of Kidney Transplant Recipients Treated With Cyclosporine
B. D. Kahan 425

The Management of Heart Transplant Recipients Treated With Cyclosporine
B. D. Kahan 433

WORKSHOPS ON PATIENT MANAGEMENT

Practical Aspects on Renal Transplant Management .... *B. D. Kahan* 449

Pancreas Transplantation .... *J. M. Dubernard and E. Bosi* 460

Practical Aspects of Cardiac Transplant Patient Management .... *C. T. Van Buren* 462

CYCLOSPORINE TOXICITY

The Nephrotoxicity of Cyclosporine in Renal Transplant Recipients
S. M. Flechner, C. Van Buren, R. H. Kerman, and B. D. Kahan 473

Renal Effects of Cyclosporine: Clinical and Experimental Observations
R. Devineni, N. McKenzie, J. Duplan, P. Keown, C. Stiller, and A. C. Wallace 479

Cyclosporine in Patients With Oligoanuria After Cadaveric Kidney Transplantation
L. A. Castro, G. Hillebrand, W. Land, B. Schneider, K. Günther, and H. J. Gurland 483

Nephrotoxicity of Cyclosporine in Combination With Aminoglycoside and Cephalosporin Antibiotics .... *P. H. Whiting, J. G. Simpson, and A. W. Thomson* 486

Renal Failure in Heart Transplant Patients Receiving Cyclosporine
J. Egel, A. Greenberg, M. E. Thompson, R. L. Hardesty, B. P. Griffith, H. T. Bahnson, R. L. Bernstein, and J. B. Puschett 490

CONTENTS
(continued)

Nephrotoxicity in Marrow Graft Recipients Treated With Cyclosporine
J. M. Hows, J. M. Smith, A. Baughan, and E. C. Gordon-Smith 492

Increasing the Hepatic Metabolism of Cyclosporine Abolishes Nephrotoxicity
C. Cunningham, P. H. Whiting, M. D. Burke, D. N. Wheatley, and J. G. Simpson 496

Demonstration of Cyclosporine in Renal Transplants by Fine Needle Aspiration Biopsy .... *E. von Willebrand and P. Häyry* 500

Cyclosporine, the Renin-Angiotensin-Aldosterone System, and Renal Adverse Reactions
H. Siegl, B. Ryffel, R. Petric, P. Shoemaker, A. Muller, P. Donatsch, and M. Mihatsch 503

Cyclosporine-Associated Hyperkalemia
R. J. Foley, C. T. Van Buren, R. Hamner, and E. J. Weinmann 510

Cyclosporine and Sodium and Potassium Excretion in the Rat
A. S. Tonnesen, R. W. Hamner, and E. J. Weinmann 514

Nephrotoxicity of Cyclosporine-An Animal Model: Study of the Nephrotoxic Effect of Cyclosporine on Overall Renal and Tubular Function in Conscious Rats
H. Dieperink, H. Starklint, and P. P. Leyssac 520

Rat Composite Tissue Allograft Recipients Demonstrate a Dose-Related Increase in Renal Toxicity With Therapeutic Doses of Cyclosporine
C. W. Hewitt, K. S. Black, L. A. Fraser, E. B. Howard, A. Ingerman, B. Philosophe, B. M. Achauer, D. C. Martin, and D. W. Furnas 526

Complications of Cyclosporine Therapy-A Comparison to Azathioprine
A. Laupacis, London, Canada, for the Canadian Transplant Study Group 532

Cyclosporine and Liver Function in Renal Allograft Recipients
R. S. C. Rodger, J. H. Turney, I. Haines, J. Michael, D. Adu, and P. McMaster 538

Cholestasis in Heart Transplant Recipients Treated With Cyclosporine
R. R. Schade, A. Guglielmi, D. H. Van Thiel, M. E. Thompson, V. Warty, B. Griffith, A. Sanghvi, H. Bahnson, and R. Hardesty 541

Cyclosporine-Associated Hepatotoxicity After Allogeneic Marrow Transplantation in Man: Differentiation From Other Causes of Posttransplant Liver Disease
K. Atkinson, J. Biggs, A. Dodds, and A. Concannon 545

Infections in Kidney, Heart, and Liver Transplant Recipients on Cyclosporine
M. Ho, C. P. Wajszczuk, A. Hardy, J. S. Dummer, T. E. Starzl, T. R. Hakala, and H. T. Bahnson 552

Infection in Renal Transplant Recipients on Cyclosporine: Pneumocystis Pneumonia
A. M. Hardy, C. P. Wajszczuk, T. R. Hakala, J. T. Rosenthal, T. E. Starzl, and M. Ho 557

Cellular Immune Response and Cytomegalovirus Infection in Renal Transplant Recipients Receiving Cyclosporine
C. R. Rinaldo, Jr., W. H. Hamoudi, R. L. DeBiasio, B. Rabin, T. R. Hakala, and M. Liebert 559

CONTENTS
(continued)

Infections in Patients on Cyclosporine and Prednisone Following Cardiac Transplantation .... *J. S. Dummer, H. T. Bahnson, B. P. Griffith, R. L. Hardesty, M. E. Thompson, and M. Ho* 563

Glomerular Thrombi and Infarction in Rabbits with Serum Sickness Following Cyclosporine Therapy .... *G. H. Neild, K. Ivory, and D. G. Williams* 566

Occurrence of Hemolytic Uremic Syndrome Under Cyclosporine Treatment: Accident or Possible Side Effect Mediated by a Lack of Prostacyclin-Stimulating Plasma Factor?
C. Leithner, H. Sinzinger, E. Pohanka, M. Schwarz, G. Kretschmer, and G. Syré 571

Lymphomas Complicating Organ Transplantation .... *I. Penn* 574

Immunoglobulin Abnormalities and Infectious Lymphoproliferative Syndrome (ILPS) in Cyclosporine-Treated Transplant Patients
J. L. Touraine, S. El Yafi, E. Bosi, C. Chapuis-Cellier, J. Ritter, N. Blanc, J. M. Dubernard, C. Pouteil-Noble, M. Chevalier, R. Creyssel, and J. Traeger 582

Histiocytic Lymphoma in Renal Transplant Patients Receiving Cyclosporine
J. T. Rosenthal, S. Iwatsuki, T. E. Starzl, R. J. Taylor, and T. R. Hakala 589

Malignant Lymphoma in Nontransplanted Cynomolgus Monkeys Receiving Cyclosporine
N. L. Garnett, H. R. Taylor, G. J. Hoffman, R. L. Heberling, R. F. Ambinder, A. C. Huber, and B. A. Valentine 592

PROBLEMS IN DIFFERENTIAL DIAGNOSIS—TOXICITY VERSUS ALLOGRAFT REJECTION

Clinical and Laboratory Signs in Nephrotoxicity and Rejection in Cyclosporine-Treated Renal Allograft Recipients
G. Klintmalm, O. Ringdén, and C. G. Groth 599

Morphological Findings in Kidney Transplants After Treatment with Cyclosporine
M. J. Mihatsch, G. Thiel, H. P. Spichtin, M. Oberholzer, F. P. Brunner, F. Harder, V. Olivieri, R. Bremer, B. Ryffel, E. Stöcklin, J. Torhorst, F. Gudat, H. U. Zollinger, and R. Loertscher 605

Morphology of Cyclosporine Nephrotoxicity and of Acute Rejection in Cyclosporine-Prednisone–Immunosuppressed Renal Allograft Recipients
R. K. Sibley, R. M. Ferguson, D. E. R. Sutherland, R. L. Simmons, and J. S. Najarian 620

Effects of Cyclosporine on Human Renal Allograft Rejection: An Ad Interim Report
P. Häyry, J. Ahonen, E. von Willebrand, B. Eklund, K. Höckerstedt, K. Salmela, E. Pettersson, A. Kauste, E. Taskinen, M. Lalla, H. Sarelin, B. Kuhlbäck, M. Kääriäinen, R. Paldanius, E. Lampainen, K. Huttunen, M. Viranta, T. Vänttinen, J. Forström, V. A. Myllyniemi, L. Tarssanen, U. M. Henttula, A. Helanterä, A. Relander, H. Borgmästars, A. Linkola, E. Leijala, P. Kunelius, A. Vartia, M. Eloranta, S. Pajunen, and H. Granlund 626

CONTENTS
(continued)

Tubular Changes in Renal Transplant Recipients on Cyclosporine .... *S. Thiru, E. R. Maher, D. V. Hamilton, D. B. Evans, and R. Y. Calne* 630

Pathology in Renal Transplant Patients Treated with Cyclosporine *A. Farnsworth, B. M. Hall, P. Kirwan, G. A. Bishop, G. C. Duggin, B. Goodman, J. Horvath, J. Johnson, A. Ng, A. G. R. Sheil, and D. J. Tiller* 636

CYCLOSPORINE CONVERSION AND USE AS ADJUNCTIVE THERAPY

Conversion Rejection Consequences by Changing the Immunosuppressive Therapy From Cyclosporine to Azathioprine After Kidney Transplantation *W. Land, L. A. Castro, G. Hillebrand, K. Günther, and J. M. Gokel* 641

The Consequences of Conversion From Cyclosporine to Azathioprine and Prednisolone in Renal Allograft Recipients .... *R. F. M. Wood, J. F. Thompson, N. H. Allen, A. Ting, and P. J. Morris* 646

The Effect of Conversion From Cyclosporine to Azathioprine Immunosuppression for Intractable Nephrotoxicity .... *S. M. Flechner, C. T. Van Buren, R. Kerman, and B. D. Kahan* 653

Cyclosporine Nephrotoxicity in Renal Allograft Recipients: Conversion to Azathioprine to Improve Renal Function ...... *D. M. Canafax, D. E. R. Sutherland, N. L. Ascher, R. L. Simmons, and J. S. Najarian* 658

Conversion Problem—Azathioprine to Cyclosporine .... *K. Rolles, R. Merion, and R. Y. Calne* 662

Total Lymphoid Irradiation and Cyclosporine .... *D. E. R. Sutherland, R. M. Ferguson, M. I. Aeder, W. I. Lewis, F. R. Bentley, N. L. Ascher, R. L. Simmons, and J. S. Najarian* 665

Use of Cyclosporine and Monoclonal Antibodies in Clinical Renal Transplantation *N. L. Tilney, R. L. Kirkman, J. L. Araujo, C. B. Carpenter, E. L. Milford, E. L. Reinherz, S. F. Schlossman, and T. B. Strom* 673

EFFECTS IN AUTOIMMUNITY, VIRAL AND FUNGAL INFECTIONS

Effect of Cyclosporine on Antigen Presentation: Relationship to Lupus *M. Fischbach and N. Talal* 683

Response of Murine Autoimmune Disease to Cyclosporine and Thiols *M. G. Jones, G. Harris, and G. Cowing* 688

The Effect of Cyclosporine on Lymphocyte Subsets in Experimental Allergic Encephalomyelitis: Functional Loss of Disease-Suppressing Cells In Vivo *L. M. Fredane, G. A. Hashim, and R. E. McCabe* 693

CONTENTS
(continued)

Cyclosporine Therapy in the Treatment of Uveitis .... *R. B. Nussenblatt, A. G. Palestine, C. C. Chan, W. C. Leake, A. H. Rook, I. Scher, and I. Gery* 698

The Effects of Cyclosporine on Viruses .... *X. E. Gui, R. W. Atchison, and M. Ho* 701

In Vitro Effects of Cyclosporine on Lymphocyte Responses to Cytomegalovirus *P. J. Converse, A. D. Hess, P. J. Tutschka, and G. W. Santos* 707

In Vitro and In Vivo Antifungal Activity of Cyclosporine .... *M. S. Osato, T. J. Roussel, K. R. Wilhelmus, and D. B. Jones* 711

EXPERIMENTAL TRANSPLANTATION

KIDNEY

Combination Immunotherapy With Low-Dose Cyclosporine and Azathioprine in Splenectomized Canine Recipients of Renal Allografts .... *M. I. Aeder, D. E. R. Sutherland, W. I. Lewis, and J. S. Najarian* 717

Cyclosporine Enhances an Effect of Donor-Specific Blood Tranfusion in Canine Renal Transplantation .... *T. Ochiai, M. Gunji, M. Nagata, T. Suzuki, K. Enomoto, T. Asano, N. Yamada, H. Sato, and M. Ohtsuka* 723

Immunosuppression of Renal Allograft Rejection by Perioperative Administration of the Combination of Histocompatibility Antigen in the Form of 3M KCl Extract or Blood Transfusion and Cyclosporine .... *T. Yasumura and B. D. Kahan* 726

Reversal of Kidney and Prevention of Pancreas Transplant Rejection With Cyclosporine in Beagles............ *G. K. Kyriakides, L. Olson, C. Flaa, and J. Miller* 734

Inhibition of Chronic Kidney Allograft Rejection by Cyclosporine *R. L. Marquet, W. Weimar, E. Heineman, and J. Jeekel* 737

HEART AND LUNG

Orthotopic Cardiac Transplantation in the Cyclosporine-Treated Neonate *L. Bailey, Z. Li, F. Lacour-Gayet, P. Perier, D. Killeen, J. Perry, C. Schmidt, H. Roost, and W. Jolley* 740

Benefit From Circadian Timing of Cyclosporine Revealed by Delay of Rejection of Murine Heart Allograft .... *M. Cavallini, G. Magnus, F. Halberg, L. Tao, M. Y. Field, R. Sibley, J. S. Najarian, and D. E. R. Sutherland* 744

Synergistic Effect of a Nucleotide-Free Diet and Cyclosporine on Allograft Survival *C. T. Van Buren, A. Kulkarni, and F. Rudolph* 751

Prolonged Heart Allograft Survival in Cyclosporine-Treated Presensitized Rats *J. A. Schulak, J. Shelby, E. Wakely, and R. J. Corry* 753

Effect of Cyclosporine on Lymphocyte Migration in Rat Cardiac Transplantation *N. Kuromoto, C. Iga, R. Fawwaz, R. Nowygrod, K. Reemtsma, and M. A. Hardy* 757

Studies With T Cells From Long-Term Surviving Canine Lung Allograft Recipients: Reduced Lymphocyte-Mediated Cytotoxicity But Not Reduced Mixed Lymphocyte Reactivity .... *A. J. Norin, E. E. Emeson, K. L. Pinsker, S. L. Kamholz, and F. J. Veith* 763

LIVER, PANCREAS, INTESTINE

Histologic Evidence of Modification of Liver Allograft Rejection in Inbred Miniature Swine by Cyclosporine .... *M. W. Flye* 767

Induction of Liver Graft Tolerance in a Primarily Nontolerant Rat Strain Combination With Temporary Treatment of Cyclosporine
R. Engemann, K. Ulrichs, A. Thiede, W. Müller-Ruchholtz, and H. Hamelmann 770

The Effect of Cyclosporine Alone and in Combination With Steroids on Experimental Segmental Pancreatic Allografts in the Baboon
D. F. Du Toit, J. J. Heydenrych, G. Louw, T. Zuurmond, L. Laker, D. Els, and S. Woolfe-Coote 776

Segmental Pancreatic Allotransplantation With High-Dose Cyclosporine and Low-Dose Prednisone
H. W. Sollinger, D. Kamps, K. Cook, T. Warner, N. R. Glass, and F. O. Belzer 781

Pancreas and Kidney Allograft Rejection Responds Differently to Cyclosporine Immunosuppression
J. Klempnauer, E. Wagner, B. Steiniger, K. Wonigeit, and R. Pichlmayr 785

Effect of Cyclosporine on Allotransplanted Pancreatic Islets in DLA-MLC-Compatible Dogs.................................. *M. D. Williams, R. Walshaw, R. W. Bull, W. D. Schall, G. A. Padgett, V. V. Gossain, and R. F. Nachreiner* 788

The Effect of Cyclosporine on Simultaneous Skin and Pancreatic Islet Allografts in the Rabbit............................*W. B. Jolley, K. Knierim, J. Ham, and J. K. Longerbeam* 795

Pharmacokinetics of Cyclosporine in a Canine Intestinal Transplantation Model
Z. Cohen, S. R. Nordgren, R. D. Mackenzie, A. G. Lossing, C. R. Stiller, and B. Langer 797

Successful Small Bowel Allografts in Piglets Using Cyclosporine
C. Ricour, Y. Revillon, F. Arnaud-Battandier, D. Ghnassia, P. Weyne, A. Lauffenburger, J. Jos, J. L. Fontaine, P. Gallix, and M. Vaiman 803

Prevention of Graft-Versus-Host Reaction Following Small Bowel Transplantation by Temporary Cyclosporine Treatment
E. Deltz, K. Ulrichs, R. Engemann, T. Schack, B. Friedrichs, W. Müller-Ruchholtz, H. K. Müller-Hermelink, and A. Thiede 811

Uptake of ^{14}C-Glucose by the Transplanted Small Intestine
S. Nordgren, Z. Cohen, R. Mackenzie, D. Finkelstein, G. R. Greenberg, and B. Langer 816

(Continued)

CONTENTS
(continued)

BONE MARROW

Studies on the Immunobiology of Syngeneic and Autologous Graft-Versus-Host Disease in Cyclosporine-Treated Rats .. *A. Glazier, P. J. Tutschka, and E. Farmer* 819

Suppressor and Cytotoxic Cells in DLA Nonidentical Canine Radiation Chimeras Given Cyclosporine and Methotrexate as Prophylaxis for Graft-Versus-Host Disease .... *H. J. Deeg, R. F. Raff, E. Severns, F. R. Appelbaum, E. D. Thomas, and R. Storb* 826

The Effect of Cyclosporine on Host-Versus-Graft Disease in Canine Bone Marrow Transplantation .... *A. M. Miller, E. P. Walma, W. Klapwijk, and D. W. Van Bekkum* 830

EFFECTS ON WOUND HEALING, COMPOSITE GRAFTS, SKIN, CORNEA, AND VEIN ALLOGRAFTS

Effects of Cyclosporine on the Healing of Vascularized and Nonvascularized Bone Allografts in Rodents .... *P. F. Halloran, M. Bushuk, and J. A. Stewart* 837

Modification of Experimental Limb Allograft Rejection With Cyclosporine and Prednisone: A Preliminary Report .... *B. H. J. Press, R. K. Sibley, and A. R. Shons* 841

Cyclosporine and Long-Term Survival of Composite Tissue Allografts (Limb Transplants) in Rats (With Historical Notes on the Role of Plastic Surgeons in Allotransplantation) .... *D. W. Furnas, K. S. Black, C. W. Hewitt, L. A. Fraser, and B. M. Achauer* 847

Diagnosis of Rejection and Functional Analysis of Composite Tissue (CT) and Skin Allografts Prolonged with Cyclosporine *K. S. Black, C. W. Hewitt, E. B. Howard, L. A. Fraser, B. J. Mah, J. C. Koumas, and B. M. Achauer* 853

Cyclosporine Prolongs Skin Allografts in a Rat Burn Model *B. M. Achauer, C. W. Hewitt, K. S. Black, B. Philosophe, R. L. Linfesty, and D. W. Furnas* 857

Concomitant Transfusion and Cyclosporine-Induced Enhancement of Rabbit Skin Allografts: Histocompatibility Requirements *G. J. A. Clunie, L. J. Dumble, H. P. King, L. G. Bowes, P. Masendycz, and A. Mirisklavos* 861

Cyclosporine and Experimental Corneal Transplantation *T. J. Roussel, M. S. Osato, and K. R. Wilhelmus* 865

Improved Survival of Venous Allografts in Dogs Following Graft Pretreatment With Cyclosporine *K. O. Bandlien, L. H. Toledo-Pereyra, M. I. Barnhart, S. P. Choudbury, A. Diaz-Velez, G. H. MacKenzie, and J. A. Cortez* 868

(Continued)

CONTENTS

(continued)

Effect of Cyclosporine on Wound Healing .... *J. Ahonen, A. Nemlander, K. Wiktorowicz, E. von Willebrand, R. Hekali, M. Lalla, and P. Häyry* 876

SUMMATION

Basic Science Summation .... *J. F. Borel and K. J. Lafferty* 881

Clinical Aspects of Cyclosporine Therapy: A Summation .... *T. E. Starzl* 887

Author Index 892

Foreword

F. G. Moody

FEW events in medicine are more gratifying than the successful transplantation of an organ from one person to another. The rapid development of this unique therapy for end-stage disease has depended upon the courage of the receivers, the generosity of the donors, and the extraordinary efforts of surgeons and their scientific health care collaborators. Although the logistics of organ procurement, preservation, and placement are in various phases of resolution, the problem of rejection has persisted as a major detractor from the safety and efficacy of the procedure. Cyclosporine, as is so elegantly expressed in the pages of this book, offers the hope for a major breakthrough in modifying the immunologic relationship between the recipients and their new organs.

The First International Cyclosporine Congress provided an appropriate forum for an in-depth analysis of the virtues and potential faults of this remarkable drug. Dr. Kahan and his colleagues have recorded in elaborate detail the context of this discussion in the pages that follow. It is likely that the book *Cyclosporine* will be for many years to come the scientific baedeker for those seeking ways to improve and extend the therapy of tissue and organ transplantation. Clearly, this is not the last word on cyclosporine. There is much that remains to be done towards reducing its toxicity, defining its mechanism of action, and extending its therapeutic usefulness. My congratulations to those who have worked so hard to bring this remarkable drug into the mainstream of medical practice.

From the Department of Surgery, The University of Texas, Health Science Center at Houston, 6431 Fannin St., Houston, TX 77030.

PREFACE

Cosmas and Damian Revisited

B. D. Kahan

THE LIVES OF THE SAINTS

COSMAS and Damian, twin brothers, were born in the second half of the third century in Arabia (presumably Asia Minor) to devout Christian parents. Their father was martyred in a persecution and their mother, Teodata, was noted for her piety. The boys, nurtured in an atmosphere of love and compassion, grew up with a strong sense of commitment to their faith. After completing their studies of letters, the brothers set off for Syria to study medicine, convinced that the Holy Spirit called them to heal the sick. Then, qualified to practice their art, Cosmas, a physician, and Damian, a surgeon, established themselves in Egea, a city in Cilicia, where they began to minister to the suffering. They did not confine their activities to Egea, however. The two young men travelled widely tending not only the suffering humanity they encountered along the way, but beasts of burden as well. Their ministrations resulted in healings too numerous to count, and where science ended, faith took over, so that people called their cures miraculous. Indeed, they were holy men, performing their services freely and living humbly.[1] Their example inspired many to embrace Christianity. Their example also established four tenets of proper conduct for the physician—to neglect no one suffering infirmity, to apply suitable treatment, to inflict no harm, and not to demand excessive fees.

In an attempt to crush the imagined danger to the Roman Empire posed by Christianity, the Emperors Diocletian and Maximo, motivated by cruelty and superstitious fear, declared war on the followers of Christ. Because of their enormous influence, Cosmas and Damian became a prime target of attack. Thus it was that Lysias, the Prefect of Egea, undertook to entice the gentle doctors to make sacrifice to his idols, thereby denouncing their faith. Flattery was used initially, and then threats, and ultimately corporal punishment. Finally, with a heavy stone tied around their necks, the brothers were submerged in the sea. But they were rescued from death by an angel of God who released their bonds and conducted them safely to shore. In a fit of rage, Lysias had them re-arrested and condemned to be burned in a fiery furnace. But the flames consumed the assassins and left the two men unharmed. They were then ordered to be crucified and wounded with arrows and stones. Both arrows and stones were mysteriously turned back upon the executioners.

Cosmas and Damian, along with their three brothers, Antimo, Leonzino, and Eurepio, were martyred in 287 A.D. by decapitation, as shown in the famous Fra Angelico panel in the monastery of Saint Mark in Florence. The holy doctors were buried in a magnificent tomb in Ciro, the home of Bishop Teodoreto, their first biographer, who eulogized them in "The Famous Heros and Glorious Martyrs."[2] They became the Christian counterparts of the Greek gemini twin brothers, Castor and Pollux. After Cosmas and Damian's deaths, a continuous procession of pilgrims and sick people visited their grave to petition them to intercede with God to heal their afflictions. They were considered particularly as healers of the kidney, throat diseases, pestilence, and dropsy.[3] Among the supplicants was the Emperor Giustiniano, who suffered from a grave and debilitating illness. Having been cured of his disease, he decreed that an exquisite basilica be erected at the gravesite in

From the Division of Immunology and Organ Transplantation, Department of Surgery, University of Texas Medical School, Houston, TX.

Address reprint requests to Dr. B. D. Kahan, Division of Immunology and Organ Transplantation, Department of Surgery, University of Texas Medical School, Houston, TX 77030.

0041–1345/83/1505–0001$01.00/0

thanksgiving and that the entire city be fortified. While this legend, originating from Arabia Minor, is the most popular, Wittman[4] has compiled other legends from Asian, Roman, and Syrian literature.

Following the establishment of the eastern capital of the Roman Empire at Constantinople, the Roman Forum came under the jurisdiction of the court of Theodoric the Great at Ravenna. Theodoric, an Ostrogoth, desiring to maintain peaceful coexistence with the native Roman majority, responded favorably to the request of Pope Felix IV (526–530) to establish a church dedicated to Saints Cosmas and Damian in two antiquated buildings at the end of the Via Sacra in the Roman Forum, namely, the main hall of the Sacra Urbis, the Library of Peace, built in 78 A.D. by Vespasius, and the pagan Temple of the Divine Romulus, said to have been built by Maxentius around 307 A.D. in honor of his son Romulus who died in childhood. This particular section of the Forum was considered a medical district: Galen himself had taught here and on this site wrote his commentaries on the Hippocratic text in 169–170 A.D. It was the pious Amalasunta, Theodoric's daughter, who, after her father's death, formally transferred the buildings to Felix for his Basilica.

Pope Felix ordered construction of the basilica in 526 A.D. and work was completed in 530.[5] The apse of the new basilica was decorated with a mosaic that is now considered to be one of the most unique and best preserved examples of Byzantine art extant. Entitled "To the Medical Martyrs, the Hope for the Salvation of the People," it depicts Christ, the Redeemer holding the scroll of the New Law standing amid multicolored clouds in the center, with Saint Felix holding a model of the basilica, Saint Cosmas bearing in his hands his crown of martyrdom, and the Apostle Paul with his hand on Cosmas' shoulder. On the opposite side stand Saint Peter, his hand on Damian's shoulder, who bears his own martyr's crown, and Saint Theodore, dressed in the colorful cloak of a Byzantine dignitary, also bearing a crown. It is interesting to note that all the figures, with the exception of Theodore are wearing Roman tunics and paliums. Palm trees, a symbol of triumph, appear on either side of the mosaic. Above one of these trees can be seen a phoenix, with rays of light emanating from its head, the symbol of resurrection and immortality. The basilica must have rendered the faithful spellbound. Leaving the squalid, littered ruins of the Roman Forum, they would enter the former Temple of Romulus and gaze in awe as the light, streaming through the round window in the ceiling, fell upon the scintillating golds of the mosaic.

Eight inlaid polychromes decorate the basilica, showing scenes from the lives of Cosmas and Damian: the healing of a dromedary; the figure of the woman, Palladia, cured of cancer praising God; the Saints' appearance before Lysias; their ordeal in the sea and their rescue; the incident of the furnace; and their decapitation and burial. The centuries old alabaster altar built in 526, now in the crypt because of the construction of a floor above, contains relics of the martyrs transported from the Middle East by Pope San Gregorio Magno (590–604) and authenticated by Pius XI (1924). Because of the gradual deterioration of the Forum, a religious order was consigned to oversee the shrine and to give spiritual aid to the faithful. In 1512, the basilica was placed under the aegis of the Third Order Regular of St. Francis, which now uses it as its international headquarters. Other relics can be found in numerous churches dedicated to these patrons of the healing professions throughout Europe.

THE MIRACLE OF THE BLACK LEG

The miracle of the black leg is the most well known of the posthumous deeds attributed to Cosmas and Damian. At the dawn of the Christian era, a popular custom was "incubation," namely, a visit by the sick to the temples of Aesculapius to pray for healing. They would sleep in the temple in the expectation that the gods would cure them as they slumbered. Temple attendants would apply oil and wax to the afflicted body parts, and perform surgery if necessary. Deubner[6] published 48 legends, recalling that miracles had occurred when sick persons made pilgrimages to the holy places dedicated to Cosmas and Damian, particularly the church in Blachernai, in front of the walls of Constantinople, where "incubation" was practiced in a fashion similar to that in temples dedicated to Aesculapius. Saints Cosmas and Damian would appear in the night to give advice, administer medication, and lay on hands. The miracle of the black leg, which was believed to have occurred in c. 348 A.D. at the site of the Roman Basilica dedicated to the saintly doctors, was first recorded in *The Leggenda Aurea* (1270) by Jacopo da Varagine.[1] After a devout prayer to the saints, the elderly sacristan of the church fell asleep near the altar and dreamt that Cosmas and Damian came to him and removed his gangrenous, cancerous leg with a saw. The leg was described as "Iam crus totum consumpserat cancer." Cancer was understood at that time to be a disease that ate away skin and flesh; therefore, each artist portrayed this in his own special way.[2] The sacristan overheard Cosmas ask: "Where will we get healthy flesh to fill up the holes since we have to cut out the rotten flesh?" To which Damian was heard to reply: "A Moor was buried today in the Cemetery of Saint Peter, his body is still fresh, bring from him what we need."[1] And so it was done. The limb of the deceased Ethiopian was removed from his body at the pagan gladiator graveyard on Vatican Hill at the Circus of Nero, where Saint Peter's Cathedral now stands; attached at the thigh of the good sacristan; and ointments applied to the site. Upon awakening the old man no longer experienced the pain that had constantly tormented him. He could no longer feel the sores that heretofore had plagued him. He excitedly struck a light and discovered that indeed his leg was whole again. There was nothing wrong with it. It was a perfectly healthy black leg. Filled with joy he recalled his dream and went to the cemetery in company with other believers. There they found his diseased limb lying in the grave beside the body of the Moor.

The concept of transplantation was totally alien to the times in which the miracle took place. Even in the 15th century most physicians, notably Hieronymus Brunchwieg, vigorously denied the possibility that appendages could ever be reattached to the body. He stated that if someone tried to reattach a part of the body it would be equivalent to "a monkey becoming a philosopher" or a man "trying to fly in the air."[7] Sommering, in his 18th century treatise, pointed out that there were many discrepancies between reality and early artistic representation.[8] But in art, nearly anything is possible; in science it is a rather different matter. Today the scientific achievement of the third century miracle continues to elude twentieth century transplant surgeons.

CYCLOSPORINE

In 1976 it could hardly have been said that, during its 20-year history, clinical transplantation had achieved consistent graft success. Advances had been painfully slow. Unsuccessful renal allotransplantation into the groin of a patient who suffered from mercury bichloride poisoning in 1936 was followed by the connection of a cadaveric kidney to the brachial artery and cephalic vein of a young woman in acute renal failure by Landsteiner, Hufnagel, and Hume in 1945. The graft was removed after 48 hr without having produced significant amounts of urine. Fortunately, the patient's own kidneys had resumed function a few hours after transplantation.[9] Lawler et al. (1950)[10] replaced a kidney in a woman with polycystic disease by orthotopic renal transplantation from a cadaver. The success of this allograft was never documented. When removed, 9.5 months after implantation, it measured 4 × 3 × 2 cm. Two years later, Michon (1955)[11] transplanted a mother's left kidney to the iliac fossa of her son who had fallen from a scaffolding, thereby rupturing an unrecognized solitary right kidney. Although the kidney was lost due to rejection, this case firmly established a secure technique of allotransplantation, as documented by Murray et al. (1955)[12] using grafts in monozygotic twins.

Progress was severely hindered by the refractoriness of the immunologic process mediating allograft rejection. Although technical advances in organ retrieval[13] and heterotopic, extraperitoneal graft placement in the pelvis reduced operative complications to less than 5% by 1970, attempts to control the immune response initially with total body irradiation and later with chemical immunosuppression using azathioprine and prednisone yielded only 50% allograft function, with a 15% patient mortality rate primarily due to infection.[14–16] In 1967, Starzl[17] began the clinical application of antilymphocyte serum (ALS), based on the scientific foundations described by Metchnikoff in 1903[18] and later tested in an animal model by Monaco et al.[19] (1964). Najarian and colleagues[20] confirmed and extended these findings, but noted that the improved graft survival was attended by an increased risk of infection caused by two factors. First, the synergistic effects of antilymphocyte serum to opsonize circulating granulocytes and platelets compounded their reduced numbers due to the myelosuppressive effects of concomitant azathioprine therapy. Secondly, ALS treatment was associated with activation of viral agents, particularly cytomegalovirus, possibly due to marked T-cell depression. Thus, 1-year renal allograft survival rates of 65% were achieved, with the penalty of a 20% mortality rate. In addition, the significance of the immunosuppressive effect of ALS was obfuscated by the practice of administering 10 blood transfusions preoperatively and splenectomizing all allograft recipients.

The transfusion policy by itself may have exerted two effects. First, it depresses the immunoreactivity of the recipients, as documented by Opelz et al.[21] Although the mechanism of the effect is uncertain, multiple transfusions were shown to convert recipients displaying strong pretransplant immunoreactivity to weak responsiveness in a prospective study.[22] Secondly, extensive transfusions may exclude the strongest immune responders, who thereafter produce such a broad spectrum of antibodies as to routinely display positive pretransplant crossmatches. In spite of the benefit of diminished immune responsiveness, transfusions increase the waiting time for some cadaveric transplant recipients, and produce donor-specific sensitization in living-related recipients,[23] although this complication may be decreased when transfusions are combined with azathioprine immunosuppression. Therefore, the benefits of a liberal transfusion policy must be balanced against the risks of pretransplant sensitization.

During this era, the annual mortality rate attending chronic maintenance hemodialysis treatment for end-stage renal disease was reduced to 10%. Although dialysis could never offer the quality of life provided by successful transplantation, only a relatively small, highly committed number of end-stage renal disease patients were prepared to accept the risks of transplantation in the face of an uncertain outcome.

The discovery of the immunosuppressive properties of cyclosporine by Borel in 1976[24] offered new hope to transplantation, since the agent possessed selectivity for T lymphocytes not obtained with the nonspecific agents azathioprine, ALS, and steroids. The initial clinical studies conducted by Calne et al. (1978)[25] suggested that the new agent was highly toxic. Several patients succumbed to infection, often accompanied by lymphoma. Although most grafts continued to function, they all displayed significant impairment. Calne's judgment that the agent was too toxic to be used in combination with other immunosuppressants has fortunately proved to be overly pessimistic. Recent work by Starzl et al.[26] indicates that effective safe immunosuppression with cyclosporine combined with steroids can be obtained (1) if other primary antiproliferative agents are withheld, (2) if evidences of toxicity are closely monitored and drug dosage reduced, and (3) if the agent is administered at more modest initial doses, namely, 14 mg/kg initially, rather than 20–25 mg/kg.[27]

Clearly, the use of cyclosporine should be restricted to patients who require potent immunosuppression. Therefore, the agent may not be necessary for patients who (1) preoperatively display a weak immune responder status, (2) have been treated with multiple blood transfusions for preexistent conditions, (3) have undergone extensive pretransplant conditioning by 10 blood transfusions and splenectomy,[28] or (4) will receive an HLA-identical graft. On the other hand, there is no evidence that patients receiving the drug under these conditions fare less well than conventionally treated recipients. However, patients who display strong responses in T-lymphocyte assays,[29] who wish to undergo transplantation as their primary form of end-stage renal disease therapy, or who wish to receive a graft from a willing, but highly mismatched, live donor, all experience appreciable improvement in kidney survival when cyclosporine is substituted for azathioprine. It may suffice to only employ induction therapy with cyclosporine and prednisone in order to achieve an unresponsive state that can be maintained with azathioprine-prednisone or with cyclosporine alone. Certainly, the most compelling application of cyclosporine is in the setting wherein rejection is fatal to the recipient, namely, hepatic,[30] cardiac,[31] and heart-lung[32] transplantation. In the setting of pancreas transplantation for diabetes mellitus, wherein the contributions of technical failures and recurrence of original disease are uncertain, cyclosporine by virtue of effectively suppressing rejection may also be helpful.

THE FUTURE OF TRANSPLANTATION

Given this promising conquest of rejection, are we finally in a position to state that we have "conquered" clinical transplantation? Such a conclusion would be as ludicrous as Baron Boyer's[33] statement in 1827 that surgery has "reached the highest degree of perfection of which it is capable." In response, Halstead[34] noted that in 1827 anesthesia had not yet been discovered, hemorrhage was poorly controlled, and infection could not be prevented. Similarly, it is clear that cyclosporine represents but one, albeit important, step on the road to successful transplantation. Cyclosporine has led to significant accomplishments. Ninety percent of cadaveric renal recipients escape even a single allograft rejection episode, and at least 80% of patients have functioning grafts at the end of 1 year. Cyclosporine has enabled older patients, high immune responders, diabetics, and untransfused recipients to enjoy the benefits of early transplantation, which had heretofore only been an optimistic hope.

A myriad of problems confront us in the use of the drug: Which in vitro and in vivo immunologic indices of drug effect predict adequate immunosuppression? What is the role of therapeutic drug monitoring? What features distinguish rejection from drug-induced nephrotoxicity? What are the long-term effects of drug administration? What is the role of corticosteroids? Can rejection be controlled by simple adjustment of the cyclosporine regimen? Could reversal of rejection be achieved by plasmalymphopheresis or ALS without steroids? Most importantly, can one minimize the length or amount of immunosuppressive therapy by the induction of specific unresponsiveness using donor bone marrow infusions, solubilized donor histocompatibility antigens, or donor blood transfusions?

Furthermore, cyclosporine may enable us to dissect the immune response, since it is probably highly selective for a limited subset of the helper T-cell population, or, if one prefers, for a specific function of many lymphocytes, namely, the response to an antigenic stimulus by the generation of lymphokines. Since the author believes cyclosporine to act primarily at the cell membrane, there may be distinctive surface properties of susceptible cells, clearly distinguishable from the capacity of the drug to nonspecifically dissolve in lipid bilayers. The possibility that the drug competes with a natural mediator of immune activation for a critical membrane function poses the prospect of defining an important agonist of the allograft response. Alternatively, the drug may act by inhibiting distinctive metabolic membrane pathways, such as calcium flux, phospholipid methylation, or generation of secondary messengers. Thus, precise definition of the site of action, as well as analysis of structural congeners, not only may lead to second, third, etc., generations of active cyclosporine compounds, as seen with the penicillins, but also afford new insights into immunosuppression. Thus, cyclosporine may be a scalpel to dissect the complex variables of immune homeostasis. Elucidation of T-lymphocyte function may then provide insight into mechanisms of immunologic unresponsiveness, thereby facilitating the design of appropriate maneuvers to achieve allograft tolerance and make the miracle of Cosmas and Damian a commonplace occurrence.

ACKNOWLEDGMENT

The author acknowledges Fr. Adalbert Wolski, TOR, Franciscan Father, Basilica of Cosmas and Damian, Rome, Italy, for ecclesiastic information; Helly Liebling for translation of original sources; and Mikki Karroll for editorial assistance.

REFERENCES

1. da Varagine J: Leggenda Aurea. Libreria Editrice Fiorentina, 1952, pp 648–652
2. Artelt W: Kosmas and Damien—Die Schutzpatrone der Artze und Apretheker. Frankfurt, Darmstadt von G. Stritt, (no date)
3. Bibliotheca Sanctorum, vol. IV, 1st Giovanni XXIII della pontifica universita lateraneuse. Roma, Vatican Press, 1964, pp 224–238
4. Wittmann A: Kosmas und Damian Kultausbreitung und Volksdevotion. Berlin, Schmidt, 1967, pp 12–21
5. Chioccioni PP: Illustrated Guide to the Basilica of Saints Cosmas and Damian. Rome, Tipolito Aurelia 1973
6. Deubner L: Kosmas and Damian (ed 1). Leipzig and Berlin, Druck and Verlag von B.G. Teubner, 1907
7. Danilevicius Z: JAMA 201:145, 1967
8. Zimmerman L, Veith I: Mod Med 28:212, 1960
9. Hume D, Merrill JP, Miller BF, et al: J Clin Invest 34:327, 1955
10. Lawler RH, West JW, McNulty PH, et al: JAMA 144:844, 1950
11. Michon P: J Urol (Paris) 58:194, 1952
12. Murray JE, Merrill JB, Harrison JH: Surg Forum 6:432, 1955
13. Belzer F, Kountz SL: Ann Surg 172:394, 1970
14. Murray JE, Merrill JP, Dammin GJ, et al: Ann Surg 156:337, 1962
15. Starzl TE, Marchioro TL, Waddell WR: Surg Gynecol Obstet 117:385, 1963
16. Hume DM, Lee HM, Williams GM, et al: Ann Surg 164:352, 1964
17. Starzl TE, Marchioro TL, Porter KA, et al: Surg Gynecol Obstet 124:301, 1967
18. Metchnikoff E: L'Immunite dans les Maladies Infectieuses. Paris, Masson, 1901 (English translation by Macmillan, New York, 1905; reprinted by Johnson Reprint, New York, 1969)
19. Monaco AP, Wood ML, Russell PS: Transplantation (Suppl)5:1106, 1967
20. Najarian JS, Simmons RL, Condie RM, et al: Ann Surg 184:352, 1976
21. Opelz G, Graver B, Terasaki PI: Lancet 1:1223, 1981
22. Kerman R, Agostino G, Van Buren CT, et al: Transplant Proc 15:1022, 1983
23. Salvatierra O, Iwaki Y, Vincenti F, et al: Transplantation 32:528, 1981
24. Borel J: Immunology 31:631, 1976
25. Calne RY, White D, Rolles K: Lancet 1:1183, 1978
26. Starzl T, Weil R, Iwatsuki S, et al: Surg Gynecol Obstet 151:17, 1980
27. Kahan BD, Van Buren CT, Lin S, et al: Transplantation 34:36, 1982
28. Ferguson RM, Rynasiewicz J, Sutherland DER, et al: Surgery 92:176, 1982
29. Kerman RH, Kahan BD: Ann Clin Res 13:244, 1981
30. Starzl TE, Klintmalm GB, Porter KA: N Engl J Med 305:266, 1981
31. Oyer P, Stinson E, Reitz B: Transplant Proc 13:199, 1981
32. Reitz BA, Wallwork J, Hunt S, et al: N Engl J Med 306:557, 1982
33. Boyer A le baron: Traite des Maladies Chirurgreales et des Operations qui deur Conviennent. Paris, V. Migneret, 1927, p 11
34. Halstead WS: Surgical Papers, vol. 2, Baltimore, Johns Hopkins Press, 1924, p 512

CYCLOSPORINE
Biological Activity and Clinical Applications

MECHANISMS OF ACTION

Cyclosporine: Historical Perspectives

J. F. Borel

LIKE all other creatures, humans have to procreate for the survival of their species. The most common transplantation procedure is the transfer of sperms into the uterus. In fertilization, the fusion of a spermatozoon with an oocyte occurs, i.e., the mixing of two incompatible tissues. Even more astounding is the fact that this histoincompatible product, the embryo and later the fetus, is tolerated in the womb for the period of 9 months. The final event, birth, might be the result of an immunologic rejection, as is suggested by some hypotheses. Much insight may no doubt be gained into the natural immunosuppressive and tolerance mechanisms involved during pregnancy from the in-depth investigation of this still unexplained, but so very reproducible phenomenon.[1,2]

One should also remember in this context the well known unspecific anergy observed in large areas surrounding tumors. It is known that a number of developing cancers produce immunosuppressive factors that are released into the patient's plasma. They have been characterized as glycoproteins, with a molecular weight of approximately 70,000 daltons.[3] Whether these so-called natural suppressor mechanisms in pregnancy and tumor growth are related, and whether they may in the future lead to new therapeutic approaches, remains to be seen.

Another type of transplantation, an imaginary puzzle compounded of parts of different animals, seems deeply rooted in the unconscious of mankind. It is represented in numerous mythical hybrid animals; one of the most familiar to us being called the Chimaera (Χίμαιρα). This very word is now used to describe any fantastic or horrible imaginary creature and is also the term applied by biologists to plants and animals that have hybrid characteristics. This monster appears in Homer's *Iliad,*[4] located in Lycia (in today's Anatolia). The Chimaera was of divine origin, being "a lion at the front, a serpent at the rear and in the middle a goat," and it breathed flashing fire from its three heads. Another more human-like chimeric state is that of certain Asian gods, such as Brahma, who are endowed with many arms as well as heads or faces. This is a symbolic expression of their many attributes and may perhaps be connected with the more common desire of man to possess additional limbs or to be able to exchange parts of his body with a view to obtaining added strength.

Leaving myths and considering more practical aspects, it is obvious that amputation of a diseased organ and its replacement by a healthy one has long haunted the fantasy of surgeons. The first reported attempt, though carried out under miraculous conditions, was performed by the holy twins Cosmas and Damian, who replaced the gangrenous leg of a verger with a leg taken from a recently deceased Ethiopian Moor. A simplified graphic version of this picture was selected as the symbol of the present cyclosporine congress. In an editorial in the *New England Journal of Medicine*[5] referring to this saintly ministration, Dr. Kahan posed the question: Will the third century legend become 20th century fact?

It seems, indeed, that the allografting of a hind limb from a hybrid Brown Norway rat to a Lewis recipient has been successfully achieved under cyclosporine treatment (25 mg/kg/day subcutaneously for 20 days, then twice weekly thereafter). The picture of such a long-term survivor at 110 days postoperative is shown in an article by Black et al.[6] Recent-

From Preclinical Research, Sandoz Ltd., Basel, Switzerland.

Address reprint requests to Dr. J. F. Borel, Preclinical Research, Sandoz Ltd., CH-4002 Basel, Switzerland.

0041-1345/83/1505-0003$02.00/0

ly, vascularized whole knee joint allografts between different strains of rabbit were successfully performed using 15 mg/kg/day of cyclosporine.[7]

The effects of cyclosporine are not confined exclusively to transplantation. Another large and promising area for any immunoregulatory agent is that of immune disorders. It may be hoped that the phenomena of autoaggression, or autoimmunity in particular, will become amenable to the action of cyclosporine. There are already a number of animal models (see Table 4) as well as some scattered clinical cases that strongly support such an approach.[8]

Finally, the fascinating work performed in parasitology with cyclosporine will also be summarized, since, as far as is known, no such article has been submitted to this congress.

APPROACHES TO IMMUNOSUPPRESSION

Most of the surgical problems of organ allografting had generally been solved (with the noticeable exception of segmental pancreas) long before it was understood how to protect the transplants from their inevitable immunologic rejection. Blood transfusions before transplantation and tissue matching have clearly been shown to be of importance in prolonging graft survival;[9,10] however, these measures were of value only if integrated into a chemotherapeutic protocol.

The immunosuppression first introduced in the late 1950s and during the 1960s acted indiscriminately, blocking or damaging all the cells that happened to be in mytosis, i.e., also normally functioning cells that are particularly important to the organism's survival. Although graft rejection could be held at bay by the use of these agents, which interfered nonspecifically with the induction or expression of the immune response, the toxic side effects were usually so severe that the overall results were not considered very satisfactory. The major drawback to the commonly used combination of steroids and cytotoxic drugs is the high risk of overwhelming infections from organisms, many of which are not normally pathogenic. It can be concluded that the concept of interference at various stages of the immune system, e.g., repression of the formation of precursor cells, destruction or blockade of immunocompetent cells, suppression of proliferation, and differentiation of lymphocytes and monocytes by inhibition of the biosynthesis of nucleic acids and proteins, was basically correct. However, the use of nonspecific drugs, i.e., drugs whose action was not limited to the immunocompetent cells, remained a "faute de mieux" approach.

The next step was, therefore, the development of lymphocytotoxic drugs or procedures, which were mostly restricted to the elimination of the immunocompetent cells. This goal could be achieved by the use of total lymphoid irradiation, thoracic duct cannulation, antilymphocyte globulin, L-asparaginase, and steroids. The last are known to possess lymphocytolytic activity, particularly with respect to the T lymphocytes, and to exert a stabilizing effect on the lysosomal membranes, along with those of other cellular organelles. Steroids not only intervene at many points of the immune response (lymphocyte recirculation, generation of cytotoxic effector cells), but they also possess a remarkable antiinflammatory potency. They inhibit neutrophil adherence to vascular endothelium in an inflammatory site and suppress monocytic functions such as microbicidal activity and monocyte response to lymphokines.

The current or third stage is that of immunopharmacology. This stage is characterized by selective immunoregulation using compounds or methods that specifically modulate defined subpopulations of immunocompetent cells. Immunopharmacology deals with new pathways toward the development of agents with selective action on the acquisition of immunologic responsiveness, recognition of immunogenic stimuli by receptor cells, induction of differentiation and maturation of lymphocytes, cellular interactions, and modulation of effector functions. Cyclosporine emerged as the first drug that fulfilled these requirements to some extent and that has proved of permanent clinical value (Fig. 1).[11,12] It is self-evident that this compound has had an impact on immunology. However, other promising and original attempts need to be mentioned here. The new technology of monoclonals has allowed the production of highly specific antibodies directed toward lymphocyte subsets. I have no doubts that further refinements of monoclonal antibodies may soon add to their therapeutic usefulness. The modulation of lymphokines is another potential approach for both immunosuppression and immunostimulation.

The final phase of immunosuppression will be the induction of antigen-specific depression of allograft reactivity. Classical transplantation tolerance has been induced in a developing immune system, but it is virtually impossible to achieve in a fully developed immune system.[13] Several experimental approaches have been successfully used in various animal models, but their practicability for clinical purposes appears still to be rather in the realms of academic significance. Thus, the presence of auto-antiidiotypic antibodies can produce prolongation of skin graft survival in certain strains of rat.[14,15] The generality of this type of reaction, however, is not yet estab-

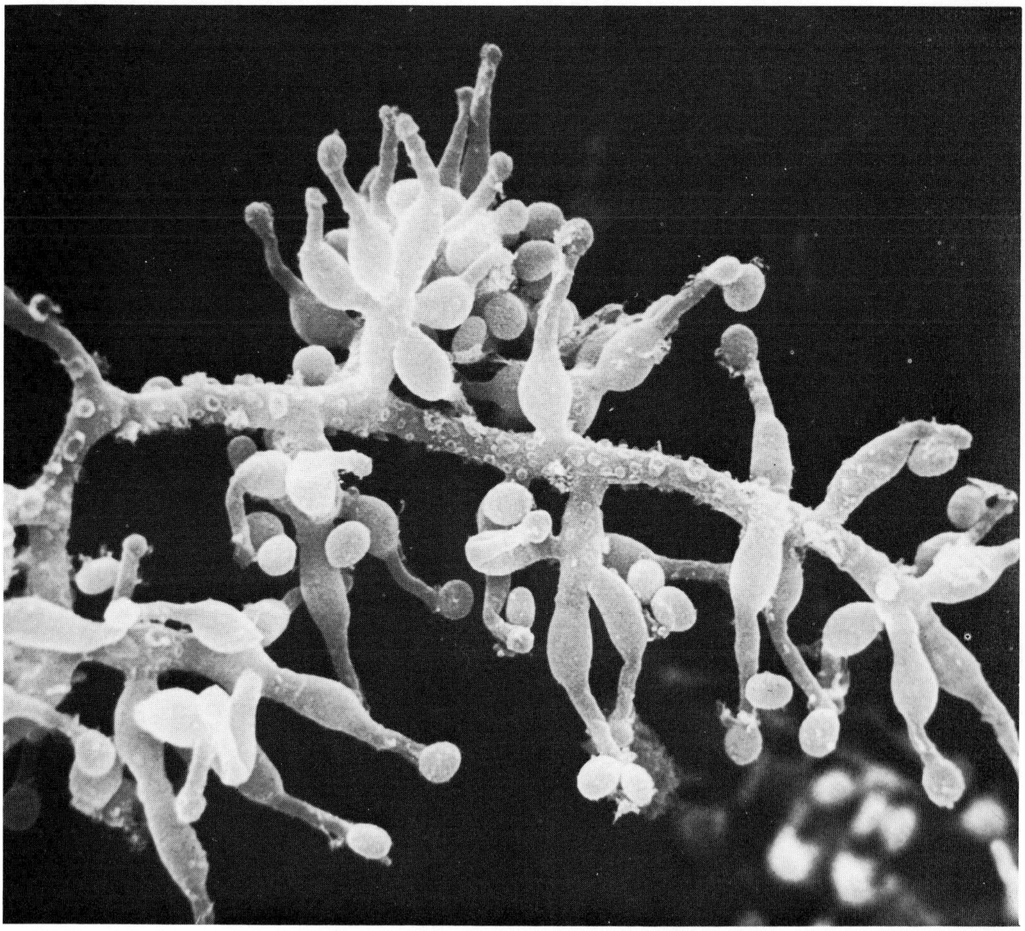

Fig. 1. Scanning electron micrograph of the producer strain *Tolypocladium inflatum* Gams. The fungus is grown by fermentation, and cyclosporine is obtained from it by extraction and costly chromatographic purification. The picture shows a conidiophore with numerous phialides and conidia ($\times$5200). (Photograph by courtesy of M. Dreyfuss and U. Strahm, Sandoz, Ltd., and R. Guggenheim and G. Lüönd, University of Basel.)

lished. Another, easier solution may be to evoke antigen-specific antibodies that protect rather than destroy a graft.[16] The precise mechanism of enhancing sera has still to be elucidated. Tentative explanations suggest, on the one hand, that the antibodies combine with the surface antigen of the target cells, which are then no longer accessible to the receptors of the cytotoxic lymphocytes, i.e., masking by antibody; on the other hand, blocking by antigen has been proposed: shedding of cell surface antigens due to complexing with antibody would spare the graft from being killed, or alternatively, the free or complexed antigens could block the receptors of the cytotoxic T cells or the antibody involved in antibody-dependent cell-mediated cytotoxicity (ADCC). Finally, it is known that the modification of the graft by culture procedures can induce prolonged survival, presumably by the removal from the graft of the passenger leukocytes that play an important role in the induction of graft rejection.[17]

HISTORY OF CYCLOSPORINE

The innovative nature of cyclosporine as an immunomodulator appears clearly from the context of the preceding section. This compound can indeed be considered as the prototype of a new generation of immunosuppressants. Cyclosporine has proved that immunopharmacology is now possible, i.e., that the immune response is amenable to modulation by drugs. Cyclosporine is a specific immunoregulator in the sense that it acts specifically and reversibly on the immunocompetent T lymphocytes or, in other words, it suppresses specifically the immune response.[18,19] Admittedly, this effect is not restricted to any particular antigen-specific response. The mode of action will be discussed at length during the basic science sessions.

The history of cyclosporine has already been published,[20] and there is not much to be added (Table 1). Following this general review on the practical as well as the experi-

Table 1. Review of the History of Cyclosporine

1970
B. Thiele: Isolation of two new strains of fungi imperfecti producing antifungal metabolites
Z.L. Kis et al.: Isolation of a metabolite mixture and characterization as novel neutral polypeptides
1971
Haerri/Ruegger: Isolation of the partially purified two-component metabolite mixture (24-556) on a preparative scale for initial biologic screening
1972
Borel: Discovery of immunosuppressive properties of metabolite 24-556 in rodents
1973
Ruegger: Purification of CsA (27-400)
Dreyfuss et al.: Culture and production of CsA
1974
Borel et al.: Animal studies of the immunosuppressive activity of CsA, in vivo and in vitro
1975
Petcher et al./Ruegger et al.: Elucidation of the structure of CsA (x-ray studies and chemical degradation)
1976
Toxicity studies (rats, monkeys) demonstrate selectivity of CsA for lymphocytes and lack of effect on hemopoiesis
World-wide confirmation of specific immunosuppressive effect of CsA in experimental transplantations and other models
1978
Calne et al./Powles et al.: First clinical trials (kidney transplantation, graft-versus-host disease)
1980
Wenger: Total synthesis of CsA. (Ruzicka Award presented in 1982)
1981
Bueding et al./Thommen: Publication of antischistosomal and antimalarial activity of CsA
CsA Symposium at Trinity Hall, Cambridge
1983
Sandimmune first registered in Switzerland

mental means and concepts of interference in the immune response, and a presentation of the history of the development of cyclosporine, the significance of this drug in three different major areas will now be dealt with.

Significance of Cyclosporine in Organ Transplantation, Including Bone Marrow

Cyclosporine was first shown to inhibit humoral immunity to T-cell-dependent antigens, but it also strongly suppresses cell-mediated immunity. Thus, it is effective in preventing allograft rejection. Prolonged graft survival under cyclosporine treatment has been achieved in a great variety of species and using a variety of organs, several of which have, as a result, been successfully grafted for the first time (e.g., nerve[21] and muscle cells,[21a] lung,[22] small bowel,[23] etc.). Both first- and second-set graft survival can be prolonged under cyclosporine treatment.[24] The prevention of rejection of concordant xenografts in rats,[25] rabbits,[26] and dogs[27] represents a further remarkable feature. The survival of pancreatic islet cells across a major histocompatibility barrier cannot be prolonged by cyclosporine; however, islet cells implanted under the renal capsule can be transplanted as a vascularized graft and rejection prevented by cyclosporine treatment.[28] Rejection of corneal grafts can also be prevented by topical administration of the drug to the rabbit eye.[29]

A special type of organ transplantation is that of bone marrow cells to reconstitute the hemopoietic tissues. Graft-versus-host reaction (GVHR) can be prevented or cured by cyclosporine in several species.[30–34] It was demonstrated in rats that the drug, given on 28 consecutive days, assists the establishment of histoincompatible marrow grafts, completely prevents GVHR, and allows the repopulation of lymphoid organs and recovery of T-dependent immune functions at 35 days posttransplantation, as compared with 150 days in control animals treated with placebo.[35] In contrast, the transplantation of bone marrow among histoincompatible unrelated dogs does not seem promising using cyclosporine alone. However, the combination of methotrexate, early after grafting, with cyclosporine permits engraftment of histoincompatible marrow, and some recipients become long-term survivors.[36] Thus, it can be concluded from the above, as well as other data, that cyclosporine can induce graft-to-host tolerance across minor, but not major (except in rodents), histocompatibility differences.

The extensive toxicologic results [acute oral and intravenous toxicity in three rodent species, several long-term toxicity studies in rodents, dogs, and cynomolgus (i.v.) or rhesus (p.o.) monkeys, carcinogenicity and teratology studies in three rodent species, fertility and reproductive performance studies in rats] have all indicated that cyclosporine was a remarkably safe drug compared with reference immunosuppressants.[37,38]

As regards further drug safety aspects, on the basis of the similarity of many pharmacokinetic parameters and the existence of the same biotransformation pathways in the toxicity species (rat, rabbit, and dog) and man, it can be concluded that the results obtained in animals are relevant for man.[39–41]

Dr. T. Beveridge (Clinical Research, Sandoz Ltd., Basel) has summarized the clinical data on kidney transplantation available up to December 1982 (Table 2).[42] His review concerns the results of five studies carried out in Europe and Australia involving 278 patients who received cyclosporine compared with 279 control patients and the results of 10 studies conducted in North America (as reported by Dr. D. Winter, Clinical Research, Sandoz Inc., East Hanover, NJ) involving 251 patients who received cyclosporine and 266 control patients.[43] In the European and Australian studies, cyclosporine was, in principle, used alone as immunosuppressant, at least initially, and steroids in the form of intravenous boluses of methylprednisolone were used only for the treatment of rejection episodes and then only up to 6 g. In the North American study, cyclosporine was combined with steroids from the beginning. Standard therapy (control patients) in all studies consisted of

Table 2. Summary of Results for Renal Transplant Patients

Group of Studies in	Cyclosporine Group No. of Patients	Cyclosporine Group One-Year Graft Survival	Control Group No. of Patients	Control Group One-Year Graft Survival
Europe and Australia	278	55%–78%	279	49%–73%
North America	251	71%–90%	266	53%–82%
Europe M/C	114	73%	114	53%
Canada M/C	103	80%	106	64%

Comparison of patients treated with cyclosporine or with conventional therapy. The results of the European and Canadian multicenter trials (M/C) are indicated separately. Graft survival probability was calculated by the Kaplan-Meier method (product limit estimate).

either azathioprine and steroids and, in a few cases, antilymphocyte globulin (ALG) in addition.

A common feature in these studies was the decrease in number of rejection episodes seen in cyclosporine-treated patients. When rejection episodes did occur, they were readily resolved with rejection therapy. In the European multicenter trial, graft failure due to rejection was markedly less common in the cyclosporine group than in the control group (23 versus 40, respectively). There were more patients who did not experience any rejection episodes in the cyclosporine group than in the control group (20% versus 11%).[44]

The main purpose of the clinical sessions will be to assess the advantages and disadvantages of cyclosporine in the different indications of organ transplantation, so they will not be discussed here. Suffice it to say that, compared with conventional therapy, this drug has produced superior results in liver,[45] heart,[46] and heart and lung transplantation.[47]

Concerning bone marrow transplantation, the situation is slightly different, in the sense that no controlled trials are available except those from Seattle, which will be reported separately at this congress. There is also an ongoing double-blind study in Baltimore (P. Tutschka, personal communication). Cyclosporine was first used in the treatment of GVHD about 5 years ago, and although not particularly successful in the first 5 patients[48] (more recently it has been used successfully to treat existing GVHD), it did lead on directly to the drug being used in the prevention of acute GVHD. The available data from 4 European centers are as shown in Table 3.

From September 1978 to May 1981 cyclosporine was given prophylactically to a series of 153 bone marrow recipients at 5 centers.[49] Overall, 90 of the 132 patients (68%) who received matched grafts were survivors (1 was lost to follow-up). Eight of the 20 patients given mismatched grafts were still alive at >109 to >508 days (median 295 days). All but 7 of the 153 patients (including 20 mismatched grafts) achieved a prompt and sustained engraftment under cyclosporine therapy. Relapse was the sole or a contributory factor in the death of 17 of 99 leukemics (17%).

Under cyclosporine treatment, GVHD still

Table 3. Pooled 1-Year Data From Four Centers Comparing Total Experience Using Cyclosporine (CsA) With a Group of 25 Patients (pts) Treated With Methotrexate (MTX) and Documented as Historical Controls. Also Shown Are the Results in Each of Different Categories of Patients Receiving Matched Grafts Only[49]

Group (Matched Grafts Only)	No. of Patients	One-Year Survival
CsA pts: total	123	68%
MTX pts: total	25	52%
CsA pts only		
Leukemia pts	93	65%
Aplastic anemia pts	29	79%
AML	65	67%
ALL	22	58%
CML/CGL	6	67%
Leukemia in first remission	57	71%
Leukemia in later remission or relapse	30	49%

occurred in more than 70% of patients, but in contrast to previous epxerience with methotrexate, the morbidity and mortality were considerably less (56% having only a rash or a grade I severity and 30% grade II). Death was associated with GVHD in 8% (10 cases of the 132) of matched grafts at 5 centers. Only 3% of episodes were chronic GVHD, and 12% of all episodes occurred after the patient had stopped cyclosporine therapy.

The main other advantages of this drug are: it has no myelotoxicity, it is associated with prompt and sustained engraftment, hematologic recovery tends to be quicker, and time in hospital is shorter.

To conclude this very incomplete clinical summary, it must be pointed out that cyclosporine is no panacea. It has, nevertheless, been shown in 638 transplant procedures included in the analysis in the registration dossier to be the most potent and specific immunosuppressant so far discovered and to have an acceptable incidence of side effects. Consistently safe and effective immunosuppression is still an elusive goal, and the future is likely to see the development of other new agents designed to modulate the immune system specifically. In the meantime, unless some as yet unrecognized side effects emerge to limit the usefulness of cyclosporine, this drug should permit significant advances in organ transplantation.

Significance of Cyclosporine in Autoimmunity

As the remaining problems concerning the optimal protocol for the use of cyclosporine in transplantation (relevance of dose range to blood levels, drug combinations, long-term safety, importance of preoperative blood transfusions or tissue type matching, etc.) are being assessed in further controlled trials, a new official research project has recently been launched. Cyclosporine has entered phase 1 of clinical trials in an important new area, namely that of diseases related to an autoimmune disorder. Since the very few clinical

Table 4. Summary of Results Obtained With Cyclosporine in Experimental Autoimmune Models

Animal Model	Species	Prev/Ther	Reference
Adjuvant arthritis (rheumatoid arthritis)	Rat	+/+	30, 51
Experimental allergic encephalomyelitis (multiple sclerosis)	Rat, guinea pig monkey	+/+*	30, 52, 53, 54, 55
Experimental allergic neuritis (Guillain-Barré syndrome)	Rat, guinea pig	+/+*	56
Experimental uveitis (human uveitis)	Rat	+/+	57, 58
Experimental ai myasthenia gravis (myasthenia gravis)	Rat	+/+*	59
Experimental ai thyroiditis (Grave's disease, Hashimoto's thyroiditis)	Rat	nd/+*	60
Spontaneous ai thyroiditis (Hashimoto's thyroiditis)	Chicken	−/nd	61
Spontaneous ai diabetes (juvenile-onset diabetes type I)	Rat	+/nd	62, 63
EMC-induced diabetes (insulin-dependent diabetes)	Mouse	−/−	64
Murine ai lupus (systemic lupus erythematosus)	NZB/W	+/nd	31, 65, 66
Murine ai lymphoproliferative disease (SLE, arteritis, arthritis)	MRL/lpr	+/nd	65, 66

The drug was used either preventively (prev) or therapeutically (ther). The human correlates to the animal models are indicated in parentheses.

*Relapse of symptoms following discontinuation of cyclosporine treatment.

ai, autoimmune.

cases reported so far are more of an anecdotal character, they will no be discussed here;[50] a few controlled trials in some autoimmune conditions, which have just been or will soon be started are in such a preliminary state that no relevant information can yet be deduced. A series of experimental results can, however, be quoted, which clearly demonstrate the effectiveness of cyclosporine in autoimmune animal models and thus offer support for a cautious approach in similar indications in man.

Table 4 summarizes the results obtained in autoimmune animal models in which cyclosporine was used either preventively or therapeutically. In the top five models listed, complete Freund's adjuvant is used in conjunction with the antigen in order to render it more immunogenic. Cyclosporine inhibited the onset of symptoms when used preventively, i.e., when treatment was started at the time of sensitization. The compound was also successful in curing the animals in all these models when treatment was started as late as when the first pathologic symptoms appeared (therapeutic treatment). However, owing mainly to the persistence of the slow release of antigen mixed with complete Freund's adjuvant, a relapse of the disease was observed after stopping the drug in experimental allergic encephalomyelitis,[30,52–55] allergic neuritis,[56] and myasthenia gravis.[59] It is unlikely that this phenomenon was due to the absence of T suppressor cells, since in the models of myasthenia gravis[59] and of experimental encephalomyelitis (Borel, unpublished results), little or no rebound was observed when cyclosporine was maintained for prolonged periods of time.

The other six animal models listed are induced without the aid of complete Freund's adjuvant. In the experimental autoimmune thyroiditis induced in rats by thymectomy and irradiation, cyclosporine led to a significant improvement in diseased animals as measured by the fall in antithyroglobulin antibodies and the concomitant normalization of the T_H:T_S ratio during treatment. Relapse occurred when the drug was stopped.[60] In contrast, the attempt to prevent spontaneous autoimmune thyroiditis in the obese strain of chicken met with failure, and early treatment of embryos increased the severity of the disease.[61]

A discrepancy was also found among the two autoimmune diabetes models. While the preventive use of cyclosporine in spontaneous autoimmune diabetes in the B/B rat completely suppressed the onset of the disease,[62] both the early (0–14 days) and the late treatment (21–35 days) produced marked detrimental effects in the encephalomyocarditis-induced diabetes model in mice.[64] Though clearly inhibiting the pancreatotropic immune reaction, the drug strongly enhanced the diabetogenic action of the virus, as demonstrated by the increase in the incidence of diabetic females, which are known to be much more resistant than the males. Promising results were observed in the two genetically determined murine lupus models. Early therapy starting at 16 weeks of life strongly reduced mortality and positively influenced other parameters in treated animals as compared with controls.[31,65,66]

Significance of Cyclosporine in Parasitology

It is self-evident that a selective compound for T cells, such as cyclosporine, immediately exerted an impact on fundamental immunology. There are, in particular, a number of basic pathologic phenomena in which the involvement of T lymphocytes is still a matter of debate. It was with the purpose of solving this very problem that the compound was originally used in several experimental models of parasitic, fungal, and viral infections.

Unexpectedly, it was discovered almost simultaneously that cyclosporine had per se a remarkable antiparasitic effect, e.g., in schistosomiasis and malaria. These discoveries represent a major landmark, since these two diseases alone are thought to affect about 10^9 people throughout the world. Moreover, the increasing resistance of parasites, especially of *Plasmodium falciparum*, to the few available drugs creates a formidable problem.

The antischistosomal activity of cyclosporine was reported by Bueding et al.[67] They demonstrated a therapeutic effect in *Schistosoma mansoni* infected mice that were treated subcutaneously with suboptimal immunosuppressive doses. A marked reduction of globinase activity and protein content was found in the female worms. Since the protective effect could not be transferred with spleen cells and the drug had no direct effect in vitro, it was suggested that the action was host mediated. A similar therapeutic effect was also found in nude mice, and it was concluded that the antiparasitic activity was independent of immunosuppression. Moreover, a strong synergistic effect was observed when cyclosporine was combined with amoscanate. Bout and co-workers[68] confirmed the protective effect of cyclosporine against *S. mansoni* and claimed that the drug rendered the mice resistant to reinfection. This protection was afforded only by cyclosporine and not by other antischistosomal drugs, such as oxaminiquine.

The antimalarial effect of cyclosporine was first reported by Thommen,[69] who investigated its effect in a murine model. Suboptimal immunosuppressive doses given orally for a few days were effective in preventing infection or in curing already parasitaemic animals infected with *Plasmodium berghei* or *chabaudi*. Moreover, a clear synergism was demonstrated between cyclosporine and pyrimethamine, a drug affecting mainly the schizonts. These results were independently confirmed and extended by Nickel, Scheibel, and Cole,[70] who showed that prevention of infection against *P. berghei* and *yoelii* led to a state of resistance to reinfection, thus indicating that immunity had developed. Cure of parasitemia was regularly followed by a self-limiting and drug-independent recrudesence of a low parasitemia that may have been due to the selection of drug-resistant parasites. Since the drug was also effective in lethally irradiated mice (850 R), it appears that the antiparasitic effect is not linked to immunosuppression. The drug, used in concentrations from 0.1 to 10 μg/ml continuously for 48 hr or longer, clearly inhibited the survival of *P. falciparum*. No cross-resistance was found between cyclosporine and chloroquine, and it appeared that cyclosporine caused a selective reduction of the ring stages (merozoites).

Furthermore, Perrudet-Badoux[71] has studied the effect of cyclosporine in an experimental mouse model using *Trichinella spiralis*. Her results led to the following conclusions: cyclosporine exerted no effect on the dissemination of the parasite from the gut to the muscles, nor did it affect the established muscular larvae. However, preventive treatment (starting at the time of infestation) resulted in inhibition of release of newborns by the females, and treatment on days −1 to 14 completely eliminated the adult parasites. The same author also studied the effect of cyclosporine in an experimental filariasis model in the cotton rat. With the use of 15 mg/kg for 5 days, not only did the number of microfilaria remain constant in the treated animals, but the female macrofilaria recovered from the pleural cavity were all dead, while the males stayed alive.

Other parasitic models are currently under investigation. It is, however, of interest to note that, in trypanosomiasis, the use of cyclosporine demonstrated the importance of the T cells, since the severity of parasitosis significantly increased in the treated animals.[72]

It is difficult to envisage the use of cyclosporine proper as an antiparasitic agent. Since there is evidence that the antiparasitic properties are not linked to the immunosuppressive activity, the search for a cyclosporine derivative possessing antiparasitic properties but devoid of immunosuppressive activity is at present underway. Provided that part of the molecule responsible for the immunosuppressive effect is not identical to that which elicits the antiparasitic effect, this should be possible.

CONCLUSIONS

This first talk, which may be regarded as a foreword to the congress, was designed to set cyclosporine in its historical perspectives. This drug is novel, because it can be considered as the prototype of a new generation of immunosuppressants, in the sense that it is probably the first one to demonstrate clearly that an immunopharmacologic approach to the modulation of the immune response by drugs is feasible. This presentation was not conceived as a summary of current knowledge on cyclosporine, but rather was meant as a survey of the impact that this drug in particular is having and, hopefully, other similar ones will have in the field of immunopharmacology.

The present story tells us that it is not sufficient to discover a new type of pharmacologic activity; its potential must be demonstrated by assessing the effect of the compound in many experimental models, and its mechanism of action has to be elucidated as far as possible. Moreover, one has to be prepared to recognize the relevance of unexpected findings, such as the antiparasitic activities in this case. The collaboration of many individuals or groups of investigators has to be sought to ensure a continuous and fruitful progress.

ACKNOWLEDGMENT

I wish to thank M. B. Maggs for assistance in preparation of the manuscript. I am also particularly grateful to a number of investigators who have graciously contributed as yet unpublished data.

REFERENCES

1. Wegmann TG, Gill TJ (eds): Immunology of Reproduction. Oxford, Oxford University Press, 1983
2. Faulk WP, Mclnyre JA: Transplantation 32:1, 1981
3. Roth JA, Grimm EA, Gupta RK, et al: Immunobiology 159:190, 1981
4. Homer: Iliad, Book 6
5. Kahan BD: N Engl J Med 305:280, 1981
6. Black KS, Hewitt CW, Fraser LA, et al: N Engl J Med 306:368, 1982
7. Siliski JM, Green CJ: N Engl J Med 307:1642, 1982
8. Beveridge T: In White DJG (ed): Cyclosporin A. New York, Elsevier Biomedical, 1982, p 561
9. van Rood JJ, Balner H: Transplantation 26:275, 1978
10. van Rood JJ, Persijn GG, Hendriks GFJ, et al: Transplant Clin Immunol 14:195, 1982
11. Woodruff M: In White DJG (ed): Cyclosporin A. New York, Elsevier Biomedical, 1982, p 569
12. Morris PJ: Transplantation 32:349, 1981
13. Streilein JW, Gruchalla RS, Wood P, et al: Ann NY Acad Sci 392:276, 1982
14. Binz H, Wigzell H: Transplant Proc 11:914, 1979
15. Binz H, Soots A, Nemlander A, et al: Ann NY Acad Sci 392:360, 1982
16. Morris PJ: Immunol Rev 49:93, 1980
17. Lafferty KJ, Prowse SJ, Simeonovic CJ, et al: Annu Rev Immunol 1:143, 1983
18. Borel JF: Heart Transplant 1:237, 1982
19. Borel JF, Lafferty KJ: Transplant Proc (in press)
20. Borel JF: In White DJG (ed): Cyclosporin A. New York, Elsevier Biomedical, 1982, p 5
21. Gulati AK, Zalewski AA: Exp Neurol 77:378, 1982
21a. Walt DJ, Partridge TA, Sloper JC: Transplantation 31:266, 1981
22. Norin AJ, Emeson EE, Kamholz SL, et al: Transplantation 34:372, 1982
23. Craddock GN, Nordgren SR, Reznick RK: Transplantation 35:248, 1983
24. Deeg HJ, Storb R, Gerhard-Miller L: Transplantation 29:230, 1980
25. Homan WP, Williams KA, Fabre JW, et al: Transplantation 31:164, 1981
26. Green CJ, Kemp E, Kemp G, et al: In White DJG (ed): Cyclosporin A. New York, Elsevier Biomedical, 1982, p 155
27. Danko I, Gebhard C, Scholz S, et al: Eur Surg Res (in press)
28. Reece-Smith H, Homan WP, McShane P, et al: Transplantation 33:452, 1982
29. Hunter PA, Wilhelmus KR, Rice NSC, et al: Clin Exp Immunol 45:173, 1981
30. Borel JF, Feurer C, Gubler HU, et al: Agents Actions 6:468, 1976
31. Borel JF: Transplant Proc 13:344, 1981
32. van Bekkum DW, Knaan S, Zurcher C: Transplant Proc 12:278, 1980
33. Gratwohl A, Forster I, Speck B: Transplantation 33:361, 1982
34. Deeg DJ, Storb R, Weiden PL, et al: Transplant Proc 13:402, 1981
35. Tutschka PJ, Beschorner WE, Allison AC, et al: Nature 280:148, 1979
36. Deeg HJ, Storb R, Weiden PL, et al: Transplantation 34:30, 1982
37. Ryffel B: In White DJG (ed): Cyclosporin A. New York, Elsevier Biomedical, 1982, p 45
38. Matter BE, Donatsch P, Racine RR, et al: Mutation Res 105:257, 1982
39. Beveridge T, Gratwohl A, Michot F, et al: Curr Ther Res 30:5, 1981

40. Beveridge T: In White DJG (ed): Cyclosporin A. New York, Elsevier Biomedical, 1982, p 35
41. Maurer G, Loosli HR, Schreier E, et al: Drug Metab Disp (in press)
42. Beveridge T: Med Bull (SANDOZ) 12:9, 1983
43. Winter DL: Med Bull (SANDOZ) 12:39, 1983
44. European Multicentre Trial: Lancet 1:57, 1982
45. Starzl TE, Iwatsuki S, van Thiel DH: Hepatology 2:614, 1982
46. Reitz BA, Stinson EB: JAMA 248:1225, 1982
47. Beveridge T: Transplant Proc 15:433, 1983
48. Powles RL, Barrett AJ, Clink H, et al: Lancet 2:1327, 1978
49. Beveridge T: Exp Hematol 10(Suppl 10):88, 1982
50. Beveridge T: In White DJG (ed): Cyclosporin A. New York, Elsevier Biomedical, 1982, p 561
51. Borel JF, Wiesinger D, Gubler HU: Eur J Rheum Inflam 1:237, 1978
52. Borel JF: Triangle 20:97, 1981
53. Ryffel B, Feurer C, Heuberger B, et al: Immunobiology 163:470, 1982
54. Bolton C, Borel JF, Cuzner ML, et al: J Neurol Sci 56:147, 1982
55. Borel JF: Transplant Clin Immunol 13:3, 1981
56. Tomkins C, King RHM, Thomas PK: Neuropathol Appl Neurobiol 6:240, 1980
57. Nussenblatt RB, Rodrigues MM, Wacker WB, et al: J Clin Invest 67:1228, 1981
58. Nussenblatt RB, Rodrigues MM, Salinas-Carmona MC: Arch Ophthal 100:1146, 1982
59. Drachman D: Personal communication
60. McGregor AM, Rennie DP, Weetmann AP, et al: Life Sci 32:97, 1983
61. Wick G, Müller PU, Schwarz S: Eur J Immunol 12:877, 1982
62. Laupacis A, Gardell C, Dupre J, et al: Lancet 1:10, 1983
63. Like AA, Anthony M, Guberski DL, et al: Diabetes 32:326, 1983
64. Vialettes B, Baume D, Charpin C, et al: J Clin Lab Immunol 10:35, 1983
65. Jones MG, Harris G, Cowing G: Transplant Proc (this issue)
66. Gozes Y, Theofilopoulos AN, Park CH, et al: Fed Proc 41:547, 1982
67. Bueding BE, Hawkins J, Cha YN: Agents Actions 11:380, 1981
68. Bout D, Deslee D, Capron A: Fed Proc 42:1246, 1983
69. Thommen-Scott K: Agents Actions 11:770, 1981
70. Nickel SP, Scheibel LW, Cole GA: Infect Immun 37:1093, 1982
71. Perrudet-Badoux A: Personal communication
72. Kierszenbaum F, Gottlieb CA, Budzko DB: Tropenmed Parasitol 34:4, 1983

Synthesis of Cyclosporine and Analogues: Structure, Activity, Relationships of New Cyclosporine Derivatives

R. Wenger

CYCLOSPORINE is a metabolite isolated from the culture broths of the fungal species *Tolypocladium inflatum* Gams, previously known as *Trichoderma polysporum* (Link ex Pers.) Rifai. The isolation of the fungus, its fermation conditions, and its taxonomy were described by Dreyfuss et al.[1]

ELUCIDATION OF THE STRUCTURE OF CYCLOSPORINE

The structure of cyclosporine was established by chemical degradation together with x-ray crystallographic analysis of an iododerivative and was first published by Rüegger et al.[2] and Petcher et al.[3]

Cyclosporine (Fig. 1) is a neutral, hydrophobic cyclic peptide composed of 11 amino acid residues, all having the S-configuration of the natural L-amino acids, except for the D-alanine in position 8, which has the R-configuration, and sarcosine in position 3. Seven amino acids are N-methylated. Ten of the amino acids are known aliphatic amino acids, they are α-aminobutyric acid in position 2, sarcosine in position 3, *N*-methylleucine in positions 4, 6, 9, and 10, valine in position 5, alanine in position 7, D-alanine in position 8, and *N*-methylvaline in position 11. These amino acids were readily characterized following acidic hydrolysis of cyclosporine.

One amino acid was hitherto unknown. This is the amino acid in position 1, which was reported as the "C-9 amino acid," being composed of 9 carbon atoms. The C-9 amino acid is also N-methylated. This amino acid, which was found for the first time in cyclosporine, has never previously been isolated or known in free from. Only the isolation of artifacts and derivatives has been reported by Rüegger et al:[2] hydrolysis of cyclosporine followed by ion-exchange chromatography produces a cyclic derivative of the *N*-methyl-C-9-amino acid as the only isolable C-9-derivative (see Fig. 2). The free *N*-methyl-C-9-amino acid was not obtained. Acidic treatment of cyclosporine in absence of water effects an *N*,*O*-acyl migration and gives isocyclosporine. Applying a modification of Edman degradation technique on isocyclosporine by use of methylisothiocyanate produces an anhydromethylthiohydantoin derivative of the *N*-methyl-*C*-9-amino acid as the only isoluble C-9-derivative and established the C-9 amino acid as the first amino acid in the sequence. The complete sequence was established by repetitive Edman degradation.

In order to determine the absolute stereochemistry of the amino acid in position 1 of cyclosporine, the preparation of a suitable derivative for x-ray crystallographic analysis was undertaken. Treatment of cyclosporine with iodine and thallium acetate, a procedure established by Cambie et al.,[4,5] gave a cyclosporine derivative in which the C-9 amino acid was present as an iodinated cyclic derivative (Fig. 2). This compound, on treatment with zinc and acetic acid, regenerated cyclosporine. X-ray analysis established the structure of the iododerivative from which the structure

From Preclinical Research, Sandoz Ltd., Basel, Switzerland.

A part of this work has already been presented at the Seventh Symposium on Synthesis in Organic Chemistry, organized by the Royal Society at Cambridge, Perkin Division in Oxford, July 21–23, 1981, and at an International Symposium on Cyclosporin A held at Cambridge (England) September 16–18, 1981. The synthesis of cyclosporine has been presented at the autumn sessions of the Swiss Chemical Society in Berne, October 16, 1981 (first part), and October 15, 1982 (second part).

Address reprint requests to Dr. R. Wenger, Preclinical Research, Sandoz Ltd., CH-4002, Basel, Switzerland.

0041–1345/83/1505–0004$02.00/0

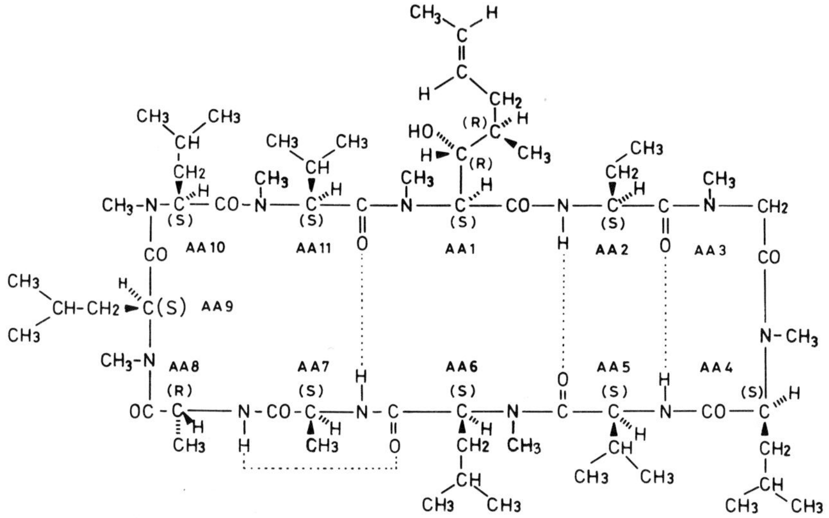

Fig. 1. Cyclosporine ($C_{62}H_{111}N_{11}O_{12}$; mol wt 1202).

of cyclosporine itself could be deduced, with the exception of the geometry of the double bond of the C-9 amino acid residue. This final problem was solved by the measurement of the coupling constant (16 Hz) between the vinyl protons from the 360 MHz NMR spectrum of cyclosporine in deuterobenzene, which characterized the trans geometry. The structural assignments have since been confirmed by an unpublished x-ray crystallographic analysis of cyclosporine itself performed by Dr. H. P. Weber in the Sandoz Research Laboratories in Basel and shows that the backbone of cyclosporine has the same conformation as the heavy atom derivative.

From the x-ray structure, the cyclosporine molecule is seen to be composed of two different parts, one of which is the antiparallel β-pleated sheet conformation of residues 1–6, and the other the open-loop of residues 7–11. The β-pleated sheet is held together, as shown in Fig. 1, by the following hydrogen bonds: NH of α-aminobutyric acid to C = O of Val-5; NH of Val-5 to C = O of aminobutyric acid; and NH of Ala-7 to C = O of MeVal-11. The remaining hydrogen bond is from NH of D-Ala-8 back to the C = O of MeLeu-6, resulting in a 7-membered ring Ala-7 conformation. These hydrogen bonds contribute significantly to the rigidity of the cyclosporine skeleton.

CYCLOSPORINE NOMENCLATURE

For practical reasons, it was previously proposed to define cyclosporine as the cyclic undecapeptide with the structure of "Cyclosporin A."[6] Now that the USAN-name CYCLOSPORINE has been accepted in the USA, this name will be adopted for the basic structure and the other fungal metabolites of the same type. Cyclosporins B, C, D, and E, published by Rüegger et al.[2] and Traber et al.[7–9] then have, according to the peptide nomenclature, the following names: [Ala[2]]cyclosporine for cyclosporin-B, [Thr[2]]cyclosporine for cyclosporin-C, [Val[2]]cyclosporine for cyclosporin-D, and [Val[11]]cyclosporine for cyclosporin-E.

The World Health Organization has adopted the INN name CICLOSPORIN for "Cyclosporin A," and in France and Great Britain, the compound is known as CICLOSPORINE.

SYNTHESIS OF AN ENANTIOMETRICALLY PURE N-METHYL-C-9-AMINO ACID (MeBmt) STARTING FROM TARTARIC ACID

The C-9 amino acid was the only unknown amino acid in cyclosporine, and there had

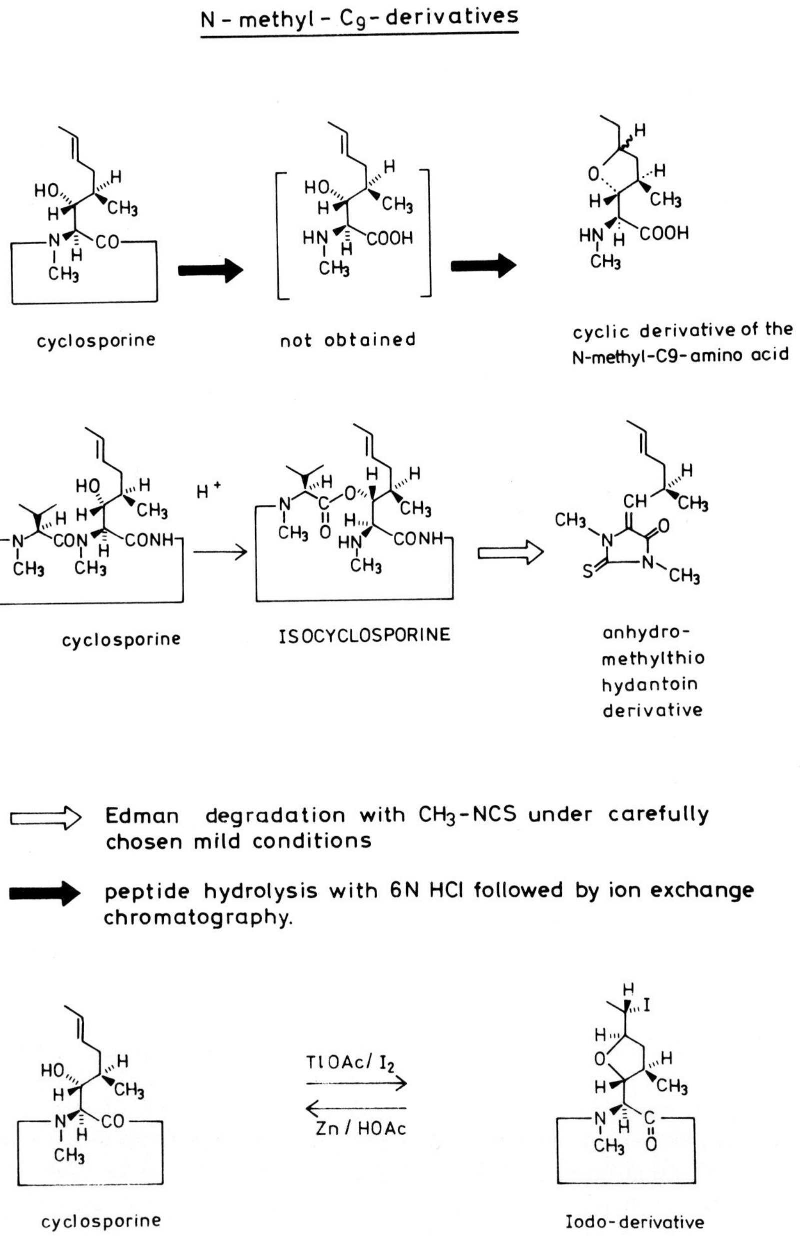

Fig. 2. ***N*-Methyl-C-9 derivatives.**

previously been no means for its isolation. For this reason, and because it is possible that the C-9 amino acid could play a significant role in determining the pharmacologic activity of cyclosporine, we decided at Sandoz to synthesize this amino acid in stereochemically pure form.

Figure 3 shows the *N*-methyl-C-9-amino acid in its staggered form (i) and as a Fischer projection (ii); it shows also the *N*-methyl-(L)-threonine amino acid in its Fischer projection (iii) as a reference. The methylamino and hydroxy groups of the *N*-methyl-9-amino acid are as in *N*-methyl-(L)-threonine in a threo-configuration; the hydroxy and methyl groups are in an erythro-configuration. The

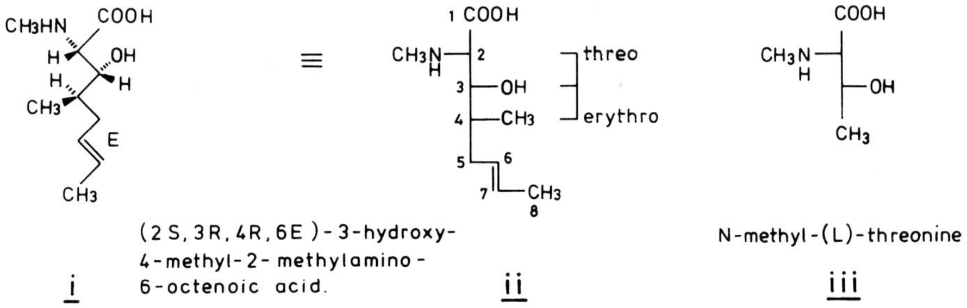

Fig. 3. ***N*-Methyl-C-9-amino acid or (2S,3R,4R,6E)-3-hydroxy-4-methyl-2-methylamino-6-octenoic acid.**

double bond is trans (E). The *N*-methyl-C-9-amino acid is in accordance with the Cahn-Ingold-Prelog nomenclature (2S, 3R, 4R, 6E)-3-hydroxy-4-methyl-2-methylamino-6-octenoic acid. It is a conventional practice for the peptide nomenclature to use three letters to describe an amino acid of the L-configuration. "Leu" as example represents (L)-leucine and "MeLeu" N-methylated (L)-leucine. It is therefore proposed to use the abbreviation MeBmt for the *N*-methyl-C-9-amino acid. The "Me" represents the N-methylated residue of Bmt, these three letters being the abbreviation of (4R)-4-but-2E-en-1-yl-4-methyl-(L)-threonine.

Strategy Used for the Synthesis of the (4R)-4-Butenyl-4-Methyl-N-Methyl-(L)-Threonine (Fig. 4)

(R,R)-(+)-Tartaric acid was used as the basic optically active building block in the synthesis and modified in three major operations to introduce successfully the features of the C-9 amino acid. In the first operation, one hydroxy group of the (R,R)-(+)-tartaric acid molecule was incorporated with the correct configuration and one hydroxy group of the original tartaric acid structure is replaced by a methyl group, accompanied by inversion of configuration. This was achieved by nucleophilic opening of the intermediate transepoxide, with methyllithium in the presence of cuprous iodide, which provides the asymmetric centers at C-3 and C-4 of the desired amino acid. The second operation consists of introducing the chain of carbon atoms containing the trans double bond. The carbon chain is first elongated by formation of an aldehyde, which is the starting material for a Wittig reaction under Schlosser and Christman[10] conditions. In the third operation, the methylamino and carboxyl groups are introduced via a cyclic intermediate, permitting stereochemical control of the asymmetric center at C-2 during hydrolysis of this intermediate to the unprotected *N*-methyl-(4R)-4-butenyl-4-methyl-threonine (MeBmt). MeBmt as the free amino acid is obtained with a yield of 7.8% starting from (*R*,*R*)-(+)-tartaric acid diethylester over 24 steps. This corresponds to an average yield of 90%/

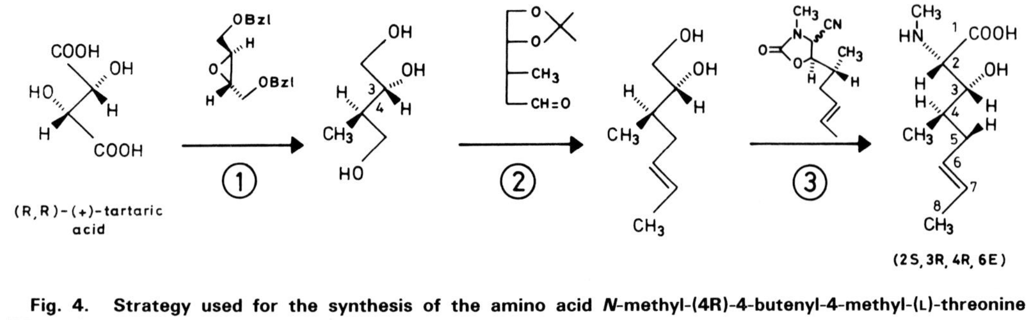

Fig. 4. Strategy used for the synthesis of the amino acid *N*-methyl-(4R)-4-butenyl-4-methyl-(L)-threonine (MeBmt).

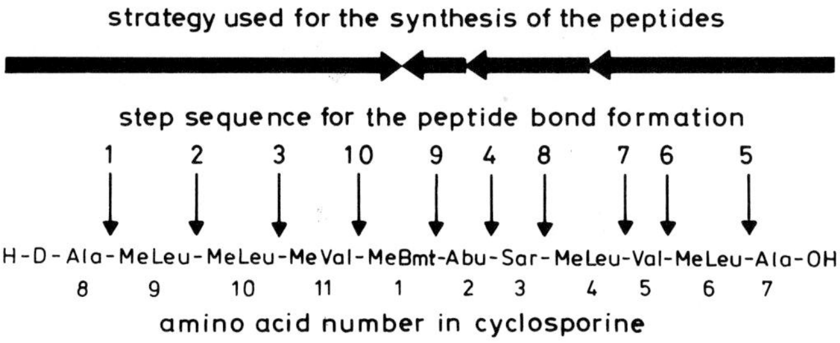

Fig. 5. Strategy used for the synthesis of the peptides.

step. This synthesis has been described elsewhere in detail.[6,11]

SYNTHESIS OF CYCLOSPORINE

Choice of the Cyclization Step (Fig. 1)

In the synthesis of cyclosporine, cyclization is effected at the peptide bond between the L-alanine in position 7 and the D-alanine in position 8. Bond formation between N-methylated amino acids presents more difficulties than for non-N-methylated derivatives. For this reason, bond formation between the only consecutive pair of non-N-methylated amino acids in cyclosporine was chosen for the cyclization step.

Strategy Used for the Synthesis of the Undecapeptide

A fragment condensation technique introducing the MeBmt amino acid at the end of the synthesis was used for the synthesis of the linear undecapeptide. In this way, the number of steps after the introduction of the MeBmt amino acid is minimized. The peptide fragments are built up in the direction shown in Fig. 5 by the arrows using the step sequence that is indicated numerically. Bonds 1,2, and 3 were first made and the tetrapeptide BOC-D-Ala-MeLeu-MeLeu-MeVal-benzylester synthesized. The benzylester of this tetrapeptide could not be made starting from the right, by making the bond 3 first, because of instantaneous formation of a diketopiperazine ring when working with the dipeptide H-MeLeu-MeVal-benzylester. Bond 4 was made, and the dipeptide BOC-Abu-Sar-benzylester synthesized.

The tetrapeptide BOC-MeLeu-Val-MeLeu-Ala-benzylester was synthesized by forming bonds 5,6, and 7 in that order. Then, by forming the bond 8, the hexapeptide BOC-Abu-Sar-MeLeu-Val-MeLeu-Ala-benzylester was prepared. Following the formation of bond 9 and the synthesis of the heptapeptide H-MeBmt-Abu-Sar-MeLeu-Val-MeLeu-Ala-benzylester, the final amide linkage—the bond 10—was made to produce the undecapeptide BOC-Ala-MeLeu-MeLeu-MeVal-MeBmt-Abu-Sar-MeLeu-Val-MeLeu-Ala-benzylester. Cyclosporine (Fig. 6) is obtained

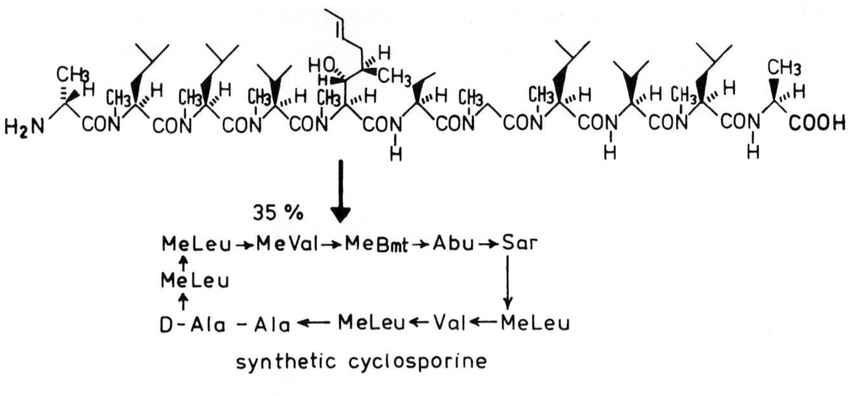

Fig. 6. Cyclization of the undecapeptide to cyclosporine.

in a yield of 35% if cyclization is effected on the undecapeptide with a free amino group and a free carboxyl group using the BOP-reagent[12] or the mixed phosphonic anhydride method.[13]

Activation of the Carboxyl Group for Peptidization

Carboxyl groups are activated using the mixed pivalic anhydride method according to Zaoral[14] and modified by us in such a way that

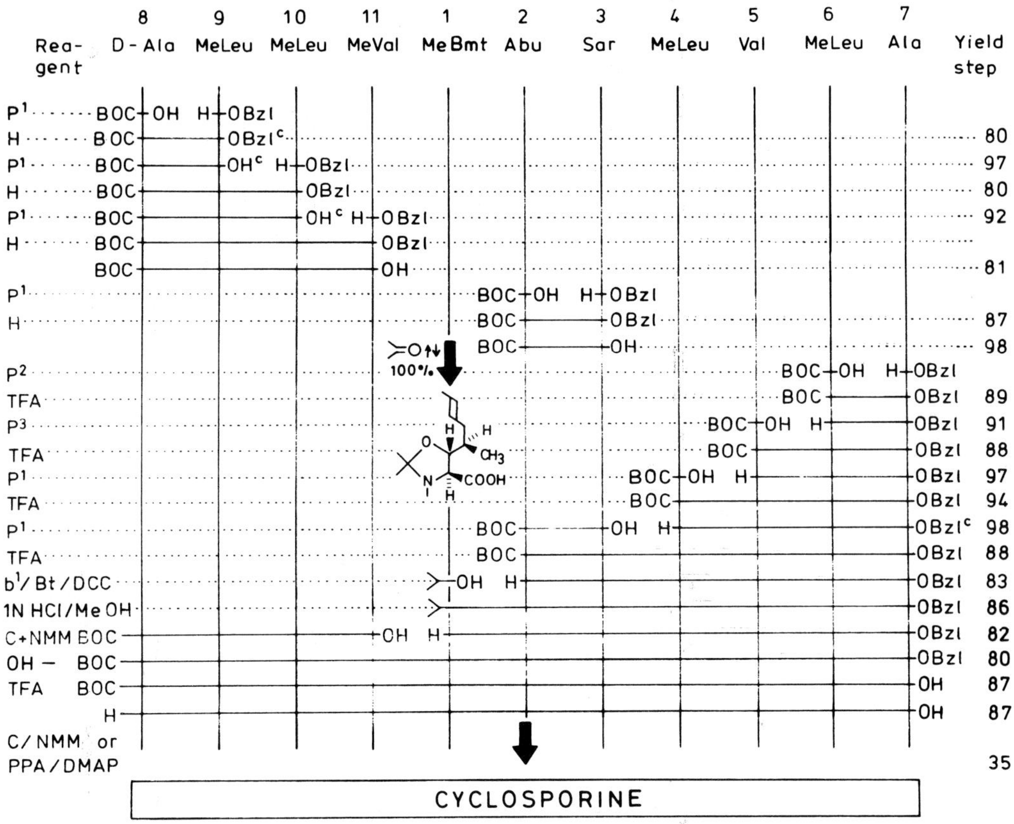

Fig. 7. Synthesis of cyclosporine. b = base; 1 = NMM = N-methylmorpholine; c = crystalline.

C = BOP = benzotriazolyl-*N*-oxy-tris (dimethylamino) phosphonium hexafluorophosphate

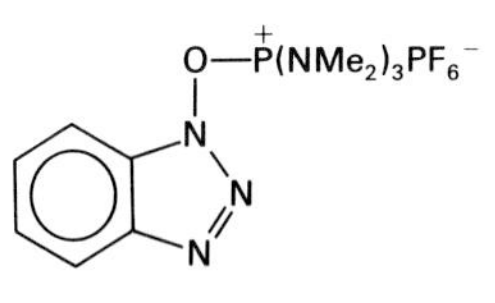

T.L. *1975,* 1219[12]

DCC = dicyclohexylcarbodiimide

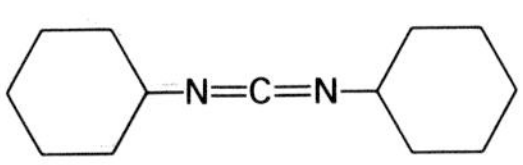

Bt = *N* = hydroxy-benztriazol

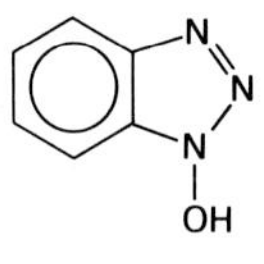

DMAP = 4-Dimethylamino-pyridine; H = Hydrogen + palladium on charcoal in EtOH;

PPA = $(CH_3CH_2CH_2\text{-}PO_2)_3$ Angew. *1980,* 129; P = mixed pivalic anhydride method (+ +COCl + base).[14]

the anhydride formation with pivaloylchloride is made at $-20°C$ to $-25°C$ during 3–6 hr in the presence of two equivalents of *N*-methylmorpholine. Strong activation of the carboxyl group—as in the case of an anhydride—is necessitated by the low reactivity of most of the usual forms of activation used in the peptide synthesis when applied to protected N-methyl-amino acids. The *N*-methyl-(4R)-4-butenyl-4-methyl-threonine is incorporated as a derivative, having a five-membered ring protecting the hydroxy and the methylamino functions. The dimethyloxazolidine-protecting group is introduced quantitatively by refluxing the amino acid in acetone and has the advantage of avoiding epimerization of the MeBmt amino acid during peptide bond formation (thermodynamically more stable trans structure). The peptide bond 9 is made using the classical dicyclohexylcarbodiimide (DCC) method in presence of HOBt.[15,16] The BOP-reagent[12] has been used for the formation of bond 10. The use of this reagent has the advantage that BOC-D-Ala-MeLeu-MeLeu-MeVal-OH (DLLL) or its diastereomer (DLLD) give selectively the same reaction product, the desired (DLLL)-(LLLLLLL)-undecapeptide.

Scheme and Yields of the Reactions

The yields of all reactions are 80% or above, with the sole exception of the cyclization step (35%). The synthesis is shown schematically in Fig. 7.

MODIFIED CYCLOSPORINES

Choice of the Variations

Some naturally occurring modifications of the cyclosporine peptide structure have been described,[2,7–9] and their contribution to our understanding of structure–activity relationships will be described in below. Using the synthetic approach, potentially any amino acid can be modified and specific aspects of the structure–activity relationships examined one after the other. Four such variations will be described here, together with the synthesis of cyclosporin-H, a naturally occurring isomer of cyclosporine.

In order to study the importance of the unusual carbon chain of the *N*-methyl-(4R)-4-butenyl-4-methyl-(L)-threonine (MeBmt) in position one, this amino acid was replaced by *N*-methyl-threonine, which retains the polar features of MeBmt but not the extended lipophilic chain.

(Threonine^2) Cyclosporine (CsC) is a potent immunosuppressant, and unlike the other natural variations of the amino acid in position 2 of cyclosporine, carries a hydroxyl group. To examine whether or not this hydroxyl group is involved in some special receptor interaction, a modified cyclosporine with a serine in position 2 (replacing Abu in CsA and Thr in CsC) was prepared.

The x-ray structure of cyclosporine indicates that the sarcosine in position 3 participates in a type I β turn. Replacement of sarcosine by D-proline would be expected to stabilize this structural feature and make it more rigid. The proline ring would be expected to take an equatorial position relative to the peptide ring and should not alter the conformation of the peptide backbone relative to that of cyclosporine.

To relieve steric crowding and to allow a little more flexibility into the peptide ring at position 11, *N*-methyl-valine was replaced by *N*-methyl-leucine, an amino acid with one additional methylene group in its carbon chain.

The above four modifications of cyclosporine also would be expected to provide information as to the sensitivity of the biologic activity of cyclosporine to minor changes at each position and indicate whether or not these amino acids are likely to be involved in interactions with the receptor.

Synthesis of (MeThr^1) Cyclosporine

Following the same strategy as used for the synthesis of cyclosporine (see above), bond 9 is made between BOC-(OBzl)Thr-OH and the hexapeptide to synthesize the heptapeptide BOC-Thr(OBzl)-Abu-Sar-MeLeu-Val-

MeLeu-Ala-benzylester. The BOC-protecting group is removed with trifluoroacetic acid at −20°C to produce H-Thr(OBzl)-Abu-Sar-MeLeu-Val-MeLeu-Ala-benzylester, which is coupled with the tetrapeptide BOC-D-Ala-MeLeu-MeLeu-MeVal-OH using the BOP-reagent,[12] resulting in the formation of bond 10 and the linear undecapeptide BOC-D-Ala-MeLeu-MeLeu-MeVal-MeThr(OBzl)-Abu-Sar-MeLeu-Val-MeLeu-Ala-benzylester. The ester- and BOC-protecting groups are removed by hydrolysis with 0.2 *N* sodium hydroxide and trifluoracetic acid, respectively. [(OBzl)Thr[1]]-cyclosporine is then formed in a yield of 32% by cyclization of the undecapeptide using the mix *n*-propylphosphonic anhydride method.[13] By removing the benzyl-protecting group with hydrogen and palladium on charcoal (MeThr[1])-cyclosporine (Fig. 8) is obtained quantitatively.

Synthesis of (Ser²) Cyclosporine

This analogue of cyclosporine is synthesized following the same fragment condensation technique as for cyclosporine (see above). Using FMOC-$(OSi(CH_3)_2C(CH_3)_3)$Ser-OH and H-Sar-OBzl as starting materials, bond 4 was formed via a mixed pivalic anhydride coupling, and the dipeptide FMOC-Ser(OSi-$(CH_3)_2C(CH_3)_3$)-Sar-benzylester obtained. The bond 8 was then formed, producing the hexapeptide FMOC-Ser(OSi$(CH_3)_2$-$C(CH_3)_3$)-Sar-MeLeu-Val-MeLeu-Ala-benzylester. Following the formation of bond 9 and the synthesis of the protected heptapeptide, the amino hydroxy protecting groups were removed by acid treatment and H-MeBmt-Ser-Sar-MeLeu-Val-MeLeu-Ala-benzylester isolated. The final amide linkage—the bond 10—was made to produce the undecapeptide BOC-D-Ala-MeLeu-MeLeu-MeVal-MeBmt-Ser-Sar-MeLeu-Val-MeLeu-Ala-benzylester. (Ser[2]) Cyclosporine (Fig. 9) is obtained in a yield of 30%, if cyclization is effected on the undecapeptide with a free amino group and a free carboxy group using the *n*-propylphosphonic anhydride method of Wissmann et al.[13]

Synthesis of (D-Pro³) Cyclosporine

For this analogue of cyclosporine, bond 4 was made starting from BOC-Abu-OH and coupling it with H-D-Pro-benzylester to form the dipeptide BOC-Abu-D-Pro-benzylester. Then, by forming the bond 8, the hexapeptide BOC-Abu-(D)-Pro-MeLeu-Val-MeLeu-Ala-benzylester was prepared. Following the formation of bond 9 and the synthesis of the heptapeptide H-MeBmt-Abu-(D)-Pro-MeLeu-Val-MeLeu-Ala-benzylester, the final amide linkage—the bond 10—was formed to produce the undecapeptide BOC-D-Ala-MeLeu-MeLeu-MeVal-MeBmt-Abu-D-Pro-MeLeu-Val-MeLeu-Ala-benzylester. Cyclization is effected on the undecapeptide with a

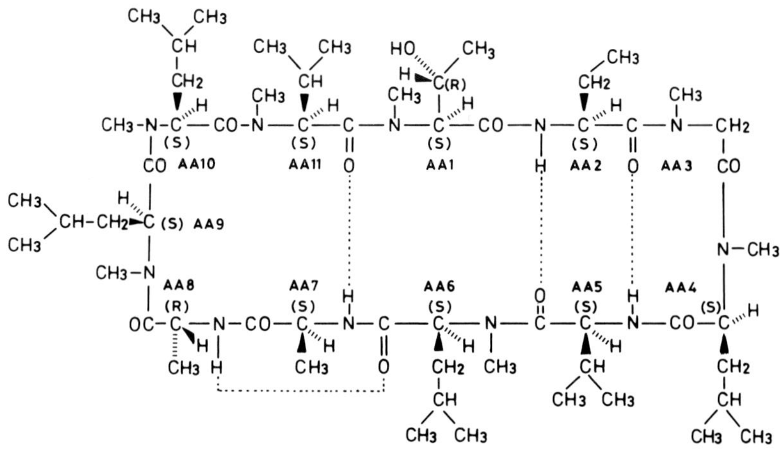

Fig. 8. (*N*-Methyl-threonine¹)Cyclosporine.

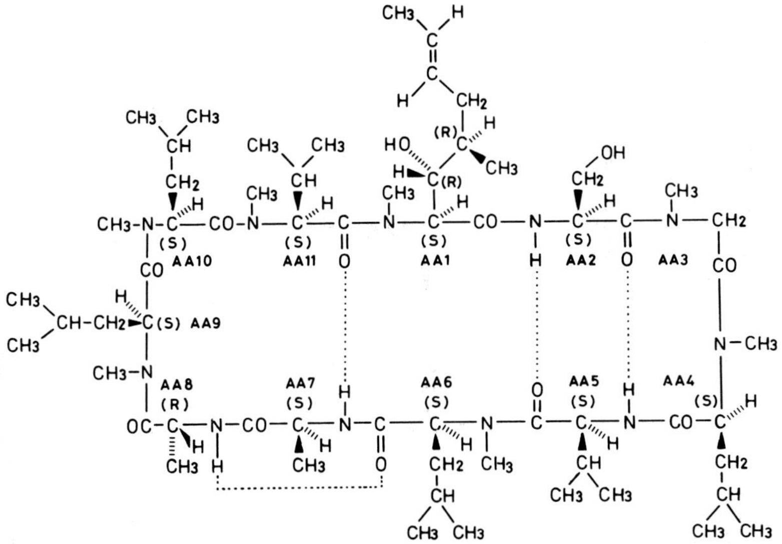

Fig. 9. (Serine[2])Cyclosporine.

free amino group and a free carboxy group using the mixed *n*propylphosphonic anhydride method developed by Wissmann et al.[13] to produce (D-Pro[3])cyclosporine (Fig. 10) in 25% yield.

Synthesis of (MeLeu[11])Cyclosporine

This *N*-methyl-(L)-leucine analogue of cyclosporine was made via the following variation of the synthesis of cyclosporine. Starting from the tripeptide BOC-D-Ala-MeLeu-MeLeu-OH, bond 3 was made, and the tetrapeptide BOC-D-Ala-MeLeuMeLeu-MeLeu-benzylester synthesized. The benzylester protecting group was removed, and the tetrapeptide acid condensed with the heptapeptide H-MeBmt-Abu-Sar-MeLeuVal-MeLeu-Ala-benzylester, forming bond 10 and

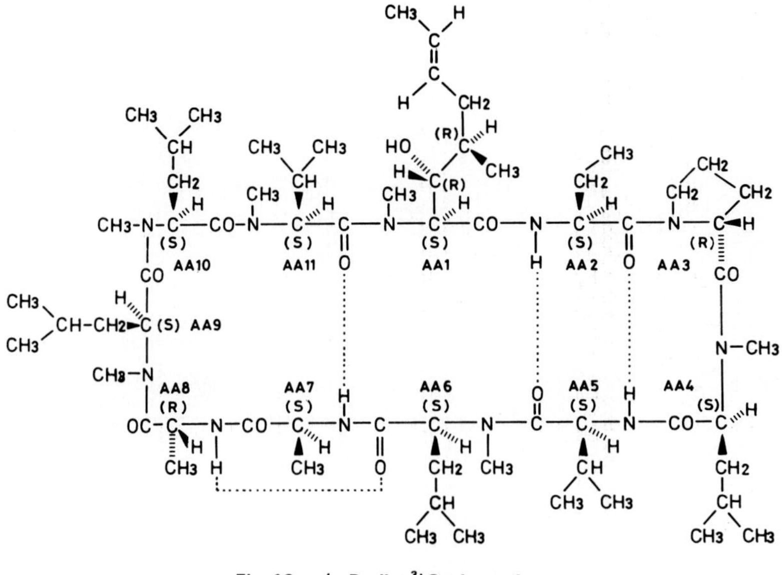

Fig. 10. (D-Proline[3])Cyclosporine.

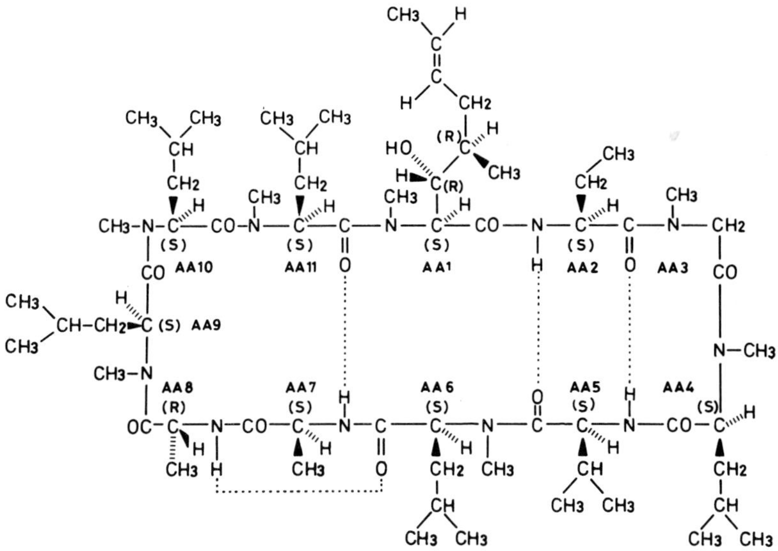

Fig. 11. (*N*-Methyl-leucine[11])Cyclosporine.

the undecapeptide BOC-D-AlaMeLeu-MeLeu-MeLeu-MeBmt-Abu-SarMeLeu-Val-MeLeu-Ala-benzylester. The benzylester and BOC-protecting groups are removed by hydrolysis with 0.2 *N* sodium-hydroxide and trifluoroacetic acid, respectively. (MeLeu[11])-cyclosporine (Fig. 11) is then obtained in a yield of 30% by cyclization, using the mixed *n*-propylphosphonic anhydride method described by Wissmann et al.[13] The structural assignments for this analogue have been supported by an x-ray crystallographic analysis of (MeLeu[11])cyclosporine performed by Dr. H.P. Weber in the Sandoz Research Laboratories in Basel. This unpublished analysis confirms the structure predicted by total synthesis and by physicochemical methods. It also shows that the backbone of (MeLeu[11])cyclosporine has practically the same conformation as cyclosporine itself in the solid state.

Synthesis of (D-MeVal[11])Cyclosporine

This analogue of cyclosporine was made with exactly the same starting materials using the same strategy as for the synthesis of cyclosporine, with the sole exception that the tetrapeptide BOC-D-Ala-MeLeu-MeLeu-MeVal-OH (DLLL) was condensed with the heptapeptide H-MeBmt-Abu-Sar-MeLeu-Val-MeLeu-Ala-benzylester using the mixed pivalic anhydride method[14] instead of the BOP-reagent[12] forming bond 10 and selectively producing the undecapeptide BOC-D-Ala-MeLeu-MeLeu-D-MeVal-MeBmt-Abu-Sar-MeLeu-Val-MeLeu-Ala-benzylester at −25°C. (D-MeVal[11])cyclosporine (Fig. 12) was obtained in a yield of 65% using the mixed *n*-propylphosphonic anhydride method[13] for cyclization. This compound is in all respects (NMR, rotation, m.p.) identical to the natural cyclosporin-H.[9]

BIOLOGIC ACTIVITY AND STRUCTURE–ACTIVITY RELATIONSHIPS OF CYCLOSPORINE ANALOGUES

The relative potency of some synthetic and naturally occurring analogues of cyclosporine are shown in Table 1. The compounds were characterized using pharmacologic models previously used to test cyclosporine.[17–22] Details of the tests used and differences in activity spectrum will be presented elsewhere (P. Hiestand, manuscript in preparation).

From the results in Table 1, it is evident that the carbon chain of amino acid 1 is important for biologic activity. Removal of the nonpolar part of the side chain, as in

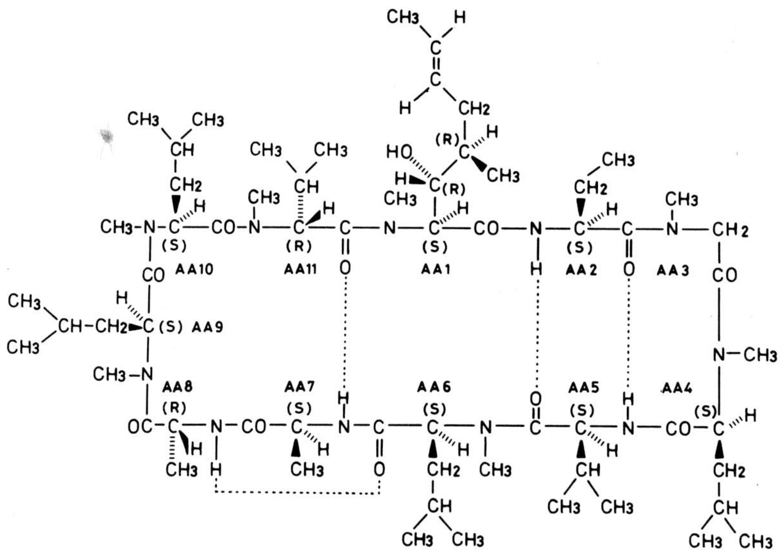

Fig. 12. [(D)-*N*-Methylvaline[11]]Cyclosporine (CS-H).

(MeThr[1])cyclosporine, reduces the immunosuppressive activity dramatically, as does modification of the hydroxy group, as seen in *O*-acetyl- and des-oxy cyclosporine. Even the double bone makes a contribution to the biologic activity, since dihydrocompounds are generally less potent.

Amino acid 2 permits some variation, with alkyl chains of 2–3 carbons showing good activity. Although (Thr[2])cyclosporine is a potent immunosuppressant, (Ser[2])cyclosporine is significantly less active, suggesting that hydrophobic interactions are more important for the interaction of the aliphatic chain of amino acid 2 with the receptor and that the OH group of (Thr[2])cyclosporine is not involved in any special binding function.

Although (D-Pro[3])cyclosporine and (MeLeu[11])cyclosporine should have almost the same conformation as cyclosporine itself, they are negative variants, suggesting that, in this case, the steric bulk of the peptide side chains

Table 1. Immunosuppressant Activity of Cyclosporine Analogues

	Activity	Natural Product or Synthetic	References
Cyclosporine	***	Nat.	2
(MeThr[1]) cyclosporine	*	Synt.	
(Thr[2]) cyclosporine	***	Nat.	7
(Ser[2]) cyclosporine	**	Synt.	
(Ala[2]) cyclosporine	**	Nat	8
(Val[2]) cyclosporine	**	Nat.	8
(nVal[2]) cyclosporine	***	Nat.	9
(D-Pro[3]) cyclosporine	*	Synt.	
(D-MeVal[11]) cyclosporine	*	Nat./Synt.	9
(MeLeu[11]) cyclosporine	*	Synt.	
(O-acetyl)-cyclosporine	*		9
3′-Desoxy-cyclosporine	*	Nat.	9
Dihydro-cyclosporine	**		2
H-MeBmt-OH	*	Synt.	

***Indicates potent immunosuppressant activity, **intermediate activity, and *little or no activity.

probably prevents efficient binding of these derivatives to the cyclosporine receptor. The loss of activity observed with (D-MeVal[11])cyclosporine, a derivative in which the conformation of the peptide ring at this position is certainly different from that of cyclosporine, also confirms that the carbon chain of amino acid 11 is important for biologic activity.

In conclusion, some structure–activity relationships for cyclosporine are now emerging from the study of specifically modified derivatives. However, much remains to be done. It is clear that the unusual MeBmt chain is intimately involved in the biologic actions of the cyclosporine molecule, but that it alone is not sufficient for immunosuppressant activity. The biologic activity is associated with a larger portion of the cyclosporine structure, and the results presented above indicated that this probably includes amino acids 1, 2, 3, and 11.

REFERENCES

1. Dreyfuss M, Härri E, Hoffmann H, et al: Eur J Appl Microbiol 3:125, 1976

2. Rüegger A, Kuhn M, Lichti H, et al: Helv Chim Acta 59:1075, 1976

3. Petcher TJ, Weber HP, Rüegger A: Helv Chim Acta 59:1480, 1976

4. Cambie RC, Rayward RC, Roberts JL, et al: J Chem Soc Perkin 1:1120, 1974

5. Cambie RC, Hayward RC, Robert JL, et al: J Chem Soc Perkin 1:1858, 1974

6. Wenger R: In White DJG (ed): Cyclosporin A. Amsterdam, Elsevier Biomedical, 1982, p 19

7. Traber R, Kuhn M, Rügger A, et al: Helv Chim Acta 60:1247, 1977

8. Traber R, Kuhn M, Loosli HR, et al: Helv Chim Acta 60:1568, 1977

9. Traber R, Loosli HR, Hofmann H, et al: Helv Chim Acta 65:1655, 1982

10. Schlosser M, Christmann KF: Ann Chem 708:1, 1967

11. Wenger R: Helv Chim Acta (in press)

12. Castro B, Dormoy JR, Evin G, et al: Tetrahedron Lett 1219, 1975

13. Wissmann H, Kleiner HJ: Angew Chem 92:129, 1980

14. Zoaral M: Coll Czech Chem Commun 27:1273, 1962

15. Khorana HG: Chem Rev 53:145, 1953

16. König W, Geiger R: Chem Ber 103:788, 1970

17. Borel JF, Feurer C, Gubler HU, et al: Agents Actions 6:468, 1976

18. Borel JF, Feurer C, Magnée C, et al: Immunology 31:631, 1976

19. Borel JF, Feurer C, Magnée C, et al: Immunology 32:1017, 1977

20. Borel JF, Wiesinger D, Gublier HU: Eur J Rheum Inflam 1:237, 1978

21. Wiesinger D, Borel JF: Immunobiology 156:454, 1979

22. Ryffel B, Goetz U, Heuberger B: J Immunol 129:1978, 1982

Cyclosporine-A (CsA): Models for the Mechanism of Action

K. J. Lafferty, J. F. Borel, and P. Hodgkin

CYCLOSPORINE-A (CsA) is the first of a new generation of immunosuppressive agents with a specific site of action within the immune system.[1] The agent is primarily lymphocyte specific and acts at an early stage of its activation.[1] It has a very low degree of myelotoxicity, a feature that has made its use in bone marrow transplantation attractive. The drug also appears to suppress lymphocyte function without damaging the phagocytic activity of the reticuloendothelial system; animals treated with CsA show a normal capacity to clear colloidal carbon or heterologous erythrocytes from the circulation. The drug does not affect the migratory capacity of phagocytic cells; human monocytes phagocytose bacteria in a normal manner in the presence of CsA.[2-5] Thus, cyclosporine-A provides the means for regulation of the lymphocytic response to a tissue graft without completely laying waste the antibacterial defenses of the recipient. It is important that we understand this drug's mechanism of action.

There is general agreement that CsA affects the function of T lymphocytes and that many of its in vivo effects stem from this modification of T-cell function.[6-11] There is little agreement beyond this point. There are a number of competing theories concerning the mechanism of T-cell activation, and these ideas have become entwined with attempts to understand just where CsA exerts its control. In this discussion, we will first consider arguments as they relate to the process of T-cell activation and then examine how well different models for the action of CsA fit the experimental findings. Having come to some conclusions about the drug's mode of action, we will consider how these ideas relate to its in vivo function.

T-CELL ACTIVATION

It was once thought that antigen alone triggered the process of lymphocyte (T-cell) activation.[12] However, it is now clear that antigen does not provide a sufficient stimulus for lymphocyte activation. Two signals are required for T-cell activation.[13-17] One signal is provided by antigen binding, and the second signal is provided by a molecule that expresses costimulator (CoS) activity.[18] Evidence for the two-signal model came initially from a study of T-cell responses to living or u.v.-killed spleen cells,[13] and from a study of the in vitro response of T cells to cultured tumor lines.[17]

Tumors fall into two categories. Those of lymphoreticular origin have the capacity to stimulate allogeneic lymphocytes in vitro and are said to express the S^+ phenotype.[17] Other tumors, such as cells of epithelial origin, are S^-. Table 1 shows some of the characteristics of S^+ and S^- tumors derived from the DBA/2 mouse strain. The P815 tumor expresses the S^+ phenotype and will activate allogeneic T cells in vitro. Inactivation of this cell line, with u.v.-irradiation, converts it to the S^- phenotype. The epithelial tumor is constitutively S^- and the γ-irradiated (metabolically active) cell fails to stimulate allogeneic T cells in vitro (Table 1). When a source of lymphokine is added to the cultures, the S^- cell lines stimulate a strong response (Table 1). Clearly, the S^- cells have all the antigenic requirements for T-cell activation, but presentation of anti-

From the Barbara Davis Center for Childhood Diabetes, Denver, CO; Preclinical Research, Sandoz Ltd., Basel, Switzerland; and the Transplantation Biology Unit, John Curtin School of Medical Research, Canberra, Australia.

Address reprint requests to Dr. K. J. Lafferty, Barbara Davis Center for Childhood Diabetes, 4200 East Ninth Avenue, Box B140, Denver, CO 80262.

0041-1345/83/1505-0005$01.00/0

Table 1. Two Signals are Required For Alloantigen-Mediated Activation of Cytotoxic T-Cell Precursors[17]

In Vitro Reaction Mixture*	Cytotoxic Activity (Log_{10} CU/Culture) No Added Lymphokine	Lymphokine Added To Cultures
P815(γ) → C57BL LN†	5.4	6.0
P815(u.v.) → C57BL LN	2.5	6.1
CaD2(γ) → C57BL LN	3.7	6.0
C57BL LN	3.7	3.7

*Technical details of this study were described by Talmage et al.[17]
†Lymph node.

gen alone is not a sufficient condition for induction of the T-cell response. Addition of lymphokine alone (Table 1) also fails to provide a sufficient stimulus for T-cell activation. Hence, the process of T-cell activation requires the provision of both signals.

These results also demonstrate that lymphocyte activation in such cultures does not *require* the processing of antigen by some accessory cell in the responsive population.[19] While such antigen processing may take place, it cannot account for the response observed. If the response was induced in this way, we would not expect to see such a marked difference between the S^+ and S^- tumors. That is not to say that antigen processing does not have an important role in the immune system. Antigen processing by a stimulator cell is seen as the normal way in which soluble antigens trigger the immune response.[19] Allogeneic interactions are simply abnormal immune reactions in which the foreign antigen is an integral part of the stimulator cell surface.[19]

The process of T-cell activation has been analyzed in some detail by Larsson et al.,[16] who showed the antigen-presenting stimulator cell of the mouse to be Ia^+, possibly the dendritic cell,[20] and that interleukin 1 (IL 1) provided the second signal required for lymphocyte activation.[11,16] That is, IL 1 expresses costimulator (CoS) activity. They also showed the activated T cell to have receptors for IL2. This molecule provides the signal required for T-cell proliferation and resultant clonal expansion.[21]

We can write these reactions in the following way,

$$T \xrightarrow[(2)]{(1)} T' \text{ -------- (a)}$$

$$T \xrightarrow{IL2} nT' \text{ -------- (b)},$$

where T is the resting T cell, and T′ is the activated T cell that carries receptors for IL2 and can express effector function.[11] Signal (1) is provided by antigen binding to the T-cell surface and signal (2) is CoS activity, which can be provided by IL1.[19]

There is controversy concerning the details of the events leading to lymphocyte activation and clonal expansion. One school of thought sees T cells as being divided into functionally distinct subsets, the helper subset and the cytotoxic/suppressor subset, which have distinct antigenic markers (Table 2) and differ in that the former is specified wholly or in part by class II MHC antigens, and the latter by class I antigens.[22] The more extreme adherents of this notion suggest that the helper subset produces helper factors, but does not respond to these factors, and that it is the cytotoxic/suppressor subset that responds to helper factors.[23,24] Others do not see such a strict division of function; they admit that T cells of both subsets respond to growth factors, but suggest that cytotoxic and helper function are properties of different subsets.[25,26] On the other hand, there is evidence that cells belonging to the different subsets, defined in terms of antigenic markers ($Lyt2^+$/$Lyt2^-$; OKT8/OKT4) and MHC antigen reactivity, can express both cytotoxic activity and produce lymphokine when appropriately triggered.[27–29] Studies of this latter type have involved the use of bulk cultures of cells, and it may be that such cultures are made up of a heterogeneous group of cells with differing function. Certainly, clonal analysis of T-cell function has shown the potential for cells to express either cytotoxic or helper function, or a combination of these functions.[9] What is clear, however, is that the strict division of T-cell populations into functionally distinct subsets on the basis of antigenic markers and MHC antigen reactivity is not warranted at this stage. We have shown that reactions (a) and (b) above also describe events involved in the activation and clonal expansion of both the $Lyt2^+$ and $Lyt2^-$ subset in the mouse.[30]

Activated T cells (T′) secrete a number of different lymphokines when appropriately stimulated.[31] These lymphokines include IL2, IL3, macrophage-activating factor (MAF), migration inhibitory factors (MIF), and interferon (IF).

Cycling T′ cells do not secrete lymphokine. In fact, biochemical studies (Granelli-Piperno, personal communication) have shown that these cells do not contain mRNA for IL2 synthesis. Within 2–4 hr of triggering with either antigen or mitogen, T′ cells begin to secrete lymphokine.[30] In marked contrast to the process of T-cell activation, triggering of T′ cells into lymphokine production requires only one signal—antigen binding to the T-cell receptor.[26]

We can write this process in the following form:

$$T' \xrightarrow{(1)} l \text{ -------- (c).}$$

Signal (1) can be provided either by the specific priming antigen or by mitogen.[30]

The reactions describing primary T-cell activation (a), clonal expansion (b), and the triggering of lymphokine release (c), apply to cells of either subset when these subsets are defined in the classical way (Table 2). Moreover, cells of each subset can express cytotoxic activity.[32] That is, there is no asymmetry in the process of T-cell activation and clonal expansion, and all activated T-cell populations have the potential to express cytotoxic activity or produce lymphokine.

Table 2. Classical Classification of T-Cell Subsets on the Basis of Alloantigen Reactivity and Surface Antigenic Markers

T ↙	↘
$T'_{(K)}$, $T'_{(K.x)}$*	$T'_{(I)}$, $T'_{(I.x)}$*
Cytotoxic/Suppressor Subset	Helper Subset
$Lyt2^+$, $OKT8^+$	$Lyt2^-$, $OKT4^+$
Class I reactive	Class II reactive

*$T'_{(K)}$: activated T cells specific for class I MHC antigens (K-type antigens).

$T'_{(K.x)}$: activated T cells specific for antigen x seen in association with class I MHC antigens.

$T'_{(I)}$: activated T cells specific for class II MHC antigens (I-type antigens).

$T'_{(I.x)}$: activated T cells specific for antigen x seen in association with class II MHC antigens.

K and I region antigens of the mouse H-2 complex are used as prototypes for class I and class II MHC antigens.

SITE OF ACTION OF CsA

Basically, two different models have been proposed to account for the biologic activity of CsA.

(1) *The subset model* postulates that different subsets show differing sensitivities to CsA. The drug inhibits the activation of the helper subset, and because "help" is required for the activation of the cytotoxic subset, the drug secondarily inhibits cytotoxic cell formation.[22] It is also proposed that CsA does not inhibit the activation of suppressor cells.[33] This model sees CsA to have a differential effect on different T-cell subsets.

(2) *The signaling model* does not discriminate between the activities expressed by subsets defined as set out in Table 2. This model postulated that CsA interferes with the transmission of the antigen-specific signal (1) to the interior of the cell at some stage following antigen binding.[28] A variant of this model is the idea that CsA interferes with signaling by preventing the binding of antigen to the cell membrane.[34]

Let us now consider how the known experimental information relates to each of these models. To carry out this analysis, it is convenient to consider the effect of CsA on each of the three steps in T-cell activation and expression of function (reaction a, b, and c above).

Clonal Expansion—Reaction (b)

There is general agreement that CsA, at concentrations of up to 1 μg/ml, does not affect IL2-dependent clonal expansion of activated T cells.[6,9,10,11,22] At concentrations higher than 4 μg/ml, the drug is inhibitory, possibly due to a toxic effect. This latter conclusion is speculative, and studies of the reversibility of the effect seen at high CsA concentrations would clarify this point.

Function of Activated T Cells (T′)

Cyclosporine-A does not inhibit the expression of cytotoxic activity by cells of the T′ class.[1,11] Since expression of cytotoxic activity requires the binding of the T′ cell to its target, it follows that the drug cannot inhibit antigen binding to the T′ cell. Palacios and Moller suggested the CsA expressed its function by inhibiting the binding of class II MHC antigen to the specific T-cell receptor in the autlogous mixed lymphocyte reaction (MLR).[34] The above evidence makes this an unlikely explanation. A close examination of the data that form the basis of this conclusion[34] shows that CsA inhibits the result of class II antigen binding to the reactive T cell. This block could be at the level of antigen binding or it could be at some stage subsequent to binding.

Reaction (c), the antigen- or mitogen-triggered release of lymphokine from the activated T cell, is inhibited by CsA in the concentration range of 10–100 ng/ml: CsA, in this concentration range, does not inhibit binding of antigen to the T′ cell population[11] or to a cloned cell line.[9] It follows, therefore, that the drug must interfere with the delivery of signal (1) at some stage after antigen binding by the T cell receptor.[9,11]

Two pieces of experimental evidence allow us to focus more sharply on the site at which CsA blocks the "helper-function" of T′ cells. Studies from our laboratory have shown that CsA at concentrations of as high as 1.0 μg/ml has no effect on lymphokine (IL2) production by the primate MLA144 cell line (unpublished).

The drug also has no effect on IL3 secretion by WEHI-3 (unpublished); CsA does inhibit IL3 production by specific antigen- or mitogen-triggered T′ cells. At face value, this evidence suggests that CsA does not inhibit the process of lymphokine synthesis and export out of the cell; the constitutive lymphokine producers are insensitive to the drug. Evidence presented at this meeting[35] suggests that this is not some odd characteristic of tumor line. Bouwer et al.[35] have demonstrated that within 8 hr of triggering by antigen, IL2 production by cells of the T′ class becomes insensitive to CsA. Thus, if CsA does not inhibit antigen binding and if it does not affect the synthesis or export of lymphokine from the T′ cell, it follows that the drug must interfere with the transmission of the antigenic signal to the nucleus of the cell. A more accurate designation of CsAs site of action on the T′ cell will require detailed biochemical investigation.

While it is clear that CsA inhibits the expression of the helper function of T′ cells,[9,10,11,22] and does not affect the expression of cytotoxic function,[1,9,11] it is not a subset-specific inhibitory agent. In the mouse, cells of both the $Lyt2^+$ and $Lyt2^-$ subset produce both IL2 and IL3, and this function of T′ cells of both subsets is equally sensitive to inhibition by CsA (unpublished data).

Primary T-Cell Activation: T → T′

The process of primary T-cell activation is more difficult to analyze because of its multifactorial nature. Two signals, antigen binding in the presence of a source of IL1, are required to shift the T cell to the T′ state.[11,16] CsA interferes with this step in the case of the generation of both lymphokine-producing T cells and cytotoxic T cells.[9,11] However, this system is inherently leaky. CsA is a reversible inhibitor of T-cell function, that is, at any given concentration of CsA, there will be a finite probability that a fraction of the cells will not be blocked by the drug. This fraction will decrease as the concentration of drug increases, but will only asymptote to zero. On the other hand, any cells that escape to the T′ state, an event that will be likely if both antigen and some exogenous source of lymphokine is present in the cultures, will be insensitive to CsA (see above). Thus, there will be a tendency for added lymphokine to compete with the effect of CsA on the primary interaction and for the system to leak toward the formation and clonal expansion of activated cells. Experimental evidence indicates this to be the case.[6,7]

The fact that CsA can inhibit the formation of cytotoxic or lymphokine-producing T′ cells, even in the presence of added lymphokine, shows that the effect of CsA on T-cell priming is not simply due to lymphokine production by "helper" cells.

In conclusion we can make the following points:

(1) Clonal expansion of activated T cells is insensitive to CsA. That is, CsA does not interfere with the signal delivered to the activated T cell by IL2.

(2) The response of the activated T cell to antigenic triggering is very sensitive to CsA, and the effect appears to result from an interference with the delivery of the immunologically specific signal to the nucleus of the cell.

(3) The process of primary T-cell activation is inhibited. However, because CsA is a reversible inhibitor of T-cell function, and because of the multifactorial nature of this reaction, there is a competitive interaction between antigen and lymphokine driving the resting T cell toward the T′ state and the inhibitory effect of CsA.

CsA is not a subset-specific drug in the sense that it affects one subset and not another. At least, this is the case when the subsets are defined in terms of antigenic markers (Table 2). However, it is also clear that CsA affects the helper function (synthesis and release of lymphokine) without interfering with other T-cell effector functions, for example, the expression of cytotoxic activity or clonal expansion under the influence of IL2.

The question of how CsA affects suppressor cell function is open to debate. There is clear in vitro evidence that both antigen-specific and antigen-nonspecific suppressor T cells can be generated in the presence of CsA.[36,37] One question still requires resolution in relation to these studies: Are the suppressor cells generated in vivo relevant to tolerance mechanisms seen in vivo?[38–40] In particular, the antigen-specific tolerance that develops in animals grafted with tissues, such as the heart, under the cover of short-term cyclosporin-A.[39,40] One would like to see evidence for the in vivo transfer of antigen-specific unresponsiveness before wholeheartedly accepting the concept that CsA treatment allows the development of suppressor cells. A better understanding of how suppressor cells function would also assist in the interpretation of this aspect of T-cell biology.

RELEVANCE TO IN VIVO FUNCTION

If we accept that CsA inhibits the pathway of primary T-cell activation, and the expression of helper function, but does not influence the expression of the cytotoxic activity of T′ cells, then we can make certain predictions concerning the in vivo function of this agent. At levels of 100–1000 ng/ml in the tissue fluids, the drug should inhibit T-cell priming and so inhibit primary immune responsiveness. The agent will inhibit lymphokine-dependent functions of T′ cells, e.g., expression of delayed-type hypersensitivity—a function that may be relevant to both allergic phenomenon[41,42] and allograft reactivity—however, the agent will not influence the expression of already activated cytotoxic T cells. Since we have good evidence that T cells of either subset (class I reactive or class II reactive) have the potential to express cytotoxic activity or to release lymphokine, CsA can provide an analytical tool to help investigate which function of a given T′ cell population is responsible for a particular in vivo effect.

REFERENCES

1. Borel JF: Triangle 20:97, 1981

2. Paavonen T, Jarvelainen H, Kontiainen S, et al: Clin Exp Immunol 43:342, 1981

3. Thomson AW, Moon DK, Geczy CL, et al: Immunology (in press)

4. McIntosh LC, Thomson AW: Transplantation 30:384, 1980

5. Tutschka PJ, Beschorner WE, Hess AD: Blut 25:241, 1980

6. Dos Reis GA, Shevach EM: J Immunol 129:2360, 1982

7. Bunjes D, Hardt C, Rollinghoff M, et al: Eur J Immunol 11:657, 1981

8. Hess AD, Tutschka PJ, Pu Z, et al: J Immunol 128:360, 1982

9. Orosz CG, Fidelus RK, Roopenian DC, et al: J Immunol 129:1865, 1982

10. Hess AD, Tutschka PJ, Santos AW: J Immunol 128:355, 1982

11. Andrus L, Lafferty KJ: Scand J Immunol 15:449, 1982

12. Medawar PB: Ciba Found Study Group 16:1, 1963

13. Lafferty KJ, Misko IS, Cooley MA: Nature 249:275, 1974

14. Lafferty KJ, Cunningham AJ: Aust J Exp Biol Med Sci 53:27, 1975

15. Cunningham AJ, Lafferty KJ: Scand J Immunol 6:1, 1977

16. Larsson E-L, Coutinho A: Nature 280:239, 1979

17. Talmage DW, Woolnough JA, Hemmingsen H, et al: Proc Natl Acad Sci USA 74:4610, 1977

18. Larsson E-L, Iscove NN, Coutinho A: Nature 283:664, 1980

19. Lafferty KJ, Prowse SJ, Simeonovic CJ: Annu Rev Immunol 1:143, 1983

20. Steinman RM, Witmer MD, Nussenzweig MC, et al: Transplant Proc 15:299, 1983

21. Larsson E-L, Coutinho A, Martinez AC: Immunol Rev 51:61, 1980

22. Bunjes D, Hardt C, Rollinghoff M, et al: Eur J Immunol 11:657, 1981

23. Wagner H, Rollinghoff M: J Exp Med 148:1523, 1978

24. Gronvik KO, Andersson J: Immunol Rev 51:35, 1980

25. Swain SL, Wetzel GD, Soubiren P, et al: Immunol Rev 63:111, 1982

26. Lafferty KJ, Andrus L, Prowse SJ: Immunol Rev 51:279, 1980

27. Luger TA, Smolen JS, Chused TM, et al: J Clin Invest 70:470, 1982

28. Andrus L, Prowse SJ, Lafferty KJ: Scand J Immunol 13:297, 1981

29. Okada M, Henney CS: J Immunol 125:300, 1980

30. Andrus L, Prowse SJ, Lafferty KJ: Behring Inst Mit 67:61, 1980

31. Prystowsky MB, Ely JM, Beller DI, et al: J Immunol 129:2337, 1982

32. Juretic A, Nagy ZA, Klein J: Nature 289:308, 1981

33. Hess AD, Tutschka PJ: J Immunol 124:2601, 1980

34. Palacios R, Moller A: Nature 290:792, 1981

35. Bouwer HGA, Hinrichs DJ: Transplant Proc (this issue)

36. Hess AD, Tutschka PJ, Santos GW: Transplant Proc 13:374, 1981

37. Wang BS, Heacock EH, Chang-Xue Z, et al: J Immunol 128:1382, 1982

38. Green CJ, Allison AC, Precious S: Lancet 2:123, 1979

39. Hutchinson IF, Shadur CA, Duarte JSA, et al: Transplantation 32:210, 1981

40. Nagao T, White DJG, Caine RY: Transplantation 33:31, 1982

41. McKenzie IFC: Transplant Proc 15:269, 1983

42. Mason DW: Transplant Proc 15:264, 1983

Effect of Cyclosporine on the Induction of Cytotoxic T Lymphocytes: Role of Interleukin-1 and Interleukin-2

A. D. Hess, P. J. Tutschka, and G. W. Santos

CONSIDERABLE interest and enthusiasm has been generated by the recent description of a new immunosuppressive agent, cyclosporine (CsA), a fungal metabolite that is highly immunosuppressive but not myelotoxic.[1] Initial studies by Borel[1] and Borel et al.[2,3] have shown that apart from mild antifungal activity, CsA had profound immunosuppressive activity. In a variety of experimental animal systems, administration of CsA resulted in the inhibition of antibody formation to T-dependent antigens and the suppression of delayed-type hypersensitivity reactions.[3,4] In addition to its ability to inhibit cell-mediated immune responses, CsA also appeared to be capable of preventing graft rejection, and in some animal systems facilitated the induction of transplantation tolerance.[5,6] The mode of action of CsA in preventing graft rejection and its role in establishing immunologic unresponsiveness to allografts remain unclear.

The present report summarizes our studies attempting to assess the role of CsA on the induction of cytotoxic T cells and on the production of soluble proliferative factors, such as interleukin-2 (IL2), in response to alloantigens using the primary mixed lymphocyte reaction (MLR), an in vitro model of the allograft response.

From the Bone Marrow Transplant Program, Oncology Center, The Johns Hopkins University, School of Medicine, Baltimore, MD.

Supported in part by NIH Grants CA-15396, AM-26502, and a gift from the Harley W. Howell Foundation. A.D.H. is a Scholar of the Leukemia Society of America, Inc.

Address reprint requests to Dr. A. D. Hess, Oncology Center, Room 3-127, Johns Hopkins Hospital, 600 North Wolfe Street, Baltimore, MD 21205.

0041-1345/83/1505-0006$02.00/0

MATERIALS AND METHODS

Lymphocyte Isolation

Human peripheral blood lymphocytes were isolated from fresh defibrinated blood from normal healthy volunteers by Ficoll-Paque (Pharmacia Fine Chemicals, Piscataway, NJ) density centrifugation as previously described.[7]

Bulk Mixed Lymphocyte Reactions (MLR)

Bulk primary and secondary MLR were established using standard techniques described in detail elsewhere.[7,8] The cultures were incubated at 37°C in a humidified 5% CO_2 in air incubator. Proliferation in bulk culture was assessed by pipetting 0.1 ml of the bulk culture cell suspension into triplicate wells of a microtiter plate and labeling with 1 μCi of ^{3}H-thymidine as detailed elsewhere.[7,8]

Cell-Mediated Lympholysis Assay (CML)

Primed cells harvested from bulk MLR cultures were incubated for 4 hr at 37°C with 10^4 3-day-old phytohemagglutinin (PHA) blast cells labeled with ^{51}Cr, as previously described.[7] Percent specific ^{51}Cr release was calculated according to the following formula:

$$\%\ \text{Specific}\ ^{51}\text{Cr release} = \frac{\text{cpm Experimental} - \text{cpm Spontaneous}}{\text{cpm Maximum} - \text{cpm Spontaneous}} \times 100.$$

Suppressor Cell Assay

The primed cells from the bulk cultures were tested for their ability to suppress the proliferative response of fresh responding cells (A; autologous to the initial responding cell) to the original sensitizing lymphocytes (B_x; arbitrarily designated specific suppression) and to unrelated third-party lymphocytes (C_x; arbitrarily designated nonspecific suppression), as previously described.[7,8] Percent of the MLR response was calculated according to the following formula:

$$\%\ \text{Suppression} = \frac{\begin{array}{c}\text{Response of test cultures}\\ [(AB_x) + \text{fresh } A + \text{fresh } B_x \text{ or } C_x]\end{array}}{\begin{array}{c}\text{Response of control cultures}\\ [AA_x)_x + \text{fresh } A + \text{fresh } B_x \text{ or } C_x]\end{array}} \times 100.$$

Irradiated (1500 rad) autologously primed lymphocytes $(AA_x)_x$ added in equal numbers as the primed lymphocytes (AB_x) were utilized as the control.[7]

Assay for IL2 and the Ability to Respond to IL2

IL2 activity in supernatants from primary MLR cultures was assessed by measuring the ability of the supernatants to stimulate proliferation and enhance cell-mediated lymphocytotoxicity (CML) activity of alloantigen-primed lymphocytes (harvested from 10-day-old control primary MLR cultures) as previously described.[9,10] IL2 activity in the primary MLR supernatants was also assessed by measuring their ability to support growth of an IL2-dependent cloned cytotoxic T-cell line as described in detail elsewhere.[11] To assess responsiveness to IL2, primed cells (10^6 cells) harvested from primary MLR on days 9–10 were plated in macrotiter wells and cultured with 2 U/ml of IL2 or the day-2 primary control MLR supernatants containing IL2 (50% v/v), as detailed elsewhere.[9,10] The cultures were allowed to incubate for 48 hr, at which time proliferation was assessed by pipetting 0.1 ml of the cell suspension into triplicate wells of a microtiter plate and labeling with 1 μCi of ^{3}H-thymidine for 16–18 hr. On day 3 of culture, the remainder of the cells was harvested and tested for CML activity.

Cyclosporine

Powdered CsA, a generous gift from Sandoz Ltd., Biological and Medical Research Division, Basel, Switzerland, was dissolved in 95% ethanol, diluted to the appropriate concentration with complete culture medium and added to the bulk MLR cultures. Control cultures received ethanol in complete medium. CsA was removed from the cultured lymphocytes prior to assessment of function by incubation in fresh medium containing 20% serum (normal human) at 37°C for 1 hr, followed by 2 washes and resuspension in fresh complete medium.

RESULTS

Effect of CsA on the Production of IL2 in Primary MLR

Initial studies were undertaken to determine the effect of CsA on the production of IL2 in primary MLR, and the results are shown in Fig. 1 and Table 1. CsA markedly reduced the production of IL2 in primary MLR, as detected by the inability of the supernatants from the CsA-treated cultures to support growth of the cloned cytotoxic T-cell line (Table 1). At the highest doses of CsA tested (0.5–2.5 μg/ml), there was a virtual absence of IL2 activity. In cultures receiving 0.1 μg/ml, detectable levels were found in the primary MLR supernatants, but were reduced compared to levels of IL2 found in control MLR cultures. It is of interest to note that addition of CsA to control MLR supernatants did not inhibit the response of the murine cytotoxic T-cell line. Another assay system that we have utilized to detect lymphocyte growth factors produced in MLR is the promotion of proliferation and enhancement

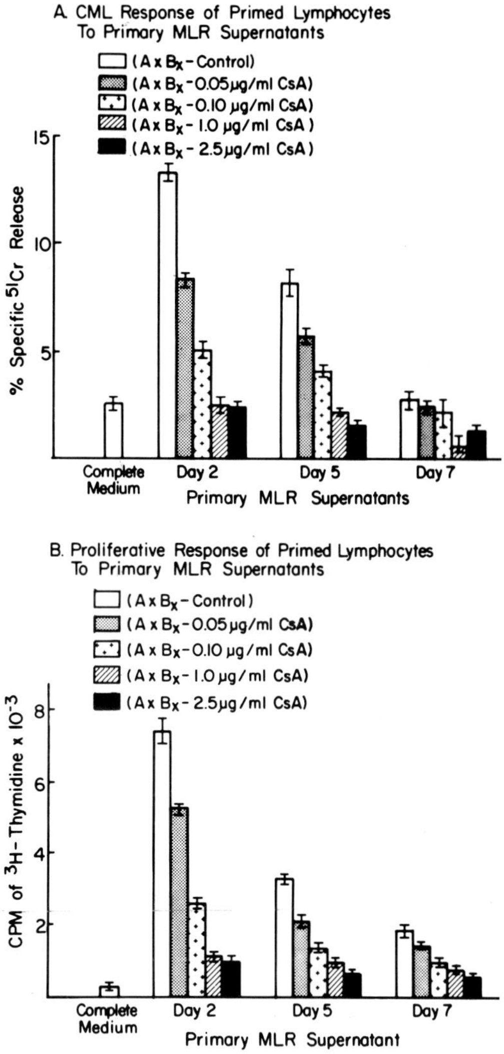

Fig. 1. The effect of CsA on the production of T-lymphocyte stimulatory growth factors in primary MLR. The CML response (A) was measured on day 3 of culture (effector-to-target ratio, 10:1) and the proliferative response (B) assessed after 48 hr of incubation. Bars in A and B indicate the SE.

Table 1. IL2 Activity in CsA-Treated and Control Primary MLR Supernatants Measured by Growth Support of a Cloned Cytotoxic T-Cell Line*

Supernatants From Primary MLR Cultures	Proliferation of Cloned Cytotoxic T-Cell Line (Mean + SD of ^{3}H-Thymidine Uptake)
$A \times B_x$—Control	12,947 ± 2,034
$A \times B_x$—Control + 2.5 μg/ml CsA	11,866 ± 2,336
$A \times B_x$—2.5 μg/ml CsA	230 ± 35
$A \times B_x$—1.0 μg/ml CsA	281 ± 8
$A \times B_x$—0.5 μg/ml CsA	451 ± 54
$A \times B_x$—0.1 μg/ml CsA	1,770 ± 100
Complete medium—Control	211 ± 29

*Cloned cytotoxic T cells (3 × 10^3 cells/well) were incubated for 18 hr in the test supernatants before labeling with 0.5 μCi of ^{3}H-thymidine for 4 hr.

of cytotoxic T-cell activity of alloantigen-primed lymphocytes from long-term MLR cultures by the supernatants from primary MLR cultures. As shown in Fig. 1 there was a general agreement between the two assay systems used for detection of T-lymphocyte growth factor activity. The production of T-lymphocyte growth factors in control primary MLR cultures was greatest in the supernatants harvested on day 2, as noted by a significant increase in the proliferative and CML response of alloantigen-primed cells cultured in the presence of this supernatant compared with the response of these cells cultured with complete medium. Substantial activity in the day-5 control supernatant was noted, and much lower levels of stimulatory activity when the control supernatant was harvested on day 7. In comparison, supernatants from CsA-treated MLR cultures had lower levels of activity. In the cultures with 2.5 and 1.0 μg/ml of CsA, very little stimulatory activity was detected when tested on alloantigen-primed lymphocytes with only a 2–3-fold increase in the proliferative response and no detectable increase in the CML response compared to the responses of primed cells cultured in complete medium. However, supernatants from the MLR cultures with 0.1 and 0.05 μg/ml did contain substantial levels of T-lymphocyte stimulatory activity, although lower than that found in control MLR supernatants. Moreover, the data indicate that the time course kinetics of production of the stimulatory factor in CsA-treated cultures was comparable to the production in control cultures, with the peak activity in the supernatants of day-2 cultures. It is important to note that this latter system may be detecting soluble factors other than IL2. The supernatants from the cultures with 2.5 and 1.0 μg/ml of CsA were capable of stimulating a weak proliferative response of the alloantigen-primed cells but failed to increase the CML activity of these cells, a property of IL2. The same supernatants failed to promote growth of the IL2-dependent cytotoxic T-cell line, the specific and most sensitive assay system for IL2. These results suggest the possibility of other growth factors produced in MLR that are apparently insensitive to CsA.

Further studies revealed that the reduced level or absence of this growth factor was not due to the presence of a soluble inhibitor of IL2 (data not shown) nor did CsA inhibit the response of primed lymphocytes from control cultures to these growth factors (Fig. 2). These observations indicate that CsA could not inhibit the action of IL2 once the lymphocytes acquired the ability to respond to this growth factor.

Development of Responsiveness to IL2 in the Presence of CsA

The primed lymphocytes from CsA-treated and control cultures were tested for their ability to respond to IL2. Figure 3 compares the response in primary MLR with the ability to respond to IL2. In the cultures with 0.5, 1.0, and 2.5 μg/ml CsA, low levels of proliferation

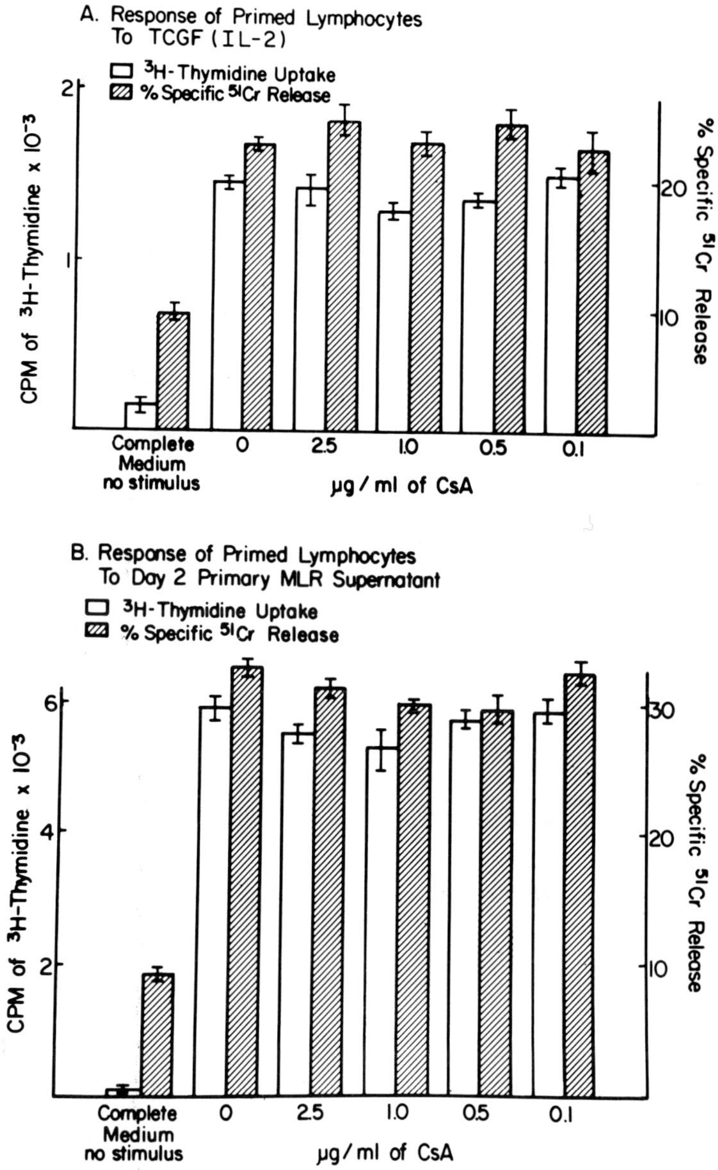

Fig. 2. The effect of CsA on the ability of primed lymphocytes to respond to TCGF (IL2) (A) or day-2 control primary MLR supernatants (B). After 48 hr of incubation, proliferation was measured, and CML activity (effector-to-target ratio, 30:1) assessed on day 3 after initiation of the cultures. The bars in A and B represent the SE.

in primary MLR with a virtual absence of detectable CML activity were observed. Primed lymphocytes from these cultures harvested on day 12 did exhibit a proliferative response upon exposure to either IL2 or day-2 control MLR supernatants compared with cells cultured in complete medium. The levels of proliferation were comparable to the primed cells harvested from the control MLR culture. However, no CML activity was detected in the CsA-treated (0.5, 1.0, and 2.5 μg/ml) cultures, whereas the control primed cells exhibited a strong CML response. It is of interest to note that the primed cells from the primary cultures containing 0.1 μg/ml, in which some CML activity was detected in primary MLR, exhibited both a proliferative and a CML response upon culture with IL2 and/or the control primary MLR supernatants. Exposure of the primed lymphocytes from the control and CsA-treated cultures to specific alloantigens (B_x) resulted in signifi-

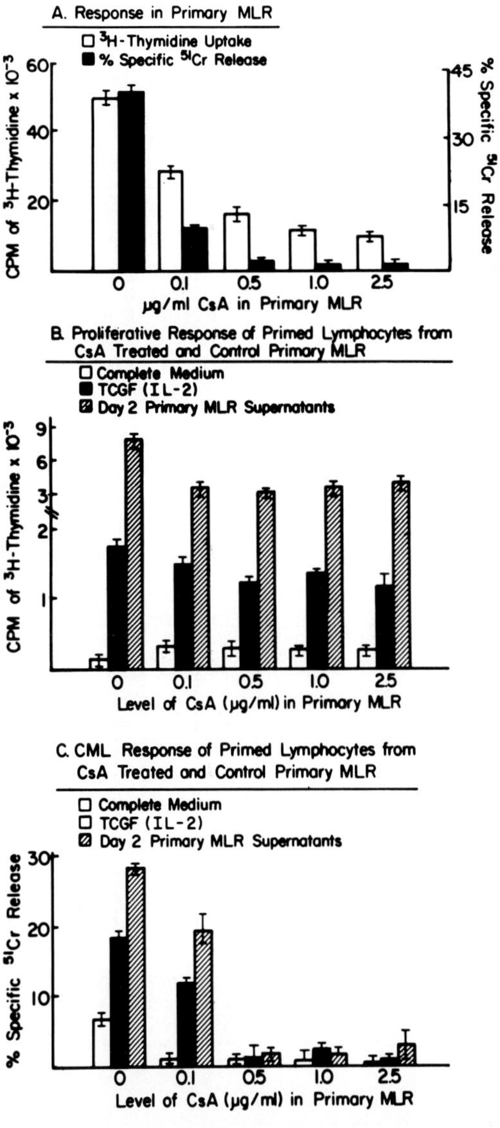

Fig. 3. Comparison of the proliferative and CML response in primary MLR with the development of the ability to respond to T-lymphocyte stimulatory growth factors. (A) Proliferation in primary MLR bulk cultures was measured on day 6, and CML activity (effector-to-target ratio, 30:1) assessed on day 8. The primed lymphocytes were harvested from MLR culture on day 10 and rechallenged with either IL2, day-2 control primary MLR supernatant, or complete medium. The proliferative response (B) was assessed after 48 hr and the CML response (C) measured on day 3 of culture (effector-to-target ratio, 30:1). Bars in A, B, and C represent the SE.

cant CML activity detected only in the cells from the control MLR cultures (50.6% ± 4.0% specific ^{51}Cr release), and the cells from the MLR cultures treated with 0.1 μg/ml of CsA (25.3% ± 2.9% specific ^{51}Cr release) when tested at an effector-to-target ratio of 30:1. In comparison, cells from the MLR cultured with 0.5, 1.0, and 2.5 μg/ml, upon restimulation with the specific alloantigen, exhibited an absence of detectable CML activity (0.8% ± 2.9%, 0.4% ± 1.2%, and 2.0% ± 1% specific ^{51}Cr release, respectively). Table 2 summarizes the results of 5 separate experiments describing the response of primed lymphocytes from CsA-treated cultures to IL2, day-2 control primary MLR supernatants and/or specific alloantigen. In each instance, stimulation of primed lymphocytes from the CsA-treated cultures with IL2, primary MLR supernatant, or specific alloantigen led to substantial levels of proliferation compared with cells cultured in complete medium. However, little if any CML activity was detected in these cultures. In comparison, cells from the control MLR exhibited strong CML responses when exposed to IL2, the primary MLR supernatant or the specific alloantigen. The proliferative response of the cells from CsA-treated MLR cultures upon exposure to IL2, the day-2 primary MLR supernatant, or the specific alloantigen was associated with substantial increases in suppressor cell activity, as demonstrated in Fig. 4, indicating that the suppressor cell subset was activated in primary MLR even in the presence of CsA.

In order to determine if the suppressor cells from CsA-treated cultures inhibited mature cytotoxic T lymphocytes from responding to IL2, accounting for the absence of CML activity, primed lymphocytes from control MLR cultures containing mature cytotoxic effector cells were cocultured with either primed lymphocytes from the CsA-treated cultures or cells from CsA-treated autologously primed cultures (to control for cell density) and exposed to IL2. The results (Table 3) demonstrate that the primed lympho-

Table 2. Response of Control and CsA-Treated Primary MLR Cells to T-Lymphocyte Growth Factors*

Primed Cell Population	Response of Primed Cell Population							
	Complete Medium		IL2		Primary MLR Supernatant		Specific Alloantigen (B_x)	
	Proliferation†	CML Activity‡	Proliferation	CML Activity	Proliferation	CML Activity	Proliferation	CML Activity
$A \times B_x$—Control	260 ± 70	8.7 ± 0.5	2,575 ± 207	20.3 ± 2.6	6,386 ± 1,393	27.3 ± 1.3	36,419 ± 5,644	33.5 ± 5.1
$A \times B_x$—2.5 μg/ml CsA	698 ± 103	−0.5 ± 1.9	1,982 ± 429	3.1 ± 1.8	4,252 ± 350	4.5 ± 0.8	3,700 ± 1,208	3.5 ± 0.9
$A \times B_x$—1.0 μg/ml CsA	616 ± 45	0.8 ± 0.4	1,734 ± 218	3.5 ± 1.6	4,845 ± 209	4.8 ± 0.3	4,969 ± 800	2.4 ± 1.7
$A \times A_x$—Control	257 ± 7	0.2 ± 2.8	558 ± 120	1.7 ± 3.2	412 ± 36	2.4 ± 1.9	NT§	NT
$A \times A_x$—2.5 μg/ml CsA	634 ± 120	−0.2 ± 0.2	715 ± 95	0.3 ± 2.3	718 ± 136	2.6 ± 1.2	NT	NT

*Lymphocytes from primary MLR cultured with and without CsA were harvested on day 12, thoroughly washed to remove CsA, and restimulated with either complete medium, IL2 (2U/ml), day-2 primary MLR supernatant (50% v:v), or specific alloantigen (B_x). Proliferation was assessed after 2 days of incubation following restimulation by pulsing with 1 μCi of ^{3}H-thymidine and allowing the cultures to further incubate 16–18 hr. CML activity was assessed on day 3 of culture, with the effector-to-target ratio being 30:1. Data represent mean ± SE of 5 separate experiments.

†Mean ± SE of ^{3}H-thymidine uptake.

‡Mean ± SE of percent specific ^{51}Cr release.

§Not tested.

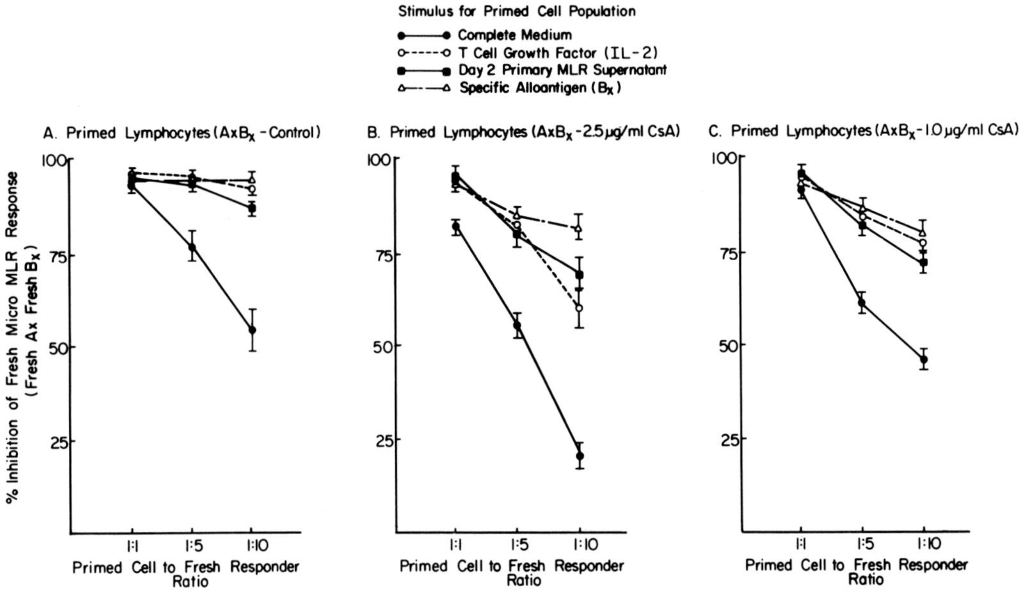

Fig. 4. The ability of IL2, day-2 control primary MLR supernatant, or alloantigen to stimulate suppressor cell activity in the primed lymphocyte population. Primed lymphocytes from MLR cultured with the control diluent (A), 2.5 μg/ml of CsA (B), or 1.0 μg/ml of CsA (C) were harvested on day 12 of culture. The cells (10^6) were cultured with IL2 (2 U/ml), day-2 control primary MLR supernatant (1 ml), specific alloantigen (10^6 irradiated B lymphocytes—1 ml), or 1 ml of complete medium. After 48 hr of incubation, the cells were harvested and tested for their ability to suppress a fresh micro-MLR response of fresh responder lymphocytes (A) to a fresh aliquot of the original stimulating lymphoyts (B_x). Percent inhibition ± SE (bars) of the micro-MLR response was based on comparison to control micro-MLR to which irradiated autologously cultured lymphocytes ($(A \times A_x)_x$) were added in equal numbers and averaged 39,697 ± 2323 (SE) of ^{3}H-thymidine uptake.

cytes from CsA-treated cultures did not inhibit the mature cytotoxic T cells from responding to IL2.

Effect of IL1 and/or IL2 on the Immunosuppressive Effects of CsA

We attempted to determine if exogenous IL1 and/or IL2 could overcome the immunosuppressive effects of CsA in the human MLR system. As shown in Fig. 5 addition of exogenous IL2 did, in part, overcome the immunosuppressive effect of CsA on the proliferative response in primary MLR even at the highest doses of CsA. In comparison, addition of exogenous IL1 (1:150 dilution of partially purified IL1, supplied by Dr. L. Lachman,

Table 3. Failure of Suppressor Cells From CsA-Treated MLR Cultures to Inhibit the Proliferative and CML Response of Primed Lymphocytes From Control Cultures to IL2*

	Response of Primed Cell Populations			
	Complete Medium		IL2 (2 U/ml)	
Cell Populations	Proliferation	CML Activity	Proliferation	CML Activity
AB_x—Control + AA_x CsA 2.5 μg/ml	274 ± 196	3.8 ± 1.2	7,935 ± 1,801	42.6 ± 3.5
AB_x—Control + AB_x CsA 2.5 μg/ml	569 ± 37	6.0 ± 0.8	8,341 ± 862	41.9 ± 2.6
AA_x CsA 2.5 μg/ml + —	448 ± 104	0.6 ± 1.2	819 ± 76	2.1 ± 0.3
AB_x CsA 2.5 μg/ml + —	467 ± 33	0.7 ± 1.0	2,497 ± 540	3.6 ± 1.4

*Primed lymphocytes (10^6) harvested from CsA-treated and control cultures were harvested on day 10, thoroughly washed to remove CsA, and cultured with complete medium or IL2. Proliferation (mean ± SD of ^{3}H-thymidine uptake) was assessed on day 2 of culture and CML activity (percent specific ^{51}Cr release at a 40:1 effector-to-target ratio) was measured on day 3 of culture.

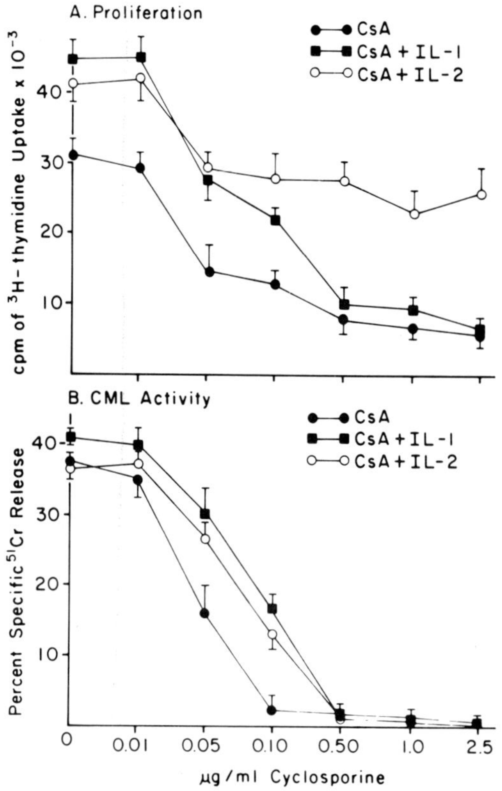

Fig. 5. Effect of exogenous IL1 and IL2 on the immunosuppressive action of CsA in primary MLR. IL2 (2 U/ml) and/or IL1 (1:150 dilution of partially purified material) were added to primary MLR at the initiation of culture. Proliferation (A) was assessed on day 6/7 of culture, while CML activity (effector-to-target ratio—40:1) was measured on day 7. Bars in A and B represent the SEM.

Immunex, Seattle, WA) did not enhance the proliferative response in MLR at doses of 0.5–2.5 μg/ml of CsA, but an enhanced proliferative response in MLR was observed at the lower doses of (0.1–0.01 μg/ml) of CsA.

Cytotoxic T-cell activity was also measured in these cultures. Significant cytotoxic T-cell activity could not be demonstrated in primary MLR cultures treated with as little as 0.1 μg/ml of CsA. Addition of exogenous IL1 or IL2 to the culture system did not promote the generation of cytotoxic T-cell activity at the highest doses (0.5–2.5 μg/ml) of CsA tested. On the other hand, cytotoxic T-cell activity could be demonstrated at 0.05 and 0.1 μg/ml of CsA when exogenous IL1 or IL2 were added to the culture. Although addition of exogenous IL2 to cultures receiving 0.5–2.5 μg/ml of CsA did show an enhanced proliferative response in the presence of this growth factor, cytotoxic T-cell activity could not be demonstrated in these cultures indicating that the precursor cytotoxic T-cell did not acquire responsiveness to IL2 at these doses of CsA. However, in cultures that received 0.1 μg/ml of CsA, a dose that resulted in complete inhibition of CML activity, addition of exogenous IL2 led to detectable levels of CML activity. These results suggested that the precursor CTL did acquire responsiveness to this growth factor, but due to the inhibition of IL2 production, could only be amplified if exogenous IL2 was added. The enhancement of proliferation and the generation of cytotoxic T-cell activity at this dose of CsA (0.1 μg/ml) in the presence of IL1 appeared to be due to the promotion of IL2 production (data not shown).

Effect of Sequential Addition of Cyclosporine and IL1 or IL2 on the Lymphocyte Response in Primary MLR

The above studies demonstrated that CsA will inhibit the precursor cytotoxic T cell from acquiring a receptor for IL2, even though the proliferative response was enhanced by addition of exogenous IL2 suggesting that cells other than the precursor cytotoxic T cell did acquire the receptor for and/or responsiveness to IL2. In an attempt to probe the induction of the development of responsiveness to IL2 by the precursor cytotoxic T cell in primary MLR, CsA, CsA + IL2, or CsA + IL1 (dose of CsA was 2.5 μg/ml) were added at various times after initiation of the MLR culture. The results, shown in Fig. 6, demonstrate that addition of CsA alone within the first 96 hr of culture resulted in significant inhibition of the proliferative response. In contrast, addition of CsA + IL2 during this time interval resulted in the enhancement of the proliferative response in primary MLR (compared to cul-

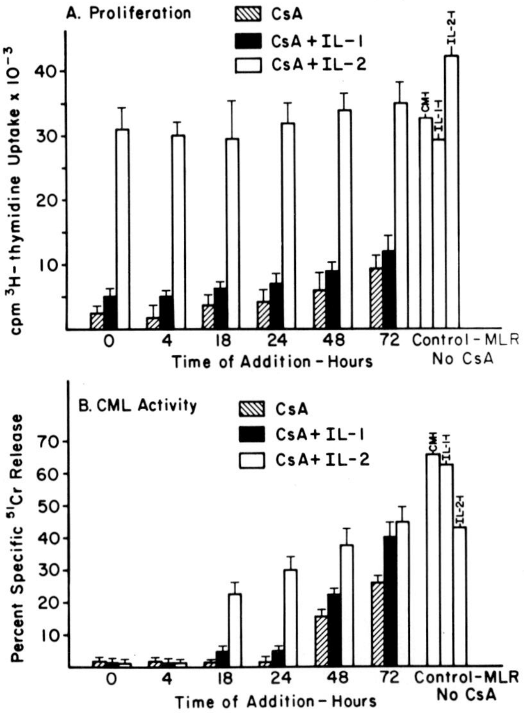

Fig. 6. Time sequential addition of CsA, CsA + IL1, or CsA + IL2 on the proliferative and CML response in primary MLR. CsA concentration was 2.5 μg/ml for all studies. Final concentrations of IL2 and IL1 were 2 U/ml and 1:150 dilution of the partially purified material, respectively. Proliferation (A) was assessed on day 6/7 of culture, while CML activity (effector-to-target ratio—50:1) was measured on day 7. Bars in A and B represent the SEM. CM, complete medium.

tures with CsA only). Addition of CsA + IL1 did not overcome the suppression of CsA on the proliferative response in MLR.

The cultures were also assessed for CML activity. Cytotoxic T-cell activity could not be demonstrated in the primary MLR cultures when CsA was added within the first 24 hr of culture. Thereafter, addition of CsA resulted in significantly reduced levels of cytotoxic T-cell activity. Comparable observations were observed when CsA + IL1 were added to the MLR cultures, with only a slight enhancement (compared to cultures without any CsA added) of CTL activity when these components were added late in culture (addition at 48 and 72 hr). However, cultures that received CsA + IL2 at different time intervals allowed for the determination of the requisite time necessary for the sensitization of the precursor CTL. Addition of CsA + IL2 at 0 and 4 hr did not result in any detectable cytotoxic T-cell activity. When the CsA + IL2 was added at 18 and/or 24 hr after the initiation of culture, significant levels of cytotoxic T-cell activity were observed, even though no CTL activity was found in cultures that received CsA alone at these time intervals. Thereafter, addition of CsA + IL2 resulted in enhanced levels of cytotoxic T-cell activity compared with cultures that received CsA alone. These results indicated that within the first 18–24 hr of culture, the precursor cytotoxic T cell must have acquired responsiveness to IL2, presumably through a receptor for this growth molecule, but could only be clonally expanded in the presence of exogenous IL2.

DISCUSSION

The activation of cytotoxic T lymphocytes (CTL) upon response to alloantigens in primary MLR is thought to be a two-signal mechanism requiring appropriate antigen presentation and the production of a soluble proliferative factor, such as IL2.[12,13] An integral component of this process is the acquisi-

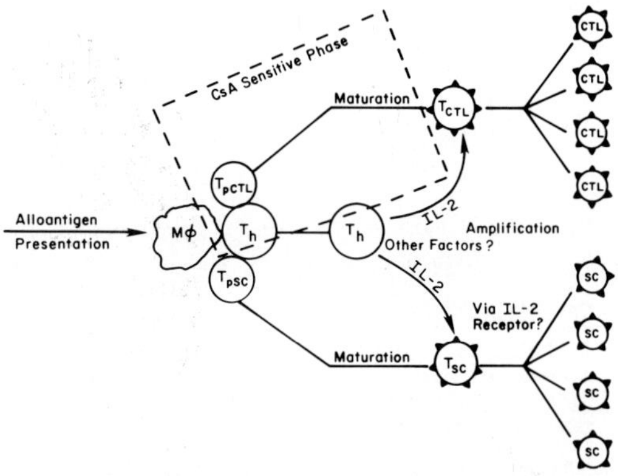

Fig. 7. Schematic representation of the cellular interactions occurring in MLR, resulting in the activation and maturation of cytotoxic and suppressor lymphocytes. Mϕ, monocyte/macrophage; CTL, cytotoxic T lymphocyte; SC, suppressor cell; Th, T helper lymphocyte; IL2, interleukin-2; p, precursor cells; ▲, IL2 receptor.

tion of responsiveness to IL2 by the precursor cytotoxic T cell, presumably mediated by a receptor to IL2.[14] The production of IL2 by the activated T helper cells drives the clonal amplification of the cytotoxic T-cell subset. The effect of CsA on this T:T cell collaborative process is schematically diagrammed in Fig. 7. The present studies indicate that CsA is capable of preventing the T helper cell from producing IL2, results that are in agreement with the findings of Bunjes et al.[15] and Wagner.[16] Another important aspect of CsA-mediated immunosuppression is its ability to inhibit the precursor cytotoxic T cell from acquiring a receptor to IL2. It must be noted that other cells must develop the receptor for IL2, since addition of IL2 to the primary mixed lymphocyte response restores a relatively normal proliferative response despite the presence of CsA, indicating the ineffectiveness of CsA in preventing IL2-dependent growth once the cells acquire responsiveness to this growth factor. Similarly, cells harvested from CsA-treated cultures will indeed respond to IL2 with an enhancement of suppressor T-cell activity. The enhancement of suppressor cell activity of primed lymphocytes from CsA-treated MLR cultures by IL2 or specific antigen would suggest that the suppressor T-lymphocyte subset is activated despite the presence of CsA, findings that are in agreement with our original observations[7] in primary MLR and with the findings of Leapman et al.[17] for Con-A-induced suppressor cell activity. However, it is unknown if the suppressor cells respond directly to IL2, thus causing clonal expansion of these regulatory cells or if this growth factor activates or expands an interacting lymphocyte subpopulation that amplifies suppressor cell function.

Previous studies in our laboratory[18] have shown that a certain percentage of T-helper cells are indeed activated in the presence of CsA, as determined by their ability to express Ia antigens, an indicator of T-cell activation. It is not known whether this T-helper cell subset is activated but inhibited from producing IL2 or whether those cells responsible for IL2 production represent a distinct T helper cell subset and are inhibited from activation by CsA. Data from Bunjes et al.[15] would suggest that the inhibition of IL2 by CsA occurs primarily through the inhibition of IL2 release by activated T-helper cells and by inhibiting the production of IL1, a macrophage-derived soluble component that is essential for T-helper cell activation and subsequent IL2 production. However, the studies by Bunjes et al.[15] were in a mitogen-drive system. In the present investigations, addition of exogenous IL1 to primary MLR cultures did not fully overcome the immunosuppressive effects of CsA, suggesting that CsA either inhibited the activation of the IL2-producing T helper cell subset or made it refractive to the effects of IL1. Clearly, further studies are required to discern the immunosuppressive effects of CsA on the T helper cell and on the events leading to IL2 production.

Of interest was the inability of the precursor cytotoxic T cell to acquire responsiveness to IL2 in the presence of CsA, as indicated by the failure of this cell from CsA-treated cultures to respond to IL2 and by the failure of exogenous IL2 to overcome the immunosuppressive effects of CsA on this T-cell subset. The precise mechanism accounting for the inhibition of the precursor cytotoxic T cell from acquiring the receptor for IL2 is not known. It may be due to a direct binding of the drug to the precursor cytotoxic T cell or it may be due to the disruption of the appropriate T:T cell collaboration in MLR required for the activation of the precursor cytotoxic T cell. Furthermore, in the present studies, CsA was used to probe the development of IL2 responsiveness by the precursor cytotoxic T cell. Our results suggest that the development of responsiveness to IL2 presumably by the acquisition of the receptor for IL2 by the precursor CTL must occur within 24 hr after the initiation of culture. More importantly, the present studies also demonstrate that once the precursor CTL acquires the ability to respond to IL2, the cells can be clonally expanded by IL2 despite the presence of CsA.

The IL2-dependent clonal amplification of the CTL is remarkably insensitive to the effects of CsA.

Taken together our results suggest that CsA has two primary functions. First, it has the ability to inhibit IL2 production, and second, it has the capacity to inhibit the precursor CTL from acquiring responsiveness to this soluble mediator. It may be possible that a CsA-sensitive inducer cell is required for both the triggering of IL2 production and for the activation of the precursor CTL, accounting for both inhibitory functions of cyclosporine. One cannot rule out a differential effect of CsA on two independent T-cell subsets. However, both the inhibition of IL2 production and/or the prevention of the development of responsiveness to IL2 by the precursor CTL would clearly result in an immunosuppressive effect in the transplant recipient. It would be most desirable to inhibit the precursor CTL from acquiring responsiveness to IL2, since when CsA is either discontinued or the dose lowered, it is conceivable that IL2 formation could be triggered either by the primary immunogenicity of the graft or by challenge with an environmental agent, leading to clonal amplification of the cytotoxic T-cell population and possible initiation of graft rejection. The present studies also point out that persistant levels of CsA capable of preventing the cytotoxic T cell from becoming activated and acquiring responsiveness to IL2 must be achieved early, since sensitization of the cell could conceivably occur within 18 hr. In addition, recent studies by Hess et al.[10] and Schwartz et al.[19] suggest that activated CTL are much less sensitive to the effects of regulatory suppressor cells than the naive precursor CTL. Since CsA permits the activation of suppressor T cells, maximal affect should be achieved at levels of CsA that prevent activation of the precursor cytotoxic T cell, thus allowing for the development of potential effective immunoregulation by suppressor T lymphocytes.

The data presented in these studies and in the reports of others[13,15,16] clearly document the role of CsA in inhibiting the production of IL2 and the development of responsiveness by the precursor CTL to this important soluble mediator of the immune response. More importantly, an understanding of the role of CsA on the T:T cell collaborative response to alloantigens will enhance the therapeutic potential of CsA. In addition, this agent and its affect on T-lymphocyte subpopulations, production of lymphokines, and development of responsiveness to these soluble mediators of the immune response makes CsA a valuable tool with which to probe T-lymphocyte activation.

REFERENCES

1. Borel JF: Immunology 31:631, 1976

2. Borel JF, Feurer C, Gubler H, et al: Agents Actions 4:468, 1976

3. Borel JF, Feurer C, Magnee C, et al: Immunology 32:1017, 1977

4. Borel JF: Transplant Proc 13:344, 1981

5. Green CL, Allison AC: Lancet 1:1182, 1978

6. Tutschka PJ, Beschorner WE, Allison AC, et al: Nature 280:5718, 1979

7. Hess AD, Tutschka PJ: J Immunol 124:2601, 1980

8. Hess AD, Tutschka PJ, Santos GW: J Immunol 126:961, 1981

9. Hess AD, Tutschka PJ, Pu Z, et al: J Immunol 128:360, 1982

10. Hess AD, Tutschka PJ, Santos GW: Transplant Proc 15:539, 1983

11. Gillis S, Mochiuzuki DY, Conlan PJ, et al: Immunol Rev 63:167, 1982

12. Synrington FW, Teh N-S: Scand J Immunol 12:1, 1980

13. Larsson E-L, Coutinho A, Martinez C-A: Immunol Rev 51:61, 1980

14. Smith KA: Immunol Rev 51:337, 1980

15. Bunjes D, Hardt C, Rollinghoff M, et al: Eur J Immunol 11:657, 1981

16. Wagner H: Transplant Proc 15:523, 1983

17. Leapaman SB, Filo RS, Smith EJ, et al: Transplant Proc 13:405, 1981

18. Hess AD, Donnenberg AD, Tutschka PJ, et al: J Immunol 130:717, 1983

19. Schwartz A, Sutton SL, Gershon RK: J Exp Med 155:783, 1982

Lack of Evidence for a Cyclosporine Receptor on Human Lymphocyte Membranes

S. J. LeGrue, A. W. Friedman, and B. D. Kahan

THE cyclosporines are a family of structurally related cyclic endecapeptides composed of predominantly hydrophobic L and D amino acids.[1] Evidence from in vitro studies suggests that cyclosporine-A (CsA) blocks an early event during T-cell activation, which restricts the release of interleukin-2 by helper T cells.[2–4] The activity of suppressor T cells is spared by CsA, indicating differential activation mechanisms of these two major T-cell lineages.[2,5,6]

Recent reports have described a specific membrane receptor for CsA on the surface of human and murine lymphocytes.[7–9] Conversely, we have been unable to confirm the existence of a specific CsA receptor.[10] This report extends our previous observations on the uptake and release of ^{3}H-CsA by human cells and phospholipid vesicles. Our results suggest that CsA partitions into phospholipid bilayers by virtue of its extremely hydrophobic character. Insertion of CsA into the lymphocyte membrane may increase membrane surface area and fluidity, leading to an upcoupling of electrochemical membrane hyperpolarization, in a manner similar to that of lipid-soluble anesthetics.[11]

MATERIALS AND METHODS

CsA, CsD, and CsH were gifts of Sandoz, Ltd. (Basel, Switzerland). Crystalline drug in ethanol (10 mg/ml) was diluted in Rosewell Park Memorial Institute Medium 1640 (RPMI 1640; Grand Island Biological Co., Grand Island, NY), as previously described.[10] A 1.6×10^{-4} M stock solution of ^{3}H-CsA in ethanol (42 mCi/mg) was kindly provided by E. Wiskott (Sandoz, Ltd.).

Human peripheral blood lymphocytes (PBL) and erythrocytes and splenocytes were prepared as described.[10] Briefly, lymphocytes of the B lineage were enriched by adsorption onto nylon wool followed by bulk SRBC rosetting. Nonrosetting cells were 85% pure by cytofluorography, using FITC-conjugated OKT3 antibody (Ortho Diagnostic Systems, Raritan, NJ). The nylon wool nonadherent T-cell population displayed 85% positive cytofluorographic reactivity with FITC-OKT3 antibody.

Helper and suppressor T-cell-enriched populations were prepared by indirect complement-mediated cytotoxicity using anti-Leu-2 or anti-Leu-3 monoclonal antibodies, respectively (Becton-Dickinson, Rutherford, NJ). Splenic T lymphocytes were suspended in RPMI 1640 medium, supplemented with 0.2% sodium azide and 5% gammaglobulin-free fetal bovine serum, at a concentration of 10^7 cells/ml. Ten micrograms of arsanilate-conjugated monoclonal antibodies were added per 10^7 cells and incubated 30 min at 4°C. Following two washes, 10 μg of a rabbit anti-arsanilate antibody (Becton-Dickinson) was added per 10^7 cells for an additional 30 min. Cells were washed twice prior to addition of undiluted rabbit complement (200 μl/10^7 cells) for 30 min, 37°C. Cells were suspended into medium supplemented with 15% human AB serum and live cells isolated by Ficoll-Hypaque centrifugation. Cytofluorographic profiles using FITC-conjugated OKT4 and OKT8 monoclonal antibodies indicated greater than 70% purity of the helper and suppressor subpopulations, respectively.

Human thymuses were surgically removed from pediatric cardiac patients as part of their operative procedure. Organs were bathed in RPMI 1640 and teased apart. After brief incubation at 1 *g*, the supernatant fluid, containing primarily single cells, was collected and washed twice prior to use. Kidney cells were isolated from a normal male cadaveric kidney donor, age 7. The cells were derived mainly from tubules and maintained in tissue culture for 3.6 doublings.

Liposomes were prepared by the reverse-phase evaporation method of Szoka and Papahadjopoulos,[12] using 65 μmole each of egg yolk phosphatidylcholine and cholesterol (Sigma Chemical Co., St. Louis, MO).

Binding assays were performed in triplicate, as previously described.[10] Briefly, the stock solution of ^{3}H-CsA was diluted with RPMI 1640 to give drug concentrations ranging from 10^{-10} to 5×10^{-7} M. A quantity of 10^6 cells in 1 ml of drug solution was incubated for 30 min at 37°C, unless otherwise indicated. Specific uptake was assessed by subtracting the amount of drug remaining with the cells or liposomes following addition of 5×10^{-5} M

From the Department of Surgery, Division of Immunology and Organ Transplantation, The University of Texas Medical School at Houston, TX.

Address reprint requests to Dr. S. J. LeGrue, Department of Surgery, Division of Immunology and Organ Transplantation, University of Texas Medical School, Houston, TX 77030.

0041-1345/83/1505-0007$01.00/0

unlabeled CsA. Free drug concentration was determined by counting the reaction supernatant fractions.

The kinetics of ^{3}H-CsA uptake by cells and liposomes was examined using cartesian, semilogarithmic, and Scatchard[13] analyses. In Scatchard diagrams, the ordinate (B/F) represents the moles of ligand specifically bound to targets divided by the moles of free (unbound) ligand and the abscissa (B) is the mole of specifically bound ligand. Application of Scatchard analyses to cell binding studies has been shown to be appropriate if certain assumptions are met.[10,14–16]

RESULTS AND DISCUSSION

Uptake of CsA by Human Cells

Normal human PBL bound significant amounts of ^{3}H-CsA, with saturation at 5×10^{-7} M CsA and half maximal uptake at 8×10^{-8} *M* (Fig. 1, left panel). An equal number of cultured human kidney cells also demonstrated sigmoidal uptake, although saturation was not achieved using CsA concentrations up to 5×10^{-7} *M* (Fig. 1, right panel). The inability to saturate 10^6 kidney cells in this experiment was probably due to the greater surface area of the kidney cells, relative to PBL.

No difference was observed in the in vitro uptake of ^{3}H-CsA by separated splenic B-cell or T-cell populations, or between splenic T-cell populations enriched for T helper or T suppressor populations (Fig. 2). Normal human thymocytes also bound equivalent amounts of ^{3}H-CsA, although decreased uptake was observed at CsA concentrations above 10^{-8} *M*. Human erythrocytes sequestered substantial amounts of drug, even at very low ^{3}H-CsA concentrations. The signifi-

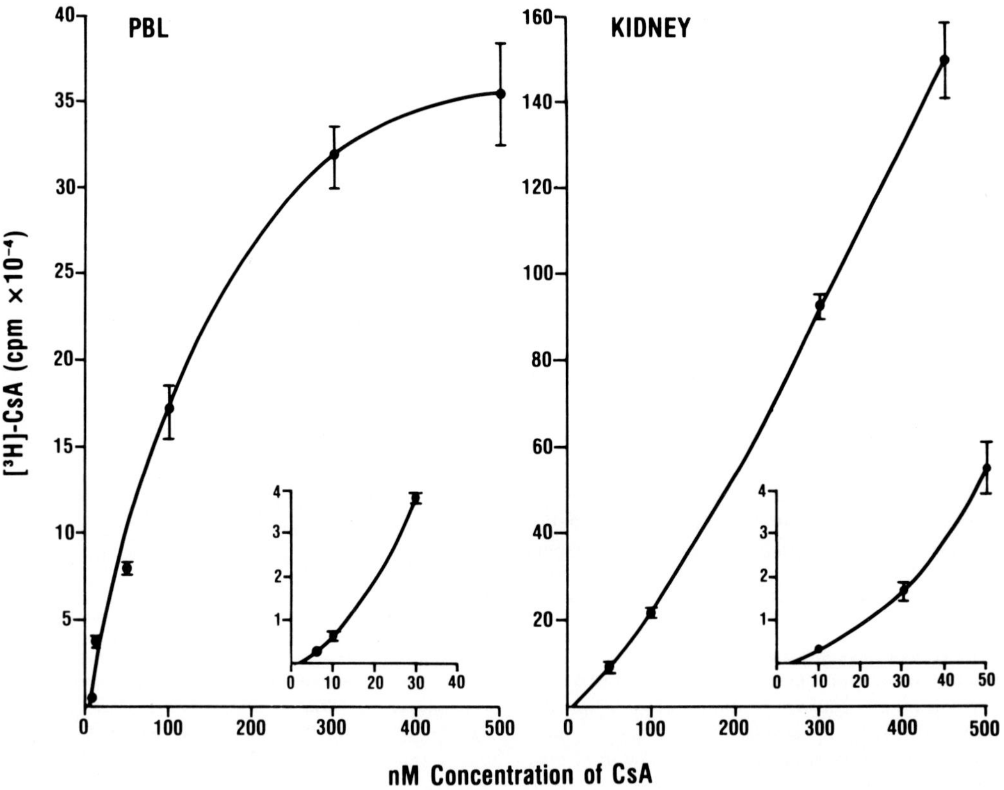

Fig. 1. Binding of ^{3}H-CsA by human PBL and kidney cells. 5×10^6 normal human PBL or cultured kidney cells were incubated for 60 min in 1 ml RPMI 1640 containing the indicated concentrations of ^{3}H-CsA. The cells were washed twice and lysed with 1 *N* NaOH prior to determination of bound radioactive ligand. (Inset) The binding of drug at very low ^{3}H-CsA concentrations. The units for the ordinate and abscissa are unchanged. Bars: standard error of the mean of triplicate assays.

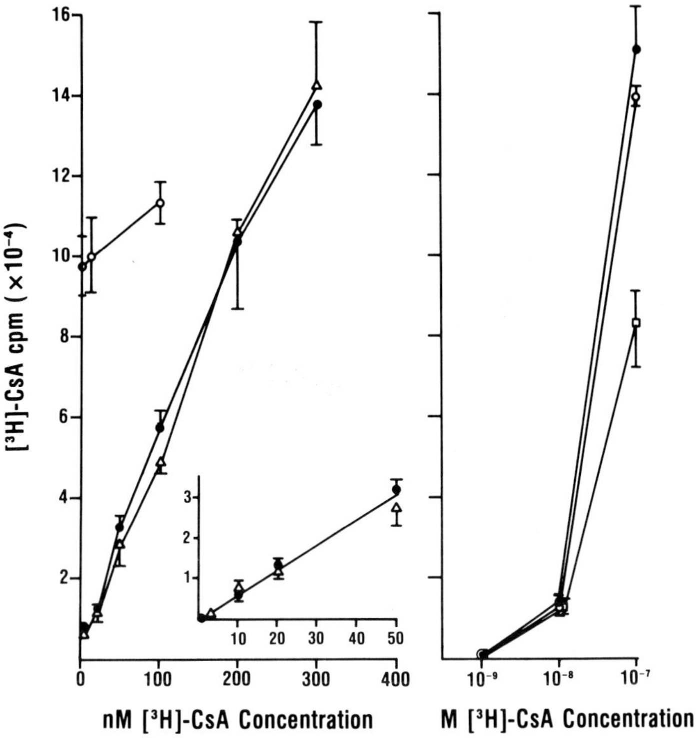

Fig. 2. Binding of ^{3}H-CsA by human B cells, T cells, thymocytes, and erythrocytes. Cells were incubated in media containing ^{3}H-CsA, as described in the legend to Fig. 1. (Left): Cartesian plot of ^{3}H-CsA binding by normal human splenic B cells (Δ), T cells (●), and erythrocytes (O). (Right): Semilogarithmic plot of ^{3}H-CsA binding by human thymocytes (□) and by splenic T cells enriched for helper T-cell (●) and suppressor T-cell (O) subpopulations using anti-Leu-2 and anti-Leu-3 monoclonal antibodies, respectively, plus complement. Bars: standard error of the mean of triplicate assays.

cance of this finding remains unclear, although it may have in vivo importance for the blood–tissue distribution of CsA.

Partially purified splenic B and T lymphocytes achieved maximum uptake of 10^{-7} *M* ^{3}H-CsA within 2 min, with no significant change over the next half hour (Fig. 3). Using that concentration of labeled drug that yielded half-maximal uptake, we were unable to identify a time at which steady state had not been achieved. Thus, lymphocytes demonstrate very rapid initial uptake, with no quantitative difference in the amount of drug associated with either B or T cells.

Scatchard analysis of the uptake of ^{3}H-CsA by partially purified splenic B-cell and T-cell

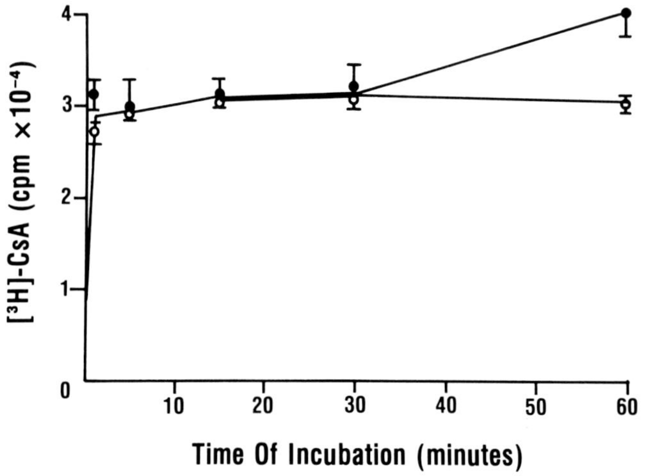

Fig. 3. Kinetics of binding of ^{3}H-CsA by normal human splenic B cells and T cells. One million cells, B cells (●) or T cells (O), were incubated in 10^{-7} *M* ^{3}H-CsA for the indicated times, washed twice, and the amount of bound radioactive ligand determined. Each centrifugation lasted for 2 min. Therefore, the earliest time point represents the time necessary to add labeled ligand and immediately remove the cells by centrifugation. Bars: standard error of the mean of triplicate determinations.

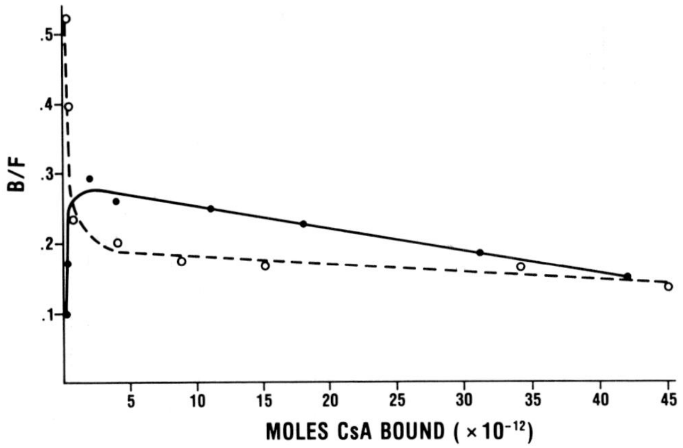

Fig. 4. Scatchard analysis of the specific binding of ^{3}H-CsA by purified splenic B cells and T cells. A single cell suspension was prepared from a normal human spleen, and the nylon-wool-nonadherent population was termed T cells (●) on the basis of an 86% positive reactivity with OKT3 monoclonal antibody. The nylon-wool-adherent cells were harvested, and the B-cell population (○) isolated to 85% purity using phagocytosis of carbonyl iron and bulk SRBC rosetting. Specific binding was defined as the amount of ^{3}H-CsA bound to 10^6 cells minus the amount bound in the presence of 5×10^{-5} *M* unlabeled CsA.

populations demonstrated a low-affinity dissociation constant (K_D) of 4–8 × 10^{-7} *M* common to both cells and a high-affinity constant of $K_D = 2 \times 10^{-9}$ *M*, which was unique to B cells (Fig. 4). Scatchard diagrams of the uptake of ^{3}H-CsA by unfractionated PBL also yielded two binding constants of $K_D = 3 \times 10^{-7}$ *M* and $K_D = 6 \times 10^{-9}$ *M*.[10] Both purified T cells from the peripheral blood of one author (S.J.L.), and cultured kidney cells displayed only a low-affinity binding constant of $K_D = 10^{-7}$ *M* and 2×10^{-7} *M*, respectively.

The extremely hydrophobic character of the CsA molecule suggested that our "binding" studies were simply measuring the partitioning of the drug into the phospholipid bilayer of the plasma membrane. To examine this hypothesis, binding studies were performed using phospholipid vesicles of defined chemical composition. Large uni- and oligolamellar liposomes were prepared using an equi-

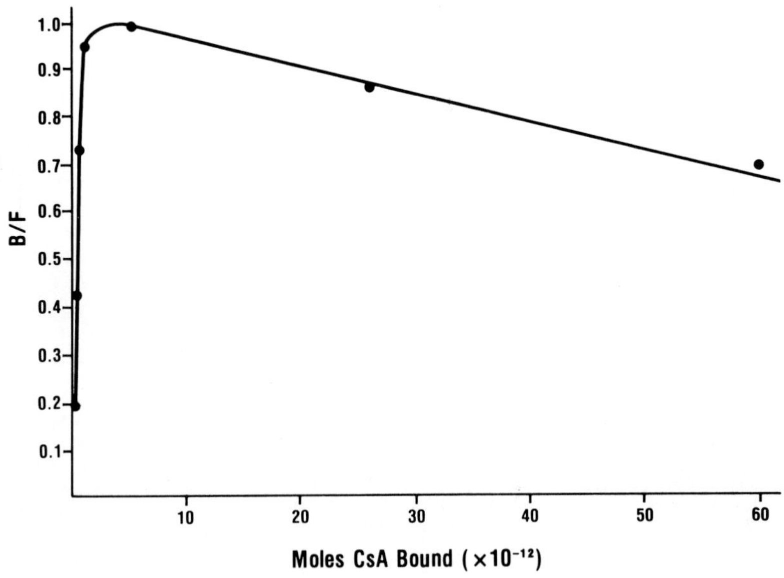

Fig. 5. Scatchard analysis of the specific binding of ^{3}H-CsA by phospholipid vesicles. Phospholipid vesicles were prepared by the reverse evaporation technique,[12] using 65 μmole each of egg yolk phosphatidylcholine and cholesterol. Vesicles (3.2 μmole total lipid) were incubated for 30 min in 1 ml RPMI 1640 containing concentrations of ^{3}H-CsA ranging from 10^{-7} to 10^{-10} *M*.

molar mixture of hen egg yolk phosphatidylcholine and cholesterol. Liposomes adsorbed ^{3}H-CsA with kinetics very similar to T lymphocyte uptake (Fig. 5). An apparent K_D of 2×10^{-8} M was calculated for the uptake of drug by liposomes. The reversal in the values of B/F observed for T cells, kidney cells, and liposomes at ^{3}H-CsA concentrations below 10^{-9} M is an unusual feature of these Scatchard diagrams. Although strong positive cooperativity of uptake by the low-affinity site could explain these results, Hill diagrams of drug uptake by T cells and liposomes provided no evidence for cooperative interactions.[10] A deviation from the assumed precondition of excess free ligand could also account for the nonlinear kinetics at low CsA concentrations. The failure of Ryffel et al.[7,8] to detect the nonspecific character of the low-affinity site and the slope changes of the Scatchard diagrams at low ligand concentrations may result from (1) their use of dihydrocyclosporin, rather than the clinically useful analog, CsA; (2) the high specific activity of our labeled ligand, which permitted investigation of binding at concentrations down to 10^{-10} M; and (3) their exclusive use of lymphocytes as targets in the binding assay.

Our previous studies have indicated that cell-associated CsA is localized in the plasma membrane[10] and may not be internalized like other immunosuppressive agents.[15,17] However, it was possible that examination of CsA uptake by resting PBL was not relevant to the mode of drug action during antigen or mitogen stimulation. To test the hypothesis that CsA exerts its immunosuppressive action at the level of the plasma membrane, the amount of nondisplaceable drug was monitored during alloantigen stimulation. In resting PBL, about 95% of labeled CsA can be competitively displaced using a 500-fold excess of unlabeled drug.[10] We reasoned that if CsA was internalized during activation, the proportion of nondisplaceable drug should progressively increase. Therefore, the CsA uptake and release by unstimulated lymphocytes in culture was compared to that of alloantigen-stimulated cells cultured in two-way mixed lymphocyte culture (MLC). No evidence was obtained to support a mechanism whereby CsA is significantly sequestered in response to activation (Fig. 6). Both stimulated and unstimulated PBL demonstrated similar net uptake and identical displacement of labeled drug during 96 hr of culture.

The results presented in this article strongly suggest that CsA associates with cells and

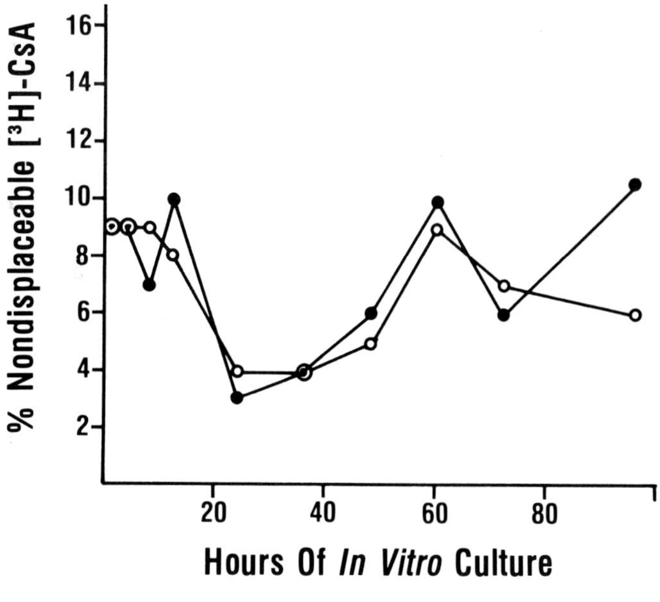

Fig. 6. Displacement of specifically bound ^{3}H-CsA during lymphocyte culture. PBL from normal donors were cultured in the presence of 10^{-7} M ^{3}H-CsA, either alone (○) or with an equal number of HLA-DR nonidentical stimulator cells, in a two-way MLC (●). At various times between 1 and 96 hr, the amount of nondisplaceable drug was determined by the addition of 5×10^{-5} M unlabeled CsA. As controls, both alloantigen-stimulated and unstimulated lymphocyte cultures were maintained in 0 or 1×10^{-7} M ^{3}H-CsA and pulsed after 96 hr with ^{14}C-dTdR to assure that lymphoproliferation did occur in the stimulated cultures and that the proliferation was suppressed in the presence of the drug.

lipid vesicles by partitioning into the phospholipid bilayer, without the participation of a specific receptor. CsA may exert its immunosuppressive action solely at the cell surface without significant internalization, although our results could also be consistent with a cytoplasmic binding protein (see Merker et al., this issue). Many lipid-soluble anesthetics and alcohols exert their pharmacologic effects at the cell surface by increasing lipid fluidity, releasing sequestered Ca^{++}, and uncoupling electrochemical action potentials.[11] Consistent with this hypothesis, (1) we have demonstrated[10] that ethanol reduces by half the incorporation of ^{3}H-thymidine into alloantigen-stimulated lymphocytes at a concentration (0.22 *M*) that fluidizes membranes and uncouples electrochemical potentials;[11] and (2) Tsien et al.[18] have reported that Ca^{++} flux and membrane hyperpolarization are very early events in lymphocyte activation. In addition, Seeman and co-workers have demonstrated that lipid-soluble compounds achieve a half maximal response when their concentration in the lipid phase is 10 m*M* or greater. We have calculated a concentration of 14 m*M* ^{3}H-CsA in the lipid phase of liposomes when half maximal drug uptake is attained, and we estimate a concentration of at least 200 m*M* ^{3}H-CsA in lymphocyte membranes.

Thus, the selective effects of CsA on T-cell subsets, and specifically on the release of interleukin-2 by helper T cells, may result from a selective disruption of membrane function related to ion flux and lipid fluidity. Specificity of CsA in the modulation of early events in immune activation would then arise from differences in electrochemical mechanisms employed by various lymphocyte populations; and not on differences in specific drug binding or net drug uptake. The model would explain the apparent resistance of suppressor T cells, NK cells, B cells, and mature effector T cells to CsA-mediated immunosuppression, while providing a mechanism for the observed blockade of interleukin-1 release by macrophages.[4] Perturbation of membrane function, particularly at high drug concentrations, would also explain the various reversible side effects reported for CsA, including hepatotoxicity, nephrotoxicity, and the disturbance of central nervous system function. The model also suggests that a new class of surface-active immunosuppressive agents may be possible, which would exhibit many of the advantageous features of CsA without the attendant toxicities.

ACKNOWLEDGMENT

We thank Dr. R. Kerman and the staff of the Immune Monitoring Laboratory for assistance in the preparation of lymphocyte populations, Dr. B. H. Tom for advice on the preparation of liposomes, and E. Vess for word processing.

REFERENCES

1. Wenger R: In White DJG (ed): Cyclosporin A. Amsterdam, Elsevier Biomedical, 1980, p 19

2. Hess AD, Tutschka PJ: J Immunol 124:2601, 1980

3. Wang BS, Heacock EH, Collins KH, et al: J Immunol 127:89, 1981

4. Bunjes D, Hardt C, Rollinghoff M, et al: Eur J Immunol 11:657, 1981

5. Hess AD, Tutschka PJ, Santos GW: J Immunol 126:961, 1981

6. Van Buren CT, Kerman RH, Agostino G, et al: Surgery 92:167, 1982

7. Ryffel B, Donatsch P, Gotz U, et al: Immunology 41:913, 1980

8. Ryffel B, Gotz U, Heuberger B: J Immunol 129:1978, 1982

9. Palacios R, Moller G: Nature 290:792, 1981

10. LeGrue SJ, Friedman AW, Kahan BD: J Immunol 131:712, 1983

11. Seeman P: Pharmacol Rev 24:583, 1972

12. Szoka F, Papahadjopoulos D: Proc Natl Acad Sci USA 75:4194, 1978

13. Scatchard G: Ann NY Acad Sci 51:660, 1949

14. DeMeyts P: In Bradshaw RA, Frazier WA, Merrell RC, et al (eds): Surface Membrane Receptors. New York. Plenum, 1976, p 215

15. Munck A: In Pasqualini IJR (ed): Receptors and Mechanisms of Action of Steroid Hormones. New York, Marcel Dekker, 1976, p 1

16. Klotz I: Science 217:1247, 1982

17. Green CJ: In Salaman JR (ed): Immunosuppressive Therapy. Philadelphia, Lippincott, 1981, p 75

18. Tsien RY, Pozzan T, Rink TJ: Nature 295:68, 1982

Cyclosporine Binding Component in BW5147 Lymphoblasts and Normal Lymphoid Tissue

M. Merker, J. Rice, B. Schweitzer, and R. E. Handschumacher

EVIDENCE that initial or triggering events in the mitogenesis of T cells are more sensitive to cyclosporine-A (CsA) than are ongoing events, including cell growth, has been documented previously[1-3] and was also presented at this meeting. However, because we were interested in studying the mechanism of action of CsA at the biochemical level, we felt that a continuous cell line with reasonable drug sensitivity would provide a more homogeneous and convenient cell source. We selected a continuous malignant T-cell line, BW5147, for these studies. Although this cell line did not display the sensitivity of thymocytes, it did enable us to discover a high-affinity binding component for the drug present in the cytosol of normal T cells as well as the malignant cell line. We have partially purified this binding component from calf thymus as well as the malignant cell line.

Initially, a number of malignant T and non-T-cell lines were surveyed for growth inhibition by CsA. Only T-cell lines were sensitive to concentrations below 10 μg drug/ml. The relative sensitivity of 3 T-cell lines is illustrative of these differences (Fig. 1). BW5147, derived from a thymoma in AKR mice, was chosen because of its relatively high sensitivity compared to the other lines. In addition, this line displayed the T-cell antigen Thy-1. It was hoped that this T lineage might preserve some of the determinants for CsA sensitivity. While this work was in progress, several reports of equivalent or greater sensitivity of selected T-cell lines have appeared.[4-6]

Because of the availability of tritiated dihydrocyclosporine-A ([^{3}H-dihydro-H_2 CsA) of high specific activity (kindly supplied by Sandoz Ltd., Basel, Switzerland, and purified on a C-18 reverse/phase HPLC system) which would subsequently be used for binding studies, we compared the growth inhibitory effects of CsA and dihydrocyclosporine-A (H_2 CsA) on BW5147 cells and found the dihydro compound to be 50%–60% as potent as CsA. This same relative potency was observed when the two compounds were compared for their ability to inhibit the concanavalin-A-induced mitogenesis of murine thymocytes.

Drug accumulation by these cells from the medium was temperature dependent (Fig. 2). At 3 μg drug/ml media, uptake was rapid and equilibrium was reached in less than 3 min at 37°C and the cells accumulated about 0.08 μg/10^6 cells. At 15°C, the time course to equilibrium was slower, but the same amount of drug was concentrated within the cells. At 0°C, there was no appreciable accumulation of drug even when the incubation was continued for 4 hr.

When the concentration of drug in the media was varied, two phases of uptake were observed: a saturating component between 0.01 and 1 μg drug/ml and a nonsaturating component at greater than 1 μg/ml (Fig. 3). At the lowest concentrations, the drug concentration in the cells is ~600-fold greater than in the media, and at the highest concentrations it is only about 10 times greater than the media. These results are comparable to those obtained by Ryffel et al. with murine and human T cells,[7,8] except that saturation occurred at a somewhat lower concentration, but it is difficult to make a direct comparison.

From the Department of Pharmacology, Yale University School of Medicine, New Haven, CT.

Supported in part by the American Cancer Society Grants CH67U and RDP22 and USPHS Grants CA 09085 and 28852.

Address reprint requests to Dr. R. E. Handschumacher, Department of Pharmacology, Yale University School of Medicine, P.O. Box 3333, New Haven, CT 06510.

0041-1345/83/1505-0008$01.00/0

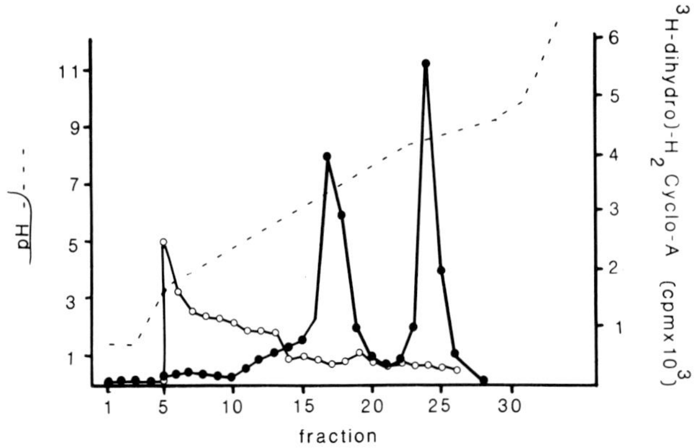

Fig. 5. [^{3}H-dihydro]-H_2CsA in BW5147 cytosol is associated with fractions that have isoelectric points of 6.8 and 8.5. A 110-ml LKB preparative isoelectric focusing column (LKB Instruments, Rockville, MD) was filled with a linear 0%–65% a sucrose gradient containing a final concentration of 1% Ampholines (LKB) Ampholines, pH 3.5–10). One milliliter serum (O—O) or cytosol (●—●) was premixed with [^{3}H-dihydrol]-H_2 CsA (0.1 μg, 3 × 10^4 cpm) and added to the dense sucrose solution before forming the gradient. Thirty fractions (3 ml) were collected and assayed for radioactivity.

in the presence of 2% serum. Thus, in the absence of the cytosol-binding component, the drug has a greater affinity for the column packing than for serum proteins.

The charge characteristics of the drug–macromolecule complex were examined on a preparative isoelectric focusing column. When cytosol complexed with radioactive drug is introduced into the apparatus, the radiolabel focuses in two discrete peaks, with isoelectric points of 6.8 and 8.5 (Fig. 5). These two forms may represent posttranslational or degradative modifications. When serum containing radiolabeled drug is subjected to the same procedure, the radiolabel remains in fractions corresponding to the region in the sucrose gradient to which it was applied, again illustrating the relatively high affinity of the drug for the cytosolic component.

Because we intended to purify the binding component in the absence of radiolabeled drug, a binding assay was developed. The assay depends on both the molecular weight difference between the drug and the binding component and the hydrophobicity of the drug. LH-20, a hydroxy-propylated Sephadex derivative was packed into pasteur pipettes. Radiolabeled drug and dextran blue were mixed with the sample to be assayed; a portion was assayed for total radioactivity and another applied to the column and elution begun with buffer. Within the range of the assay, the amount of radiolabel that was present in the effluent containing blue dextran was directly proportional to both the amount of binding component and the concentration of radiolabeled drug.

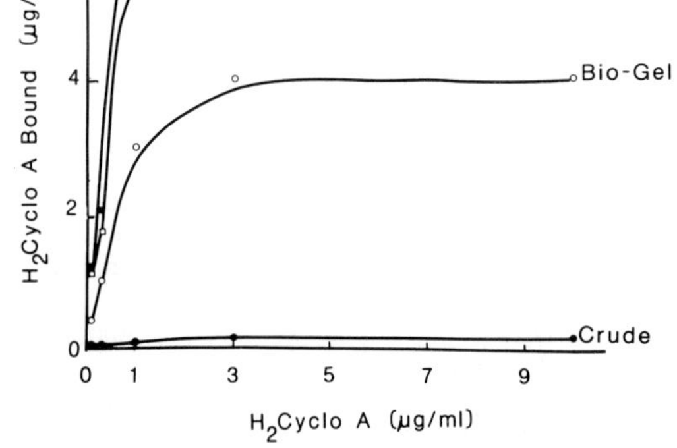

Fig. 6. Binding activity of BW5147 cytosol and partially purified fractions. Samples were assayed for H_2CsA binding using the LH-20 binding assay described in the text.

Molecular weight exclusion columns (P-150, Bio-Gel), isoelectric focusing, and $(NH_4)_2SO_4$ precipitation were employed to begin purification of the binding activity. The crude cytosol, the peak of activity from gel filtration, and the two peaks from isoelectric focusing are compared for their relative binding at saturation (Fig. 6). The molecular

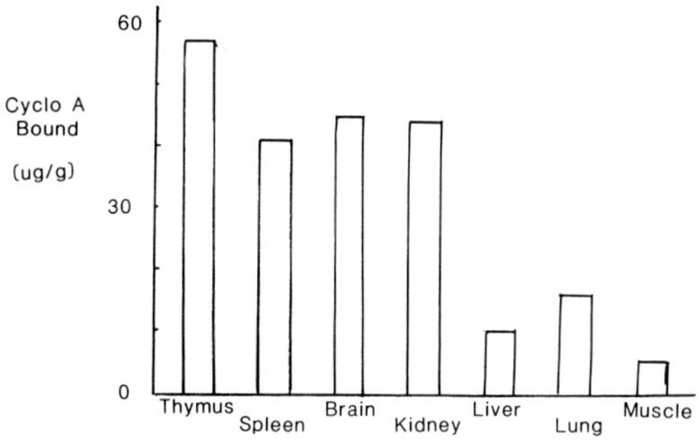

Fig. 7. Survey of CsA binding activity in the cytosol of murine tissues. Tissues were homogenized in 0.25 *M* sucrose, 10 m*M* Tris, pH 7.0, and centrifuged for 60 min at 100,000 *g*. Binding activity was assayed using LH-20 columns, as described in the text.

weight separation yielded a 20-fold purification, with 90% recovery of activity. Each of the peaks from isoelectric focusing contained 17% of the original activity, and more than a 40-fold overall purification was achieved.

To extend these findings to the possible role of the binding component in sensitive lymphoid tissue, the cytosol fractions from a variety of mouse tissues were assayed for the presence of the binding activity (Fig. 7). Using the LH-20 binding assay, cytosol from the thymus was found to contain the highest concentration. As expected, the splenic cytosol contained high activity. The high binding activity in renal cytosol might relate to the CsA toxicity observed in this organ. It is also interesting to note that the brain, an organ that expresses considerable Thy-1 antigen, also has high binding capacity.

Comparable amounts of binding component were found in homogenates of calf thymus, with a similar molecular weight to that from BW5147 cells. However, the activity showed only 1 isoelectric point at 9.4–9.7, in contrast to the activity from BW5147 cells (Fig. 8). The stability of this activity was greatly increased by addition of 5 m*M* β-mercaptoethanol or dithiothreitol. Further purification is in progress by two chromatographic methods and gel electrophoresis. If one molecule of drug binds per molecule of cytosolic component, the best preparations at this time are ~10% pure, based on protein content.

Although we have not established the role of the binding component in the mechanism of action of CsA, the high affinity and concentration of this component in target tissues assures its ultimate importance to the pharmacologic activity of the drug. When homoge-

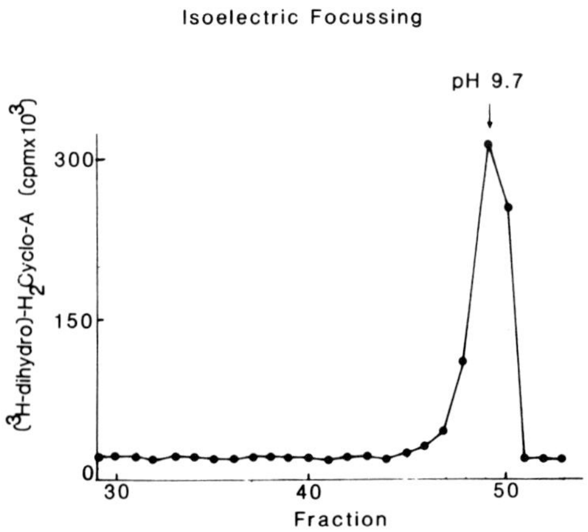

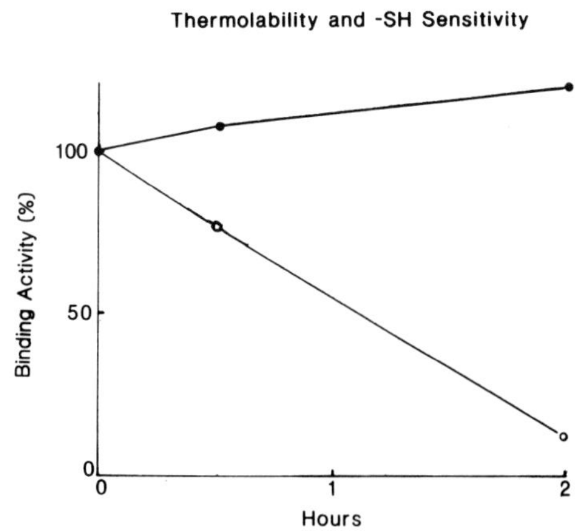

Fig. 8. Characteristics of the CsA-binding component from homogenates of calf thymus. (Left) [^{3}H-dihydro]H_2CsA in the cytosol of calf thymus (100,000 *g* supernatant from a 20% homogenate prepared as in Fig. 7.) is associated with a fraction that has an isoelectric point of 9.7 when focused as in legend to Fig. 5, with a 1% solution of pH 11–8 Pharmalytes. (Right) Stabilization of binding component by dithiothreitol. Binding component was incubated at 37°C in the presence (●—●) or absence (○—○) of dithiothreitol (5 m*M*) and assayed for binding activity by the LH-20 binding assay described in the text.

neous preparations of the binding component are available, the kinetics of binding and turnover will be studied to assess the importance of these parameters to tissue sensitivity. We are currently preparing monoclonal antibodies to the binding component that will aid mapping of the activity at intracellular loci and among cell types.

It is also attractive to consider what might be a natural ligand for this cytosolic component. If such a ligand can be isolated by affinity chromatography, it would provide important clues as to the molecular mechanism of action of the drug and may lead to a clearer understanding of the fundamental mechanism involved in T-cell activation.

REFERENCES

1. White DVG (ed): Cyclosporin A. Amsterdam, Elsevier Biomedical, 1982.

2. Wiesinger D, Borel JF: Immunobiology 156:454, 1979

3. Larsson EL: J Immunol 124:2828, 1980

4. Berger R, Majdic O, Meingassner JG, et al: Immunopharmacology 5:123, 1982

5. Totterman TH, Danersund A, Nilsson K, et al: Blood 59:1103, 1982

6. Fidelus RK, Ferguson RM, Widmer MB, et al: Transplantation 34:308, 1982

7. Ryffel B, Donatsch P, Gotz U, et al: Immunology 41:913, 1980

8. Ryffel B, Gotz U, Heuberger B: J Immunol 129:1978, 1982

Effects of Cyclosporine on Experimental Infections

G. A. Cole, S. P. Nickell, F. Mokhtarian, and L. W. Scheibel

CYCLOSPORINE (CsA) selectively and reversibly inhibits a number of T-cell functions normally expressed after antigen-priming without depressing bone marrow or causing structural damage to lymphoid tissues.[1] These properties distinguish CsA from other commonly used immunosuppressants that are lymphocytotoxic and often impair hemopoiesis.[2,3] Having these rather unique properties, CsA may be used as a tool for assessing the importance of immune effector functions, mediated directly or indirectly by T cells, in animal models of infections, especially those produced by agents that parasitize cells of bone marrow origin.

In this context, several assumptions can be made. First, animals undergoing continuous treatment with CsA should exhibit a drug dose-dependent decrease in resistance to primary infections that normally are controlled or eliminated by T-cell-dependent defense mechanisms. Second, in such animals, local inflammatory responses consequent to these infections should be reduced or absent if recruitment of the participating mononuclear cells requires the presence of antigen-triggered T cells or their products.[4] Third, withdrawal of CsA treatment during active infection should permit the reestablishment of specific immunocompetence, as reflected by the development of relatively normal, albeit delayed, humoral or cellular responses to the causative agent.

In this article are summarized the salient findings from a series of studies in which the effects of CsA treatment were compared in several well studied animal models of viral and parasitic infections. These consisted of vaccinia virus (VAC), lymphocytic choriomeningitis virus (LCMV), and Sindbis virus (SIN) infections of mice as well as malarial infections of mice and owl monkeys (*Aotus trivirgatus*) produced with the asexual blood stages of, respectively, *Plasmodium yoelli* (*Py*), or *P. berghei* (*Pb*) and *P. falciparum* (*Pf*). Our findings indicate that the foregoing assumptions are essentially correct, but with some notable exceptions.

MATERIALS AND METHODS

Animals

Inbred mice of the C3H/He and BALB/c strains were purchased from the Jackson Laboratories, Bar Harbor, ME. Outbred ICR mice were purchased from Blue Spruce Farms, Altamont, NY. All mice were females and were 6–8 weeks of age when used. Owl monkeys (karyotypes 2 and 3) of both sexes and ranging in age from 8 months to 13 years were purchased either from Dr. P. Heltne, who owned a breeding colony at the Johns Hopkins University, Baltimore, MD, or from the Charles River Research Primates Corp., Port Washington, NY. None of the monkeys had been infected previously with plasmodia and all were seronegative for *P. falciparum* when received.

Experimental Infections

In previous publications, we have described in detail both the procedures for initiating murine infections with either VAC (WR strain)[5] LCMV (E-350 strain),[6] SIN (AR339 strain)[7] *Py* (17XL strain),[8] or *Pb* (NK65 strain)[8] and the characteristics of the disease produced by each of these agents. The course and lethal outcome of untreated *Pf* infections of susceptible owl monkeys has been described extensively by others.[9] Employed in the present study was the chloroquine-sensitive FCR-3/Gambia strain of *Pf*. Levels of parasitemia were determined by microscopic examination of Giemsa-stained blood films.

From the Department of Microbiology, University of Maryland School of Medicine, Baltimore, MD, and the Department of Preventive Medicine, Uniformed Services University of the Health Sciences, Bethesda, MD.

Supported in part by Public Health Service Grant NS-17741 from the National Institute of Neurological and Communicative Disorders and Stroke, and a gift from Sandoz Ltd., Basel, Switzerland.

Address reprint requests to Dr. G. A. Cole, Department of Microbiology, University of Maryland School of Medicine, Baltimore, MD 21201.

0041-1345/83/1505-0009$01.00/0

Measurements of Immune Responses and Inflammation

Most of the methods used have been published previously. Primary VAC- and LCMV-specific splenic cytolytic T lymphocyte (CTL) activity was measured in vitro using an 18-hr ^{51}Cr-release assay.[5,6]

Indirect immunofluorescence was used to detect antibodies reactive specifically with methanol-fixed LCMV-infected Vero cells or *Pf*-parasitized human erythrocytes on glass slides. Bound antibodies in sera from infected mice and monkeys were visualized using fluorescein-isothiocyanate-conjugated rabbit and goat antisera specific for, respectively, mouse and human immunoglobulins (Cappel Laboratories, Cochranville, PA).

Mononuclear cell inflammatory responses within the cerebral compartment that invariably accompany LCMV[4] and SIN[10] infections of the murine central nervous systems (CNS) were monitored by enumeration of cells in samples of cerebrospinal fluid (CSF) from individual mice. Approximately 10–12 μl of CSF were obtained per animal, by cisternal puncture, from groups of 3–5 mice previously inoculated intracerebrally (i.c.) with virus or with saline diluent (as controls). Samples were centrifuged at 600 *g* for 10 min; the pelleted cells were resuspended in an appropriate volume of saline and counted immediately.

Preparation and Use of CsA

Powdered CsA (Sandoz Ltd., Basel, Switzerland), was dissolved in either undiluted Emulphor EL620 (GAF Corp., New York, NY) or undiluted Miglyol 812 (Kay-Fries Inc., Montvale, NJ) at concentrations of 50–100 mg/ml. Depending on whether mice or monkeys were to be treated, these stock solutions were diluted to obtain desired drug doses (in mg/kg body weight) in volumes suitable for inoculation subcutaneously. Using Emulphor as the solvent, stock solutions could be diluted up to 10-fold with distilled water.

RESULTS

Effect of CsA on Induction of VAC-Specific CTL

The outcome of infections produced in mice inoculated intravenously with the poxvirus, VAC, is virus dose-dependent.[5] Inocula containing less than 2×10^5 plaque-forming units (PFU) are usually nonlethal. Greater virus doses often lead to fatal liver damage, but induce specific splenic CTL responses that peak 6 days later and differ very little between individual animals. To determine whether CsA suppressed these responses, 7 daily doses of 5, 25, or 50 mg/kg were given to corresponding groups of 4–6 C3H/He (H-2^k) mice, beginning 2 days before they received 5×10^6 PFU of VAC. Normal and infected mice given a course of drug diluent (10% Emulphor) served as controls. On the sixth day postinfection, spleens from mice without each group were pooled and made into suspensions that were assayed at various effector:target ratios (E/T) for cytolytic activity against 2×10^4 ^{51}Cr-labeled VAC-infected and uninfected L-929 (H-2^k) cells.[5] As expressed in percent VAC-specific lysis or in lytic units per spleen[11] (Table 1), activity correlated inversely with CsA dose and was insignificant in mice treated with 50 mg/kg.

Interestingly, spleen cells from mice infected with sublethal doses of VAC during CsA treatment, if stimulated in vitro with VAC several weeks after treatment was discontinued, yielded apparently normal levels of secondary virus-specific CTL activity (data not shown). This observation suggested that, while inhibiting the expression of CTL function (Table 1), CsA did not prevent T-cell priming.

Inhibition by CsA of LCMV-Induced T-Cell-Mediated Neurologic Disease

Immunocompetent mice of all conventional strains, when inoculated i.c. with the arenavirus, LCMV, develop an acute inflammatory process localized to the meninges and choroid plexi. Such animals exhibit a convulsive diathesis secondary to choriomeningitis and, within 8 days, all die during a seizure. The disease (LCM) is mediated solely by a virus-specific T-cell response having a CTL component.[6,12]

Given extraneurally, LCMV induces a qualitatively similar response which, in the spleen, reaches a maximum 9–10 days later.[6] All animals survive, because infection and the accompanying viremia are eliminated before virus can invade the CNS. Being noncytolytic, LCMV replicates benignly in most tissues of mice whose T cells are nonfunctional or absent;[12] infections of such mice persist in the absence of LCM and induce a chronic viremia.

Table 1. Suppression by Cyclosporine of Primary Splenic CTL Responses to Vaccinia Virus

CsA Treatment* (Days −2 through 4)	VAC-Specific Lysis at E/T (%)† 40	10	2.5	Lytic Units per Spleen
None	60.2	45.1	18.6	2,040 (100%)
5 mg/kg	64.6	47.6	20.0	2,080 (102%)
25 mg/kg	33.4	18.0	4.8	210 (10.3%)
50 mg/kg	9.6	4.7	2.1	15 (0.7%)
Unprimed	6.1	4.7	3.0	5 (0.2%)

*Given subcutaneously in 10% Emulphor.

†Lysis on 6th day postinfection of C3H/HE mice with 5 × 10^6 PFU of vaccinia virus (VAC) i.v., at effector:target ratios (E/T) indicated.

Using daily subcutaneous 50-mg/kg doses (in Miglyol), the effects of CsA were compared between groups of C3H/He mice in which treatment—begun 1 day before either i.c. or i.p. inoculation of 5 × 10^2 PFU of LCMV—was continued for 4, 7, or 10 days (Table 2). Of untreated animals, all that were infected i.c. died of immune-mediated CNS disease after a mean survival time (MST) of 6.5 days; those infected i.p. remained asymptomatic and, by day 10, they were free of viremia and had developed splenic CTL responses. In contrast, the MST of i.c. infected mice given CsA increased in rough proportion to treatment length, indicating that T-cell-mediated choriomeningitis was delayed rather than prevented. As expected, the magnitude of CTL responses in i.p. infected mice was inversely related to the length of CsA treatment. Prolonged treatment maintained viremia and led eventually to lethal disease, presumably because infection had extended to the CNS by the time these animals regained their ability to mount virus-specific T-cell responses. In contrast to the temporary T-cell-suppressive activity of CsA, a single 175-mg/kg dose of cyclophosphamide given to mice 3 days after they were inoculated with LCMV either i.c. or i.p. prevented both virus-specific T-cell priming and CNS disease.[4] Such mice survived as persistent virus carriers.

In a similar experiment (Table 3), BALB/c mice were subjected to daily treatment with CsA (75 mg/kg) in 10% Emulphor, beginning 1 day before, and continuing for 12 days after, their inoculation i.c. with LCMV. By day 7 postinfection, these animals (but not those untreated) had developed neither the convulsive diathesis nor the pronounced influx into CSF of mononuclear cells that typify unmodified LCM. Drug-treated mice also failed to develop detectable LCMV-specific antibodies.

Table 2. Delayed Development of Fatal Lymphocytic Choriomeningitis and LCM Virus-Specific CTL Responses in C3H/HE Mice Treated With Cyclosporine

Days of CsA Treatment* (50 mg/kg)	Route of Virus Inoculation: i.c. MST ± SD	i.c. S/T†	i.p. Lytic Units per Spleen	i.p. Viremia	i.p. S/T†
Untreated	6.6 ± 0.5	0/10	3,420	−	10/10
−1 to 4	9.7 ± 2.7	0/10	2,760	−	10/10
−1 to 7	11.8 ± 4.3	0/10	530	+	7/10
−1 to 10	17.9 ± 7.8	0/10	4	+	0/10
Cyclophosphamide (Day 3, 175 mg/kg)		10/10	2	+	10/10

*Given s.c. in Miglyol.

†Surviving (S) mice of total (T) inoculated intracerebrally (i.c.) or intraperitoneally (i.p.) 30 days previously; CTL activity and viremia measured on day 10.

Table 3. Suppression of LCM Virus-Induced Symptomatic Disease, CNS Inflammation, and Specific Antibody Responses in BALB/c Mice Treated With Cyclosporine

Day Postinfection	CsA* Days −1 through 12 (75 mg/kg)	Convulsions (%)	CSF Cells/μl† (× 10²)	Anti-LCMV Antibody
5	+	0	3 ± 3	−
	−	0	42 ± 19	−
7	+	0	3 ± 3	−
	−	100	437 ± 237	+

*Given s.c. in 10% Emulphor.
†Mean ± SD in groups of 4–5 mice.

Suppression of Sindbis-Virus-Induced CNS Inflammation With CsA

Sindbis virus (SIN) is the prototype of the alphavirus group and a close relative of the viruses causing eastern, western and Venezuelan equine encephalitis.[13] The immunologic and pathologic features of acute CNS infection and inflammation produced by alphaviruses in man are very similar to those seen during SIN infections of mice. BALB/c mice infected i.c. with SIN (10^3 PFU) develop a necrotizing meningoencephalitis; most or all animals develop frank paralysis, and about 30%–50% die within 10 days.[14] Between days 4 and 6 postinfection, mononuclear inflammatory cells appear in the meninges and CSF. Inflammation is mediated by SIN-specific T cells,[10] and it can be both accelerated and enhanced by the passive administration of certain monoclonal anti-SIN antibodies[7] during the first 2 days of infection.

Based on CSF cell numbers on days 3 and 5 postinfection (Table 4), treatment of infected mice with CsA (50 mg/kg, days −1 through 4) suppressed the development of CNS inflammation as well as its augmentation by antibody. Treatment with CsA appeared to hasten the onset of paralysis, although the frequency of this symptom was reduced in animals that had received antibody.

Effect of CsA on Infections Produced by Rodent and Human Malarial Parasites

We recently reported that lethal murine malaria caused by *P. yoelii* (*Py*) or *P. berghei* (*Pb*) was preventable by treating outbred mice with CsA at the time of parasite inoculation.[8] This finding, as summarized in Table 5, was the unexpected result of an attempt to potentiate *Py* and *Pb* infections by suppressing, with CsA, host T-cell functions that are known to be important in immune elimination of these agents.[15] Upon further investigation, it was found that established parasitemias fell precipitously to undetectable levels in mice that were treated with 25 mg/kg of CsA for 2 consecutive days. Low-level parasitemias reappeared after 3–5 days, but were self-

Table 4. Suppression of Sindbis-Virus-Induced Encephalitis in BALB/c Mice Treated With Cyclosporine

Treatment: CsA* Days −1 through 4 (50 mg/kg)	Treatment: Anti-SIN Antibody Day 2 (~0.1 mg)	Paralysis† by Day 5 (%)	CSF Cells/μl × 10²‡ Day 3	CSF Cells/μl × 10²‡ Day 6
−	−	46	10 ± 7	26 ± 12
−	+	13	40 ± 18	51 ± 20
+	−	67	11 ± 6	4 ± 1
+	+	22	14 ± 4	5 ± 2
Sham-infected (untreated)		0	11 ± 5	3 ± 2

*Given s.c. in 10% Emulphor.
†In groups of 20 mice infected i.c. with 1000 PFU of Sindbis virus (SIN).
‡Mean ± SD in groups of 3–5 mice.

Table 5. Prevention of Lethal Murine Malaria With Cyclosporine

Plasmodial Species	CsA* Days 0 Through 3	Mean No. Days to ≥ 25% P†	P† (%)	D† (%)	MST ± SEM (Days)
P. yoelii	None	7	100	100	13.0 ± 1.6
	1 mg/kg	9	100	80	13.3 ± 2.3
	5 mg/kg	16	100	80	20.5 ± 1.9
	25 mg/kg	—	0	0	—
P. berghei	None	16	100	100	20.2 ± 1.4
	25 mg/kg	26	10	10	36.0 ± 0.0

*Administered s.c. in 10% Emulphor.

†Parasitemia (P) and Death (D) in groups of 5–10 mice after i.p. inoculation with 10^6 parasitized erythrocytes.

limiting. Furthermore, when CsA was added to cultures of human erythrocytes actively infected with *P. falciparum* (*Pf*), drug concentrations as low as 0.1 μg/ml of culture medium cuased significant inhibition of parasite growth.

The above findings confirmed and extended those of an earlier study,[16] and they prompted a limited exploration of CsA's potential therapeutic value in the owl monkey model of human falciparum malaria. Because of their restricted availability and high acquisition cost, only 5 monkeys were used. After determining that baseline blood chemistries of all monkeys were normal, each was inoculated i.v. (day 0) with 2×10^6 *Pf*-parasitized homologous erythrocytes that had been infected in vitro several days previously. Beginning 1 week postinfection, blood was obtained routinely from finger/toe-sticks and used for hematologic measurements and also to prepare daily Giemsa-stained blood films that were examined microscopically for parasites. At intervals of 1–2 weeks, venous blood samples were collected from each monkey for detection of *Pf*-specific antibodies as well as for monitoring the changes in blood chemistries (to be reported elsewhere) that occur in these animals during falciparum malaria.[17]

The results of this study are summarized in Table 6. Four monkeys (nos. 1–4) began receiving CsA daily when their parasitemias reached 0.1%–1.0% (10–100 parasitized erythrocytes in a total of 10^4), between days 10 and 25 postinfection. One monkey (no. 5) was used initially to establish that an other-

Table 6. Cyclosporine Treatment of Falciparum (*PF*) Malaria in Owl Monkeys

Monkey*	Parasitized RBC per 10^4 RBC (Begin CsA)	(Stop CsA)	Dose/kg†	Anti-*PF* Antibody‡	Relapse	Epilogue
1	100 (Day 25)	<1 (Day 36)	50 mg (×8) 25 mg (×4)	+	No	Died (day 57) nephritis pneumonia
2	85 (Day 17)	11 (Day 24)	50 mg (×4) 75 mg (×3)	+	—	Died (day 24) nephritis colitis
3	65 (Day 10)	<1 (Day 19)	50 mg (×9)	+	Yes	Died (day 63) nephritis
4	10 (Day 10)	<1 (Day 20)	50 mg (×10)	+	Yes	Died (day 49) nephritis
5	160 (Day 39)	<1 (Day 46)	150 mg (×1) 100 mg (×1) 50 mg (×2) 25 mg (×3)	+	No	Alive and well

*Inoculated i.v. (day 0) with 2×10^6 parasitized owl monkey erythrocytes (RBC).

†Drug given s.c. in Emulphor.

‡Measured on day 14.

wise lethal *Pf* infection could be controlled with chloroquine if CsA treatment proved ineffective in the others. On day 13, a rising parasitemia of about 10% disappeared in this monkey after a course of 5 daily 20-mg/kg doses i.m. of chloroquine (not shown); it relapsed after 2 weeks and, upon reaching $160/10^4$, treatment with CsA was begun (day 39).

Parasitemias in all 5 monkeys began to fall within 2–3 days after the first dose of CsA (50 mg/kg) was given. Subsequent doses varied as to number and size between individual monkeys, based on the course of infection in each (Table 6). In 4 monkeys, circulating parasites became undetectable between 7 and 11 days; one monkey (no. 2) died suddenly while its parasitemia was still falling. All monkeys developed *Pf*-specific antibodies by day 14. Relapses occurred in 2 monkeys (nos. 3 and 4) within 3 days of discontinuing CsA treatment. Although not shown, resumption of treatment kept parasites at a relatively constant 1% level but did not eliminate them (no. 3). Relapsing parasitemia in no. 4 appeared to develop complete resistance to CsA; it rose too rapidly to be checked by chloroquine and was fatal.

As indicated in Table 6, all but one monkey (no. 5) died from what seemed, at autopsy, to be renal failure due to the combined effects of malaria[17,18] and CsA.[19]

DISCUSSION

The impressive success of CsA in controlling allograft rejection in both experimental animals and man[1,19] provided the rationale for its use in the present studies. We assessed the effects of CsA by using a variety of animal models of viral and parasitic infections in which the expression of agent-specific T-cell functions had been shown to be either beneficial (VAC,[5] SIN,[10] and plasmodia[15]) or detrimental (LCMV[6]) to host survival. In sufficient concentrations and doses, ongoing CsA treatment of acute viral infections suppressed or delayed specific T-cell-mediated effector and inflammatory responses and virus clearance (Tables 1–4). Similar results have been reported by others who used CsA to treat mice infected with influenza virus[20] and herpesvirus.[21] The reversibility of CsA-induced suppression of effector T-cell function was illustrated in the murine model of LCM (Table 2). Infected mice developed fatal T-cell-mediated choriomeningitis shortly after cessation of CsA treatment.

The mechanism by which CsA exerts its antiplasmodial activity is unknown. Because CsA inhibits parasite growth in vitro[8] as well as in vivo (Tables 5 and 6), this activity is almost certainly not an indirect result of immunosuppression. Neither does it appear to be associated with that portion of the CsA molecule affecting T-cell functions (J. Borel, personal communication). This might explain why, in monkeys, relatively large doses of CsA were required to eliminate preexisting parasitemias. Alternatively, subcutaneous injection in Emulphor may have been an inefficient method of CsA delivery; this point should be clarified when blood samples from monkeys have been assayed for CsA levels.

As an antimalarial, CsA was considerably more effective in mice than in owl monkeys. In the latter, it is probable that the nephrotoxic property of Cs contributed significantly to mortality. In kidneys of all monkeys that died, the histopathologic changes were too severe to be attributed to malaria alone.[17,18] Another point to be noted is that CsA treatment seemed to favor the emergence of drug-resistant parasites. As seen previously while using CsA to treat rodent malaria,[8] relapsing parasitemia occurred in 2 monkeys, and it could not be cleared with CsA. These negative aspects are offset by the fact that the antiparasitic activity of CsA is not limited to plasmodia. Recent studies have shown that, in mice, all developmental stages of *Schistosoma mansoni* are strikingly sensitive to 5 daily 25-mg/kg doses of CsA.[22]

Although cyclosporine's immunosuppressive properties preclude its clinical use in treatment of parasitic infections, it is exciting to contemplate that current attempts to modify the CsA molecule (J. Borel, personal communication) may result in a drug suitable for this purpose.

REFERENCES

1. Borel JF: Transplant Proc 13:344, 1981

2. Turk JL, Poulter LW: Clin Exp Immunol 10:285, 1972

3. Heyworth MF: Immunol Rev 65:79, 1982

4. Cole GA, Nathanson N, Prendergast RA: Nature 238:335, 1972

5. Hapel AJ, Bablanian R, Cole GA: J Immunol 121:736, 1978

6. Johnson ED, Cole GA: J Exp Med 141:866, 1975

7. Schmaljohn AL, Johnson ED, Dalrymple JM, et al: Nature 297:70, 1982

8. Nickell SP, Scheibel LW, Cole GA: Infect Immun 37:1093, 1982

9. Schmidt LH: Am J Trop Med Hyg 27:671, 1978

10. Park MM, Griffin DE, Johnson RT: Infect Immun 34:306, 1981

11. Cerrotini JC, Brunner KT: Adv Immunol 18:67, 1974

12. Johnson ED, Monjan AA, Morse HC: Cell Immunol 36:143, 1978

13. Calisher CH, Shope RE, Brandt W, et al: Intervirology 14:229, 1980

14. Griffin DE, Johnson RT: J Immunol 118:1070, 1977

15. Jaywardena AN, Targett GA, Carter RL, et al: Immunology 32:849, 1977

16. Thommen-Scott K: Agents Actions 11:770, 1981

17. Wellde BT, Johnson AJ, Williams JS, et al: Am J Trop Med Hyg 21:260, 1972

18. Jervis HR, Sprinz H, Johnson AJ, et al: Am J Trop Med Hyg 21:272, 1972

19. White DJG, Calne RY: Immunol Rev 65:115, 1982

20. Amerding D: Infect Immun 32:1164, 1981

21. Amerding D, Scriba M, Hren A, et al: Antiviral Res 2:3, 1982

22. Bueding E, Hawkins J, Cha J-N: Agents Actions 11:380, 1981

Potential for Tolerance Induction With Cyclosporine

D. J. G. White, H. ff. S. Davies, N. Kamada, and T. Nagao

SINCE the earliest experimental use of cyclosporine-A in organ grafting, it has been apparent that, under certain circumstances, withdrawal of cyclosporine-A immunosuppression from the recipient of an allograft is not inevitably followed by graft rejection.[1–4] This observation is not unique to cyclosporine-A immunosuppression.[5] Indeed, any clinician charged with the long-term management of kidney transplant recipients knows that, as the years pass, the graft can be maintained in situ with the use of homeopathic doses of immunosuppression. However, unlike other immunosuppressive regimens, cyclosporine-A, at least experimentally, is able to induce easily long-term graft acceptance in a wide range of animals. The first report on cyclosporine-A-induced graft acceptance was by Green and Allison using kidneys grafted between outbred rabbits.[2] However, Dunn, using the same animal model, cast some doubt on the specificity of the effect of cyclosporine-A in this graft acceptance. This has been resolved by a detailed kinetic study performed by combined heart and skin grafts in rats.

AN ANALYSIS OF POST-CYCLOSPORINE-A GRAFT ACCEPTANCE

DA rat heart grafts implanted heterotopically into the neck of PVG recipients, which are then treated for 14 days with cyclosporine-A intramuscularly at 15 mg/kg, will, barring technical mishaps, survive for the life-time of the recipient.[6]

From the Department of Surgery, University of Cambridge, Addenbrooke's Hospital, Cambridge, U.K.

Supported in part by the Medical Research Council.

Address reprint requests to Dr. D. J. G. White, Department of Surgery, University of Cambridge, Addenbrooke's Hospital, Hills Road, Cambridge CB2 2QQ, U.K.

0041–1345/83/1505–0010$01.00/0

Nagao has studied the stability of these heart transplants by placing grafts of either donor (DA, $RT1^a$) or third-party (WAG, $RT1^u$) skin onto these recipients (PVG) at differing times after heart transplantation, as shown in Fig. 1. To control for the effect of cyclosporine-A, we skin grafted ungrafted normal PVG rats that had received the same cyclosporine-A regimen as the heart graft recipients.

The results of these experiments (Figs. 2 and 3) showed that, in those groups of non-transplanted PVGs where the skin, either WAG or DA, was placed after cessation of cyclosporine-A therapy, no immunosuppressive effect due to residual drug or residual influence on the immune system could be observed, the skin grafts being rejected in the same tempo as those on unmodified controls. In those animals where the skin was grafted while cyclosporine-A was still being administered, some prolongation of survival (14.8 days for DA and 14.2 days for WAG skin) was achieved. If the time during which the cyclosporine-A was administered when these skin grafts were placed (6 days) is subtracted from these times then the survival of the grafts after cessation of cyclosporine-A therapy is not significantly different from that of untreated skin graft controls, indicating that it is the cyclosporine-A therapy that is producing the prolongation, and no extra "tolerizing" effect can be seen in these groups of rats.

The results of placing donor skin grafts onto heart graft recipients were as follows. In experimental group 1 (DA skin challenge at 1 week after DA heart graft) the survival of skin grafts was greatly prolonged (median survival time 43.5 days), with 2 of these grafts surviving for the lifetime of the animal (>200 days). Rejection of the heart grafts occurred in two of these rats in this group within 7 days of skin graft rejection. The other 4 heart grafts sur-

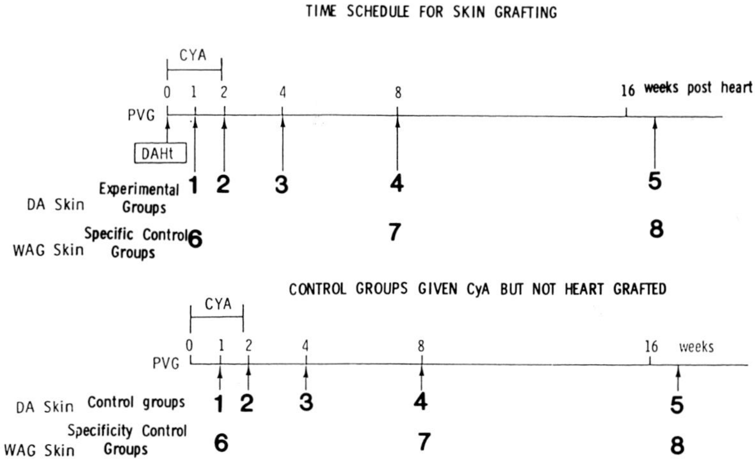

Fig. 1. The timing of the skin and CsA-treated non-heart grafted third-party (WAG) on CsA-treated recipients of DA heart grafts (top) PVG rats (bottom).

vived indefinitely. The ungrafted cyclosporine-A-treated control group had a median skin graft survival of 15 days. The skin grafts in experimental group 2 (DA skin challenge 2 weeks after DA heart grafting) also survived longer (median survival time 20 days) than those in the specificity control group (median survival time 9 days), but the extent of the prolongation was much less than that observed in experimental group 1. In addition, all the heart grafts were rejected within 7 days of skin graft loss.

In experimental group 3 (DA skin challenge at 4 weeks postgrafting), the skin grafts were rejected as quickly as their controls (median survival time 9.5 days versus control

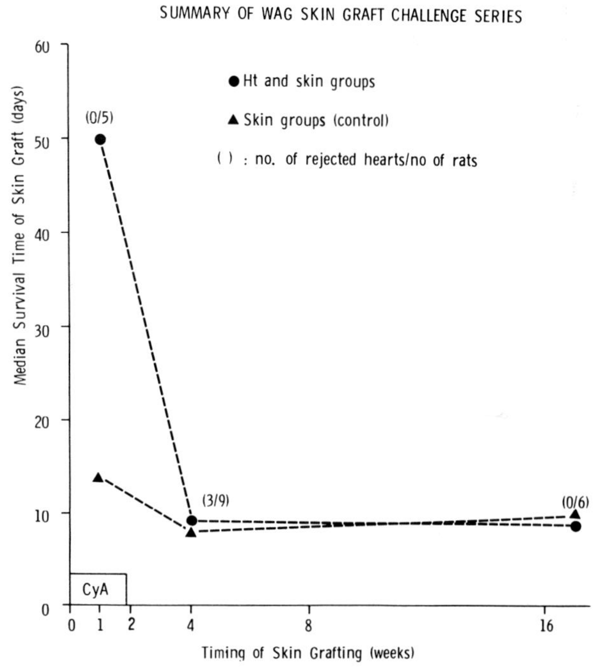

Fig. 2. Rejection times of DA skin grafts on either DA heart graft recipients (PVG) (●----●) or CsA-Treated ungrafted PVGs (▲----▲).

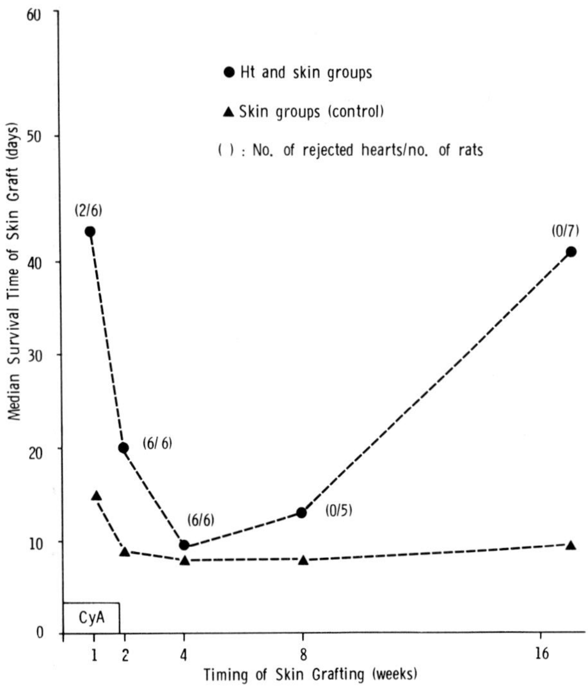

Fig. 3. Third-party control rejection times of WAG skin grafts on either DA heart graft recipients (PVG) (●-----●) or CsA-treated ungrafted PVGs (▲------▲).

group median survival of 8 days). Not only did this schedule fail to produce skin graft prolongation but, as in the previous group, the rejection of the skin graft was invariably followed by the rejection of the original heart graft.

In experimental group 4 (DA skin challenge at 8 weeks postgrafting), the skin grafts were rejected more slowly (median survival time 13 days) than those in the control group (median survival time 8 days). However, unlike the previous experimental groups, the rejection of the skin grafts in this group failed to induce the rejection of the heart graft. In group 5 (DA skin challenge at 16–21 weeks following heart grafting), the DA skin graft survived for a very prolonged period (median survival time 41 days). One skin graft from this group survived for the lifetime of the animal (>200 days), whereas controls of this group rejected normally (median survival time 9.5 days). In this group none of the original heart grafts were affected by the eventual loss of the skin graft, all being retained for the lifetime of the animal.

Specificity controls of WAG skin grafted onto the recipients of DA heart grafts showed that the prolonged survival of skin grafts placed 1 week after DA heart grafting (experimental group 1) was not specific, in that the WAG skin grafts (specificity control group 6) survived much longer than their controls. However unlike the DA skin grafts placed in experimental group 1, the eventual rejection of the WAG skin failed to induce the rejection of any of the DA hearts. In the remaining two specificity control groups WAG skin grafts on the DA heart graft recipients were rejected in the same tempo as their relevant controls. In the specificity control group, where WAG skin was placed 4 weeks after DA heart grafting, 3 of 9 of the DA heart grafts were rejected about 3 weeks after the loss of the WAG skin graft. This (23.3 ± 0.5 days) is significantly slower than the rate at which a DA skin graft can induce the loss of a DA heart graft in the comparable group (3.7 ± 1.8 days).

These data show that both the form and degree of responsiveness in these heart graft

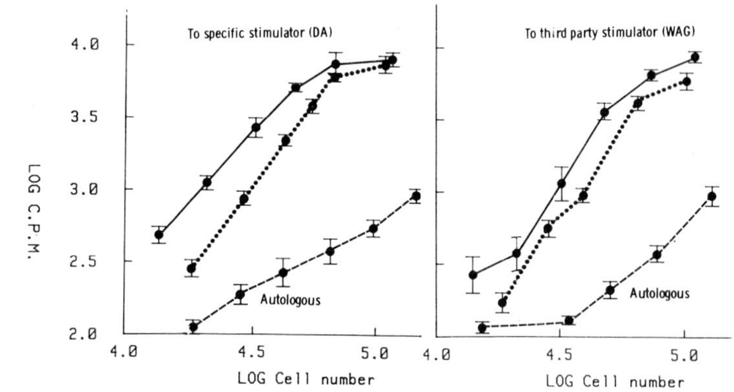

Fig. 4. The responses to both specific and third-party stimuli in mixed lymphocyte culture of lymphocytes taken from the lymph nodes of normal PVG rats (.......) and PVG recipients of a DA heart graft (_____).

recipients varies with time and can be conveniently subdivided into three stages. Stage 1 overlaps the period of cyclosporine-A treatment. The recipients are highly unresponsive, giving very prolonged skin graft survival. The nonresponsiveness is relatively stable, nonspecific, and is induced by the presence of the heart graft not solely as a consequence of cyclosporine-A therapy. The second stage in this process probably represents a transitional phase between two different mechanisms. Characteristic of this period is a decline in unresponsiveness. Skin graft survival is not prolonged, and rejection of the DA skin graft is inevitably followed by the loss of the DA heart graft. Indeed, some DA hearts are lost after the rejection of the third-party WAG skin grafts. In the third stage of this process, recipients become specifically nonresponsive to skin grafts from the heart donor strain. These survive for a very prolonged period and are eventually rejected chronically, whereas the third-party WAG skin grafts are rejected in a normal, acute, first-set fashion. This phase of nonresponsiveness is highly stable, and eventual rejection of the skin graft is not able to induce the rejection of the accompanying specific heart graft.

ALLOREACTIVE REPERTOIRE OF NONRESPONSIVE STAGE III HEART GRAFT RECIPIENTS

White investigated the ability of lymph node cells taken from these "stage III" long-term nonresponsive rats to proliferate in mixed lymphocyte culture and their ability to produce cytotoxic lymphocytes in these cultures.[7] The results of these studies are shown in Figs. 4 and 5. These data show that the animals mount normal responses both for mixed lymphocyte culture (MLC) and cell-mediated lympholysis (CML) against the

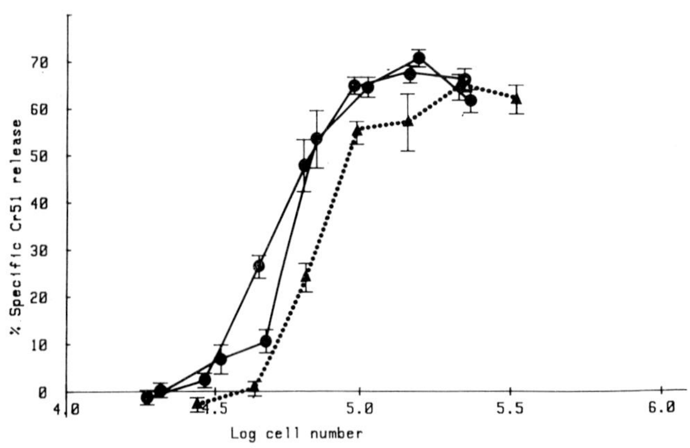

Fig. 5. A titrated cell-mediated lysis of specific DA targets by lymph node lymphocytes from normal PVG (.....) or PVG recipients of a DA heart graft (_____) (2 experiments shown).

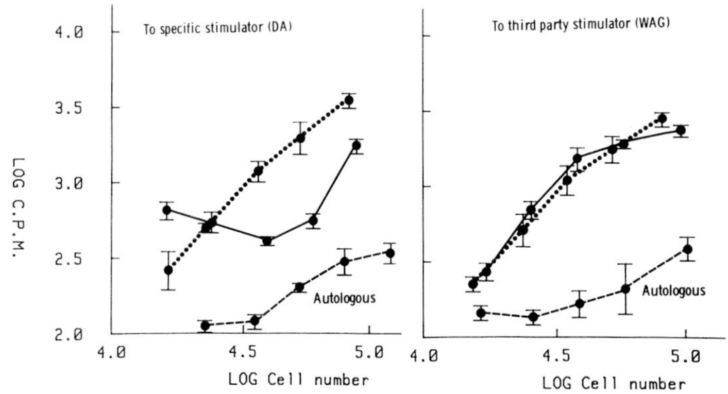

Fig. 6. **The titrated MLC responses of PBL from normal PVG (.......) and a PVG recipient of a DA heart graft responding to specific (DA) stimulation (left-hand graph) and third-party (WAG) stimulation (righthand graph).**

antigens of the heart graft donor. However, when we look at the ability of peripheral blood lymphocytes (PBL) to proliferate in MLC in response to antigens from the heart donor, we obtain a different result. Figure 6 shows that while the response of titrated PBL from a long-term nonresponsive heart graft recipient is entirely normal toward third-party stimulus, there is a marked hyporesponsiveness toward donor-specific stimulation. We also tested the ability of PBL from PVG recipients of a DA heart to mount a graft-versus-host (GVH) response, as measured by popliteal lymph node assay, when injected into the footpad of a (DA × PVG) F_1. The results show that these PBL are unable to mount a substantial GVH response to donor antigens compared to that produced by the PBL from unmodified animals (Fig. 7). We have previously shown that lymph node cells from long-term cyclosporine-A animals mount normal GVH responses in this system.

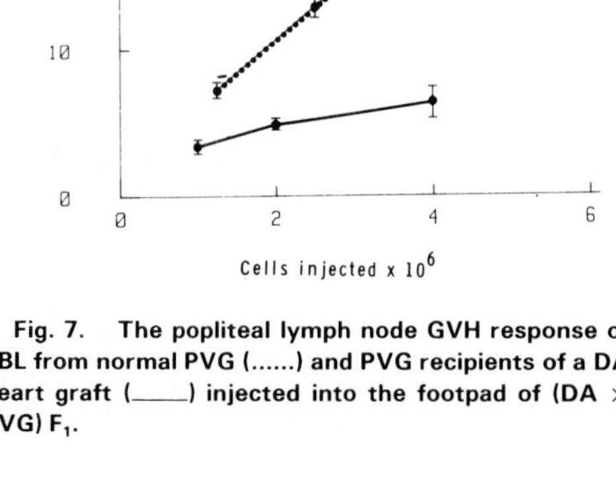

Fig. 7. **The popliteal lymph node GVH response of PBL from normal PVG (......) and PVG recipients of a DA heart graft (_____) injected into the footpad of (DA × PVG) F_1.**

Transfer of Tolerance By Serum

A possible interpretation of these data is that they demonstrate a clonal elimination taking place in the peripheral lymphocyte population but not in the lymph node compartment. This might occur as a result of the phagocytosis of complexes of antigen, antibody, and alloreactive cells, as suggested by Hutchinson.[8] If this were so, then it might be reasonable to suppose that there was sufficient excess complex in the serum of tolerant animals to permit the transfer of clonal elimination, and hence tolerance to untreated recipients. Accordingly, we harvested 500 ml of rat serum by repeatedly bleeding 51 PVG rats that had been tolerating DA grafts for more than 16 weeks. A similar volume of serum was also obtained from 48 normal PVG rats at sacrifice. Five milliliters of serum per day was then transferred intravenously to naive PVG recipients of DA hearts starting the day prior to grafting. The serum taken from the tolerant rats failed to prolong the heart graft survival compared with controls (Table 1). Two rats received 10 ml of tolerant serum (5 ml intravenously and 5 ml intraperitoneally) per day,

Table 1. Results of Serum Transfer Into PVG Rats Bearing DA Hearts

Treatment	Number	Graft Survival in Days
Normal serum (5 ml/day)	6	7, 7, 8, 8, 8, 8
"Tolerant" serum (5 ml/day)	4	7, 8, 8, 9
Tolerant serum (10 ml/day)	2	11, 11

The survival time in days of DA hearts implanted into PVG rats that have received either normal serum or "tolerant" serum, 5 ml a day, until the time of graft rejection.

and in these animals, a mild graft prolongation was observed. However, daily transfer of this volume is hemodynamically unsound, and failure to prevent graft rejection, even with these large volumes of sera, make us believe that this effect cannot be transferred by serum.

Transfer of Tolerance by Cells

Kamada has tested whether graft acceptance could be transferred by cells.[9] A quantity of 50 × 10^6 lymphocytes taken from the thoracic duct of PVG rats tolerating DA hearts for more than 16 weeks (primary recipient) were transferred to 800–850 rad irradiated PVG recipients (secondary host). This amount of irradiation is insufficient to totally remove the secondary host's immune system, so that an unrepopulated grafted secondary host will eventually recover enough immunity to reject the allograft. In our particular strain combination, many test heart grafts were permanently accepted, whereas all skin grafts were rejected (at about 1 month). Animals repopulated with 50 × 10^6 "normal" thoracic duct lymphocytes (TDL) reject skin grafts in 9 days. Roser and Dorsch[10] have shown that repopulation from a neonatally tolerant primary recipient (i.e., suppressor T cells) will retain specific skin grafts indefinitely, while rejecting third-party grafts at normal time. Repopulation with TDL that have been specifically clonally deleted causes the secondary host to reject third-party grafts normally, whereas the specific graft is rejected as the secondary host's own immune system recovers. In our experiments (Tables 2 and 3), we found transferred TDL from animals accepting DA hearts gave neither of these options. We observed a small specific prolongation of graft survival when the test graft was either heart or skin. These data could be interpreted as showing either a weak suppressor cell population or partial clonal elimination. These results are similar to those achieved by Hall et al.,[11] who transferred lymph node cells to irradiated hosts.

Bordes-Aznar et al.[12] have recently shown that T cells from the spleen of cyclosporine-A tolerant rats transferred to *unmodified* secondary hosts give the same extent of prolongation of test heart grafts as we have observed and that this activity resided in the T cytotoxic/suppressor subpopulation. These data strongly support the role for suppressor cell activity in this system. However, these authors have also shown a sequestration of the helper cell population into the liver of the secondary

Table 2. Results of Cell Transfers to 850-Rad Irradiated PVGs With Test Skin Grafts (DA and WAG)

Cells Transferred	Number	Origin of Test Graft	MST
None	8	DA	28.4 ± 1.8
		WAG	26.3 ± 1.7
50 × 10^6 normal PVG	6	DA	9.8 ± 0.5
TDL		WAG	9.3 ± 0.3
50 × 10^6 TDL from	6	DA	12.5 ± 0.9
PVG tolerating DA heart		WAG	10.1 ± 0.8

The mean survival time of skin grafts of both DA and WAG placed on 850-rad irradiated PVG recipients with cell transfer from tolerant PVGs, normal PVG, or no cell transfer.

Table 3. Results of Cell Transfers to 850-Rad Irradiated PVGs With Test Heart Grafts

Cells Transferred	Number	Origin of Test Graft	MST
None	8	DA	>100
	8	WAG	>100
50×10^6 normal PVG	6	DA	9.6 ± 0.5
TDL	6	WAG	9.1 ± 0.4
50×10^6 TDL from	6	DA	12.5 ± 0.9
PVG tolerating DA heart	6	WAG	9.5 ± 0.5

The mean survival time of heart grafts of both DA and WAG placed on 800-rad irradiated PVG recipients with cell transfer from tolerant PVGs, normal PVG, or no cell transfer.

host implying that perhaps clonal elimination is also taking place. Of course the two possibilities are not mutually exclusive, and it may well be as Bordes-Aznar suggests, that a shift in balance due to selective sequestration away from helper cells toward suppressor cells is sufficient to induce prolonged graft survival.

CONCLUSIONS

It is difficult to appreciate that small shifts of emphasis between one cell subpopulation and another can result in the acceptance of an allograft. As we accumulate knowledge about the mechanisms of graft rejection and how this process changes with time, it is to be hoped that the principles of donor-specific nonresponsiveness described here can be applied to man.

REFERENCES

1. Kostakis AJ, White DJG, Calne RY: IRCS Med Sci 5:243, 1977
2. Green CJ, Allison AC: Lancet 1:1182, 1978
3. Calne RY, White DJG, Rolles K, et al: Lancet 1:1183, 1978
4. Dunn DC, White DJG, Herbertson BM: Transplantation 29:349, 1980
5. Goodnight JE, Coleman DA, Steinmulller D: Transplantation 22:391, 1976
6. Nagao T, White DJG, Calne RY: Transplantation 33:31, 1982
7. White DJG, Nagao T, Davies HffS: Transplant Clin Immunol 13:21, 1982
8. Hutchinson IV: Immunol Rev 49:167, 1980
9. Kamada NE, White DJG: (in preparation)
10. Roser B, Dorsch S: Immunol Rev 46:83, 1979
11. Hall BM, Jelbart ME, Dorsch SE: Transplant Proc 15:504, 1983
12. Bordes-Aznar J, Kupiec-Weglinski JW, Duarte AJS, et al: Transplant 35:185, 1983

ble to nonspecific killing by macrophages and NK cells. The percentage of ^{51}Cr released as a consequence of cell-mediated cytotoxicity was calculated using the formula

$$\% \, ^{51}\text{Cr release} = \frac{\text{Experimental release} - \text{Spontaneous release}}{\text{Total release} - \text{Spontaneous release}} \times 100.$$

As shown in Fig. 1, which illustrates one experiment, the killing shown by cells from untreated animals exhibits both a specific and a nonspecific component, whereas the cells from animals treated with CsA show only nonspecific killing. In other words, in treated animals the killing of the Y3 target is comparable to that of the NS1 target. Depletion of the cells of macrophages by carbonyl iron removed about ⅔ of the nonspecific killing in both groups. Thus it is apparent that CsA does little to alter the infiltration of the allografts with mononuclear lymphoid cells, but it does markedly suppress killer-cell activity in the grafts of treated animals, which is in keeping with the in vitro data that we have mentioned previously. CsA does not appear to influence nonspecific killing in the rat that is due presumably to both macrophages and NK cells.

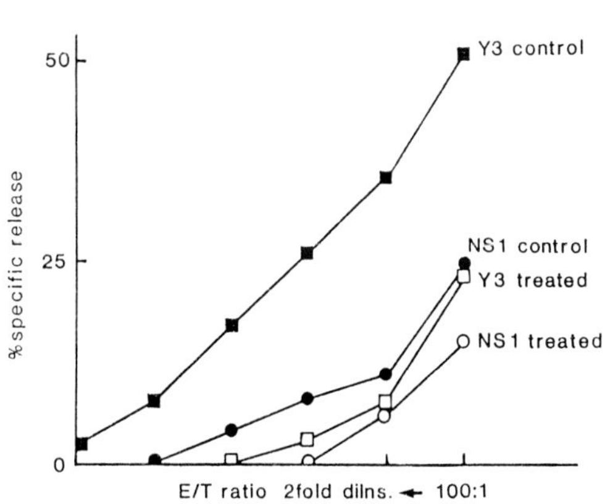

Fig. 1. The specific and non specific cytotoxic activity of mononuclear cells harvested from kidney allografts in cyclosporine A–treated or untreated (control) rats. The Y3 target expresses the same MHC antigens as the kidney allografts, so the cytotoxicity represents specific and nonspecific killing, while nonspecific killing is represented by the ^{51}Cr release from the mouse myeloma NS1.[9]

Furthermore, it would seem that nonspecific killing does not play a significant role in rejection of a renal allograft in the rat.

CsA AND THE MAINTENANCE PHASE OF ALLOGRAFT SURVIVAL

In the rat, a short course of CsA results in prolonged survival of most vascularized organ allografts, as shown in the case of a renal allograft in Table 1. But in other outbred species (e.g., dog, primate), CsA needs to be continued to prevent graft rejection.[1,2] Thus, in discussing mechanisms associated with maintenance of an allograft as a result of CsA treatment, it is possible that there are differences in the mechanism responsible for the maintenance of an allogeneic graft between, for example, the rodent renal allograft model and the dog renal allograft model. However, we are inclined to think that the difference is likely to be a quantitative one in the alteration of the immunoregulatory mechanism rather than two entirely different mechanisms.

The specificity of the tolerance produced by CsA in the rodent appears to be related to the time at which it is tested after cessation of administration of the drug. Both specificity and lack of specificity of the tolerant state have been shown in rats and rabbits challenged with third-party grafts,[10,11] while in our own laboratory, rats with long-surviving renal allografts rejected third-party renal allografts 100 days after cessation of CsA but did not mount a humoral response against the third-party histocompatibility antigens.[12] As complete serological cross-reactivity between the donor strain and the third-party strain is most unlikely, it is possible that this represents a quantitative difference in the mechanism of suppression of the cellular and humoral arms of the immune response.

White and colleagues have demonstrated, in a heterotopic cardiac allograft model, that the specificity of the tolerance induced by CsA passes through three phases after cessation of CsA treatment (Table 3).[13] Immediately after cessation of CsA, nonspecific tolerance to donor-strain and third-party skin allografts is demonstrable, followed by a

Table 3. DA (RT1[a]) Allografts Were Implanted Heterotopically in PVG (RT1[c]) Recipients Given CsA 15 mg/kg for 14 Days. DA or WAG (RT1[u]) Skin Allografts Were Placed at Various Times after Cardiac Transplantation[13]

Skin Graft	Time of Skin Grafting after Cardiac Transplantation	Median Survival (days)	
		Skin Grafts	Cardiac Grafts after Skin Grafting
DA	1 week	43	>100
	4 weeks	9	12
	20 weeks	41	>100
WAG	1 week	50	>100
	4 weeks	9	>100
	20 weeks	9	>100

period of normal reactivity to donor-strain skin and heart grafts, passing finally to a state of specific tolerance. The different conclusions drawn about the specificity of CsA-induced tolerance in different models might well be explained by these findings.

The evidence available suggests that this tolerant state in the rodent is actively maintained. For example, in the rat it is not possible to cause rejection of an established cardiac or renal allograft in a recipient given a short course of CsA with either normal or sensitized lymphocytes,[14,15] and, in general, animals with an established graft show normal reactivity to donor histocompatibility antigens in the MLR or popliteal GVH node assay.[13,14] These findings are not compatible with a mechanism of clonal deletion in these animals treated with CsA. In other words, not only does CsA prevent rejection of an allograft by preventing the generation of T_c, but it also allows the development of an active mechanism of suppression, which might be due to suppressor T cells (T_s).

What then is the evidence for the presence of suppressor T cells following CsA treatment in allograft models in animals? Again, most of the data apply to rodents, especially the rat. For example, in a bone-marrow transplant model in the rat, Tutschka and colleagues have shown that GVH disease is prevented by CsA and that specific suppressor cells can be demonstrated in vitro in the chimeric rat soon after transplantation.[16] However, data showing that suppression can be adoptively transferred are slender. In studies by the Brigham group, spleen or thymus lymphocytes were transferred from LEW rats bearing long-surviving (L × BN)F1 cardiac allografts after CsA treatment to naive LEW recipients who were challenged with a fresh (L × BN)F1 cardiac allograft.[17,18] This resulted in a modest but significant prolongation of graft survival for several days in these animals. The immunosuppressive effect could be transferred with unseparated spleen and thymic lymphocytes and their $T_{c/s}$ subpopulations, and with thymic T_h cells but not the splenic T_h subpopulation. Furthermore, passive transfer of serum from the same animals did not produce any prolongation of survival.

In our own laboratories, we have not been able to demonstrate convincingly T_s by adoptive-transfer experiments. We have transferred 2×10^8 spleen lymphocytes to naive normal DA hosts from syngeneic rats bearing long-surviving LEW grafts without any evidence of suppression of rejection of a LEW kidney. In the same model, we have also transplanted a whole spleen in case the functional structure of the spleen was in some way related to the suppressor-cell mechanism, but again this was ineffective. In more recent experiments, spleen and thymus lymphocytes were transferred from LEW recipients with a DA renal allograft maintained by a 14-day course of CsA (10 mg/kg) into naive LEW recipients that had been given a sublethal dose of 500 rad irradiation, which by itself does not lead to prolonged renal allograft survival. However, as can be seen from Table 4, although prolonged survival was seen in sublethally irradiated LEW rats given lymphocytes from LEW rats bearing long-surviving DA

Table 4. Adoptive Transfer of Spleen and Thymus cells (2×10^8) from Lewis Recipients Bearing DA Kidneys after CsA Treatment (10 mg/kg) for 14 Days to Naive LEW Recipients Given a Sublethal Dose of Irradiation (500 rad)

Treatment of Recipient	Cells Transferred	Time after Transplant	Survival (days)
500 rad	CsA Spleen	2 weeks	6*, 7*, 10
	CsA Thymus	2 weeks	12, 14
	CsA Spleen	6 weeks	10, 11, 13, 140, >140, 147
	CsA Thymus	6 weeks	6*, 14, 21, 70
	CsA Spleen	12 weeks	16, 16, 25
	CsA Thymus	12 weeks	8*, 14
500 rad	Normal Spleen	—	7*, 12, 13, 14, 24, 26
	Normal Thymus	—	10, 12, 13, 56, 56, >140
None	Normal Spleen	—	10, 11, 11, 13, 14
	Normal Thymus	—	11, 11, 12, 13, 14
500 rad	—	—	8*, 10, 10, 10, 11, 11, 12, 12, 13, 15, 16, 19, >100

All animals had a delayed nephrectomy on day 7.

*These animals died of causes unrelated to rejection.

kidneys, some of the irradiated control animals that received normal lymphocytes showed prolonged survival. Although these experiments are inconclusive, they certainly do not suggest that adoptive transfer of suppression has been achieved in this model.

However, in further support of a suppressor-cell mechanism are recent experiments by Kupiec-Weglinski and colleagues in which they have failed to cause rejection of (LEW × BN) F1 hearts established in LEW rats by a 7-day course of CsA (15 mg/kg), either with sensitized splenic lymphocytes, IL-2, or a combination of both.[18] However, treatment of the rats with cyclophosphamide (50 mg/kg i.p.) before infusing them with sensitized splenic lymphocytes with or without IL-2 did produce acute rejection. Irradiation of animals (750 rad) before infusion of sensitized splenic lymphocytes with IL-2 did not result in graft rejection. These findings suggest that suppression is maintained by a radiation-resistant but cyclophosphamide-sensitive cell population, findings that would be compatible with the active agent's being a T_s.[19,20]

On balance, one feels that the maintenance phase of a graft after CsA treatment is produced by suppressor cells, even though they are difficult to demonstrate convincingly. And there is some evidence that T_s, at least in the mouse, are insensitive in vitro to CsA.[21] It should also be noted (although not strictly belonging to our brief, which concerns animal lymphocytes) that the generation of specific suppressor cells in the MLR has been demonstrated with human cells.[22] It is also of interest to note that in our dose-response studies (see Table 1), a high dose of CsA (20 mg/kg) failed to produce indefinite survival of renal allografts, whereas lower doses (5 and 10 mg/kg) did. It is possible that T_s, which do not appear to be susceptible to CsA at optimal dose levels, may be sensitive at higher doses, at least in the rat. This phenomenon is obviously worthy of further investigation. Finally, are these findings in the rodent relevant to the clinical action of the drug? We suspect that they are, although this remains to be clearly demonstrated.

CONCLUSIONS

In animal models, there is sound evidence that CsA prevents the production of lymphokines such as IL-2 from T_h after exposure to antigen, thus preventing the generation of specific T_c. That this also allows the proliferation of T_s, which must be less sensitive to CsA and which are responsible for the continuing suppression of rejection of tissue allografts, is not so soundly based. However, the evidence available makes this the most attractive explanation. Many of these findings in experimental models of tissue transplantation are relevant to the clinical use of the drug.

REFERENCES

1. Morris PJ: Transplantation 32:349, 1981

2. Morris PJ: Advances in Surgery (in press)

3. Bunjis D, Hardt C, Röllinghoff M, et al: Eur J Immunol 11:657, 1981

4. Wagner H: Transplant Proc 15:523, 1983

5. Andrus L, Lafferty K: Scand J Immunol 15:449, 1982

6. Duayte AJ, Carpenter CB, Strom TB: J Immunol 128:580, 1982

7. Gilman SC, Rosenberg JS, Feldman JD: J Immunol 129:1012, 1982

8. Cantrell DA, Robins RA, Brooks CG, et al: Immunology 45:97, 1982

9. Mason DW, Morris PJ: Transplantation (in press)

10. Green CJ, Allison AC: Lancet 2:123, 1979

11. Dunn DC: Transplant Proc 13:383, 1981

12. Homan WP, Fabre JW, Morris PJ: Transplantation 28:439, 1979

13. White DJG (ed): Cyclosporin A. New York, Elsevier Biomedical, 1982

14. Hall BM, Jelbart ME, Dorsch SE: Transplant Proc 15:504, 1983

15. Homan W, Morris PJ: (unpublished data)

16. Tutschka PJ, Beschorner WE, Alison AC, et al: Nature 20:148, 1979

17. Bordes-Aznar J, Kupiec-Weglinski JW, Durarte AJ, et al: Transplantation 35:185, 1983

18. Kupiec-Weglinski JW, Lear PA, Bordes-Aznar J, et al: Transplant Proc 15:531, 1983

19. Askenase PW, Hayden BJ, Gershon RK: J Exper Med 141:697, 1975

20. Röllinghoff M, Starzinski A, Pfizen-Maier K, et al: J Exp Med 145:455, 1977

21. Hutchings PR, Cooke A, Gunn HC: J Immunol 130:1071, 1983

22. Tutschka P, Beschorner WE, Hess AD: Blut (Suppl) 25:242, 1980

Cyclosporine Effects on Immunoregulatory Cells in Man

C. T. Van Buren, R. Kerman, S. Flechner, and B. D. Kahan

SINCE ITS EMERGENCE from a promising immunosuppressant in the animal laboratory to its current status as the next breakthrough in clinical organ transplantation, cyclosporine has been the focus of many laboratory investigative efforts. Most studies indicate that cyclosporine seems most to exert its influence on the T lymphocyte, leaving B cells and macrophages relatively unimpaired.[1,2] Moreover, the agent does not appear to lead to clonal deletion of T lymphocytes, since in most animal species cessation of cyclosporine therapy will lead to recovery of normal immune responsiveness.[3] The mechanism of action of the drug is not yet well defined, although two major hypotheses have been advanced: (1) cyclosporine exerts its effects by interfering with the function of subsets of T lymphocytes; (2) cyclosporine interferes with the second signal, which leads to proliferation of immunopotent clones of T lymphocytes.[4]

While merits of these hypotheses have been debated, several points have emerged from the data that have been presented. First, cyclosporine therapy leads to varying degrees of immunosuppression in different animal species.[5-7] Thus, observations in animal models may not be directly applicable to man. Second, in clinical renal transplantation, the side effect of cyclosporine-induced nephrotoxicity often leaves the physician monitoring the allograft recipient with renal dysfunction on the horns of a dilemma: Should the dose of cyclosporine be reduced to treat drug toxicity, or should immunosuppression be increased to treat rejection?

These practical considerations have focused attention upon the clinical course of allograft recipients treated with cyclosporine. After completion of 100 consecutive cadaveric renal transplants at The University of Texas Medical School at Houston, the Organ Transplantation Division reviewed serial immune monitoring in these patients to determine whether any characteristic shifts in phenotypic ratios of OKT4$^+$/OKT8$^+$ lymphocytes in peripheral blood could be detected in patients treated with prednisone and cyclosporine following transplantation. Concurrently, in a series of 50 consecutive living related allograft recipients receiving cyclosporine and prednisone, patients receiving HLA identical renal allografts were studied to determine helper T-lymphocyte activity both prior to and following renal transplantation.

METHODS

From October 1981 through April 1983, 170 patients received renal transplants at The University of Texas Medical School at Houston. Of this number, 100 patients received cadaveric renal transplants and 50 patients experienced living related renal transplantation using cyclosporine and prednisone immunosuppressive therapy. Immunosuppressive therapy was the same for cadaver and living related kidney transplant recipients. Recipients of renal allografts received 120 mg prednisone/day immediately following transplantation; the steroid dose was rapidly tapered to ~0.5 mg/kg/day over the next month. Cyclosporine therapy was started 5 days prior to transplantation in living related allograft recipients at an oral dose of 14 mg/kg/day. This dose was tapered to 12 mg/kg/day 1 week following surgery and further decreased to 10 mg/kg/day in the third postoperative week. Cadaveric renal allograft recipients received 14 mg/kg/day of oral cyclosporine immediately prior to surgery and were treated with the same dose-reduction regimen used for living related transplant recipients. Daily cyclosporine trough levels were available for clinical use, and cyclosporine doses were regularly reduced to achieve a trough level of less than 200 ng/ml. Low 24-hr serum trough levels (<100 ng/ml) were treated by supplemental intravenous cyclosporine (2 mg/kg/day) during the first 2 weeks following transplantation and by

From the Division of Immunology and Organ Transplantation, Department of Surgery, The University of Texas Medical School, Houston, TX.

Reprint requests should be addressed to C. T. Van Buren, Department of Surgery, The University of Texas Medical School, 6431 Fannin, Houston, TX 77030

0041-1345/83/1505-0012$01.00/0

Table 1. Sequential Enumeration of OKT4⁺/OKT8⁺ Cells in Cadaveric Renal Allograft Recipients Treated with Cyclosporine

	Pretreatment	0–7 Days	8–14 Days	> 14 Days
N	65	62	62	53
$OKT4^+/OKT8^+$	1.98 ± 0.1	1.52 ± 0.1	1.53 ± 0.1	1.58 ± 0.1
Pretreatment vs.	—	$p < 0.001$	$p < 0.05$	$p < 0.005$

gradually increasing the oral cyclosporine dose later in the postoperative course. Rejection episodes were diagnosed clinically, based on decreased renal function and a deteriorating renal scan; clinical suspicions were usually confirmed by renal biopsy. Rejection episodes in both living related and cadaveric renal allograft recipients were treated with 1500 mg of intravenous methylprednisolone over 24 hr and an increase in oral prednisone therapy to 3 mg/kg/day.

Sixty-five cadaveric renal transplant recipients were monitored pre- and postoperatively with monoclonal OKT antibodies using the Spectrum III cytofluorometer as previously described.[8] $OKT3^+$, $OKT4^+$, and $OKT8^+$ lymphocyte subpopulations were determined daily on these patients during hospitalization and on subsequent clinic visits. Average percentages of $OKT4^+$ and $OKT8^+$ lymphocytes and $OKT4^+/OKT8^+$ ratios were determined for each patient for the following time periods: preoperative, 0–7 days, 8–14 days, and greater than 14 days following transplantation. Mean values and standard errors for lymphocyte phenotypic subpopulations were calculated for each of these four periods. Differences in variance were determined by Student-Newman-Kuel analysis. The patient group was further subdivided into groups that preoperatively had relatively high (<2.5) or relatively low (<1.5) ratios of $OKT4^+/OKT8^+$ cells. Postoperative shifts in lymphocyte subpopulations for these two patient groups were determined, and differences were analyzed by Student's t test for significance.

Helper-Cell Assay

Molinaro's reverse hemolytic plaque assay was used to determine helper-cell activity.[9] Since helper-cell activity in this system is genetically restricted,[10] helper-cell activity was only determined between a living related renal donor and his or her respective HLA identical sibling who was a renal allograft recipient. Percentage of helper-cell activity is expressed by the following formula:

$$\%\ \text{Helper-cell activity} = \frac{(T_R + B_D)}{(T_D + B_D)} \times 100,$$

where T_R represents T cells from the recipient, T_D represents T cells derived from the HLA identical donor, and B_D represents donor B cells. Values for these cell groups are hemolytic plaques derived from the designated cocultured cells. Helper T-lymphocyte activity in HLA identical renal allograft recipients immunosuppressed with cyclosporine and prednisone was compared to activity in HLA identical renal allograft recipients treated with azathioprine and prednisone. In addition, four patients treated with cyclosporine and prednisone were followed pre- and postoperatively for changes in helper-cell activity.

RESULTS

Preoperative $OKT4^+/OKT8^+$ ratios of T lymphocytes in cadaveric renal allograft recipients were within the range previously reported by our laboratory for both normal individuals and patients on dialysis (Table 1.)[11] During the first week following transplantation, there was a significant decrease in the $OKT4^+/OKT8^+$ ratio of peripheral blood lymphocytes ($p < 0.001$). This decrease persisted following discharge from the hospital. No significant difference was noted in the phenotypic ratio during any of the periods of observation postoperatively.

The decrease in $OKT4^+/OKT8^+$ lymphocyte ratios was due primarily to a decrease in the number of $OKT4^+$ cells (Table 2). There was a significant decrease in $OKT4^+$ lymphocytes immediately following transplant, and this population remained depressed during all periods of observation postoperatively ($p < 0.001$). In contrast, no discernible change was noted in $OKT8^+$ cells postoperatively.

Table 2. Sequential Analysis of Percentage of OKT4⁺ Lymphocytes in Cadaveric Renal Allograft Recipients Treated on Cyclosporine (UTMSH)

	Pretreatment	0–7 Days	8–14 Days	> 14 Days
N	65	62	62	53
$OKT4^+$	42.2 ± 1.4	27.7 ± 1.2	30.3 ± 1.3	33.4 ± 1.2

Pretreatment vs. all other groups $p < 0.001$

0–7 group vs. > 14 group $p > 0.005$

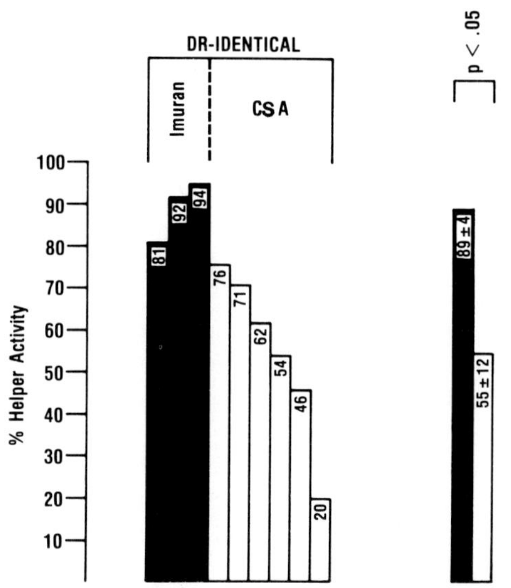

Fig. 1. Helper-cell activity in HLA identical recipients receiving either Imuran or CsA. The graph on the left represents individual values for the groups. The graph on the right represents average helper-cell activity plus or minus standard SEM for each group.

Functional activity of helper cells was also decreased in the HLA identical living related renal allograft recipients studied. Helper-cell activity following renal transplantation was significantly depressed in cyclosporine-prednisone–treated individuals compared with a similar group of patients receiving azathioprine-prednisone (Fig. 1, $p < 0.05$). Sequential assay of helper-cell activity in patients receiving cyclosporine-prednisone demonstrate a decrease in activity posttransplantation in 3 of 4 patients followed sequentially (Table 3).

DISCUSSION

Cyclosporine has led to a marked improvement in allograft survival in heart, heart-lung, liver, and renal transplantation.[12–15] Cadaveric graft survival at The University of Texas Medical School at Houston has improved to 81% in 100 consecutive cadaveric renal allograft recipients.[16] This success has been achieved even though many patients received poorly matched grafts and though 20% of the total received no preoperative blood transfusions. Flechner et al. have previously reported similarly improved allograft survival results using cyclosporine in high-MLC haploidentical living related renal allograft recipients without the benefit of donor-specific blood transfusion.[17]

The mechanism of cyclosporine's action remains a matter of dispute. Hess favors the hypothesis that cyclosporine exerts its influence primarily upon helper T-cell lymphocytes.[18] Suppressor T-cell function in both animals and man remains largely intact, while helper-cell function is depressed.[18,19] Lafferty favors the hypothesis that cyclosporine primarily interferes with the response to the second-signal triggering of lymphocyte proliferation.[20] Matters are further complicated by the fact that phenotypic markers, often used to define helper and suppressor T-lymphocyte subpopulations, may not be specific. In the mouse, Lafferty has demonstrated Lyt-1^+ cells with suppressor activity, and Lyt-1^-, Lyt-$2,3^+$ cells with helper function.[20] Thus, any conclusions drawn upon shifts in lymphocyte subpopulations should be supported by corresponding changes in lymphocyte functional activities.

Several centers have used monoclonal antibodies to monitor human T-lymphocyte subsets in renal allograft recipients receiving cyclosporine-prednisone immunosuppression. Hakala et al. were unable to demonstrate a postoperative change in $OKT4^+/OKT8^+$ ratios in 30 cadaveric renal allograft recip-

Table 3. Sequential Study of Helper-Cell Activity in HLA-DR Identical Transplants

P. M. and J. M.		R. B. and C. B.		L. W. and C. W.		J. S. and D. F.	
02/07/83	97%*	10/29/82	41%*	10/08/82	31%*	09/21/82	66%*
02/17/83	80%	11/11/82	40%	11/05/82	13%	09/29/82	41%
05/03/83	71%	05/03/83	46%	05/03/82	20%	05/03/83	54%

*The first value for each recipient-donor pair represents preoperative recipient T helper-cell activity.

ients; only 6 of these patients were followed sequentially, and all patients received blood transfusions prior to transplantation.[21] The University of Minnesota has previously reported no change in OKT4$^+$/OKT8$^+$ lymphocyte ratios in cyclosporine patients after renal transplantation.[22] However, all cadaveric renal allograft recipients entered into the Minnesota randomized protocol received at least 10 third-party blood transfusions, received well-matched renal allografts, and were subjected to pretransplant splenectomy. In contrast, Stiller's prospective immune monitoring of 19 cadaveric renal allograft recipients randomly assigned into the cyclosporine treatment arm of the Canadian trial revealed a decrease in OKT4$^+$/OKT8$^+$ lymphocytes in peripheral blood of these patients following transplantation.[23] Moreover, the effect was more marked the longer the patient received cyclosporine.

Data from The University of Texas Medical School at Houston reveals a marked post-transplant decrease in OKT4$^+$/OKT8$^+$ lymphocytes in 65 cadaveric renal allograft recipients immunosuppressed with cyclosporine and prednisone. These results confirm previous reports from this center of such a phenotypic shift in T lymphocytes; this alteration in OKT4$^+$/OKT8$^+$ ratios was not noted in azathioprine-treated patients with stable allograft function.[8,24] The present study also demonstrates that the decreased ratio in cyclosporine patients is primarily due to a drop in the percentage of OKT4$^+$ lymphocytes following transplantation. The proportion of OKT8$^+$ lymphocytes remains largely unaffected. The hypothesis that this phenotypic shift reflects a decrease in helper-cell numbers is supported by the decreased helper-cell activity observed in HLA identical living related allograft recipients compared to similarly matched azathioprine-treated recipients. As noted in the cyclosporine patients sequentially followed for helper-cell activity, however, other factors may suppress helper-cell activity in the uremic patient. Sequential analysis of helper-cell activity in correlation with changes in phenotypic helper T-lymphocyte populations will be most helpful in clarifying the relationship between phenotype and function in the transplant patient.

Although a significant postoperative decrease in the proportion of OKT4$^+$ T lymphocytes in peripheral blood is observed in cadaveric renal allograft recipients treated with cyclosporine and prednisone, these results do not necessarily support the subset T-lymphocyte hypothesis of cyclosporine's action. Successful renal transplantation may be observed in cyclosporine-treated individuals with a relatively high preoperative OKT4$^+$/OKT8$^+$ lymphocyte ratio that remains unaltered after transplantation. C. B. in the HLA identical series (Table 3) revealed no significant decrease in OKT4$^+$ lymphocytes and also had no decrease in helper-cell activity postoperatively. Thus, a shift in OKT4$^+$/OKT8$^+$ ratios is not necessary for cyclosporine to be an effective immunosuppressant. Cyclosporine combined with prednisone therapy may have a different influence upon lymphocyte subpopulations than the effect of cyclosporine alone. This remains to be further clarified in animal studies. Different T-lymphocyte subpopulations may have differing susceptibility to cyclosporine's adverse influence upon IL-2 responsiveness. Thus, changes in phenotypic T-lymphocyte subpopulations may be directly due to cyclosporine's suppression of the expansion of immunopotent T-lymphocyte clones.

The observed postoperative decrease in OKT4$^+$/OKT8$^+$ lymphocyte ratios seen in cyclosporine-treated cadaveric renal allograft recipients is at present probably most useful in revealing a cyclosporine effect. If during the induction of immunosuppressive therapy a shift is observed from a high preoperative to a low postoperative OKT4$^+$/OKT8$^+$ ratio, one may feel relatively secure that the patient is adequately immunosuppressed. Further follow-up of these patients will be necessary to determine whether such a shift may be useful in distinguishing postoperative renal dysfunction due to cyclosporine nephrotoxicity from that due to acute rejection. Analysis of the fate of patients who fail to reflect a shift in lymphocyte subpopulations following cyclosporine treatment may also reveal whether such a shift is of prognostic importance. These studies will determine the ultimate value of immune monitoring in the cyclosporine-treated renal allograft recipients.

REFERENCES

1. Lindsey MJ, Harris KR, Norman HB, et al: Transplant Proc 12:252, 1980

2. Drath DB, Kahan BD: Transplant Proc (in press)

3. White DJG, Plumb A, Pawelec G: Transplantation 27:55, 1979

4. Bunjes D, Hardt C, Röllinghoff M, et al: Eur J Immunol 11:657, 1981

5. Calne RY, White DJG: IRCS Med Sci 5:595, 1977

6. White DJG, Nagao, T, Davies H: In White DJG (ed): Cyclosporin A. New York, Elsevier Biomedical, 1982, p 89

7. Gratwohl A, Forster I, Speck B: Transplant Proc 15:497, 1983

8. Van Buren CT, Kerman R, Agostino G, et al: Surgery 92:167, 1982

9. Molinaro GA, Maron E, Dray S: Proc Natl Acad Sci USA 71:1229, 1974

10. Strelkauskas AJ, Wilson BS, Callery RT, et al: J Exp Med 146:1765, 1977

11. Kerman RH, Van Buren CT, Payne WD, et al: Transplant Proc 15:1170, 1983

12. Baumgartner WA, Reitz BA, Oyer PE, et al: Curr Probl Surg 16:1, 1979

13. Reitz BA, Wallwork JL, Hunt SA, et al: N Engl J Med 306:557, 1982

14. Starzl TE, Klintmalm GBG, Porter KA, et al: N Engl J Med 305:266, 1981

15. Najarian JS, Ferguson RM, Sutherland DER, et al: Transplant Proc 15:438, 1983

16. Kahan BD, Van Buren CT, Flechner SM, et al: Transplant Proc (in press)

17. Flechner SM, Kerman RH, Van Buren CT, et al: Transplant Proc 15:442, 1983

18. Hess AD, Tutschka PJ, Santos GW: In White DJG (ed): Cyclosporin A. New York, Elsevier Biomedical, 1982, p 209

19. Hutchinson IF, Shadur CA, Duarte A, et al: Transplantation 32:210, 1981

20. Lafferty K, Borel JF: Transplant Proc (in press)

21. Hakala TR, Starzl TE, Rosenthal JT, et al: Transplant Proc 15:465, 1983

22. Ferguson RM, Fidelus RK, Sawchuk RJ, et al: Transplant Proc (in press)

23. Stiller C: Transplant Proc (in press)

24. Van Buren CT, Kerman RH, Agostino G, et al: Transplant Proc 15:527, 1983

Analysis of Lymphocytes Concerned in Spontaneous Blastogenesis During Acute Rejection

T. Oka, N. Yoshimura, Y. Ohmori, I. Aikawa, T. Matsumura, T. Usui, K. Arakawa, and I. Hashimoto

MANY CLINICAL STUDIES have demonstrated that spontaneous blastogenesis (SB) assay using a small amount of peripheral blood is an efficient immunological monitor of acute rejection.

We have found a good correlation between the SB values of peripheral blood or perpared lymphocytes and rejection in human renal allografts immunosuppressed with a combination of azathioprine and steroids.[1]

Little has been reported about the association between SB values and rejection in patients treated with cyclosporine (CsA).

We tried to determine whether the assay of SB value is useful for assessing and predicting rejection and what subpopulation of lymphocytes is involved during the rejection period in CsA-treated patients.

MATERIALS AND METHODS

Patients

Twenty patients were treated with CsA after renal transplantation from a living related or cadaveric donor. Postoperatively, CsA was given in a single daily dose of 14 mg/kg, tapering by 2 mg/kg each month until a maintenance dose of 8 mg/kg was reached. All patients were treated with the same corticosteroid regimen in which the daily dose of prednisolone was progressively reduced from 50 mg to 10 mg.

Episodes of acute rejection were diagnosed on the basis of fever, graft swelling, and laboratory data, and were treated with bolus doses of methylprednisolone.

SB Assay

To perform the SB assay, 50 μl of heparinized blood or $2 \times 10^5/50$ μl of separated lymphocytes was taken from patients and mixed with 200 μl of RPMI 1640 medium and 1 μCi of ^{3}H-thymidine in a U-bottomed microtiter plate. After 2 hr incubation at 37°C, the tray was harvested and the filter strips were counted by a liquid scintillation counter.

Discontinuous Gradient of Percoll[2]

Nine parts of Percoll were mixed with one part of (10×) concentrated phosphate-buffered saline (PBS) and progressively diluted in PBS (normal concentration) to obtain solutions containing the desired percentage of Percoll.

Two milliliter volumes of each of the Percoll solutions were layered carefully in 15-ml plastic tubes, and, finally, 2×10^7 lymphocytes in PBS were layered on top of this gradient. The gradient was spun at 2300 *g* for 12 min at room temperature. After centrifugation, each fraction contained the cells banded at the interface between two different densities. The cells were carefully removed and washed twice with minimal essential medium (MEM).

Cell Surface Characterization

Rosette formation with SRBC (E rosette) was assessed by the method of Jondal et al.[3] Leu phenotype was examined by indirect immunofluorescence with monoclonal antibodies anti-Leu-1, Leu-2a, and Leu-3a.[4] 5×10^5 cells were incubated at 4°C for 30 min with 100 μl of appropriately diluted monoclonal antibody. After washing, the cells were stained with FITC-conjugated rabbit anti-mouse IgG.

RESULTS

Correlation Between SB Values and Episodes of Acute Rejection in the CsA-Treated Patients

Episodes of acute rejection, which were diagnosed by clinical symptoms and laboratory data, occurred seven times in 20 recipients. The consequent elevation of SB values on two or more determinations at any time in the course of the rejection reaction was observed in 6 episodes (86%) and was not observed in 1 (14%) (Table 1). The mean value of 21 assays in acute rejection was 10,998 ± 1665 dpm (Fig. 1), significantly higher than that of quiescent periods and control samples (data not shown).

From the Second Department of Surgery, Kyoto Prefectural University of Medicine, Kyoto.

Reprint requests should be addressed to Dr. Takahori Oka, Second Department of Surgery, Kyoto Prefectural University of Medicine, Hirokoji Kawaramachi Kamikyoku, Kyoto 602, Japan.

0041-1345/83/1505-0013$01.00/0

Table 1. Association Between SB Values and Episodes of Acute Rejection in CsA-Treated Patients[1]

No. of Patients	Rejection	SB Value	
		Elevation	No Change
20	7	6 (86%)	1 (14%)

SB Value of Each Fraction from Discontinuous Gradient of Percoll

2×10^5 cells of each fraction separated by discontinuous gradient of Percoll, in the patients undergoing rejection, were incubated with 1 μCi of ^{3}H-thymidine for 2 hr, and incorporation of ^{3}H-thymidine was measured. The lymphocytes from fraction IV at the interface between 55% and 60% Percoll concentration showed the highest incorporation of ^{3}H-thymidine, 11,998 ± 1334 dpm (Fig. 1). In the other five fractions, incorporation of ^{3}H-thymidine ranged from 200 to 4498 dpm. Lymphocytes of fraction IV from post-transplant patients during the quiescent period, from patients on hemodialysis, and from healthy subjects showed no higher incorporation of ^{3}H-thymidine than any other fraction (Fig. 2).

These results suggest that the lymphocytes concerned in SB at the rejection period are densely populated in fraction IV.

Characterization of Lymphocytes from Fraction IV

In order to investigate what subpopulation of lymphocytes is included in fraction IV, E-rosette testing or immunofluorescent staining using monoclonal antibody (Leu series) was performed (Table 2). Unseparated cells contained 40% or 45% of T cells. This subpopulation was greatly increased in fraction IV but not in fraction V. The Leu phenotype of unfractionated lymphocytes and lymphocytes from fraction 4 were examined by monoclonal anti-Leu antibody. Unseparated cells contained 18% to 26% of Leu-2a antigen-positive cells. The number of this subpopulation was increased in fraction IV. However, Leu-3a antigen positive cells, which were 34% or 40% in unfractionated lymphocytes, were decreased in fraction IV (Table 2).

DISCUSSION

A good correlation between elevated SB values and allograft rejection has been

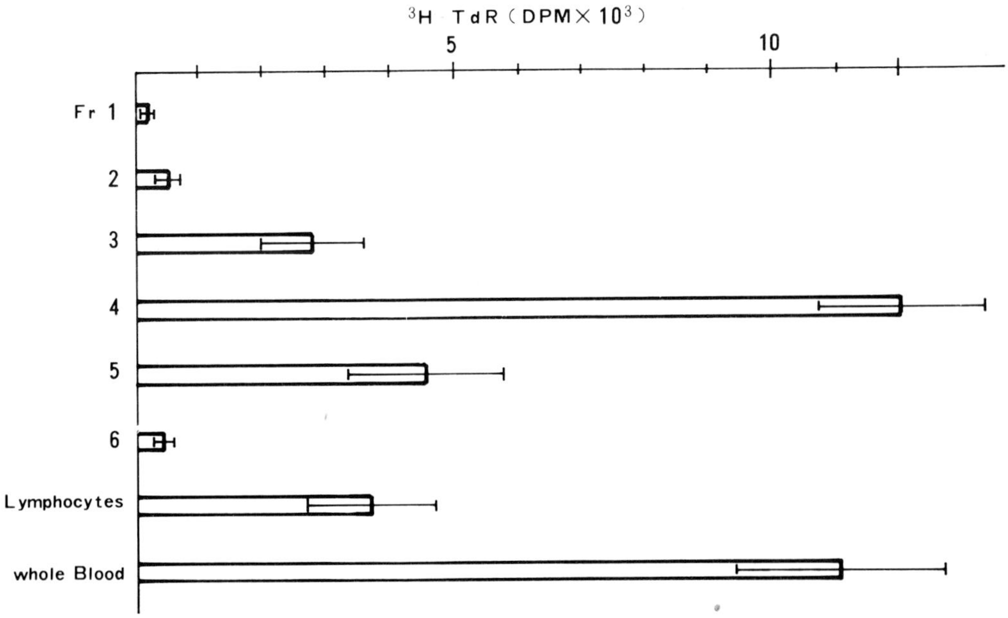

Fig. 1. Spontaneous blastogenic activity of each Percoll fraction at acute rejection.[1]

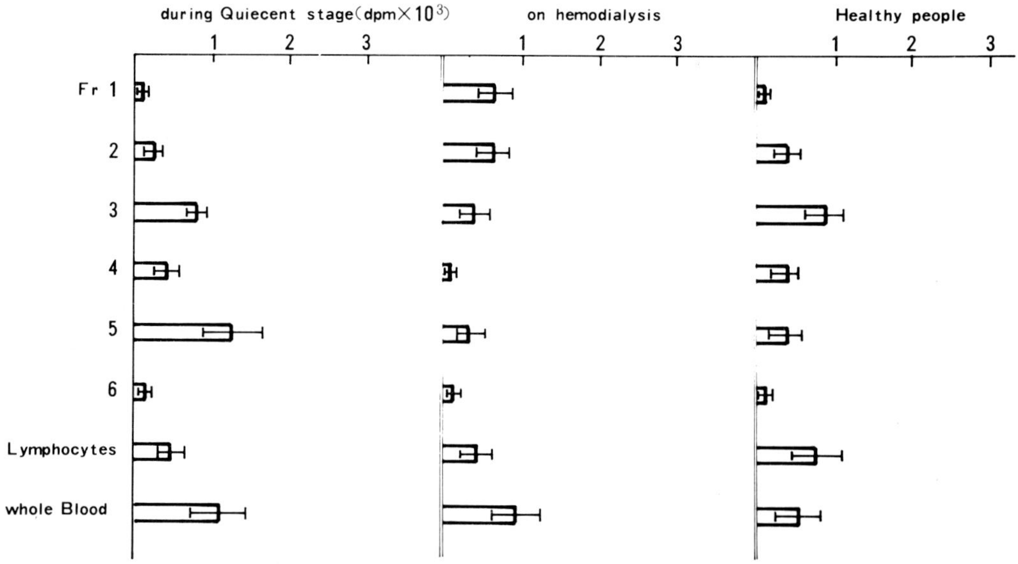

Fig. 2. **SB activity in post-transplant patients during quiescent stage, patients on hemodialysis, and healthy people.**[1]

reported by many investigators in patients mainly on azathioprine and steroids. In the present study, the association between SB values and acute rejection in the CsA-treated patients was investigated.

As shown in Table 1, an elevation of SB values was observed in 6/7 (86%) during acute rejection episodes. These results suggest a good correlation between elevated SB values and rejection crises in the CsA-treated patients as well.

Several investigators have reported that CsA-treated patients displayed a significantly decreased ratio of percentage of helper/inducer T cells to percentage of suppressor/killer T cells (T_h/T_s)[5].

They speculated that this decreased ratio observed in recipients treated with CsA was due to a decreased number of T_h cells and that the increased ratio observed in acute rejection was due to an increased number of T_h cells. In our experiments also, this ratio decreased during the quiescent period and increased during the rejection episodes (Table 2). However, from the experiments using a discontinuous gradient of Percoll during the rejection period, the ratio decreased markedly in fraction IV, from which lymphocytes displayed the highest value of SB during the rejection episodes (Fig. 1).

Because SB is thought to be the result of an in vivo mixed lymphocytes reaction (MLR) between donor and recipient, we speculate that the lymphocytes in fraction IV play an

Table 2. Characterization of Lymphocytes from Percoll Fractions at Rejection Period[1]

	ExP 1				ExP 2			
SB (dpm)	10,990 ± 493				5,248 ± 1,724			
	E	Leu (%)			E	Leu (%)		
Monoclonal Ab	Rosette	1	2a	3a	Rosette	1	2a	3a
Whole lymphocytes	34	40	18	34	43	45	26	40
Fr. IV	81	83	59	24	70	69	55	4
Fr. V	37	39	22	22	—	—	—	—

important role in acute rejection. From our experiments, the percentage of helper/inducer T cells decreased and the percentage of killer/suppressor T cells increased in fraction IV. Active blastogenic lymphocytes in the acute rejection may not be helper/inducer T cells but killer/suppressor T cells. An analysis of function of the lymphocytes from fraction IV will be necessary in further study.

REFERENCES

1. Oka T, Matsumura T, Ohmori Y, et al: Jap J Surg 13:196, 1983
2. Guitierrez C, Bernabe RR, Vega J, et al: J Immunol Methods 29:57, 1979
3. Jondal M, Holm G, Wigzell H: J Exp Med 136:207, 1972
4. Ledbetter JA, Evans RL, Lipinski M: J Exp Med 153:310, 1981
5. Van Buren CT, Kerman R, Agostino G, et al: Surgery 92:167, 1982

Immunologic Monitoring of Renal Allograft Recipients Treated with Cyclosporine

R. H. Kerman, S. M. Flechner, C. T. Van Buren, W. Payne, and B. D. Kahan

IMMUNOLOGIC monitoring of transplant recipients may detect donor-specific and nonspecific host-immune events leading to renal allograft damage.[1] Early diagnosis of graft injury could permit immediate therapeutic intervention with resolution of the injury process and prolonged allograft survival.[2] Moreover, serial evaluation of immune parameters, correlated with clinical indices, may allow discrimination between drug-induced nephrotoxicity and immune injury leading to graft loss. Renal allograft recipients were therefore subjected to post-transplant immune evaluation for (1) donor-specific immunity including complement-dependent antibody (CDA), lymphocyte-dependent antibody (LDA), and lymphocyte-mediated cytotoxicity (LMC), and (2) nonspecific immunity including spontaneous blastogenesis (SB), percentage (%) active thymus rosette-forming cells (A-T RFC), T helper/inducer cells ($OKT4^+$, T_h), and T suppressor/cytotoxic ($OKT8^+$, T_s) cells.[3-5] The present study analyzed the results of both nonspecific and donor-specific postoperative immune monitoring of cadaveric renal allograft recipients treated with either azathioprine (Aza) and steroids or cyclosporine (CsA) and steroids. Our data confirm the potent immunosuppressive action of CsA to dampen recipient immune responsiveness and suggest that post-transplant immune monitoring of T_h/T_s ratios may help in discriminating between CsA nephrotoxicity or immune injury.

From the Department of Surgery, Division of Immunology and Organ Transplantation, The University of Texas Medical School, Houston, TX.

Reprint requests should be addressed to R. H. Kerman, Department of Surgery, The University of Texas Medical School, 6431 Fannin, Houston, TX 77030.

0041-1345/83/1505-0014$01.00/0

MATERIALS AND METHODS

Patients

Some 211 recipients of cadaveric donor allografts were postoperatively evaluated for % A-T RFC, SB, T_h, and T_s cell levels and donor-specific immunity including LDA, CDA, and LMC. These parameters were correlated with clinical indices of (1) diagnosed rejection episodes based on the presence of clinical signs of rejection, diffuse mononuclear cell infiltrates on renal biopsy, and either a response to steroid pulse therapy or progression to graft loss, or (2) episodes of CsA nephrotoxicity based on creatinine elevations of $>25\%$ of baseline and lacking in the above criteria defining rejection.

Nonspecific Immune Tests

Postoperative monitoring of nonspecific immune events described by increased SB and decreased A-T RFC were enumerated daily, as previously described.[3]

Enumeration of T-Cell Subsets

T-cell subsets were analyzed using xenoantisera to human lymphocyte surface antigens and flow cytometry (T helper/inducer (T_h) and T suppressor/cytotoxic (T_s) cells identified by OKT4 and OKT8 reagents, respectively (Ortho Diagnostics, Inc., Raritan, NJ). Briefly, 10 μl of fluoresceinated monoclonal antibody (OKT4 or OKT8, Ortho-mune is added to 100 μl of EDTA-treated whole blood and incubated for 30 min. To the solution is added 2 ml of lysing reagent (to lyse red blood cells); the mixture is then centrifuged for 5 min at 800 rpm at 4°C. Following centrifugation, the supernatant is discarded, and the cell pellet is resuspended in 2 ml of PBS and centrifuged for 10 min at 800 rpm at 4°C. The supernatant is again discarded, the cell pellet is resuspended in 2 ml of PBS, and the sample then analyze on the Spectrum III flow cytometer.[6] Differences between the ratios of T_h/T_s in various groups were assessed using a Wilcoxon signed-rank sum test.

Donor-Specific Immune Tests

Three donor-specific immune assays were performed approximately every 7 days postoperatively as previously described, utilizing recipient serum and lymphocytes for CDA, LDA, and LMC assays against ^{51}Cr-labeled donor PBL.[5]

Therapy

Of the 211 patients, 111 received conventional immunosuppressive therapy including azathioprine (1–3 mg/

kg) and tapering dosages of corticosteroids (120–30 mg every day). Rejection crises were treated with increased steroid dosage and local graft irradiation.[7] The other 100 patients received (CsA (instead of Aza), distributed in olive oil, orally at dosages of 14 mg/kg for 7 days, 12 mg/kg for 2 weeks, 10 mg/kg for 1 month and tapered to 8 mg/kg at 3 months (provided by Sandoz Co., East Hanover, NJ). Dosages were adjusted to maintain plasma trough CsA levels at less than 200 ng/ml.[8]

RESULTS

Renal allograft recipients were monitored daily for alterations in % A-T RFC, SB, and T-cell subsets (T_h and T_s). CsA did not interfere with postoperative immune monitoring. Characteristic postoperative changes experienced by both CsA- and Aza-treated patients included (1) increases in T_h/T_s ratios associated with nonspecific immune events (increased SB and decreased % A-T RFC) and clinical rejections which reversed following increased steroid therapy (Tables 1 and 2); (2) high T_h/T_s ratios associated with nonspecific immune events in the absence of clinical rejection, possibly indicating subclinical immune injury; and (3) stable T_h/T_s ratios during periods of clinical quiescence. Table 1 summarizes the post-transplant nonspecific immune monitoring data for Aza-treated allograft recipients. During the first 30 postoperative days, 25 Aza-treated recipients experienced 28 clinical rejection episodes accompanied by 48 episodes of increased T_h/T_s ratios, increased SB, and decreased % A-T RFC. All rejections were associated with nonspecific immune events (↑ T_h/T_s ratios and ↑ SB ↓ A-T RFC). Twenty nonspecific immune events occurred in the absence of clinical rejection; 6 of the 20 were associated with infectious episodes. We have previously reported that these extra nonspecific immune events occurring in the absence of rejection or infection were associated with subclinical immune injury.[3] Table 2 summarizes the posttransplant nonspecific immune monitoring data for CsA-treated allograft recipients. During a mean follow-up period of 11 ± 5 months, the 100 CsA-treated recipients experienced only 19 rejection episodes accompanied by increased T_h/T_s ratios (53 times) and increased SB and decreased A-T RFC (61 times). All 19 rejection episodes were associated with nonspecific immune events (↑ T_h/T_s ratios and ↑ SB ↓ A-T RFC). Forty-eight increased T_s ratios occurred concomitantly with 48 increased SB and decreased A-T RFC in the absence of clinical rejection, possibly indicating infection or subclinical immune events.[3] The remaining 5 T_h/T_s ratios and 13 SB and A-T RFC events represent a false positive rate of 7% (5/72) and 16% (13/80) for T_h/T_s ratios and SB and A-T RFC, respectively. The relative changes in T-cell subsets served as a better indication of immune events than arbitrary absolute values.

Table 1. Immunologic Monitoring Results of 28 Treated Rejection Episodes During the First 30 Postoperative Days in 25 Aza-Treated Recipients of Cadaveric Renal Allografts

↑ T_h/T_s	↑ SB ↓ A-T RFC	Rejections
48	48	28
20	20	0
14*	14*	0

*20 immune events less 6 infection episodes = 14 nonspecific immune events, possibly indicating subclinical injury.

Table 2. Immunologic Monitoring Results of 19 Treated Rejection Episodes in 100 CsA-Treated Recipients of Cadaveric Renal Allografts

↑ T_h/T_s	↑ SB ↓ A-T RFC	Rejections
72	80	19
53*	61*	0
5†	13*	0

*48 concomitant T_h/T_s and SB and A-T RFC events due to subclinical events or infections.

†False positive rate of 7% (5/72) and 16% (13/80) for T_h/T_s ratios and SB and A-T RFC, respectively.

Compared to Aza patients, CsA patients experienced fewer clinically diagnosed rejection episodes (0.19 vs. 1.1, $p < 0.01$) and fewer instances of postoperative nonspecific immune events, increased SB, and decreased A-T RFC (0.8 vs. 1.9, $p < 0.01$) and displayed less donor-specific immunity (16% vs. 45%, $p < 0.05$ for positive LDA, CDA, or LMC, postoperatively).

The potent immunosuppressive activity of CsA has been shown to be accompanied by nephrotoxicity.[9,10] Because CsA is toxic to the kidney, it is questionable whether changes would be expected to occur in peripheral blood immune parameters similar to those seen in rejection. In a preliminary evaluation of 11 patients diagnosed as experiencing CsA-induced nephrotoxicity, we were unable to find concomitant significant changes occurring in T_h/T_s ratios. The patients were evaluated for T_h/T_s ratios several days prior to and following the CsA nephrotoxicity. Of the 11 patients evaluated 10, (91%) did not display significant changes in T_h/T_s ratios either several days prior to or following the diagnosis of CsA-induced nephrotoxicity. However, the remaining patient did experience a change in T_h/T_s ratio of 0.4 to 1.1 to 0.7 prior to, during, and following CsA nephrotoxicity, respectively.

We have previously reported pretransplant parameters defining immunologically high-risk recipients with poor allograft survival, including poor HLA A, B, and DR matching and recipients with <5 random blood transfusion (BT) and strong immune responders.[11–13] We evaluated our data to determine whether pretransplant levels of T helper and T suppressor cells also correlated with and could be additive in delineating risk groups. Evaluation of 100 normal individuals revealed them to have a T_h of 42 ± 8%, a T_s of 26 ± 7%, and a T_h/T_s ratio of 1.9 ± 0.5 (mean ±1 SD). For data analysis, the 95% confidence interval (±2 SD) was obtained for each parameter (T_h = 26%, T_s = 12%, and T_h/T_s = 0.9), and groups were compared with regard to being above or below this interval. Interestingly, appropriate pretransplant T_h and T_s levels correlated with these risk factors and could therefore be seen also to delineate preoperative immunologically high-risk recipients. For example, 96% (42/44) of strong immune responders displayed T_h/T_s ratios greater than 2 SDs from normal (>1.9), compared to 18% of weak responders ($p < 0.01$).

Postoperative evaluation of T-cell subset levels in CsA patients also correlated with pretransplant immune high-risk parameters. Some 67% (16/24) of patients receiving 0 blood transfusions and 61% (27/44) of strong immune responders had high levels of T_h cells (>26%), compared to 37% (12/35) and 32% (4/11) of patients who received >5 transfusions or were weak immune responders preoperatively (both $p < 0.05$). In contrast, 69% (24/35) of patients receiving >5 transfusions and 64% (7/11) of weak immune responders and high levels of T_s cells (>12%), compared to 25% (6/24) and 36% (16/44) of patients receiving 0 transfusions who were strong immune responders preoperatively (both $p <$ 0.05). Yet, in spite of this association of high postoperative T_h cells with preoperative immune risk factors, CsA profoundly altered postoperative T_h/T_s ratios in preoperatively strong but not weak immune responders. Of strong immune responders, 73% (32/44) displayed preoperative T_h/T_s ratios greater than 2 SD from normal (>1.9), compared to only 32% (14/44) of the patients postoperatively (Table 3). No comparable changes were seen in CsA-treated weak immune responders.

DISCUSSION

The nonspecific and donor-specific immune assay results demonstrate the potent immunosuppressiveness of CsA compared to Aza. The postoperative monitoring results obtained utilizing the T_h/T_s ratios do no more than confirm the immune-event changes detected by the % A-T RFC and SB. Thus, the currently available reagents (OKT4 and OKT8) do not afford a reliable index of rejection. Other reagents identifying different lymphocyte activation receptors may allow for better discrimination of lymphocyte subsets and afford better clinical correlations.

Pre- and postoperative immune evaluation successfully delineated individuals who are

Table 3. Effect of CsA on Strong Responder T_h/T_s Ratios

	T_h/T_s ratio			
	>1.9	1.9–1.4	1.4–0.9	<0.9
Pretransplant	73%	23%	—	—
Post-transplant	32%	21%	27%	20%

immunologically high-risk renal allograft candidates. Our results confirm the immunosuppressive potenct of CsA to dampen host immunity and clearly point out the major effect of CsA on high-risk patients.

Preoperative immune evaluation has successfully delineated immunologically high-risk renal allograft candidates who may benefit the most from CsA immunosuppression.[11-13] Preoperative identified high-risk patients displayed higher T_h/T_s ratios than low-risk patients. Most important, however, CsA affected significant decreases in T_h and T_s cells postoperatively, thus allowing for reduced donor and nonspecific immunity and significantly improved graft survival in these high-risk patients. Finally, preliminary results suggest that postoperative delineation of T_h/T_s ratios may allow for discrimination between CsA-induced nephrotoxicity and immune renal injury. Of 11 patients experiencing CsA-induced nephrotoxicity, 10 (91%) did not display significant changes in T_h/T_s ratios, whereas all recipients experiencing rejection episodes did. A much larger series will allow us to confirm this finding.

REFERENCES

1. Stiller CR, Keown PA: Transplant Proc 13:1699, 1981

2. Cosimi AB, Colvin RB, Burton RC, et al: N Engl J Med 305:308, 1982

3. Kerman RH, Floyd M, Van Buren CT, et al: Transplantation 32:16, 1981

4. Kerman RH, Van Buren CT, Payne W, et al: Transplant Proc 15:1170, 1983

5. Kerman RH, Kahan BD: Ann Clin Res 13:244, 1981

6. Hoffman RA, Kung PC, Hansen WP, et al: Proc Natl Acad Sci 77:4914, 1980

7. Kahan BD: In Goldsmith H (ed): Lewis Practice of Surgery. Hagerstown, Md., Harper & Row, 1978, p 1077

8. Kahan BD, Van Buren CT, Lin S, et al: Transplantation 34:36, 1982

9. Calne RY, Thiru S, McMaster P, et al: Lancet 2:1323, 1979

10. Flechner SM, Van Buren C, Kerman RH, et al: Transplant Proc (in press)

11. Kerman RH, Floyd M, Van Buren CT, et al: Transplantation 30:450, 1980

12. Kerman RH, Flechner S, Van Buren CT, et al: Transplant Proc, (in press)

13. Kerman RH, Van Buren CT, Payne W, et al: Transplantation 36:50, 1983

Cyclosporine Effects on Mitogen-Induced T- and B-Cell Proliferation

H. G. A. Bouwer and D. J. Hinrichs

THE MAJORITY of lymphocytes present in a host exist in a resting state. Following an antigen stimulus, a cascade of regulatory events occur, leading to lymphocyte activation. Monokines, such as interleukin-1 (IL-1), and lymphokines such as interleukin 2 (IL-2) and B-cell growth factor (BCGF), are reportedly involved as cell communication signals.[1-6]

Borel, in 1976, reported the discovery of a fungal metabolite, cyclosporine A (CsA), with lymphocyte-specific immunosuppressive properties.[7] Many papers have been published in an attempt to understand the mechanism of action of CsA.[8-13] It appears that the CsA mode of action is the interruption or cessation of early activation events and/or cell communication signals. The purpose of this report is to assess CsA-mediated immunosuppression of T- and B-cell responses, using mitogen activation to initiate the cell response. We focused our studies on the factors associated with early cell communication that lead to proliferation and have found that CsA alters these signals in terms of proliferation and recognition.

MATERIALS AND METHODS

Animals

Female inbred Lewis rats (obtained from Microbiological Associates) were used at 3–5 months of age. Female BALB/c inbred mice raised in the Washington State University vivarium were used at 6–8 weeks of age. Athymic animals were obtained from heterozygote matings and were maintained in our vivarium.

From the Department of Bacteriology and Public Health, Washington State University, Pullman, WA.

Reprint requests should be addressed to H. G. A. Bouwer, Department of Bacteriology and Public Health, Washington State University, Pullman, WA 99164-4340.

Supported by PHS Grant NS16731.

0041-1345/83/1505-0015$01.00/0

Lymphocyte Proliferation Assay

Spleen cells were washed and resuspended in serum-free modified DMEM (Gibco Laboratories, Grand Island, 430-2100) as previously described by Iscove and Melchers.[14] Cells were added at 1×10^5 cells/well to 96 well round-bottomed microtiter plates (NUNC) with lipopolysaccharide (LPS, *S. typhimurium,* Difco Laboratories, Detroit, MI, 3125-25) 2.5 μg/well, concanavalin A (Con A, Sigma, St. Louis, MO) 0.1 μg/well, or CsA (gift provided by Dr. Borel, Sandoz, Ltd., Basel) added with the final well volume adjusted to 200 μl. For the last 4 hr of culture, the cells were pulsed with 1 μCi/well ^{3}H-thymidine (^{3}H-TdR, New England Nuclear, Boston, MA, 6.7 Ci/mmole). Cells were collected onto glass-fiber filter paper using a multiwell cell harvester. Incorporation of ^{3}H-TdR was determined by standard liquid scintillation techniques.

IL-2 Production

Spleen cells were washed and resuspended at 1×10^7 cells/ml in serum-free Iscove and Melchers–modified DMEM in tissue-culture-quality tubes (Falcon Labware, Oxnard, CA, 3033). Cells were stimulated with Con A (5 μg/ml) with or without CsA. Supernatants were collected by centrifugation 24 hr following lectin stimulation. Supernatants were frozen (−20°C) until assayed for IL-2 activity.

IL-2 Assay

Supernatants were assayed as previously reported.[15] Doubling dilutions of the supernatants were prepared and assayed for IL-2 activity on 6×10^3 cells of the IL-2–dependent continuous cell line, HT-2. A 24-hr culture period was used with a 1-μCi/well ^{3}H-TdR pulse during the last 4 hr of culture. One unit of IL-2 is defined as the dilution that gives 50% maximal proliferation as determined by probit analysis.

RESULTS AND DISCUSSION

Published data concerning IL-2 production in the presence of CsA are conflicting. Larsson demonstrated that CsA did not block IL-2 production,[11] while Wagner has shown that CsA blocked or prevented IL-2 production.[12] The kinetics of IL-2 production from Con A–stimulated rat spleen cells is shown in Fig. 1(A). IL-2 activity progressively accumulated in supernatants over a 24-hr period, with no

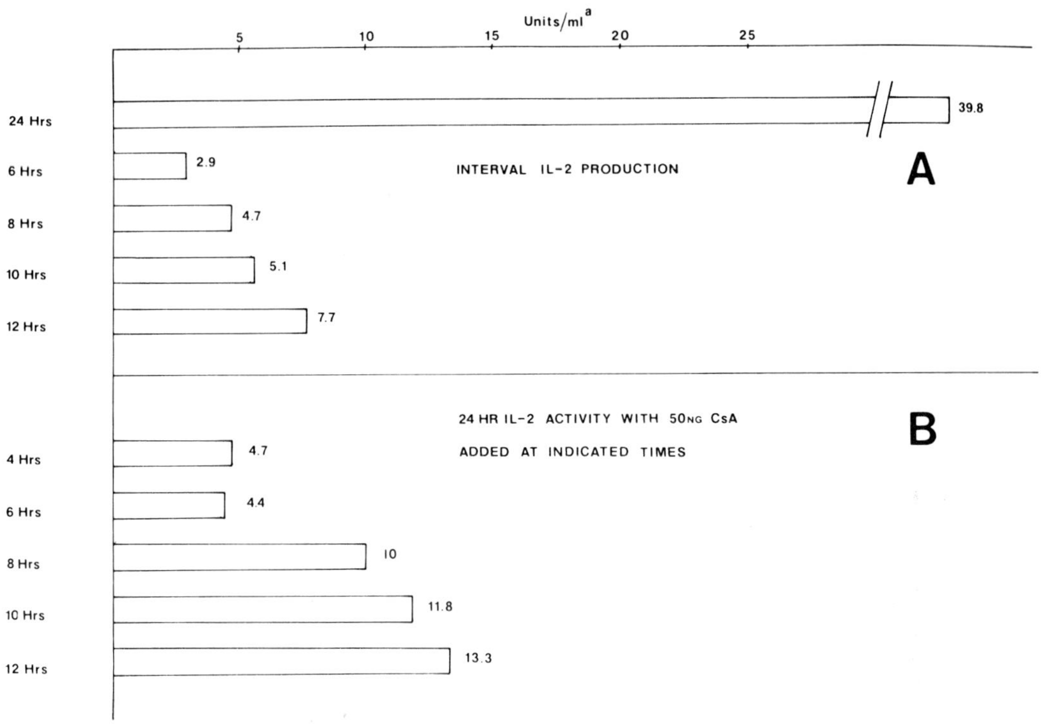

Fig. 1. IL-2 production in the presence of CsA[a]. Supernatants from 1-ml cultures of Con A–stimulated spleen cells were assayed utilizing the IL-2–dependent continuous cell line, HT-2. Doubling dilutions were prepared and assayed as described in Methods. (A) Kinetics of IL-2 production. IL-2 activity found in culture supernatants at the times indicated following lectin stimulation were measured. No IL-2 activity was detected within the first 4 hr following lectin stimulation. (B) IL-2 activity found in a 24-hr lectin-stimulated cell supernatant with 50 ng CsA added at the indicated times. When CsA was added at initiation of culture 2 hr following stimulation, no 24-hr IL-2 activity was detected.

IL-2 activity detectable during the first 4 hr of culture. This increase in IL-2 activity was most likely the result of recruitment of IL-2–producing cells into the activation process rather than increased IL-2 production on a cell-to-cell basis from a select subpopulation of lymphocytes. As shown in Fig. 1(B), IL-2 production from lectin-stimulated cells was altered in the presence of CsA: Production of IL-2 was inhibited, and the effect was time-dependent. Addition of CsA at the time of Con A stimulation resulted in no measurable 24-hr IL-2 activity. However, by delaying the addition of CsA following lectin stimulation, increased levels of 24-hr total IL-2 activity were detected. After the delayed addition of CsA, approximately twice the IL-2 activity was found in the 24-hr supernatant than was present prior to CsA addition. This would imply that cells already committed to IL-2 production prior to CsA addition continued IL-2 production following CsA addition. In the presence of CsA, cells capable of IL-2 production that would normally be recruited into the activation process were not activated to a state of IL-2 production. The role of IL-1 in this process is not clear.

Lymphocyte responsiveness to exogenous IL-2 in the presence of CsA is not clearly defined in the literature.[11,12] It was determined in our study that CsA diminished the responsiveness of lymphocytes to exogenous IL-2 (Fig. 2). This was most evident when CsA was added concurrently with mitogen. IL-2 present in conditioned medium did not reverse CsA-mediated inhibition of proliferation. Proliferation in response to exogenous IL-2 by lymphocytes previously stimulated with lectin

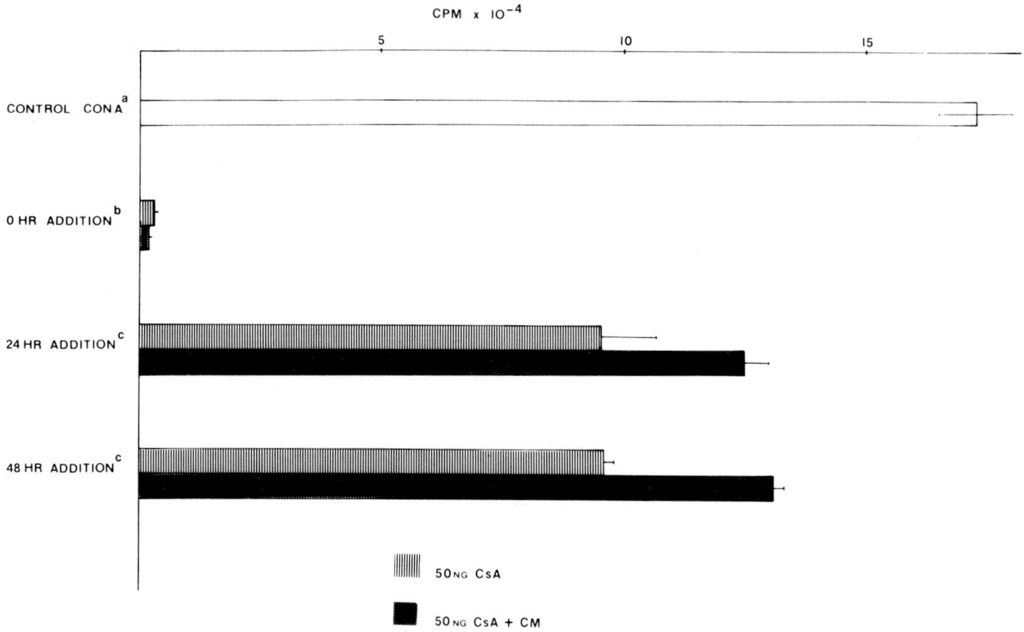

Fig. 2. Responsiveness to exogenous IL-2 in the presence of CsA.[a] Control Con A indicates control proliferation of 72-hr Con A–stimulated spleen cells.[b] At hour 0, 50 ng CsA/well was added with or without conditioned medium at culture initiation. Proliferation was measured at 72 hr.[c] At 24 and 48 hr, Con A–stimulated spleen cells (1 μg/l × 10^6 cells) were washed and resuspended in tissue culture medium. Cells were placed in microtiter wells at 1 × 10^5 viable cells/well in the presence of 50 ng CsA with or without conditioned medium. Total culture period was 72 hr. Cells in tissue culture medium alone or conditioned medium resulted in the same proliferation as the control cultures.

for 24 or 48 hr was still altered by the addition of CsA; however, the effect was less evident than time 0 CsA addition. Perhaps a cell cycle stage does exist (i.e., IL-2 receptors already present) that allows for responsiveness to exogenous IL-2 even in the presence of CsA. This is supported indirectly because the presence of CsA did not alter the proliferation of HT-2 cells in response to exogenous IL-2 (data not shown). A cell not in this cell cycle stage (i.e., pre–IL-2 receptor display) may be sensitive to CsA treatment. In the presence of CsA, Il-2 receptors are not displayed, and the lymphocyte is not capable of a proliferative response in the presence of exogenous IL-2.

LPS-induced proliferation has previously been shown to be resistant to CsA treatment.[10,13,16] Our study did not correlate with these findings. When LPS was used to stimulate spleen cells obtained from an athymic (rnu/rnu) rat, CsA (50 ng/1 × 10^5 cells) inhibited the proliferative response [Fig. 3(A)]. As the addition of CsA was delayed after culture initiation, the CsA-mediated suppression of LPS-induced proliferation was less evident. This would suggest that inhibition of proliferation was not due to CsA-mediated lymphocyte toxicity. CsA-mediated suppression was not due to altered T-lymphocyte function because athymic rat spleen cells lack T-cell function. CsA-mediated inhibition of the LPS-induced response was not restricted to athymic rat spleen cells or to the type of LPS used for stimulation. Similar results were obtained for CsA suppression when LPS derived from *E. coli* was used to stimulate normal Lewis rat spleen cells [Fig. 3(B)].

If LPS functions as an accessory cell-independent polyclonal B-cell activator, the CsA inhibition results are difficult to explain. However, Mosier and Sabbarao have sug-

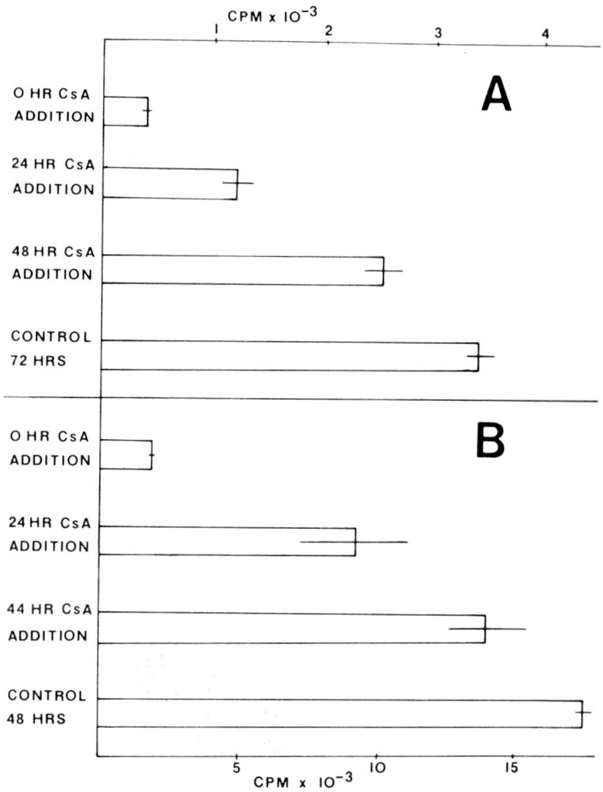

Fig. 3. Time-dependent inhibition of LPS-induced proliferation by CsA. (A) Response of athymic (rnu/rnu) rat spleen cells to stimulation with 2.5 μg *S. typhimurium* LPS per 1 × 10^5 cells. At the indicated times, 50 ng CsA was added to the stimulated cells and 72-hr proliferation measured. (B) Response of normal Lewis rat spleen cells to stimulation with 2.5 μg *E. coli* LPS per 1 × 10^5 cells. At the indicated times, 50 ng CsA was added and 48-hr proliferation measured.

gested a role of macrophage-derived factors for all B-cell activation.[17] The signal may be IL-1, as well as other factors. It was then of interest to investigate the influence of macrophage factors in LPS-induced proliferation.

Glucose polymers have previously been reported to increase macrophage activity.[18] Dextran sulfate (DxS), a glucose polymer, was shown to augment a proliferative response in concert with LPS (Table 1). Increased macrophage activity was measured indirectly by determining the IL-1 levels found in the culture supernatants. The increased IL-1 activity found in LPS+DxS culture supernatants correlated with the increased proliferation from LPS+DxS–stimulated spleen cells. However, it must also be considered that other macrophage-derived factors may play a role in the augmentation of the proliferative response.

It is possible, then, that the CsA inhibition of an early activation event in LPS-induced proliferation is mediated via an alteration in the macrophage derived cell communication signal. This mechanism may be altered macrophage factor production (IL-1?) or diminished factor responsiveness (IL-1 recep-

Table 1. Costimulator Properties of Dextran Sulfate (DxS)

Mitogen*	SI†	IL-1 Activity‡ (U/ml)
—	1	not detected
LPS	6.9	1.3
LPS + DxS	16.6	3.1
DxS	not mitogenic	not determined

*LPS added at 2.5 μg/well with or without DxS at 2.5 μg/well, or 2.5 μg/well DxS alone.

†Stimulation index determined as cpm stimulated cultures ÷ cpm nonstimulated cultures.

‡IL-1 activity determined by a previously reported thymocyte proliferation assay.[19] 5 × 10^5 Lewis thymocytes/well were activated with 0.5-μg/well PHA and doubling dilutions of IL-1–containing supernatant with a 4-hr 1-μCi/well ^{3}H-TdR pulse before cell harvesting at 72 hr.

tor?] by the LPS-responding population of B cells.

In conclusion, these studies have shown that CsA (1) alters the production of Il-2 from lectin-stimulated spleen cells, (2) diminishes the responsiveness of activated lymphocytes to exogenous IL-2, (3) inhibits LPS-induced B-cell activation, and (4) has its greatest effect on early lectin-induced lymphocyte-activation events.

REFERENCES

1. Solbach W, Barth S, Röllinghoff M, et al: Clin Exp Immunol 49:167, 1982
2. Palacios R: Immunol Rev 63:41, 1982
3. Mizel MB: Immunol Rev 63:51, 1982
4. Watson J, Gillis S, Marbrook J, et al: J Exp Med 150:849, 1979
5. Muraguchi A, Kasahara T, Oppenheim JJ, et al: J Immunol 129:2486, 1982
6. Howard M, Farrar J, Hilfiker M, et al: J Exp Med 155:914, 1982
7. Borel JF, Feurer C, Gubler HU, et al: Agents and Actions 6:468, 1976
8. Andrus L, Lafferty KJ: Scand J Immunol 15:449, 1982
9. Britton S, Palacios R: Immunol Rev 65:5, 1982
10. Dongworth DW, Klaus GGB: Eur J Immunol 12:1018, 1982
11. Larsson EL: J Immunol 124:2828, 1980
12. Bunjes D, Hardt C, Röllinghoff M, et al: Eur J Immunol 11:657, 1981
13. Fernandez C, Palacios R, Möller G: Scand J Immunol 16:33, 1982
14. Iscove NN, Melchers F: J Exp Med 147:923, 1978
15. Gillis S, Ferm MM, Ou W, et al: J Immunol 120:2027, 1978
16. Borel JF, Feurer C, Magnee C, et al: Agents and Actions 6:1017, 1976
17. Mosier DE, Sabbarao B: Immunol Today 3:217, 1982
18. McNamee R, Jones E, Cook JA, et al: In Fink MA (ed): The Macrophage in Neoplasia. New York, Academic Press, 1976, p 181
19. Gillis S, Mizel SB: Proc Natl Acad Sci 78:1133, 1981

Cyclosporine Selectively Inhibits Certain Mitotic Responses of Thymocytes

I. Gery, W. R. Benjamin, S. Jones, and R. B. Nussenblatt

THE INHIBITORY EFFECT of cyclosporine (CsA) on the T-lymphocyte population has been shown to be largely related to the effect of this drug on the interleukin (IL) system. In particular, CsA was found to inhibit two processes that are essential for the T-lymphocyte response: (1) the release of IL-2[1,2] and (2) the formation of receptors for IL-2 on "resting" T lymphocytes.[2,3] Many studies concerning the biologic activities of both IL-1 and IL-2 have been carried out in cultures of murine thymocytes.[4–7] Both ILs stimulate these thymocytes in two ways: (1) direct mitogenicity and (2) potentiation of the response to other stimuli such as lectins.[4–7] It is generally accepted that IL-2 acts directly on the "activated" population of thymocytes.[5,8] On the other hand, the "direct" mitogenic activity of IL-1 was reported to be mediated by newly formed IL-2, similar to the potentiating activity of the ILs.[5–8] The present study was aimed at analyzing the effects of CsA on the various responses of thymocytes to IL-1 and IL-2.

MATERIALS AND METHODS

Lymphocyte Stimulants

Phytohemagglutinin P (PHA) and lipopolysaccharide W from *S. typhimurium* (LPS) were purchased from DIFCO, Detroit, MI, while concanavalin A (Con A, 3× crystallized) was supplied by Miles-Yeda, Rehovot, Israel. Two preparations of human IL-1 were used in experiments reported here: (1) a supernatant of a human monocyte monolayer,[9] which was incubated for 5 hr with LPS at 20 μg/ml, and (2) a partially purified preparation obtained by Sephadex chromatography;[9] the fraction making the 15,000 dalton peak was used. The preparations of IL-2 used here included (1) crude murine IL-2, prepared from spleen cultures, as described by Larsson,[3] and (2) a partially purified human IL-2, kindly provided by B. Sredni (NIAID, NIH), which was prepared by gel chromatography followed by isoelectrofocusing.

Drugs

CsA (kindly provided by J. R. Borel, Sandoz, Ltd., Basel, Switzerland) and dexamethasone (DEX, Sigma, St. Louis, MO) were dissolved in ethanol to 10 mg/ml and 4 mM, respectively, and further diluted in the culture medium. Ethanol, diluted similarly to CsA, was used for control cultures.

Lymphocyte Cultures

Thymocytes were obtained from CBA/N (the breeding facilities, NIH) or CBA/J mice (Jackson Laboratories, Bar Harbor, ME), 6–9 weeks of age. After gentle teasing, the thymocytes were washed once and used without further treatment or after fractionation with peanut agglutinin (PNA), as described by Reisner et al.[10] Only PNA$^-$ thymocytes were used in the present study.

CT6, an IL-2–dependent cell line, was originally obtained from J. Watson (University of California, Irvine). Cells used for test cultures were collected after 3–4 days of logarithmic growth.

Cultures were set up in triplicate in flat-bottomed Micro Test II plates (Falcon, Oxnard, CA) and consisted of 1.5×10^6 unfractionated thymocytes, 3×10^5 PNA$^-$ thymocytes, or 2×10^4 CT6 cells in 0.2 ml of RPMI-1640 medium with HEPES (GIBCO, Grand Island, NY), with 100 U/ml penicillin and 100 μg/ml streptomycin and 5% fetal calf serum (GIBCO).

The stimulants and drugs were added at time 0, and the cultures were incubated at 37°C with 5% CO_2 in air for a total period of 48 hr. The cultures were pulsed with ^{3}H-thymidine (Amersham, Arlington Heights, IL, 2 Ci/mM, 0.5 μCi/10 μl/well) during the last 6 hr of incubation. The cultures were harvested by MASH II (Whittaker M.A. Bioproducts, Walkersville, MD), and the results are presented as mean cpm values; SEM values were usually <10% of the means.

RESULTS

Selective Effects of CsA on Thymocyte Cultures

Table 1 summarizes two typical experiments in which the effects of CsA or DEX

From the Laboratory of Vision Research (I. G., S. J.), the Clinical Branch, National Eye Institute (R. B. N.), and the Laboratory of Microbiology and Immunology, National Institute for Dental Research (W. R. B.), National Institutes of Health, Bethesda, MD.

Reprint requests should be addressed to Igal Gery, Laboratory of Vision Research, National Eye Institute, Bldg 6, Rm 232, National Institutes of Health, Bethesda, MD 20205.

0041-1345/83/1505-0016$01.00/0

were examined on thymocyte cultures stimulated with Con A, PHA, IL-1, IL-2, and the combination of PHA and the ILs. The tested ILs included both crude and partially purified preparations. CsA inhibited markedly the response to Con A; more than 80% inhibition was evoked by CsA at 40 ng/ml. On the other hand, the direct mitogenic responses to both IL-1 and IL-2 were found to be essentially resistant to CsA at doses of ≤200 ng/ml; slight to moderate inhibitory effects were induced by CsA at 1000 ng/ml (data not shown). In contrast to the direct mitogenic activity of the ILs, their potentiating activities on the PHA response were found to be highly susceptible to CsA. The potentiating activities are best demonstrated when the ILs are added at low concentrations that give clear synergy with PHA. Thus, the synergistic responses were considerably inhibited by CsA at 40 ng/ml, whereas at higher CsA doses the responses to the ILs plus PHA were reduced to the levels obtained by the ILs alone.

The selectivity of the CsA effect on the thymocyte responses was further underscored by the comparison with the pattern of effects of DEX (Table 1). Conversely to CsA, DEX was found to inhibit the direct mitogenic responses to the ILs more than the responses to the combinations of ILs and PHA or to Con A.

Effects of CsA on Cocultures of Thymocytes and CT6 Cells

The direct mitogenic activity of IL-1 on thymocytes is assumed to be mediated by newly formed IL-2.[5–8] Thus, the data of Table 1 could be interpreted to show that IL-2 release in this system is resistant to CsA. This hypothesis was examined by testing the CsA effect on the release of IL-2 by thymocytes stimulated with IL-1. Since the levels of IL-2 released by these thymocyte cultures were found to be low and variable (data not shown), we chose to assess the IL-2 release by coculturing the thymocytes with cells of the IL-2–dependent cell line, CT6. Thus, any increase in thymidine uptake in excess of the additive values of the two cell types was interpreted to be the result of IL-2 being produced and released by the thymocytes and stimulating the CT6 cells.

A typical experiment is shown in Table 2. The thymocytes used here were of the PNA^- population, which are known to produce high levels of IL-2.[8] The PNA^- cells resembled the unfractionated thymocytes in their pattern of susceptibility to CsA (compare Tables 1 and 2).

Cocultures without added stimulants incorporated thymidine in excess of the additive values found in the individual cultures of thymocytes or CT6 cells alone, thus suggesting that the PNA^- thymocytes released spontaneously moderate levels of IL-2, which stimulated the CT6 cells. Cocultures stimulated with Con A, PHA, or IL-1 also incorporated more thymidine than the additive values of the two corresponding individual cells, or more than the levels incorporated by the unstimulated cocultures, thus suggesting that IL-2 release by the thymocytes was enhanced by these stimuli. CsA inhibited moderately the thymidine uptake by unstimulated cocultures but markedly suppressed the cocultures stimulated with Con A or PHA, reducing their responses to levels similar to those of the unstimulated cocultures. On the other hand, CsA had a small effect on cocultures stimulated with IL-1, reducing their response by the same extent as that found in the corresponding cultures of thymocytes alone.

DISCUSSION

The results recorded here demonstrate that CsA at ≤200 ng/ml inhibits selectively the potentiating effect of both IL-1 and IL-2 but has no effect on the direct mitogenic activity of these ILs on murine thymocyte cultures. The selectivity of the CsA effect is further underscored by the findings with DEX, which, contrary to CsA, inhibited more the direct mitotic response to the ILs than the potentiated responses to the combination of ILs and PHA.

Most of the data recorded here are in line

Table 1. Effects of CsA and DEX on Mitotic Responses of Murine Thymus Cells

Exp. No.	Stimulant*	Drug added: None	CsA (ng/ml) 40	CsA (ng/ml) 200	DEX (4nM)
I	None	110†	169	227	179
	Con A	152,018	17,513	3,563	118,755
	PHA	350	122	73	111
	IL-1 (1:40)	50,918	50,096	47,631	1,446
	+PHA	43,247	36,390	24,334	11,952
	IL-1 (1:2000)	3,985	3,594	3,167	162
	+PHA	29,962	7,327	4,743	2,118
	IL-2 (1:15)	16,874	13,783	14,507	2,865
	+PHA	34,077	15,913	9,631	9,591
II	None	132	183	160	112
	Con A	173,902	7,217	1,223	58,647
	PHA	859	82	264	193
	IL-1 (1:15)	8,774	7,916	7,213	658
	+PHA	31,093	6,817	5,812	4,856
	IL-2 (1:15)	14,998	16,972	14,321	2,798
	+PHA	148,451	73,885	26,377	43,450
	IL-2 (1:150)	3,818	4,174	3,519	503
	+PHA	18,843	5,508	4,309	2,117

*Con A was added to a final concentration of 2 μg/ml and PHA to 0.1%. The interleukin preparations are described in detail in Materials and Methods; the crude preparations were used in experiment I and the partially purified ones in experiment II.

†Mean cpm values of ^{3}H-thymidine incorporation. The standard error of the mean values was usually lower than 10% of the mean value.

with the generally accepted assumptions concerning the mode of action of CsA. Thus, the potentiated response to ILs and PHA was expected to be highly susceptible to CsA, because mainly "resting" lymphocytes react to this stimulus, and the reaction is mediated by newly formed IL-2.[2,5] Also expected was the resistance to CsA of the direct mitotic response of thymocytes to IL-2, since only "activated" lymphocytes react to this mediator, and this response has been shown to be CsA-resistant.[2,3] On the other hand, the resistance to CsA of the direct mitotic response to IL-1 was unexpected; this response was reported to be mediated by newly formed IL-2,[5–8] and, therefore, one could expect it to be inhibited by CsA. The CsA resistance of the response to IL-1 was further analyzed by using cocultures of thymocytes and the IL-2–dependent (CT6 cells (Table 2). The results with this system (1) support the notion that IL-1 stimulation increases the release of IL-2 by cultured thymocytes and (2) indicate that this increased IL-2 release is resistant to CsA.

Table 2. Selective Effects of CsA on Cocultures of Thymocytes (PNA$^-$) and CT6 Cells

Cells	CsA (100 ng/ml)	Stimulant: None	Con A (8 μg/ml)	PHA (0.1%)	IL-1* (1:100)
Thymocytes	No	502†	27,895	39,078	32,138
	Yes	274	805	3,421	23,713
CT6	No	6,238	4,716	5,852	9,239
	Yes	6,068	5,155	5,978	8,575
Thymocytes + CT6	No	17,001	63,315	64,664	62,572
	Yes	12,841	14,765	14,605	48,310

*The "crude" preparation, as described in Materials and Methods.

†Incorporation of ^{3}H-thymidine, as mean cpm.

The notion that IL-2 release may be resistant to CsA in certain systems is consistent with findings from another system, that is, the resistance to CsA of the mitotic response[2,11] and the IL-2 release by human lymphocytes stimulated with phorbol myristate acetate (PMA).[2]

The mechanism underlying the resistance to CsA of the thymocyte response to IL-1 is not known. It is suggested, however, that the biochemical processes that bring about this response, including the production and release of IL-2, are different from those bringing about the responses to the combinations of ILs and lectins. This notion is in accord with the assumption that different subpopulations of thymocytes participate in the different responses; namely, "preactivated" thymocytes react to IL-1 alone, while "resting" ones respond to the combination of IL-1 and lectins.[12]

REFERENCES

1. Bunjes JD, Hardt C, Röllinghoff M, et al: Eur J Immunol 11:657, 1981
2. Britton S, Palacios R: Immunol Rev 65:5, 1982
3. Larsson EL: J Immunol 124:2828, 1980
4. Gery I, Gershon RK, Waksman BH: J Exp Med 136:128, 1972
5. Smith KA, Ruscetti FW: Adv Immunol 31:137, 1981
6. Oppenheim JJ, Stadler BM, Siraganian RP, et al: Fed Proc 41:257, 1982
7. Oppenheim JJ, Gery I: Immunol Today 3:113, 1982
8. Conlon PJ, Henney CS, Gillis S: J Immunol 128:797, 1982
9. Gery I, Zigler JS, Brady RO, et al: J Clin Invest 68:1182, 1981
10. Reisner Y, Linker-Israeli M, Sharon N: Cell Immunol 25:129, 1976
11. Gordon D, Nouri AME: Clin Exp Immunol 44:287, 1981
12. Beller DI, Unanue ER: J Immunol 123:2890, 1979

Cyclosporine Modulates the Human In Vitro T-Dependent Antigen-Induced Synthesis of Specific Antibody

J. B. Harley and A. S. Fauci

CYCLOSPORINE A (CsA) is a cyclic undecapeptide extracted from the fungi *Tricoderma polysporum* and *Cylindrocarpon lucidium booth.*[1] The discovery during routine screening that humoral and cell-mediated immune responses (including graft vs. host disease) were prevented by CsA[2,3] focused subsequent studies upon the interaction of CsA with the immune system, in general, and its potential usefulness in transplantation, in particular.[4] Using CsA, Kostakis et al.[5,6] were able to achieve allogeneic cardiac engraftment in mice, and Green and Allison reported spectacular results with renal transplantation across major histocompatibility barriers in dogs.[7] CsA is a promising immunosuppressive for use in human tranplantation and is being evaluated for use in transplants of kidney, bone marrow, liver, and, more recently, lung and heart.[8]

Many cellular and molecular details of the mechanism of CsA action are known. The earliest studies demonstrated that CsA inhibited blastogenesis in response to mitogens.[2] Subsequent workers have shown that the mixed lymphocyte response, antigen-induced proliferation, and the primary generation of allogeneic cytotoxic cells are all inhibited by CsA.[4] T cells previously established in culture, however, are resistant to the action of CsA, especially in the presence of exogenous IL-2. It appears that CsA prevents the expression of the IL-2 receptor in the unstimulated T cell and that exogenous IL-2 bypasses the inhibited step in previously established cultures,[9–11] though suppressor cells may not be as sensitive to CsA as are some other T-cell types.[12] Ryffel et al. described a receptor for CsA analogs in both mouse and man that is present in greater quantities on T cells than on B cells with first-order binding kinetics and an apparent equilibrium dissociation constant of $\sim 10^{-7} M$.[13,14]

CsA prevents primary immunization with T cell–dependent antigens. On the other hand, secondary responses to these antigens have also been inhibited in some experiments, but in others the secondary response proceeds without an apparent effect.[3,15] Data have been collected showing enhancement, no effect, and even suppression of T cell–independent responses in the presence of CsA.[3,15] Finally, recent in vitro studies with CsA have shown the inhibition of antibody synthesis after stimulation with PWM.[16]

The development of an in vitro model of antigen-induced production of specific antibody production in man[17,18] has made possible the study of B-cell–terminal differentiation and of specific antibody synthesis in PBMNC from normal human donors. We have used this model system to study the influence of CsA upon the T cell–dependent induction of specific antibody.

MATERIALS AND METHODS

Immunizations

Normal volunteers were immunized with 5 mg KLH (Calbiochem-Behring, La Jolla, CA) and boosted with the same dose 2 weeks later, as has been described.[17,18] Other normal donors were boosted with 5 mg of tetanus toxoid (TT; Wyeth Laboratories, Marietta, PA). Blood was collected 2–3 weeks after either immunization.

Cell Separations

PBMNC were obtained from heparinized venous blood by Hypaque-Ficoll (Winthrop Laboratories, New York,

From the Laboratory of Immunoregulation, National Institute of Allergy and Infectious Diseases, National Institutes of Health, Bethesda, MD, and the Department of Medicine, University of Oklahoma, and the Oklahoma Medical Research Foundation, Oklahoma City, OK

Reprint requests should be addressed to John B. Harley, National Institute of Allergy and Infectious Diseases, National Institutes of Health, Bethesda, MD 20205.

0041-1345/83/1505-0017$01.00/0

NY) density gradient centrifugation. Purified T cells were prepared from PBMNC by sheep red blood cell rosette formation followed by Hypaque-Ficoll density centrifugation. The rosette positive cells were then passed through a nylon wool column.[19] Populations of B lymphocytes and monocytes (hereafter referred to as B cells) were prepared by treating the unfractionated PBMNC with the mouse monoclonal antihuman T-cell hybridoma antibody Leu-1 (Becton-Dickinson, Sunnyvale, CA) and rabbit complement (Dutchland, Denver, PA), as described.[20,21] T-cell kill was considered adequate when <3% of the cells either formed sheep red blood cell rosettes or were leu-1 or OKT3 (Ortho Pharmaceuticals, Raritan, NJ) positive. The functional purity of T cells and B cells was assessed relative to unfractionated PBMNC and appropriately reconstituted populations. Neither purified T cells nor purified B cells synthesized specific antibody above background levels when stimulated with antigen. Also, PWM-induced total immunoglobulin (Ig) secretion from the purified populations was decreased by more than 90% in the experiments presented below.

Cell Cultures

Cultures were established in 10% FCS and RPMI 1640 with 2 m*M* glutamine and 10 μg/ml gentamycin in 1 ml. Twenty-four-well Costar dishes (Costar, Cambridge, MA) were used at an optimal cell density of 1.5×10^6 cells/well for antigen-stimulated cultures and at 0.75×10^6 cells/well for PWM-stimulated cultures. Certain individual experiments were also performed using 12 × 75 mm tubes (2058, Falcon, Oxnard, CA) at 0.5×10^6 cells/tube or flat-bottomed microtiter dishes (3596, Costar, Oxnard, CA) at 0.2×10^6 cells/well. No consistent difference in the results reported here was appreciated by using these alternative culture methods. Various concentrations of CsA, KLH, TT (dialyzed against PBS), or PWM (1:200 of stock solution; Grand Island Biological Company, Grand Island, NY) were added to cultures. CsA (gift of J. F. Borel, Sandoz, Basel, Switzerland), diluted 1:1000 from a 50-mg/ml CsA suspension in ethanol:PBS (1:1) into medium. Ethanol (1:10,000) was added as a control to all other cultures. Ethanol (1:10,000) had no effect on specific antibody or polyclonal Ig production in control experiments.

Assays for Antibody or Ig Production

Culture supernatants were harvested between days 10 and 12 and assayed for antigen-specific and total Ig production (IgM or IgG) by an enzyme-linked immunoabsorbent assay (ELISA) technique, as previously described.[17,18] Briefly, supernatants or dilutions of supernatants were incubated in plates that had been coated with either KLH, TT, the IgG fraction of goat antihuman $F(ab')_2$, or the IgG fraction of goat antihuman IgM. After washing, alkaline phosphatase conjugated goat antihuman IgG or IgM was incubated in the wells. Finally, this was replaced by a solution of substrate, *p*-nitrophenylphosphate, and development of the chromophore was monitored at 405 mm. Antibody production was quantified by direct comparison with standard sera for anti-KLH and anti-TT and with known standards of human IgG and IgM.

Pulsing Experiments

Cultures were pulse with CsA for 4 hr at the beginning of the culture period or after 24, 48, 72, or 96 hr. Unfractionated PBMNC were incubated at a constant cell density of 1.5×10^6 cells/ml with 1 or 10 μgm/ml CsA or with an ethanol control. At the end of the pulse period, cells were washed three times in medium, and cultures were initiated or continued.

RESULTS

Effect of CsA on Specific Antibody Production.

CsA inhibited specific anti-KLH antibody production in antigen-stimulated cultures from all KLH-immunized normal volunteers who were shown to be in vitro responders to antigen stimulation (8 experiments). In these responders, the lowest concentration of CsA required to inhibit the response varied over a broad range, from 0.1 to 1000 ng/ml CsA. This range was similar whether specific IgG or IgM was measured. Two typical experiments are presented in Fig. 1. The concentration of CsA needed to inhibit polyclonal Ig production was less variable and varied from 100 to 1000 ng/ml CsA. The concentrations of CsA required to inhibit the antigen-specific response in any single experiment were always less than or equal to, but not greater than, those needed to inhibit the polyclonal response.

Kinetics of CsA-Induced Suppression

In order to determine the CsA-sensitive period of culture, CsA was added to culture at various times after culture initiation (Fig. 2). CsA inhibited specific antibody production when added from time of intiation of culture (0 hr) to 72 hr afterward, whether stimulated with either antigen (KLH) or PWM. Total Ig production stimulated by PWM also showed similar kinetics. Since specific anti-KLH antibody production does not begin until ~96 hr in culture and since CsA addition at this time did

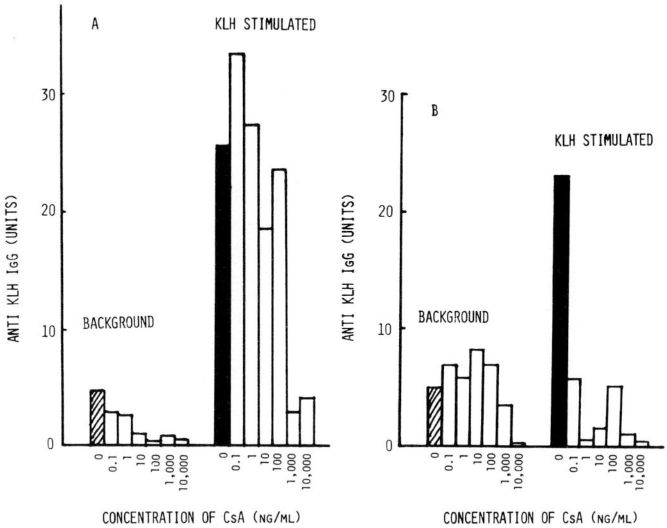

Fig. 1. **CsA inhibits the in vitro antigen-induced production of specific antibody. Examples (A and B) from two different donors are presented, showing the range of variation in the minimal CsA concentration required for inhibition after stimulation with KLH (50 ng/ml). Data are the log mean average of three determinations.**

not prevent specific antibody production, it was concluded that CsA does not directly prevent mature B cells from synthesizing and secreting antibody.

Other experiments had shown that pulsing the cultures with 1 μg/ml CsA for only 4 hr followed by washing of cells was sufficient to inhibit the production of antibody. This result indicated that cultures were sensitive to CsA from their inception to as late as 3 days afterward. When these pulsed cells were mixed with cells that had not been pulsed, an intermediate response was observed [Fig. 3 (A)]. These results led to the conclusion that a pulse of CsA was sufficient to prevent irreversibly antibody production and that the pulsed cells apparently did not affect the unpulsed cells (or at least not to great extent) in the mixed culture.

The foregoing results also suggested that it would be possible to determine which lymphocyte population, B cells or T cells, was pri-

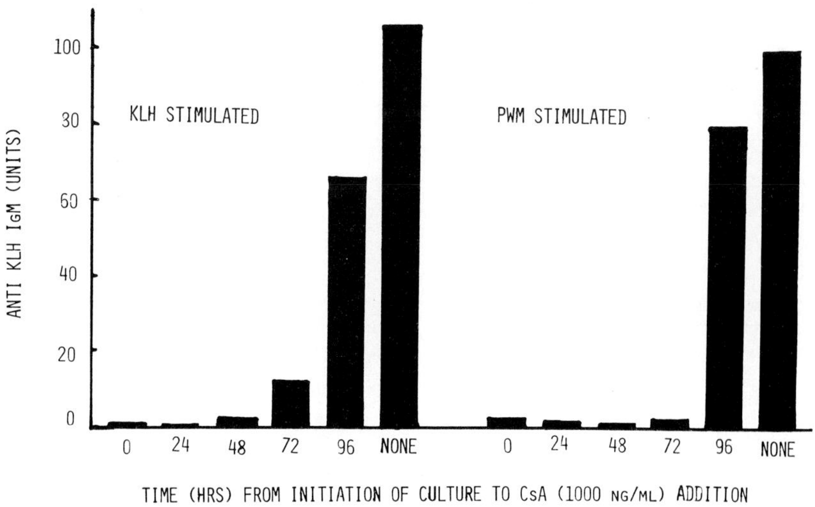

Fig. 2. **CsA inhibits specific antibody production up to 72 hr after initiation of culture whether stimulated by low-dose antigen (50–200 ng/ml KLH) or PWM. Data are the log mean average of two experiments, each done in triplicate).**

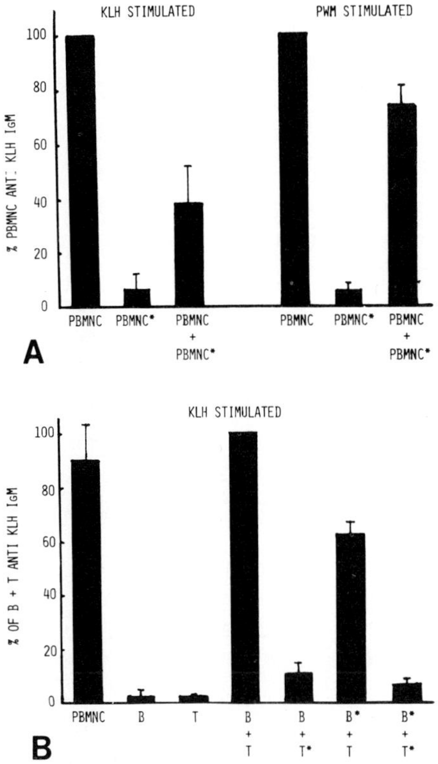

Fig. 3. Specific antibody production is suppressed by a 4-hr pulse of CsA (PBMNC*), while mixed populations (PBMNC + PBMNC*) generate intermediate amounts of specific antibody. Data are averaged from four experiments ± SEM. Average maximal response stimulated by KLH was 62 units anti-KLH-IgM and by PWM was 135 anti-KLH-IgM units. (B) T cells (T) are more sensitive than B cells (B) to a pulse (*) of CsA. Data represent the log mean average of two experiments (± SEM), each done in triplicate.

marily affected by CsA in this in vitro model system. Accordingly, T-cell and B-cell/monocyte populations were prepared and pulsed with 1 or 10 μg/ml CsA for 4 hr (see Materials and Methods). Reconstituted cultures were established and antibody production assayed. These data [Fig. 3(B)] demonstrated that the pulsed T-cell population was more profoundly affected by treatment with CsA and was unable to reconstitute the B-cell response. Pulsed B cells, on the other hand, were relatively less affected by CsA, since they were able to reconstitute the antigen-induced synthesis of specific antibody when mixed with unpulsed autologous T cells.

A small percentage of the KLH-immunized and a slightly larger proportion of the TT-boosted volunteers did not respond to in vitro antigen stimulation. PBMNC of most of these nonresponders, however, made specific antibody after stimulation with PWM. During the course of these studies, five individuals were found who did not initially synthesize specific antibody after antigen stimulation but who did synthesize specific antibody after the addition of CsA to their antigen-stimulated cultures. In these individuals, the optimal response was found over a broad range of CsA concentrations, from 1 to 1000 ng/ml. Examples are presented in Fig. 4. The reversal of the nonresponder state was observed only for the antigen-induced synthesis of antigen-specific IgG. It was not seen in the antigen-specific

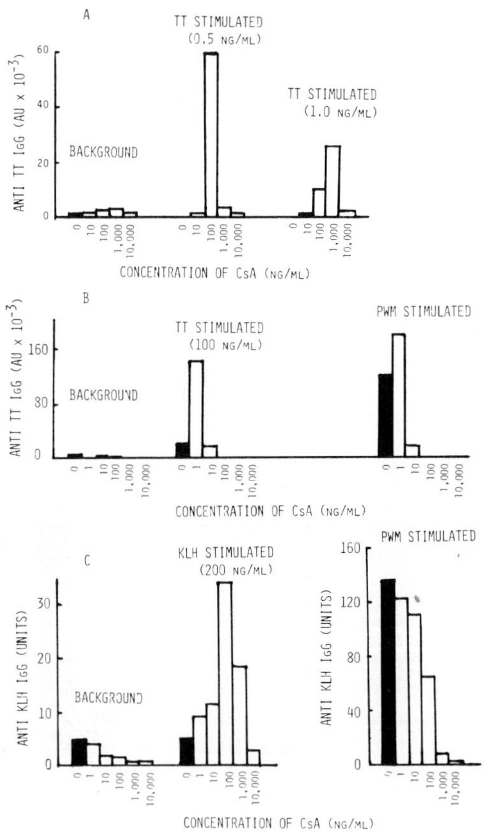

Fig. 4. Low doses of CsA can reverse the in vitro state of nonresponsiveness to low-dose antigen. Three examples (A, B, C) are presented.

IgM response. In all instances but one, there was no increase in the background total IgG or total IgM production after antigen stimulation, leading to the conclusion that this reversal of the nonresponder state was antigen-specific and not due to a polyclonal triggering of Ig production by CsA.

DISCUSSION

In the present study it has been demonstrated that CsA inhibits the secondary in vitro antibody response in man directed against the T lymphocyte–dependent antigens KLH and TT. In some individuals, specific antibody production is inhibited at extremely low concentrations of CsA (0.1 ng/ml), while in others antibody production is relatively resistant (1000 ng/ml) (Fig. 1). The inhibition of specific antibody production to the T cell–dependent antigen KLH is more dependent on interaction of CsA with T cells, since CsA-pulsed T cells inhibit specific antibody production, while CsA-pulsed B cells are less effective (Fig. 3). These experiments and most of the published data from other workers amply demonstrate the effects of CsA upon T cells. These include the CsA-dependent inhibition of T-cell mitogens,[20–22] the mixed and autologous mixed lymphocyte response,[11,12,23,24] the primary generation of cytotoxic lymphocytes,[10–12,23] and the abrogation of Epstein-Barr virus outgrowth suppression.[16,24,25] This interpretation is further supported by the observations that the proliferation of B cells transformed by Epstein-Barr virus[25] proceeds unimpeded by CsA. However, many issues concerning the effect of CsA on normal B-cell proliferation and differentiations have not been directly addressed by these experiments and definitive studies remained to be performed.

The data presented here support the findings of other investigators that the predominant immunosuppressive effect of CsA is on T cells. Others working in animal models have shown the prevention of the primary in vivo B-cell response to T-dependent responses and enhancement or no change in the T-independent responses.[3,15] In vivo T cell–dependent secondary responses have been reported either to be inhibited or to not be changed by CsA.[3,15] This study suggests that in man, in vivo CsA may be able to influence early secondary responses (KLH as used here predominantly induces an IgM response) as well as late secondary responses (TT induces an IgG response).

Specific antibody production was inhibited with the addition of CsA as late as 72 hr after culture initiation. Previous work has shown that antibody production is first detectable on the fourth day of culture.[18] Taken together, our results suggest that a T-cell function is required between 72 and 96 hr in order for antibody secretion to occur in this system. The finding that PWM and low-dose antigen have very similar kinetics suggests that this T-cell function need not be antigen-specific. In other lymphocyte response assay systems, CsA can also be added after the initiation of the culture without changing the extent of inhibition.[3,10,16,21,23] The prevention of Epstein-Barr virus outgrowth suppression was also found to occur even though CsA was added up to 3 to 4 days after the cultures were initiated.[6] Also, CsA could be added to the autologous mixed lymphocyte cultures after at least 48 hr of culture and still inhibit the proliferative response.[23] When assaying for polyclonal antibody production after stimulation with PWM under somewhat different experimental conditions, it was reported that CSA was required within 36 hr of culture initiation for suppression to occur.[16] Substantial differences in methodology could explain the apparent minor differences from our data. For example, these authors[16] used a 250-fold higher concentration of ethanol in their cultures. Indeed, 10-fold differences in the concentration dependence of CsA inhibition have been shown to be due to differences in the solvent used to deliver CsA to the culture.[10] But our data agree with the fundamental finding that CsA fully inhibits antibody production when added some time after stimulation with PWM.

The complexity of the interaction of CsA with mixed populations of mononuclear cells in unfractionated PBMNC is further demonstrated with the reversal of the nonresponder state (Fig. 4). The reversal of the responder state is usually antigen-specific, since changes in the total Ig production were not detected except in one donor.[26] Also, the induction of Ig production in nonresponders was only detected for specific antibody of the IgG isotope. In no case was an increase of specific IgM antibody detected. Both the enhancement of antigen-specific immunoglobulin production and the restriction of the finding of the IgG isotype in those nonresponders suggest that CsA affects either different subpopulations or that it affects a subpopulation with both an inhibitory (Fig. 1) and an enhancing (Fig. 4) effect on antigen-specific immunoglobulin production. The enhancing effect occurs at lower CsA concentrations than the inhibitory effect (Fig. 4).

Thus, CsA interacts in very complex ways with the immune system. The clinical use of the drug in transplantation may influence specific antibody production in response to T cell–dependent antigens in a variety of ways, and the net effect is difficult to predict.

REFERENCES

1. Dreyfuss M, Harri E, Hoffman H, et al: Eur J Appl Microbiol 2:125, 1976
2. Borel JF, Feuer C, Gubler HU, et al: Agents and Actions 6:468, 1976
3. Borel JF, Feuer C, Magnee C, et al: Immunology 32:1017, 1977
4. Klauss GGB: Immunol Today 5:83, 1981
5. Kostakis AJ, White DJG, Calne RH: J Med Sci 5:243, 1977
6. Kostakis AJ, White DJG, Calne RH: J Med Sci 5:280, 1977
7. Green CJ, Allisoni AC: Lancet 1:1183, 1978
8. Kahan BD: N Engl J Med 305:280, 1981
9. Larsson EL: J Immunol 124:2828, 1980
10. Bunjes D, Hardt C, Röllinghoff M, et al: Eur J Immunol 11:657, 1981
11. Hess AD, Tutschka PJ, Santos GW: J Immunol 128:355, 1982
12. Hess AD, Tutschka PJ, Pu Z, et al: J Immunol 128:360, 1982
13. Ryffel B, Donatsch P, Gotz U, et al: Immunology 41:913, 1980
14. Ryffel B, Gotz U, Heuberger B: J Immunol 129:1978, 1982
15. Kunkl A, Klaus GGB: J Immunol 125:2556, 1980
16. Tosato G, Pike SE, Koski IR, et al: J Immunol 128:1285, 1982
17. Volkman DJ, Lane HC, Fauci AS: Proc Natl Acad Sci USA 78:2558, 1981
18. Lane HC, Volkman DJ, Whalen G, et al: J Exp Med 154:1043, 1981
19. Werner C, Klouda PT, Correa MC, et al: Tissue Antigens 9:227, 1977
20. Burkhardt JJ, Guggenheim B: Immunology 36:753, 1979
21. Leoni P, Garcia RC, Allison AC: J Clin Lab Immunol 1:67, 1978
22. White DJG, Plumb AM, Powalec G, et al: Transplantation 27:55, 1979
23. Hess AD, Tutschka PJ: J Immunol 124:2601, 1980
24. Bird AG, McLachlan SM: Lancet 2:418, 1980
25. Bird AG, McLachlan SM, Britton S: Nature 289:300, 1981
26. Harley JB, Fauci AS: (unpublished observations)

Dissociation of T Helper-Cell Function and Helper-Cell Priming by Cyclosporine

G. G. B. Klaus and A. Kunkl

THERE IS NOW considerable evidence for the hypothesis that T helper (T_h) cells are the primary targets in the immunosuppression induced by cyclosporine A (CsA) in a variety of experimental systems.[1] During a study of the effects of CsA on antibody responses in the mouse, we found that primary T-dependent responses were suppressed by CsA, whereas secondary responses were not.[2] This appeared to be due to the emergence of CsA-resistant T_h cells after priming with antigen. We subsequently extended this study to examine the effects of CsA on the induction of T_h-cell memory; the results of these experiments are summarized here. Full details of the data are presented elsewhere.[3]

MATERIALS AND METHODS

Helper-cell function and priming were studied in a hapten-carrier adoptive transfer system: In brief, T_h cell donor mice were immunized with keyhole limpet hemocyanin (KLH), and groups of these were given CsA (generally 50 mg/kg s.c.) from days −1 to 1 or daily throughout priming. After 7–21 days, spleen cells from these mice were transferred together with spleen cells or B cells from mice given dinitrophenylated ovalbumin (DNP-OVA; 1–3 months previously) to irradiated syngeneic recipients, which were challenged with soluble DNP-KLH. Anti-DNP IgG hemolytic plaque-forming cells in the spleens of these recipients were assayed 7 days later. In certain experiments, some of the recipients also received CsA (50 mg/kg, days −1 to 1 relative to transfer).

RESULTS AND DISCUSSION

In an initial transfer experiment, irradiated mice were given DNP-primed B cells and either normal spleen cells or cells from mice immunized with KLH >1 month previously as sources of virgin or primed T_h cells, respectively: CsA treatment of the recipients suppressed the help given by the unprimed cells but not that provided by the primed cells. This directly confirmed earlier experiments showing that T_h cells become CsA-resistant at some time (in fact, within 7 days) after immunization.

Subsequently, mice were given KLH with or without CsA daily, either from day −1 through 1, or daily until day 6. Cell transfer on day 7 showed that donors treated with CsA throughout had developed a normal level of help, while cells from those receiving a 3-day course of CsA gave significantly enhanced help compared with controls. T_h-cell titration experiments from donors given this short course of CsA showed that this "overshoot' effect is due to the emergence of supranormal numbers of T_h cells.

The results indicate that doses of CsA that abrogate help in situ do not diminish priming of T_h cells as assayed by adoptive transfer. Higher doses of CsA (150–300 mg/kg) do abolish T_h-cell priming. However, in marked contrast, doses as low as 12.5 mg/kg cause 50% suppression of a primary antibody response to DNP-KLH. It is therefore clear that in this system there is a marked discrepancy between the dose of CsA needed to suppress help during a primary response vs. that required to suppress helper-cell priming.

Because help normally becomes CsA-resistant soon after immunization, we next wished to study what effects CsA treatment has on the appearance of drug-resistant T_h memory cells. In a series of experiments, mice were given 50 mg/kg CsA for varying periods of time; spleen cells from these were transferred together with B cells as before but into CsA-treated recipients. The results showed that

From the Division of Immunology, National Institute for Medical Research, London.

Reprints requests should be addressed to G. G. B. Klaus, Division of Immunology, National Institute for Medical Research, Mill Hill, London NW7 1AA, U.K.

0041-1345/83/1505-0018$01.00/0

T_h-cell donor mice treated with CsA throughout the priming period (7–14 days) produced helper cells that were able to help B cells in control but not in CsA-treated recipients. Further, although spleen cells from donors given a short course of CsA again gave supranormal levels of help, this overshoot phenomenon remained CsA-sensitive for some time after the cessation of drug treatment. These data suggest that although normal or even elevated numbers of T_h cells can develop under cover of CsA, these T_h cells are not fully mature memory cells, if we define these as cells providing CsA-resistant help.

Taken together, our findings define certain novel properties of CsA. First, they confirm that secondary T-cell responses are significantly more resistant to suppression than primary responses, a conclusion in line with data from other systems.[4,5] Since CsA is known to be potently antiproliferative for T cells in vitro, this could indicate that T memory cells (especially T_h cells) do not need to proliferate in order to exert their effector functions. However, T-cell priming presumably involves precursor proliferation. If so, the observation that normal (or even supranormal) numbers of T_h cells can emerge under cover of an immunosuppressive regimen of CsA remains an unexplained paradox. A similar effect has been described in monkeys subjected to experimental allergic encephalomyelitis,[6] so it appears that the phenomenon does not represent an idiosyncracy of the drug in the mouse. In addition, the fact that T_h cells that develop in CsA-treated mice are somehow abnormal in that they remain drug-sensitive is a further inexplicable finding. In the present state of knowledge, we cannot offer a satisfactory explanation for our findings in terms of the known actions of CsA on lymphocyte proliferation or lymphokine release in in vitro systems. Nevertheless, regardless of the mechanisms involved, if CsA has similar effects on human T cells in vivo, this could have serious implications for its clinical usefulness.

REFERENCES

1. Morris PJ: Transplantation 32:349, 1981
2. Kunkl A, Klaus GGB: J Immunol 125:2526, 1980
3. Klaus GGB, Kunkl A: Transplantation (in press)
4. Homan WP, Fabre JW, Williams KA, et al: Transplantation 29:361, 1980
5. Horsburgh T, Wood P, Brent L: Nature 286:609, 1980
6. Borel JF: In Touraine JL, Traeger J, Betuel H, et al (eds): Transplantation and Clinical Immunology (vol XIII). Amsterdam, Excerpta-Medica, 1981, p 3

Differential Effect of Cyclosporine on the Generation of Allogeneic Versus Syngeneic Cytotoxic T Lymphocytes

Z. K. Ballas and W. E. Schulte

ALLOGRAFT REJECTION and tumor immunity are generally considered to be manifestations of cell-mediated immune mechanisms. Of the cellular immune phenomena, the cytotoxic T lymphocytes (CTL) are perhaps the best understood. Allogeneic CTL can be easily generated, in vivo and in vitro, against alogeneic stimulator cells that differ from the responding cells across part or all of the major histocompatibility complex (MHC).[1] CTL can also be generated against syngeneic cells that have been virally infected or chemically modified.[2] Such CTL show dual specificity in that they preferentially lyse target cells expressing both syngeneic MHC products and the antigen used for sensitization, for example, virus, hapten, or minor histocompatibility gene products.[2-4] Among the chemical haptens, 2,4,6-trinitrobenzene sulfonic acid (TNBS) has been studied most extensively. MHC-restricted CTL (henceforth referred to as syngeneic CTL) are thought to be of importance in autoimmunity and in surveillance against autologous neoplastic cells and infections. Allogeneic CTL, on the other hand, are thought to be of importance in allograft rejection. The relationship between these two kinds of CTL is far from clear. It appears, however, that the precursors of in vitro–generated allogeneic and syngeneic CTL may reside in different lymphocyte clones[2,5,6] and be distinguishable on the basis of cell surface-marker display.[7] Similarly, the precursors of these two kinds of CTL seem to have a different susceptibility to the in vivo administration of large doses of cyclophosphamide.[8,9]

The fungal metabolite cyclosporine A (CsA) is a potent immunosuppressive agent with relatively little myelotoxicity. CsA has been demonstrated to inhibit the generation of allogeneic CTL, graft-vs.-host reaction, and delayed type hypersensitivity.[10-13] CsA has also been shown to inhibit natural killer (NK)–cell activity.[14-16] The experiments presented in this report were undertaken to examine the effect of CsA on the generation of syngeneic, TNBS-specific CTL and on the NK-like activity, termed anomalous killer (AK)–cell activity, present in allogeneic mixed lymphocyte cultures (MLC).[17] Additionally, we wanted to compare the doses of CsA needed to inhibit the generation of syngeneic CTL to those needed to inhibit the generation of allogeneic CTL. Our data demonstrated that CsA inhibits the generation of TNBS-specific CTL at doses at least an order of magnitude less than those needed to inhibit the generation of allogeneic CTL. Similarly, AK-cell activity was inhibited at doses less than those needed to inhibit allogeneic CTL generation. In contrast, CsA had no effect on the lytic activity of differentiated CTL.

MATERIALS AND METHODS

Mice

Female C57BL/6 (B6), CBA, and BALB/c mice were obtained from the Frederick Cancer Center (Frederick, Md.) through the VA Central Animal facility and were used when 6–8 weeks of age.

Cyclosporine A

CsA was a kind gift of Dr. J. F. Borel (Sandoz Ltd., Basel, Switzerland). A stock solution of CsA was prepared by dissolving 10 mg of the hydrophobic powder in

From the Department of Internal Medicine, the Iowa City VA Medical Center, and the University of Iowa, Iowa City, IA.

Supported by the Veterans Administration and by grant CA 31982 from the National Cancer Institute. Z.K.B. is the recipient of a Research Associate Career Award from the Veterans Administration.

Reprint requests should be addressed to Zuhair K. Ballas, Department of Internal Medicine, University of Iowa, Iowa City, IA 52240.

0041-1345/83/1505-0019$01.00/0

1.0 ml 95% ethanol, 0.2 ml Tween 80, and dropwise addition of culture medium to a final volume of 10 ml. This stock solution was stored at 4°C for a maximum of 3 weeks. Fresh dilutions from the stock solution were made immediately before use. A solvent solution consisting of ethanol and Tween 80 was prepared and stored identically.

Cell Cultures

The generation of allogeneic and syngeneic, TNBS-specific CTL was described in detail previously.[18] Briefly, 7×10^6 responder spleen cells were cultured with 3×10^6 irradiated (2,000 rad) stimulator spleen cells that were unmodified or modified with 10 m*M* TNBS, in RPMI 1640 supplemented with 5% FCS, $5 \times 10^{-5} M$ 2-mercaptoethanol and antibiotics, for 5 days at 37°C in 5% CO_2 humidified-air atmosphere.

Target-Cell Preparation

LPS-induced (2 to 3 days) spleen cell blasts were used as target cells. Modification of the target cells was described in detail previously.[18] Briefly, the target cells were labeled with $Na^{51}CrO_4$, washed, and incubated with 10 m*M* final concentration of TNBS at 37°C for 10 min at a cell density of 10^6/ml.

For assay of AK-cell activity, an NK-susceptible clone of the L5178Y lymphoma, termed C127V, maintained in vitro, was used.[19]

Cell-Mediated Cytolysis

A short-term ^{51}Cr release assay was performed as previously described.[18] Briefly, the effector cells were harvested from 5-day cultures, washed, added to 10^4 ^{51}Cr-labeled target cells in V-bottomed microtiter plates (Cooke Laboratory Products, Alexandria, Va.) in a final volume of 0.2 ml, and incubated in 5% CO_2-humidified atmosphere for 4 hr at 37°C. After 4 hr, the paltes were briefly centrifuged (450 *g*, 2 min), and an aliquot of the supernatant was collected and assessed for radioactivity. Percent specific lysis was calculated as follows:

$$\% \text{ Specific cytolysis} = \frac{E - N}{T - N} \times 100,$$

where E was ^{51}Cr released in the presence of effector cells, N was ^{51}Cr released in the presence of normal spleen cells, and T the total counts obtained after lysis of the labeled target cells with 2% acetic acid.

For calculation of lytic units (LU), a dose-response curve was generated for the effector-cell population in question. Percent specific lysis was plotted vs. the log of the effector-to-target-cell ratio. The linear portion of such a curve was used to calculate the number of effector cells needed to lyse 30% of 10^4 target cells. This number was arbitrarily assigned the value of one lytic unit.

RESULTS

Effect of CsA on the Generation of CTL

We first examined the effect of adding CsA at the onset of culture on the generation of CTL. Thus, spleen cells from C57BL/6 (B6) mice were cultured either with irradiated TNBS-modified syngeneic spleen cells or with irradiated BALB/c spleen cells. CsA, or its solvent, was added at the onset of culture. After 5 days, the cells were harvested and assayed for their ability to lyse their specific target cells. As shown in Table 1, CsA at 10 ng/ml (final concentration) completely abolished the generation of TNBS-specific CTL with little or no effect on the generation of allogeneic CTL. At 100 ng/ml, CSA caused significant inhibition, but not complete ablation, of the generation of allogeneic CTL. Solvent, in equivalent dilutions, had no effect on either kind of CTL. CsA inhibition of both kinds of CTL was dose-dependent, with some inhibition of the TNBS-specific CTL seen at doses as little as 2.5 ng/ml. A typical dose-response experiment is shown in Fig. 1. Again, complete inhibition of TNBS-specific CTL was seen at 10 ng/ml of CsA, whereas some allogeneic CTL activity remained at a dose of 160 ng/ml, at all the effector-to-target-cell ratios tested. Indeed, in at least 20 experiments using different preparations of CsA stock solutions, complete inhibition of TNBS-specific CTL was seen at doses of 10–20 ng/ml, whereas comparable inhibition of allogeneic CTL was seen at doses of 100–200 ng/ml.

Table 1. Effect of CsA on the Generation of Allogeneic vs. TNBS-Specific CTL

		% Specific Lysis*	
Effectors	CsA	TNBS-60	BALB/c
B6 + TNBS-B6	—	55.0	ND†
	10 ng/ml	−0.9	ND
	Solvent	50.8	ND
B6 + BALB/c	—	ND	80.7
	10 ng/ml	ND	73.9
	100 ng/ml	ND	31.9
	Solvent	ND	84.5

*Effector-to-target-cell ratio was 10:1.

†Not determined.

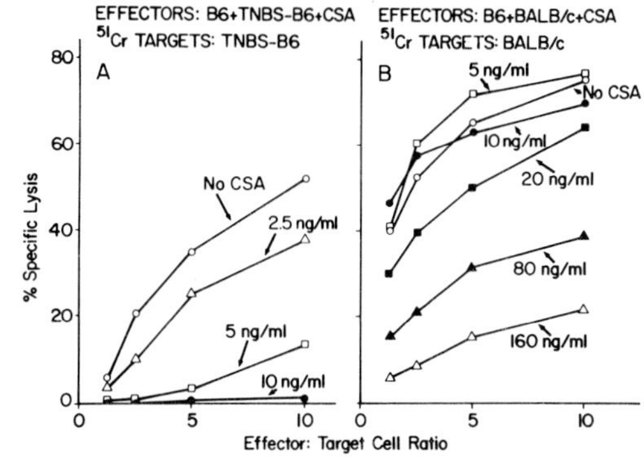

Fig. 1. Differential effect of CsA on TNBS-specific vs. allogeneic CTL. Spleen cells from C57BL/6 mice were cultured with TNBS-B6 (A) or BALB/c (B) spleen cells in the absence or in the presence of the indicated final concentrations of CsA. The effector cells were harvested after 5 days in culture and assayed against their specific targets in a 4-hr ^{51}Cr-release assay.

Effect of Preincubation with CsA

In the above experiments, CsA was present throughout the 5-day culture period. We then examined the effect of pretreating the responder cells with CsA. Thus, B6 spleen cells were incubated with 100 ng/ml, or equivalent solvent dilution, at 37°C for 3 hr, after which they were washed extensively, adjusted as to viable cell concentration, and used as responders. As shown in Table 2, such treatment was sufficient to abolish the ability of these lymphocytes to generate TNBS-specific CTL with little effect on their ability to mount an allogeneic CTL response, again suggesting an exquisite sensitivity of the syngeneic CTL precursors to CsA.

Table 2. Effect of Preincubation with CsA

		% Specific Lysis†	
Responders R_x*	Stimulators	TNBS-B6	BALB/c
Solvent	TNBS-B6	40.4	ND‡
CsA	TNBS-B6	− 1.7	ND
Solvent	BALB/c	ND	52.6
CsA	BALB/c	ND	41.4

*C57BL/6 spleen cells were incubated with 100 ng/ml CsA or equivalent solvent dilution at 37°C. After 3 hr, the cells were washed extensively, adjusted as to viable cell concentration, and used as responders in a 5-day culture.

†Effector-to-target-cell ratio on TNBS-B6 and BALB/c was 40:1 and 20:1, respectively.

‡Not determined.

Effect on Differentiated CTL

A trivial explanation of these findings could be that the observed differential effect of CsA was due to some carry-over of the CsA into the ^{51}Cr-release assay, in which case the effect would be on the CTL themselves rather than on the cells involved in CTL induction. This was tested by generating both kinds of CTL in the classical manner, that is, in the absence of CsA, then adding CsA directly to the ^{51}Cr-release assay. As shown in Fig. 2, CsA in doses as high as 200 ng/ml had no effect on the lytic activity of either kind of CTL.

Effect on AK Cell Generation

It has been previously reported that in allogeneic MLC an NK-like activity termed anomalous killer (AK)–cell activity is observed.[17] Whereas the allogeneic CTL response is maximal on day 5 of culture, AK cell activity is maximal on day 3 or 4. We thought it interesting to examine the CsA dose needed to inhibit AK cell activity as compared to allogeneic CTL. Thus, spleen cells from B6 (H-2^b) mice were cultured with irradiated CBA (H-2^k) spleen cells. The cultures were harvested either on day 3 or day 5 of culture and assayed for their AK-cell activity against an NK-susceptible cell line, C127V (H-2^d),

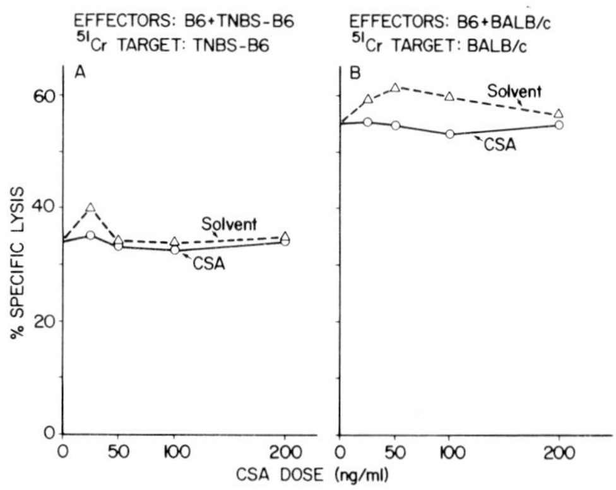

Fig. 2. CsA has no effect on differentiated CTL. CTL vs. TNBS-B6 (A) or BALB/c (B) were generated in the absence of CsA from B6 responder spleen cells. CsA, at the indicated concentrations, was added directly to the individual wells of the ^{51}Cr-release assay. Effector-to-target-cell ratio was 20:1 for TNBS-B6 (A) and 10:1 for BALB/c (B).

Table 3. Effect of CsA on AK vs. Allogeneic CTL

	% Specific Lysis		
	CL27V*		CBA†
CsA (ng/ml)	Day 3	Day 5	Day 5
0	43.4 (5.2)‡	30.0 (5.1)‡	40.1 (120.2)‡
5	29.1 (2.6)	15.4 (1.8)	31.6 (91.8)
10	18.2 (1.3)	ND§	31.9 (84.3)
20	8.9 (0.1)	9.1 (0.9)	20.2 (43.4)

*Effector-to-target-cell ratio was 40:1.

†Effector-to-target-cell ratio was 1.25:1.

‡LU/10^6 effector cells.

§Not determined.

and for their CTL activity against CBA target cells. It appeared that AK-cell activity was more susceptible to inhibition by CSA than CTL activity (Table 3). The differential sensitivity was not as clear-cut nor as dramatic as that between allogeneic and TNBS-specific CTL. Nevertheless, at 5 ng/ml, CsA caused 50% and 64.7% inhibition (inhibition was calculated on basis of lytic units) of AK-cell activity when assayed on day 3 and day 5 of culture, respectively. In contrast, CsA at 5 ng/ml caused 23.6% inhibition of allogeneic CTL activity.

DISCUSSION

It has been previously reported that CsA inhibits the generation of allogeneic CTL.[10–13] The data presented here confirmed those findings and extended them to include MHC-restricted, TNBS-specific CTL. Indeed, our data demonstrated that the generation of TNBS-specific CTL is inhibited far more readily than allogeneic CTL. Complete inhibition of TNBS-specific CTL was obtained at 10 ng/ml of CsA, whereas comparable inhibition of the generation of allogeneic CTL was obtained at doses at least 10–20 times as much (Table 1, Fig. 1). Moreover, preincubation of the responder lymphocytes with CsA for as little as 3 hr resulted in abrogation of their ability to mount a cytotoxic response against TNBS-modified syngeneic stimulator cells, while their ability to mount an allogeneic CTL response remained intact (Table 2). We believe that this differential sensitivity to CsA was not due to the susceptibility of differentiated CTL to CsA carried over from the culture to the ^{51}Cr-release assay, since direct addition of CsA to the ^{51}Cr-release assay had no effect on the lytic ability of preformed CTL (Fig. 2).

We also examined the effect of CsA on the induction of AK cell activity. As shown in Table 3, CsA seemed to inhibit the generation of AK cell activity at doses smaller than those needed to inhibit the generation of allogeneic CTL. The dose differential, however, was not as dramatic as that between syngeneic and allogeneic CTL. AK cells have been shown to be closely related to NK cells,[17] which are thought to be of importance in tumor surveillance in vivo. This finding is in agreement with the findings of Yanaghira and Adler,[15] who showed that CsA inhibited the Con A–induced augmentation of NK-cell activity in vitro. Yanaghira and Adler, however, found that this inhibition could be reversed by the addition of the supernatants of mouse spleen cells cultured with Con A, suggesting that CsA acts by preventing the release of NK-augmenting lymphokines by T cells in response to antigenic or mitogenic signals.

It has also been suggested that CsA inhibits the generation of allogeneic CTL by preventing the release of the lymphokines interleukin 1 and interleukin 2[13] or by preventing the induction of receptors for interleukin 2.[20] In data not shown, we found that CsA impaired the release of interleukin 2 in the supernatants of allogeneic MLC in a dose-dependent fashion that paralleled the inhibition of allogeneic CTL generation. However, the doses of CsA needed to effect a significant inhibition of IL-2 generation were again much more than those needed to inhibit the generation of TNBS-specific CTL. It thus appeared that CsA may act by mechanisms other than its ability to inhibit the elaboration of Interleukin 2.

An interesting finding was that preincubation of responder lymphocytes with CsA for as little as 3 hr was sufficient to inhibit the generation of syngeneic CTL. This finding is surprising in the context that similar treatment had little or no effect on the generation of allogeneic CTL. It has been suggested that CsA prevents the activation of T cells by inhibiting the expression of cell-surface "activation" antigens, namely the receptors for interleukin 2 or Ia antigens.[20-22] The doses needed for such inhibition, however, were much larger than the doses employed in this study. It is conceivable that the lymphocytes involved in the generation of syngeneic CTL reside in a subset distinct from the subsets involved in allogeneic CTL and that these lymphocytes (be they precursor or helper lymphocytes) are exquisitely sensitive to CsA. Alternatively, the soluble mediators involved in the generation of syngeneic CTL, and their receptors, may be different from those involved in the generation of allogeneic CTL. Obviously, more experimentation is needed to clarify these points.

Finally, these data may have significant clinical implications. Thus, the inhibition of syngeneic CTL may be beneficial in the treatment of autoimmune diseases, and small doses of CsA may be sufficient. In transplant recipients, however, the inhibition of allogeneic CTL may prolong graft survival, but the concomitant inhibition of syngeneic CTL and AK-cell activity may lead to an increased incidence of infections and tumors. Indeed, an increased incidence of lymphomas in transplant patients receiving CsA has been reported.[23,24]

REFERENCES

1. Cerottini JC, Brunner KT: Adv Immunol 18:67, 1974
2. Zinkernagel RM, Doherty PC: Adv Immunol 27:52, 1979
3. Zinkernagel RM, Doherty PC: Nature 248:701, 1974
4. Shearer GM: Eur J Immunol 4:527, 1974
5. Janeway CA, Murphy PD, Kemp J, et al: J Exp Med 147:1065, 1978
6. Pang T, McKenzie IFC, Blanden RV: Cell Immunol 26:153, 1976
7. Cantor H, Boyse EA: Cold Spring Harbor Symp Quant Biol 41:23, 1977
8. Hurme M: J Exp Med 149:290, 1979
9. Hurme M, Shivola M, Bang B: J Exp Med 155:327, 1982
10. Borel JF: Immunology 31:631, 1976
11. Borel JF, Feurer C, Magnee C, et al: Immunoloy 32:1017, 1977
12. Nemlander A, Hayry P: Scand J Immunol 12:493, 1980
13. Bunjes D, Hardt C, Röllinghoff M, et al: Eur J Immunol 11:657, 1981
14. Yanagihara RH, Adler WH: Immunology 45:325, 1982
15. Yanagihara RH, Adler WH: Immunopharmacology 4:243, 1982
16. Introna M, Allavena P, Spreafico F, et al: Transplantation 31:113,
17. Karre K, Seeley JK, Eriksson E, et al: J Exp Med 156:385, 1983
18. Ballas ZK: J Immunol 127:1589, 1981
19. Durdik JM, Beck BN, Clark EA, et al: J Immunol 125:683, 1980
20. Larsson EL: J Immunol 124:2828, 1980
21. Palacios R, Möller G: Nature 290:792, 1981
22. Leapman SB, Strong DM, Filo RS, et al: Transplantation 34:94, 1982
23. Calne RY, Rolles K, Thiru S, et al: Lancet ii:1033, 1979
24. Crawford DH, Thomas JA, Janassy G, et al: Lancet 2:1356, 1980

Differential In Vitro Action of Cyclosporine on Non-T-Cell and T-Cell Responses to Non-HLA Alloantigens: Significance for MHC-Independent Graft-Versus-Host Disease

L. Delmonte

THE FUNGAL METABOLITE cyclosporine A (CsA) is a potent immunomodulator that reversibly blocks early events in T-cell responses to alloantigens[1–6] as well as some B-cell[7] and natural-killer (NK)-cell[8] responses, while selectively sparing monocyte functions[5] and myeloproliferative activity.[1] This differential action renders the drug uniquely useful for preventing MHC-dependent alloreactions in transplant patients. In clinical trials, CsA has been reported to reduce the incidence or severity of alloreactions in recipients of MHC-matched and -mismatched solid organ transplants[9–14] and bone marrow transplants (BMT).[15–19] However, CsA is not uniformly effective in abrogating MHC-independent alloreactions.

Non-HLA allodisparities that may contribute to the induction of MHC-independent graft-vs.-host disease (GvHD) in BMT recipients can be detected with a high degree of accuracy in the MO/NK-cell assay, an allosensitizing coculture of radioresistant Ia$^-$ third-population responder cells (MO/NK cells) and third-population sensitizer cells from bone marrow (BM) and peripheral blood (PB) of HLA-matched prospective donor-host pairs.[20–22] MO/NK cells sensitized to non-HLA alloantigens in this assay can, in turn, induce autologous cytotoxic/suppressor T cells.[22] This may be a mechanism whereby engrafted donor-type T cells are induced to initiate MHC-independent GvHD.

In the present studies, we probed the problem of CsA-resistant MHC-independent GvHD, using two approaches: First, we examined the in vitro action of CsA on MO/NK-cell functions, including MO/NK–T cell interactions, in an attempt to shed light on cellular mechanisms involved in GvHD resistant to CsA. Second, we examined the correlation between MO/NK-cell responses before BMT and GvHD development in CsA-treated engrafted BMT recipients.

From the Memorial Sloan-Kettering Cancer Center, New York.

Reprint requests should be addressed to Dr. Lilian Delmonte, 440 East 62 St., New York, NY 10021.

0041–1345/83/1505–0020$01.00/0

MATERIALS AND METHODS

We evaluated 43 BMT recipients with acute leukemia, their HLA-matched sibling donors, and 57 unrelated third-party controls for non-HLA allodisparities. Two anti-GvHD regimens were compared: 33 recipients received methotrexate (MTX) as per the Seattle protocol;[23] 10 received CsA (8–16 mg/kg, p.o.) in two divided doses beginning on the day of BMT. Prior to BMT, all prospective donor-recipient pairs and all donor–third-party control combinations were evaluated for non-HLA allodisparities, using the two-step MO/NK-cell assay.[20,22] Twenty-one of the prospective donor-host pairs and 14 of the MO/NK(+) donor–third-party control combinations were also evaluated for T cell–inducing activity of MO/NK cells allosensitized in vitro in the presence or absence of CsA. After engraftment, recipients were evaluated for GvHD by the clinical criteria of Glucksberg et al[24] and the histopathologic criteria of Woodruff et al.[25]

Cell Purification

Mononuclear cells (MNC), separated from BM or PB on a 1.071-g/mm^2 Percoll gradient, were rosetted with neuraminidase-treated sheep erythrocytes (E rosetting).[26] E-positive (E^+) T cells were recovered from E rosettes by hypotonic lysis with NH_4Cl-Tris, pH 7.65, 2 min, 37°C. MNC were further purified by reaction with monoclonal antibodies for ½ hr at 4°C and lysing with rabbit complement (C) (Gibco) for 1 hr at 37°C. The antibodies used were (1) anti-HuLyt-3 (New England Nuclear), a pan-T antibody that reacts with E^+ T cells and with E^+ NK cells cytotoxic for K562 erythroleukemia cells, (2) anti-Ia (New England Nuclear), which reacts with B cells, the majority of monocytes, activated T cells, and NK cells cytotoxic for HSV-1-infected human fibroblasts, and (3) OKM2 (donated by Ortho), which reacts with mature monocytes and a minor subset of NK cells. Radioresistant Ia^- $OKM2^+$ non-T cells (MO/NK cells: HuLyt-$3^-Ia^-OKM2^+$) served as responders/inducers; radioresistant Ia^+ $OKM2^-$ non-T cells (HuLyt-$3^-Ia^+OKM2^-$), as sensitizers. Purity of cell preparations was controlled by indirect immunofluorescence of antibody-reacted cells developed with FITC (Cappel Laboratories, Cochranville, PA), using a fluorescence-activated cell sorter (FACS-IV).[27]

Aliquots of E^-MNC from donor BM were cryopreserved in McCoy's 5A medium supplemented with 10% DMSO and 10% fetal calf serum (FCS) and stored in the liquid phase of nitrogen until needed as myeloid progenitor cell-rich (CFUc) target cells.

Media

For suspension culture, McCoy's 5A medium was supplemented with 10%–20% FCS, glutamine, and antibiotics. For cloning, the medium was further enriched with 1% methylcellulose and a cell-free source of myeloid colony stimulating factor.[20]

MO/NK-Cell Assay

The one-way MO/NK-cell assay has been described in detail elsewhere.[22] Briefly, equal numbers of 1500-rad-irradiated donor MO/NK cells and host sensitizer cells, derived prior to BMT, are placed in 1º suspension coculture at 37°C, 5% CO_2-air. Five days later, the cocultured cells are washed, reacted with anti-Ia + C to delete residual sensitizers, mixed with equal numbers of cryopreserved CFUc-rich target cells, incubated overnight in suspension, and plated in semisolid 2º coculture at 37°C in a humidified 5% CO_2-air atmosphere. The assay endpoint is inhibition of 7-day myeloid colony growth. Significant inhibition—MO/NK(+) response—is defined as ≧25% decrease in colony numbers generated by target CFUc cloned alone. Negative controls are autologous cultures of donor, host, or third-party cells; positive controls, donor–third-party-cell combinations.

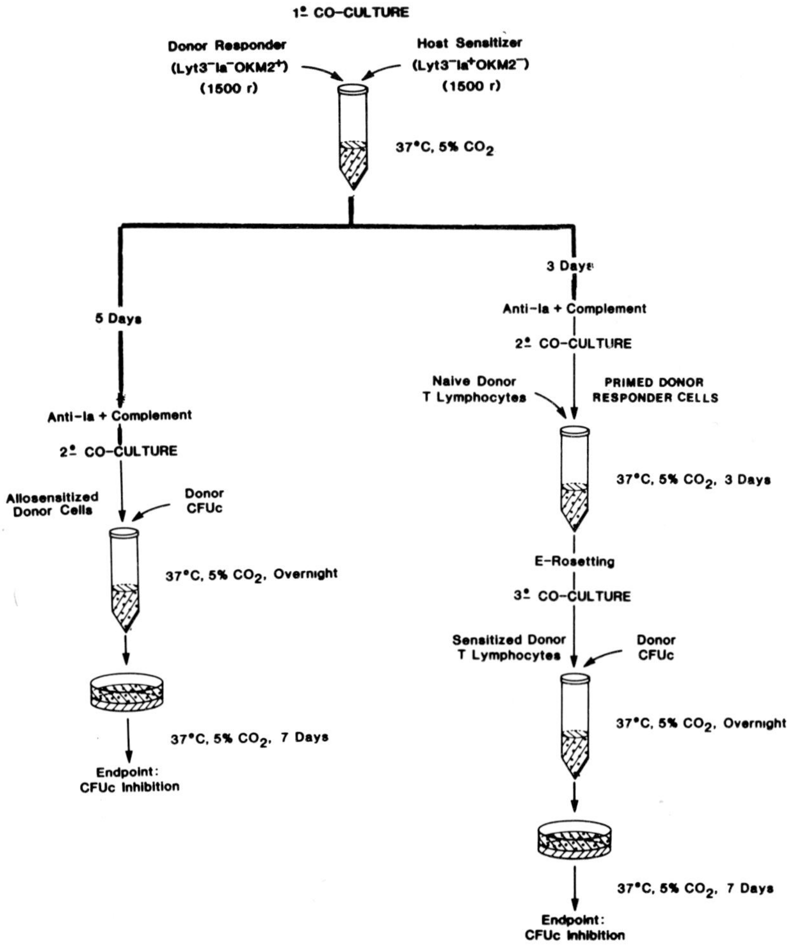

Fig. 1. Dual-assay system for evaluating action of CsA on MO/NK-cell functions; medium supplemented with CsA (1–50 μg/ml) or DMSO (carrier: 0.05%) during 1º coculture only.

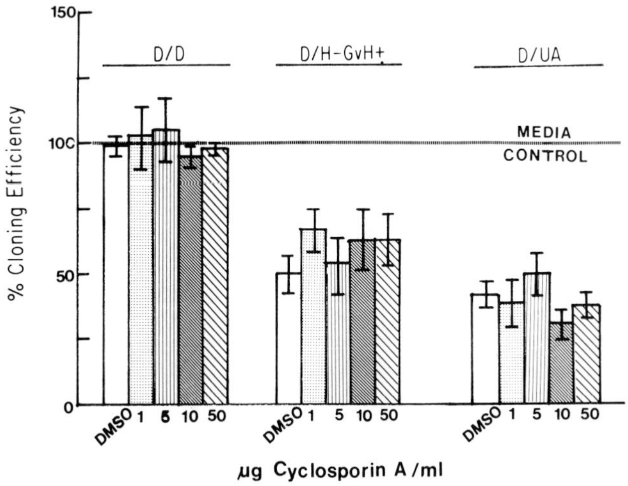

Fig. 2. MO/NK cells allosensitized in CsA-supplemented medium develop CFUc-inhibitory activity (mean ± SD). Donor MO/NK cells were sensitized in 1° coculture with autologous control (D/D), MO/NK(+) HLA-matched prospective host [D/H-GvH(+)], or MO/NK(+) HLA-mismatched unrelated allogeneic (D/UA–third party control) Ia$^-$ non-T sensitizers. CsA (1–50 μg/ml) or DMSO (carrier control: 0.05%) added to 1° coculture medium only. Normalized cloning efficiency: 100% represents cloning efficiency (colony growth) of CFUc cloned alone in unsupplemented medium (media control).

Dual MO/NK–T-Cell Assay

As reported elsewhere,[22] donor MO/NK cells sensitized for at least 3 days with HLA-matched non-T sensitizers develop the capacity to induce CFUc-inhibitory activity in autologous T cells, in a three-step variant of the MO/NK-cell assay.

We assessed the in vitro action of CsA on MO/NK-cell functions in a dual-assay system (Fig. 1) using the principles of both the two-step MO/NK-cell assay and the three-step T cell–induction variant. MO/NK cells and Ia$^-$ non-T sensitizer cells were placed in 1° preculture in either unsupplemented suspension medium (medium control) or in suspension medium supplemented with 0.05% DMSO (carrier control) or CsA (donated by Sandoz). Gradated doses of CsA ranging from 1–50 μg/ml were tested.

To assay for direct CFUc-inhibitory activity, the allosensitized MO/NK cells were harvested after 5 days' preculture, washed three times, treated with anti-Ia + C, mixed with CFUc, incubated overnight in suspension, and cloned in CsA-free semisolid medium. To assay for T cell–inducing function, the allosensitized MO/NK cells were harvested after 3 days' preculture, washed three times, treated with anti-Ia + C, and recultured with equal numbers of autologous T cells in CsA-free suspension medium. Three days later, the T cells were recovered by E-rosetting, mixed with target CFUc, incubated overnight in suspension, and cloned in CsA-free semisolid medium. For both arms of the assay, the endpoint was inhibition of 7-day myeloid colony growth. As in the original assay, significant inhibition was defined as ≧25% decrease in colony numbers generated from target CFUc cloned alone. Paired CsA- and DMSO-treated cultures were considered evaluable only if the DMSO control did not significantly inhibit colonies. (Fig. 1.)

RESULTS

CsA Actions on MO/NK-Cell Functions In Vitro

MO/NK cells did not become sensitized in medium control or CsA-supplemented cultures of autologous controls (25/25 and 11/11, respectively) or of donor-host-GvHD(−) combinations (7/7 and 2/2, respectively). In contrast, MO/NK cells became allosensitized in both medium control and CsA-supplemented cocultures of donor-host-GvHD(+)

Table 1. MO/NK Cells Allosensitized in CsA-Supplemented Medium Fail to Develop T Cell–Inducing Function (Mean ± SD)

Cell Combinations in Primary Coculture	Medium Control		DMSO (0.05%)*		CsA (1 μg/ml)*	
	N	% CE†	*N*	% CE	*N*	% CE
Donor-Donor	25	104.3 ± 18.7	11	99.0 ± 14.3	11	99.3 ± 11.0
Donor-Host-GvH(−)	7	107.5 ± 23.0	2	105.2 ± 3.8	2	100.9 ± 7.8
Donor-Host-GvH(+)	14	55.8 ± 20.8	8	50.7 ± 25.2	8	102.5 ± 23.7
Donor-Third Party	14	53.7 ± 21.7	12	53.4 ± 21.6	12	107.9 ± 22.3

*CsA or DMSO present in 1° coculture medium only. DMSO is carrier control.

†CE = Normalized cloning efficiency. 100% is CE of CFUc cloned alone in unsupplemented medium.

combinations (14/14 and 8/8, respectively) or donor–third-party combinations (14/14 and 12/12, respectively). CsA doses as high as 50 μg/ml failed to prevent development of direct CFUc-inhibitory activity by the allosensitized MO/NK cells, whereas doses as low as 1 μg/ml 1º coculture medium completely abrogated the capacity of allosensitized MO/NK cells to induce autologous T cells in CsA-free 2º coculture. (Fig. 2, Table 1.)

Correlation of MO/NK-Cell Assay with GvHD in Engrafted Recipients

MO/NK-cell assay responses before BMT and development of GvHD after engraftment showed high overall correlation (90.9%: $X^2 = 8.5333$, $p = 0.005$) in the MTX-treated group but low overall correlation (60.0%: $X^2 = 0.6667$, $p =$ NS) in the CsA-treated group. Of the 8 CsA-treated recipients who had MO/NK(+) responses to their donors and were predicted to develop GvHD, 4 failed to do so and engrafted uneventfully. Response or resistance of the 8 high-risk [MO/NK(+)] patients to CsA was not dose dependent.

DISCUSSION

The present studies have shed some light on the cellular basis for variability in the anti-GvHD efficacy of CsA. Crucial to this variability appear to be differential effects of CsA on MO/NK-cell functions and on MO/NK–T cell interactions in response to non-HLA alloantigen stimulation.

The MO/NK cell, which recognizes non-HLA alloantigens expressed on HLA-matched cells, may be an inducer of MHC-independent GvHD.[22] The cell has been partially identified by surface-marker analysis as a subset of either monocytes or NK cells—hence the acronym MO/NK cell.[21] Functional studies suggest a monocyte rather than NK lineage, since some MO/NK-cell functions resist CsA levels five times in excess of doses inhibiting NK cytotoxicity against K562 erythroleukemia cells[8] but comparable to doses to which monocytes participating in mixed lymphocyte reaction are resistant.[5]

MO/NK cells sensitized by non-HLA alloantigens appear to have two separate functions detectable in vitro: a direct CFUc-inhibitory activity and a T-cell–inducing activity. The significance of the CFUc-inhibitory function has not yet been established. It could reflect a direct role of the MO/NK cell in a T-cell–independent induction mechanism of MHC-independent GvHD. It almost certainly reflects a regulatory function of MO/NK cells in hemopoietic recovery after BMT. The T cell–inducing function of allosensitized MO/NK cells may well be a mechanism whereby engrafted donor-type T cells become initiators of MHC-independent GvHD.

We have shown that CsA neither inhibits in vitro sensitization of MO/NK cells nor prevents the allosensitized MO/NK cells from developing CFUc-inhibitory activity but that the drug does interfere with in vitro communication between allosensitized MO/NK cells and naive T cells. Since CsA inhibits T-cell responses to alloantigens controlled by the MHC[4,6] but does not inhibit MO/NK-cell

Table 2. Correlation of MO/NK-Cell Assay with GvHD in MTX- and CsA-Treated Bone Marrow Transplant Recipients

Treatment	Clinical Outcome	MO/NK-Cell Assay* –	MO/NK-Cell Assay* +	Correlation with GvHd	Intragroup Differences X^2	Intragroup Differences p
MTX	GvHD(–)	7	1	87.5%	8.5333	0.005
	GvHD(+)	2	23	92.0%		
CsA	GvHD(–)	2	4	33.3%	0.6667	NS
	GvHD(+)	0	4	100.0%		
Intergroup Differences					12.3023	0.005

*MO/NK(+) response defined as ≧25% inhibition of myeloid colony growth in CFUc–MO/NK cell cocultures, as compared to colony growth from CFUc cloned alone.

allosensitization by non-HLA alloantigens, allosensitized MO/NK cells may well be inducers of GvHD resistant to CsA. Further studies will be necessary to determine whether MO/NK–T cell interactions are inhibited in vitro due to failure of CsA-treated MO/NK cells to produce or elaborate a stimulator signal—possibly interleukin-1[5]—or whether CsA bound to the MO/NK-cell membrane leaches out during 2º coculture and acts on T cells directly.

Our studies have shown that, whereas the MO/NK-cell assay is a reliable prognosticator of MHC-independent GvHD in MTX-treated BMT recipients, it does not predict for GvHD in CsA-treated recipients. This is not surprising, in view of our present findings and previous observations by others[1–8] that CsA has divergent actions on T-cell and non-T-cell components of the GvH reaction. It is interesting that the expected incidence of GvHD in CsA-treated BMT recipients, based on MO/NK(+) responses, coincides with the incidence of GvHD reported for BMT recipients treated with other anti-GvHD modalities,[23] whereas the observed incidence of GvHD in the CsA-treated group is four times lower than expected. Thus, our data suggest that the MO/NK-cell assay may identify patients at high risk of MHC-independent GvHD who are likely to benefit from CsA therapy.

SUMMARY

A dual-assay system has been described for detecting non-HLA allodisparities between prospective BMT donor–host pairs and for evaluating differential effects of CsA on functions of non-T cells that may be involved in the induction of MHC-independent GvHD. The assay consists of (1) an allosensitizing coculture of Ia$^-$ third-population responders (MO/NK cells) and monocyte-depleted third-population sensitizers from BM or PB of prospective donor–host pairs; (2) a T cell–inducing coculture of allosensitized MO/NK cells and naive autologous T cells; and (3) cloning of target CFUc in coculture with either allosensitized MO/NK cells or induced T cells. Inhibition of 7-day myeloid colony growth (≧25%) using either arm of this dual-assay system is indicative of non-HLA allodisparities between responder and sensitizer cells.

High-dose CsA (50 μg/ml) failed to inhibit MO/NK-cell allosensitization or development of CFUc-inhibitory activity, whereas low-dose CsA (1 μg/ml) during 1º coculture totally abrogated the allosensitized MO/NK cells' capacity to induce CFUc-inhibitory T cells in CsA-free 2º coculture. It is proposed that MHC-independent GvHD in CsA-treated BMT recipients may be initiated by CsA-resistant alloreactive MO/NK cells and that CsA-induced impairment of the allosensitized MO/NK cells' T cell–inducing function may be a mechanism involved in reducing the severity of GvHD in these patients.

Alloreactivity between prospective donor–host pairs, as detected in the two-step MO/NK-cell assay, correlates well (90.9%) with GvHD development in engrafted MTX-treated patients but poorly (60.0%) with GvHD development in engrafted CsA-treated patients. Of 8 high-risk [MO/NK(+)] patients treated with CsA, 4 failed to develop GvHD. Possibly, the MO/NK-cell assay could be used to identify high-risk recipients most likely to benefit from CsA therapy.

ACKNOWLEDGMENT

HLA-matching was established by Drs. M. Pollack, K. Sullivan, and B. Dupont. Bone marrow and blood specimens were kindly provided by Drs. R. J. O'Reilly, D. Kirkpatrick, R. Dinsmore, and S. Goulati. The author wishes to thank Dr. D. Kirkpatrick for help in evaluating the clinical correlates.

REFERENCES

1. Borel JF: Immunology 31:632, 1976

2. Borel JF, Wiesinger D: Br J Pharmacol 66:66, 1979

3. Hess AD, Tutschka PJ: J Immunol 124:2601, 1980

4. Wang BS, Heacock EH, Collins KH, et al: J Immunol 127:89, 1981

5. Bunjes D, Hardt C, Röllinghoff M, et al: Eur J Immunol 11:657, 1981

6. Palacios R, Möller G: Nature 290:792, 1981

7. Kunkl A, Klaus GGB: J Immunol 125:2526, 1980

8. Introna SB, Allavena P, Spreafico F, et al: Transplantation 31:113, 1981

9. Starzl TE, Klintmalm GBC, Weil R, et al: Surg Gynecol Obstet 151:17, 1981

10. Starzl TE, Iwatsuki S, Van Thiel DH, et al: Hepatology (in press)

11. Calne RY: Transplant Proc 15:1263, 1983

12. Sutherland DER, Goetz FC, Elick BA, et al: Transplant Proc 15:1322, 1983

13. Oyer PE, Stinson EB, Jamieson SE, et al: Transplant Proc 15:1247, 1983

14. Griffith BP, Hardesty RL, Bahnson HT, et al: Transplant Proc 15:1241, 1983

15. Powles RL, Clink AM, Spence D, et al: Lancet 1:327, 1980

16. Speck B, Gratwohl A, Nissen C, et al: In Baum SJ, Ledney GD, Khan A (eds): Experimental Hematology Today. New York, Springer-Verlag, 1981

17. Hows JM, Palmer S, Gordon-Smith EC: Transplantation 33:382, 1982

18. Deeg HJ, Storb R, Thomas ED, et al: Transplant Proc 15:1384, 1983

19. Powles RL, Evans B: Transplant Proc (in press)

20. Delmonte L, O'Reilly RJ, Kirkpatrick D, et al: Transplantation 34:100, 1982

21. Delmonte L: Blood 60:166a, 1982

22. Delmonte L: In Cohen E, Singal DP (eds): Non-HLA Antigens in Health, Aging, and Malignancy. New York, Alan R. Liss, 133:235–242, 1983

23. Thomas ED, Storb R, Clift RA, et al: N Engl J Med 299:832, 1975

24. Glucksberg RP, Storb R, Fefer A, et al: Transplantation 18:675, 1974

25. Woodruff JM, Hansen JA, Good RA, et al: Transplant Proc 8:675, 1976

26. Wahl SN, Rosenstreich D, Oppenheim JJ: In Vitro Methods of Cell-Mediated Immunity 16:231, 1976

27. Herzenberg LA, Herzenberg LA: In Weiss DM (ed): Handbook of Experimental Immunology. Oxford, Blackwell Scientific Publications, 1978

Induction of Suppressor T Lymphocytes in Mice Treated with Cyclosporine

N. Yoshimura, T. Oka, Y. Ohmori, I. Aikawa, M. Fukuda, Y. Kondoh, and I. Hashimoto

IN RECENT YEARS, cyclosporine (CsA), a fungal metabolite with a potent immunosuppressive effect, was investigated in a variety of experimental animal models and clinical studies. Calne et al. had first described its suppressive effect on organ allograft rejection in dogs and humans.[1] Kahan et al. described the immunopharmacologic monitoring of CsA-treated recipients of cadaveric kidneys.[2]

Studies of the mechanism of action of CsA suggest that CsA suppresses the helper T-cell function by blocking the production of interleukin-2 (IL-2) and the appearance of the receptor for IL-2. In the present experiments, we attempted to show the presence of suppressor T cells in mice treated with CsA and to analyze the mechanism of these suppressor T cells. The results showed that suppressor T cells that are radiosensitive and nylon-wool-nonadherent are involved in CsA-mediated immunosuppression and that this suppressor activity of T cells is mediated by one or more soluble factors as well.

MATERIALS AND METHODS

Animal and Cell Line

Seven to 10-week-old C57BL/6(H-2^b) mice were used in our studies. P815 mastocytoma cells (H-2^d) were kindly provided by Dr. Amagai (Department of Microbiology, Kyoto Prefectural University of Medicine) and maintained in RPMI 1640 media, supplemented with 10% fetal calf serum (FCS) and 5×10^{-5} 2-mercaptoethanol (2-ME).

From the Second Department of Surgery, Kyoto Prefectural University of Medicine, Kyoto, Japan.

Reprint requests should be addressed to Norio Yoshimura, Second Department of Surgery, Kyoto Prefectural University of Medicine, Hirokoji Kawaramachi Kamikyoku, Kyoto 602, Japan.

0041–1345/83/1505–0021$01.00/0

Reagents

CsA, provided by Sandoz, Ltd., Basel, was initially dissolved in olive oil at 50 mg/ml and adjusted to 10 mg/ml with olive oil before use. Monoclonal antibody, anti-Thy-1.2, was obtained from Olak, Ltd. (England).

Treatment of Mice with CsA

B6 mice were immunized by intraperitoneal injection of 1×10^7 P815 cells. Some mice were injected intramuscularly with 1 mg of CsA in 0.1 ml for 5 consecutive days. After 10 days the mice were killed, and lymphocytes were prepared from their spleens.

Fractionation of Spleen Cells on Nylon-Wool Columns

Prepared spleen cells were passed through nylon-wool columns according to the methods of Julius et al.,[3] and a T cell–enriched spleen-cell population was obtained.

In Vitro Generation of Cytotoxic T Lymphocytes (CTL)

10^7 B6 lymphocytes were cultured with 5×10^5 Mitomycin C (MMC)-treated (100 μg/ml, 1 hr, 37°C) P815 cells in 2 ml of culture medium in NUNC plates. These cultures were incubated for 5 days at 37°C in an atmosphere of 95% air, 5% CO_2.

Cytotoxic Assay

The cytolytic activity of cultured lymphocytes was assayed using a micro-cytotoxicity assay employing ^{51}Cr-labeled P815 targets. Approximately 4 and 40×10^4 effector cells were mixed with 10^4 ^{51}Cr-labeled target cells in a V-bottomed microtiter plate. After incubation at 37°C for 4 hr, an aliquot of cell-free supernatant was taken and its ^{51}Cr content was determined. The cytolytic activity was determined from triplicate cultures and calculated as follows:

$$\%\ \text{Specific lysis} = \frac{\text{Experimental release} - \text{Spontaneous release}}{\text{Maximum release} - \text{Spontaneous release}} \times 100.$$

Treatment of Lymphocytes with Monoclonal Antibody

6×10^6 spleen cells were incubated in 1.2 ml of minimal essential medium (MEM) with monoclonal anti-Thy-1.2 antibody (2×10^3 dilution) for 30 min at 4°C.

After incubation, 0.6 ml of guinea pig complement (C 1/20 dilution) was added and incubated for 30 min at 37°C in CO_2 incubator. After incubation, cells were washed three times with MEM and suspended in RPMI 1640 containing 10% FCS.

RESULTS

Suppressor Cells Induced in Alloantigen-Sensitized and CsA-Treated Mice

Lymphocytes prepared from allo-sensitized and CsA-treated mice were tested for cytotoxicity to ^{51}Cr-labeled P815 target cells. As a result, these lymphocytes did not show any cytotoxic effect on target cells. To determine whether these noncytotoxic lymphocytes contain suppressor cells, these noncytolytic spleen cells were added in varying numbers to conventional MLR between normal B6 lymphocytes and MMC-treated P815 cells. After 5 days' incubation, effector cells were harvested and tested for cytotoxic activity. As a result, spleen cells from alloantigen-sensitized and CsA-injected mice significantly inhibited the induction of CTL (Fig. 1). This result suggested the existence of suppressor cells in alloantigen-sensitized and CsA-injected mice.

Nylon-Wool Fractionation and Dish Separation

To identify the suppressor cells induced in this system, 1 × 10^8 spleen cells from both allo-sensitized and CsA-treated mice were fractionated on nylon-wool columns or plastic dishes. 2.8 × 10^7 nylon-wool-passed cells or 7.1 × 10^7 plastic-dish-nonadherent cells were obtained, and the suppressor effect of these cells was tested. Nylon-wool-passed cells or

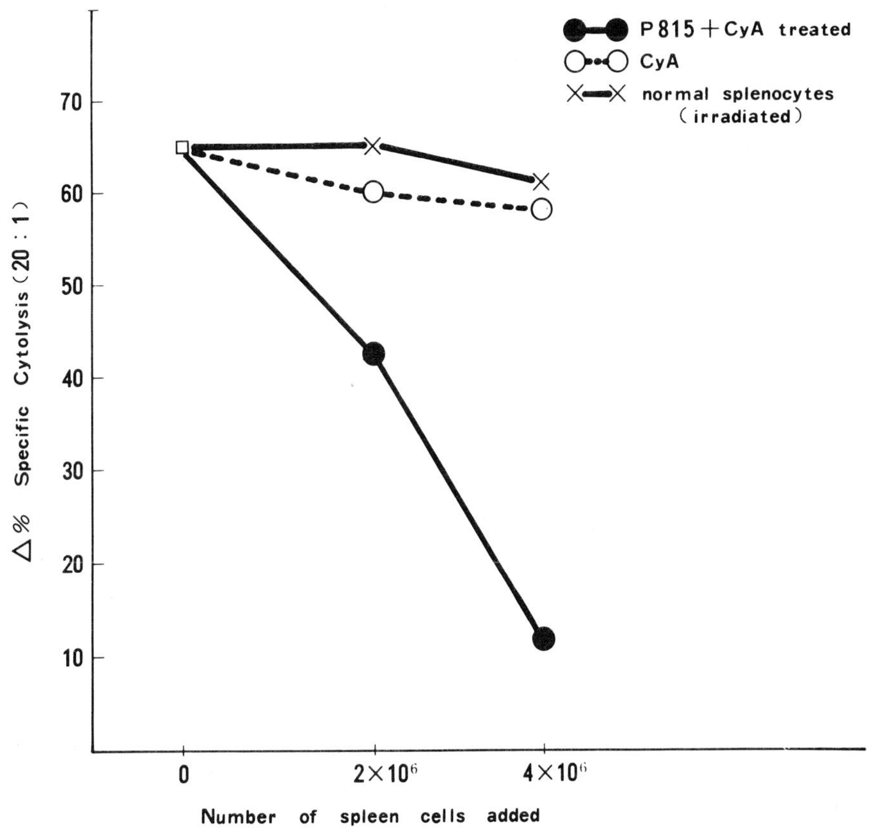

Fig. 1. Suppressor activity of spleen cells from CsA-treated mice.

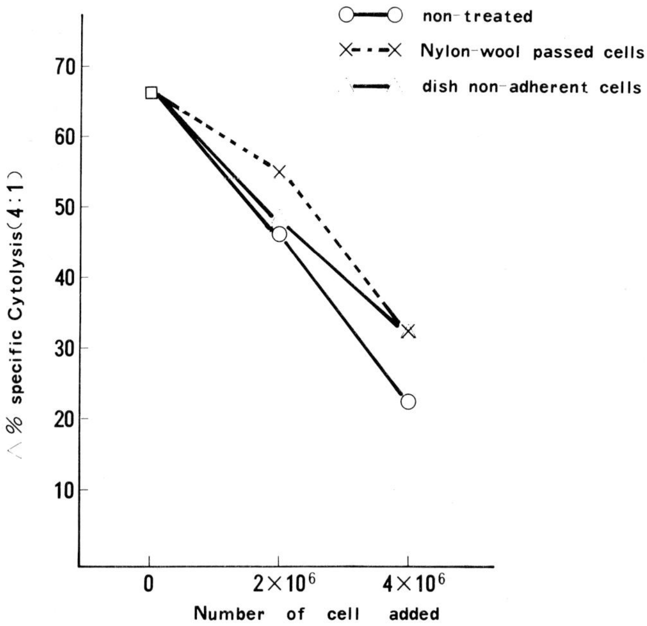

Fig. 2. Suppressor activity of nylon-wool-passed cells or dish-nonadherent cells.

dish-nonadherent cells suppressed the induction of CTL in the same magnitude of unfractionated cells (Fig. 2). These results suggest that this suppression was mediated by T cells.

Treatment of Suppressor Cells with Monoclonal Anti-Thy-1.2 Antibody

In order to confirm the cell type responsible for the suppressor effect, spleen cells from allo-sensitized and CsA-treated mice were incubated with monoclonal anti-Thy-1.2 antibody + C. After treatment, spleen cells were added into the conventional MLR system. As a result, the suppressor effect of spleen cells was diminished (Fig. 3). This result clearly showed that the suppressor cells induced in this system were T cells.

Radiosensitivity of Suppressor T Cells

To determine whether the suppressor T cells in this system were radioresistant or not, spleen cells from treated mice were irradiated (1500 rad) and added to the conventional MLR system. As indicated in Fig. 4, 1500-rad-irradiated spleen cells did not inhibit the induction of CTL. This suggested that the suppressor T cells in this system were radiosensitive.

Suppressor Effect Mediated by Soluble Factor(s)

To determine whether the suppressor effect of CsA-induced suppressor T cells is mediated by one or more soluble factors, the supernatant, after the culture of 5×10^6 spleen cells for 48 hr was added to the MLR system and cultured for 5 days. After 5 days' incubation, cytotoxicity of responder B6 lymphocytes to the original stimulator P815 cells was tested. As shown in Fig. 5, the culture supernatant showed a suppressive effect on the induction of cytotoxic T cells. However, culture supernatant from lymphocytes prepared from only CsA-injected mice or only P815-sensitized mice or from 1500-rad-irradiated suppressor cells did not show any suppressive activity. This shows that the suppressor activity of CsA-induced suppressor T cells was mediated by soluble factors as well.

DISCUSSION

The present study showed that suppressor T cells are involved in CsA-mediated immuno-

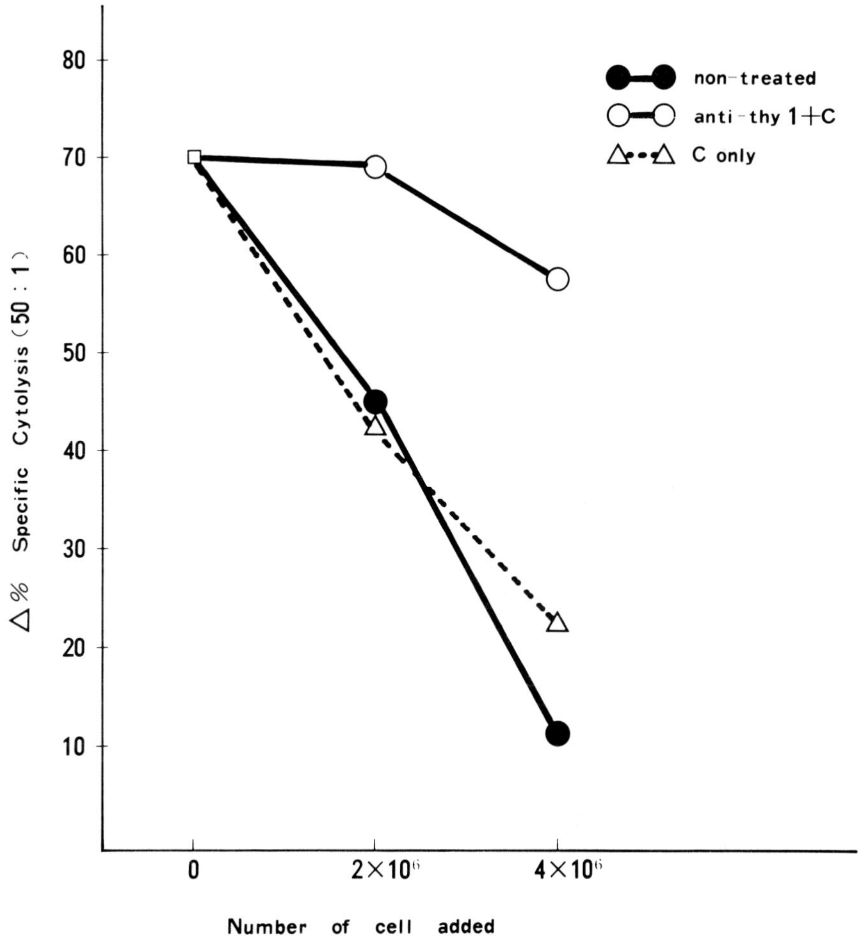

Fig. 3. **Effect of monoclonal anti-Thy-1 antibody on suppressor activity.**

suppression. Many investigators have already reported the immunosuppressive effect of CsA. Studies by Larsson have shown that CsA inhibits the appearance of a receptor for IL-2 without intefering with the production of IL-2.[4] In contrast, Bunjes et al. have shown that CsA inhibits not only the appearance of a receptor for IL-2 but also the production of IL-2 in MLR.[5] In the analysis of soluble factors involved in the generation of CTL, it has been suggested that IL-2 is essential for the induction of CTL.[6] From these reports, there seems to be little doubt that the immunosuppressive effect of CsA results partially from the inhibition of helper T-cell activity, that is, IL-2 production. Wang et al. reported the presence of suppressor T cells in CsA-mediated immunosuppression.[7] The suppressor T cells, they reported, are radioresistant. Conversely, in our experiments, suppressor T cells are radiosensitive. It is not known why this discrepancy occurred. One possibility may be that the differences of dosages of CsA and antigen induced a different subset of T cells. Rich et al. demonstrated that the presence of suppressor T cells inhibited CTL induction in other systems.[8] They injected C57BL/6 spleen cells into the footpads of allogeneic BALB/c mice. Four days after sensitization, suppressor T cells were detected in spleen cells from these mice. However, they reported that no suppressive activity was

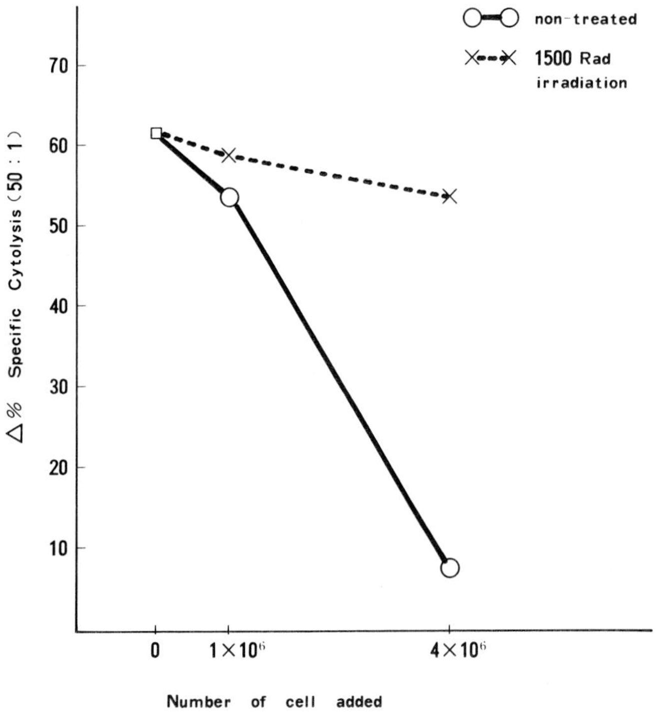

Fig. 4. **Radiosensitivity of suppressor T cells induced by CsA.**

detected at 7 days or at later times, and no suppressor T cells were detected in i.p.-sensitized mice. Therefore, it is not known whether their suppressor T cells and those in our system belong to the same subset of T cells.

Klimpel et al. have shown that macrophage-like suppressor cells are induced in the BCG-injected mice.[9] However, as shown in the present results (Figs. 2 and 3), CsA-induced suppressor cells are not macrophages, because the suppressive activity was diminished by the treatment of Thy-1 antibody + C, and remained on the dish-nonadherent population. In our experiments, culture supernatant from CsA-induced suppressor cells inhibited in vitro CTL generation. However, culture supernatant from irradiated CsA-induced suppressor cells did not show any inhibitory activity on CTL induction. From these results, the possibility of a carry-over of CsA into MLR was ruled out; this suggests that CsA-induced suppressor T cells mediate the suppressor effect with soluble factors as well. Thus, by employing our system, we will be able to analyze not only the cellular mechanism of CsA-mediated immunosuppression but also the soluble suppressor factor produced by suppressor T cells.

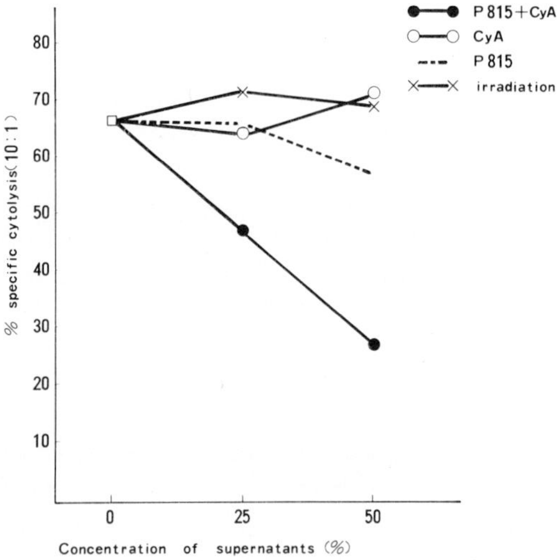

Fig. 5. **Suppressor activity of culture supernatants from CsA-induced suppressor cells.**

REFERENCES

1. Calne RY, Rolles K, Thiru S, et al: Lancet 1:1033, 1979

2. Kahan BD, Van Buren CT, Lin S, et al: Transplantation 34:36, 1982

3. Julius MH, Simpson E, Herzenberg LA: Eur J Immunol 3:645, 1973

4. Larsson EL: J Immunol 124:2828, 1980

5. Bunjes D, Hardt C, Rollinghoff M, et al: Eur J Immunol 11:657, 1981

6. Gillis S, Gillis AE, Henney CS: J Exp Med 154:983, 1981

7. Wang BS, Heacock EH, Chang-Xue Z, et al: J Immunol 128:1382, 1982

8. Rich SS, Rich RR: J Exp Med 142:1391, 1975

9. Klimpel GR, Okada M, Henney CS: J Immunol 123:350, 1979

Suppressor Cells in Cyclosporine-Induced Long-Term Graft Acceptance in the Rat

K. Sakamoto, T. Ochiai, N. Shinohara, T. Asano, and H. Sato

CYCLOSPORINE (CsA) has been shown to be a powerful agent to suppress graft rejection in organ transplantation.[1] In the rat, it induces virtually indefinite acceptance of allogeneic heart or kidney grafts by short-term treatment of hosts at the initial stage of transplantation.[2] The indefinite survival of the allogeneic heart grafts in CsA-treated hosts should involve certain mechanisms for maintenance of the unresponsiveness. We intended to analyze the mechanisms underlying the stable acceptance of allografts induced by CsA.

MATERIALS AND METHODS

Animals

WKA ($RT1^k$), F344 ($RT1^{lvl}$), and BN ($RT1^n$) rats of both sexes, 10 to 16 weeks old, were used in this study. WKA and F344 strains were obtained from commercial sources (WKA: Matumoto Experimental Animal Inc.; F344: Charles River, Japan), and BN rats were originally obtained from Hokkaido University and maintained in our animal facility. Male animals were used exclusively as recipients in heart-grafting experiments.

Cyclosporine (CsA)

CsA was supplied from Sandoz Corporation, Basel, as a powder and dissolved in olive oil at 60°C for 1 hr to make a 10-mg/ml solution. It was administered orally to rats using an orogastric stainless tube.

Cardiac Allografts

Heterotopic heart transplantation was performed by infrarenal anastomosis of donor aorta and pulmonary artery to recipient aorta and inferior vena cava, respectively, according to Ono and Lindsey.[3] Rejection was determined by daily palpation of the graft and confirmed by histological study when necessary.

Skin Graft

A full-thickness tail skin graft (1 cm × 1 cm) was placed on the posterolateral chest wall of the recipient rats, fixed by sutures at four corners. Grafts were inspected daily, technical failure was excluded on day 6, and rejection was judged as the day on which there was 90% necrosis of the graft.

Cell Transfer

Single cell suspensions were prepared from spleens of normal WKA rats and CsA-treated WKA recipients bearing long-term surviving F344 heart grafts. The cells were transferred into sublethally irradiated syngeneic rats intravenously immediately after heart transplantation.

RESULTS

Administration of CsA 10 mg/kg/day p.o. for 14 successive days resulted in a marked prolongation of F344 heart allografts, and the majority of the grafts survived virtually indefinitely in the CsA-treated WKA recipients, whereas they were rejected within less than 10 days in control recipients. In order to analyze the nature of long-term graft acceptance by CsA, the long-term acceptors were challenged with skin grafts of the donor and the third-party strains without any additional immunosuppressive treatment (Table 1). In contrast to the effect on heart grafts, administration of CsA exerted much less effect on primary skin grafts on normal recipients. Skin-graft survival time was only moderately prolonged by treatment with CsA after grafting. Survival of F344 skin grafts transplanted to the heart graft–bearing WKA hosts on day 30 was significantly prolonged, compared with those on the normal recipients. Such prolongation of graft survival was donor-specific, as skin grafts of the third-party strain (BN) were normally rejected. Nevertheless, the F344 skin grafts on day-30 recipients were eventu-

From the Department of Surgery, School of Medicine, Chiba University, Chiba, Japan.

Supported by a grant from the Ministry of Education, Japan.

Reprint requests should be addressed to K. Sakamoto, Department of Surgery, School of Medicine, Chiba University, 1-8-1 Inohana, Chiba 280, Japan.

0041–1345/83/1505–0022$01.00/0

Table 1. Skin Graft Survival Time on Long-Term Heart-Graft-Accepting WKA Rats

Recipient of the Skin Graft	Skin Graft Survival in Days (Mean ± SD) F344 Skin	BN Skin
Normal WKA	9.6 ± 0.5	11.0 ± 1.7
CsA-treated WKA for 14 days	25.6 ± 2.2	—
WKA bearing F344 heart graft for 30 days	32.2 ± 11.0 ($p = 0.008$*)	9.8 ± 1.2
WKA bearing F344 heart graft for 210 days	85.5 ± 24.2 ($p = 0.016$*)	12.8 ± 0.8

*Mann-Whitney's U test.

ally rejected. Interestingly, the original heart grafts were not rejected even after skin had been completely rejected. In contrast to the day-30 recipients, day-210 recipients showed striking prolongation of the F344 skin-graft survival. In this case also, the unresponsiveness was donor-specific. Considering the relative failure of CsA treatment to directly induce skin-graft acceptance and the specific nature of the unresponsiveness, these results strongly suggest that the host immune system was modulated by the long-term presence of the allograft rather than by the direct effect of the CsA. Alloreactivity of the lymphocytes of the long-term acceptors was further analyzed by cell-transfer experiments. Splenic and lymph-node lymphocytes of normal and long-term heart-graft acceptors (210 days after transplantation) were transferred into sublethally irradiated (500 rad) WKA rats. The reconstituted animals received F344 and BN skin grafts immediately after cell transfer. As shown in Table 2, irradiation caused delay of skin-graft rejection. Reconstitution of the irradiated animals with normal lymphocytes resulted in partial recovery of rapid rejection. Transfer of lymphocytes from the day-210 acceptors, however, did not recover the reactivity. Rather, it caused a tendency for further prolongation of skin-graft survival time, as evidenced by the two recipients that rejected the specific skin later than 70 days. This prolongation of skin-graft survival was specific to the F344, and the rejection time of the third-party (BN) skin was comparable to that in the animals that had received normal lymphocytes. This result supports the existence of F344-specific suppressor cells among lymphocytes of the long-term acceptors. When the mixture of lymphocytes from normal and long-acceptor rats were transferred, skin rejection time of the recipients was almost comparable to that of the recipients of the normal lymphocytes. This result indicated that the suppressor activity, if any, of the lymphocytes of long-term accepters was not strong enough to inhibit the response of normal lymphocytes.

DISCUSSION

Indefinite graft acceptance requires at least two essential conditions: inhibition of induction of immune response to the allogeneic antigens of the graft, and maintenance of the unresponsiveness state.

A short course of treatment with CsA induced long-term heart-graft acceptance in the rat, which accepted skin grafts syngeneic to the heart grafts. This striking low respon-

Table 2. Skin Graft Survival Time on the X-Irradiated, Lymphocyte-Transferred Rat

	Cell Source	X-Irradiation (500 rad)	Skin Graft Survival in Days (Mean ± SD) F344 Skin	BN Skin
1	—	—	11.5 ± 1.3	11.0 ± 1.7
2	—	+	20.8 ± 1.8	21.0 ± 1.7
3	Normal WKA	+	14.3 ± 2.5	14.8 ± 2.3
4	WKA bearing F344 heart graft for 210 days	+	74.0 ± 66.0	16.6 ± 0.8
5	3 + 4	+	17.0 ± 2.4	14.3 ± 1.9

3 vs. 4: $p = 0.032$ (Mann-Whitney's U test).

siveness was shown to be specific to the heart-donor strain, because these animals rejected skin grafts from the third-party strain in an almost normal fashion. This low responsiveness was shown to be enforced in a time-dependent manner. The almost identical observation was reported by Nagao et al.[4] These results indicate that the long-term acceptance of allogeneic grafts by CsA-treated hosts involves certain autonomic mechanisms of the host immune system in addition to the direct effect of CsA.

The rejection of skin by the acceptor hosts may indicate action directed against the antigens expressed on the skin but not on the heart. This speculation is based on the fact that the heart grafts remained stable even after rejection of the syngeneic skin grafted on the 30th day of heart transplantation. If the rejection in this case was directed to the antigens shared by both organs, it would be difficult to explain the failure of the host effector cells to reject the original heart grafts, since the majority of the accepted hearts were shown to be fully immunogenic in untreated second hosts. Thus, the feasible explanation would be that the skin-graft rejection by the 30-day heart acceptors is attributable to unshared minor (skin-specific?) antigens. If this is truly the case, then how can the specific prolongation of survival of the syngeneic skin by 210-day heart acceptors be explained? The host immune system should not have experienced the unshared antigen until skin grafting. The observed enforcement of low responsiveness of the heart acceptors to the syngeneic skin cannot be due to the deletion of specific clones, which were shown to be capable of rejecting the skin transplanted on the 30th day after heart transplantation. Therefore, the involvement of suppressor cells was suspected. In hapten-carrier systems, suppressor cells induced against the carrier protein are known to be capable of suppressing immune responses to unexperienced haptens if the haptens are introduced as conjugates to the carrier. The induction of low responsiveness to skin grafts observed in the heart acceptors may well be explained by such suppressive cellular interactions. In the cell-transfer equipment, the result obtained suggested involvement of such cells with suppressive function. Although irradiation of the recipients caused marked prolongation of the skin-graft survival time, recipients could still reject the allogeneic skin. The lymphocytes of 210-day acceptors not only failed to recover the specific allograft rejection of the sublethally irradiated hosts but also caused further delay of rejection of the specific grafts. Nevertheless, these lymphocytes had only a marginal suppressive effect, if any, on the response of normal lymphocytes co-transferred to irradiated hosts. These results suggest that the suppressive effect of these cells is not strong enough to inhibit the vigorous immune responses of the normal cells to MHC antigens and that they are nevertheless capable of suppressing immune responses to weak antigens or already suppressed responses. The nature of the suppressor cells is yet to be studied.

REFERENCES

1. Morris PJ: Transplantation 32:349, 1981

2. White DJG, Rolles K, Ottawa T, et al: Transpl Proc 12:261, 1980

3. Ono K, Lindsey ES: J Thorac Cardiovasc Surg 57:225, 1969

4. Nagao T, White DJG, Calne RY: Transplantation 33:31, 1982

Suppressor-Cell Amplification Circuitry in Cyclosporine-Treated MLR Cultures

A. D. Hess, A. D. Donnenberg, P. Engel, P. J. Tutschka, and G. W. Santos

CYCLOSPORINE (CsA) is an immunobiologically active fungal metabolite that appears to have unique immunosuppressive properties without the significant myelotoxicity associated with other immunosuppressive regimens.[1,2] CsA acts predominantly on T lymphocyte–dependent responses and appears to facilitate the induction of transplantation tolerance in a variety of experimental model systems.[3–5] The mode of action of CsA and its role in establishing this state of immunological unresponsiveness remains unclear. Recent studies in our laboratory have demonstrated that this agent inhibits the induction of cytotoxic effector T lymphocytes but permits the activation and expression of suppressor cells in primary MLR, a process that leads to a state of specific alloantigen tolerance that is maintained by a nylon-wool-adherent suppressor cell.[6,7] Further studies have indicated that CsA prevents the precursor cytotoxic T cell from acquiring the ability to respond to interleukin 2 (IL-2), an event that appears to be required for the maturation and proliferation of cytotoxic T lymphocytes.[8–10] Furthermore, CsA significantly inhibits the production of IL-2 in primary MLR and limits the activation of T helper cells.[11] It is of interest to note that despite the absence of significant levels of IL-2 production and the limited activation of T helper cells in CsA-treated primary MLR, suppressor cell activity is amplified to near normal levels. Although T suppressor cells can be amplified by IL-2, our results suggest that an alternative mechanism accounts for suppressor-cell amplification that is relatively insensitive to the effects of CsA. The present studies were undertaken to determine what mechanisms account for suppressor-cell amplification in CsA-treated primary MLR cultures.

MATERIALS AND METHODS

Lymphocyte Isolation

Human peripheral blood lymphocytes were isolated from fresh defibrinated blood from normal healthy volunteers by Ficoll-Paque (Pharmacia Fine Chemicals, Piscataway, NJ) density centrifugation as previously described.[6,7]

Bulk MLR

Bulk primary and secondary MLR were established using standard techniques described in detail elsewhere.[6,7] The cultures were incubated at 37°C in a humidified 5% CO_2-in-air incubator. Proliferation in bulk culture was assessed by pipetting 0.1 ml of the bulk culture cell suspension into triplicate wells of a microtiter plate and labeling with 1 μCi of ^{3}H-thymidine as detailed elsewhere.[6,7]

Cell-Mediated Lympholysis Assay (CML)

Primed cells harvested from bulk MLR cultures were incubated for 4 hr at 37°C with 1×10^4 3-day-old PHA blast cells labeled with ^{51}Cr as previously described.[6] Percent specific ^{51}Cr release was calculated according to the following formula:

$$\% \text{ Specific } ^{51}\text{Cr release} = \frac{\text{cpm Experimental} - \text{cpm Spontaneous}}{\text{cpm Maximum} - \text{cpm Spontaneous}} \times 100.$$

Lytic units were calculated according to the methods of Brunner et al.[12] by plotting percent specific ^{51}Cr release vs. the log of the number of effector cells, with the estimated number of effector cells required for 20% lysis arbitrarily defined as one unit.

From the Bone Marrow Transplant Program, Oncology Center, The Johns Hopkins University, School of Medicine, Baltimore, MD.

Supported in part by NIH Grants CA 15396, AM 26502, and CA 31687 and a gift from the Harley W. Howell Foundation. A.D.H. is a scholar of the Leukemia Society of America, Inc.

Reprint requests should be addressed to Dr. A. D. Hess, Oncology Center, Rm. 3-127, Johns Hopkins Hospital, 600 N. Wolfe St., Baltimore, MD 21205.

0041–1345/83/1505–0023$01.00/0

Suppressor-Cell Assay

The primed cells from the bulk cultures were tested for their ability to suppress the proliferative response of fresh responding cells (A; autologous to the initial responding cell) to the original sensitizing lymphocytes, (B_x; arbitrarily designed specific suppression) and to unrelated third-party lymphocytes (C_x; arbitrarily designated nonspecific suppression) as previously described.[7,8] Percent of the MLR response was calculated according to the following formula:

$$\% \text{ Suppression} = \frac{\text{Response of test cultures } [(AB_x) + \text{Fresh A} + \text{Fresh } B_x \text{ or } C_x]}{\text{Response of control cultures } [(AA_x)_x + \text{Fresh A} + \text{Fresh } B_x \text{ or } C_x]} \times 100$$

Irradiated (1500 rad) autologously primed lymphocytes $(AA_x)_x$ added in equal numbers as the primed lymphocytes (AB_x) were utilized as the control.[6] Suppressor cell units were calculated according to the method of Hess et al.[13] by plotting percent suppression vs. the log of the number of effector cells, with the estimated number of effector cells required for 50% suppression arbitrarily defined as one unit.

Assay for Interleukin 2 (IL-2) and the Ability to Respond to IL-2

IL-2 activity in supernatants from primary MLR cultures was assessed by measuring the ability of the supernatants to stimulate proliferation and enhance CML activity of alloantigen-primed lymphocytes (harvested from 10-day-old control primary MLR cultures) as previously described.[8] IL-2 activity in the primary MLR supernatants was also assessed by measuring their ability to support growth of an IL-2–dependent cloned cytotoxic T-cell line as described in detail elsewhere.[14] To assess responsiveness to IL-2, primed cells (1×10^6 cells) harvested from primary MLR on days 9–10 were plated in macrotiter wells and cultured with 2 units/ml of IL-2 or the day-2 primary control MLR supernatants containing IL-2 (50% v/v) as detailed elsewhere.[8] IL-2 used in these studies was prepared from a 50%–70% ammonium sulfate cut of MLA 144 culture supernatant. MLA 144 is a cell line derived from a spontaneous Gibbon ape T-cell lymphoma that secretes IL-2 constitutively.[15] MLA 144 supernatants are devoid of IL-1, IL-3, CsA, MIF, and interferons.[16] The cultures were allowed to incubate for 48 hr, at which time proliferation was assessed by pipetting 0.1 ml of the cell suspension into triplicate wells of a microtiter plate and labeling with 1 μCi of ^{3}H-thymidine for 16–18 hr. On day 3 of culture, the remainder of the cells were harvested and tested for CML activity.

Ab + C′ Treatment

Lymphocyte subpopulations were depleted by using monoclonal antibody techniques as detailed elsewhere.[11] Briefly, the primed lymphocytes were harvested from MLR and washed thoroughly with phosphate-buffered saline. Cells (2×10^6 cells/ml) were incubated with the OKT4 or OKT8 (Ortho Pharmaceutical Corp., Raritan, NJ) monoclonal antibody for 1 hr at 4°C, at which time the cells were pelleted by centrifugation and 0.4 ml of rabbit complement (diluted ⅓ in Dulbecco's PBS) added to the cells. The cells were incubated for 1 hr at room temperature, pelleted, and subjected to another round of antibody-plus-C lysis.

Cyclosporine

Powdered CsA, a generous gift from Sandoz Ltd. (Biological and Medical Research Division, Basel, Switzerland), was dissolved in 95% ethanol, diluted to the appropriate concentration with complete culture medium, and added to the bulk MLR cultures. Control cultures received ethanol in complete medium. CsA was removed from the cultured lymphocytes prior to assessment of function by incubation in fresh medium containing 20% serum (normal human) at 37°C for 1 hr, followed by two washes and resuspension in fresh complete medium.

Lymphocyte Colony Cultures

The ability of culture supernatants to support lymphocyte colony formation of MLR-primed lymphocytes was tested using a modification of the whole-blood technique described by Knox et al.[17] and Donnenberg et al.[18] MLR-primed lymphocytes were resuspended (4.5×10^5 cells/ml) in RPMI 1640 medium containing 2 m*M* L-glutamine, 25 m*M* HEPES buffer, 50 μg/ml gentamicin, 100 U/ml penicillin, and 5×10^{-5} *M* 2-mercaptoethanol. Test supernatant (1.0 ml) MLR cell suspension (0.9 ml), pooled human serum (0.8 ml), x-irradiated (1500 rad) whole blood from the subject used as a stimulator in MLR (0.1 ml), and 0.2 ml 6 × RPMI 1640 medium were aliquoted in 12 × 75 mm snap-cap tubes and warmed to 40°C, and 1.0 ml 2% Agarose (Agarose indubiose A37, Accurate Chemical Co., Hicksville, NY) was added per tube to a final concentration of 0.5%. Cell suspensions were plated in triplicate (1 ml/well) in 35 mm wells (Costar 3506).

After 6 days of incubation at 37°C in a humid atmosphere of 5% CO_2 in air, cultures were cleared of red blood cells by the addition of 30% acetic acid (0.1 ml/well) and fixed with 20% paraformaldehyde (0.1 ml/well). Cultures were allowed to air-dry, washed with distilled water, and stained with toluidine blue. Colonies were counted on an inverted microscope.

RESULTS

Proliferative Response of Cloned CTL and Alloantigen-Primed Lymphocytes to MLR Supernatants

Initial studies were undertaken to determine if supernatants from CsA-treated and control primary MLR cultures contained

Table 1. Proliferative Response of Cloned Cytotoxic T Cells and Alloantigen-Primed Lymphocytes to MLR Supernatants

Supernatants from Primary MLR Cultures*	Proliferative Response in Test Supernatants: Cloned Cytotoxic T Cells†	Alloantigen-Primed Lymphocytes‡
Control MLR	12,947 ± 2,034	5,747 ± 109
Control MLR + 2.5 μg/ml CsA	11,436 ± 1,089	5,548 ± 281
2.5 μg/ml CsA-treated MLR	230 ± 35	465 ± 57
1.0 μg/ml CsA-treated MLR	281 ± 78	522 ± 81
Complete medium	201 ± 69	210 ± 52

*Supernatants were harvested from primary MLR on day 2.

†Cloned CTL cells (3 × 10^3 cells in 0.1 ml) were incubated for 18 hr in the test supernatants (0.1 ml) prior to labeling with 0.5 μCi of ^{3}H-thymidine for 4 hr.

‡Alloantigen-primed lymphocytes (1 × 10^6/ml) harvested from control primary MLR on day 10 were incubated for 48 hr in the supernatants (1.0 ml) prior to labeling a 0.1-ml aliquot (in triplicate) with 0.5 μCi of ^{3}H-thymidine.

IL-2. As demonstrated in Table 1, supernatants of control MLR cultures promoted a vigorous proliferative response of an IL-2–dependent cloned cytotoxic T-cell line. More important, the addition of CsA to the control MLR supernatant did not result in a significant inhibition of the cloned CTL proliferative response. This supernatant also enhanced the proliferative response of alloantigen-primed lymphocytes harvested from day-10 primary MLR cultures. In contrast to the findings from control MLR supernatants, supernatants from CsA-treated MLR cultures were not able to promote the proliferative response of the cloned CTL line. However, the supernatants from the CsA-treated cultures did stimulate a very weak proliferative response of the alloantigen-primed lymphocytes. The proliferative response was approximately twice that of the background of the primed lymphocytes cultured in complete medium.

Functional Activity of the Primed Lymphocytes After Culture in Supernatants from Primary MLR Cultures

CML activity and suppressor-cell function of the primed lymphocytes after culture in the primary MLR supernatants were assessed, and the results of a representative experiment are shown in Table 2. The data demonstrate that culture of alloantigen-primed lymphocytes harvested from control primary MLR on day 10 in the presence of supernatant from a primary MLR culture resulted in the enhancement of both cytotoxic T-cell activity and of suppressor-cell activity compared to cells cultured in complete medium. The addi-

Table 2. Suppressor Cell–Specific Enhancing Activity in Supernatants from CsA-Treated Primary MLR Cultures

Day-2 Supernatants from Primary MLR Cultures	CML Activity of Primed Lymphocytes After Culture in Test Supernatants: % Specific ^{51}Cr-Release Effector-to-Target Ratio 40:1	20:1	10:1	Lytic Units/10^7 Primed Cells	Suppressor-Cell Activity of Primed Lymphocytes After Culture in Test Supernatants: % Suppression of Fresh Micro MLR Primed Cell–to–Fresh Responder Ratio 1:1	1:5	1:10	Suppressor-Cell Units/10^7 Primed Cells
A × B_x (Control)	30.3	19.6	13.2	54.8	97.6	95.3	67.3	1,553
A × B_x (Control) + 2.5 μg/ml CsA	29.9	19.9	14.3	56.5	98.3	94.2	69.6	1,737
A × B_x (2.5 μg/ml CsA)	13.3	12.8	12.9	<1	95.5	85.9	55.7	1,139
A × A_x	12.7	13.1	10.9	<1	79.3	20.1	3.0	156
Complete medium	12.5	11.3	10.4	<1	81.7	17.9	1.0	161

Response of Primed Lymphocytes to Test Supernatant*

*Primed lymphocytes (1 × 10^6/ml) harvested on day 10 from control primary MLR were cultured with 1.0 ml of the test supernatants. After 72 hr of incubation, the cells were harvested and tested for CML and suppressor-cell activity.

†Suppressor-cell activity expressed in terms of percent suppression based on comparison to control MLR cultures which received irradiated autologously cultured cells and averaged 55,658 ± 4,328 (SE) of ^{3}H-thymidine uptake.

Table 3. Specificity of Suppressor-Cell Activity After Culture in CsA-Treated and Control MLR Supernatants*

Test Supernatants	Specific Suppression of Fresh Micro-MLR (A × B_x) Primed Cell-to-Fresh Responder Ratio			Nonspecific Suppression of Fresh Micro-MLR (A × C_x) Primed Cell-to-Fresh Responder Ratio		
	1:2	1:5	1:10	1:2	1:5	1:10
Complete medium	67.8†	36.7	4.6	3.7	5.1	−2.3
A × B_x (Control)	93.0	89.8	77.6	11.7	11.4	0.3
A × B_x (CsA 2.5 μg/ml)	95.6	83.9	64.9	24.5	−1.0	−8.9
IL-2 (2 units/ml)	92.4	89.1	88.9	32.9	32.3	13.0

*Primed lymphocytes (1 × 10^6/ml) harvested from 10-day-old control primary MLR cultures were incubated for 72 hr with the test supernatants. After the 3-day incubation period, the cells were assessed for specific and nonspecific suppressor-cell activity in the fresh micro-MLR system.

†Percent suppression based on comparison to the control responses to which irradiated autologously cultured cells were added. Mean cpm ± SE of ^{3}H-thymidine uptake for the [A × B_x + $(AA_x)_x$] control cultures was 47,902 ± 3,474 (SE) and for the [A × C_x + $(AA_x)_x$] cultures, 35,532 ± 1,159.

tion of CsA to the control MLR supernatants did not inhibit the ability of the soluble growth factors (IL-2) to enhance either CML activity or suppressor-cell function. In contrast, cells cultured with the supernatants from the CsA-treated MLR cultures did not show an enhanced CML response compared to cells cultured in control supernatants. However, there was a significant ($p < 0.01$) enhancement of suppressor-cell function. Further studies demonstrated that the failure to enhance cytotoxic T-cell function of the alloantigen-primed cells was not due to a soluble inhibitor of IL-2 (data not shown). The specificity of the suppressor-cell activity after culture in the CsA-treated in control MLR supernatants was assessed. As shown in Table 3, culture of the alloantigen-primed lymphocytes in either control MLR supernatant, supernatant from a CsA-treated MLR culture, or IL-2 resulted in an enhancement of suppressor-cell function compared to cells cultured in complete medium. The cells were capable of mediating specific suppression of a fresh micro-MLR consisting of fresh autologous responder cells (A) stimulated with the original sensitizing antigen (B_x). In contrast these cells were not capable of mediating suppression of the fresh micro-MLR response to a third-party alloantigen (C_x). The data rule out the possibility that a nonspecific suppressive effect accounted for the observed enhanced suppression.

To identify the cells that were responsive to

Table 4. Enhancement of OKT8$^+$ Suppressor-Cell Activity by IL-2 and/or Supernatants from CsA-Treated MLR Cultures*

Cell Population	Test Supernatants	Percent Suppression of Fresh Micro MLR Primed Cell-to-Fresh Responder Ratio		
		1:5	1:10	1:20
AB_x—Unfractionated	Complete medium	60.9†	27.7	−17.7
	IL-2 (2 units/ml)	96.5	96.0	82.9
	2.5 μg/ml CsA-treated MLR	92.4	87.4	75.8
AB_x—OKT8-enriched (OKT4-depleted)	Complete medium	78.5	45.3	22.2
	IL-2 (2 units/ml)	97.5	95.2	94.4
	2.5 μg/ml CsA-treated MLR	96.8	89.6	71.1
AB_x—OKT4-enriched (OKT8-depleted)	Complete medium	54.8	45.1	24.5
	IL-2 (2 units/ml)	58.9	48.9	36.0
	2.5 μg/ml CsA-treated MLR	39.9	35.0	−13.6

*Primed lymphocytes (1 × 10^6 cells/ml) harvested from 10-day-old control primary MLR were left unfractionated or depleted of the OKT4 (OKT8-enriched population) or the OKT8 (OKT4-enriched population) subsets by antibody-plus-complement treatment. The respective cell populations were cultured for 72 hr in the test supernatants and assessed for suppressor-cell activity.

†Percent suppression based on comparison to the control response to which irradiated autologously cultured cells were added. This control averaged 43,078 ± 2,068 (SE) of ^{3}H-thymidine uptake.

the suppressor-cell-enhancing activity in the supernatants from CsA-treated MLR cultures as well as to identify the cells capable of mediating suppression of fresh micro-MLR cultures, alloantigen-primed cells harvested from primary MLR on day 10 were left unfractionated or depleted of the $OKT4^+$ or $OKT8^+$ lymphocytes by treatment with monoclonal antibody and complement. The respective cell populations were cultured for 72 hr in either complete medium, complete medium plus IL-2 (2 U/ml), or the supernatants from CsA-treated MLR and assessed for suppressor-cell activity after culture. The results (Table 4) demonstrate that the OKT8-enriched population (depleted of the OKT4 subset) responded to both IL-2 and the supernatants from CsA-treated MLR cultures, with the resultant enhancement of suppressor-cell function, as compared to this population cultured in completed medium. In contrast, the OKT4-enriched subset (depleted of the OKT8-cell population) did mediate some residual suppression of the fresh micro-MLR but was not enhanced after culture with either IL-2 or the supernatants from CsA-treated MLR cultures.

Lymphocyte Colony Formation (LCF) of MLR-Primed Lymphocytes

To determine if the MLR supernatants from CsA-treated MLR cultures will support LCF, lymphocytes from ongoing MLR cultures were harvested on day 5 of culture and plated in *Agarose* with the supernatants from CsA-treated MLR cultures or IL-2 as growth-promoting activity. The results in Table 5 demonstrate that IL-2 supports colony growth of MLR-activated cells and that LCF is not inhibited by the presence of exogenous CsA. Similarly, the supernatants from CsA-treated cultures also support growth of MLR-activated cells, but to a much lesser extent, approximately 1/10 the number of colonies as compared to the cultures that received IL-2. This lack of support of colony growth was not due to a soluble inhibitor, since mixing of supernatant from the CsA-treated cultures with known IL-2 did not result in the reduction of colony growth supported by IL-2. Of interest is the morphology of the colonies in cultures supported with the supernatants from the CsA-treated cultures. Figure 1 compares the colonies grown in the presence of IL-2 and colonies grown in the presence of only the supernatant from CsA-treated MLR cultures. Colonies grown in IL-2 formed very large clusters of cells, densely packed in the center and more diffuse on the periphery. In contrast, the colonies from the cultures supported by the CsA-treated MLR supernatants were smaller and less tightly packed and contained fewer cells than those from IL-2–treated cultures.

Table 5. Effect of MLR Supernatants on Lymphocyte Colony Formation of MLR-Primed Lymphocytes

Test Supernatant	Mean Colonies/Well (SEM)
A × B_x CsA 2.5 μg/ml	24 (4)
A × B_x CsA 0.1 μg/ml	34 (4)
IL-2*	348 (14)
IL-2 + CsA 2.5 μg/ml	402 (56)
Complete medium	0
Complete medium + CsA 2.5 μg/ml	0
AB_x CsA 2.5 μg/ml + IL-2†	400 (10)
A × B_x CsA 0.1 μg/ml + IL-2	392 (18)

*Final concentration 10 half-maximal units/ml in complete medium.

†Test supernatant plus exogenous IL-2 (final concentration = 10 units/ml).

DISCUSSION

Initial studies with CsA in primary MLR have revealed that CsA preferentially inhibits the induction of cytotoxic T lymphocytes but permits the activation of suppressor cells. It appears that suppressor cells are fully amplified in the presence of CsA despite the fact that there is a virtual absence of IL-2, a soluble factor capable of promoting cytotoxic T-cell growth and apparently of promoting the clonal expansion of suppressor lymphocytes. In the present studies, supernatants from CsA-treated MLR cultures were capable of enhancing $OKT8^+$ suppressor-lymphocyte function in alloantigen-primed cells. No

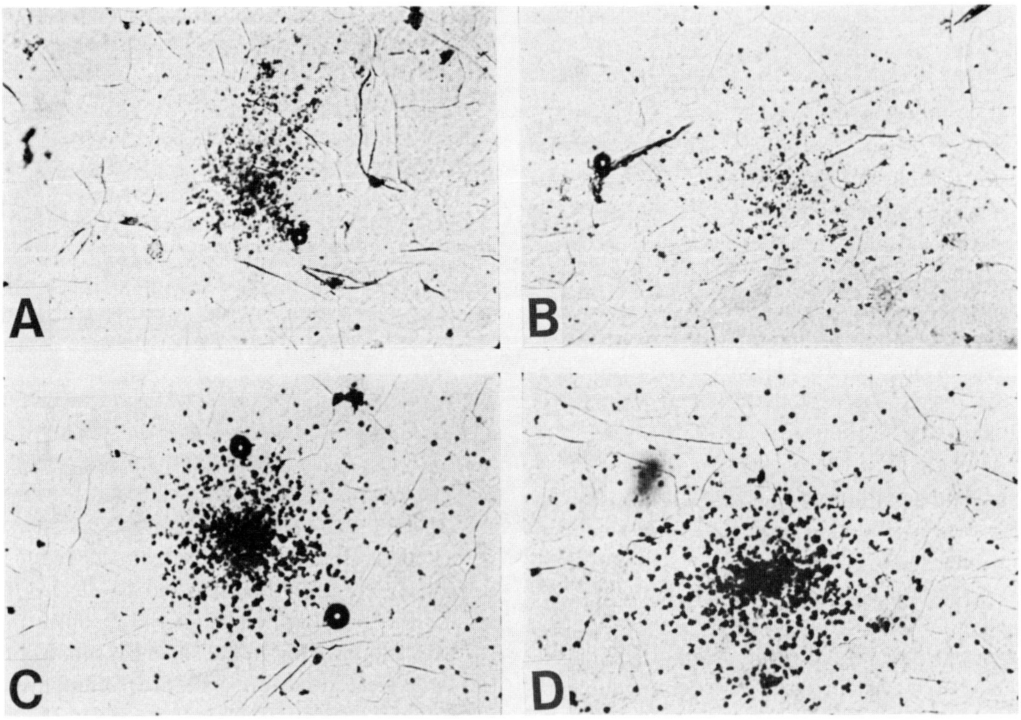

Fig. 1. Lymphocyte colonies derived from MLR-primed lymphocytes. (A, B) Primed lymphocytes grown with 25% MLR supernatant prepared in the presence of 1.0 μg/ml CsA. (C, D) Primed lymphocytes grown in the presence of 1 U/ml IL-2.

IL-2 could be detected in these supernatants, suggesting that this activity represents a moiety distinct from IL-2, although IL-2 also was demonstrated to amplify suppressor T-cell function. Three distinct explanations can account for our findings. First, it is possible that the suppressor cells are much more sensitive to IL-2 than the cytotoxic T cells, a process that would result in the enhancement of suppressor-lymphocyte function in supernatants where the IL-2 concentration is too low to be detected by the classical assay system. In preliminary studies attempting to absorb the CsA-treated MLR supernatants with a cloned IL-2–dependent cytotoxic T-cell line, the suppressor cell–enhancing activity could not be removed even after two rounds of absorption. The second possibility is that we are detecting a molecular variant of IL-2. Such a precedent is provided by the studies of Robb Smith[19] and by Meier and Gallo,[20] who showed that there are different variants of IL-2 based on the degree of glycosylation. It is intriguing to speculate that there is a distinct IL-2–like molecule specific for suppressor but not cytotoxic T cells. Such an explanation could also account for the inability to absorb out the suppressor cell–enhancing activity with a cloned cytotoxic T-cell line. The third possibility is that the suppressor cell–enhancing activity found in the CsA-treated MLR supernatants is a differentiation factor that allows the suppressor T cell to attain full suppressor-cell function. Of interest are the findings of Wagner et al.,[21] who recently reported a differentiation factor required for the maturation of cytotoxic T lymphocytes. In his studies, both IL-2 and this differentiation factor were required for the complete activation, maturation, and clonal amplification of the cytotoxic T-cell response. It is conceivable that we have observed an analogous mechanism involved in the regulation of the suppressor-cell arm of the immune response. If this last interpretation holds, it would appear that the suppressor cell–enhancing factor is distinct from the differentiation factor for cytotoxic T lymphocytes, since in no instance was CML activity enhanced in the presence of the CsA-treated primary MLR supernatant.

Although the lymphocyte colony data indicate that our soluble factor is capable of promoting growth of MLR-primed lymphocytes, the identity of the cell population(s) comprising these colonies is not known. Current studies are under way to clonally expand the T-cell colonies grown in this system and to determine their functional status. Colonies grown in the presence of our soluble factor are morphologically distinct from those grown in the presence of IL-2. It is tempting to speculate that we have observed preferential growth of the suppressor-cell population and that the reduced colony size and density reflects an autoregulatory mechanism. The observation that there is a low degree of tritiated thymidine uptake of the primed lymphocytes exposed to the CsA-treated MLR supernatants is also consistent with this interpretation. Furthermore, if one cultures MLR-primed lymphocytes in the presence of our "growth factor" for longer than 3 days (standard assay conditions), one finds that suppressor-cell activity increases as a function of time.

In summary, our data suggest that there is an alternative mechanism that allows for suppressor-cell amplification in CsA-treated MLR cultures. This alternative mechanism appears to be independent of IL-2, but it is conceivable that in the absence of CsA the two may act in concert or synergistically. The molecular nature of this suppressor cell–enhancing activity is not known and awaits initial biochemical characterization. However, initial studies rule out IL-1 and alpha interferon, since addition of partially purified preparations of these lymphokines to the alloantigen-primed lymphocytes did not result in enhancement of suppressor-cell activity. Clearly, further studies are necessary to characterize the suppressor cell–enhancing activity both biochemically and immunobiologically and to assess its importance in the induction and clonal expansion of suppressor T-cells.

ACKNOWLEDGMENT

We acknowledge the excellent secretarial assistance of Ms. C. Rutter in the preparation of this manuscript.

REFERENCES

1. Borel JF: Immunology 31:631, 1976
2. Borel JF, Feurer C, Buler HU, et al: Agents and Actions 4/6:468, 1976
3. Borel JF, Feurer C, Magnee C, et al: Immunology 32:1017, 1977
4. Green CL, Allison AC: Lancet 1:1182, 1978
5. Calne RY, White DJC, Rolles K, et al: Lancet 1:1183, 1978
6. Hess AD, Tutschka PJ: J Immunol 124:2601, 1980
7. Hess AD, Tutschka PJ, Santos GW: J Immunol 126:961, 1981
8. Hess AD, Tutschka PJ, Pu Z, et al: J Immunol 128:360, 1982
9. Symington FW, Teh N-S: Scand J Immunol 12:1, 1977
10. Larsson EL, Coutinho A, Martinez CA: Immunol Rev 51:61, 1980
11. Hess AD, Donnenberg AD, Tutschka PJ, et al: J Immunol 130:717, 1983
12. Brunner KT, Engers ND, Cerottini JC: In Bloom BR, Davis JE (eds): In Vitro Methods of Cell Mediated and Tumor Immunity. New York, Academic Press, 1976, p 423
13. Hess AD, Tutschka PJ, Santos GW: Exp Hematol 9:415, 1981
14. Gillis S, Mochiuzuki DY, Conlan PJ, et al: Immunol Rev 63:167, 1982
15. Rabin H, Hopkins RF, Ruscetti FW, et al: J Immunol 127:1852, 1982
16. Henderson LE, Hewetson JF, Hopkins RF, et al: J Immunol (in press)
17. Knox SJ, Shifrine M, Wilson FD, et al: Exp Hematol 9:926, 1981
18. Donnenberg AD, Elfenbein GJ, Santos GW: J Immunol 129:1080, 1982
19. Robb RJ, Smith KA: Fed Proc 40:1163, 1981
20. Meier JW, Gallo RC: Proc Natl Acad Sci USA 77:6134, 1980
21. Wagner H, Hardt C, Bartlett R, et al: J Exp Med 153:1517, 1981

The Immunosuppressive Action of Cyclosporine in Man

R. M. Ferguson and R. Fidelus-Gort

CYCLOSPORINE (CsA) is a cyclic endecapeptide that has been shown to elicit potent immunosuppressive action both in vivo and in vitro.[1-3] As an immunosuppressive agent it has been associated with prolonged allograft survival in both animals and man.[4-6] How CsA manifests its immunosuppressive action in vivo is unknown. Numerous investigators have described selective effects of CsA on specific T-cell subpopulations.[6-9] Donor-specific immunologic tolerance and clonal detection have been suggested as the mechanism responsible for prolonged allograft survival in the CsA-treated transplant patient. In vitro evidence, however, demonstrates a rapidly reversible immunosuppressive effect on lymphocytes.[8] Also, the data of Deeg et al. showing graft rejection immediately following the discontinuance of cyclosporine therapy supports the lack of tolerance induction with CsA therapy.[5] Thus, the ability of CsA to cause a permanent immunosuppressive effect on lymphocytes remains controversial.

In order to utilize CsA effectively in the transplant population, a clearer understanding of its action in the prevention of allograft rejection would be useful. We investigated whether the inhibition of lymphocyte proliferation was associated with absorption and metabolism of CsA following a single oral dose. Further, we studied whether a plasma inhibitory factor or a direct effect on lymphocyte responsiveness and proliferation was associated with CsA therapy and if these depressed responses were permanent or reversible. Through these studies we hoped to delineate the site of CsA action in the prevention of allograft rejection.

From the Ohio State University College of Medicine, Columbus, OH.

Reprint requests should be addressed to R. M. Ferguson.

0041-1345/83/1505-0024$01.00/0

The immunosuppressive effect of CsA was monitored by assaying the proliferative responses of both patient and normal lymphocytes cultured in the presence of patient plasma obtained at various intervals following an oral dose of CsA. Serial monitoring over a 24-hr period of the whole blood and plasma CsA levels by high-pressure liquid chromatography (HPLC) facilitated the correlation of blood level with the inhibition of lymphocyte proliferation assessed in patient cells and in patient plasma following an oral dose of CsA. Lymphocyte proliferation was determined by culture in both patient plasma and pooled normal plasma.

Through these studies we hoped to determine (1) to what extent metabolism and absorption of CsA was necessary for the detection of plasma inhibitory activity, (2) whether the clearance of inhibitory activity in the circulation was cyclic and reversible, (3) the duration of time in which an inhibitory factor could be detected in plasma and its association with CsA blood levels, (4) whether depressed lymphocyte responses seen in patient cells on CsA therapy was permanent, and (5) if a suppression of normal lymphocyte proliferation could be induced when cultured in the presence of plasma obtained from patients following CsA therapy.

MATERIALS AND METHODS

Patient Population

These studies were performed on patients receiving CsA in a prospective randomized clinical trial comparing a regimen of CsA and prednisone with conventional immunosuppressive therapy of anti-lymphocyte globulin (ALG), azathioprine, and prednisone. All kinetic studies were carried out within the first 10 days following transplantation. All patients were receiving a single oral dose of CsA at 12 mg/kg with concomitant prednisone therapy at ~1 mg/kg.

CsA Blood Levels

CsA whole blood and plasma levels were determined by high-pressure liquid chromatography (HPLC) according to the method of Sawchuk and Cartier.[10] Trough blood levels are determined just prior to the administration of the daily oral dose of CsA. Subsequently, heparinized blood is drawn every 3 hr over a 24-hr period and evaluated for blood level of CsA and inhibitory capacity as assessed in a mixed lymphocyte culture and mitogen-response assay.

Mitogen Stimulation in Alloantigen Stimulation

Patient peripheral blood lymphocytes (PBL) were isolated on Ficoll-Hypaque from blood drawn at trough and analyzed for the proliferative response to mitogenic stimulation with phytohemagglutinin 1% (PHA) and 20 μg of concanavalin A (Con A). Cells are cultured in the presence of either 20% patient autologous plasma drawn at each 3-hr interval or 20% pooled normal plasma. Cultures were incubated for 72 hr at 37°C and at 5% CO_2. Eighteen hours prior to the termination of the cultures, 0.1 μCi of tritiated thymidine was added to each well. Lymphocytes were harvested, and the tritium incorporation was determined using liquid scintillation. The mixed lymphocyte responses (MLR) were determined by culturing (10^5) patient lymphocytes with an irradiated (2000 rad) pool of lymphocytes from three normal individuals as stimulators. Cells were cultured for 5 days in the presence of either 20% patient autologous plasma or 20% normal pooled plasma. In order to evaluate the effectiveness of plasma from patients treated with CsA or inhibiting the proliferation of patient PBL following stimulation, the percentage of inhibition of the MLR and PHA responses was determined using patient or normal PBL cultured in the presence of patient plasma obtained at trough versus the proliferation detected when cells were in the presence of patient plasmas obtained following oral dose. The percentage of inhibition in the proliferative response occurring with the patient plasma at each 3-hr interval was then calculated. Also assessed was inhibitory activity detected with trough plasma by comparing it with proliferation of cells cultured in the presence of pooled normal plasma.

RESULTS

Twenty patients receiving oral CsA therapy were assessed in a 24-hr kinetic profile for the presence of inhibitory activity in plasma by determining the proliferative response of cells cultured in the presence of patient plasma obtained at serial 3-hr intervals post oral dose. Patient PBL (drawn at trough) and normal cells were isolated and stimulated with alloantigens and mitogens in the presence of 20% patient plasma obtained at each 3-hr interval. Of the 20 patients assessed for the presence of an inhibitory factor in plasma following oral CsA therapy, 12 additionally had whole-blood and plasma CsA levels determined by HPLC on each sample. Of these 12 patients, 11 had a single peak in CsA blood level at 3–6 hr post oral dose; CsA values returned to trough levels by 9–12 hr post oral dose. One patient indicated an absence of absorption of oral CsA with no detectable changes in blood level following a 12-mg/kg dose.

In following the detection of an inhibitory factor present in patient plasma following an oral dose of CsA, two patterns of inhibitory

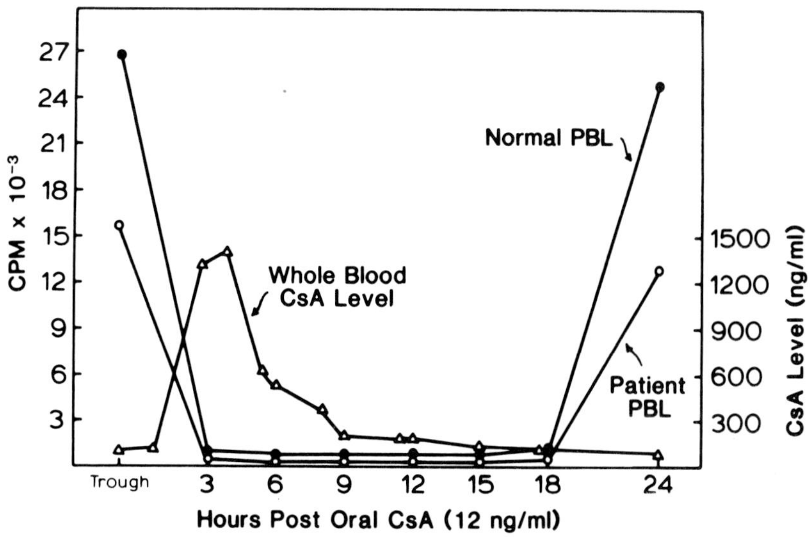

Fig. 1. Representative kinetic profile showing a single cycle of inhibitory activity. Whole-blood CsA levels (Δ) are compared to each plasma sample's ability to inhibit the proliferation (^3H incorporation) of normal PBL. (●) and patient PBL (O) stimulated with a pool of allogeneic stimulator cells.

activity were noted. Seven patients showed a single cycle of inhibitory activity detected in plasma samples drawn 3–21 hr post oral dose. Biphasic inhibitory kinetics were noted in 4 patients. The patient with no detectable CsA blood levels also showed no indication of inhibitory activity present in any of the plasma samples tested. Figure 1 is a representative kinetic profile for 7 patients taking 12 mg/kg of CsA orally in which whole-blood and plasma CsA levels were analyzed and which indicated a single cycle of inhibitory activity. Initially, CsA levels were low and rose to a peak 4–6 hr post oral dose. The level of CsA detected in the peripheral blood then rapidly decreased, returning to trough levels by 12 hr post oral dose. CsA blood levels remained low until the next oral dose was administered. In contrast, the proliferative responses of both patient and normal PBL stimulated with a pool of allogeneic cells in the presence of trough plasma were normal when compared to the response in pooled normal plasma. However, plasmas obtained 3–21 hr post oral dose were consistently inhibitory to the proliferation of both patient and normal cells. Lymphocyte proliferation remained suppressed by patient plasma despite declining levels of native CsA as measured by HPLC. The proliferative ability of lymphocytes was unaffected with plasma samples obtained ~20–24 hr post oral dose, similar to the proliferation detected in the presence of trough plasma. Thus, it appears that initially, CsA has potent immunosuppressive ability, which is correlated with a rapid increase in the CsA levels detected in peripheral blood as measured by HPLC. However, as CsA levels return to trough levels (12 hr post oral dose), the inhibition of lymphocyte proliferation by patient plasma samples obtained 15–21 hr post oral dose continues to be detected. A summary of these first seven patients is seen in Fig. 2, which indicates the presence of inhibitory activity in patient plasma following a single oral dose of CsA. CsA blood levels had returned to trough blood levels by 12 hr post oral dose in all seven patients. In addition, trough plasma was also inhibitory when compared to pooled normal plasma, averaging 65% of the response detected with pooled normal plasma. In all patients, the inhibition of patient lymphocytes was strongly correlated with inhibitory effects on normal PBL proliferation.

In examining the proliferative response of patient lymphocytes when compared to the response of normal lymphocytes, both cultured in pooled normal plasma, the relative response of patient lymphocytes was only mildly suppressed, averaging ~64% of normal. This depressed lymphocyte reactivity was probably due to steroids, since it was not detected in the absence of steroid therapy.

Several important conclusions can be drawn as a result of these observations. (1)

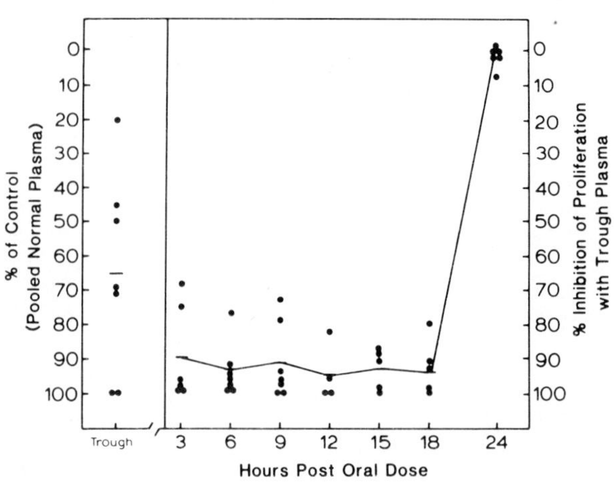

Fig. 2. **Summary of the inhibitory activity detected in the plasma of seven patients who showed a single cycle of inhibitory activity following a single oral dose of CsA. The left side compares the proliferation of patient cells in autologous plasma drawn at trough with the proliferation detected in pooled normal plasma. The right side indicates the percent of inhibition in the proliferation of patient cells cultured in the presence of plasma obtained just prior to oral dose compared with plasma samples obtained at 3-hr intervals post oral dose.**

Plasma obtained from patients receiving CsA has the ability of inhibiting the proliferative responses of *both* patient and normal peripheral blood lymphocytes. This inhibition was closely correlated in all of the patients studied ($r = > +0.90$). (2) These data suggest a plasma-inhibitory component present following oral CsA in the peripheral blood that may be responsible for the immunosuppressive action of CsA and the prolongation of graft survival. (3) There was no correlation between CsA blood levels and the presence of inhibitory activity detected in the plasma of all patients described in Fig. 2. This lack of correlation was probably due to the low CsA blood levels that occur at 12–24 hr post oral dose, while at the same time inhibitory activity remains present in the circulation for an extended 8–10 hr irrespective of blood levels. (4) These data suggest an alternate immunosuppressive agent present in the peripheral blood 18–24 hr post dose that is not measured by HPLC.

Further to document the presence of an alternate immunosuppressive agent (other than native drug) present in the peripheral blood following the oral dose of CsA, 4 of the 12 patients in whom blood levels were correlated with inhibitory activity had suggestive evidence of a biphasic distribution of inhibitory activity detected in the plasma following a single oral dose of CsA. This is represented by Fig. 3. As in the earlier patients, there is an initial phase of inhibitory activity that corresponds directly with increasing CsA blood levels as measured by HPLC. As the CsA blood levels declined (8–10 hr post oral dose), the inhibitory activity also began to decline, almost to trough levels by 12 hr post dose. This was the first cycle of inhibitory activity. By 15 hr post oral dose, however, strong inhibitory activity was again detected in the patient's plasma. This inhibitor was detected at 18 hr post oral dose but not in the 24-hr post oral dose sample. (The 24-hr plasma was drawn just prior to CsA administration the following day). This second cycle of inhibitory activity was associated with low levels of CsA as detected by HPLC.

In conclusion, (1) inhibitory activity as detected in patient plasma samples drawn post oral dose do not correlate with CsA blood levels as measured by HPLC. (2) The second cycle of inhibitory activity demonstrated in patient plasma, which was not measured by

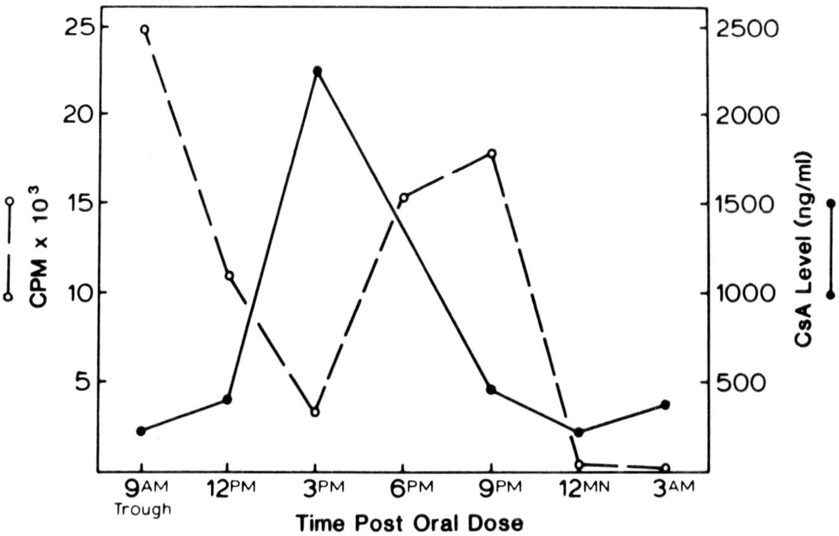

Fig. 3. Representative kinetic profile showing a dual cycle of inhibitory activity detected in a 24-hr period. Whole-blood CsA levels (●) are compared to each plasma sample's ability to inhibit the proliferation (^{3}H incorporation) of normal PBL (O) stimulated with a pool of allogeneic stimulator cells.

HPLC, suggests a second immunosuppressive agent (other than native drug) present in the circulation 15–20 hr after oral dose. This suggests that the metabolism of the drug is important for the demonstration of inhibitory activity and possibly for its immunosuppressive action in allograft survival.

Because of the large discrepancy in inhibitory activity vs. CsA blood level, we next tested whether CsA, when added to plasma at the same concentrations as detected in patient plasma, would inhibit the proliferation of normal PBL in a similar pattern as the patient plasma samples. Figure 4 compares the plasma CsA blood level of a patient over a 24-hr period as measured by HPLC, with the inhibitory activity detected in those particular plasma samples. Also plotted is the inhibitory activity demonstrated by normal plasma to which CsA was added at the same concentrations as detected in the patient plasma. As expected, there is a strong correlation between the inhibitory activity detected in spiked normal plasma and the actual CsA blood levels as measured by HPLC. Once again, very poor correlation was demonstrated with plasma CsA levels and inhibitory activity detected in patient plasma following a single oral dose of CsA. We conclude that the prolonged immunosuppressive activity detected in patient plasma following an oral dose of CsA suggests an additional mechanism of immunosuppressive action by CsA not associated with the native drug as detected by HPLC.

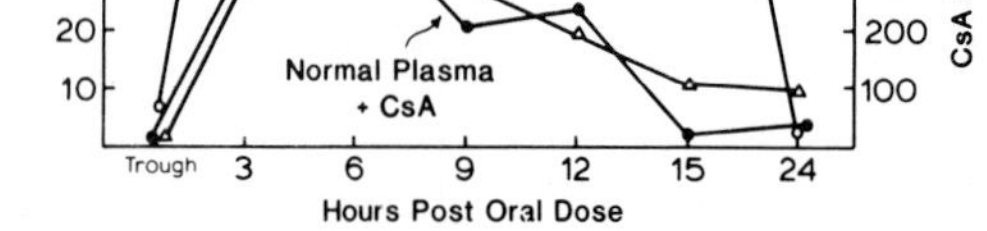

Fig. 4. A comparison of the inhibitory activity detected in patient plasma following oral CsA with inhibitory activity detected with normal plasma samples to which CsA was added at the same concentrations detected in the patient plasma samples with the use of HPLC. Plasma levels of CsA detected by HPLC (Δ) are compared to the percent of inhibition in lymphocyte proliferation when cultured with pooled normal plasma vs. patient plasma samples obtained following oral CsA (O) or normal plasma to which CsA was added (●).

DISCUSSION

Clinical studies have shown CsA to be effective in the prevention of allograft rejection, but how this immunosuppressive effect manifests itself at the cellular level is unknown. In this study, we have tried to compare the absorption and metabolism of CsA as reflected in the whole-blood and plasma drug levels measured by high-pressure liquid chromatography with the direct effects of CsA in abrogating patient immune responsiveness. How CsA blocks the events responsible for allograft rejection are not addressed here, but rather the immediate effects of CsA in patient plasma following an oral dose. Whole blood levels of CsA, which are inhibitory, correspond directly to concentrations that in vitro cause inhibition of MLC and mitogen responses. As the native drug levels decrease, a persistent blockade of lymphocyte reactivity is detected in the plasma. The presence of inhibitory activity in patient plasma is detected for an additional 8–10 hr beyond the time when blood levels have returned to those detected at trough. Some patients indicate a biphasic clearance of inhibitory activity present in the peripheral blood following a 12-mg/kg oral dose. In conjunction, Keown et al. also noted a rapid rise in the CsA blood levels occurring 1–3 hr after the oral dose, while the biological effect—suppression of MLC proliferative responses—was not detected until 6 hr post oral dose.[11] This also demonstrates the lack of correlation between actual blood levels and the biological suppression of lymphocyte proliferation.

The cyclic behavior of the inhibition of lymphocyte proliferation by patient plasma indicates a reversible effect on lymphocytes. Further, the proliferation of lymphocytes in patient plasma drawn at trough when compared to proliferation in the presence of pooled normal plasma is only mildly suppressed, occurring in both patient and normal PBL. This again is evidence that the immunosuppressive effect of CsA as seen in patients is demonstrable in plasma and not a permanent effect on the lymphoid cells themselves. The mild suppression of the lymphocytes' ability to proliferate can be explained by the effect of steroids[12] (known to significantly affect lymphocyte function) over prolonged periods of time rather than from CsA. Our patient data are supported by the in vitro findings of Larsson[8] and Borel,[1] who showed rapidly reversible effects of CsA on lymphocyte function.

The data presented here showing the lack of correlation of blood level and with the inhibitory activity present in the plasma suggest the formation of a CsA metabolite occurring ~12–18 hr post oral dose that has potent immunosuppressive activity and is not detected by HPLC. Donatsch et al. (Sandoz)[13] report that 10–15 metabolites of CsA have been detected in the blood and urine of patients receiving CsA. Further evidence supporting the presence of a metabolite is the fact that the clearance of the native CsA molecule occurs within 27 hr post dose as measured by HPLC. The clearance of the radiolabeled CsA molecule (both the native drug and metabolites) is 110 hr.[14] This again suggests that residual CsA metabolites remain in the circulation long after the native drug has been cleared. Since Sandoz has reported some cross-reactivity between native CsA and one of its metabolites as measured by the radioimmunoassay,[13] it may be possible to better correlate the second cycle of inhibitory activity with the radioimmunoassay. Further, since many institutions currently utilizing CsA in clinical trials are administering it twice daily, the second and prolonged phase of inhibitory activity would remain undetected, being overshadowed by the presence of native drug.

These data demonstrate the potential importance of CsA metabolism in maintaining its immunosuppressive activity. The association of demonstrable immunosuppressive activity in vitro with allograft survival is not completely clear. It is interesting to note that 1 remaining patient of the 12 in which both inhibitory activity and CsA blood levels were analyzed showed no change in CsA blood level following a 12-mg/kg oral dose, as well as no detectable inhibitory activity present in the plasma. This is the only patient of the 12 who subsequently lost the allograft to rejection. In addition, the inability to detect inhibitory activity in the plasma, even with concomitant steroid therapy, further emphasizes that the presence of inhibitory activity in plasma is due to CsA and not steroids.

The mechanism of immunosuppression in CsA that causes the lack of lymphocyte reactivity is unknown. More important is the existence of an alternative to native CsA that also blocks cell-mediated responses. Whether both the native drug and the metabolite have similar effects on helper T-cell function will require further investigation. We speculate as to its generation and its effects on preventing allograft rejection.

To summarize, the presence of CsA in patient plasma can block in vitro cell-mediated responses of both patient and normal cells. The strong immunosuppressive effect on lymphocyte proliferation seen 4–6 hr post oral dose returns to normal by 20–24 hr after the initial dose. A cyclic behavior of plasma inhibitory activity was demonstrated in the patient's circulation following an oral dose as emphasized by the inhibition of proliferative response of lymphocytes stimulated with alloantigens and/or mitogens. This suggests that the presence of CsA in plasma is necessary for its blockage of lymphocyte responsiveness and thus the prevention of allograft rejection. The questions of absorption, metabolism, and immunosuppressive action need further investigation, but the suggestion of a secondary immunosuppressive agent following CsA therapy extends the complexity in our understanding of the in vivo mechanism of CsA's immunosuppressive action.

ACKNOWLEDGMENTS

We wish to thank Mr. Tom Cunningham, Ms. Janet Conway, and Ms. Sheryl Olson for their excellent technical assistance and Ms. Jean Hume for her secretarial help.

REFERENCES

1. Borel JF: Immunology 31:631, 1976
2. Keown PA, Essery GL, Stiller CR, et al: Transplant Proc 3:380, 1981
3. White DG, Plumb AM, Pawelec G, et al: Transplantation 27:55, 1979
4. Dunn DC, White DJG, Herbertson BM, et al: Transplantation 27:359, 1979
5. Deeg HJ, Storb R, Gerhard-Miller L, et al: 1980
6. Fidelus RK, Ferguson RM, Widmer MB, et al: Transplantation
7. Palacios R: Cell Immunol 161:453, 1981
8. Larsson EL: J Immunol 124:2828, 1980
9. Tutschka PJ, Beschorner WE, Allison AC, et al: Nature 280:148, 1979
10. Sawchuk R, Cartier LL: Clin Chem 27:1368, 1981
11. Keown PA, Stiller CR, Ulan RA, et al: Lancet 1:686, 1981
12. Cupps TR, Fauci AS: Immunol Rev 65:133, 1982
13. Donatsch P, Abisch E, Hamberger M, et al: J Immunoassay 2:19, 1981
14. Beveridge T, Gratwohl A, Michot F, et al: Current Therapeutic Res 30:5, 1981

Population of Cyclosphosphamide-Sensitive T Suppressor Cells Maintain Cyclosporine-Induced Allograft Survival

J. W. Kupiec-Weglinski, P. A. Lear, T. B. Strom, and N. L. Tilney

CYCLOSPORINE (CsA), a biologically active fungal metabolite, leads a new generation of drugs possessing remarkable immunosuppressive properties in clinical and experimental organ transplantation.[1] However, its complex mechanism of action has not been clearly defined. CsA appears effective in the early stages of T-lymphocyte activation.[2] Specifically, it may inhibit selectively induction of T helper cells (T_h)[3,4] and the generation of T cytotoxic effector cells (T_c).[3,5] Alternatively, the ability to facilitate transplantation tolerance following a limited period of treatment in graft recipients suggests that this agent favors the suppressor-regulatory arm of the immune response.[6-8] Additionally, inhibition of the secretion of essential lymphocyte-dependent biologic amplification factors may play a pivotal role in the mechanism of CsA action. Thus, the drug appears to inhibit the production and/or release of interleukin 2 (IL-2) by T_h and prevents activation of T_h by reducing the availability of interleukin 1 (IL-1) from adherent cells.[9-11]

Previous studies in our laboratory have demonstrated that 7 days of CsA therapy only inevitably result in permanent acceptance of cardiac allografts in the strongly histoincompatible (LEW × BN)F1 → LEW rat strain combination. The data from in vivo and in vitro investigations support the concept that CsA-mediated unresponsiveness is created at least in part by sparing and/or amplification of alloantigen-specific T suppressor lymphocytes (T_s).[5,12-14] In the present report, attempts have been made to re-create the events of acute rejection toward long-standing cardiac allografts in CsA-treated hosts, and further supportive evidence for this concept is presented.

MATERIALS AND METHODS

Animals and Grafting Procedures

Inbred adult male Lewis rats (LEW, $RT1^l$), weighing 200–300 g, served as recipients of heterotopic abdominal cardiac allografts from Lewis × Brown Norway hybrids (LEW × BN)F1 (Microbiological Associates, Walkersville, Md.). Orthotopic full-thickness skin allografts from Brown Norway (BN, $RT1^n$) were grafted into unmodified LEW in order to generate alloimmune lymphocytes.

Therapeutic Host Manipulation

CsA (Sandoz Inc., Basel, Switzerland) was dissolved in olive oil and administered to cardiac allografted animals (15 mg/kg i.m.) for 7 days beginning the day of transplantation. In the (LEW × BN)F1 → LEW rat strain combination this regimen produces indefinite allograft survival.[12-14] CsA-modified recipients of cardiac allografts functioning well for at least 20 days were used throughout the studies. CR-rat T-cell growth factor (partially purified IL-2–rich conditioned medium, IL-2CM; Collaborative Research Inc., Waltham, Mass.) was dissolved in RPMI 1640/10% FCS medium to appropriate concentration and stored at 4°C until use. 25–100 half-maximal units (U) of IL-2CM was inoculated i.v. into experimental animals for 5 consecutive days. Cyclophosphamide (CY; Sigma Chemical Co., St. Louis, Mo.) was dissolved in sterile saline immediately before use and injected i.p. as a single dose of 20–100 mg/kg.

Cell Suspensions

Specifically sensitized splenic leukocytes (SSL) or thoracic duct lymphocytes (STDL) were obtained from unmodified LEW that had acutely rejected BN skin grafts. SSL were prepared by mincing and expressing the

---

From the Departments of Surgery and Medicine at Brigham and Women's Hospital and the Surgical Research Laboratory, Harvard Medical School, Boston, Mass.

Supported by Grant AI 19071-09.

Reprint requests should be addressed to Dr. J. W. Kupiec-Weglinski, Department of Surgery, Brigham and Women's Hospital, Boston, MA 02115.

0041-1345/83/1505-0025$01.00/0

spleens through a 60-gauge stainless steel mesh into RPMI 1640/5% FCS medium. Erythrocytes were lysed by a brief treatment with Tris-buffered ammonium chloride (0.83%, pH 7.21), as described.[14] STDL were collected fresh from the donor,[15] centrifuged, and resuspended in medium to appropriate concentrations.

SSL Labeling with ^{111}Indium-oxine

SSL were incubated with ^{111}Indium-oxine (^{111}In; Medi-Physics Inc., San Francisco, CA, sp. act 20 mCi/ml, 10–15μCi/10^8 cells) for 15 min at room temperature.[16] The cells were then washed three times, counted, and infused i.v. at a concentration of 3–4 $\times$ 10^7/ml into the groups of CsA- and CsA + CY-treated graft recipients. More than 80% of the radioactivity was consistently incorporated in the cell fraction, and the viability of labeled cells was greater than 90%. Twenty-four hours after transfer, the radioactivity of excised organs and tissues was determined in a well-type gamma counter and expressed as a percentage of total injected dose per gram of tissue sample.

Measurement of IL-2 Inhibitor

The activity of circulating T_s-derived IL-2 inhibitor[17] was measured in serum by its ability to inhibit proliferation of a strictly IL-2–dependent Kendall-Smith–type murine cytolytic T-cell line (CTLL-2).[18] CTLL-2 were harvested from the cell line, washed twice, and resuspended in RPMI 1640 medium containing 5 m*M* HEPES acid buffer, 5 $\times$ 10^{-5}-*M* 2-mercaptoethanol, and 10% FCS to a final concentration of 8 $\times$ 10^4/ml. 4 $\times$ 10^3 cells (50 μl) were then incubated with 2 U of IL-2CM in each well of a flat-bottomed Micro Test II tissue culture plate (Falcon Products, Oxnard, CA). When measuring IL-2 inhibitor, 0.1 ml of serially diluted and filter-sterilized (0.22 μm) experimental sera were added at the initiation of cultures. Triplicate cultures were incubated for 18 hr at 37°C in a humidified atmosphere of 5% CO_2 in air, then pulsed with methyl-^{3}H-thymidine (^{3}H-TdR; New England Nuclear, Boston, MA, sp. act 6.7 C/m*M*, 1 μCi/well), and harvested 4 hr later on glass-fiber strips by using an automatic cell harvester.[18] ^{3}H-TdR uptake by CTLL-2 cells was measured in a liquid scintillation spectrophotometer.

Statistics

Statistical significance was ascertained using Student's paired t test.

RESULTS

Re-creation of Immune Responsiveness Toward Cardiac Allografts in CsA-Treated Rats

In an attempt to restore acute rejection of long-standing cardiac allografts, groups of 4–10 CsA-modified recipients were subjects for various treatment protocols (Fig. 1). Passive transfer of 10^8 SSL, which contains ± 60% T cells (W3/13+) and which can be subdivided equally into T_h(W3/25+) and T cytotoxic/suppressor ($T_{c/s}$, MRC OX8$^+$) fractions by monoclonal antibody flow cytometry,[14] did not influence otherwise indefinite graft survival, even if multiple doses totaling 5 $\times$ 10^8 cells were transferred [Fig. 1 (A)]. Infusion of 25–100 U of IL-2CM alone produced eventual late rejection after 4–7 weeks in only 30% of animals. Similarly, SSL administered concomitantly with IL-2CM could not reproducibly induce graft destruction, even if combined with total body x-radiation (750 rad) applied to destroy host lymphoid cells. As the spleen is a poor source

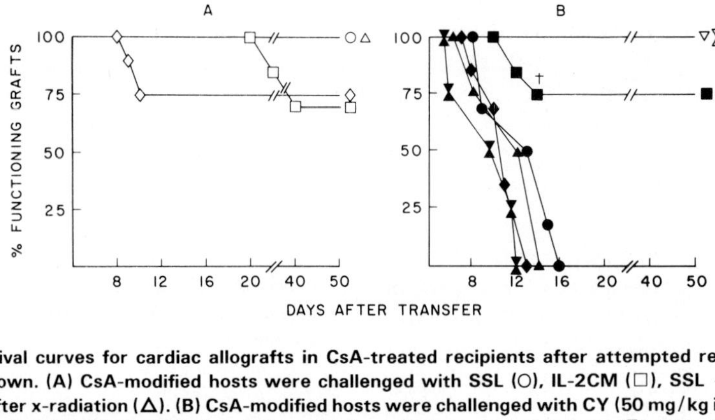

Fig. 1. Survival curves for cardiac allografts in CsA-treated recipients after attempted re-creation of acute rejection are shown. (A) CsA-modified hosts were challenged with SSL (○), IL-2CM (□), SSL + IL-2CM (◇), and SSL + IL-2CM after x-radiation (△). (B) CsA-modified hosts were challenged with CY (50 mg/kg i.p., ■), followed by SSL (●), SSL + IL-2CM (♦), IL-2CM (▽), SSL + SL from CsA-treated recipients (⧖), SSL + SL from CsA + CY-treated recipients (⧗), and SSL + SL from normal rats (▲).

of recirculating lymphocytes capable of generating delayed-type hypersensitivity responses such as graft rejection,[19] the potency of transferred STDL was next evaluated. Infusion of 10^8–10^9 STDL (W3/13+ > 85%, W3/25+/MRC OX8$^+$ ratio = 2.5–3.0) was no more effective in restoring immune responsiveness in CsA-treated hosts than SSL. These results suggest that under in vivo conditions, CsA-modified hosts are capable of negating the potential of both alloimmune lymphocytes and exogenous lymphokine to induce allograft rejection.

Therefore, in the second series of experiments, CsA-treated and grafted hosts were challenged with CY, which inactivates T_s and increases an apparent sensitization by converting a state of low responsiveness into one of high responsiveness in vivo.[17,20] Administration of CY (20–100 mg/kg i.p.) was followed 2 days later by infusion of SSL and/or IL-2CM [Fig. 1 (B)]. CY (20 mg/kg) failed to abrogate CsA-mediated appearance of T_s. Thus, 2 days later, despite a sharp fall in the white blood cell count (WBC, $\pm 4 \times 10^6$/ml, vs. $\pm 9 \times 10^6$/ml in CsA-modified hosts), transfer of SSL ± IL-2CM could not induce graft rejection. CY at 50 mg/kg was the lowest dose that apparently abolished T_s such that all allografts in recipients given this dose underwent acute rejection following infusion of 10^8 SSL alone or combined with 50 U of IL-2CM (MST ± SD = 12.8 ± 3.1 and 11.0 ± 1.9 days, respectively). Although treatment of CsA-modified hosts with 80 or 100 mg/kg of CY initially produced the same degree of leukopenia as 50 mg/kg ($\pm 2.3 \times 10^6$/ml), IL-2CM proved to be an essential factor in this model for restoring full immune responsiveness in addition to alloimmune cells (MST ± SD = 11.5 ± 1.8 and 9.4 ± 0.9 days, respectively). The failure to restore immunocompetence in recipients challenged with high doses of CY without further treatment coincided with severe irreversible leukopenia, inevitably resulting in death within 10 days. Although administration of IL-2CM alone into the rats inoculated with high doses of CY again could not induce graft rejection, such treatment considerably prolonged recipient survival. Possibly multiple factors in the conditioned medium sustain and support the growth of residual lymphoid and myeloid cells in these severely depleted animals.[21]

We can assume that CY facilitates immune responsiveness by destroying the cellular mechanism preventing i.v.-infused SSL from expressing their cytotoxic function. If this anticytotoxic activity is mediated by a population of CY-sensitive T_s, it should be possible to counteract CY therapy and transfer of SSL by repopulating with putative T_s from CsA-treated and grafted hosts. The fate of the grafts was thus assessed in CsA-modified hosts receiving the optimal dose of CY(50 mg/kg) and SSL (10^8) followed 1 day later by i.v. infusion of 10^8 splenic leukocytes (SL) from CsA-treated hosts bearing well-functioning grafts [Fig. 1 (B)]. Such passive transfer of SL completely inhibited graft rejection. In contrast, administration of SL from normal untreated rats had no effect on the outcome of combined CY + SSL therapy (MST ± SD = 12.3 ± 2.9 days). Additionally, treatment of CsA hosts with CY 1 day before harvesting the cells completely ablated the capacity of their SL to suppress CY-facilitated rejection (MST ± SD = 9.75 ± 2.6 days). This represents direct proof that CsA-modified recipients of organ allografts contain a population of CY-sensitive T cells that suppress the action of passively transferred SSL. Finally, SL (10^6) from CsA-treated and grafted hosts adoptively transferred into normal syngeneic secondary recipients improved (LEW × BN)F1 test-graft survival to ±16 days. In contrast, SL from CsA + CY (50 mg/kg)–treated hosts had apparently lost suppressor activity and were totally ineffectual following transfer (test-graft survival = 6.8 ± 1.0 days, $p < 0.001$).

Lymphocyte Migration Studies

Having demonstrated that the CsA-mediated unresponsive state could be reproducibly abolished only after treatment with CY, the traffic of adoptively transferred ^{111}In-labeled SSL was followed in these complex recipients (Table 1). These experiments were designed to test the hypothesis that CY therapy might induce an alteration in lymphoid cell migration, and a return to normal trafficking might be responsible for inducing graft rejection. In normal rats, SSL homed preferentially to the spleen ("ecotaxis") when compared to the other peripheral lymphoid tissues. CsA-modified graft recipients showed a profound alteration of this physiological phenomenon, with SSL localized in much higher numbers in lymph nodes, accompanied by a concomitant fall in splenic accumulation. Interestingly, a fall in bone marrow sequestration was also noted. CsA-treated and grafted hosts further modified by CY therapy demonstrated in some aspects a return toward normal physiologic migration patterns; specifically, there was an increase in SSL uptake by spleen and marrow. However, there was a further increase in lymph node sequestration, probably due to prior CY-induced severe depletion of the lymphocyte recirculating pool. The findings of these migration studies might be explained on the basis of different debris clearance from these anatomically dissimilar organs. Thus, the spleen is aptly suited to clear dead cells via its venous drainage, whereas the lymph nodes become "clogged" by cell debris in the efferent channels. Although it is purely conjecture, we feel that overall CY therapy does induce a return toward normal cell migration, and that cannot be easily reflected because of anatomic disparities. Finally, in both CsA- and CsA+CY-treated hosts, SSL showed initially equal and preferential accumulation in the allograft when compared to the native heart (grafted heart/native heart activity ratio = 5.4 ± 2.4 and 7.8 ± 2.8, respectively). As CsA has been shown not to alter the immunogenicity of the graft over time,[14] high accumulation of SSL is not unexpected. Furthermore, CY treatment may alter the "immunologic microenvironment" of the graft. Thus, in both treatment protocols there was high graft sequestration of SSL, but with abrogation of a CY-sensitive

Table 1. Accumulation of ^{111}In-Labeled SSL in Organs and Tissues of Experimental Animals*

Organ or Tissue	CsA-Treated Graft Recipient (I)	CsA + CY-Treated Graft Recipient† (II)	Normal Rat (III)
Peripheral blood	0.17	0.15	0.19
Peripheral lymph nodes‡§	11.50††	16.57††	7.55††
Mesenteric lymph nodes‖	11.64††	15.69††	7.38‡‡
Spleen¶	27.46††	34.06	37.09‡‡
Bone marrow**	0.45††	0.83	0.72††
Lung	0.85††	1.22	1.05‡‡
Kidney	0.67	0.58	0.64
Liver	3.75	3.67	4.11
Native heart	0.07	0.06	0.07
Grafted heart	0.34	0.44	—
	I vs. II	II vs. III	I vs. III

*There were 4–7 animals in each group. Results are expressed as a percentage of total dose injected per gram of tissue. Means are shown.

†CsA-modified hosts were treated with CY (50 mg/kg i.p.); 2 days later ^{111}In-labeled SSL were infused i.v.

‡Radioactivity of iliac, brachial, and cervical lymph nodes.

§The weight of peripheral lymph nodes in CsA-treated hosts = 0.3 ± 0.08 g; after CY treatment, 0.23 ± 0.04 g ($p < 0.025$).

‖The weight of mesenteric lymph nodes in CsA-treated hosts = 0.2 ± 0.09 g; after CY treatment, 0.09 ± 0.03 g ($p < 0.01$).

¶The weight of the spleen in CsA-treated hosts = 0.69 ± 0.1 g; after CY treatment, 0.4 ± 0.04 g ($p < 0.0001$)

**Radioactivity of the femur.

††$p < 0.005$.

‡‡$p < 0.01$.

population, transferred cells were capable of expressing full functional reactivity.

IL-2 Inhibitor in Experimental Animals

In order to monitor the activity of a circulating IL-2 inhibitor, inhibition of proliferation of an IL-2–dependent CTLL-2 cell line by sera from CsA- or CsA+CY-treated and grafted hosts was used as a test system (Fig. 2). CTLL-2 cultured without IL-2CM showed only background incorporation of ^{3}H-TdR. In contrast, the cells proliferated progressively in increasing concentrations of IL-2CM; the maximum cpm response occurred when CTLL-2 were cultured with 1–5 U of IL-2CM/well. Sera from CsA-treated hosts added at the start of cultures profoundly inhibited the proliferation of CTLL-2 in a dose-dependent manner, suggesting a high level of circulating IL-2 inhibitor in vivo. Next, the concept of IL-2 inhibitor activity being under the control of CY-sensitive T_s[17] has been investigated. Indeed, pretreatment of CsA-modified recipients 2 days earlier with CY (50 mg/kg i.p.) resulted in reduction of IL-2 inhibitor; consequently, the ability of these sera to exert suppression of CTLL-2 proliferation in vitro became significantly diminished, and virtually abrogated at lower concentrations of sera. Similarly, increasing concentration of IL-2CM lessened the effects of IL-2 inhibitor. Some disparity was observed in the CTLL-2 responsiveness from different batches of sera, probably due to variability in the level of inhibitor activity in individual rats. However, the general pattern was as described.

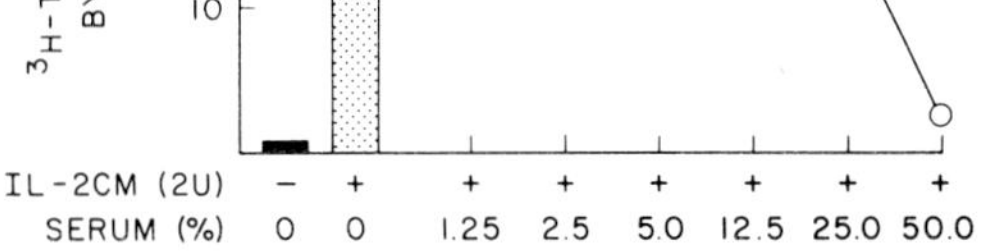

Fig. 2. Titration of IL-2 inhibitor in serum of CsA (O)- or CsA + CY (●)-treated and grafted hosts. CTLL-2 (4 × 10^3) were incubated for 18 hr with 2 U of IL-2CM. ^{3}H-TdR incorporation was determined 4 hr later, and the data from a representative experiment are presented. The SD of a triplicate culture did not exceed 10%. Similar results were obtained in four separate trials.

DISCUSSION

The studies presented have sought to recreate the events of acute rejection of longstanding cardiac allografts in CsA-treated rats by overriding the immunologic mechanisms governing their acceptance. This could only be reproducibly achieved through abrogation of T_s by a combined therapy, comprising CY and alloimmune cells. Thus, it can be concluded that CY-sensitive T_s are crucial in the acquisition and maintenance of transplantation tolerance after CsA treatment.

The anticancer action of CY, with particular reference to the delayed hypersensitivity reactions in tumor systems, has been well established.[22,23] Previously there have also been reports that CY could abolish the effect of immunologic enhancement of liver allografts in baboons[24] and cardiac allografts in rats.[25] The efficacy of CY depends on its dose and the timing with respect to antigen challenge. CY probably facilitates cellular immune responses by the destruction of active T_s or their precursors; this results in conversion of the state of low responsiveness to one of sensitivity in vivo.[9,17,20,22,23] It has also been recently postulated that natural killer (NK)–cell activity can be strongly augmented by CY treatment. However, the role of NK cells in allograft immunity is uncertain; neonatal thymectomy results in supranormal NK activity, yet organ allografts invariably survive indefinitely in these individuals.[26]

CsA may play a passive role in the emergence of T_s, since the driving force for their activation is alloantigen. Indeed, the evidence for T_s involvement in mediating transplantation tolerance in humans and animal models is becoming increasingly well founded.[3,8,12–14] In the present studies as well as those by others,[27]

T_s have been shown to be potent in suppressing huge numbers of transferred mature alloimmune cells. Most recently, we have noted that in CsA-treated hosts, cortical thymocytes (presumably T_s) migrate preferentially to cardiac allografts and may act locally to prevent rejection. Additionally, the generation and amplification of CsA-induced CY-sensitive T_s in vivo was demonstrated by the success of thymic grafts from CsA- but not from CsA+CY-modified hosts to improve significantly the survival of specific cardiac allografts in otherwise untreated secondary hosts (unpublished data).

It has been postulated that after CsA administration, T_c precursors fail to differentiate into full effector cells, distorting the relative numbers of T_c and T_s lymphocytes; this may correlate with T_c inability to respond to T_h-derived IL-2.[3] On the other hand, activated T_s may severely limit the function of IL-2 by elaborating a lymphokine that specifically inhibits its action.[17] Sera of CsA-treated and grafted hosts did in fact contain high levels of an IL-2 inhibitor, whereas sera of CsA- and CY-treated hosts did not. Thus we can assume that CY eliminated a T_s population that elaborates IL-2 inhibitor, subsequently allowing transferred alloimmune cells to express fully their cytotoxic function. The inability of exogenous IL-2CM to modify the immune unresponsiveness of CsA-treated hosts correlates with other studies that have shown that inoculated lymphokine is rendered inactive in only a few minutes, even in unmodified animals.[28] However, we do have strong evidence that IL-2 works in vivo by augmenting immune responsiveness toward cardiac allografts in T cell–depleted B rats;[15] this is closely associated with marked cellular infiltration of the graft (absent if cells alone are transferred). The varying levels of IL-2 inhibitor between these two experimental models (high in CsA-treated, low in B rats) confirms the different manner in which allografts are accepted. T-cell subpopulations appear necessary for elaboration of IL-2 and IL-2 inhibitor. Indeed, the concept of circulating IL-2–inhibitory factors is an attractive one, which would have the effect of checking any spurious peripheral activity. Thus, IL-2 producers and responders need to exist in close proximity for optimal cooperation. CsA may work (partially) in vivo by modifying lymphokine production; a population of CY-sensitive T_s present within the graft produce suppressor factors that are locally active and are ultimately responsible for allograft survival.

REFERENCES

1. Bordes-Aznar J, Tilney NL: J Clin Surg 1:53, 1982
2. Wiesinger D, Borel JF: Immunobiology 156:454, 1979
3. Hess AD, Tutschka PJ: J Immunol 124:2601, 1980
4. Leapman SB, Filo RS, Smith EJ, et al: Transplant Proc 13:405, 1981
5. Wang BS, Heacock EH, Collins KH, et al: J Immunol 127:89, 1981
6. Borel JF, Feurer C, Magnee C, et al: Immunology 32:1017, 1977
7. Green CL, Allison AC: Lancet 1:1182, 1978
8. Tutschka PJ, Beschorner WE, Allison AC, et al: Nature (Lond) 280:5718, 1979
9. Bunjes D, Hardt C, Röllinghoff M, et al: Eur J Immunol 11:657, 1981
10. Larsson EL: J Immunol 124:2828, 1980
11. Palacios R: Cell Immunol 61:453, 1981
12. Baldwin WM III, Hutchinson IF, Meijer CJ, et al: Transplantation 31:117, 1981
13. Hutchinson IF, Shadur CA, Duarte AJS, et al: Transplantation 32:210, 1981
14. Bordes-Aznar J, Kupiec-Weglinski JW, Duarte AJS, et al: Transplantation 35:185, 1983
15. Clason AE, Duarte AJS, Kupiec-Weglinski JW, et al: J Immunol 129:252, 1982
16. Oluwole S, Wang T, Fawwaz R, et al: Transplantation 31:51, 1981
17. Hardt C, Röllinghoff M, Pfizenmaier K, et al: J Exp Med 154:262, 1981
18. Gautan SC, Hilfiker ML, Battisto JR: J Immunol 130:533, 1983
19. Hall BM, Dorsch S, Roser B: J Exp Med 147:878, 1978
20. Röllinghoff M, Starzinski-Powitz A, Pfizenmaier K, et al: J Exp Med 145:455, 1977
21. Lipton JM, Nathan DG: Progress in Clinical and Biological Research 58:57, 1981
22. North RJ: J Exp Med 155:1063, 1982

23. Yu S, Lannin DR, Tsui-Collins AL, et al: Cancer Res 40:2756, 1980

24. Myburgh JA, Smit JA: Transplantation 14:227, 1972

25. Marquet R, Heysteek G: J Immunol 115:405, 1975

26. Herberman RB: Hospital Practice 4:83, 1982

27. White DJG, Timmerman W, Davies MS, et al: Transplant Proc 13:379, 1981

28. Donohue JM, Rosenberg SA: J Immunol 130:2203, 1983

Effects of Cyclosporine on the Efferent Limb of the Immune Response

M. Mochizuki, R. B. Nussenblatt, T. Kuwabara, and I. Gery

MOST STUDIES ON cyclosporine (CsA) have focused on its effect on the afferent limb of the immune response, namely, the capacity of the drug to suppress processes such as the sensitization against foreign antigens[1,2] or development of experimental autoimmune diseases.[2,3] However, recent studies on experimental animals[4,5] and our data on uveitic patients[6] indicate that CsA is also capable of inhibiting processes of the efferent limb, which are mediated by presensitized lymphocytes. The present study is aimed at further examining the CsA effect on two immune processes of the efferent limb: (1) the delayed-type skin hypersensitivity (DTH) and (2) the adoptive transfer of experimental autoimmune uveitis (EAU), an ocular disease that is actively induced in rats by immunization with the retinal S-antigen (S-Ag).[7] This EAU is believed to be an animal model for certain human ocular entities.[8]

MATERIALS AND METHODS

Animals

Lewis rats of both sexes, 8–12 weeks of age, purchased from M.A. Bioproducts (Walkersville, MD), were used.

Immune Responses to Bovine Gamma Globulin (BGG)

Rats were immunized with a single injection into one hind footpad consisting of 100 μg BGG (Miles Laboratories, Elkhart, IN) emulsified in complete Freund's adjuvant (CFA; DIFCO Laboratories, Detroit, MI, with 2 mg/ml *Mycobacterium tuberculosis* H37), in a volume of 0.1 ml. The animals were skin-tested 12 days after immunization by an intracutaneous injection of BGG, 60 μg in 0.1 ml phosphate-buffered saline (PBS), and their responses were read after 3 hr (Arthus) or 20 hr (delayed). The responses were assessed according to the size of induration (diameter, in mm). Some of the rats were also tested on the following day for their immediate hypersensitivity reactions: 5 μg BGG in 50 μl PBS was injected into the dermis of the dorsal side of one ear, while the second ear was injected with PBS for control. Five minutes later, 0.5 ml of 1% Evans blue solution was injected intravenously, and the response was read after 10 min.

Adoptive Transfer of EAU

Donor rats were immunized with 30 μg S-Ag (kindly provided by Drs. Wacker, Shichi, and El-Saied and prepared as described by Wacker et al.[7]) emulsified in CFA and injected into both hind footpads, 0.1 ml per footpad. Twelve days after immunization, the draining popliteal lymph nodes were removed and cell suspensions were prepared and washed twice. Cultures were set up in multiwell plates (Linbro, Hamden, CT, 24 × 17 mm) and consisted of 4×10^6 cells in 2 ml RPMI 1640 medium with HEPES (GIBCO, Grand Island, NY) supplemented with streptomycin (100 μg/ml), penicillin (100 U/ml), 2-mercaptoethanol (5×10^{-5} *M*) and 5% heat-inactivated fetal calf serum (FCS; GIBCO). The cultures were stimulated with S-Ag at 2 μg/ml. After incubation for 72 hr at 37°C with 5% CO_2, the cells were collected and washed twice with RPMI 1640 medium. The cells were injected intraperitoneally to normal recipient rats. Development of EAU was determined by daily clinical examination, and changes were further evaluated histologically after the rats were sacrificed. Blood samples were collected by heart puncture before sacrifice, and levels of antibodies to S-Ag in the sera were kindly determined by Dr. J. P. Faure, using the ELISA as described.[9] Levels of both IgG and IgE antibodies were determined.

Treatment with Drugs

CsA (a generous gift from Sandoz Ltd., Basel, Switzerland) and dexamethasone (DEX; Sigma, St. Louis, MO) were dissolved in olive oil and administered subcutaneously. Control rats were injected with olive oil alone. Rats tested for skin responses to BGG were injected with a daily drug dose 20 hr before being tested and with half daily doses 4 hr before and 4 hr after the skin test. Recipients of EAU were treated on days −1 to +6 post cell transfer.

From the Laboratory of Vision Research and Clinical Branch, National Eye Institute, National Institutes of Health, Bethesda, MD.

Supported in part by the U.S.-Japan Exchange Scientist Program in Vision Research.

Reprint requests should be addressed to Dr. M. Mochizuki, National Eye Institute, NIH, Bldg. 6, Rm 232, Bethesda, MD 20205.

0041-1345/83/1505-0026$01.00/0

RESULTS

Effects of CsA on Skin Responses

Figure 1 summarizes data of six experiments in which CsA and DEX were tested for their effect on skin responses of immunized rats. Treatment with CsA had no effect on the Arthus skin responses but markedly suppressed the DTH responses in a dose-dependent manner. Histologic examination of the tested skin sites of CsA-treated rats showed suppression of the infiltration by mononuclear cells. Unlike the selective effect by CsA, treatment with DEX suppressed both the Arthus and the DTH responses. Subgroups of the immunized rats (4 each) were also tested for immediate hypersensitivity reaction. CsA treatment did not affect this reaction, while DEX inhibited it (data not shown).

Effects of CsA on Adoptive Transfer of EAU

Table 1 summarizes the results concerning the CsA effects on adoptive transfer of EAU. All recipients treated with olive oil developed EAU within 5–7 days and exhibited moderate levels of antibodies to S-Ag. Treatment of recipients with CsA completely inhibited the appearance of EAU in these rats clinically as well as histologically. Yet the treated recipients demonstrated antibodies (both IgG and IgE) to S-Ag with levels similar or just slightly lower than those in the control recipients.

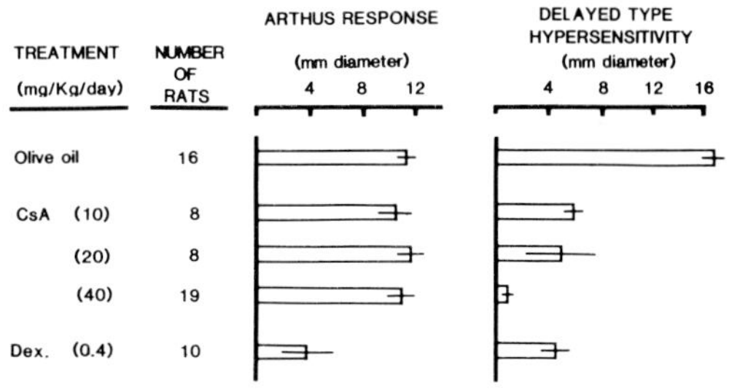

Fig. 1. Effect of CsA and DEX on skin responses of rats immunized with BGG (summary of six different experiments).

DISCUSSION

The data reported here demonstrate that CsA could efficiently inhibit the two tested immune responses of the efferent limb, i.e., the skin DTH response and the adoptive transfer of EAU. These findings confirm and extend those reported by Borel and his colleagues showing that CsA inhibits the adoptive transfer of another disease, experimental allergic encephalomyelitis.[4,5] Our results with the skin responses of rats further underlined the selectivity of the CsA effect: This drug inhibited only the cell-mediated DTH, having no effect on the immune complex–mediated inflammation of the Arthus type or on the immediate hypersensitivity mediated by mast-cell products. The selectivity of the CsA effect was further exhibited by the effect of DEX, which inhibited all three skin responses.

Of interest also was the finding that CsA

Table 1. Inhibition by Cyclosporine of Adoptively Transferred EAU

Rat No.	Cells Transferred (× 10^6)	Cyclosporine (10 mg/kg/day)	EAU		Serum Antibodies to S-Antigen*	
			Onset (days)	Severity	IgG	IgE
1	32	No	5	+++	0.95	0.15
2	22	No	6	++	0.80	0.08
3	20	No	5	+++	0.66	0.07
4	20	No	7	++	0.61	0.07
5	14	No	5	++	0.87	0.13
6	32	Yes	—	0	0.98	0.08
7	22	Yes	—	0	0.89	0.08
8	20	Yes	—	0	0.40	0.03
9	20	Yes	—	0	0.38	0.04
10	14	Yes	—	0	ND†	ND†

*Measured by ELISA. Values are absorption at 490 nm with sera diluted 1:100.

†Not determined.

had essentially no effect on the formation of specific antibodies in the recipients of S-Ag–sensitized lymphocytes. The cellular mechanisms involved in the antibody production by the recipient rats are not known, and more studies are needed to determine whether the resistance to CsA is due to the lack of involvement of helper T cells in this immune reaction.

The findings reported here further suggest that the tested experimental systems may be used as models for investigating the mode of action of CsA on immunopathogenic processes in man, in particular those that are mediated by presensitized lymphocytes.

CONCLUSIONS

CsA inhibited two immune responses of the efferent limb. (1) Delayed-type skin hypersensitivity in rats immunized previously with BGG was inhibited by CsA given 20 hr and 4 hr before skin testing and 4 hr thereafter. (2) Adoptive transfer of EAU by lymphocytes from rats immunized with S-antigen was completely suppressed by daily injections of CsA into recipients on days −1 to +6. The CsA effect was selective for the cell-mediated immune response; Arthus skin reaction and antibody production were not suppressed in the treated rats.

ACKNOWLEDGMENTS

We are grateful to Ms. Mary Alice Crawford for excellent technical help and to Ms. Joyce McIntyre for typing the manuscript.

REFERENCES

1. Borel JF, Feurer C, Magnée C, et al: Immunology 32:1017, 1977

2. White DJG, Calne RY: Immunol Rev 65:115, 1982

3. Nussenblatt RB, Rodrigues MM, Wacker WB, et al: J Clin Invest 67:1228, 1981

4. Ryffel B, Feurer C, Heuberger B, et al: Immunobiology 163:470, 1982

5. Bolton C, Borel JF, Cuzner ML, et al: In White DJG (ed): Cyclosporin A. New York, Elsevier Biomedical Press, 1982, p 135

6. Nussenblatt RB, Palestine AF, Chan CC, et al: Transplant Proc (this issue)

7. Wacker WB, Donoso LA, Kalsow CM, et al: J Immunol 119:1949, 1977

8. Nussenblatt RB, Gery I, Ballintine EJ, et al: Am J Ophthalmol 89:173, 1980

9. Tuyer VV, Fauer J-P, Thillaye B, et al: Current Eye Res 2:7, 1982

Pulmonary Macrophage and Polymorphonuclear Leukocyte Function in Response to Immunosuppressive Therapy

D. B. Drath and B. D. Kahan

PHAGOCYTIC CELLS, particularly pulmonary alveolar macrophages (PAM) and polymorphonuclear leukocytes (PMN), are most responsible for maintaining the sterility of the lower respiratory tract.[1] Since pulmonary infections are common in renal allograft recipients on immunosuppressive drug therapy, the effects of drugs on PAM and PMN may provide an overall indication of the integrity of the immune response of the lung.[2] The studies presented here compared the effect of 30 days of i.p. administration of a new immunosuppressive agent, cyclosporine (CsA), on critical cellular elements of host defense with the effects of azathioprine and prednisolone, the conventionally used immunosuppressive drugs. Chemotaxis, phagocytosis, and superoxide release were measured as indices of the phagocytes' ability to localize and engulf microorganisms and to generate reactive microbicidal oxygen metabolites.

Preliminary results suggested that in vitro addition of 10^{-8} *M* CsA caused marked inhibition of PAM superoxide release; incubation periods as short as 30 min resulted in 40% inhibition of release of this oxygen metabolite.[3] On the other hand, azathioprine at concentrations 1000-fold higher had no effect on superoxide release. Prednisolone had to be used at 10-fold higher concentrations than CsA to produce comparable levels of inhibition. This report extends those studies to include another phagocytic cell, the PMN, and evaluates the effects of in vivo immunosuppressive drug administration.

MATERIALS AND METHODS

Animals and Drug Administration

Male rats of the Fischer 344 strain (Timco Breeding Co., Houston, TX.) weighing 150 g at the onset of drug treatment received a daily intraperitoneal injection of either azathioprine, 20 mg/kg (Burroughs-Wellcome Co., Research Triangle Park, NC); cyclosporine, 5 or 15 mg/kg (a gift of Sandoz Inc., Basel, Switzerland); prednisolone, 2 or 0.5 mg/kg (Upjohn Co., Kalamazoo, MI); or drug vehicle. Azathioprine and prednisolone were dissolved in bacteriostatic water, and CsA was dissolved in a 1/10 mixture of a 95% ethanol and intralipid 10% (Cutter Medical, Berkeley, CA). Drugs were administered as either the sole immunosuppressive agent or in combination with prednisolone (0.5 mg/kg) for a 30-day period. Nine groups of rats were subjected to the drug regime, of which the first six groups consisted of those given a primary immunosuppressant, those given the primary agent combined with prednisolone, and those given drug vehicle alone. Groups 7–9 were given either the lower prednisolone dose, the higher dose, or the drug vehicle.

Cell Isolation

On the final day of drug administration, rats were given an i.p. injection of 15 ml of 12% sodium caseinate. Fourteen hours later, PMN were harvested from the peritoneal cavity. Pulmonary macrophages were harvested from treated and control rats by bronchopulmonary lavage on the day following the final drug administration. Briefly, after rats were anesthetized with sodium pentobarbitol (30 mg/rat), the abdominal aorta was severed, the trachea was cannulated, and 7 ml of 0.9% sodium chloride was instilled and removed seven times. In all instances (including drug treatment), the cells obtained following centrifugation and washing were greater than 95% PAM or PMN and were 95% viable. Depending on the particular experiment, cells were used either as suspensions (chemotaxis) or as monolayers (superoxide release and phagocytosis), prepared as described by Michell and coworkers.[4]

Chemotaxis

The chemoattractants included 10^{-8}-*M* synthetic tripeptide FMLP (Sigma Biochemicals, St. Louis, MO) or 10% C5a activated serum prepared by incubating homologous rat serum with zymosan particles at 37°C for 15 min. The attractant was added to the lower half of modified Boyden chambers containing M199 and 0.1%

From the Division of Immunology and Organ Transplantation, Department of Surgery, The University of Texas Medical School, Houston, TX.

Reprint requests should be addressed to Dr. Kahan.

0041-1345/83/1505-0027$01.00/0

albumin. The upper half of the chamber contained 1.5 × 10^6 PAM or PMN harvested from control or drug-treated rats and suspended in medium 199 containing 0.1% albumin. Control chambers contained only M199 and albumin in the lower half to assess random migration. The upper and lower halves of the chambers were separated by an 8-μm-pore, gelatin-coated polycarbonate filter (Nucleopore Corp., Pleasanton, CA). After the chambers were incubated for 2 hr at 37°C in 95% air, 5% CO_2, the filters were removed, fixed, stained using a Dif-Quik staining kit (Scientific Products, McGraw Park, IL), mounted on glass slides, and allowed to dry overnight before placing coverslips.[5] Migration was assessed by enumerating the PAM or PMN that had moved through the filter in 15 randomly selected oil power fields (1000×).

Phagocytosis of Labeled Bacteria

The live bacterial particle was used at levels consistent with biological reality (10 bacteria/macrophage). Monolayers consisting of 3 × 10^6 cells (when added) were formed at 37°C as previously described.[4] After 1 hr, nonadherent cells were washed off (~35%). Fresh Hanks' balanced salt solution containing glucose (1 mg/ml) was added to the monolayers followed by the ^{14}C-labeled *S. aureus* (strain 209P) at a ratio of 10 particles/phagocyte. At the indicated time, the particles were removed; the monolayers were vigorously washed in saline and dried in preparation for counting. Zero time counts were subtracted from subsequent measurements.[6] Protein determinations were performed on the monolayers as well as on the bacteria.

Superoxide Release

Superoxide release was measured on monolayers consisting of 3.0 × 10^6 PAM as previously described.[7] Superoxide-dependent cytochrome c reduction was determined spectrophotometrically at 550 nm in the presence or absence of superoxide dismutase (Sigma Chemicals), both on cells at rest and following phagocytosis of opsonized zymosan. Pulmonary macrophage or PMN monolayers used in these studies were prepared from cells harvested from rats subjected to the drug regimen as well as their controls.

Statistical Analysis

The results obtained for superoxide release and for chemotaxis are expressed as mean values ± SEM. The statistical significance between immunosuppressive drug and control groups was determined using Student's t test.

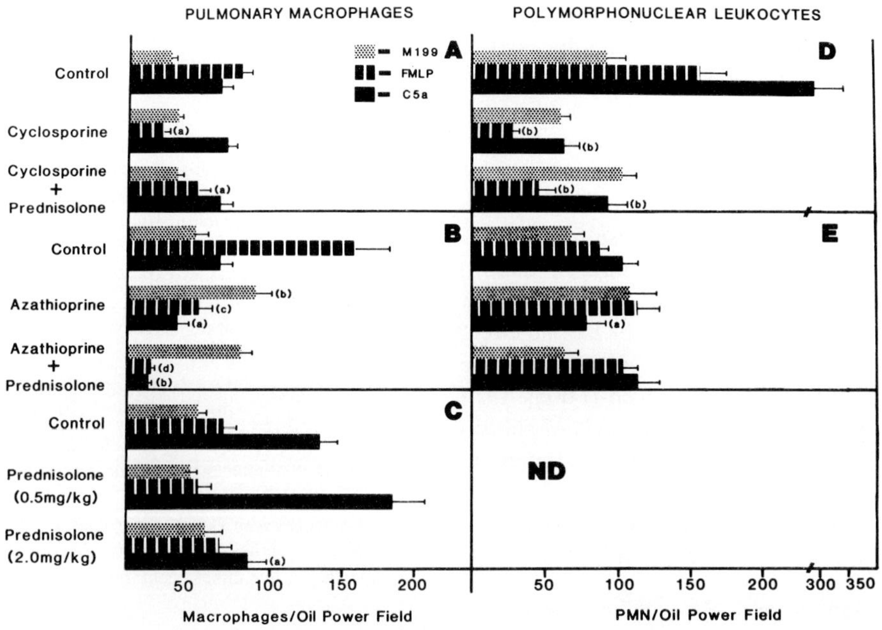

Fig. 1. Chemotaxis was measured in modified Boyden chambers with either 10^{-8}-*M* FMLP or 10% C5a-activated serum as the chemoattractant. Pulmonary macrophages or PMN were placed in the upper compartments of the chamber in M199 with 0.1% albumin. Either M199 (random migration) or attractant (chemotaxis) was added to the lower compartment. Results are expressed as the mean number of phagocytes per oil power field (1000×) ± SEM. Statistical significance between control and drug-treated groups is indicated at the end of each relevant bar. (a) $p<.05$; (b) $p<.025$; (c) $p<.001$; (d) $p<.0001$.

RESULTS

The most pronounced effect of the immunosuppressive drug therapy was on phagocyte chemotaxis toward FMLP or C5a. Cyclosporine with or without prednisolone had no effect on PAM random migration or chemotaxis toward C5a but did have a marked inhibitory effect when FMLP served as the chemoattractant [Fig. 1 (A)]. CsA affected PMN chemotaxis even more severely and blocked migration toward C5a-activated serum as well [Fig. 1 (D)].

In contrast, azathioprine induced more dramatic effects on PAM [Fig. 1 (B)] than on PMN [Fig. 1 (E)]. In fact, following an initial stimulation of PAM random migration, directed migration (chemotaxis) was depressed. The inhibitory effects were amplified by combined azathioprine-prednisolone therapy. Neutrophil chemotaxis, on the other hand,

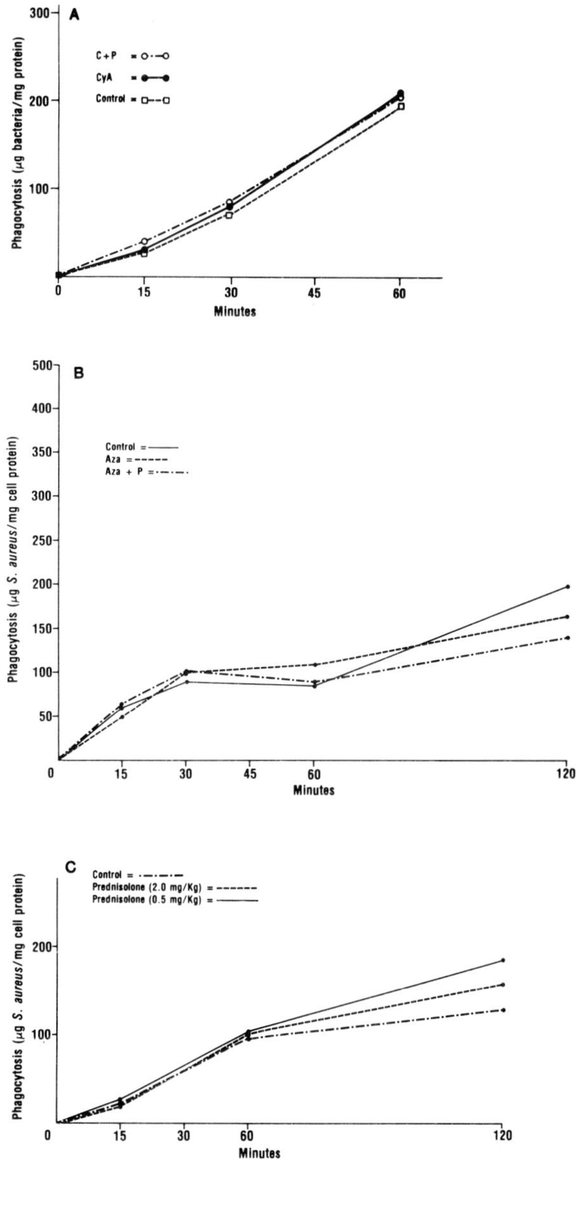

Fig. 2. Phagocytosis of ^{14}C-labeled *S. aureus* was assessed over a 60-min (A) or 2-hr (B, C) period. Control rats were treated with drug vehicle. All injections were i.p., and immunosuppressive drugs were administered for 30 days. Pulmonary macrophages were harvested from rats treated with (A) cyclosporine (5 mg/kg) and cyclosporine + prednisolone (0.5 mg/kg), (B) azathioprine (20 mg/kg) or azathioprine + prednisolone (0.5 mg/kg), or (C) 2 mg/kg or 0.5 mg/kg prednisolone.

cell than was seen with PAM. Since azathioprine caused an inhibition of responsiveness toward both attractants, it may exert a more general membrane effect on PAM than CsA. On the other hand, PMN were largely spared from the inhibitory effects of these drugs.

Since guinea pigs whose chemotaxis was blocked by immunosuppressive drugs display significantly reduced survival from experimental pneumonia compared to animals with unimpaired chemotaxis,[10,11] these observations suggest that the more pronounced inhibition of chemotaxis by azathioprine, particularly when combined with prednisolone than for cyclosporine (±prednisolone), may correlate with the increased incidence of pulmonary infection in azathioprine-treated vs. cyclosporine-treated hosts.

On the other hand, phagocytosis of *S. aureus* by pulmonary macrophages was unaffected by the drugs, suggesting that this critical process remains intact in these immunosuppressed hosts. Except for a transient inhibition caused by azathioprine, PMN phagocytosis remained operational throughout the assay period.

The most surprising results was the unimpaired superoxide release. Previous investigations suggested that CsA and to a lesser extent prednisolone effectively inhibited in vitro superoxide release.[3] At concentrations as low as $10^{-8}M$, CsA caused a 35% inhibition of superoxide release after contact with PAMs for as little as 30 min. The results described here, however, indicate that 30-day in vivo administration of immunosuppressive drugs was without effect on both PAM and PMN superoxide release. Thus either CsA (±prednisolone) is not achieving high enough concentrations in the appropriate environment of these phagocytes (alveoli, lung parenchyma, bronchi, bloodstream), or the cells are not sensitive to the circulating form of the drug, which may in fact be a metabolite of the native molecule that is not an effective inhibitor of superoxide release. Thus, chemotaxis may be more sensitive to lower concentrations of active drug molecule than superoxide release.

These results suggest additional studies to assess the effects of immunosuppressive drugs on other properties of PAM and PMN, including their ability to release lysosomal enzymes and demonstrate antifungal and antiviral activity. Furthermore, it will be important to assess the functional activity of macrophages obtained from other sites, including the spleen and the bloodstream.

REFERENCES

1. Green GM, Kass EM: J Exp Med 119:167, 1964
2. Munda R, Alexander JW, First MR, et al: Ann Surg 187:26, 1978
3. Drath DB, Kahan BD: Transplantation (in press)
4. Michell RH, Pancakee SJ, Noseworthy J, et al: Cell Biol 40:216, 1969
5. Gallin JI, Quie PG (eds): Methods Physiology and Clinical Implications. New York, Raven Press, 1978
6. Drath DB, Karnovsky ML, Huber GL: Inflammation 3:281, 1979
7. Drath DB, Karnovsky ML: J Exp Med 141:257, 1975
8. Chatterjee SN, Gottlief L, Berne TV: Surg Gynecol Obstet 147:583, 1979
9. Pennington JE, Harris EA: Annu Rev Respir Dis 123:299, 1981
10. Dale DE, Fauci AS, Wolff SM: N Engl J Med 291:1154, 1974
11. Pennington JE, Ehrie NG: J Infect Dis 137:764, 1978

Effect of Cyclosporine Alone or Combined with Prednisolone or Azathioprine on Macrophage Phagocytosis

A. Rios, L. H. Toledo-Pereyra, and S. Buscetta

CYCLOSPORINE A (CsA) is a potent immunosuppressive agent[1] that appears to spare macrophage function.[2,3] Its effects when combined with prednisolone or azathioprine have not been determined,[4] though such combinations are being either used or considered for use in clinical transplantation.[5] We therefore initiated a series of studies to determine the effect of CsA in combination with prednisolone or azathioprine on murine macrophage function.

Our objectives were (1) to determine the effect of CsA alone or combined with prednisolone or azathioprine on phagocytosis by normal resident murine macrophages and (2) to investigate whether CsA alone or in combination with prednisolone or azathioprine would modify the mortality of intraperitoneal *E. coli*.

MATERIALS AND METHODS

Normal resident peritoneal macrophages of BALB/c female mice were allowed to adhere, were washed extensively to remove nonadherent cells, and then were incubated with CsA in the appropriate concentration for 2 hr. CsA was dissolved in anhydrous ethanol (0.1 ml/mg CsA), and appropriate ethanol controls were always included. Following this incubation, the adherent cells were again washed, and prednisolone (10 μg/ml) or azathioprine (10 μg/ml) was added for 90 min. Cells were washed free of drug, and latex beads (Dow Corning) were added for 30 min. All incubations were carried out in minimal essential medium (MEM) with 5% fetal calf serum (FCS) at 37°C with 5% CO_2. Phagocytosis of latex beads was determined by visual counts of 200 cells/well with all groups in triplicate in at least two separate in vitro experiments. Phagocytosis is presented as the percent adherent cells that ingested three or more latex beads. All experiments included the following groups: untreated control, ethanol control, CsA, prednisolone, azathioprine, P + A, C + P, and C + A. Optimal drug concentrations and incubation times were determined in preliminary experiments.

In vivo treatment of BALB/c mice was carried out with daily injections of CsA (15 mg/kg s.c.), prednisolone (1.0 mg/kg i.p.), or azathioprine (2.5 mg/kg i.p.). CsA treatment started on day 0 and prednisolone and azathioprine on day 1 for a total of 12 daily injections. Groups used the same drug combinations as the in vivo experiments. Peritoneal macrophages were harvested 30 hr after the last drug injection from six individual mice per group, and phagocytosis was determined as above.

Mortality due to *E. coli* was determined in immunosuppressant-pretreated BALB/c mice by intraperitoneal injection of *E. coli* (ATCC 29552) 30 hr after the last drug injection. Drug dose and schedule were identical to the in vivo phagocytosis experiments described above. Bacterial counts were confirmed with pour plates. Initial experiments by direct counts and pour-plate technique determined that CsA did not inhibit *E. coli* growth in vitro. Mortality of intraperitoneal *E. coli* was determined daily, and all deaths occurred within 1 week.

RESULTS

Effect of In Vitro Treatment with Cyclosporine, Prednisolone, or Azathioprine on Peritoneal Macrophage Phagocytosis

CsA did not affect phagocytosis of latex beads by peritoneal macrophages (Fig. 1). Prednisolone or azathioprine alone or combined significantly inhibited phagocytosis ($p \leq 0.05$ when compared to control, CsA alone, or CsA + P). Incubation with CsA followed by azathioprine inhibited phagocytosis to the same extent as azathioprine alone. The opposite results were obtained with incubation with CsA followed by prednisolone: CsA abrogated the inhibition of phagocytosis by prednisolone.

From the Department of Surgery, Section of Transplantation and Surgical Research, Mount Carmel Mercy Hospital, Detroit, MI.

Supported by an Institutional Grant from the Mount Carmel Research and Education Corporation.

Reprint requests should be addressed to Dr. Luis H. Toledo-Pereyra, Department of Surgery, Mount Carmel Mercy Hospital, 6071 West Outer Drive, Detroit, MI 48235.

0041-1345/83/1505-0028$01.00/0

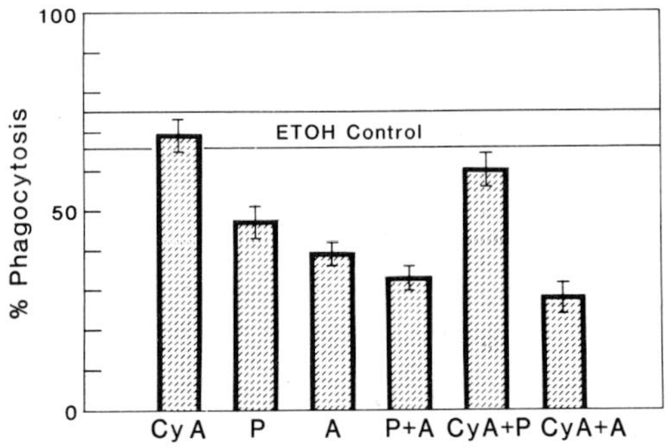

Fig. 1. It is evident that CsA and CsA combined with prednisolone (P) did not inhibit phagocytosis. All other combinations including prednisolone alone or combined with azathioprine (A) inhibited phagocytosis. Data are mean ± SD (*N* = 12 per group).

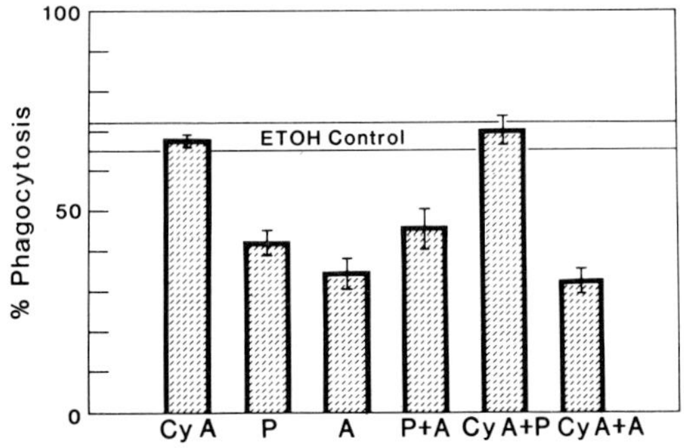

Fig. 2. Again the administration of CsA alone or combined with prednisolone (P) did not inhibit phagocytosis. However, all other combinations including prednisolone alone or combined with azathioprine (A) inhibited phagocytosis. Data are mean ± SD (*N* = 6 per group).

The effects of varying concentrations of CsA are shown in Table 1. CsA alone had no effect on phagocytosis except at levels of 50 μg/ml, at which a slight inhibition was seen and the peritoneal macrophages themselves became less adherent. The inhibitory effect of CsA plus azathioprine was seen at all CsA concentrations. The ability of CsA to abrogate the deleterious effect of prednisolone was also maintained until the concentration of 50 μg/ml, at which point CsA itself interferes with this aspect of macrophage function. We then examined whether the in vitro effect of CsA on phagocytosis could be reproduced by in vivo pretreatment of BALB/c mice.

Effect of In Vivo Administration of Cyclosporine, Prednisolone, or Azathioprine on Peritoneal Macrophage Phagocytosis

Initially we used two doses of CsA, 15 mg/kg and 150 mg/kg. We chose to study the dose of 15 mg/kg because the higher dose of CsA caused severe weight loss, diarrhea, and near mortality at 10 days. The results are shown in Fig. 2. Peritoneal macrophages harvested from mice pretreated with CsA were not different from those of control animals receiving ethanol or from untreated normal mice (65.1 ± 2.6). Pretreatment with prednisolone or azathioprine or the two combined again significantly inhibited phagocytosis ($p \leq 0.05$ when compared to control, CsA, or CsA + P). CsA combined with azathioprine inhibited phagocytosis ($p \leq 0.05$). CsA again

Table 1. Effect of Varying Concentrations of Cyclosporine A on Phagocytosis

CsA Dose (μg/ml)	% Phagocytosis: CsA Alone	CsA + Prednisolone (10 μg/ml)	CsA + Azathioprine (10 μg/ml)
0	67.0 ± 5.1	45.0 ± 4.0	38.4 ± 5.1
1	62.7 ± 3.2	59.0 ± 7.5	31.6 ± 5.7
10	66.4 ± 5.6	58.0 ± 4.5	39.2 ± 4.8
20	60.7 ± 1.5	64.7 ± 6.8	44.5 ± 13.4
50	50.2 ± 2.8	29.5 ± 4.9	31.0 ± 3.5

Data are mean ± SD (*N* = 6 per group).

Table 2. Mortality Due to Intraperitoneal *E. Coli* in BALB/c Mice Pretreated with Cyclosporine A Alone or Combined with Prednisolone or Azathioprine

Group No.	Pretreatment*	Mortality Rate 2×10^7	Mortality Rate 3×10^7
1	None	2/10	10/10
2	Control	5/10	9/10
3	Cyclosporine A	2/10	3/10‡
4	Prednisolone	4/10	9/10
5	Azathioprine	7/10	10/10
6	Prednisolone + Azathioprine	5/10	8/10
7	Cyclosporine A + Prednisolone	6/10	7/10
8	Cyclosporine A + Azathioprine	2/10	3/9‡

*BALB/c female mice were given 12 daily injections of cyclosporine A 15 mg/kg s.c., prednisolone 1.0 mg/kg i.p., or azathioprine 2.5 mg/kg i.p.

†2×10^7 or 3×10^7 *E. coli* inoculated intraperitoneal 30 hr after injection of day-12 immunosuppressants. Mortality equals number of animals dead/number per group 21 days after *E. coli* inoculum.

‡$p \leq 0.05$ when compared to groups 1, 2, 4, 5, and 6 (chi squares).

reduced the inhibitory effects of prednisolone. The in vivo pretreatment produced the same pattern as in vitro incubation.

Mortality Due to Intraperitoneal E. coli in BALB/c Mice Pretreated with Cyclosporine Alone or Combined with Prednisolone or Azathioprine

All deaths occurred within 7 days, and we did not observe any difference in pattern between early and late mortality in any group. Ethanol pretreatment increased mortality due to intraperitoneal *E. coli* (Table 2). BALB/c mice pretreated with CsA demonstrated a significant resistance to intraperitoneal *E. coli.* Pretreatment with prednisolone, azathioprine, prednisolone plus azathioprine, or CsA plus prednisolone did not affect the mortality rate. Pretreatment with CsA and azathioprine produced a reduction in mortality equal to that of CsA alone.

CONCLUSIONS

This study examined the effect of CsA when combined with prednisolone or azathioprine on peritoneal macrophage phagocytosis and mortality due to intraperitoneal *E. coli.* Inhibition of latex-bead phagocytosis was seen in all drug combinations except CsA alone and CsA with prednisolone. In mortality due to intraperitoneal *E. coli,* all groups demonstrated mortality equal to or greater than normal except animals pretreated with CsA or CsA combined with azathioprine. The results show that while the effects of CsA on peritoneal macrophage phagocytosis are consistent and reproducible, they are not predictive in the more complex model of mortality due to intraperitoneal *E. coli.* The mechanism for the divergent and modulating effects of CsA alone or in combination with prednisolone or azathioprine is unknown.

REFERENCES

1. Kahan BD: Texas Heart Inst J 9:253, 1982
2. Borel JF, Feurer C, Gubler HU, et al: Agents and Actions 6:468, 1976
3. McIntosh LC, Thomson AW: Transplantation 30:384, 1980
4. Starzl TE, Iwatsuki S, Klintmalm G, et al: Surg Gynecol Obstet 151:17, 1980
5. Rinehart JJ, Sagone AL, Balcerzak SP, et al: N Engl J Med 292:236, 1975

Inhibitory Effect of Cyclosporine on Adherent Cells in Oxidation-Induced Lymphocyte Proliferation

K. Uyemura, J. F. P. Dixon, and J. W. Parker

IN BOTH EXPERIMENTAL models and clinical trials, cyclosporine A (CsA) has proved to be a potent immunosuppressive agent. Reports to date indicate that CsA acts predominantly or exclusively on lymphocytes.[1-3] Early exposure to CsA effectively inhibits the proliferative response of both animal and human lymphocytes to phytohemagglutinin (PHA),[4,5] Concanavalin A (Con A),[1,6,7] and pokeweed mitogen (PWM).[4,8] Inhibition of the mixed lymphocyte reaction has also been demonstrated,[8-10] and such findings have led investigators to conclude that CsA exerts a selective action on T lymphocytes or a specific subpopulation of T lymphocytes. It has been suggested that the action of CsA may also be directed against B cells, as it inhibits both T-dependent and T-independent B-cell responses.[11,12] However, other workers have found that only T-dependent responses are blocked.[13]

Detailed studies of the effects of CsA on macrophages and their immunologic functions have not been reported, although it has been demonstrated that CsA does not block phagocytosis of colloidal carbon by murine Kupffer cells,[14] chemotactic migration of rabbit peritoneal macrophages,[1] or enzyme secretion of plasminogen activator and acetylglycosaminidase.[1] However, these functions may have little relevance to macrophage immunoregulatory functions.

Most studies of the effects of CsA on lymphocyte transformation have involved cell preparations containing both lymphocytes and macrophages, thus obscuring the effect this agent might have on each cell type separately. In view of the critical role of the macrophage in mitogen- and antigen-induced in vitro lymphocyte proliferation and in graft rejection, we decided to explore the effects of CsA on macrophage functions.

Populations of adherent cells highly enriched for macrophages and of highly purified lymphocytes were oxidized with the mitogen neuraminidase–galactose oxidase (NAGO), then independently treated with CsA, and recombined to assess their ability to proliferate. We found that lymphocyte proliferation was inhibited only when the adherent cells were exposed to CsA, regardless of whether or not the lymphocytes were treated with CsA. Our studies indicate that in oxidation-induced lymphocyte proliferation, macrophages are the cellular target of CsA action, and this suggests that this effect may also be involved in the demonstrated immunosuppressive action of CsA.

MATERIALS AND METHODS

Preparation of Cells

Human peripheral blood was collected from healthy adult donors into heparinized tubes. Following centrifugation, the plasma was collected and used to prepare culture medium (RPMI 1640 supplemented with 2 m*M* L-glutamine, 50 IU penicillin/ml, 50 μg streptomycin/ml, and 10% autologous plasma). Heterogeneous mononuclear (HM) cells were obtained by Ficoll-Paque (Pharmacia Fine Chemicals, Piscataway, NJ) density centrifugation and incubated for 2 hr in 75-cm^2 plastic flasks (Corning, Corning, NY). Nonadherent cells were removed from the flasks and passed through a nylon-wool column[15] and a Sephadex G-10 (Pharmacia) column[16] as previously described.[17] These cells (referred to as PL)

From the Department of Pathology, University of Southern California School of Medicine, Los Angeles, CA.

Supported by the Robert E. and May R. Wright Foundation. K. U. is a recipient of a Fieger Leukemia Research Fellowship from the USC Comprehensive Cancer Center.

Reprint requests should be addressed to Dr. J. F. P. Dixon, Department of Pathology, USC School of Medicine, 2025 Zonal Ave., Los Angeles, CA 90033.

0041-1345/83/1505-0029$01.00/0

were resuspended at 10^6/ml culture medium. These PL and the adherent cells remaining on the flasks were incubated separately overnight in culture medium. The following day, the flasks containing the adherent cells were thoroughly rinsed with RPMI 1640 to remove any residual nonadherent cells that were then discarded. The adherent cells were recovered from the flasks with cold 0.2% EDTA in PBS. These cells (now referred to as AC) were counted and evaluated for viability with trypan blue, adjusted to 10^6/ml culture medium, and exposed to 1000 rad/min for 3 min from a ^{60}Co source.

Characterization of Cell Populations

Cytocentrifuge preparations of HM, PL, and AC were stained with Wright's stain for differential counts. Nonspecific esterase activity was demonstrated with alpha-naphthyl acetate[18] (Sigma, St. Louis, MO). Immunoperoxidase staining[19] was performed utilizing anti-Leu-4 (Becton Dickinson, Mountain View, CA) or OKM-1 (Ortho Diagnostics, Raritan, NJ) for identification of T lymphocytes and monocytes/macrophages, respectively. Ingestion of 1.1-μm-diameter latex particles[20] (Dow Diagnostics, Indianapolis, IN) and 0.1% neutral red[21] (J. T. Baker Chemical Co., Phillipsburg, NJ) identified phagocytic cells.

Cell Treatment with NAGO

Cells treated with NAGO were suspended in a 1-ml solution of 20 U/ml NA (Calbiochem-Behring, La Jolla, CA) and 0.5 U/ml GO (Worthington, Freehold, NJ) in RPMI 1640[20] for 30 min at 37°C, washed twice with RPMI 1640, and placed in fresh culture medium.

Cell Treatment with CsA

One milligram CsA (kindly provided by Sandoz Ltd., Basel, Switzerland) was dissolved in 0.1 ml ethanol containing 20% Tween 80.[1] To this solution, 0.9 ml of warm RPMI 1640 was added dropwise with constant stirring. The final concentration of CsA was adjusted to 1 μg/ml with culture medium. Cells were treated with CsA solution for 6 hr, washed three times with RPMI 1640, and resuspended in culture medium.

Experimental Design

PL and AC were treated separately with NAGO, and CsA was added to either one or both cell populations. After 6 hr, the cells were washed with RPMI 1640 and placed in fresh culture medium. PL, AC, or PL combined with 10% AC were placed in Micro Test culture plates (Becton Dickinson) and incubated in a CO_2 incubator at 37°C for 66 hr.[22] Two hours prior to the termination of culture, 0.2 μCi of tritiated thymidine (^{3}H-TdR, 20 μCi/ml, 0.5 Ci/m*M*; New England Nuclear, Boston, MA) was added to each culture well. The cultures were harvested on a Titertek Cell Harvester (Flow Laboratories, Rockville, MD) onto glass-fiber filters which were then placed in Econofluor (New England Nuclear) and counted in a liquid scintillation counter (Beckman, Fullerton, CA).

RESULTS

Composition of Test Populations

Following separation procedures, the recovered cells were evaluated for purity, utilizing the procedures for identification of lymphocytes and macrophages described above. HM were mixtures of lymphocytes and macrophages and as expected showed a strong proliferative response to NAGO. PL contained more than 99% lymphocytes and fewer than 0.4% macrophages as determined by nonspecific esterase and phagocytic activity. Over 94% of the lymphocytes in PL were T lymphocytes (Leu-4$^+$). In all of our experiments, oxidation of PL resulted in <5% of the proliferative response given by the reconstituted oxidized control cultures containing PL and AC, indicating depletion of accessory cell function. The AC population contained more than 93% macrophages, based on morphology, esterase activity, OKM - 1$^+$ immunoperoxidase staining, and phagocytosis, and did not respond to mitogen treatment. AC also contained granulocytes (<3%) and T lymphocytes (<1.4%).

Inhibition of Proliferation with Early CsA Treatment

Treatment of oxidized HM with CsA during the first 6 hr of culture resulted in an 85% inhibition of the proliferative response. Six-hour CsA exposures at later periods of culture resulted in progressively less inhibition of the mitogenic response. A 6-hr treatment with CsA of both PL and AC together or AC alone significantly reduced the mitogenic response to 6%–16% of the positive control (oxidized PL and AC without CsA treatment). However, when oxidized PL were treated with CsA, they were still capable of proliferating, in the presence of oxidized AC, to 69%–89% of controls (Table 1). These results demonstrated that CsA treatment of AC signifi-

Table 1. Effect of CsA on PL and AC in NAGO-Induced Lymphocyte Proliferation

	% Maximal Proliferative Response*		
	—	AC_{NAGO}	$AC_{NAGO/CsA}$
—	—	5.6 ± 2.6	2.8 ± 1.7
PL_{NAGO}	2.8 ± 1.4	100	8.3 ± 2.6
$PL_{NAGO/CsA}$	2.5 ± 1.1	74.8 ± 5.1	2.5 ± 1.3

*Data are expressed as percentages of maximal proliferative response of control PL and AC. Proliferation was assessed by ^{3}H-TdR incorporation. Data represent the mean ± SEM of 5 experiments.

cantly reduces the mitogenic response to NAGO but has little direct effect on lymphocytes.

DISCUSSION

There are few reports in the literature on the action of CsA on macrophage function, and these describe the absence of effect on functions such as phagocytosis and chemotaxis.[1,13] Since other macrophage functions may play a more important role in the immune response, specifically in graft rejection, it seemed to us that the effect of CsA on other, more pertinent macrophage functions should be evaluated. With that in mind, we utilized a familiar model in which the macrophage is evaluated as a necessary cell in the lymphocyte response to mitogen.

Other investigators have used lymphocyte populations depleted of accessory cells to study the effect of CsA on in vitro mitogenesis. Paavonen and Hayry[12] and White et al.[3] found that the macrophage-depleted cell preparations were still responsive to PWM and PHA. Since mitogen stimulation requires accessory cells to produce a lymphocyte proliferative response, it is clear that their lymphocyte-enriched populations contained some residual accessory cells.

Our ability to prepare highly purified PL and AC populations and to expose only one or the other to CsA allowed us to conclude that, in the oxidative mitogenesis model, the principal inhibitory action of CsA is on adherent cells (macrophages) and that the effect on lymphocytes is minimal. In preliminary results on PHA- and Con A–induced lymphocyte transformation, we have obtained results that are almost identical to those obtained with NAGO.

At this time, we have not yet defined the precise cellular and molecular action of CsA on macrophage functions. CsA may exert its immunosuppressive action by alteration of macrophage metabolism, membrane receptors, or production or secretion of soluble factors. Studies to determine the mechanisms of action of CsA on macrophages should enhance our understanding of macrophage biology, and they may also point to other ways of altering macrophage function for immunosuppressive purpose.

REFERENCES

1. Weisinger D, Borel JF: Immunobiology 156:454, 1979

2. Burckhardt JJ, Guggenheim B: Immunology 36:753, 1979

3. White DJG, Plumb AM, Pawelec G, et al: Transplantation 27:55, 1979

4. Leoni P, Garcia RC, Allison AC: J Clin Lab Immunol 1:67, 1978

5. Calne RY, White DJG: IRCS J Med Sci 5:595, 1977

6. Larsson EL: J Immunol 124:2828, 1980

7. Borel JF: Transplant Proc 13:344, 1981

8. Leapman SB, Filo RS, Smith EJ, et al: Transplant Proc 13:405, 1981

9. Hess AD, Tutschka PJ: J Immunol 124:2601, 1980

10. Keown PA, Essery GL, Stiller CR, et al: Transplant Proc 13:386, 1981

11. Dongworth DW, Klaus GGB: Eur J Immunol 12:1018, 1982

12. Paavonen T, Jarvelainen H, Kontianinen S, et al: Clin Exp Immunol 43:342, 1981

13. Fernandez C, Palacios R, Moller G: Scand J Immunol 16:33, 1982

14. McIntosh LC, Thomson AW: Transplantation 30:384, 1980

15. Julius MH, Simpson E, Herzenberg LA: Eur J Immunol 3:645, 1973

16. Ly IA, Mishell RI: Immunol Methods 5:239, 1974

17. Yam LT, Li CY, Crosby WH: Ann J Clin Pathol 55:283, 1971

18. Dixon JFP, Bruszewski WB, Uyemura K, et al: J Reticuloendothel Soc 49:61, 1981

19. Hofman FM, Billing RJ, Parker JW, et al: Clin Exp Immunol 49:355, 1982

20. Johnson WD Jr, Mei B: J Exp Med 146:1613, 1977

21. Gresner BM, Howard JG: In Weir DM (ed): Handbook of Experimental Immunology. Philadelphia, FA Davis, 1967

22. Dixon JFP, Parker JW, O'Brien RL: J Immunol 116:575, 1976

HUMORAL MEDIATORS

Effect of Cyclosporine on Human Leukocyte Interferon Production: Selective Inhibition of IFN-Gamma Synthesis

J. Abb and H. Abb

INTERFERONS (IFNs) are a heterogenous group of glycoproteins produced by animal cells in response to viral and nonviral stimuli.[1] Antigenic, biologic, and physicochemical properties allow the distinction of three major classes of human IFN: IFN alpha (leukocyte), IFN beta (fibroblast), and IFN gamma (immune).[2] IFNs inhibit the replication of most DNA or RNA viruses,[1] suppress the proliferation of malignant cells in vitro,[3] and exert immunomodulatory activities. Thus it has been demonstrated that IFNs regulate the activity of nonspecific cytotoxic (NK) effector cells.[4] These findings have led to the suggestion that the IFN/NK system may participate in host defense mechanisms against viral infections or neoplastic disease.[5]

The possible importance of IFNs and/or NK cells in limiting the spread or viral agents and the growth of tumors has caused intensified efforts in the search for pharmacological substances that modulate nonspecific effector functions. Among these agents, cyclosporine A (CsA) has become the subject to growing interest because of its well-documented immunosuppressive properties.[6] We have studied the effect of CsA on human leukocyte IFN production and IFN-induced activity of NK cells. We report that CsA markedly decreased the synthesis of IFN gamma but had no significant effect on the production of IFN alpha. In addition, CsA inhibited the activation of human NK cells by treatment with inducers of IFN gamma, but not by treatment with inducers of IFN alpha.

From the Max von Pettenkofer-Institute, Munich, Germany.

Supported by the Gertrud-Hagmann-Stiftung für Malignomforschung, Basel, Switzerland.

Reprint requests should be addressed to Jochen Abb, Max von Pettenkofer-Institute, Pettenkoferstraße 9a, D-800 Munich 2, Germany.

0041-1345/83/1505-0030$01.00/0

MATERIALS AND METHODS

Cyclosporine A

Powdered CsA (Sandoz, Basel, Switzerland) was kindly provided by Dr. H. Rodt, Institute of Hematology, FRG. Solutions of CsA were made in 95% ethanol to a final solvent concentration in the culture medium of 0.2%.

IFN Production

Nonadherent leukocytes were induced to produce IFN by the addition of purified phytohemagglutinin (PHA-P), protein A of *Staphylococcus aureus* (SpA), staphylococcal enterotoxin B (SEB), *Corynebacterium parvum* (CP), influenza A/X31 virus (A/X31), Sendai virus (SV), polyinosinic-polycytidilic acid (poly I-C), Epstein-Barr virus (EBV)-transformed human lymphoblastoid cell lines (LCL), or allogeneic leukocytes in secondary mixed leukocyte cultures (MLC).

IFN Assay and IFN Characterization

Leukocyte culture supernatants were assayed for antiviral activity by measuring the inhibition of the cytopathic effect (CPE) of vesicular stomatitis virus on human WISH amnion cells are previously described.[7] Antiviral units are expressed as the reciprocal of the highest culture supernatant dilution inhibiting 50% of the CPE and are equivalent to approximately 1 reference unit of the WHO Human Leukocyte Reference IFN B 69/19. Antiviral activity induced by stimulation of leukocytes with PHA-P, SpA, SEB, or alloantigens in secondary MLC was characterized as IFN gamma. Antiviral activity produced in response to stimulation with CP, A/X31, SV, or poly I-C shared the characteristics of IFN alpha. Culture supernatants of leukocytes stimulated with allogeneic EBV-LCL contained a mixture of IFN gamma and IFN alpha.

Interleukin 2 (IL-2)

Supernatants of cultured gibbon lymphosarcoma cells[8] served as the source for IL-2.

Assay for NK-Cell Activity

NK-cell activity was tested in a standard 4-hr ^{51} chromium-release assay with K562 target cells as previously described.[9]

RESULTS

Preliminary experiments demonstrated that CsA suppressed the SEB-induced synthesis of IFN gamma in a dose-dependent fashion. Maximal inhibition of IFN-gamma yields occurred at a CsA concentration of 1 μg/ml. The A/X31-induced production of IFN alpha was not significantly affected by CsA. In addition, CsA inhibited the augmentation of NK-cell activity by treatment with inducers of IFN gamma but had no effect on the spontaneous or IFN alpha–induced activity of NK cells (data not shown).

Figure 1 gives a summary of the effects of CsA on the production of antiviral activity in leukocyte cultures. CsA markedly inhibited the production of IFN gamma in response to stimulation with a lectin mitogen, bacterial products, and alloantigens in secondary MLC. In contrast, the secretion of IFN alpha induced by CP, viruses, or a synthetic polynucleotide was not changed by CsA. Antiviral activity induced by EBV-LCL was decreased by approximately 50%. Decreased IFN yields appeared to be due to CsA-mediated interference with IFN-gamma production, because the remaining IFN activity in CsA-treated cultures could be completely neutralized by incubation with antibody against IFN alpha.

Further experiments were designed to determine whether the inhibition of IFN-gamma synthesis was due to a direct effect of CsA on IFN-producing cells or to a CsA-mediated suppression of IL-2 production. As illustrated in Table 1, the addition of exogenous IL-2 to CsA-treated cultures did not restore the IFN-gamma response to normal levels. Thus, the inhibitory action of CsA appeared to be the result of a direct effect on IFN gamma–producing leukocytes.

DISCUSSION

Clinical trials have confirmed the potential usefulness of CsA as a selective immunosuppressive drug.[10] However, there have been disturbing reports of EBV-associated lymphomas presenting in renal allograft recipients

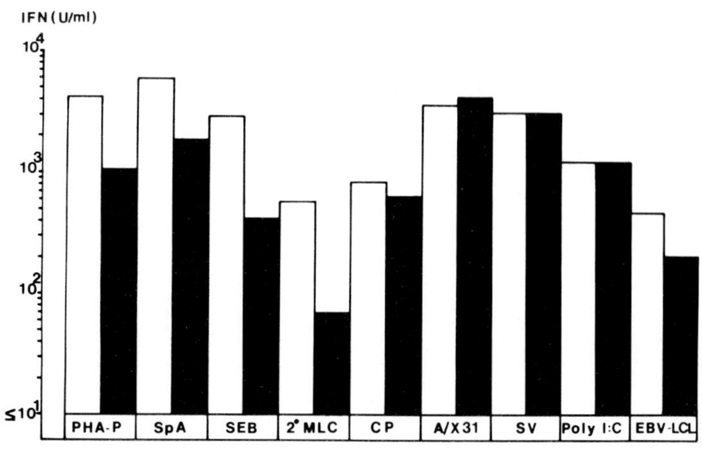

Fig. 1. Effect of CsA (1 μg/ml) on human leukocyte IFN-gamma or IFN-alpha production. Results are given as mean yields of IFN (U/ml) in untreated □ or CsA-treated ■ leukocyte cultures.

Table 1. Effect of Exogenous IL-2 on the CsA-Mediated Inhibition of Human Leukocyte IFN-Gamma Production

Inducer	CsA	IL-2*	Yield of IFN Gamma (U/ml)
PHA-P	—	—	1280
PHA-P	—	50%	1280
PHA-P	—	25%	1280
PHA-P	1 μg/ml	—	160
PHA-P	1 μg/ml	50%	160
PHA-P	1 μg/ml	25%	160

*Supernatants of cultured MLA 144 gibbon lymphosarcoma cells.

treated with CsA.[11,12] Defects of IFN-gamma production have been described in patients with primary infection with EBV or with EBV-associated lymphoma.[13] Our results demonstrate that CsA causes a selective inhibition of IFN-gamma synthesis in human leukocyte cultures. These observations provide further evidence for the previous assumption the CsA predominantly acts on T lymphocyte–dependent immune responses.[14,15] Inhibition of the production of T-cell factors appears to be a general feature of CsA activity. Abrogation of lymphokine-regulated cytotoxic effector-cell control may explain the reported promotion of the spontaneous outgrowth of EBV-induced LCL by CsA in vitro.[16] In the presence of CsA, inhibition of effector mechanisms results in a polyclonal proliferation of EBV-infected B cells that in vitro form lymphoblastoid cells but in vivo manifest as the immunoblastic proliferation characteristic of immunosuppressed patients.[17]

REFERENCES

1. Stewart WE II: The Interferon System. Vienna and New York, Springer-Verlag, 1980

2. Stewart WE II: Nature 286:110, 1980

3. Gresser I, Maury C, Brouty-Boyé D: Nature 239:167, 1972

4. Trinchieri G, Santoli D, Koprowski H: J Immunol 120:1849, 1978

5. Santoli D, Koprowski H: Immunol Rev 44:125, 1979

6. Borel JF: Immunology 31:631, 1976

7. Abb J, Abb H, Deinhardt F: Immunopharmacology 4:303, 1982

8. Rabin H, Hopkins RF III, Ruscetti FW, et al: J Immunol 127:1852, 1981

9. Abb J, Abb H, Deinhardt F: Int J Cancer 30:307, 1982

10. Calne RY, Rolles K, White DJG, et al: Lancet 2:1033, 1979

11. Crawford DH, Thomas JA, Janossy G, et al: Lancet 1:1355, 1980

12. Nagington J, Gray J: Lancet 1:536, 1980

13. Virelizier JL, Lenoir G, Griscelli C: Lancet 2:231, 1978

14. Hess DA, Tutschka PJ: J Immunol 124:2601, 1980

15. Palacios R, Möller G: Nature 290:792, 1981

16. Bird AG, McLachlan SM, Britton S: Nature 289:300, 1981

17. Purtilo DT: Lancet 1:300, 1980

Effects of Cyclosporine on the Production of Various Interferons

V. K. Kalman and G. R. Klimpel

CYCLOSPORINE A (CsA) is a hydrophobic undecapeptide fungal metabolite with potent immunosuppressive effects on T cell–mediated immune responses.[1] Although the exact mechanism of action of CsA is presently unknown, CsA has been shown to act primarily on early events of lymphocyte activation.[2,3] The production and action of different interleukins (IL-1, IL-2) is inhibited by CsA,[4–7] however, the effects of CsA on the production and action of various interferons (IFNs) is unclear. Thus, the purpose of this study was to investigate what effects CsA has on the production and action of immune (IFN gamma), leukocyte (IFN alpha), and fibroblast (IFN beta) interferons. Results from these studies show that CsA inhibited the production of IFN gamma by mitogen- or alloantigen-stimulated T cells. This inhibition of IFN-gamma production was evident even when early events in lymphocyte activation were allowed to take place and was reversible. In contrast, CsA had no effect on the production of virus-induced IFN alpha or beta or on the antiviral activity of already formed IFN gamma, alpha, or beta.

MATERIALS AND METHODS

Female C57Bl/6 mice, male DBA mice, and female Sprague-Dawley rats were obtained from Timco Breeding Laboratories, Houston, TX.

A stock solution of CsA at 200 μg/ml was prepared in ETOH/20% Tween 80 as previously described.[2] CsA was kindly provided by Dr. W. Flye (Department of Surgery, The University of Texas Medical Branch, Galveston, TX).

For IFN-gamma production, mononuclear cells were obtained from the peripheral blood of laboratory personnel by centrifugation on Ficoll-Hypaque gradients.[8] Sterile suspensions of murine spleen cells were prepared, and red blood cells were osmotically lysed as previously described.[9] Human peripheral blood lymphocytes (PBLs) and mouse spleen cells were cultured as previously described in flat-bottomed Linbro plates.[9] Supernatants were collected at varying times and stores at −70°C until tested for IFN activity.

For IFN-alpha and IFN-beta production, cultures were established as previously described[10] using mouse spleen cells, human PBLs, and L929 cells infected with Newcastle disease virus (NDV) at an input multiplicity of five plaque-forming units (PFU)/cell.

IL-2 containing supernatants from concanavalin A (Con A)–stimulated lymphocyte cultures was prepared by stimulating Timco rat spleen cells with 5 μg/ml Con A in 200 ml of RPMI 1640 supplemented with 5% fetal calf serum, 100 U/ml penicillin, 100 μg/ml streptomycin, and 5×10^{-5}-*M* 2-mercaptoethanol. After 24 hr, the supernatant was harvested, absorbed with Sephadex G-200 to remove Con A, filtered, and stored at −70°C until used.

IFN units were determined using L929 or human amniotic WISH cells in a microplaque-reduction assay according to Campbell et al.[11] One unit of IFN was defined as that amount required to reduce the number of PFU per well by 50% compared to the virus control.

RESULTS AND DISCUSSION

Inhibition of IFN-Gamma Production by CsA

C57Bl/6 spleen cells and human PBL stimulated with staphylococcal enterotoxin A (SEA) or spleen cells stimulated with alloantigen (irradiated DBA spleen cells) produce IFN gamma. The addition of CsA at ≥ 0.1 μg/ml totally inhibited IFN-gamma production (Tables 1 and 2). This inhibition mediated by CsA was not due to the amount of mitogen or alloantigen required for stimulation nor to the possibility that CsA was blocking the antiviral action of IFN gamma (data not presented). Inhibition of IFN-gamma production by CsA was also not due to an alteration in the kinetics of IFN produc-

---

From the Department of Microbiology, The University of Texas Medical Branch, Galveston, TX.

Supported by Public Health Service Grant CA 30183.

Address reprint request to Dr. G. R. Klimpel, Department of Microbiology, The University of Texas Medical Branch, Galveston, TX 77550.

0041–1345/83/1505–0031$01.00/0

Table 1. Inhibition of IFNγ Production by CsA*

Culture Conditions	IFN U/ml
C57b1/6 spleen plus:	
SEA	570
SEA + CsA	<10
DBA spleen irradiated	60
DBA spleen irradiated + CsA	<10
Human PBL plus:	
SEA	170
SEA + CsA	<10

*Human PBL (6×10^6) or C57B1/6 spleen cells were cultured with either SEA (0.4 μg/ml) or irradiated DBA spleen cells (10^7). CsA at 1 μg/ml was added to these cultures. Supernatants from these cultures were harvested at day 3 and assayed for IFN activity.

tion. Peak IFN production was seen on days 3 and 4 of cultures stimulated with SEA. Furthermore, the solvent (ETOH/20% Tween 80) without CsA had no effect on IFN-gamma production (Table 2). The addition of CsA at 24 hr post culture initiation to spleen cells stimulated with SEA also inhibited IFN-gamma production. This indicates that CsA-mediated inhibition occurs even when early events in lymphocyte activation are allowed to take place. Next, we looked at whether or not this inhibition of IFN-gamma production by CsA was reversible. C57B1/6 spleen cells were stimulated with SEA in the presence or absence of CsA. Supernatants were harvested every 24 hr and assayed for IFN activity. To test for reversibility, spleen cells were obtained from some cultures and then washed three times with Hanks' medium to remove CsA. These cells were then recultured with SEA. Results from a representative experiment can be seen in Fig. 1. When spleen cells from cultures containing SEA + CsA were washed and then recultured in the presence of SEA, they produced IFN gamma, but at lower levels than control cultures. Thus, removal of CsA from these cell cultures restores the ability of these lymphocytes to produce IFN gamma. Therefore, it seems that the effects of CsA on IFN-gamma production are partially reversible. It has been previously shown that murine spleen cells stimulated with mitogen produce IFN gamma, and this production is dependent on IL-2 produced by Lyt-1$^+$ cells.[12] Other studies have shown that the addition of IL-2 directly to spleen cell cultures induces IFN-gamma production.[13] We next looked to see what effect CsA has on IL-2–induced IFN-gamma production. Surprisingly, when CsA was added at culture initiation to spleen cells stimulated with IL-2, it did not inhibit IFN-gamma production at 24 hr. However, when supernatants from these cultures were harvested at 48 hr and assessed for IFN activity, an inhibition in IFN-gamma production was observed. The amount of IFN present on day 2 was equivalent to or less than the amount present on day 1 (Table 2). Inhibition mediated by CsA was dependent on the amount of IL-2 present in these cultures. CsA added initially to spleen cells stimulated with low doses of IL-2 inhibited IFN-gamma production at 24 hr (data

Table 2. C57B1/6 Spleen Cells Cultured With SEA (0.4 μg/ml) as Previously Described*

Culture Conditions	IFN U/ml Days Post Culture Initiation 1	2	3	4	5
C57B1/6 spleen and SEA plus:					
Medium	30	150	270	280	130
Alcohol/Tween 80	15	165	265	160	110
CsA at culture initiation	<10	<10	<10	<10	<10
CsA added at 24 hr postculture initiation†	15	65	30	<10	<10
C57B1/6 spleen and IL-2 plus:					
Medium	115	320	115	NT‡	NT
CsA at culture initiation	120	115	115	NT	NT

*CsA (0.1 μg/ml) or solvent (absolute alcohol/20% Tween 80) without CsA, or IL-2 (0.5 ml/well), was added to different cultures.

†IFN activity present in cultures before the addition of CsA at 24 hr post culture initiations.

‡Not tested.

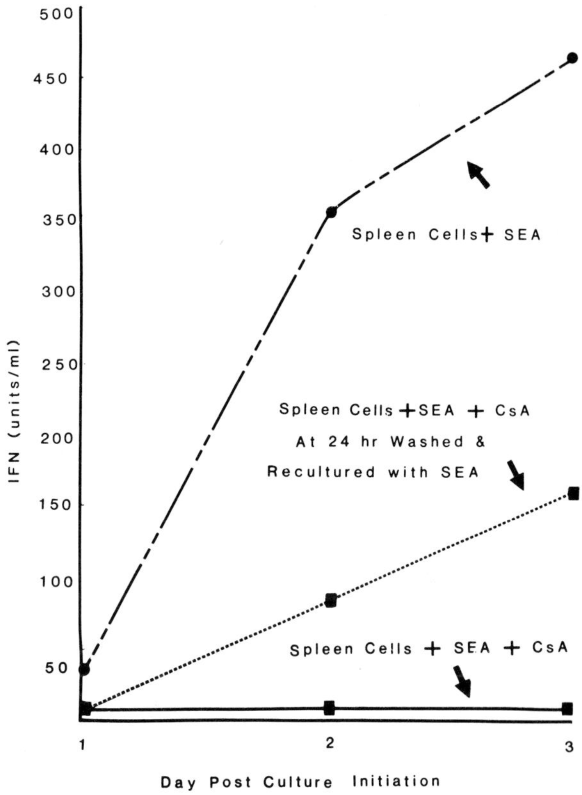

Fig. 1.

not shown), whereas CsA did not significantly inhibit IFN-gamma production when high doses of IL-2 were used.

CsA was shown to inhibit mitogen-induced IFN-gamma production even when added 24 hr post culture initiation. When we tested what effects CsA had on IL-2–induced IFN-gamma production, we found that CsA did not inhibit IFN-gamma production during the first 24 hr using a high concentration of supernatant that contained IL-2. It did, however, inhibit any further IFN-gamma production. Thus, CsA may act by inhibiting both IL-2 production and/or IL-2 action. Alternatively, CsA may act by inhibiting one or more events that occur after 24 hr of culture that are independent of IL-2.

Table 3. Virus-Induced IFNα/β Production Is Not Inhibited by CsA*

Culture Conditions	Type of IFN Induced	IFN /U/ml
L cells and NDV plus:	IFNα/β	
Medium		350
CsA (0.1 μg/ml)		345
C57B1/6 spleen and NDV plus:	IFNα/β	
Medium		230
CsA (0.1 μg/ml)		210
C57B1/6 spleen and SEA plus:	IFNγ	
Medium		460†
CsA (0.1 μg/ml)		<10
Human PBL and NDV plus:	IFNα	
Medium		5,500
CsA (0.1 μg/ml)		6,000

*Supernatants were obtained at 24 hr from cultures containing the cell types indicated as assessed for IFN activity.

†Supernatants harvested at day 2.

The next question we addressed was what effect CsA has on virus-induced IFN-alpha and IFN-beta production. IFN alpha and beta are produced by virus-infected fibroblasts and lymphocytes. CsA was added to different cultures of NDV-infected C57B1/6 spleen cells, mouse L cells, and human PBLs. After 24 hr of culture, supernatants were collected, dialyzed at pH 2, and assayed for IFN activity. Results can be seen in Table 3. The addition of CsA to both mouse and human cells had no effect on virus-induced IFN-alpha and/or IFN-beta production.

To summarize, our findings demonstrate that the addition of CsA to either human or murine lymphocytes stimulated with mitogen or alloantigen totally inhibited the production of IFN gamma. This inhibition was evident even when CsA was added at 24 hr post culture initiation to spleen cells stimulated with mitogen. However, CsA did not inhibit IL-2–induced IFN-gamma production at 24 hr. Thus, CsA may inhibit IFN-gamma production in a manner that is independent of IL-2 production and/or action. This inhibition of IFN-gamma production was also partially reversible.

In contrast to IFN-gamma production, virus-induced IFN-alpha and IFN-beta production was not inhibited by the addition of CsA. This was observed even when CsA was added at concentrations (0.1–5 μg/ml) that totally inhibited IFN-gamma production by T cells. These data provide further evidence that CsA acts predominantly on T lymphocytes and also extend the number of lymphokines whose production is inhibited by CsA.

REFERENCES

1. Calne RY: Immunol Rev 46:113, 1979
2. Wiesinger D, Borel JF: Immunobiology 156:454, 1979
3. Hess AD, Tutschka PJ: J Immunol 124:2601, 1980
4. Bunjes D, Hardt C, Röllinghoff M, et al: Eur J Immunol 11:657, 1981
5. Hess AD, Tutschka PJ, Zhang P, et al: J Immunol 128:360, 1982
6. Palacios R: Immunol Rev 63:19, 1982
7. Dos Reis G, Sherach E: J Immunol 129:1978, 1982
8. Klimpel GR, Dean JH, Day KD, et al: Cell Immunol 32:293, 1977
9. Dorshkind K, Klimpel GR, Rosse C: J Immunol 124:2584, 1980
10. Klimpel GR, Fleischmann WR, Baron S, et al: J Immunol 129:946, 1982
11. Campbell JB, Grunber MA, White SL: Can J Microbiol 21:1247, 1975
12. Torres BA, Yamamoto JK, Johnson, HM: Infect Immun 35:770, 1982
13. Yamamoto JK, Farrar WL, Johnson HM: Cell Immunol 66:331, 1982

Cyclosporine Inhibits Interleukin-2 and Interferon Gamma Synthesis by Human Thymocytes

G. H. Reem, L. A. Cook, and M. A. Palladino

THE AIM OF THIS study was to investigate the effect of cyclosporine A (CsA) on the synthesis of lymphokines by human thymocytes and on thymocyte proliferation. Studies from our laboratory have shown that human thymocytes synthesize interferon (IFN) gamma and interleukin 2 (IL-2) after induction with two or more of the following agents: concanavalin A (Con A), B lymphoblastoid cells (B_l cells), and 12-*O*-tetradecanoylphorbol-13-acetate (TPA).[1-3] IFN-alpha synthesis could be induced by Sendai virus.[4]

The present study provides evidence that CsA inhibits the synthesis of IFN gamma and IL-2 but not of virus-induced IFN alpha.

MATERIALS AND METHODS

CsA was a gift from Dr. J. F. Borel (Sandoz Pharmaceuticals, Basel, Switzerland)[5] and purified IL-2 from Dr. K. A. Smith.[6] Con A was purchased from Miles Laboratory (Elkhart, IN) and TPA from Consolidated Midland Corp. (Katona, NY).

Human thymocytes were isolated from sections of thymus obtained in the course of cardiac surgery of infants and very young children. Thymocytes were immediately suspended in RPMI 1640 medium supplemented with 5% heat-inactivated fetal-calf serum (FCS), 2 m*M* L-glutamine, 100 U/ml penicillin, 100 μg/ml streptomycin, and 0.25 μg/ml amphotericin B (complete medium). Thymocytes (6×10^6/ml) were cultured in 96-well flat-bottomed microtiter plates (Costar 3596 Costar Data Packaging, Cambridge, MA) containing complete medium (200 μl/well) in a humidified atmosphere with 5% CO_2 at 37°C. Irradiated (4,800 rad) B_l cells (3×10^5/ml) and Con A were added as indicated. For some experiments, thymocytes were preincubated with TPA (5 ng/ml) for 3 hr at 37°C, washed with complete medium, and cultured. Supernatants were harvested after a 48-hr incubation period and stored at −80°C until assayed for IL-2[3,7] and IFN activity. The type of the IFN synthesized was determined by neutralization with the appropriate antibody.[1,4] Proliferative rates were determined by pulsing cells with ^{3}H-thymidine (specific activity 6.7 Ci/mmole; New England Nuclear, Boston, MA) for the last 18 hr of the incubation period.

RESULTS

CsA added at the start of cultures (Table 1) inhibited both IL-2 and IFN-gamma synthesis induced with Con A and irradiated B_l cells, with Con A and TPA, or with all three inducing agents. Con A–induced proliferation was inhibited by CsA following 120 hr culture, while proliferation induced with B_l cells and TPA or B_l cells, TPA, and Con A was more resistant to the inhibitory effect of CsA (Table 1). At 48 hr of culture, thymocytes proliferated spontaneously, and this proliferation was resistant to inhibition by CsA (data not shown).[3] The inhibitory effect of CsA on IL-2 and IFN synthesis was dose-dependent (Table 2) and was apparent even in TPA-treated thymocytes. Addition of IL-2 and Con A at the start of culture enhanced IFN-gamma synthesis and proliferation; however, IL-2 did not reverse CsA inhibition of IFN-gamma synthesis and thymocyte proliferation (Table 3). The proliferation of thymocytes preincubated with Con A for 7 hr and subsequently cultured with IL-2 was not inhibited by CsA (Table 3). Proliferation induced by TPA, IL-2, and TPA in combination with IL-2 was refractory to inhibition by CsA. The combination of these agents did not result in the synthesis of detectable levels of IFN gamma in the medium (Table 4).

CsA did not inhibit Sendai virus–induced synthesis of IFN alpha by thymocytes (data not shown).

DISCUSSION

Our studies indicate that CsA inhibits IL-2 and IFN-gamma synthesis by human thymo-

---

From the New York University Medical Center (G. H. R., L. A. C.) and the Memorial Sloan Kettering Cancer Center (M. A. P.), New York.

Supported by a grant of the Sandoz Foundation and by American Cancer Society Grants IM-310 and JFRA-30.

Address reprint requests to Dr. Reem, New York University Medical Center, 560 First Avenue, New York, NY 10016.

0041-1345/83/1505-0032$01.00/0

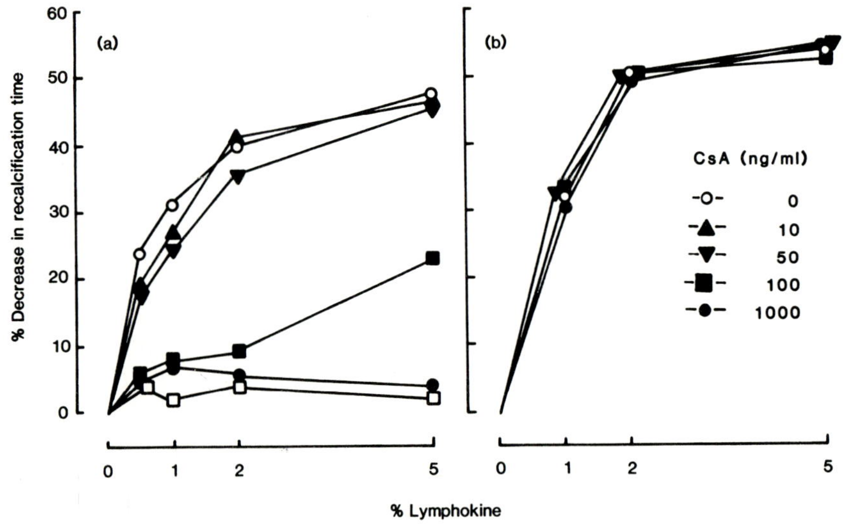

Fig. 2. Effect of CsA on production by mouse spleen cells of the lymphokine-inducing MPCA. (A) Procoagulant activity of PU5 cells induced by incubation with i Con A–induced lymphokine, produced in the presence of various CsA concentrations. The effect of control supernatant to which the mitogen was added at the end of the culture period is also shown (□). (B) Procoagulant activity of PU5 cells induced by incubation with preformed i Con A–induced lymphokine in the presence of various CsA concentrations.

using the MPCA assay, was observed over a similar range of CsA concentrations [Fig. 2 (A)]. In contrast, 16–20 hr incubation of the macrophage-like (PU5) indicator cells with CsA, followed by washing, did not affect their basal procoagulant activity or their ability to respond to preformed lymphokine [Fig. 2 (B)].

Lymphocyte-Derived Chemotactic Factor (LDCF)

Similar observations were made with regard to LDCF. Whereas lymphokine production by mouse spleen cells in response to PHA was inhibited by CsA in a dose-related manner, neither the spontaneous migration of peritoneal macrophages nor their ability to migrate toward preformed LDCF was affected (Fig. 3).

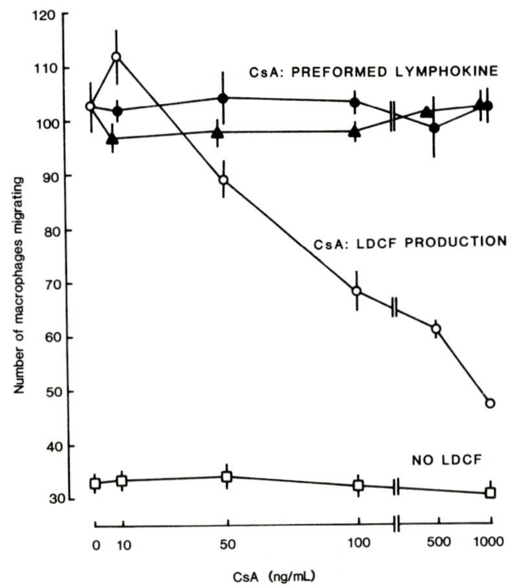

Fig. 3. Effect of CsA on LDCF production by mouse spleen cells in response to phytohemagglutinin. Symbols show mean numbers of macrophages migrating (±1 SE) in response to LDCF produced in the presence of various CsA concentrations (○) or in the absence of lymphokine (□). The response of macrophages to preformed LDCF when CsA was added to the upper (●) or lower (▲) wells of the chemotaxis chamber is also shown.

IL-1 Production

In comparison with the results on lymphokine production, studies on IL-1 secretion by LPS-stimulated guinea pig or mouse peritoneal macrophages revealed that much higher CsA concentrations (of the order 5 mg/ml) were required to consistently achieve an inhibitory effect (data not shown).

DISCUSSION

We have shown in these in vitro studies that CsA inhibits the production by guinea pig LNC or mouse spleen cells of lymphokines affecting macrophage behavior; in contrast, the response of macrophages to these lymphokines was unaffected in the presence of the drug. These results complement those of other workers who have demonstrated that CsA impairs production of IL-2 by alloantigen-activated T cells in vitro[7–10] and the release of MAF in antigen-challenged mice.[11] Thus, by inhibiting T-cell activation, CsA not only reduces availability of factors (IL-2) essential in maintenance of T-cell proliferation but also inhibits secretion of those soluble mediators responsible for the participation of macrophages in cell-mediated immunity.

It has been suggested that CsA may interfere with the acquisition of responsiveness by T cells to interleukins.[12] In the case of macrophages, our data clearly show that the drug does not affect the capacity of these cells to respond to interleukins. Moreover, other macrophage activities, such as spontaneous migration, phagocytic responses,[13,14] and basal procoagulant activity, are not affected by CsA. We have also failed to show inhibition of IL-1 production by peritoneal macrophages at concentrations of CsA that block lymphokine production. Others, however, using different test systems, have reported that IL-1 production is depressed by CsA.[7,8]

Similar changes in lymphokine responses to those reported in this study have been observed in CsA-treated guinea pigs and mice that exhibit depressed delayed-type hypersensitivity responses.[15,16] Inhibition of lymphokine production in these animals cannot be attributed to T-cell depletion; the mechanism by which CsA selectively inhibits T-cell activation has yet to be resolved.

REFERENCES

1. Geczy CL, Hopper KE: J Immunol 126:1059, 1981
2. David JR, Al-AsKari S, Lawrence HS, et al: J Immunol 93:264, 1964
3. Friedrich W, Lazary S, Geczy C, et al: Int Arch Allergy Appl Immunol 49:504, 1975
4. Farram E, Geczy CL, Moon DK, et al: J Immunol 130:2750, 1983
5. Falk W, Goodwin RH, Leonard EJ: J Immunol Methods 33:239, 1980
6. Farram E, Nelson M, Nelson DS, et al: Immunology 46:603, 1982
7. Andrus L, Lafferty KJ: Scand J Immunol 15:449, 1982
8. Bunjes D, Hardt C, Röllinghoff M, et al: Eur J Immunol 11:657, 1981
9. Hess AD, Tutschka PJ, Santos GW: J Immunol 128:355, 1982
10. Palacios R, Möller G: Nature 290:792, 1981
11. Alberti S, Boraschi D, Luini W, et al: Int J Immunopharmacol 3:357, 1981
12. Britton S, Palacios R: Immunol Rev 65:5, 1982
13. McIntosh LC, Thomson AW: Transplantation 30:384, 1980
14. Paavonen T, Järveläinen H, Kontiainen S, et al: Clin Exp Immunol 43:342, 1981
15. Thomson AW, Moon DK, Inoue Y, et al: Immunology 48:301, 1983
16. Thomson AW, Moon DK, Nelson DS: Clin Exp Immunol 52:599, 1983

Relationship Between IL-2 Receptors and Cyclosporine-Induced Suppression of T Leukemia and T Helper Cells

C. C.-Y. Shih, R. L. Truitt, P. Abramoff, and M. M. Bortin

CYCLOSPORINE A (CsA), an immunosuppressive agent, has been shown to preferentially abrogate cell-mediated immune responses, presumably by blocking early events in T helper cell activation.[1-3] T-cell suppression by CsA has been shown to be reversed by the addition of exogenous interleukin 2 (IL-2).[3,4] Although many studies have shown the cytostatic effects of CsA on T-malignant cells,[5-7] little has been done to compare the mechanisms of suppression on malignant vs. normal T cells. We have therefore undertaken studies on the effects of CsA on IL-2–dependent and IL-2–independent tumor cells and on T helper cell clones in order to elucidate the mechanism of suppression by CsA.

MATERIALS AND METHODS

Murine Tumor Cell Lines

AKR spontaneous T leukemia cell lines, AKIL-20 and AKIL-3.H5, were maintained in Dulbecco's modified Eagle's medium (DMEM) containing 5% fetal calf serum, 2-mercaptoethanol, and additional amino acids. The other AKR T-cell leukemia clones, AKIL-1.E8, AKIL-6.A3, and AKIL-6.D12 were maintained in IL-2 conditioned medium.[8]

From the Winter Research Laboratory, Mount Sinai Medical Center, Department of Biology, Marquette University, and the Medical College of Wisconsin, Milwaukee, WI.

Supported in part by grants from Kearney and Trecker Foundation. Rexnord Foundation, Todd Wehr Foundation, and the Apollo Fund. Cyclosporine A was a gift from Dr. Jean Borel, Sandoz Ltd., Basel, Switzerland. R. L. Truitt is a Scholar of the Leukemia Society of America, Inc.

Address reprint requests to Dr. C.-Y. Shih, Winter Research Laboratory, Mount Sinai Medical Center, P.O. Box 342, Milwaukee, WI 53201.

0041–1345/83/1505–0034$01.00/0

T Helper Cell and Clones

A T helper cell line "A9" was obtained from an SJL anti-AKR limiting-dilution microcytotoxicity assay and has been maintained in IL-2 conditioned medium for more than one year (authors unpublished observations). A9 and its clones, A9.2 and A9.12, produced IL-2 and interferon gamma (IFN gamma) when treated with mitogen (Con A).

Preparation of CsA

A CsA stock solution of 400 μg/ml in 2% Tween 80 and 5% alcohol was diluted with medium to the final testing concentration. Control cultures always contained equivalent amounts of Tween 80 and alcohol in the medium.

Production of IL-2 Conditioned Medium

A modification of the method of Gillis and Smith[9] was used to produce the IL-2 conditioned medium. In brief, W/Fu rat spleen cells were incubated with 5 μg/ml of Con A for 2 hr at 37°C. Cells were then washed free of Con A and suspended in DMEM medium with a cell concentration of 1×10^6/ml. After 48 hr, the supernatant of the culture was collected, filtered (0.45 μm), and designated IL-2 conditioned medium.

Proliferation Assay

A three day proliferation assay was used. Test cells were washed free of IL-2, then 1×10^4 cells suspended in 100 μl of culture medium were distributed to microculture wells. Various concentrations of CsA, IL-2, Con A, and/or stimulator cells were added to triplicate wells and made up to a final volume of 200 μl/well. The cultures were incubated for 72 hr at 37°C in a 10% Co_2 humidified incubator. The cells were labeled 24 hr before harvesting with 1 μCi of ^{3}H-TdR in 50 μl. The cells were harvested on filter paper, dried, and counted on a liquid scintillation counter.

IL-2 Activity Test

A standard IL-2 activity test described by Gillis et al.[10] was carried out using A9 cells as indicator cells. Cells were washed free of IL-2, and 1×10^4 cells in 100 μl were distributed into microculture wells. Another 100 μl of twofold serially diluted test medium was added. The proliferative response was measured as described above.

RESULTS

IL-2–Dependent and IL-2–Independent T Leukemia Cells

Three AKR spontaneous T leukemia cell lines (AKIL-1.E8, AKIL-6.A3, and AKIL-20) were tested for sensitivity to CsA in the presence or absence of IL-2. The data in Table 1 show that both AKIL-1.E8 and AKIL-6.A3 were IL-2–dependent, since their proliferation, if any, in the absence of IL-2 was minimal compared to cultures containing IL-2. In comparison, AKIL-20 cells were highly proliferative in the medium without IL-2. Of interest is the fact that when IL-2 was added without CsA, proliferation of AKIL-20 tumor cells was depressed. This could be attributed to the fact that IL-2 conditioned medium contains IFN gamma. CsA suppressed the proliferation of three tumor-cell lines in a dose-dependent manner and had 50% suppression at 625 ng/ml (1/8) for IL-2–dependent AKIL-20 cells. IL-2–dependent tumor cells were highly sensitive to CsA when IL-2 was absent (more than 50% suppression was detected at dilution as low as 1/64, or 78 ng/ml). When IL-2 was added to AKIL-20 cultures with CsA, the cytostatic effects of CsA was unchanged (at 50% suppression). However, when IL-2 was added to IL-2–dependent cells, 625 and 312.5 ng/ml of CsA were necessary to suppress the 50% response in AKIL-1.E8 and AKIL-6.A3 cells, respectively. These results indicated that the suppression by CsA on IL-2–dependent tumors could be reversed by exogenous IL-2, whereas exogenous IL-2 was unable to reverse the suppression by CsA on IL-2–independent tumor cells.

IL-2 Receptors

Absorption tests were used to show that IL-2–dependent tumor cells carried IL-2 receptors. The assumption was that cells carrying IL-2 receptors should absorb a significant amount of IL-2 activity in a relatively short period of time. AKIL-1.E8 or AKIL-20 cells were incubated with IL-2 conditioned medium for 2 hr at 37°C, and residual IL-2 activity was assayed in an IL-2 activity test (Fig. 1). IL-2–dependent AKIL-1.E8 cells absorbed more than 50% of IL-2 activity, whereas twice as many IL-2–independent AKIL-20 cells did not absorb any significant amount of IL-2 activity. These data indicated that IL-2–dependent cells carried IL-2 receptors and that IL-2–independent cells did not. These results also raise the possibility that the CsA suppression of IL-2–independent cells cannot be reversed with exogenous IL-2 because they lacked IL-2 receptors.

Reversal of CsA Suppression Is IL-2 Dose-Dependent

Two clones of AKR spontaneous leukemia, one IL-2–dependent (AKIL-6.D12) and the other IL-2–independent (AKIL-3.H5), were tested in the presence of a constant dose of CsA (1 μg/ml) and various concentrations of IL-2. Proliferation of IL-2–independent cells

Table 1. Effect of CsA on Proliferation (^{3}H-TdR Uptake) of IL-2–Dependent and IL-2–Independent AKR T Leukemia Cells

Cells (10^4/well)	IL-2 (50 Std. U)	% Suppression* in Medium with Various Dilutions of CsA† 1/2	1/4	1/8	1/16	1/32	1/64	Proliferation in Medium Without CsA (cpm ± SD)
AKIL-1.E8	−	98.0	95.3	93.9	89.0	84.6	66.1	11,400 ± 1,150[e]
	+	85.0	71.4	51.4	29.8	27.9	18.8	137,258 ± 14,116
AKIL-6.A3	−	98.1	95.6	95.6	93.9	90.8	83.6	5,619 ± 815
	+	92.2	86.1	70.7	54.7	35.0	28.3	100,729 ± 11,462
AKIL-20	−	99.3	93.5	66.1	27.6	17.4	11.9	65,411 ± 5,464
	+	99.3	96.0	83.6	43.7	23.9	16.1	48,243 ± 4,018

*%Suppression = (cpm without CsA − cpm in CsA)/cpm without CsA × 100.

†Initial concentration of CsA = 5 μg/ml.

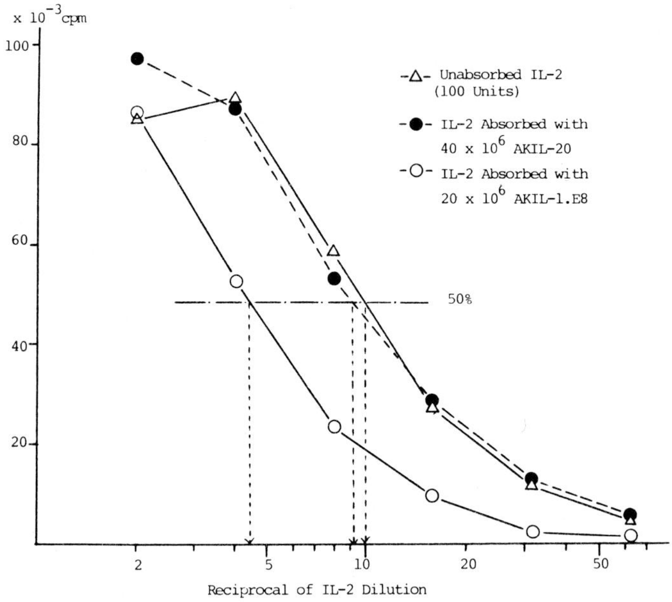

Fig. 1. Microculture wells were plated with 1 × 10^4 A9 (IL-2–dependent) T-helper cells in 100 μl of culture medium. 100 μl of serially diluted IL-2 conditioned media was added to each well. Cultures were labeled with ^{3}H-TdR 24 hr before harvesting. Incorporation of ^{3}H-TdR at 72 hr is shown.

was suppressed by CsA and could not be reversed with increasing amounts of IL-2 [Fig. 2 (A)]. In contrast, the effect of CsA on IL-2–dependent tumor cells was IL-2 dose-dependent [Fig. 2 (B)].

IL-2–Dependent T-Helper and Cloned Cells

The T helper cell line A9 and two clones, A9.2 and A9.12, were tested for their proliferative response to IL-2, alloantigen (AKR_x), and mitogen (Con A). The results of a three-day proliferation assay are shown in Table 2. Cloned and noncloned T helper cells all responded to the different stimuli as well as to exogenous IL-2 in a similar manner. However, when CsA was added to each culture, the response to alloantigen and mitogen was completely abrogated, while the response to IL-2

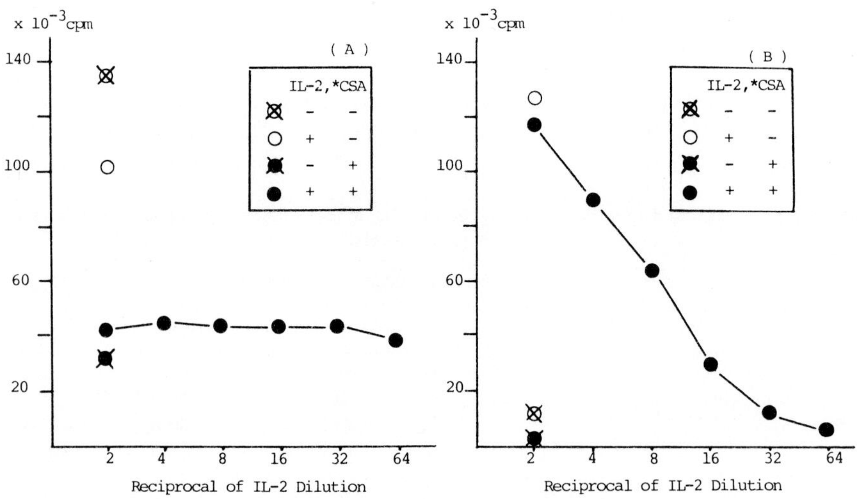

Fig. 2. Incorporation of ^{3}H-TdR in three-day microcultures containing 1 × 10^4 AKIL-3.H5 (IL-2–independent) cells (A) and AKIL-6.D12 (IL-2–dependent) cells (B) in media with no IL-2 and no CsA (⊠); IL-2 but no CsA (○); no IL-2 and 1 μg/ml CsA (✖); and serially diluted IL-2 with 1 μg/ml CsA (●). The initial concentration of IL-2 was 100 standard units. Cells were labeled with ^{3}H-TdR 24 hr before harvesting.

Table 2. Effect of CsA on Proliferation (^{3}H-TdR Uptake) of Cultured and Cloned SJL T Helper Cells in Response to Alloantigen or Mitogen (Con A) With or Without Added IL-2*

Responder Cells (0.25 × 10^5/well	CsA (0.1 μg/ml)	Medium Only	IL-2 Only (50 Std. U)	AKR_x Only (1.25 × 10^5/well)	AKR_x + IL-2	Con A Only (2.5 μg/ml)	Con A +IL-2
A9	−	434	124,901	80,011	107,099	32,966	17,812
	+	431	129,836	2,333	84,276	496	18,429
A9.2	−	569	100,657	72,638	85,125	18,512	7,500
	+	371	105,507	339	63,823	291	10,767
A9.12	−	358	97,404	68,251	111,807	28,534	10,123
	+	355	90,635	788	93,465	278	20,743

*Values shown are counts per minute of ^{3}H-TdR uptake.

remained intact. Exogenous IL-2 added to the cultures with alloantigen or Con A reversed the suppression by CsA; however, their proliferation did not reach the same level as when CsA was absent.

DISCUSSION

The results demonstrated that all tumor cells tested were sensitive to CsA, regardless of whether they carried putative IL-2 receptors or not. In those tumors with IL-2 receptors, the cytostatic effects of CsA were reversible in a dose-dependent manner by exogenous IL-2. However, exogenous IL-2 could not reverse the cytostatic effect of CsA on tumor cells presumed to be lacking IL-2 receptors. The proliferation of T helper cells in response to exogenous IL-2 was not affected by CsA. This probably was due to the presence of IL-2 receptors; that is, the suppression by CsA could be reversed by exogenous IL-2 in a manner similar to that observed with IL-2–dependent tumor cells. CsA suppression of T helper cells in response to alloantigen and mitogen may be due to the inhibition of IL-2 production, a finding similar to that of others using bulk mixed leukocyte cultures.[11-13] Based on the results presented here, it seems unlikely that CsA suppresses the generation of IL-2 receptors, as suggested by some investigators.[1,2] The ability of IL-2 to reverse CsA-induced suppression of T helper cells responding to alloantigen and mitogen (Table 2) was most likely due to the activation of existing IL-2 receptors rather than restoration of their response to alloantigen or mitogen.

REFERENCES

1. Larsson EJ: J Immunol 124:2828, 1980
2. Palacios R, Möller G: Nature 290:792, 1981
3. Bunjes D, Hardt C, Röllinghoff M, et al: Eur J Immunol 11:651, 1981
4. Bunjes D, Hardt C, Solbach W, et al: In White DJG (ed): Cyclosporin A. New York: Elsevier Biomedical Press, 1982, p 261
5. White DJG, Plumb AM, Pawelec G, et al: Transplantation 27:55, 1979
6. Fod P, Maiolo At, Baldini L, et al: Lancet 1:838, 1981
7. Fidelus RK, Orosz C, Ferguson RM: Transplant Proc 15:554, 1983
8. Shih CY, Truitt RL, Abramoff P, et al: In Vitro (in press)
9. Gillis S, Smith KA: Nature 268:154, 1977
10. Gillis S, Ferm MM, Du W, et al: J Immunol 120:202, 1978
11. Andrus L, Lafferty KJ: Scand J Immunol 15:449, 1982
12. Britton S, Palacios R: Immunol Rev 65:5, 1982
13. Wagner H: Transplant Proc 15:523, 1983

Effect of Cyclosporine on Prostacyclin Synthesis by Vascular Tissue in Rabbits

G. H. Neild, G. Rocchi, L. Imberti, F. Fumagalli, Z. Brown, G. Remuzzi, and D. G. Williams

BONE MARROW RECIPIENTS treated with cyclosporine (CsA) may develop renal failure associated with thrombocytopenia and fragmented red cells. Histologic examination of the kidney from such patients shows glomerular capillary thrombi and tubular necrosis.[1] This syndrome appears to be similar to the hemolytic-uremic syndrome (HUS), an acute illness of unknown etiology associated with endothelial damage and thrombosis in the microvasculature.[2] A failure of vascular prostacyclin (PGI_2) synthesis has been demonstrated in some of these patients,[3] and this failure has been associated with deficiency[3] of a normally occurring plasma factor that stimulates vascular PGI_2 synthesis.[4]

During experiments in which we examined the effect of CsA on acute serum-sickness nephritis in rabbits,[5] we noted that CsA-treated rabbits developed a new renal lesion characterized by glomerular capillary thrombosis and cortical infarction,[6] strikingly similar to the changes seen in HUS. As part of our investigation into the pathogenesis of this lesion, we examined the effect of CsA on vascular PGI_2 synthesis and PGI_2-stimulating factor (PSF) in rabbits.

MATERIALS AND METHODS

Animals

Female New Zealand white rabbits (1.8–2.4 kg) were used. Animals were bled from the marginal vein of the ear. Venous blood was anticoagulated with 3.8% sodium citrate (1:9, v/v) and centrifuged at 2,700 *g* for 10 min to obtain platelet-poor plasma. Plasma was stored at −70°C. Plasma taken before treatment was used as a normal control. Rabbits were killed by i.v. pentobarbitone, and their thoracic aortas were removed immediately and kept at −70°C.

From the Renal Unit, Department of Medicine, Guy's Hospital, London (G.H.N., Z.B., D.G.W.) and the Department of Nephrology, Ospedali Riuniti, Bergamo, Italy (G.R., L.I., F.F., G.R.).

Supported and financed by the Medical Research Council.

Address reprint requests to Dr. Neild.

0041-1345/83/1505-0035$01.00/0

Cyclosporine

CsA (100 mg/ml) for i.m. injection was dissolved in a solvent vehicle of Miglyol 812 and 100% ethanol. For in vitro incubation, CsA (1 mg/ml) was prepared as 1 mg CsA in 100 μl ethanol plus 20 μl Tween 80 plus 880 μl 0.05-*M* tris-saline buffer (pH 9.0).

PGI_2 Assay

PGI_2 was assayed both by radioimmunoassay of its stable, nonenzymatic degradation product 6-keto-$PGF_{1\alpha}$ (New England Nuclear, Boston, MA; NEK-008)[7] and biologically by its ability to inhibit platelet aggregation.[8] Platelet aggregation was performed in an Elvi 840 aggregometer (Elvi Logos, Milan), using human platelet-rich plasma (PRP). The human PRP was prepared from citrated blood by differential centrifugation, and for each batch the threshold aggregation concentration of adenosine diphosphate (ADP) was determined.

Vascular PGI_2 Synthesis

Pieces of thawed aorta were cut into 1-mm-thick rings (wet weight, 4–5 mg), and 4–5 pieces were incubated in 1-ml volumes of 0.05-*M* Tris-saline buffer (pH 9.0) at 22°C for two 60-min periods separated by a wash in buffer. PGI_2 production was expressed as ng 6-keto-$PGF_{1\alpha}$/ml buffer/mg wet weight of aorta. In addition, aortas from untreated rabbits were incubated with CsA in Tris buffer.

PGI_2-Stimulating Factor (PSF) Activity

Pieces of aorta were first exhausted of PGI_2 by alternate incubation with 100 μg angiotensin II (Hypertensin, Ciba Pharmaceuticals, Summit, NJ) in 1 ml Tris buffer, and Tris buffer alone at 22°C, until no PGI_2 activity was detectable in the washings.[7] Exhausted aorta was incubated with 0.3-m*M* arachidonic acid (AA, sodium arachidonate; Sigma Chemical Co., St. Louis, MO) in buffer for 25 min at 37°C, was washed three times in buffer, and was then incubated with 400 μl of rabbit plasma in water bath at 37°C. After 30 min, 100 μl of incubated plasma was mixed with 250 μl of human PRP, and platelet aggregation was initiated by ADP. As a control for each experiment, 100 μl of unincubated plasma was added to 250 μl of PRP, and platelet aggregation was recorded. By comparing the initial platelet aggregation velocities, the percentage inhibition of platelet aggregation could be calculated. The capacity of rabbit plasma to stimulate PGI_2 synthesis by vascular tissue was compared with a reference pool of normal human plasma and measured as a percentage of that pool.[7] PSF activity was also measured after plasma from normal rabbits had been incubated with CsA in Tris buffer.

Rate of PGI_2 Degradation

The rate of PGI_2, degradation was measured by monitoring the period of the antiplatelet aggregating activity of 6–23 nmole/liter synthetic PGI_2 (Farmitalia-Carlo Erba, Milan) added to plasma samples.[9,10]

Experimental Protocol

Six rabbits were given CsA 25 mg/kg for five days. Four rabbits received an equivalent volume of solvent alone. Rabbits were bled on alternate days and were killed on day 12.

RESULTS

Vascular PGI_2 Synthesis

We examined first the effect of CsA on spontaneous PGI_2 synthesis by aortic tissue. Aortas from CsA-treated and untreated rabbits generated PGI_2 in equal amounts: CsA-treated—1st hr 61 ± 6.4, 2nd hr 21.8 ± 2.2; controls—1st hr 57.7 ± 7.2, 2nd hr 20.5 ± 2.3 ng 6-keto-$PGF_{1\alpha}$/ml/mg wet weight (mean ± SEM). To investigate the direct effect in vitro of CsA on PGI_2 synthesis, aortas from four normal rabbits were incubated with CsA in Tris buffer. Concentrations of CsA from 0.1–10 μg/ml did not affect the generation of PGI_2 (data not shown). These experiments indicate that neither CsA nor its metabolites act as specific inhibitors of PGI_2 synthesis in vascular tissue.

PSF Activity

When exhausted aorta from normal rabbits was incubated with plasma from rabbits treated with CsA, its ability to convert exogenously added AA into PGI_2 was profoundly inhibited (Fig. 1). This effect was apparent by 24 hr and persisted for seven days after CsA therapy was stopped. In a separate control experiment, solvent given to four normal rabbits had no effect on PSF activity (data not shown). When CsA was added to normal plasma in vitro (0.1–10 μg/ml), it did not affect PSF activity (data not shown). Moreover, when varying amounts of plasma from CsA-treated animals were mixed with normal plasma (1:4, 1:1, 4:1), there was no inhibition of the PSF activity of normal plasma. These results suggest that neither CsA nor its metabolites act as inhibitors of PSF activity.

PGI_2 Degradation

We found that plasma from CsA-treated rabbits had no effect on the rate of PGI_2 degradation: The degradation time in plasma from four CsA-treated rabbits was 83.3 ± 4.4

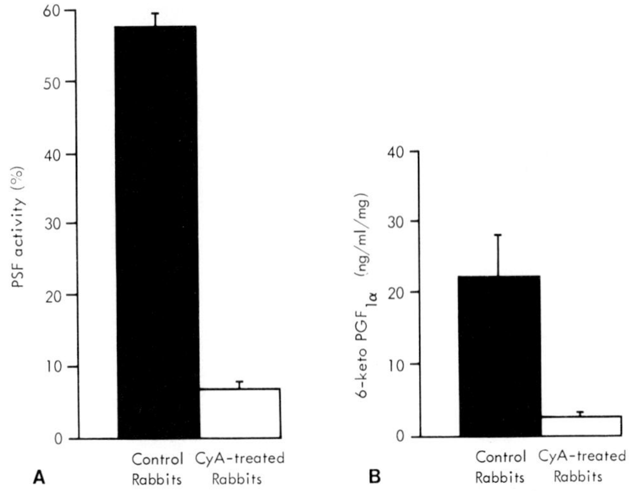

Fig. 1. Six rabbits received 25 mg/kg CsA i.m. for five days, and blood was taken during days 1–12 after the start of treatment. Plasma taken from rabbits before treatment was used as a control. (A) Rabbit plasma was compared with a pool of normal human plasma and expressed as a percentage of that pool. The figure shows the mean ± SEM of the results of all samples taken during the period of study (days 1–12). (B) The PGI_2 produced from vascular tissue after stimulation by rabbit plasma was also measured as 6-keto-$PGF_{1\alpha}$ (ng/ml/mg of vascular tissue; mean ± SEM).

min, and for the four normal controls 83 ± 6 min (mean ± SEM).

DISCUSSION

Plasma contains one or more factors that stimulate PGI_2 synthesis by endothelial cells in culture[4,11] and aortic tissue that has been exhausted of its ability to produce PGI_2.[3] Remuzzi showed that some patients with a HUS lacked this PGI_2-stimulating factor (PSF) activity in their plasma.[3] We found that there was a profound loss of PSF activity in plasma from rabbits treated with CsA. PSF is poorly characterized,[4,11] but we conclude that CsA acts by preventing either its production or release into the circulation, rather than acting as an inhibitor of its action.

PGI_2 is both a vasodilator and a potent inhibitor of platelet aggregation, and it limits excessive platelet aggregation and thrombus formation at sites of endothelial injury.[8,12] We believe that in the absence of PSF, synthesis of PGI_2 is impaired and endothelial injury can progress to capillary thrombosis and necrosis of the vessel wall. The new glomerular lesion we noted in our CsA-treated rabbits with acute serum sickness (ASS)[6] is similar to that recently reported in patients receiving CsA after allogeneic marrow transplantation,[1] and these patients also developed other features of HUS. We believe that CsA-treated rabbits with ASS, CsA-treated marrow transplantation, and HUS are three conditions in which there are different mechanisms of endothelial injury, and when they occur in the absence of PSF, they result in the same final vascular injury.

Could the effect of CsA on PSF be related to the T cell–specific inhibiting action of the drug? The origin of PSF is unknown. Since CsA inhibits the release of lymphokines from lymphocytes,[13,14] its effect on PSF could be explained if PSF were a lymphokine regulating PGI_2 synthesis. The prostaglandins play an important role in immune function,[15,16] and PSF might provide a regulating effect on the immune response by controlling mononuclear cell production of PGI_2.

ACKNOWLEDGMENTS

We thank Dr. Jean Borel and Sandoz AG for their gift of Cyclosporine A, and Prof. Stewart Cameron and Dr. G. de Gaetano for valuable discussion.

REFERENCES

1. Shulman H, Striker G, Deeg HJ, et al: N Engl J Med 305:1392, 1981

2. Alfrey AC: In Brenner BM, Rector FC (eds): The Kidney (2nd ed.). Philadelphia, W.B. Saunders, 1981, p 1668

3. Remuzzi G, Misiani R, Marchesi D, et al: Lancet 2:871, 1978

4. MacIntyre DE, Pearson JD, Gordon JL: Nature 271:549, 1978

5. Neild GH, Ivory K, Hiramatsu M, et al: Transplant Proc (in press)

6. Neild GH, Ivory K, Williams DG: Translant Proc (in press)

7. Remuzzi G, Zoja C, Marchesi D, et al: Br Med J 282:512, 1981

8. Moncada S, Higgs EA, Vane JR: Lancet 1:18, 1977

9. Chen YC, McLeod B, Hall ER, et al: Lancet 2:267, 1981

10. Remuzzi G, Imberti L, de Gaetano G: Lancet 2:1422, 1981

11. Seid JM, Jones PBB, Russel RGG: Clin Sci 64:387, 1983

12. Moncada S, Vane JR: Phil Trans Roy Soc Lond B 294:305, 1981

13. Borel JF, Feurer C, Magnee C, et al: Immunology 32:1017, 1977

14. Wiesinger D, Borel JF: Immunobiology 156:454, 1979

15. Bray MA: Immunol Today 3:65, 1980

16. Hadden JW, Coffey RG: Immunol Today 3:299, 1982

PHARMACOKINETICS

Methods to Measure Cyclosporine Levels—High Pressure Liquid Chromatography, Radioimmunoassay, and Correlation

W. T. Robinson, H. F. Schran, and E. P. Barry

SEVERAL methods have been developed for the analysis of cyclosporine in plasma and/or blood. The first method reported was the radioimmunoassay (RIA) of Donatsch (Table 1), which is now available as a kit and has been used extensively during the clinical development for cyclosporine. The method was initially developed for plasma, and as shown later, is also applicable to blood samples. The main criticism of the RIA method has been the cross-reactivity of the antisera with some of the circulating metabolites of cyclosporine.

Subsequent to the introduction of the RIA method, Niederberger et al.[2] developed a high-pressure liquid chromatography (HPLC) method based on gradient elution. The technical complexity of this method encouraged several investigators,[3–10] as well as Dr. Niederberger himself (Nussbaumer et al.), to reinvestigate the method. The results of these activities are shown in Table 1.

In designing a pharmacokinetic study to investigate the dose-proportionality of cyclosporine, we were faced with the problem of choosing a suitable method. Aside from the RIA method, only three methods had detection limits below 25 μg/liter. The extensive sample preparation associated with these methods and the long chromatography time was considered a serious drawback in the use of HPLC. We, therefore, elaborated a semiautomated method[10] based on Niederberger's,[2] Nussbaumer's,[5] and Sawchuk's[4] work. This method was designed for high sample throughput and for a minimum of technical work. The design of the method allowed for the quantitation of cyclosporine to a limit, stated conservatively, of 8 μg/liter in plasma and 20 μg/liter in blood.

Application of the semiautomated method, as well as the RIA method, in a dose-proportionality study offered a unique opportunity to better define the performance of the RIA method vis-à-vis the HPLC method.

MATERIALS AND METHODS

The clinical study was conducted in 12 normal healthy men (age, 18–43 yr; mean, 31 yr) who received a single dose of 350, 700, and 1,400 mg of cyclosporine (Sandimmune Oral Solution). The study design was a replicated 3 × 3 Latin Square with a one week washout interval between doses. Heparinized blood was collected immediately prior to dosing and at 0.5, 1, 2, 3, 4, 6, 8, 12, 24, 48, 72, and 96 hr after each dose. Both blood and plasma were analyzed by HPLC (Smith and Robinson) and by RIA.

The HPLC method involved deproteination of plasma or blood (0.5 ml) with acetonitrile (1.2 ml; hydrated with 2.5% water), and the supernatant was sampled by the Technicon/HPLC system shown in Fig. 1. After the hexane wash, the sample was loaded into a 2-ml loop, injected, and developed on the LC-8 column (Supelcosil, Supelco, Inc., Bellefonte, PA, 5 μm held at 75°C) with acetonitrile:water (55:45, v/v; 3.0 ml/min). The segment containing cyclosporine was automatically diverted by a second valve to the LC-18 column (Supelcosil, 5 μm held at 75°C), which was developed with acetonitrile:water (75:25, v/v; 1 ml/min). Detection was by ultra violet absorption at 202 nm. The precision of the method was ±8% (coefficient of variation) in plasma and ±9% in blood. The average coefficient of variation across days was ±6% and ±10% for blood and plasma, respectively. The accuracy of the method was such that any single analysis would fall (95% confidence level) within ±20% and ±27% of its true value for plasma and blood, respectively.

The RIA method of Donatsch et al.[1] was applied using the reagent kit consisting of ditritiocyclosporine, cyclosporine standard and antisera obtained via a cyclosporine-C-hemisuccinate-IgG conjugate. The lower limit of detection was 20 μg/liter when analyzing a 2-μl aliquot of blood or plasma. Larger volumes provide a proportionate increase in assay sensitivity. The precision and reproducibility of the method in blood and plasma was ±5%–7% and ±8%–12%, respectively. The accuracy was such that

From Sandoz, Inc., East Hanover, NJ.

Address reprint requests to Dr. W. T. Robinson, Sandoz, Inc., Route 10, East Hanover, NJ 07963.

0041–1345/83/1505–0036$01.00/0

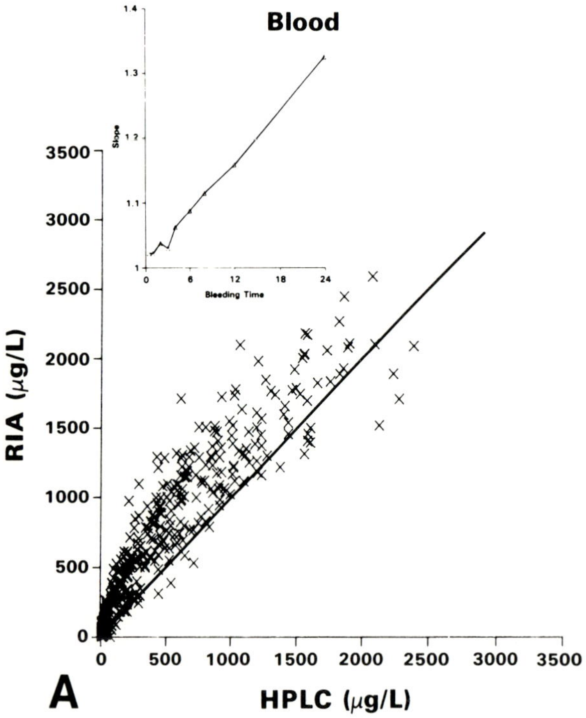

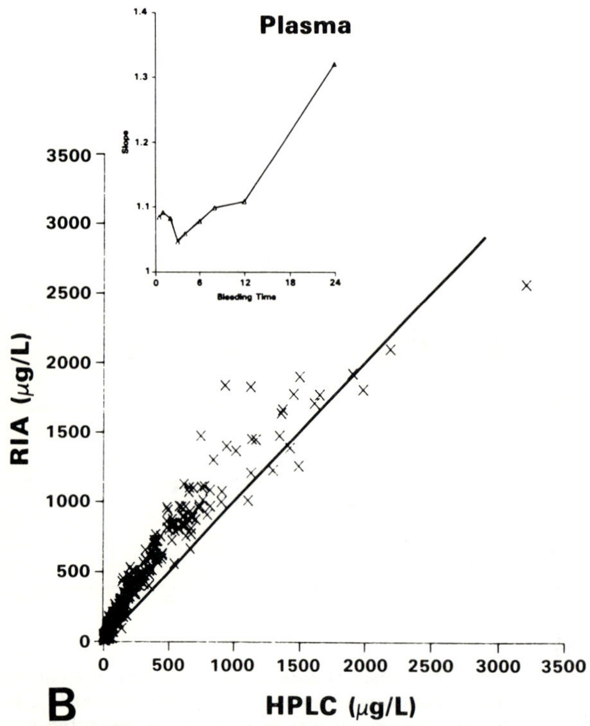

Fig. 3. Scatter diagrams of (A) blood and (B) plasma data as measured by HPLC and RIA. Insert shows temporal affect.

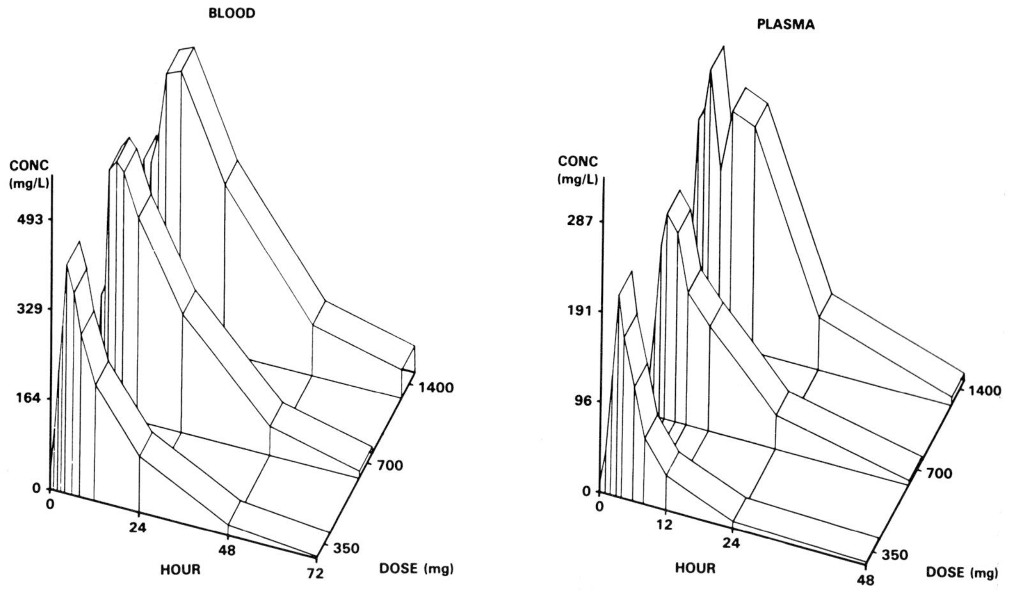

Fig. 4. **Blood and plasma concentrations/time profile for "cross-reacting" metabolites in the RIA method (see text).**

approximately 1. The slope of this envelope was independent of the administered dose. The differences between the two methods becomes clearer if this regression analysis includes a time of bleeding component. The slope of the regression line steadily increased with time from dosing (Fig. 3). If the differences between RIA and HPLC methods are averaged over subjects at each bleeding time, the curves shown in Fig. 4 are obtained. These concentrations (RIA–HPLC) represent, on a relative basis, the blood (plasma) concentration/time profile for the metabolites that crossreact in the RIA method. The T_{max} for these data is similar to the T_{max} for unchanged drug, and it is apparent that a dose-propor-

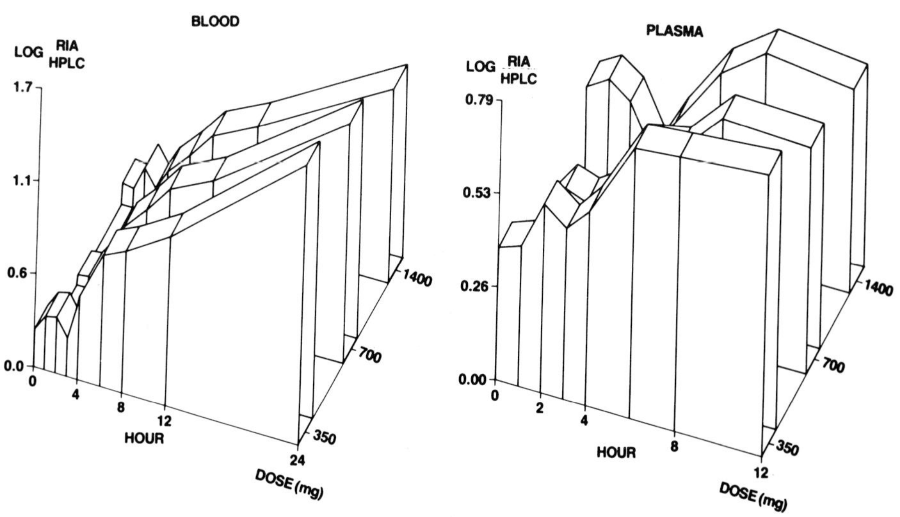

Fig. 5. **Temporal effect on the average value for log (RIA/HPLC) calculated for each bleeding time for each individual subject.**

tionality exists for AUC and C_{max}. A calculation of the half-life for the disappearance of the "crossreacting metabolites" gave results similar to the calculated terminal half-life for unchanged drug. This is shown better in Fig. 5. If the RIA data parallel the HPLC data, then the difference between log RIA and log HPLC (i.e., log [RIA/HPLC]) should be a constant. Figure 5 shows that the relationship log (RIA/HPLC) approaches a constant value between 8 and 24 hr. The earlier changes in this relationship stem from the differences in the disposition profile of unchanged drug and "crossreacting metabolites." The disposition of unchanged drug is biphasic, whereas the disposition of the "crossreacting metabolites" appears to be monophasic, with a half-life no longer than that for the terminal phase in the disposition of cyclosporine.

Since a pseudo-steady state between "crossreacting metabolites" and unchanged drug is approached at about 24 hr after dosing, only the C_{min} (trough) values for RIA data (assuming once a day dosing) reflect the change in cyclosporine concentration with any accuracy. As Carruthers et al.[9] have already demonstrated, the C_{min} values at steady state (during chronic administration) as determined by RIA and HPLC parallel each other and, therefore, either method adequately reflects a change in plasma or blood concentration.

CONCLUSIONS

In summary, the following conclusions on the value of the RIA and HPLC methods can be made: (1) Both the HPLC and RIA methods lead to the same pharmacokinetic interpretations. (2) The crossreacting metabolites in RIA have half-lives similar to that for cyclosporine. (3) Use of either RIA or HPLC is appropriate for clinical monitoring; however, different reference scales must be used. (4) When using RIA, C_{min} (trough) values should be used in clinical monitoring.

REFERENCES

1. Donatsch P, Abisch E, Homberger M, et al: Immunoassay 2:19, 1981

2. Niederberger W, Schaub P, Beveridge T: J Chromatogr Biomed Appl 182:454, 1980

3. Lawrence R, Allwood MC: J Pharm Pharmacol 32(Suppl): 100P, 1980

4. Sawchuk RJ, Cartier LL: Clin Chem 27:1368, 1981

5. Nussbaumer K, Niederberger W, Keller HP: J High Resolut Chromatogr Chromatogr Commun 5:424, 1982

6. Leyland-Jones B, Clark A, Kreis W, et al: Res Commun Chem Pathol Pharmacol 37:431, 1982

7. Kahan BD, Van Buren CT, Lin SN, et al: Transplantation 34:36, 1982

8. Yee GC, Gmur DJ, Kennedy MS: Clin Chem 28:2269, 1982

9. Carruthers SG, Freeman DJ, Koegler JC, et al: Clin Chem 29:180, 1983

10. Smith HT, Robinson WT: (submitted for publication)

11. Abisch E, Beveridge T, Gratwohl A, et al: Pharm Weekbl Sc 4:84, 1982

Cyclosporine: Pharmacokinetics, Metabolism, and Drug Interactions

A. J. Wood, G. Maurer, W. Niederberger, and T. Beveridge

THE usefulness of cyclosporine (CsA) in transplantation is now well established. However, its relatively narrow therapeutic index and the fact that there are interindividual differences in response to given doses mean that an understanding of the pharmacokinetics of CsA is required in designing optimal therapeutic regimens. The availability of a sensitive and specific high-pressure liquid chromatography method for the measurement of CsA concentrations in biologic fluids[1] has allowed several pharmacokinetic studies to be performed. This article is a review of the present knowledge of the pharmacokinetics and metabolism of CsA.

ABSORPTION

Because of its very low water-solubility, the oral dose form of CsA is an olive-oil–based solution. In one of the first pharmacokinetic studies,[2] six patients were given a single oral dose of 600 mg CsA, and serum CsA concentrations were measured at intervals over the following 48 hr (Fig. 1). Analysis of the concentration–time data showed that after a lag-time of 0.65 hr, absorption occurred with a half-life of about 1 hr. Peak serum concentrations were attained 3–4 hr after administration, and the maximum concentration measured varied from 240 to 1,250 ng/ml (mean, 538 ng/ml). There were two disposition phases; the corresponding mean elimination half-lives were 1.2 hr and 27 hr.

The absolute bioavailability of CsA from the oral solution (in steady state) was determined in five bone marrow transplant recipients by calculating the area under the blood concentration–time curve (AUC) after an intravenous infusion of the drug, and comparing this with the AUC from blood concentrations measured 30 days later after an oral dose.[3] In these five subjects, bioavailability varied from 20% to 50% (mean, 34%).

DISTRIBUTION

The distribution and binding of CsA to blood components in vitro has been studied in the concentration range from 25 to 500 ng/ml.[4] The uptake by erythrocytes was about 50%, whereas the uptake by leukocytes was 10%–20%. Of the total amount of drug in the plasma, approximately 90% was protein-bound. Most of the protein-bound drug was associated with lipoproteins, with relatively little being bound to other plasma proteins. In this concentration range, the binding to erythrocytes and lipoproteins was apparently linear, while the leukocyte accumulation appeared to be saturable.

Administration of ^{3}H-CsA to rats revealed a high tissue affinity of drug-related radioactivity (tissue-to-blood ratios, 2:10), with relatively slow elimination from tissues.[5] These observations are consistent with the high lipid solubility of CsA and its metabolites. Following single doses, the highest concentrations of radioactivity were found in liver, kidney, adrenals, pancreas, thymus, thyroid, and renal fat. With continued administration, accumulation was observed in skin and fat. This pattern of distribution has been recently confirmed in postmortem tissue samples taken from patients who had received CsA.[6,7]

The compartmental distribution of CsA has been studied in four patients with advanced renal failure who received an intravenous infusion of CsA (3.5 mg/kg over 4 hr).[8] The blood concentration–time data could be described by a three-compartment model.

From the Clinical Research and Biopharmaceutical Departments, Sandoz Ltd., Basel, Switzerland.

Address reprint requests to Dr. A. J. Wood, International Clinical Research, Sandoz Ltd., CH-4002, Basel, Switzerland.

0041-1345/83/1505-0037$01.00/0

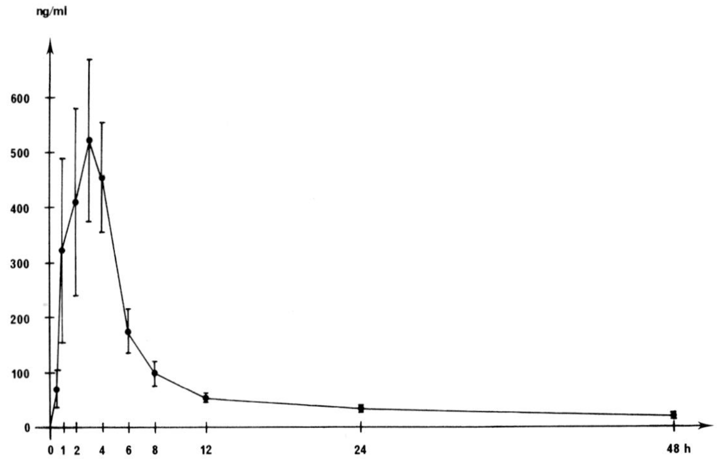

Fig. 1. Mean (±SEM) plasma concentrations after a single 600-mg dose of CsA (n = 6). Reproduced with permission from Curr. Therap. Res. (Beveridge, T. et al., 1981, 30:5–18).

Elimination of the drug from blood occurred triexponentially, with half-lives of 0.1, 1.1, and 16 hr. Tissue distribution was extensive, as indicated by a mean apparent volume of distribution of 3.5 liter/kg.

METABOLISM

The metabolism of CsA has been studied in rat, rabbit, dog, and man.[9] The biotransformation pathways are similar in all species. CsA is slowly but extensively metabolized. In pooled plasma (2–8 hr) from human subjects given ^{3}H-CsA, about 27% of the radioactivity was associated with CsA itself. Apart from the parent drug, 10–12 minor radioactive components were detected; the proportions of the individual peaks ranged from 2% to 12% of the plasma radioactivity.

From a total of 10–17 radioactive components found in different species, nine metabolites have been isolated and identified. All identified metabolites contained the intact cyclic oligopeptide structure of the parent drug. Structural modification consisted of mono- and dihydroxylation and *N*-demethylation at various sites on the CsA molecule (Fig. 2).

ELIMINATION

From numerous studies, terminal elimination half-lives from blood or plasma of 14–17 hr have been calculated. The major route of elimination of CsA and its metabolites is biliary excretion. Following intravenous administration of ^{3}H-CsA to bile-duct cannulated rats, 59% of the radioactivity was eliminated in the bile.[10] In man, the total urinary excretion of radioactivity in the period up to 96 hr following a single dose was 6% of the administered dose; unchanged CsA accounted for only 0.1% of the oral dose.[9]

INTERACTIONS

Some important or potentially important effects of other drugs on the pharmacokinetics of CsA have been reported. Ketoconazole causes a substantial increase in CsA concentrations.[11,12] Phenytoin, in maintenance anticonvulsant doses, reduces the area under the CsA concentration–time curve by 50%.[13] The intravenous administration of sulphadimidine and trimethoprim to a cardiac transplant recipient also receiving CsA resulted in a marked reduction in serum CsA concentration. This effect was not seen when sulphadimidine and trimethoprim were given orally.[14] Since the magnitude of the effect of these compounds on blood concentrations of CsA is difficult to predict, it is recommended that their coadministration with CsA be avoided. If coadministration is unavoidable, careful monitoring of CsA blood levels and appropriate modification of CsA dosage are essential.

Other reported interactions appear to be due to pharmacologic rather than pharmacokinetic mechanisms (that is, no change in CsA concentrations, but additive pharmacologic

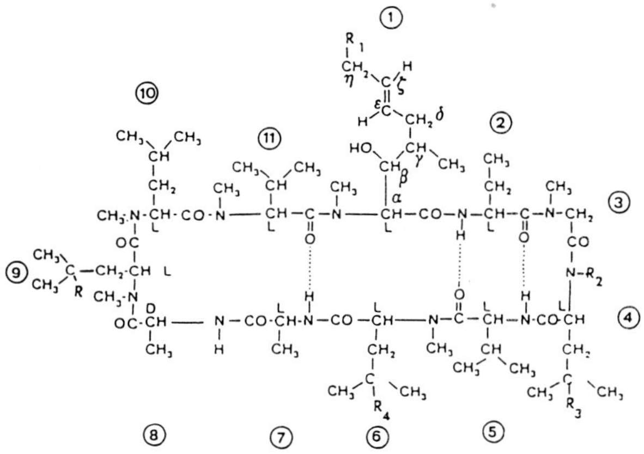

Metabolite No.	R	R_1	R_2	R_3	R_4	other modification
OL 27-400	H	H	CH_3	H	H	
1	OH	H	CH_3	H	H	
8	OH	OH	CH_3	H	H	
9	OH	H	H	H	OH	
10*	OH	H	CH_3	OH	H	
16*	OH	H	CH_3	H	OH	
17	H	OH	CH_3	H	H	
18	H	OH	CH_3	H	H	CH_{β}–O–CH_{ε} – $CH_{2\,\zeta}$ of ①
21	H	H	H	H	H	
13	hydroxylated and N-demethylated derivative of OL 27-400					

○ numbering of the amino-acids
* : metabolites not found in man.

Fig. 2. Metabolites of cyclosporine for which a structure has been proposed.

effects of the two compounds). Such interactions include the coadministration of CsA with other nephrotoxic agents, such as aminoglycosides,[15] amphotericin-B,[16] and melphalan.[17]

SUMMARY AND CONCLUSIONS

After oral administration of the olive-oil–based solution, the bioavailability of CsA is 20%–50%. Peak blood concentrations are usually reached after 3–4 hr. Because of its high lipid solubility, CsA is extensively distributed to extravascular tissues. Within the blood, approximately 50% of the drug is associated with erythrocytes and 10%–20% with leukocytes. Of the 30%–40% in the plasma, approximately 90% is bound to lipoproteins. The drug is eliminated primarily by biliary mechanisms; the terminal elimination half-life is 14–27 hr. The parent drug is metabolized to approximately 15 metabolites, all of which are present in considerably lower plasma concentrations than CsA itself. Ketoconazole and cimetidine cause an increase in CsA plasma concentrations, whereas phenytoin administration decreases CsA concentrations. Where coadministration of these compounds is unavoidable, careful monitoring of CsA plasma or blood concentrations is essential.

REFERENCES

1. Niederberger W, Schaub P, Beveridge T: J Chromatogr Biomed Appl 182:454, 1980

2. Beveridge T, Gratwohl A, Michot F, et al: Curr Ther Res 30:5, 1981

3. Beveridge T, Gratwohl A, Niederberger W: Sandoz Document 301–004, 1982

4. Lemaire M: Sandoz Document 303–026, 1981

5. Wagner O, Rietsch D: Sandoz Document 303–029, 1981

6. Kahan BD, van Buren CT, Boileau M, et al: Transplantation 35:96, 1983

7. Atkinson K, Biggs JC, Britton K: Lancet 2:1165, 1982

8. Follath F, Wenk M, Vozeh S, et al: Clin Pharmacol Ther (in press)

9. Maurer G, Loosli HR, Schreier E, et al: Drug Metab Disposit (in press)

10. Wagner O, Rietsch D: Sandoz Document 303–015, 1981

11. Ferguson RM, Sutherland DER, Simmons RL, et al: Lancet 2:882, 1982

12. Lokiec F, Poirier O, Gluckman E, et al: In White DJG (ed): Cyclosporin A. Amsterdam, Elsevier Biomedical, 1982, p 497

13. Keown PA, Stiller CR, Laupacis AL, et al: Transplant Proc 14:659, 1982

14. Wallwork J, McGregor CGA, Wells FC: Lancet 1:376, 1983

15. Hows JM, Palmer S, Want S, et al: Lancet 2:145, 1981

16. Kennedy MS, Deeg HJ, Siegel M, et al: Transplantation 35:211, 1983

17. Morgenstern GR, Powles R, Robinson B, et al: Lancet 2:1342, 1982

Cyclosporine Pharmacokinetics in Man

J. Newburger and B. D. Kahan

CYCLOSPORINE-A (CsA), a novel immunosuppressant agent, is being used clinically to avert organ rejection in human renal allograft transplantation.[1-3] It has been shown to have potent immunosuppressant properties. At the present time, CsA is administered orally on an empirical basis. This can result in problems associated with organ rejection if the dose is too low or manifestations of nephrotoxicity, hepatotoxicity, gingival hyperplasia, hirsutism, or tremor if the dose is too large.[4] If the pharmacokinetic parameters of CsA could be identified, it might be possible to suggest a more rational dosing regimen to maintain the patients in a safe clinically effective therapeutic range and avoid these problems. In this preliminary investigation, CsA was administered both orally and by i.v. infusion to both kidney transplant candidates and kidney transplant recipients. The data of patients were selected whose plasma-serum versus time profiles of CsA suggested that biliary cycling was not occurring during the single 24-hr dosing period. All data were analyzed using the NON-LIN computer program.[5]

MATERIALS AND METHODS

CsA Determination

Blood samples were immediately chilled and the plasma or serum was separated. The radioimmunoassay (RIA) for CsA, which used materials provided by the Sandoz Co. (Basel, Switzerland), was performed and analyzed as previously reported.[6]

Oral Studies

Posttransplant data were selected from those patients receiving the drug during the first 20 postoperative days. CsA was administered orally to all patients in chocolate milk at 5:00 AM before eating. Samples were withdrawn at time zero, every hour up to 6 hr, and then every 2 hr.

Infusion Studies

Data were selected from posttransplant patients who received CsA during the first 20 postoperative days. CsA was infused into a forearm vein using an IMED infusion pump at a rate of 150 mg/hr for 1 hr and then discontinued. Samples were withdrawn from the forearm opposite to that in which the infusion was administered at time zero and every 15 min up to 1 hr during the infusion. At the termination of the infusion, samples were withdrawn every half hour for 2 hr and then every hour for 24 hr.

RESULTS

Table 1 shows the results of the posttransplant patients who received CsA orally. The data were best fit to a two-compartment open model with first-order absorption and two disposition constants. The absorption half-life varies from 0.60 to 2.3 hr. The first disposition phase (α) half-life varied from 0.65 to 2.8 hr, while the terminal disposition phase (β) half-life varied from 5.6 to 34.6 hr. Our results for K_a and α are similar to those reported by Beveridge et al.[7] from patients receiving allogeneic bone marrow transplants. However, our results for β show a very large variation. It seems reasonable to suggest that one might expect a much larger variation among kidney transplant patients.

Kahan et al.[6] have reported that the fraction of the dose absorbed increases during the treatment period, resulting in an increase in the area under the curve (AUC). The AUC is defined as follows

$$\text{AUC} = \frac{(F)(\text{Dose})}{(V_B)(\beta)}$$

where F is the fraction of the dose absorbed, V_B is the total body volume, and β is the elimination phase rate constant. It can be seen that the AUC will not only increase with an

From the Department of Surgery, Division of Immunology and Organ Transplantation, University of Texas Medical School at Houston, TX.

Address reprint requests to Dr. B. D. Kahan, Department of Surgery, Division of Immunology and Organ Transplantation, University of Texas Medical School, Houston, TX 77030.

0041-1345/83/1505-0038$01.00/0

Table 1. Posttransplant Patients Receiving a Single Oral Dose of Cyclosporine

Patient	Day	Dose (mg)	K_a (hr^{-1})	α (hr^{-1})	β (hr^{-1})	AUC (ng · hr/ml)	Cp_{max} (ng/ml)	T_{max} (hr)
S.L.	1	825	0.59	0.68	0.099	5,931	443	5
T.G.	2	900	0.89	1.06	0.13	8,403	830	4
G.N.	4	900	0.33	0.16	0.021	5,683	416	4
A.G.	6	800	0.60	0.46	0.065	6,048	816	2
R.W.	7	700	0.70	0.44	0.035	6,399	649	3
W.L.	8	1,000	0.30	0.31	0.13	10,242	703	4
S.L.	8	700	0.58	0.41	0.020	9,385	1,116	3
N.V.	8	1,050	0.62	0.69	0.12	8,497	705	6
R.C.	11	1,000	0.37	0.48	0.12	8,756	630	6
T.G.	11	750	0.64	0.80	0.097	8,324	616	4
H.A.	18	850	0.42	0.24	0.048	17,835	1,543	5
J.S.	20	800	1.16	0.73	0.071	6,566	1,096	2
R.C.	20	875	0.70	0.50	0.048	16,322	1,624	3

Table 2. Posttransplant Patients Receiving an i.v. Infusion of Cyclosporine

Patient	Day	Dose (mg)	Infusion Rate (mg/hr)	α (hr^{-1})	β (hr^{-1})
J.C.	1	150	150	2.82	0.23
C.B.	10	150	150	2.58	0.097

increase in F, but also with a decrease in β. Table 1 shows that patient R.C. had a large increase in AUC and Cp_{max} (maximum blood level) on day 20 as compared to day 11, with a decrease of ~12.5% in dose. It is noted that β had a considerable decrease on day 20 as compared to day 11. This suggests that changes in AUC and Cp_{max} might be due to changes in both F and β. This same trend is observed in patient T.G. on days 2 and 11.

Table 2 shows the results for two posttransplant patients who received CsA by i.v. infusion. The postinfusion data best fit a two-compartment model. There was a rapid decline in blood levels during the first hour, followed by a slower decline up to 9 hr, after which drug levels were not detectable. The α phase rate constants were considerably larger than those observed after the oral dosing of posttransplant patients. In the case of patient J.C. on day 1, the β phase rate constant was considerably larger than that observed for the posttransplant patients dosed orally.

Table 3 shows the results of two pretransplant patients who received oral doses of CsA. These data also fit a two-compartment model, with first-order absorption as was observed in the posttransplant patients. The K_a and α rate constants were in the range observed for the posttransplant patients, but the β values were larger and similar to the value observed for patient J.C., who received an i.v. infusion on day 1.

Table 4 shows the results of three pretransplant patients who received CsA by i.v. infusion. The preinfusion data fit the same model as those observed for the posttransplant patients. There was also a rapid decline in drug levels over the first hour, followed by a slower decline up to 10 hr, after which drug levels were not detectable. The α rate constants were much larger than any previously observed, while the β rate constants were in good agreement with those observed in the pretransplant patients who received CsA orally. These large values observed for α in both pre- and posttransplant patients who received

Table 3. Pretransplant Patients Receiving a Single Oral Dose of Cyclosporine

Patient	Day	Dose (mg)	K_a (hr^{-1})	α (hr^{-1})	β (hr^{-1})	AUC (ng · hr/ml)	Cp_{max} (ng/ml)	T_{max} (hr)
D.F.	−2	1,500	0.76	1.08	0.22	15,311	2,115	4
W.L.	−2	1,500	0.37	0.42	0.28	6,593	602	5

Table 4. Pretransplant Patients Receiving an i.v. Infusion of Cyclosporine

Patient	Day	Dose (mg)	Infusion Rate (mg/hr)	α (hr^{-1})	β (hr^{-1})
C.B.	−4	150	150	9.73	0.14
D.F.	−4	150	150	5.03	0.26
J.C.	−17	150	150	5.48	0.27

i.v. infusions suggest the possibility of a second peripheral compartment that is in rapid equilibrium with the central compartment. Because of the rapid fall in blood levels and the inability to detect the drug after 10 hr, it may not be possible to observe a second distribution rate constant in the case of i.v. infusion. The large differences observed in the fast distribution phase between pre- and posttransplant patients might be due to changes in the degree of equilibration of the drug between the various compartments due to the new physiologic state of the transplanted patient.[8]

The β phase rate constants observed for all pretransplant patients were different from those observed for the posttransplant patients with one exception. Patient J.C., on day 1, had a β rate constant similar to that observed for the pretransplant patients. It may be possible that, at day 1, the patient is still handling the drug like a pretransplant patient.

SUMMARY

Differences in the fraction of the drug absorbed and the elimination phase rate constants make it very difficult to recommend a standardized dosing regimen during the initial posttransplantation stage. Attempts will be made to see if individual dosing regimens can be developed from these parameters.

Intravenous infusion studies suggest that there is a second peripheral compartment that is in rapid equilibrium with the central compartment but is not observed during oral dosing.

REFERENCES

1. Calne RY, White DJG, Evans DB, et al: Br Med J 282:934, 1981

2. Starzl TE, Klintmalm GBG, Iwatsuki S, et al: Surg Gynecol Obstet 153:377, 1981

3. Van Buren CT, Kerman R, Agostino G, et al: Surgery 92:167, 1982

4. Calne RY, Rolles K, White DJG, et al: Lancet 1:1033, 1979

5. Metzler CM: NON-LIN Program. Kalamazoo, MI, Upjohn Company

6. Kahan BD, Reid M, Newburger J: Transplant Proc 15:446, 1983

7. Beveridge T, Gratwohl A, Michot F, et al: Curr Ther Res 30:5, 1981

8. Gibaldi M, Perrier D: Pharmacokinetics, vol 1. New York, Marcel Dekker, 1975

Pharmacokinetics and Toxicity of Cyclosporine in Marrow Transplant Patients

M. S. Kennedy, G. C. Yee, H. J. Deeg, R. Storb, and E. D. Thomas

RECENT widespread use of cyclosporine in experimental and clinical trials has confirmed that it is an effective immunosuppressive drug.[1] With more widespread use, it is also apparent that many questions require answering to maximize the desired effects and minimize the toxicity associated with the drug. Marrow graft recipients present several problems that are unique among the types of patients who are treated with cyclosporine. These could be considered as risk factors, predisposing patients to adverse reactions to cyclosporine, and include: (1) preexisting organ damage from previous chemotherapy; (2) toxic effects of the transplant conditioning regimen; (3) morbidity related to infectious agents and their treatment; and (4) systemic effects of the graft-versus-host reaction. We report the current results of pharmacokinetic studies and observations regarding adverse effects of cyclosporine in patients undergoing marrow transplantation.

MATERIALS AND METHODS

Patients included in this analysis received marrow transplants in Seattle at the Fred Hutchinson Cancer Research Center and the Swedish Hospital Medical Center between October 1980 and March 1983. The conditioning regimen for patients has been published previously.[2,3] During this time, cyclosporine was given to 23 patients with aplastic anemia and 87 with hematologic malignancy according to protocols to prevent graft-versus-host disease. In addition, 47 patients received the drug as initial therapy for established graft-versus-host disease and 19 received it as supplemental therapy after failing to respond to glucocorticoids and/or antithymocyte globulin. Factors addressed in this analysis of cyclosporine kinetics and toxicity are the variation in results related to heterogeneity of patients and differences related to the method of serum level determination.

Concentration–pharmacokinetic data refer to serum values obtained by radioimmunoassay (RIA)[4] or, when indicated, high-pressure liquid chromatography (HPLC).[5] Blood was routinely drawn through double-lumen indwelling right atrial catheters (with precautions to avoid taking samples from the lumen used for infusion).[6] Blood was allowed to clot at room temperature (22 ± 2°C) for more than 2 hr prior to removal of serum. Samples were refrigerated at 4°C and assayed within three days or frozen at −70°C for future analysis.

Pharmacokinetic calculations were performed using Drug Model and statistics were computed using the statistics package, both available through BBN-Prophet.[5]

RESULTS

Variable Kinetics According to Hepatic Function and Patient's Disease Category

There were 52 oral cyclosporine time courses analyzed in 32 patients with leukemia and 13 patients with aplastic anemia. All received the drug for prophylaxis of graft-versus-host disease. The patients ranged in age from 11 to 44 yr (median, 28 yr). The dosage of oral cyclosporine was 6–20 mg/kg of body weight per day, but 85% of the courses were 11–15 mg/kg of body weight per day. Ninety percent of the courses analyzed were in the first three weeks after marrow grafting. Analysis of the above groups showed a trend toward an increase in the serum half-life in patients with elevated bilirubin. The half-life was 5.3 hr in 23 patients, with serum bilirubin <1.2 mg/dl, and 10.6 hr in six patients, with values between 2 and 5 mg/dl ($p = 0.07$). When analyzed according to disease category, there were also differences between leukemic patients and those with aplastic anemia. The

---

From the Fred Hutchinson Cancer Research Center and the University of Washington School of Medicine, Seattle, WA.

Supported in part by Grants CA 15704, CA 30924, CA 18221, and CA 18029, awarded by the National Cancer Institute, DHHS. E.D.T. is the recipient of Research Career Award AI 02425 from the National Institute of Allergy and Infectious Diseases.

Address reprint requests to Dr. M. S. Kennedy, Fred Hutchinson Cancer Research Center, 1124 Columbia Street, Seattle, WA 98104.

0041-1345/83/1505-0039$01.00/0

cyclosporine elimination half-life was 5.9 hr in 32 leukemic patients and 4.8 hr in 13 patients with aplastic anemia ($p = 0.18$). The most notable difference was in the ratio of maximum serum concentration (ng/ml) to dose (mg/kg), which was 75 ± 10 SEM in leukemic patients and 46 ± 10 in aplastic anemia patients ($p = 0.08$). These differences are thought to be due to hepatic as well as intestinal dysfunction related to prior chemotherapy or the radiation that the leukemic patients receive during preparation for transplant.

Analysis of Kinetics After Intravenous Administration: Difference Between Levels Assayed by RIA and HPLC

The currently used RIA is known to cross-react with several of the metabolites of cyclosporine. When samples were assayed by HPLC, serum concentrations both at 4 and 11 hr after a dose (oral or intravenous) were 53% ± 15% SD of the value determined by RIA. This difference was reflected in the kinetic parameters obtained by immunoassay. In 10 patient courses analyzed by both methods, the RIA value at steady-state for volume of distribution was 2.22 ± 1.1 liter/kg, the total plasma clearance was 7.7 ± 3.3 ml/min/kg, and the terminal half-life was 5.8 ± 1.79 hr. The corresponding values for the same patients' sera assayed by HPLC gave results of 3.6 ± 2.9 liter/kg, 12.2 ± 5.6 ml/min/kg, and 6.08 ± 4.6 hr ($p < 0.05$ for clearance only).

Toxicity in Patients Receiving Prophylactic Cyclosporine

The major toxicity was renal. We observed a gradual rise in serum creatinine in the majority of patients receiving the drug. Significant renal toxicity requiring withholding of cyclosporine doses and dialysis continues to be associated with use of amphotericin-B[8] or development of hepatic veno-occlusive disease. In the largest homogeneous patient group (patients with acute nonlymphoblastic leukemia in first remission or chronic myelogenous leukemia in chronic phase), there is a significant relationship by regression analysis between the preceding week's trough cyclosporine concentration and the maximum percent change from baseline in serum creatinine within the first five weeks of therapy ($r = 0.52$, $p = 0.047$).

Toxicity in Patients Receiving Cyclosporine for Treatment of Established Graft-Versus-Host Disease

Two major toxic effects have been noted in this subgroup of patients. The first is severe burning and pain in hands and feet during drug infusion, especially during initiation of treatment. This problem resulted in severe limitation or discontinuation of the drug in four of 31 patients. Slowing the infusion rate was helpful in reducing the severity of this problem in others. Long-term consequences of this reaction were not observed.

The second problem in this patient group was hypertension and grand mal seizures. Seizures were observed in two patients receiving prophylactic cyclosporine alone; both patients were receiving treatment for seizure disorders prior to transplant (seizure frequency did not increase with cyclosporine therapy). In 41 patients receiving cyclosporine as initial treatment of graft-versus-host disease, there was one seizure episode. In contrast, of 70 patients with grade II graft-versus-host disease who received concomitant cyclosporine and glucocorticoid for at least seven days, there were 10 patients who experienced seizures. All patients with seizures were hypertensive (diastolic blood pressure, 90 mm Hg). The cyclosporine serum concentrations were not significantly different in the patients with seizures, but a steroid dose effect on blood pressure was observed in at least three patients. In these patients, reduction of steroids to 1 mg/kg/day of prednisone or alternate-day administration was associated with a reduction in blood pressure in spite of continued or increased cyclosporine concentrations. Cerebrospinal fluid samples from these patients revealed barely detectable cyclosporine concentrations (<50 ng/ml).

DISCUSSION

Our data suggest that, in marrow graft recipients, absorption and elimination of cyclosporine differ among patients with different diseases, which may reflect differences in the conditioning regimens. Differences are also present if one compares pharmacokinetic data obtained by RIA and HPLC in the same patient. Certain states, such as hepatic and renal dysfunction, result in a greater discrepancy between the RIA and HPLC values (data not shown). Renal toxicity continues to be a problem in patients who also receive other nephrotoxins. Control of serum levels may allow uniform immunosuppression and also reduce the number of patients having unacceptable elevations in serum creatinine. Whether the RIA or HPLC assay should routinely be used awaits further information on the pharmacodynamics of the metabolites of cyclosporine.

The problems of hypertension and seizures are clearly manifested more frequently in patients treated with cyclosporine and glucocorticoids, as has been suggested.[9] Hypertension has been reduced in some patients by decreasing the dose of glucocorticoids in spite of continued use of cyclosporine.

REFERENCES

1. Kahan BD: Clin Haematol 11:743, 1982

2. Deeg HJ, Storb R, Thomas ED, et al: Transplant Proc 15:1385, 1983

3. Storb R, Thomas ED, Buckner CD, et al: Ann Intern Med 92:30, 1980

4. Donatsch P, Abisch E, Hamberger M, et al: J Immunoassay 2:19, 1981

5. Yee GC, Gmur DJ, Kennedy MS: Clin Chem 28:2269, 1982

6. Ford R: Transplant Proc (in press)

7. Holford N, Reid-Miller: Bolt Beranek and Newman Inc., Cambridge, MA, 1982

8. Kennedy MS, Deeg HJ, Siegel M, et al: Transplantation 35:211, 1983

9. Durrant S, Chipping PM, Palmer S, et al: Lancet 2:829, 1982

Distribution and Binding of Cyclosporine in Blood and Tissues

W. Niederberger, M. Lemaire, G. Maurer, K. Nussbaumer, and O. Wagner

DATA on the pharmacokinetics and metabolism of cyclosporine (CsA) are presented in a preceding paper of this meeting by Wood et al. This article reports the distribution, as well as the metabolite pattern, of CsA in various animal tissues or organs. In addition, the factors affecting the distribution and binding of the drug in blood are described using in vitro data.

DISTRIBUTION IN TISSUES

Studies with tritium-labeled cyclosporine in rats, mice, and rabbits have shown that the drug distributes widely into the organs and tissues. The absorption following an oral application of the drug in olive oil is in the range 27%–40% of the administered dose. The concentration of radioactivity (parent drug and metabolites) rises slowly in tissues, reaching a maximum between 4 and 8 hr after an oral dose. High-tissue affinity of drug-related radioactivity is evident from the large tissue-to-blood ratios, in the range of 2 to 10, found after both oral and i.v. administration. After multiple oral doses of 10 mg/kg of body weight per day for three weeks to rats, the highest concentrations of radioactivity were found in the secretory organs, liver, and kidney, followed by renal fat, the endocrine glands (adrenals, pancreas, thymus, thyroid), lymph nodes, spleen, and bone marrow. Lower values than in blood were only observed in muscle and brain (see Fig. 1).

Tissue concentrations of radioactivity declined from peak levels biphasically, with terminal half-lives between 60 and 120 hr. As a consequence of the relatively slow elimination, skin and fat in particular accumulate the drug and its metabolites compared to blood and most likely act as a storage depot. The metabolite pattern in blood, kidney, liver, lymph nodes, renal fat, skin, and testes of rats were studied after single and multiple oral doses of 10 mg/kg of body weight per day. The parent drug was found to be the major component in blood and in all organs analyzed. Cyclosporine represented up to 95% of total radioactivity in renal fat. Skin and lymph nodes contained a large proportion of the unchanged drug, and even in liver and kidney, cyclosporine still predominated up to 48 hr after the last dose. The metabolite pattern of CsA remains unaltered after multiple dosing: Comparable profiles are found in blood and urine after single and multiple dose, with metabolite 1 (monohydroxylated derivative) being the major metabolite.

The animal data show that tissue levels of CsA are high compared to blood or plasma levels, that they persist for a long time, and that unchanged drug is predominant in all tissues. Although results from human post-mortem tissue samples[1,2] give less detailed information, it seems that the distribution of cyclosporine is similar in both animal and man.

DISTRIBUTION AND BINDING IN BLOOD

The distribution of CsA in blood components (plasma, leukocytes, and erythrocytes) has been studied in vitro. The uptake of CsA by erythrocytes is found to be around 60%, the fraction bound to lymphocytes and granulocytes each 5%, and the remaining 30% distributed in plasma (for a blood concentration of 500 ng/ml and a temperature of 21°C).[3]

We will describe how the distribution of CsA in blood depends on temperature, drug

---

From the Biopharmaceutical Department, Sandoz Ltd., Basel, Switzerland.

Address reprint requests to Dr. W. Niederberger, Biopharmaceutical Department, Sandoz Ltd., CH-4002 Basel, Switzerland.

0041-1345/83/1505-0040$01.00/0

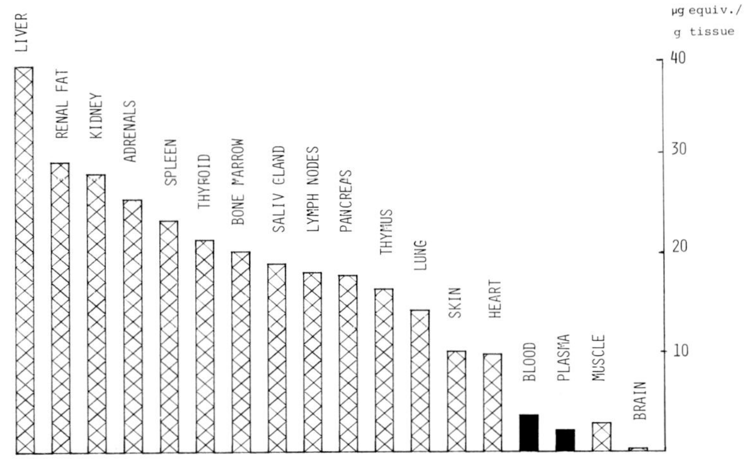

Fig. 1. Maximal concentrations of total radioactivity of cyclosporine in various organs and tissues after multiple oral doses of 10 mg/kg of body weight per day to rats for 21 days.

concentration, hematocrit, and lipoprotein concentration and composition.

When the temperature is lowered from 37°C to 21°C, CsA diffuses from plasma into the blood cells so that only about 50% of the initial concentration is found in plasma. The new equilibrium is reached within 2 hr. After cooling to 6°C, the same equilibrium value is observed, but it is reached only after 18 hr. After heating the blood samples back to 37°C, the initial plasma concentration of 100% is found, indicating that the temperature-dependent process is reversible.

The fraction found in plasma also depends on CsA concentration, since blood cells become saturated at blood concentrations above 5 µg/ml. The concentration dependence is more pronounced at lower temperatures, because the binding affinity of blood cells is higher at lower temperatures (Fig. 2). In the therapeutic range of 0.02–2 µg/ml, the plasma concentration at 21°C is only half of that at 37°C. For concentrations higher than 4 µg/ml, only small differences are observed, due to an identical saturation process (same binding capacity) at both temperatures.

The influence of hematocrit on CsA distribution is shown in Fig. 3. At low (therapeutic) plasma concentrations, an increase in hematocrit (from 25% to 45%) results in a higher increase of the blood-to-plasma ratio at 6°C compared to 37°C (50% and 20%, respectively). Because hematocrit variations can even be larger in clinical samples (between 16% and 46% observed in our laboratory), the influence of this factor cannot be neglected.

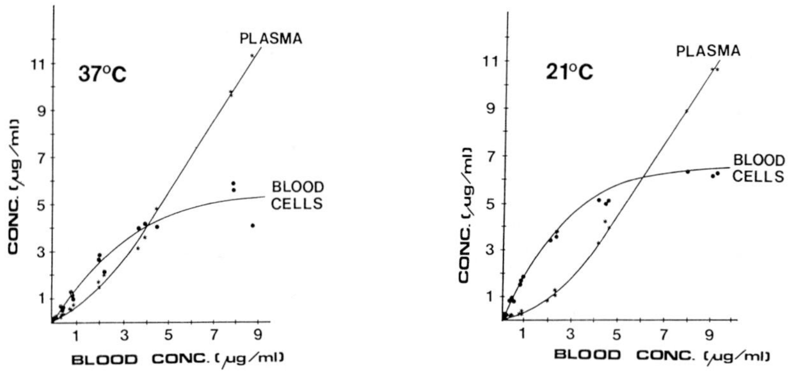

Fig. 2. Relation between equilibrium cyclosporine concentration in blood cells and plasma as a function of whole blood concentration at 21°C and 37°C.

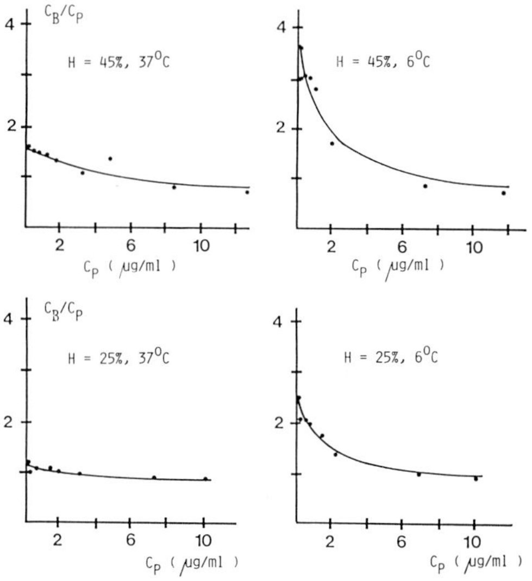

Fig. 3. Blood-to-plasma concentration ratio of cyclosporine for two hematocrit values and two temperatures.

Binding of cyclosporine to plasma proteins has been shown to be independent of concentration between 0.02 and 20 µg/ml of plasma. On the other hand, binding depends strongly on temperature: around 70% of the drug is bound at 4°C, 93% at 20°C, and about 98% at 37°C. Nevertheless, the influence of temperature on blood distribution cannot be fully described in terms of plasma protein binding. The differences observed in blood distribution between 6° and 21°C are small, although the percentage of cyclosporine unbound in plasma is considerably higher at 6°C. Preliminary experiments with erythrocyte ghosts have shown that CsA is not bound to the erythrocyte membrane. Therefore other temperature-dependent processes, such as changes in the permeability of the erythrocyte membrane, are of importance.

Fractionation of plasma by ultracentrifugation showed that about 80% of the cyclosporine is associated with lipoproteins. The high density lipoprotein (HDL) fraction binds 57% of the drug compared to 25% of the low density lipoprotein (LDL) and ~2% in the very low density (VLDL) fraction. The amount bound to chylomicrons is negligible at 1%. Since the HDL fraction varies considerably in a normal population, one would expect the lipoprotein concentration and its composition to be an additional factor influencing the distribution of cyclosporine between blood cells and plasma.

The in vitro experiments described so far show that the ratio blood versus plasma concentration reaches a maximal value of 2 at 37°C and 4 at 21°C or 6°C for small (therapeutic) concentrations. In clinical trials, these upper limits show large variations from patient to patient. Ratios as low as 2 and as high as 15 were observed at 21°C, using either RIA or HPLC for drug determination. More clinical data are needed to see whether additional factors besides the ones found in vitro influence the blood-to-plasma ratio in patients and to determine the blood level range corresponding to the now recommended therapeutic plasma level range of 50 to 400 ng/ml.

REFERENCES

1. Kahan BD, van Buren CT, Boileau M, et al: Transplantation 35:96, 1983

2. Atkinson K, Biggs JC, Britton K: Lancet 2:1165, 1983

3. Lemaire M, Tillement JP: J Pharm Pharmacol 34:715, 1982

In Vitro Stability and Storage of Cyclosporine in Human Serum and Plasma

J. Smith, J. Hows, and E. C. Gordon-Smith

EARLY reports of the use of cyclosporine-A (CsA) in human renal[1] and bone marrow transplantation[2] described nephrotoxicity as a frequent side effect of CsA. Some workers have monitored plasma or serum CsA levels to prevent toxicity and to optimize the immunosuppressive effect.[3] Opinion on the clinical relevance of pharmacologic monitoring of CsA therapy has varied. Some investigators have not been able to correlate serum or plasma levels with clinical events,[4] whereas others have shown clear correlations between serum levels, toxicity, and immunosuppressive effect.[3]

From our recent work on the in vitro stability of CsA in human blood, we have become aware of a number of factors that may interfere with the success of pharmacologic monitoring of patients receiving CsA. We have attempted to work out a simple system for the treatment of blood samples containing CsA that minimizes in vitro fluctuations in plasma and serum CsA levels. Using this system, we have found a good correlation between clinical nephrotoxicity in CsA-treated marrow transplant patients and trough serum CsA levels.[5]

MATERIALS AND METHODS

Cyclosporine-A Dose Schedule

A loading dose was begun orally on day −1; 12.5 mg/kg of body weight was given twice daily. On day +3, maintenance treatment was started orally with 6.25 mg/kg of body weight twice daily.

Pharmacologic Monitoring

Patients receiving oral CsA were monitored three times weekly. Twelve-hour trough venous samples were taken. Details of processing blood samples are given in the relevant sections below.

Measurement of CsA in Plasma or Serum

CsA was measured by radioimmunoassay using reagents supplied by Sandoz Ltd. (Basel, Switzerland). Determinations were performed in triplicate using 20-μl serum samples, diluted 1/50 with 0.05 *M* Tris buffer, pH 8.5.[6] The interassay variation was ±5%, and the assay was sensitive in the range of 60–4,000 ng/ml. The standard error and 95% confidence limits (± 2 SEM) were calculated for each result.

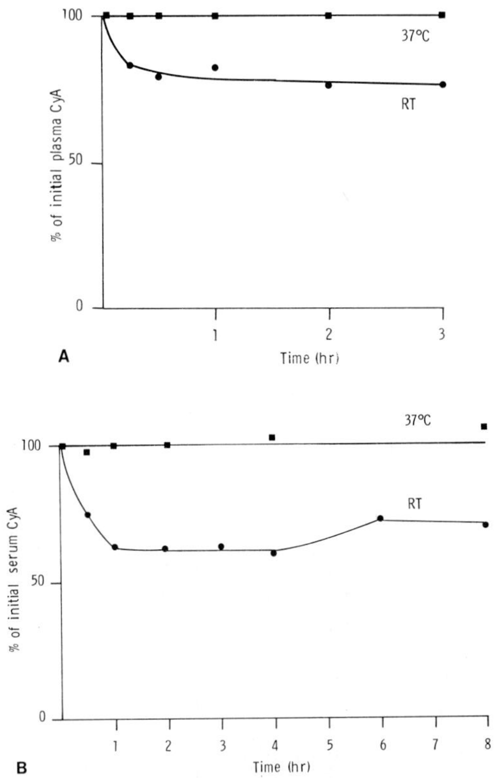

Fig. 1. (A) Decrease of plasma levels of cyclosporin A (CsA) after storage of whole blood at room temperature (20°C) and 37°C. The initial plasma CsA concentration was 445 ng/ml. (B) Decrease of serum levels of CsA after storage of whole blood at room temperature (20°C) and 37°C. The initial serum CsA concentration was 235 ng/ml.

From the Department of Hematology, Royal Postgraduate Medical School, Ducane Rd., London W12 OHS, UK.

Address reprint requests to Miss J. Smith.

0041–1345/83/1505–0041$01.00/0

Table 1. Stability of CsA in Serum After Storage of Whole Blood at 4°C or 20°C for 24 Hr

	Serum CsA (ng/ml ± 2 SEM)				
Sample*	WB at 20°C	Percent Change	Sample	WB at 4°C	Percent Change
1			7		
a	170 ± 27	42	a	76 ± 29	7
b	242 ± 13		b	81 ± 37	
2			8		
a	130 ± 1	2	a	140 ± 1	4
b	133 ± 5		b	135 ± 3	
3			9		
a	162 ± 20	17	a	204 ± 3	15
b	189 ± 28		b	174 ± 62	
4			10		
a	74 ± 20	14	a	340 ± 1	4
b	84 ± 16		b	215 ± 5	
5			11		
a	112 ± 33	36	a	98 ± 10	2
b	152 ± 26		b	100 ± 3	
6			12		
a	117 ± 1	38	a	117 ± 13	2
b	162 ± 11		b	119 ± 13	

*a: Serum separated after 2 hr at 20°C and stored at −20°C; b: serum separated after 24 hr at 4°C or 20°C.

Stability of Plasma and Serum CsA In Vitro

The effect of storage temperature before separation of the blood sample. Venous blood in lithium heparin was kept at 20°C (room temperature) or at 37°C after collection. Samples were separated at 20°C or 37°C at various times 0.5–8 hr after collection. The CsA plasma concentration was measured. The procedure was repeated using serum samples, and the results are shown in Fig. 1.

Six venous blood samples were clotted after collection and stored at 20°C for 2 hr. The serum was then separated and frozen. Paired aliquots were stored at 4°C for 24 hr before separation. The procedure was repeated, but the unseparated aliquots were stored at 20°C for 24 hr before separation. The serum CsA concentration in the samples stored for 24 hr at 4°C and 20°C before separation was compared with the paired samples separated after 2 hr (Table 1).

The effect of storage temperature after separation of blood sample. (1) A venous blood sample was clotted after collection and stored at 20°C for 2 hr. The sample was separated and the serum aliquoted. Aliquots were stored for 2 hr to 7 days at 20°C before assay. Results are shown in Table 2.

(2) Two venous blood samples were processed as in (1). The serum obtained was freeze-thawed 1–5 times before assay. The results are shown in Table 2.

(3) Two venous blood samples were processed as in (1). Aliquots of serum were stored at −20°C for 2–8 months before assay. The results are shown in Fig. 2.

RESULTS AND DISCUSSION

Figure 1 indicates that there is a fall in plasma and serum CsA in the first hour when

Table 2. Stability of CsA in Serum

(A) Serum stored at 20°C (Days)*

	1	2	3	4	5	6	7	8
Sample 1	399 ± 175	342 ± 87	394 ± 31	401 ± 32	396 ± 54	374 ± 21	385 ± 44	331 ± 52

(B) Times Serum Freeze/Thawed*

	1	2	3	4	5
Sample 2	242 ± 31	259 ± 14	259 ± 14	289 ± 44	286 ± 14
Sample 3	557 ± 50	581 ± 49	532 ± 54	542 ± 92	542 ± 77

*Serum CsA (ng/ml ± 2 SEM). Sample stored at 20°C for 1 hr before separation.

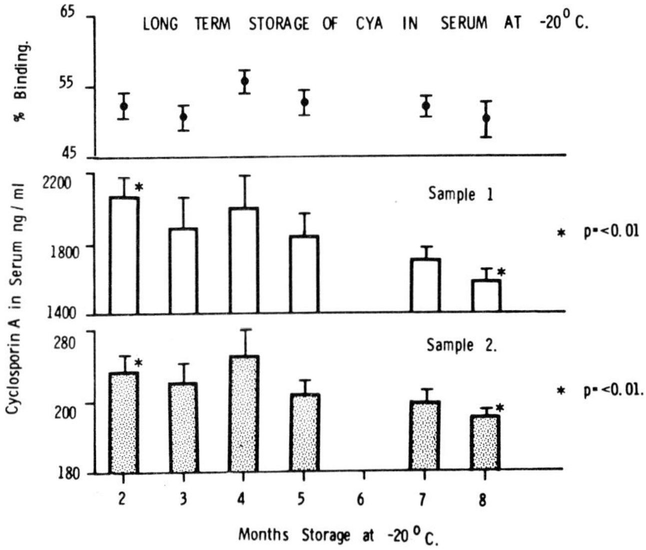

Fig. 2. Long-term storage of cyclosporine A in serum at −20°C.

unseparated blood samples are stored at 20°C prior to separation. After 1 hr, a plateau occurs in the CsA concentration in both plasma and serum samples. Experiments carried out at Sandoz Research Laboratories give similar results (Dr. A. Woods, personal communication). The molecular basis for the temperature-dependent redistribution of CsA in whole blood samples is unknown. Because of the practical difficulties of keeping routine blood samples strictly at 37°C after collection and during separation, we have standardized our sample handling by allowing all samples to remain at room temperature (20°C) for 2 hr prior to centrifugation at the same temperature. When blood samples are stored for 4°C for 24 hr before separation, the serum CsA level remains the same as in samples separated after 2 hr (Table 1). If blood samples are kept at room temperature for 24 hr before separation, a rise in the serum CsA concentration occurs presumably due to leakage of cellular CsA into the serum. These results indicate that if blood samples for CsA estimation cannot be separated 2 hr after collection, they should be stored at 4°C.

Table 2 shows that serum CsA, as measured by radioimmunoassay, remains stable after separation and storage at room temperature for several days and is unaffected by repeated freeze-thawing. These findings indicate that serum samples may be sent by mail for CsA assay without freezing.

Figure 2 shows that serum samples containing CsA deteriorate after 8 months storage at −20°C. This finding indicates that all test samples stored at −20°C should be assayed within 3–4 months of collection. Quality control sera should be replaced every 3–4 months if stored at −20°C.

Our results indicate that, provided blood samples containing CsA are carefully handled after collection, in vitro fluctuations should not affect the correlation between serum and plasma CsA measurements and the effect of the drug in vivo. If unseparated samples are equilibrated for 2 hr after collection at 20°C, the concentration of CsA in the serum or plasma becomes stable. By handling samples in this way, consistent results can be achieved for serum and plasma CsA measurements (Fig. 1). It is not practical to keep all blood samples strictly at 37°C before and during centrifugation in a routine monitoring program.

Using the system described above, we have found good correlations between clinical episodes of nephrotoxicity and high trough serum CsA levels[5] and have been able to safely increase the dose of CsA in patients with low serum CsA levels.[7] In the future, the measurement of whole blood CsA concentration may simplify pharmacologic monitoring of patients receiving the drug.[8] However, as yet, there are insufficient data available on correlations between whole blood CsA and in vivo toxicity and the immunosuppressive activity of CsA.

REFERENCES

1. Calne RY, Rolles K, White DJ, et al: Lancet 2:1033, 1979

2. Powles RL, Clink HM, Spence D, et al: Lancet 1:327, 1980

3. Keown PA, Stiller CR, Ulan RA, et al: Lancet 1:686, 1981

4. Tutschka PJ, Hess AD, Baschorner WE, et al: In White DJG (ed): Cyclosporin A. Amsterdam, Elsevier Biomedical, 1982, p 519

5. Hows JM, Chipping PM, Fairhead SM, et al: Br J Haematol 54:1983

6. Donatsch P, Abisch E, Homberger M, et al: J Immunoassay 2:19, 1981

7. Hows JM, Palmer S, Gordon-Smith EC: Transplantation 33:382, 1982

8. Kahan BD, Buren CT, Lin SN, et al: Transplantation 34:36, 1982

Distribution and Transfer of Cyclosporine Among the Various Human Lipoprotein Classes

W. Mraz, R. A. Zink, A. Graf, D. Preis, W. D. Illner, W. Land, W. Siebert, and H. Zöttlein

CYCLOSPORINE-A (CsA) is a fungal cyclic oligopeptide with an immunosuppressive action in different animal species as well as in man.[1] Since this molecule exhibits a strong hydrophobicity,[2,3] it may be supposed that CsA is mainly associated with proteins in blood serum.

In this article, evidence is presented for the exclusive association of CsA with lipoproteins in serum from renal transplant patients. Furthermore, it could be demonstrated in vitro that there is an exchange/transfer of CsA among the different serum lipoprotein classes and a transfer of the compound from nonlipoprotein proteins to lipoproteins. The physiologic implications of these findings are discussed.

MATERIALS AND METHODS

Sources of Blood Serum and Plasma

Blood plasma samples for the preparative isolation of lipoproteins were obtained from normolipidemic volunteers (Blood bank, Klinikum Grosshadern, University of Munich). For the CsA distribution studies, blood was obtained from renal transplant patients receiving an oral dose of 12–17 mg/kg of body weight of the drug.[4] The time interval between administration of CsA and blood sampling was 10 hr, unless otherwise stated. Patients who had fasted 8–15 hr were sampled.

Chemicals

Agar, bovine, and human serum albumin and antisera to apolipoprotein A and B were obtained from Behringwerke (Marburg, F.R.G.); antisera to apolipoproteins A-I, A-II, and B from Immuno Diagnostica (Heidelberg, F.R.G.). Metrizamide was purchased from Nyegaard (Oslo, Norway); the scintillation solution Pico-Fluor 30 and tritiated water as internal standard was obtained from Packard Instruments (Frankfurt, F.R.G.). All other chemicals were of reagent grade and were obtained from Merck (Darmstadt, F.R.G.).

CsA and ^{3}H-dihydro-CsA were gifts of Dr. R. Voges, and the CsA radioimmunoassay kit was provided by Dr. E. Abisch, both from Pharmaceutical Division, Sandoz Ltd. (Basel, Switzerland).

Analytical Methods

Total cholesterol, triglycerides, and choline-containing phospholipids in serum and ultracentrifugal fractions were determined enzymatically by standard methods,[5–8] using an automatic analyzer (Hitachi, model 705). Total protein was measured according to the method of Lowry et al.,[9] using bovine serum albumin as a standard.

Quantitative determination of the main lipoprotein fractions was performed by measuring their cholesterol contents after separation by semimicro-ultracentrifugation (Airfuge, Inc., Beckman Instruments, Palo Alto, CA) at densities of 1.006 and 1.063 g/ml for very low density lipoprotein (VLDL) and high density lipoprotein (HDL), respectively. Low density lipoprotein (LDL) was calculated from the values of total, VLDL, and HDL cholesterol. The required densities were adjusted according to Havel et al.[10]

Agarose-gel electrophoresis[11] was used for the qualitative analysis of serum lipoprotein distribution as well as for the establishment of the purity of isolated lipoprotein fractions.

To evaluate the serum protein and serum apolipoprotein distribution after ultracentrifugation, double diffusion analysis in agarose gel[12] was performed with antisera to albumin, apolipoprotein A-I, A-II, and B, and antiserum to total serum protein.

CsA concentrations in total serum and fractions obtained after ultracentrifugation of serum were determined by radioimmunoassay.[13] The measurement of radioactivity was performed in a LKB-Wallac liquid scintillation counter (model 1210 Ultrabeta) with Pico-Fluor 30 as scintillation liquid. Internal standardization with $^3H-H_2O$ was used for quench correction.

Preparative Isolation of Lipoprotein Density Classes

Lipoproteins were isolated from normal human plasma by sequential preparative ultracentrifugation according to Havel et al.,[10] using a model L5-65B ultracentrifuge with a rotor 60Ti (Beckman Instruments, Fullerton, CA).

From the Institute of Clinical Chemistry, the Transplantation Center Munich, and the Urological Clinic and Policlinic, Klinikum Grosshadern, University of Munich, Federal Republic of Germany.

Address reprint requests to Dr. W. Mraz, Institute of Clinical Chemistry, Klinikum Grosshadern, University of Munich, Federal Republic of Germany.

0041-1345/83/1505-0042$01.00/0

Isolated lipoproteins were dialyzed exhaustively against 0.05 mol/liter Tris/HCl buffer, pH 7.4.

Preparation of ^{3}H-Dihydro-CsA-Loaded Serum Proteins and Serum Lipoproteins

^{3}H-dihydro-CsA, dissolved in dimethyl sulfoxide (DMSO), was rapidly injected into a vigorously stirred Tris/HCl buffer (0.05 *M*/liter, pH 7.4) containing the desired protein (albumin, lipoprotein, and total serum proteins). The mixture was subsequently equilibrated for 1 hr at 20–22°C by gentle shaking. The final concentration of DMSO in the protein solution did not exceed 70 μmol/liter. The protein and CsA concentrations used are given under Results.

Incubation Conditions for the CsA Exchange/Transfer Experiments

Equal amounts of protein solutions previously loaded with ^{3}H-dihydro-CsA and unloaded protein solutions were mixed and incubated under gentle shaking for 1 hr at 20–22°C. Subsequently, aliquots of the incubation mixtures were subjected to rate zonal ultracentrifugation, followed by analysis of ^{3}H-dihydro-CsA distribution. Experimental details concerning protein and CsA concentrations are given under Results.

Analytical Separation of the Major Lipoprotein Classes

For the analysis of both the distribution and the exchange/transfer of CsA or ^{3}H-dihydro-CsA among the serum lipoproteins and proteins, two different methods were used.

(1) Fractionated precipitation of the major lipoprotein classes was performed according to the method described by Burstein et al.[14] with the following modifications.[15] To the aliquots of serum, sodium phosphotungstate and magnesium chloride were added to give final concentrations of 0.55 g/liter and 0.065 mol/liter, 3.0 g/liter and 0.065 mol/liter, and 40 g/liter and 0.4 mol/liter, resulting in the precipitation of VLDL, VLDL plus LDL, and VLDL plus LDL plus HDL, respectively. The clear infranatants or supernatants obtained after low-speed centrifugation were used to measure the CsA contents.

(2) Separation of the main lipoprotein classes by rate zonal ultracentrifugation was performed analogous to Chapman et al.[16] using an SW 40 Ti swinging bucket rotor (Beckman Instruments). Aliquots of the serum sample were layered on top of, or, after appropriate adjustment of the serum density, on the bottom of a discontinuous gradient. The gradients were formed from solutions of NaCl/KBr, sucrose or Metrizamide, varying in density from 1.006 g/ml to 1.25 g/ml, buffered with 0.005 mol/liter Tris/HCl, pH 8.0. After centrifugation (150,000 *g* at 4°C for 60 hr), fractions were collected from the bottom of the tubes, and the CsA content was measured.

A detailed description of both procedures will be published elsewhere.[17]

RESULTS

Relationship Between CsA Concentration and the Concentrations of Different Blood Constituents in Serum of Patients After Cadaver Kidney Transplantation

Though the lipoprotein patterns of our renal transplant patients showed individual differences, the lipid and lipoprotein composition of each patient remained constant over a period of at least several weeks, as could be shown by different methods (lipid analysis, lipoprotein electrophoresis, and quantitative lipoprotein determination). After administration of a standardized dose of CsA[4] and using a standardized sampling procedure, no correlation between the serum concentrations of total cholesterol, triglycerides, lipoproteins, or erythrocytes and the levels in serum of the drug could be observed.

Distribution of CsA Among the Different Lipoprotein Fractions of Human Serum

Separation by rate zonal ultracentrifugation of serum from patients receiving CsA revealed a close association of CsA with the different serum lipoprotein density classes—VLDL, LDL, and HDL. When the serum sample, after appropriate adjustment of the density, is layered on the bottom of the density gradient, approximately 30% of the recovered CsA is found to be associated with the non-lipoprotein proteins, whereas 70% is found floating in association with HDL and LDL. In this case, only minute amounts of the drug were associated with VLDL. On the other hand, when the serum specimen is layered on top of the density gradient, the total recovered CsA is associated with the lipoproteins, including VLDL. Analogous results were obtained with gradients formed by potassium bromide, Metrizamide, or sucrose. An example is presented in Fig. 1, (A and B). Using fractionated precipitation for the separation of the different lipoprotein classes, it could be demonstrated that 90%–95% of the recovered

Blood and Tissue Distribution of Cyclosporine in Humans and Mice

K. Atkinson, J. Boland, K. Britton, and J. Biggs

CYCLOSPORINE is a potent immunosuppressive agent that has proven effective in minimizing both graft rejection after solid organ transplantation and acute graft-versus-host disease after bone marrow transplantation. It is, however, associated with considerable toxicity to the kidneys,[1,2] liver,[3,4] and central nervous system.[5] In spite of its considerable clinical usage to date, there is limited information on its distribution in blood and none on its distribution in tissues. In this study we have examined the effect of factors influencing the concentration of cyclosporine (CsA) detected in the serum of patients that are receiving the drug after allogeneic marrow transplantation. Further, we determined the influence of a number of factors on the distribution of CsA in blood components when whole blood was incubated with the drug in vitro. Finally, we report tissue levels of the drug in patients receiving the drug after marrow transplantation and in mice.

MATERIALS AND METHODS

Patients

All patients were receiving CsA as immunosuppression to minimize graft-versus-host disease after allogeneic marrow transplantation as treatment for hematologic malignancy or severe aplastic anemia. The protocol for marrow transplantation has been previously described.[6,7] Blood samples were collected from patients receiving CsA immediately prior to their taking a regular 12 hourly dose of CsA (trough concentration), and were allowed to clot at either room temperature or 37°C. The clotted blood was separated at 1,200 *g* for 12 min at the respective temperatures. All serum samples were stored at −20°C prior to assay by radioimmunoassay.[8] To evaluate the effect of the temperature at which the blood was separated on subsequent CsA serum concentration, aliquots of clotted blood were allowed to stand for 1 hr at room temperature or 37°C prior to separation. To investigate the effect of delaying blood separation, aliquots of clotted blood were allowed to stand at room temperature or 37°C for 1, 4, 7, or 22-hr intervals prior to separation.

In Vitro Studies

CsA pure substance was dissolved in ethanol and Tween 80 and diluted with 0.9% sodium chloride solution to give concentrations in the range of 0.625 μg/ml to 8 μg/ml. Fresh blood (containing the anticoagulant EDTA) from normal individuals was used. The desired concentration of CsA was added to whole blood at 37°C and incubated with gentle mixing for 1 hr.

Isolation of the plasma, mononuclear cell fraction, and red cell/granulocyte fraction was performed on a Ficoll gradient. Two milliliters of incubated blood was diluted 1:3 with phosphate-buffered saline (PBS) and the diluted blood carefully layered onto 4 ml Ficoll-Paque (Pharmacia; Uppsala, Sweden) and the sample centrifuged at 400 *g* for 35 min at room temperature. The top layer of diluted plasma was drawn off and retained for CsA assay. The mononuclear layer was then removed, leaving the red cell pellet. Both the mononuclear layer and the red cell pellet were resuspended separately in PBS and centrifuged at 1,200 *g* for 10 min at room temperature. After two further washes, the cells were lysed to recover the CsA. The mononuclear cells were resuspended in 50:50 ethanol:PBS and lysed by rapid freeze-thawing in liquid nitrogen and hot water. After centrifugation, the supernatant was retained for CsA assay. The red cells were resuspended in 50:50 distilled water:ethanol and vortexed; the lysed cells were centrifuged to remove stroma and the supernatant was retained for CsA assay. To evaluate the effect of the temperature at which the blood was separated, diluted blood was separated on Ficoll at either room temperature or 37°C. To evaluate the effect of increase in CsA concentration during incubation, increasing concentrations of CsA were added to the incubation tube; concentrations used were 0.062, 0.125, 0.25, 0.5, 1, 2, 3, 4, 6, 7, and 8 μg CsA/ml of blood. To evaluate the effect of the duration of incubation, the incubation period was varied; blood was incubated with CsA for 30, 60, 90, and 120 min before separation on Ficoll.

From the Department of Haematology, St. Vincent's Hospital, Sydney, Australia.

Supported in part by grants from the National Health and Medical Research Council of Australia and the New South Wales State Cancer Council.

Address reprint requests to Dr. K. Atkinson, Department of Haematology, St. Vincent's Hospital, Sydney, Australia.

0041-1345/83/1505-0043$01.00/0

Experimental Animals

Inbred BALB/c mice of both sexes (6–10 weeks old) and weighing 15–25 g, were used. They were housed in conventional facilities and fed and watered ad libitum. CsA was given by daily subcutaneous injections at concentrations of 12.5 mg/kg, 50 mg/kg, or 200 mg/kg body mass. Groups of mice were killed at intervals of 7, 21, and 42 days after the beginning of CsA administration. At the end of each time period, at least five mice were taken from each group and killed by decapitation and exsanguination. Brain, spleen, thymus, mesenteric lymph nodes, lungs, liver, kidney, and intestines (including duodenum, jejunum, ileum, colon, and rectum) were collected from each animal, weighed, homogenized in cold 100% ethanol, and the CsA concentration of each organ measured by radioimmunoassay.

The concentration of CsA in autopsy tissues of three patients who received CsA as immunosuppression after an allogeneic marrow transplant was also measured by the same technique.

RESULTS

Patient Studies

Effect of temperature at which blood was separated. The mean CsA serum concentration when the serum was separated at room temperature was 132 ng/ml, while it was 283 ng/ml when the serum was separated at 37°C ($p < 0.0001$, two-way analysis of variance; mean of 12 experiments). There was thus approximately 50% more CsA in the serum component when separation occurred at 37°C than when separation occurred at room temperature.

Effect of delaying blood separation. The mean serum CsA concentrations after 1, 4, 7, and 22 hr when the serum was separated at room temperature or at 37°C are shown in Table 1. When the blood separation was delayed, there was a gradual increase in the CsA serum concentration at both temperatures at which serum was separated.

In Vitro Studies

Effect of temperature at which blood was separated. The proportion of CsA recovered from the plasma, mononuclear cell, and red cell components when blood was separated at room temperature or 37°C is shown in Table 2. Partitioning of CsA between plasma and red cells is thus temperature dependent, and it appears that some CsA is taken up from the serum into red cells at room temperature.

Table 1. Effect of Delay in Serum Separation on Serum Cyclosporine Concentration

Temperature at Which Serum Separated	Cyclosporine Serum Concentration (ng/ml) — Duration of Delay in Serum Separation (hr): 1	4	7	22
Room temperature	62	67	78	89
37°C	166	191	198	228

Effect of increasing the concentration of CsA during incubation. When the concentration of CsA present during incubation with blood was increased, it was found that red cells showed an apparent linear uptake until 4 μg/ml, after which their uptake appeared saturable. Both the plasma and the mononuclear cell components showed an apparent linear uptake to 7 μg/ml. On a per cell basis, it was calculated that a mononuclear cell contained approximately 1,000 times more CsA than an erythrocyte.

Effect of duration of incubation. There was no change in the distribution of CsA between blood components when CsA and blood were incubated for increasing periods of time (30–120 min). A distribution equilibrium had thus been reached within 30 min of incubation.

Tissue distribution of CsA in mice. The CsA content in the organs of mice receiving 50 mg/kg/day CsA subcutaneously is shown in Table 3. CsA was detected in every organ assayed at each concentration administered. In every organ, the mean concentration of CsA was consistently highest in mice receiving 200 mg/kg/day and lowest in those given 12.5 mg/kg/day. After the first week,

Table 2. Effect of Temperature at Which Blood Separated on Distribution of Cyclosporine in Plasma, Red Cells, and Mononuclear Cells

Temperature at Which Blood Separated	Relative Distribution of Cyclosporine (%): Plasma	Red Cells	Mononuclear Cells
Room temperature	46	51	3
37°C	60	36	4

Table 3. Tissue Distribution of Cyclosporine in Mice Given Cyclosporine 50 mg/kg/day Subcutaneously (ng Cyclosporine/mg Tissue)*

Organ	Duration of Administration of Cyclosporine (Days)		
	7	21	42
Thymus	41.8 ± 16.0	45.6 ± 28.8	33.8 ± 21.9
Mesenteric lymph node	33.9 ± 12.3	26.5 ± 12.3	24.9 ± 5.4
Spleen	26.0 ± 10.7	14.5 ± 5.8	26.0 ± 11.0
Kidney	28.3 ± 11.3	22.7 ± 11.7	18.6 ± 5.6
Lung	12.6 ± 4.1	27.7 ± 46.7	23.9 ± 24.35
Liver	18.3 ± 3.2	27.1 ± 15.8	25.1. ± 11.9
Intestine	10.9 ± 0.7	17.0 ± 7.1	26.4 ± 17.2
Brain	1.9 ± 1.3	1.0 ± 0.8	1.9 ± 1.6

*Values represent means ± SD for groups of at least five mice.

repeated daily injections of CsA at each concentration did not further elevate concentration of CsA. There was pronounced variability in the concentration of CsA between individual mice within each group.

Tissue distribution of CsA in humans. The tissue distribution of CsA in three recipients of allogeneic marrow transplants who received CsA as immunosuppression post-transplant is shown in Table 4. It should be noted that CsA was readily detectable in all organs assayed even in two patients in whom administration of CsA had ceased 6 and 16 days prior to death.

DISCUSSION

We conclude from these studies that serum should be separated at 37°C without delay after venesection when serum concentrations of the drug (measured by radioimmunoassay) are being used for immune monitoring, since it would appear that such methodology would allow the closest approximation to the serum level obtaining in the patient's circulation. A falsely low serum concentration is obtained if the blood is separated at room temperature, and from our in vitro studies, it appears that this is due to an uptake by the red cells of plasma CsA. Significant delay in blood separation after venesection results in an increasing serum CsA concentration, possibly due to release of CsA from hemolyzed erythrocytes. We conclude further from the in vitro blood studies that the distribution of CsA between blood components is also dependent on the concentration of CsA with which the blood is incubated. Distribution, however, does not seem to be markedly dependent on the duration of incubation, since equilibrium was achieved within 30 min of incubation. CsA was found in all the lymphoid and nonlymphoid tissues examined, both in humans and mice. In the mouse it appeared that tissue concentrations reached a plateau after one week of CsA administration, indicating that a balance was maintained between the rate of administration and its rate of clearance from the tissues. This feature presumably indicates why many of the side effects of CsA are rapidly reversible on lowering the dose of, or stopping, the drug. Finally, it was evident from the studies of tissue distribution in humans that the drug remains in the tissues for a considerable duration after administration of the drug has ceased.

Table 4. Tissue Distribution of Cyclosporine in Humans

Tissue	Patient 1	Patient 2	Patient 3
Renal fat	7.7	1.0	0.2
Lymph node	3.5	0.6	0.7
Spleen	3.2	0.5	0.3
Thymus	ND	0.6	ND
Liver	4.2	0.5	0.2
Kidney	ND	0.6	0.2
Lung	1.7	0.35	0.3
Brain	0.24	ND	0.3
Small intestine	ND	0.3	ND

Note: Values represent ng cyclosporine/mg of tissue. Patient no. 1 received CsA (1.1 mg/kg of body weight per day) i.v. until the day of death; patient no. 2 received CsA (1.6 mg/kg of body weight per day) i.v. that was stopped six days before death; and patient no. 3 received CsA (12.5 mg/kg of body weight per day) p.o. that was stopped 16 days before death. ND = not done.

REFERENCES

1. Atkinson K, Biggs JC, Hayes J, et al: Br J Haematol 54:59, 1983

2. Shulman H, Striker G, Deeg HJ, et al: N Engl J Med 305:1392, 1981

3. Klintmalm GBG, Iwatsuki S, Starzl TE: Transplantation 32:488, 1981

4. Atkinson K, Biggs JC, Dodds AJ, et al: Transplant Proc (this issue)

5. Atkinson K, Darveniza P, Boland J, et al: (submitted for publication)

6. Atkinson K, Biggs JC, Ting A, et al: Br J Haematol 53:265, 1983

7. Biggs J, Atkinson K, Concannon A, et al: Med J Aust 2:120, 1983

8. Donatsch P, Abisch E, Homberger M, et al: J Immunol Assay 2:19, 1981

Cyclosporine Levels in Human Tissues of Patients Treated for One Week to One Year

M. Ried, S. Gibbons, D. Kwok, C. T. Van Buren, S. Flechner, and B. D. Kahan

CALNE et al.[1] demonstrated the clinical efficacy of cyclosporine (CsA) therapy in transplantation. Subsequent studies have documented deleterious side effects of CsA administration, including nephrotoxicity, hepatotoxicity, hirsutism, gingival hyperplasia, tumors, tremors, and flushing.[2] The pharmacokinetics of CsA therapy were investigated to discover parameters that optimize the immunosuppressive activity of CsA while minimizing its toxic manifestations. For example, these studies revealed an initially low drug bioavailability in the immediate posttransplant period, followed by a steady increase within the first two weeks.[3] The present report describes the tissue levels encountered in four recipients after various lengths of therapy.

MATERIALS AND METHODS

Patients

L.T. was a 45-year-old white female whose case history has been presented elsewhere in detail.[4]

A.S. was a 48-year-old white male afflicted with end-stage renal disease secondary to polycystic kidney disease who has required chronic hemodialysis since 1977. Splenectomy, bilateral nephrectomy, and triple aortocoronary artery bypass were performed in preparation for transplantation. In September 1982, he (B+; A3,11;B7,w35;Cw4,–;DR2,3) received a renal allograft from a cadaveric donor (B+;A3,11;B7,w35; C–,–;DR2,3) Although the kidney immediately diuresed, it then became anuric. Adjuvant hemodialysis was required on day 2. At this time, on a CsA dosage of 13.5 mg/kg of body weight (950 mg), the serum CsA trough was 82 ng/ml, but he suffered extreme hypertension. By day 8, his hypertension was properly managed and his creatinine clearance was 4.5 ml/min, with a serum creatinine of 7.3 mg/dl, a blood urea nitrogen of 81 mg/dl, and a serum CsA trough value of 174 ng/ml. The CsA dosage was lowered to 11.5 mg/kg (750 mg), and his prednisone therapy, which had been tapered by 5 mg daily, was lowered to 1.0 mg/kg. On day 11, he developed a fever of 101.4°F and a white blood cell count of 23,000/mm^3. The chest roentgenogram revealed a lingular infiltrate in the left lower lobe. The pneumonia was unresponsive to antibiotic therapy; his condition progressively deteriorated. After three cardiac arrests, he died on day 15. In the preterminal period, he displayed a serum creatinine level of 8.3 mg/dl, a blood urea nitrogen of 109 mg/dl, and a CsA trough of 368 ng/ml. Postmortem examination showed no evidence of either allograft rejection or CsA toxicity, but did reveal acute bronchopneumonia, severe coronary artery sclerosis, cardiomegaly, moderate abdominal aortic arteriosclerosis, and multiple liver cysts.

D.H. was a 43-year-old white male, who suffered from diabetic nephropathy and received a renal allograft from an HLA-, DR-identical sibling in July 1982. The graft function progressively improved while on a CsA dosage of 14.0 mg/kg of body weight (950 mg) and an initial prednisone dosage of 2.0 mg/kg, which was lowered by 5 mg daily. Eight days after transplantation, the patient displayed atrial fibrillation, which initially was poorly, but later was completely, controlled by digoxin. On day 35, he was discharged from the hospital with a serum creatinine level of 0.9 mg/dl, a blood urea nitrogen of 30 mg/dl, and a serum CsA trough value of 80 ng/ml, while maintained on a CsA dosage of 14.0 mg/kg and a prednisone dosage of 1.0 mg/kg. Thirty-six days later, he was seen in the outpatient clinic, displaying a fever of 101°F and a white blood cell count of 8,900/mm^3. Chest roentgenograms revealed bilateral, interstitial lower lobe infiltrates. The patient's condition was unresponsive to therapy with nafcillin, gentamycin, and bactrim. Four days later, on day 75, he experienced a fever of 103.9°F and a white blood cell count of 11,500, leading to discontinuance of his CsA therapy. However, despite aggressive antibiotic therapy, his condition progressively worsened, and 20 days later he died.

C.P. was a 40-year-old white male afflicted with emphysema secondary to an α-1-antitrypsin deficiency. In November 1982, he (A+;A1,2;B7,8;C–,–;DR2,–) received a combined heart-lung transplant from a donor of ABO type A+ and HLA type A25,28;B7,w39;C–,–;DR1,2. Graft function was monitored by electrocardiogram, arterial blood gases, and transvenous endomyocardial biopsy. On the first day posttransplant on 14.0 mg/kg of CsA (100 mg i.v.; 700

From the Division of Immunology and Organ Transplantation, Department of Surgery, University of Texas Medical School, Houston, TX.

Address reprint requests to Dr. M. Ried, Division of Immunology and Organ Transplantation, Department of Surgery, University of Texas Medical School, Houston, TX 77030.

0041–1345/83/1505–0044$1.00/0

mg orally, p.o.) and 2.4 mg/kg of methylprednisolone, he displayed an elevated total bilirubin (2.8 mg/dl) and lactic dehydrogenase (LDH, 476 U/liter), with a normal alkaline phosphatase, serum glutamic-pyruvic transaminase (SGPT), serum creatinine, and blood urea nitrogen. On day 3, displaying good graft function, he developed a fever of 101.6°F with a white blood cell count of 17,700/mm^3. Chest roentgenograms revealed a right lower lobe infiltrate. Antibiotic therapy was begun with nafcillin, tobramycin, piperacillin, and cephamandole. The elevated bilirubin (3.0 mg/dl) and lactic dehydrogenase (LDH) (338 U/liter) persisted, but since his alkaline phosphatase, serum glutamic-oxaloacetic transaminase (SGOT), SGPT, and LDH remained within normal limits, while displaying a serum CsA trough of 119 ng/ml, he was maintained on a CsA dosage of 14.0 mg/kg of body weight (100 mg i.v.; 700 mg p.o.) and a tapered methylprednisolone dosage of 2.0 mg/kg. On day 7, he defervesced and was extubated. Because his chest roentgenogram demonstrated a residual interstitial infiltrate, the antibiotic therapy was continued. Three days later, with a serum creatinine level of 0.6 mg/dl and a blood urea nitrogen of 44 mg/dl, laboratory results revealed an elevated total bilirubin (5.7 mg/dl), alkaline phosphatase (238 U/liter), LDH (523 U/liter), and SGOT (46 U/liter). Since the previous serum CsA trough was reported as 574 ng/ml, CsA hepatotoxicity was suspected. The CsA therapy was altered to a twice daily infusion of 150 mg with a methylprednisolone dose of 48 mg daily. By day 13, the total bilirubin increased to 8.9 mg/dl. Although his serum CsA trough level was 155 ng/ml, the CsA dose was further adjusted to a single daily infusion of 150 mg, with a methylpredisolone maintenance dose of 45 mg daily. At this time, in spite of the same antibiotic therapy, he displayed a fever of 101.5°F, a white blood cell count of 20,500/mm^3, and bilateral pulmonary infiltrates on chest roentgenograms. On day 17, because sputum cultures were positive for *Escherichia coli* and *Klebsiella pneumoniae* and because pleural fluid cultures were positive for *Legionella pneumoniae,* the antibiotic

Table 1. CsA Levels in Tissues Obtained at Postmortem Examinations

	Patients			
Tissue	L.T.	A.S.	C.P.	D.H.
Fat	2,913* (1.0)†	2,068 (0.27)	2,870 (1.0)	439 (1.00)
Esophagus	—	2,453 (0.32)	—	—
Stomach	—	7,617 (1.00)	—	—
Large bowel	—	6,354 (0.83)	—	—
Jejunum	—	210 (0.03)	1,010 (0.35)	—
Gallbladder	—	1,695 (0.22)	—	—
Liver	719 (0.25)	530 (0.07)	2,206 (0.77)	36 (0.08)
Pancreas	1,500 (0.52)	3,643 (0.48)	2,811 (0.98)	50 (0.11)
Lymph node	—	3,041 (0.40)	807 (0.28)	26 (0.06)
Spleen	—	—	1,118 (0.39)	14 (0.03)
Accessory spleen	273 (0.09)	—	—	—
Bone	—	693 (0.09)	787 (0.27)	—
Adrenal	713 (0.24)	2,468 (0.32)	1,570 (0.55)	37 (0.08)
Kidney	276 (0.09)	758 (0.10)	1,418 (0.49)	30 (0.07)
Heart	—	191 (0.02)	1,079 (0.38)	—
Aorta	143 (0.05)	835 (0.11)	290 (0.10)	7 (0.02)
Atrium	798 (0.27)	—	—	15 (0.03)
Ventricle	—	—	—	7 (0.02)
Lung	396 (0.14)	145 (0.02)	760 (0.26)	13 (0.03)
Skin	—	—	1,722 (0.60)	10 (0.02)
Muscle	205 (0.07)	—	607 (0.21)	16 (0.04)
Prostate	—	—	—	10 (0.02)
Testicle	—	—	849 (0.30)	13 (0.03)
Ovary	108 (0.04)	—	—	—
Uterus	94 (0.03)	—	—	—
Breast	1,244 (0.42)	—	—	—
Brain	129 (0.04)	—	117 (0.04)	1 (0.01)
Spinal cord	21 (0.01)	283 (0.04)	—	—
Serum‡	260	368	208	—

*CsA levels in tissues obtained at postmortem examinations in ng/g of tissue wet weight.

†Relative concentration (*r*) expressed as the ratio that tissue's drug content (ng/g) to the highest drug content of that patient's tissues.

‡Concomitant serum CsA levels in ng/ml are also shown.

therapy was changed to bactrim and erythromycin. He was electively reintubated. On day 18, in the face of an elevated serum creatinine (1.6 mg/dl) and blood urea nitrogen (61 mg/dl) levels, with a serum CsA trough of 158 ng/ml, the CsA dose was lowered to 100 mg i.v. and the methylprednisolone was adjusted to 15 mg. Subsequently, dopamine was administered to aid perfusion. Four days later, during an unsuccessful attempt to repair a tracheal dehiscence exacerbated by positive-pressure ventilation, the patient died. In the preterminal period, he displayed an elevated blood urea nitrogen (101 mg/dl), serum creatinine (2.8 mg/dl), uric acid (8.6 mg/dl), total bilirubin (5.6 mg/dl), conjugated bilirubin (4.4 mg/dl), alkaline phosphatase (200 U/liter), LDH (690 U/liter), and SGOT (50 U/liter). Postmortem examination not only confirmed acute bronchopneumonia in the absence of allograft rejection, but also revealed congestion and fatty degeneration of the liver and acute tubular necrosis in the kidney.

CsA Tissue Levels

Small fragments of tissues obtained at postmortem examinations were weighed and placed in a clean 16 × 100 mm glass tube containing 2 ml of normal saline. After the tissue fragments were treated with a Polytron homogenizer using a microprobe, the homogenate was extracted twice with 5 ml of diethyl-ether and centrifuged at 3,000 rpm for 10 min. The ether phases were pooled and evaporated to dryness. The extracted drug was resuspended in 1 ml of 0.5 *M* Tris buffer (pH 8.5) containing 0.03% Tween-20. Resuspension of CsA was facilitated by placing the samples in a 50°C water bath for 30 min. CsA determinations were then made using the radioimmunoassay for CsA,[5] employing materials provided by the Sandoz Company (Basel, Switzerland), and analyzed by computer as previously described.[6]

RESULTS

Tissue Levels

The CsA levels of tissues obtained at postmortem examinations are summarized in Table 1. D.H., who had been on CsA for 75 days prior to its discontinuance 20 days prior to death, displayed only trace quantities of drug in his tissues, indicating reversible binding of the drug. Appreciable drug levels were only present in the fat. Similarly, the results from the other patients consistently demonstrated fat to contain among the highest deposits of drug, a finding concordant with the lipophilic nature of CsA.

Other tissues exhibiting a large drug deposition included the adrenal glands (713, 2,468, and 1,570 ng/g), breast (1,244 ng/g), stomach (7,617 ng/g), large bowel (6,354 ng/g), gall bladder (1,695 ng/g), esophagus (2,453 ng/g), and pancreas (1,500, 3,643, and 2,206 ng/g). The reason for the consistent large accumulation of CsA in the pancreas is uncertain, particularly since all of the patients were asymptomatic for pancreatitis. The high CsA levels in breast and adrenal glands most probably reflect the high fat content of these organs. The relative CsA content of esophagus (0.32), stomach (1.0), and large bowel (0.83) appeared to be significantly higher than in the jejunum (0.03), possibly due to the small intestine's physiologically active role of adsorption and transport of CsA across its epithelium, as opposed to the more passive functions of the other organs of the gastrointestinal tract.

The drug levels measured in the cardiopulmonary recipient's tissues were much higher than those in the renal recipients, for example, muscle (607 versus 205 ng/g), lung (760 versus 145 and 396 ng/g), heart (1,079 versus 191 ng/g), kidney (1,418 versus 758 and 276 ng/g), jejunum (1,010 versus 210 ng/g), and liver (2,206 versus 530 and 719 ng/g). Although this may reflect poor bioavailability

Table 2. Lymph Node CsA Levels and Concomitant Serum CsA Pharmacokinetics

Patient	Drug administration		CsA*	*F*(%)†
	p.o.	i.v.		
B.L.‡	14 (×3)	0	750	6.2
W.P.‡	14 (×3)	0	1,000	11.9
J.M.‡	14 (×3)	0	1,398	6.4
V.M.§	14 (×1)	3.5 (×7)	357	5.4
R.G.‖	14 (×3)	2.2 (×1)	1,018	11.4
J.V.‖	14 (×3)	2.2 (×1)	1,343	8.9

*Lymph node CsA levels in ng/g of tissue wet weight.

†The percentage of drug bioavailability (*F*) determined the day before transplantation, as described previously.[3]

‡Drug therapies in these patients receiving allografts from living-related donors was 14.0 mg/kg CsA (p.o.) for three days prior to transplantation.

§Therapy in this patient was constant CsA i.v. infusion for seven days (3.5 mg/kg/24 hr) prior to transplantation, followed by a single p.o. dose (14.0 mg/kg) 24 hr before transplant.

‖Therapy in these patients was 14.0 mg/kg CsA p.o. for three days followed by a single i.v. dose (2.2 mg/kg) prior to transplant.

or conjugation or metabolic conversion to a form not reactive in the radioimmunoassay in renal recipients, more comparative data are needed, particularly in recipients not displaying the multiple signs of toxicity observed in C.P. In this regard, C.P.'s high hepatic drug content probably reflects the hepatotoxicity. Since the liver is a highly perfused organ, performing the functions of both metabolizing and extracting CsA from the peripheral blood with subsequent elimination into the biliary tract, this organ would be expected to bind moderate amounts of drug. On the other hand, the hepatic levels in samples of L.T. and A.S. probably better represent the expected liver CsA content. Additionally, since C.P. exhibited a prolonged period of liver dysfunction, the higher drug values observed in the muscle, lung, heart, kidney, and jejunum may have arisen from hepatic impairment of CsA metabolism and excretion, resulting in an increased tissue accumulation. Therefore, high drug levels observed in C.P.'s spleen, testicle, and skin should be viewed with caution.

The consistently low CsA levels observed in the brain (129 and 117 ng/g) and spinal cord (21 and 283 ng/g) suggest that little drug crosses the blood–brain barrier. This observation is not consistent with the clinically evident CNS toxicity widely observed. Further analysis of drug metabolism may be necessary to dissect this discrepancy.

Tissue Levels and Pharmacodynamics

To assess the rate of tissue accumulation of CsA, iliac lymph nodes were obtained from recipients of living-related donor kidneys at the time of transplantation. These patients had received three different pretransplant CsA regimens. The lymph node tissue CsA content was compared with the absolute bioavailability determined on the day prior to transplantation. The results confirm the low calculated bioavailabilities previously reported in patients within the first few days posttransplant. The lymph node drug content after all three drug regimens appeared high and comparable. Detailed simultaneous analysis of CsA content and lymph node lymphocyte functions in vitro may discern whether these tissue levels correlate with immunosuppression.

DISCUSSION

The studies presented here indicate that tissue binding of CsA is a major consequence of drug therapy. In an effort to understand the relationship between tissue uptake and CsA pharmacokinetics, tissue levels were performed at autopsy in four patients. There was a high drug content in fat, attributable to the lipophilicity of CsA, and a moderate hepatic drug content, consistent with the known role of the liver in CsA elimination. Additionally, our data indicate that hepatic dysfunction results in excessive accumulation in other tissues. There was no CNS accumulation. Therefore, CNS toxicity in the presence of low levels observed within the central nervous system requires further study. Our preliminary results suggest that lymph node samplings may afford a ready site to assess CsA tissue pharmacokinetics. Further analysis of tissue profiles may permit formulation of an appropriate drug protocol that achieves selective lymphoid tissue uptake in the absence of total body saturation.

REFERENCES

1. Calne RY, Thiru S, McMaster P, et al: Lancet 2:1323, 1978

2. Calne RY, Rolles K, White DJG, et al: Lancet 1:1033, 1979

3. Kahan BD, Ried M, Newburger J: Transplant Proc 15:446, 1983

4. Kahan BD, Van Buren CT, Boileau M, et al: Transplantation 35:96, 1983

5. Donatsch P, Abisch E, Homberger M, et al: J Immunoassay 2:19, 1981

6. Kahan BD, Van Buren CT, Lin SN, et al: Transplantation 34:36, 1982

The Clinical Relevance of Cyclosporine Blood Levels As Measured by Radioimmunoassay

P. A. Keown, C. R. Stiller, N. R. Sinclair, G. Carruthers, W. Howson, M. Stawecki, J. McMichael, J. Koegler, N. McKenzie, and W. Wall

CYCLOSPORINE A (CsA) is a novel immunosuppressive agent derived from the fungal strains *Trichoderma polysporum* and *Cylindrocarpon Lucidum*. It exhibits relative specificity in its effect, inhibiting intercellular communication at the level of the T lymphocyte,[1] and thus preventing the development of humoral and cell-mediated effector mechanisms. The potency of immunosuppressive effect combined with its relative immunological specificity has rendered CsA an important advance in organ transplantation. Both patient and graft survival have improved significantly following renal transplantation,[2,3] and the transplantation of other organs including liver, heart and heart/lung has become both clinically and financially viable.[4,5]

The clinical use of CsA is rendered difficult, however, by the narrow therapeutic window between inadequate immunosuppression that occurs at low doses, and the adverse effect of hepatotoxicity, nephrotoxicity, and sepsis resulting from overadministration. Therapeutic efficacy and safety is not clearly related to the dosage administered, which varies between individuals depending upon multiple factors. In an effort to establish the parameters influencing CsA pharmacokinetics and more clearly define the therapeutic range measurements of the CsA concentration within the blood compartment have been performed sequentially both prior to and following organ transplantation in patients receiving this drug.

From the Departments of Medicine and Surgery, University Hospital, and the University of Western Ontario, London, Ontario, Canada.

Supported in part by grants from the MRC, The Ontario Ministry of Health, and The Richard and Jean Ivey Foundation.

Address reprint requests to Dr. Keown, Department of Medicine, University Hospital, and the University of Western Ontario, London, Ontario, Canada.

0041-1345/83/1505-0045$01.00/0

MATERIALS AND METHODS

Pharmacologic measurements were performed in 45 patients at intervals before or after renal or cardiac transplantation. Pharmacokinetic courses were determined upon serial blood measurements performed prior to, and 1, 2, 3, 4, 6, 8, and 12 hr after drug administration. The elimination half-life was calculated by the method of feathering, and the area under the time/concentration curve was determined by integration using a computer program.

Cyclosporine concentrations were measured both in serum, and in whole blood following erythrocyte lysis using the following two methods: (1) radioimmunoassay (RIA)—this was performed as described[6] using the kit provided by Sandoz Limited, Basel; (2) high-pressure liquid chromatography (HPLC)—this was performed using a Waters HPL chromatograph (Waters Associates, Bedford, MA), after acid and basic extraction to remove contaminating substances.[7] The flow rate was 1.5 ml/min, and the CsA peak was read at 210 nm wavelength.

The posttransplant course was monitored sequentially, and clinical and laboratory data recorded using a PDP 10 computer program. Statistical analysis of the data was performed using Student's t test, and by analysis of variance and covariance.

RESULTS

Concentrations of CsA Within the Blood Compartment

CsA is absorbed rapidly following oral administration with a peak concentration (C_{max}) time in both serum and whole blood of 2–4 hr (mean 2.8 hr). There is extensive enterohepatic recirculation,[8] and elimination occurs according to first order kinetics with an elimination half-life of 4–6 hr. Within the blood compartment, 61% of CsA is bound to the erythrocytes at C_{max}, and 5% to the leukocytes. The remainder is in the serum and is highly protein bound (~90%) predominantly to the lipoprotein fraction. The concentration of parent molecule in either serum or whole blood, as measured by HPLC, is ~73% of the total immunoreactive material (reflecting parent compound plus metabolites) at C_{max}, and 12 hr later has declined to 38%. The concentration of CsA in whole blood is dependent upon the hematocrit. Binding of CsA to the RBC is temperature dependent, increasing in inverse proportion to the temperature of incubation. Following separation of serum at 22°C or less, there was a mean of 22% reduction in the measured serum concentration compared with separation at 37°C. However the measured concentration within the separated serum was subsequently stable and independent of temperature. For these reasons we have selected serum measurement of CsA by RIA as the most reliable and practical assay for clinical studies.

Clinical Factors That Influence CsA Blood Levels

A number of factors have been examined that have a potential influence upon CsA pharmacokinetics.

The effect of food was examined using a standard test protocol.[9] CsA was administered either in the fasting state, or following a standard test breakfast, and serum CsA levels measured sequentially over the ensuing 12 hr. Food had no consistent effect in influencing CsA absorption and neither peak concentration nor elimination half-life were significantly altered (C_{max}: 770 ± 220 ng/ml fasting, 745 ± 285 ng/ml nonfasting). Within the individuals examined there was also a day to day variation in CsA that was independent of diet.

In contrast, liver dysfunction had a major impact upon CsA pharmacokinetics. CsA levels were measured sequentially following a single oral dose of 15 mg/kg in 5 potential cardiac recipients with minimal hepatic dysfunction due to passive hepatic congestion. The C_{max} remained unchanged at 664 ± 119 μg/ml, but the time taken to achieve peak serum CsA concentration was markedly increased in these patients (6.3 ± 2.9 hr) compatible with a prolonged elimination half-life.

Drug interaction has a major effect on the pharmacokinetics of certain medications. The hepatic elimination of CsA appears to be dependent upon the microsomal oxidase system within the liver. In patients receiving CsA in the stable state, the commencement of phenytoin treatment results in a marked fall in serum CsA levels (308 ± 38 ng/ml to 147 ± 18 ng/ml), despite a threefold increase in the daily CsA dose. Intravenous pharmacokinetic studies performed prior to and following the commencement of phenytoin demonstrated an ~50% reduction in the area under the CsA time/concentration curve. This effect occurred within 72 hr of commencing phenytoin therapy and persisted for 2 weeks following withdrawal of treatment.

The distribution of CsA appears to conform to a multicompartment model, in which continued administration of the drug leads to eventual saturation of the peripheral compartment. This is reflected clinically by a decreased dosage requirement with long term administration to maintain constant serum CsA levels. On commencement of therapy, trough CsA levels of 200–300 ng/ml were achieved with an oral dose of 17.5 mg/kg/day. After 8 weeks of therapy, the same levels were maintained with a mean of 9.0 mg/kg/day. Pharmacokinetic profiles performed in five patients following administration of a test dose of 17.5 mg/kg at the initiation of therapy revealed a mean peak concentration of 687 ± 62 ng/ml, whereas the same test dose after 8 weeks or more of therapy resulted in a mean peak concentration of 2675 ± 375 ng/ml. This difference was not explained by a change in the elimination half-life, but rather appeared to reflect either a change in bioavailability or the saturation of a peripheral body compartment.

CsA Blood Levels and Clinical Events

The importance of serum CsA levels has been examined in relation to both the adverse effects of hepatotoxicity and nephrotoxicity, and to the immunosuppressive effect of this medication.

We have previously suggested an apparent association between CsA levels and hepatotoxicity. Other supportive evidence has been provided by additional groups. We have now reexamined this association in 72 patients who have received CsA following organ transplantation. Six patients, all of whom had normal liver function prior to transplantation developed evidence of hepatotoxicity as evidenced by an elevation in the serum bilirubin. This was transient, with a mean duration of 35 ± 14 days, and in all cases occurred during the first 3 weeks following transplantation and resolved on adjustment of CsA dose. The serum levels in these patients rose prior to the onset of hyperbilirubinemia from a mean of 65 ± 66 ng/ml to 630 ± 112 ng/ml. After appropriate reduction in the oral dose, the serum CsA levels fell to a mean of 236 ± 66 ng/ml, which was followed shortly thereafter by a return of serum bilirubin to normal. Regression analysis plotting serum bilirubin against serum CsA level revealed a straight line relationship with an r^2 value of 0.58, and a significance value of $p = 0.001$.

The nephrotoxicity of CsA is complex, and may appear in three forms: (a) prolongation of posttransplant ATN, (b) acute reversible nephrotoxicity, and (c) chronic progressive deterioration in graft function that resolves partly or completely upon withdrawal of the agent. The toxic effect of CsA appears to act synergistically with other factors that potentiate renal damage to produce the observed dysfunction. Two such factors identified as influencing the toxic effect of the drug in the Canadian Multicentre Study have been a prolonged machine perfusion time (>24 hr)($p = 0.005$) and prolonged surgical reanastomosis (>45 min) ($p = 0.002$). The overall incidence of ATN in this study was 49% in patients receiving CsA. In those recipients with the risk factors described, this incidence rose to 80%, and was independent of the serum concentration of the drug. In patients in whom the risk factors were absent, however, the incidence of ATN was directly related to the serum CsA level during the first 3 days posttransplant, rising from 18% in those with mean trough CsA levels less than 100 ng/ml to 70% in those with levels of over 400 ng/ml during this time.[3] Chronic nephrotoxicity, in contrast, is characterized by a slow and progressive rise in serum creatinine often associated with hypertension and a histological picture of intersitital fibrosis, patchy cellular infiltration, and destruction of the proximal tubular epithelial cells. These findings may be accompanied by thickening of the wall of medium and small-sized vessels, and a decrease in luminal diameter. In the 70 patients receiving CsA, 8 (11%) exhibited such progressive nephrotoxicity confirmed by a marked fall in serum creatinine upon withdrawal of the drug. Comparison of this group with 21 unaffected subjects demonstrated a marked increase in the preponderance of risk factors within these patients. All grafts with chronic nephrotoxicity had undergone machine perfusion with a mean perfusion time of 1920 ± 216 min. In contrast, only 15 out of 21 in the comparison group had received machine perfusion, with a mean time of 1072 ± 113 min ($p < 0.01$). Furthermore, 5 of 8 patients with nephrotoxicity had a prolonged (>45 min) reanastomosis time, compared with only 5 out of 21 in the comparison group ($p = 0.05$). Poorer graft function was observed throughout the whole posttransplant course in the 8 patients who ultimately developed nephrotoxicity. The lowest serum creatinine achieved was in this group was 2.82 ± 0.25 mg%, compared with 1.66 0.11 mg% in the nonaffected subjects. Serum CsA levels were also higher during this period of time (mean 530 ± 97 ng/ml versus 231 ± 28 ng/ml). In concert, these factors suggest that nephrotoxicity is more common in those renal allografts at risk from the time of transplantation, suggesting a synergistic nephrotoxic effect of multiple factors. The mean serum CsA level during the phase of nephrotoxicity was 248 ± 84 ng/ml. In these 8 patients, CsA was either withdrawn, or temporarily withheld and reinstituted at 50% of the original dose. Serum creatinine fell in all cases and was maintained with a mean CsA level of 78 ± 37 ng/ml.

The examination of acute rejection is rendered more complex by the lack of clear criteria to differentiate this from acute nephrotoxicity. The role of serum levels was examined in 25 patients where clear clinical and histological criteria were available, and where the CsA dose was not reduced simultaneously with commencement of antirejection therapy, thus confusing the clinical picture. Six patients had unequivocal histological and clinical evidence of acute graft rejection within the first 21 days, which responded satisfactorily to antirejection therapy. Mean serum CsA levels at the time of rejection in these patients was 165 ng/ml. In 19 patients, there was no evidence of acute rejection, and the mean CsA level was 228 ng/ml. Because of the obscuring nature of ATN within this group it was difficult to isolate the nephrotoxic effects of this drug within the first 3 weeks with certainty. After 90 days, only 3 patients exhibited unequivocal evidence of acute rejection. All three episodes occurred during a deliberate reduction in the dose in an attempt to achieve lower serum drug levels and occurred with a mean CsA level of 42 ng/ml. Quiescence during this period was maintained in 20 patients. The mean CsA level in those patients was 101 ng/ml. Eight cases of chronic nephrotoxicity occurred, with mean serum levels of 240 ng/ml. Thus the therapeutic window appears to change with time, being from ~150–300 ng/ml during the first few weeks of therapy and decreasing to between 50 and 150 ng/ml after 90 days or more posttransplant.

SUMMARY

CsA is a potent immunosuppressive agent with a major potential clinical use in man. The bioavailability and pharmacokinetics of the drug do not appear to be influenced by food, but the elimination and hence serum concentration of the drug are modified by liver dysfunction, and drug interactions. The adverse effects of hepatotoxicity and acute nephrotoxicity appear to be related to elevated serum concentrations of CsA. Chronic nephrotoxicity may occur in association with trough levels of 200–400 ng/ml, and appears to develop particularly in those grafts prejudiced by the risk factors of prolonged machine perfusion and warm ischemia. The immunosuppressive effect of CsA also appears to be related to the serum concentration of the drug, although the levels required to maintain immunological quiescence decrease with time reflecting an alteration in the therapeutic window.

REFERENCES

1. Bunjes D, Hardt C, Rollinghoff M, et al: Eur J Immunol 11:657–661, 1981

2. European Multicentre Transplant Study Group: Lancet 2:57–60, 1982

3. Canadian Transplant Study Group: Submitted for publication.

4. Starzl TE, Klintmalm GBG, Porter KA, et al: N Engl J Med 305:266–269, 1981

5. Oyer P, Stinson EB, Jamieson SW, et al: Transplant Proc 15:1247–1252, 1983

6. Keown PA, Stiller CR, Ulan RA, et al: Lancet 1:686–689, 1981

7. Carruthers SG, Freeman DJ, Koegler JC, et al: Clin Chem (in press)

8. Kahan BD, Ried M, Newburger J: Transplant Proc 15:446–453, 1983

Pharmacologic Monitoring in the Clinical Use of Cyclosporine

F. Lokiec, A. Devergie, O. Poirier, and E. Gluckman

THE beneficial use of cyclosporine (CsA) in the prevention and treatment of graft-versus-host disease (GVHD) after bone marrow transplantation is now well established.[1-3] Unfortunately, the nephrotoxic side effect of CsA is also well known.[4,5] Furthermore, CsA interacts with many other drugs, such as ketoconazole, which increase serum levels of CsA;[6] sulphadimidine and trimethoprim, which decrease serum levels of CsA[7] melphalan, which enhances the nephrotoxicity of CsA;[8] and methylprednisolone, which, in combination with CsA, precipitates convulsions in young patients.[9]

The individual sensitivity of the patients to CsA is a major problem for its clinical use; furthermore, the relation between nephrotoxicity and high serum levels of CsA seems very close, according to the results reported by Hows et al.[10] The combination of these two facts leads to a fundamental question about the dose of cyclosporine to administer to the patient in order to obtain a clinical benefit without surpassing the therapeutic range and reaching nephrotoxicity.

Our transplant team decided not to administer CsA according to the body surface or the body weight of the patients, but according to the pharmacokinetic profile of the drug in each patient.

In the present study, we have reported the results we obtained using this technique in 38 patients treated by bone marrow transplantation.

From the Pharmacology and Pharmacokinetics Laboratory, René Huguenin Center, Saint-Cloud, and the Bone Marrow Transplant Unit, Saint-Louis Hospital, Paris, France.

Address reprint requests to Dr. F. Lokiec, Pharmacology and Pharmacokinetics Laboratory, René Huguenin Center, 5 G. Latouche Street, F92211 Saint-Cloud, France.

0041-1345/83/1505-0046$01.00/0

MATERIALS AND METHODS

Patients

We studied 38 patients suffering from aplastic anemia (14 patients), Fanconi's anemia (6 patients), chronic myeloid leukemia (12 patients), and acute myeloblastic leukemia (6 patients).

The patients were separated in two groups: group 1 of anemic patients (20), and group 2 of leukemic patients (18). In group 1 14 were male with a median age of 16.4 years (range, 8–34 years) and six were female with a median age of 15.7 years (range, 8–33 years). In group 2 nine were male with a median age of 16.3 years (range, 12–33 years) and nine were female with a median age of 18.4 years (range, 2–37 years).

All of the patients received allogeneic bone marrow transplantation for treatment of their disease.

CsA Assay

Estimation of CsA levels in the plasma of the patients were determined using a radioimmunoassay kit kindly supplied by Sandoz Laboratories (Basel, Switzerland and Rueil-Malmaison, France). The detection limit of this technique was 62.5 ng/ml as plasma CsA concentration.

Pharmacokinetic Study

An i.v. and p.o. pharmacokinetic study of CsA was performed in each patient. The i.v. pharmacokinetic profile was realized after an intravenous injection of 4 mg of CsA/kg of body weight of CsA. Blood samples were collected 5, 10, 20, 30 min, 1, 2, 3, 6, and 12 hr after CsA administration. The p.o. pharmacokinetic profile was realized after the oral administration of 15 mg of CsA/kg of body weight. Blood samples were collected 1, 2, 3, 4, 6, 12, and 24 hr after CsA administration.

Curves were constructed by the least-square method. The analytical pharmacokinetic program had been written for a 4341 IBM computer, and for CsA we used a classic two open compartment model. The pharmacokinetic data were compared by the Student's t test. In all cases, data were expressed as mean ± SE.

Test-Dose Technique

The calculation of the CsA dose to be administered to the patient was based on a very simple formula:

$$Q = Cl \times C \times 24$$

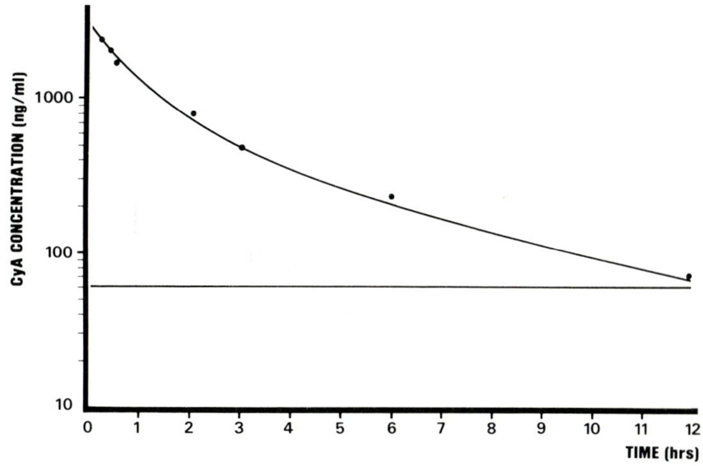

Fig. 1. Intravenous pharmacokinetic profile of CsA (4 mg/kg).

where Q was the dose of CsA to be administered to the patient, Cl was the plasmatic clearance of the drug, and C was the required plasma level; 24 signified that Q was calculated for a 24-hr course in our study.

RESULTS

After statistical analysis, we did not notice any significant difference for the i.v. and p.o. pharmacokinetic parameters in the two groups of patients.

The i.v. and p.o. typical pharmacokinetic profiles of CsA are shown, respectively, in Fig. 1 and Fig. 2. In all the patients, the maximum CsA oral absorption appeared between 3 and 4 hr postadministration.

Table 1 and Table 2 show, respectively, the i.v. and the p.o. pharmacokinetic parameters obtained after computing the radioimmunoassay data. It can be seen that the individual sensitivity to CsA was an important factor. The large variations of the C_{max}, (C_{max} represents the extrapolated CsA concentration to zero time), indicated the large variations of the distribution and/or the tissue binding of

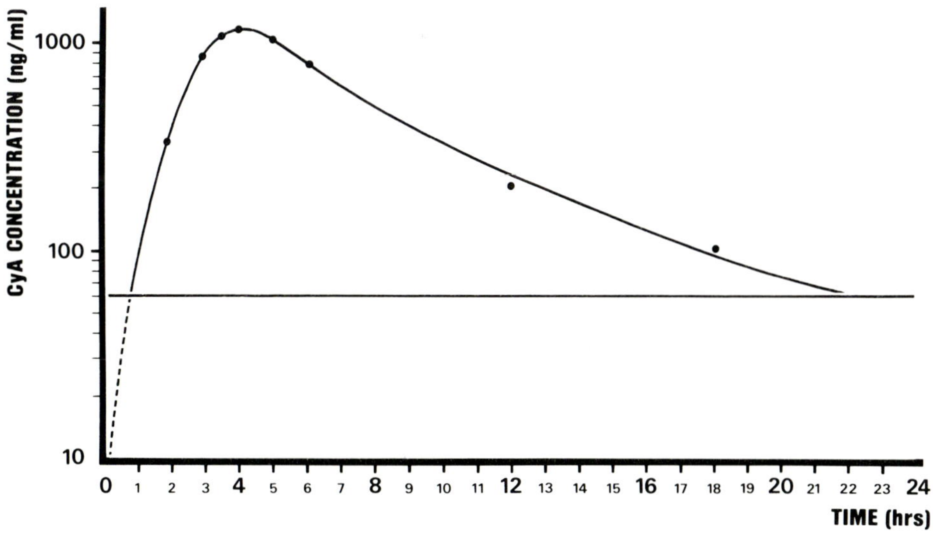

Fig. 2. Oral pharmacokinetic profile of CsA (15 mg/kg).

Detrimental Effect of Intestinal Disease on Absorption of Orally Administered Cyclosporine

K. Atkinson, K. Britton, P. Paull, C. Farrell, A. Concannon, A. Dodds, and J. Biggs

BONE marrow transplantation from an HLA-identical sibling donor is a viable therapeutic option for acute leukemia and severe aplastic anemia. Unfortunately, graft-versus-host disease (GVHD) is common posttransplant and is a cause of both morbidity and mortality. The new immunosuppressive agent, cyclosporine A (CsA), has both advantages and disadvantages when compared to methotrexate, the conventional agent used to minimize GVHD posttransplant. CsA is associated with faster engraftment and less oropharyngeal mucositis than methotrexate,[1] but it is nephrotoxic,[2] hepatotoxic,[3] and neurotoxic.[4] In a prospective randomized trial,[5] there was no significant difference in the incidence of acute GVHD posttransplant between patients receiving CsA and those receiving methotrexate. In all studies reported thus far, CsA has been administered predominantly by the oral route. We have given CsA to 56 patients receiving allogeneic transplants for treatment of hematologic malignancy or severe aplastic anemia. We report the poor absorption of orally administered CsA in the presence of clinical intestinal dysfunction and our attempts to overcome this by the use of intravenous CsA.

From the Departments of Haematology and Clinical Pharmacology, St. Vincent's Hospital, Sydney, Australia.

Supported in part by grants from the New South Wales State Cancer Council and the National Health and Medical Research Council of Australia.

Address reprint requests to Dr. K. Atkinson, Department of Haematology, St. Vincent's Hospital, Sydney, Australia.

0041-1345/83/1505-0047$01.00/0

MATERIALS AND METHODS

Patients with severe aplastic anemia were conditioned with high-dose cyclophosphamide and those with hematologic malignancy with cyclophosphamide and fractionated total body irradiation, as previously described,[1,6] prior to an allogeneic marrow transplant from a family member. Each patient was given a unique patient number (UPN). The day of marrow transplant was designated day 0. Orally administered CsA was given to all patients in milk in two 12-hr divided doses. Thirty-six patients received oral CsA (25 mg/kg/day from day −1 to day +4, and 12.5 mg/kg/day from day +5 onwards) while 10 received oral CsA, (25 mg/kg/day from day −7 to day +4, and then 12.5 mg/kg/day from day +5 onwards). The dose of oral CsA was tapered by 5% per week from day 50 onwards, unless suspected CsA toxicity occurred earlier. During periods when they were unable to tolerate or absorb the oral preparation, six patients received i.v. CsA (2–4 mg/kg/day in 2 12-hr divided infusions of 5% dextrose or normal saline given over 30 min each) while a further four patients received CsA (1–3 mg/kg/day as a continuous i.v. infusion). CsA serum values were assayed by radioimmunoassay.[7] Single-dose pharmacokinetic studies were carried out on samples drawn before and at 3, 4, 6, and 10 hr after an oral morning dose of CsA. The area under the serum concentration–time curve (AUC) over the dosage intervals was calculated by the trapezoid method,[8] and the calculated AUC values were adjusted

Table 1. CsA Trough Serum Concentration (ng/ml)* After an Oral Dose of CsA

	Time in Relation to Oral Dose of CsA					
Patient Group	Before	2 hr After	3 hr After	4 hr After	6 hr After	10 hr After
No clinical intestinal dysfunction ($n = 11$)	380 ± 327	424 ± 260	910 ± 503	879 ± 480	660 ± 446	428 ± 332
Chemoradiation enteritis ($n = 22$)	181 ± 167	312 ± 250	341 ± 265	354 ± 313	248 ± 146	165 ± 156
Acute GVHD of intestine ($n = 6$)	93 ± 61	108 ± 55	132 ± 68	121 ± 60	153 ± 59	102 ± 57

*Values represent mean ± 1 SD.

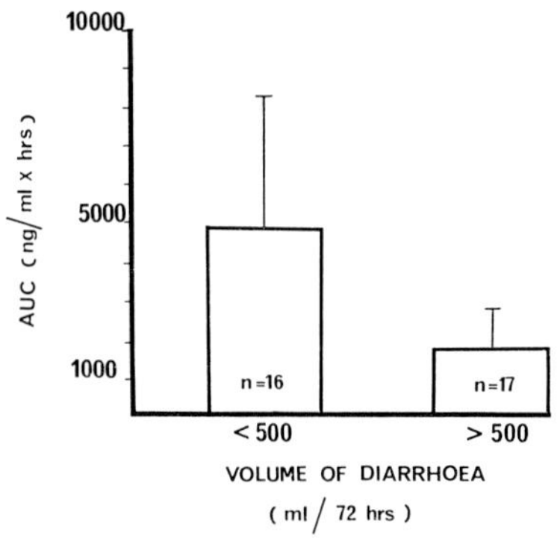

Fig. 1. Relationship between diarrhea volume and amount of CsA absorbed (area under the CsA serum-concentration time curve).

for a constant dose of 12.5 mg/kg of body weight per day. In patients receiving the 30-min i.v. infusion of CsA, serum samples were drawn at 1, 3, 6, 9, 12, 15, and 60 min, as well as at 2 and 4 hr, after the termination of the infusion, while in patients receiving a continuous i.v. infusion of CsA, serum samples were drawn at 4–6-hr intervals during the infusion. The stability of CsA in 5% dextrose in water and normal saline vehicles for intravenous infusion was assessed by high-performance liquid chromatography (HPLC).[9] Immunosuppressive capacity of CsA given by continuous intravenous infusion was assessed by the ability of the intravenous infusion fluid containing CsA to inhibit a third-party mixed lymphocyte reaction (MLC).[9] The inhibition of MLC reactivity caused by the CsA-containing solution was calculated as follows:

$$\text{Percent inhibition} = \frac{\text{cpm control culture} - \text{cpm test culture}}{\text{cpm control culture}} \times 100$$

RESULTS

Poor Absorption of Orally Administered CsA in the Presence of Clinical Intestinal Dysfunction

Patients with no clinical intestinal dysfunction (no vomiting or diarrhea) consistently showed CsA serum values peaking 3 or 4 hr after an orally administered dose of CsA (Table 1). In contrast, patients with clinical dysfunction of any cause (chemoradiation enteritis secondary to the conditioning regimen for marrow transplantation, acute GVHD of the intestine, candida enteritis) showed poor or minimal absorption of orally administered CsA (Table 1). Furthermore, when the amount of absorbed drug over a given time period (area under the CsA serum concentration–time curve) was correlated with diarrhea volume, patients with greater than 500 ml diarrhea/72 hr had a significantly lower AUC (Fig. 1).

The Effect of Initiating CsA Therapy Seven Days Instead of One Day Pretransplant

In an attempt to overcome the malabsorption of CsA associated with the chemoradiation enteritis consistently experienced by all transplant recipients in this series, we initiated CsA therapy in 10 patients seven days rather than one day pretransplant. CsA trough serum concentration values were only minimally greater in the former group (Table 2), and the overall incidence of acute GVHD and of fatal GVHD was the same in each group.

Chemical Stability of CsA in Intravenous Infusion Vehicles

We concluded from the above results that it was necessary to administer CsA intravenously during periods when malabsorption of the oral preparation occurred. We felt it first necessary to ensure that CsA remained chemically stable throughout the duration of a 12-hr infusion. CsA concentrate for infusion solution was dissolved in both normal saline and 5% dextrose in water. Throughout the duration of a 12-hr infusion, there was no significant trend toward lower concentrations of the drug as detected by HPLC (Table 3).

Table 2. Sequential CsA Trough Serum Concentrations (ng/ml)* in Patients Starting CsA on Day −1 or Day −7

Day of Initiation of CsA Administration	Day Posttransplant 0	3	6	12	15	18	21
Day −1	96 ± 64	95 ± 92	98 ± 116	129 ± 68	213 ± 177	147 ± 91	239 ± 96
Day −7	148 ± 163	118 ± 115	145 ± 98	261 ± 263	183 ± 43	143 ± 70	132 ± 110

*Values represent mean ± 1 SD.

Table 3. Chemical Stability and Immunosuppressive Capacity of CsA Administered as a Continuous Intravenous Infusion of 5% Dextrose in Water

Datum	Hours After Starting Infusion										
	0	0.5	1	2	4	6	8	10	12	22	24
Concentration of CsA in infusion solution (μg/ml)	183	179	179	173	180	174	179	181	181	ND	ND
Inhibition of MLC by CsA at culture fluid concentration of 167 ng/ml (%)	62	ND	76	ND	ND	66	ND	77	ND	67	70

ND, not done.

Immunosuppressive Capacity of CsA During Intravenous Infusion

We also felt it necessary to determine if CsA retained its immunosuppressive capacity consistently during an intravenous infusion. As judged by the capacity of the drug in solution to inhibit a third-party mixed lymphocyte reaction, we could detect no significant decrease in immunosuppressive capacity throughout the duration of a 24-hr infusion (Table 3).

CsA Serum Values in Patients Receiving Intravenous Infusions of CsA

Since the oral preparation is routinely administered on a 12-hr basis, we initially administered intravenous CsA as 30-min infusions every 12 hr. Serum values at the end of the infusion were high, but declined rapidly. An example from a representative patient is shown in Table 4. Since CsA is not cytotoxic to lymphocytes,[10] and since T lymphocytes regain their reactivity once removed from the CsA-containing milieu,[11,12] we felt that the serum values obtained by this type of infusion most likely provided suboptimal immunosuppression. We subsequently administered CsA to six patients as a continuous i.v. infusion. Serum concentrations of CsA during such infusions were constant. An example from a representative patient is shown in Table 4. During periods when the drug was administered intravenously, the trough serum concentration of CsA gradually increased (Fig. 2).

CONCLUSIONS

CsA is finding clinical utility as an immunosuppressive agent after kidney,[13] liver,[14] heart-lung,[15] and marrow transplantation.[16] In this article, we document the important detrimental effect that intestinal dysfunction has on absorption of the orally administered preparation. Further, we have documented the chemical stability of the drug and the consistency of its immunosuppressive capacity when infused intravenously over 12–24 hr intravenously in 5% dextrose in water or normal saline. Constant serum levels were obtained when the drug was infused as a continuous infusion, but not when it was infused as a 30-min infusion every 12 hr. Furthermore, with continued infusion, the trough serum concentration of CsA gradually increased over a period of time. These data indicate that

Table 4. Serum Concentration of CsA When Given by Intravenous Infusion (ng/ml)

Type of infusion	Time After Termination of Infusion					
	Pre	6 mins	12 mins	45 mins	2 hrs	4 hrs
CsA given by 30-min infusion every 12 hr	110	2,050	1,166	989	210	155
	Time of Day (hr)					
	0600	1500	1800	2300		
CsA given by continuous infusion	92	90	123	98		

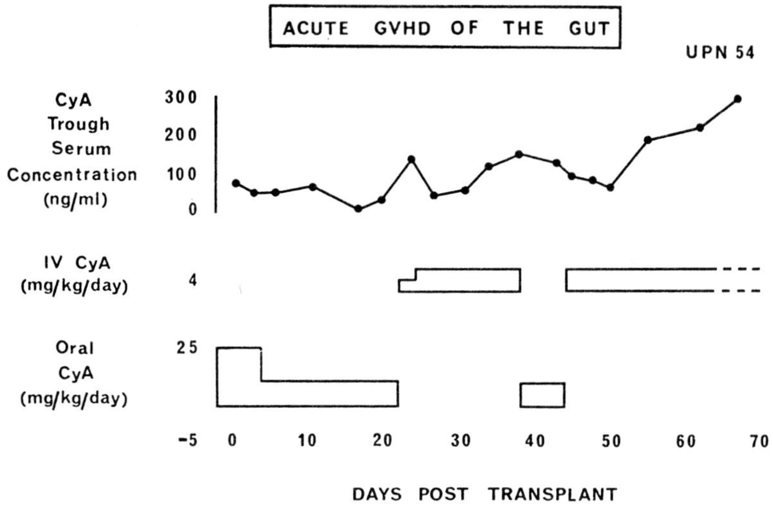

Fig. 2. Sequential CsA trough serum values in a patient receiving CsA intravenously.

the continuous intravenous infusion of CsA in 5% dextrose or normal saline is reliable and is the indicated route when malabsorption or intolerance of the oral preparation occur. A prospective randomized trial is currently in progress at our center comparing intravenous and oral routes of administration during the first 10 days after allogeneic marrow transplantation.

ACKNOWLEDGMENT

We thank Deirdre Nix for help in preparing this manuscript and Drs. Peter Isaac and Robert Mrongovius for their support during the period of these studies.

REFERENCES

1. Atkinson K, Biggs JC, Ting A, et al: Br J Haematol 53:265, 1983
2. Shulman H, Striker G, Deeg HJ, et al: N Engl J Med 305:392, 1981
3. Klintmalm GBG, Iwatsuki S, Starzl T: Transplantation 32:488, 1981
4. Atkinson K, Biggs JC, Concannon A, et al: Transplant Proc (this issue)
5. Deeg HJ, Storb R, Thomas ED: Transplant Proc 15:1385, 1983
6. Biggs JC, Atkinson K, Concannon A, et al: Med J Aust 2:120, 1983
7. Donatsch P, Abisch H, Homberger E, et al: J Immunoassay 2:19, 1981
8. Foster TS, Bourne DW: Am J Hosp Pharmacol 34:70, 1977
9. Atkinson K, Britton K, Farrell C, et al: Transplantation (in press)
10. White DJG, Carlne F, Plumb A: Transplant Proc 11:855, 1979
11. Wiesinger D, Borel JF: Immunol Biol 156:454, 1979
12. Deeg HJ, Storb R, Gerhard-Miller L: Transplantation 29:230, 1980
13. Calne RY, Rolles K, White DJG, et al: Lancet 2:1033, 1979
14. Starzl TE, Klintmalm GB, Porter KA, et al: N Engl J Med 305:266, 1981
15. Reitz BA, Wallwork JL, Hunt SA, et al: N Engl J Med 306:557, 1982
16. Powles RL, Clink HM, Spence D, et al: Lancet 1:327, 1980

Variable Tempo of Cyclosporine Peaks and Troughs in a Lung Transplant Recipient: Importance of Frequent Monitoring

S. L. Nehlsen-Cannarella, F. J. Veith, S. L. Kamholz, C. M. Montefusco, F. P. Mollenkopf, J. Goldsmith, and R. Kaleya

CYCLOSPORINE (CsA) is a new form of immunosuppressive agent that is specific for T lymphocytes, thus making this drug particularly useful in the field of organ transplantation. It has already been established that CsA prolongs allograft survival[1] and modifies autoimmune responses[1,2] in several animal species and in humans. In both experimental and clinical lung transplantation, the rejection that occurs in the presence of CsA immunosuppression is both milder and more easily reversed than classic modes of lung allograft rejection.[3] CsA does not, however, prevent lung transplant rejection absolutely. This fact, coupled with potentially serious side effects, including nephrotoxicity and hepatotoxicity,[4] indicates that the optimal methods of utilization and monitoring of CsA remain to be determined.

In the present report we describe clinical and laboratory experiences with both oral and intravenous formulations of CsA and the importance of monitoring the pharmacologic dynamics of these circumstances closely.

MATERIALS AND METHODS

Patient History

A 25-year-old male accidentally ingested 1-1′-dimethyl-4-4′-bipyridylium dichloride (paraquat). Despite treatment with activated charcoal hemoperfusion (to remove circulating paraquat) and intensive respiratory support, his pulmonary status rapidly deteriorated. On the 25th day following the accident, the patient was given a single left lung allograft from a cadaver donor.

The recipient and donor histocompatibility profiles were as follows: blood type O+, HLA-A1,A3,B7,B35,Cw4, and O+, HLA-A26,A33,B14,B39,Cw6,DR1,DR2,Le2,Le5, respectively. Using two pretransplant recipient serum samples (obtained nine days apart) and isolated B and T lymphocytes in a lymphocytotoxic crossmatch, the recipient was found to be compatible with his donor (no antibody detected at 37° C, 25° C, or 5° C in the modified Amos assay). Immunosuppressive therapy included CsA, azathioprine (1.5 mg/kg of body weight per day for the first 14 days only), and low-dose prednisone (25–40 mg daily). Large bolus doses of methylprednisolone (1 g per day for 3–5 days) and antithymocyte globulin (10–25 mg/kg for 5 days) were given to treat four episodes of lung allograft rejection. Except for the last two days, CsA was given as an oral preparation through a nasogastric tube. Sixteen days posttransplant, a right pneumonectomy was performed because of multiple abscesses due to *Pseudomonas* in the patient's remaining, damaged lung. Twenty-three days after right pneumonectomy, a bronchopleural fistula was repaired in the right bronchial stump. Eight days after repair and despite intensive antibiotic therapy, the fistula again opened and the patient died of respiratory failure 28 hr later, seven weeks after allotransplantation.[5] Figure 1 illustrates the total drug therapy schedule used in this complex case.

During the first postoperative week, blood samples were obtained 2–5 hr (peak) and 20–22 hr (trough) after administration of CsA. Daily CsA dosage was based on daily serum creatinine, the last CsA dose, and peak and trough serum CsA levels determined by radioimmunoassay (RIA) (see below). However, on several days, the peak and trough values were not spread apart as expected. Rather, they approached each other closely and sometimes inverted. As this drug was administered orally and blood levels were dependent on intestinal absorption, the patient's intestinal function was carefully observed. Periods of intestinal dysfunction correlated with unusual characteristics in peak and trough levels. Thus, on selected days, we quantitated the serum CsA levels on blood samples drawn every 2 hr in order to define the actual, rather than the assumed peaks and troughs.

RIA

Samples of peripheral venous blood were drawn for serum CsA level determinations. Reagents for the RIA (supplied by Sandoz, Ltd., Basel, Switzerland) consisted

From the Departments of Medicine and Surgery, Montefiore Medical Center–Albert Einstein College of Medicine, New York, NY.

Address reprint requests to Dr. S. L. Nehlsen-Cannarella, Transplantation Immunology, VCP 301, Montefiore Medical Center, 111 East 210th Street, New York, NY 10467.

0041-1345/83/1505-0048$01.00/0

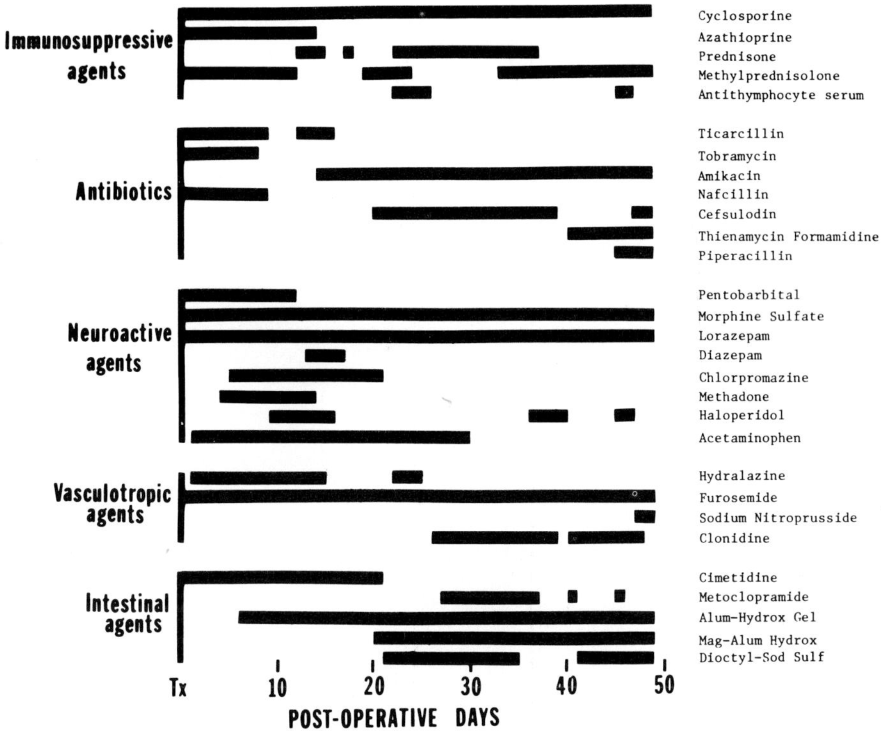

Fig. 1. Concurrent drug therapy used in treating paraquat-poisoned victim after receipt of a single lung allotransplant.

of (1) polyvalent antibody raised in New Zealand white rabbits against the hapten-protein conjugate of cyclosporine-C (threonyl) hemisuccinate coupled to free amino groups of guinea pig IgG, supplied at a titer of 2,000 in 0.15 *M* NaCl solution containing 1% dextran and 0.2% sodium azide and cross-reacting with some metabolites and CsC, (2) ^{3}H-dihydrocyclosporin A, and (3) standard reference material (cyclosporine-A). In addition, we used normal human serum (Normlcera, Medical Specialties Laboratory, Inc.), TRIS (Trizma-8.5, Sigma Chemical Co., St. Louis, MO) buffer A (0.05 *M*, pH 8.5 at 25°C), buffer B (buffer A with 0.03% Tween 20 added) used to dilute reagents and sera, and serum-coated charcoal (Sigma Chemical Co.) for separating free from bound antigen (1% solution with 0.5% serum).

Reaction mixtures were made by adding 100 μl diluted (1:20) serum (known standards, controls, or patient "unknown" samples) and 100 μl of ^{3}H-CsA to 500 μl buffer B, then adding 100 μl antibody, mixing, and incubating at 25°C for 60 min. After cooling the reaction mixtures in an ice bath for 10 min, 500 μl of cold charcoal solution was added to each tube and incubated on ice for another 10 min. The mixtures were centrifuged to sediment the charcoal and absorbed antigen. Each supernatant was decanted into 10-ml aqueous scintillation fluid (Scinti Verse I, Fisher Scientific Co., Pittsburgh, PA) and radioactivity levels determined on a Packard 3255 liquid scintillation counter (Packard Instrument Co., Inc., Downers Grove, IL). All samples were tested in triplicate. The daily standard curve, made by adding reference material to normal serum, allowed determinations of patient serum values between 25 and 2,000 ng/ml. We used controls of 250 and 1,000 ng/ml, and one or more of 11 predetermined patient sera, all of which were provided by the laboratory of Dr. Wong, Toronto General Hospital. The controls were from the quality control program of the Canadian Cyclosporine clinical trials (originating in London, Ontario). The "turn-around-time" using this assay is about 3–3.5 hr, and therefore, we assumed trough time points of 21 hr to allow time for the assay to be completed before giving the next CsA dose.

Linearization of the nonlinear standard curve was made by logit-log transformation of the raw data.[6,7] The percentage of ^{3}H-CsA not bound to charcoal in the absence of antibody was about 4%, and the ratio of bound to total activity in the presence of antiserum was 48%.

RESULTS

Radioimmunoassay

Daily CsA serum levels determined on samples taken at assumed peak (mean, 3 hr) and

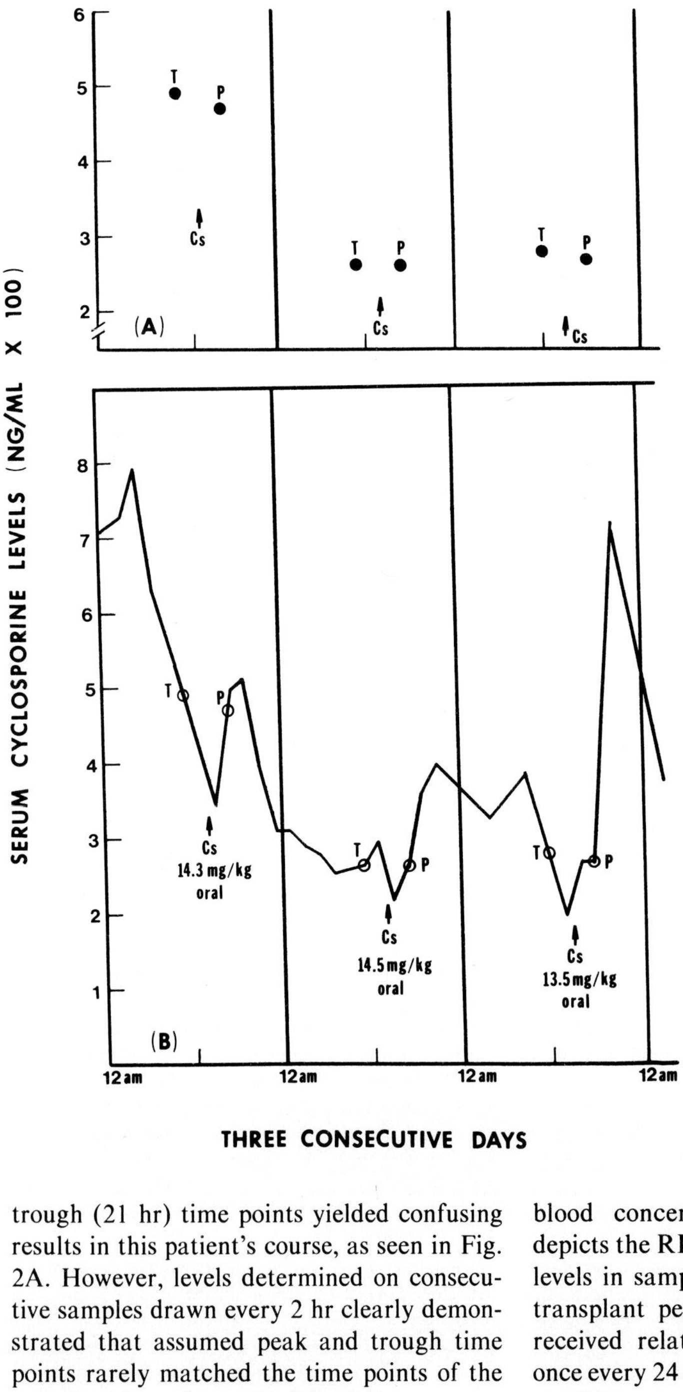

Fig. 2. Demonstration of difficulty encountered in interpreting CsA serum levels of "assumed" peak and trough time points (A) versus interpreting the information derived from testing samples obtained at frequent intervals (B).

trough (21 hr) time points yielded confusing results in this patient's course, as seen in Fig. 2A. However, levels determined on consecutive samples drawn every 2 hr clearly demonstrated that assumed peak and trough time points rarely matched the time points of the actual peaks and troughs (Fig. 2B).

Frequent monitoring of blood levels further demonstrated the lack of correlation between the dose of CsA administered and the actual blood concentrations achieved. Figure 3 depicts the RIA determinations of serum CsA levels in samples taken throughout the posttransplant period, during which the patient received relatively consistent doses of CsA once every 24 hr. On some occasions, only very small increments in blood levels were achieved (small peak-to-trough ratios); on other days, we found the expected peak-to-trough ratio (>3.0).

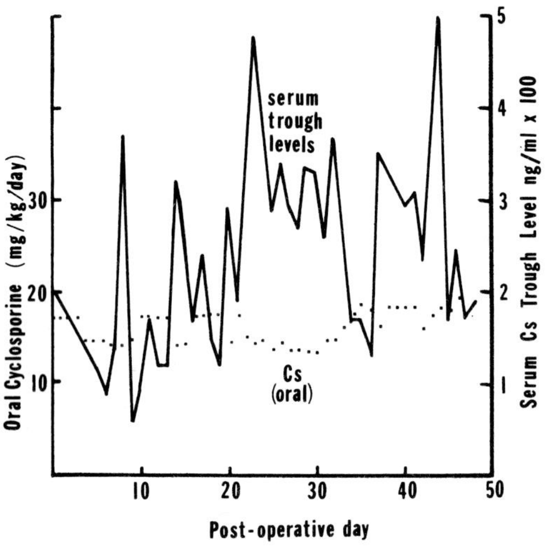

Fig. 3. Lack of correlation of serum CsA trough levels (determined by RIA) with dosage of orally administered cyclosporine.

Finally, at the end of the patient's course, low nonfluctuating CsA serum levels were observed, in spite of giving in excess of 15 mg/kg/day CsA by oral administration. Thus, for two days (postoperative days 48 and 49), CsA was given intravenously and blood levels were monitored every 2 hr. On day 48, the first intravenous dose of 315 mg was given over a period of 8 hr, and 7 hr later, 385 mg were given over another 6-hr period. A peak serum value of 750 ng/ml was achieved in the seventh hour during the first administration and 1242 ng/ml 2 hr after the second administration was completed (Fig. 4). During both of these intravenous administrations, urine output temporarily stopped and only returned 4 hr after cessation of the intravenous CsA infusion.

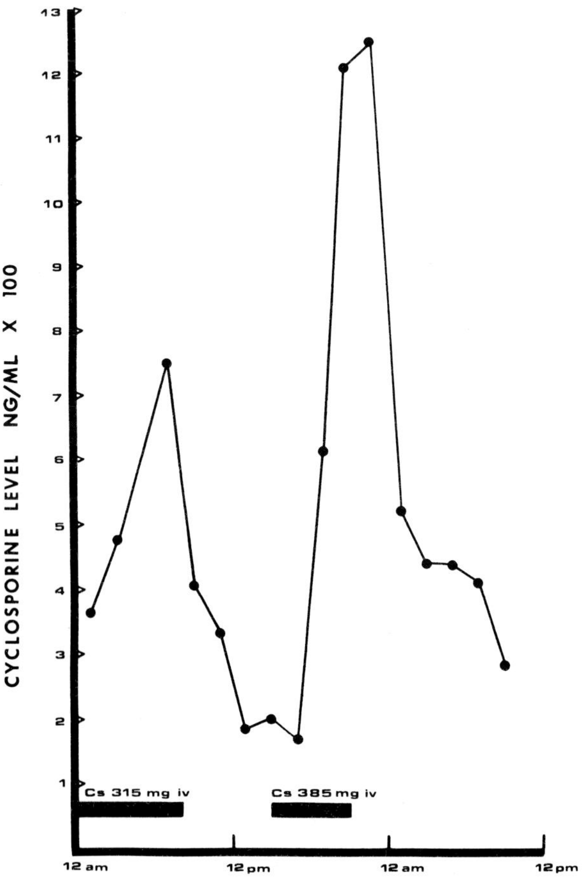

Fig. 4. Serum CsA levels obtained by administering CsA intravenously.

CsA Effects on Lung Allograft

Four episodes of lung allograft rejection occurred on posttransplant days 9, 19, 33, and 45. These were characterized by the presence of infiltrates in the transplanted lung, as seen on plain chest roentgenogram, increased pulmonary artery pressures, decreased arterial oxygen tension, and increased numbers of polymorphonuclear leukocytes on sputum gram stain without evidence of change in bacterial flora. All of these rejection phenomena improved rapidly following treatment with high-dose intravenous methylprednisolone (Fig. 1) and, on two occasions (the second and fourth rejection episodes), with concomitantly administered equine antibody to human thymocytes (ATGAM, University of Minnesota).

Concomitant Drug Therapy

Figure 1 shows the immunosuppressive agents, antibiotics, neuroactive and vasculotropic drugs, and gastrointestinal agents with which the patient was treated at various times during the posttransplant period. Throughout the 49 days that the patient survived following left lung transplantation, renal and liver functions were closely and carefully monitored. Figure 5 shows the results of daily single-channel serum creatinine measurements plotted with cyclosporine trough levels. Despite periodic increases in CsA trough levels, no evidence of renal toxicity possibly due to CsA or other drugs was ever noted.

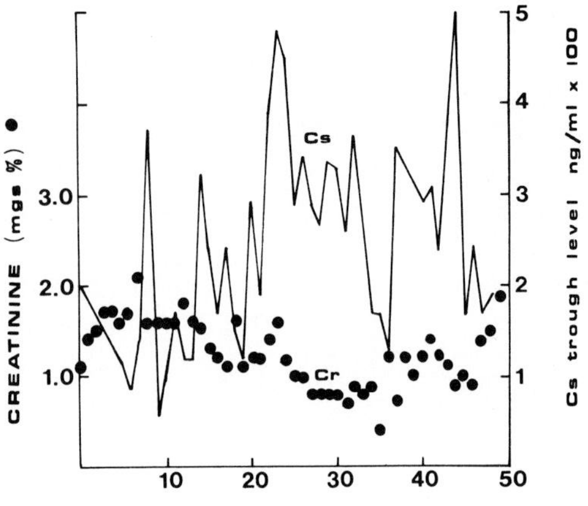

Fig. 5. Serum CsA trough levels plotted with concurrent daily serum creatinine levels. This patient had no apparent nephrotoxicity.

Figure 6 is a plot of CsA trough levels with daily liver function studies, including determinations of total bilirubin (Fig. 6A), alkaline phosphatase (Fig. 6B), serum glutamic oxalacetic transaminase (SGOT) (Fig. 6C), and serum glutamic pyruvic transaminase (SGPT) (Fig. 6D). Established liver function abnormalities were present prior to transplantation and, in the posttransplant period, this patient never exhibited normal (0.2–1.1 mg/dl) levels of total bilirubin. Alkaline phosphatase levels remained 1.5–2 times normal (10–115 IU/liter) and 2–5-fold elevations of both SGOT and SGPT (normal 5–40 IU/liter) persisted throughout most of the posttransplant period.

CsA Pharmacokinetics

The relatively low serum concentrations of CsA, taken together with the fact that our patient was receiving several barbiturates and corticosteroids, prompted us to suspect that increased hepatic catabolism of CsA may have occurred. Thus, using the serum CsA concentrations of the two hourly samples drawn throughout the two days of intravenous CsA administration, we attempted the calculation of the half-life of CsA. We found it to be approximately 2 hr on postoperative days 48 and 49, consistent with that found in dogs and humans.[9]

DISCUSSION

CsA immunosuppression has been used in a variety of clinical organ transplant systems, resulting in disagreement concerning the importance of CsA serum levels in the management of specific organ graft recipients. Thus, there is no consensus as to the appropriate CsA trough level denoting "adequate" immunosuppression. We have, however, noted a pattern of decreased trough levels, antedating clinically apparent episodes of rejection in this single lung transplant recipient. Despite our efforts to adjust the daily dose of CsA

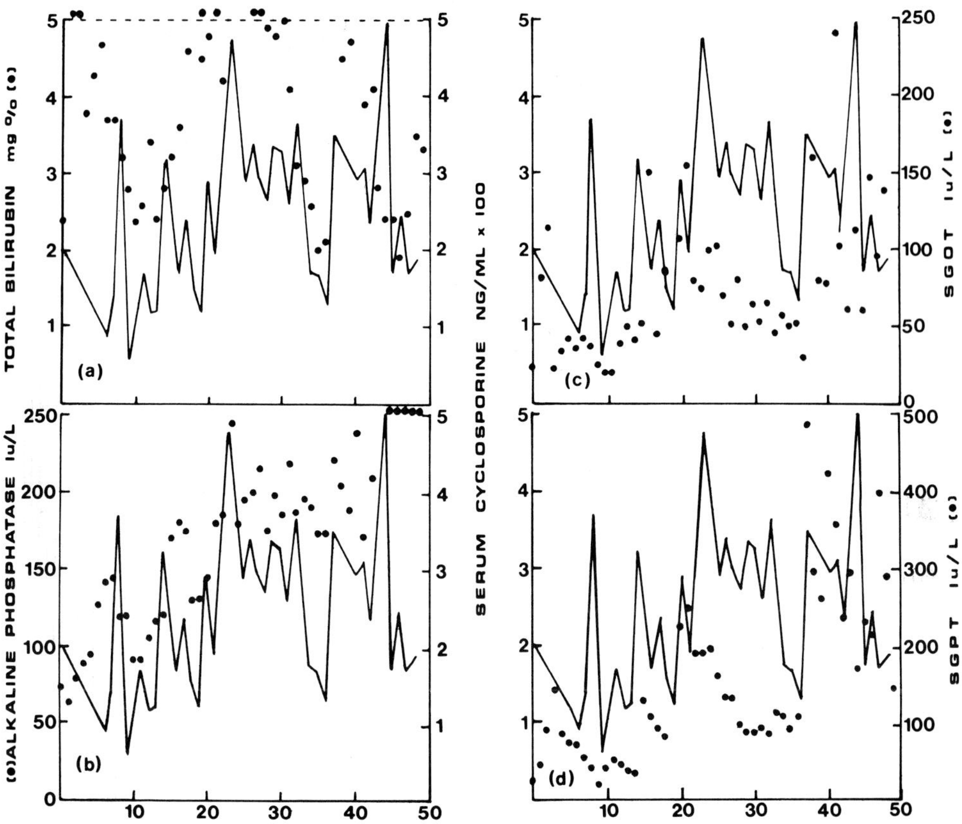

Fig. 6. Daily liver function tests plotted with daily serum CsA trough levels, indicating hepatotoxicity.

based on the availability of morning trough levels, it was still not possible to predictably achieve trough levels ≥200 ng/ml. Possible explanations for this include the following factors.

(1) Variable gastrointestinal absorption of CsA was undoubtedly related to frequently recurring episodes of small bowel ileus. These variations in intestinal motility could be attributed to concomitant drug therapy, especially with narcotic analgesics, barbiturates, antacids, and benzodiazepenes. Fluctuations in intrathoracic pressure resulting from continuous, mechanically assisted ventilation[8] may also inhibit gastrointestinal motility and delay drug absorption.

(2) Increased hepatic catabolism of CsA may have occurred as a result of induction of hepatic microsomal enzyme systems by barbiturates, corticosteroids, or persistent systemic infection, but our calculations of the half-life of CsA seem to indicate that this was not the case.[9]

(3) Protein binding to endogenous plasma protein, administered blood products, or equine antithymocyte globulin could account, in part, for variably decreased CsA levels.

(4) Increased renal clearance of CsA may have occurred on certain occasions, as a result of increased crystaloid administration, diuretic or cardiotonic drug therapy.

(5) Although a potential mechanism involved in alteration of CsA levels, it is unlikely that high renal tubular concentrations of nonreabsorbable anions (the semisynthetic penicillin antibiotics) had a significant effect on CsA excretion, since CsA is a nonpolar drug.

Renal toxicity was not seen in our patient throughout his course, but hepatotoxicity was apparent. However, it remains unclear as to whether the toxicity seen was a result of damage from the paraquat ingestion, CsA accumulation, or both. Kahan[7] has pointed out that low peak-to-trough ratios (less than 3.0) are associated with drug accumulation and toxic manifestations, in particular, elevated bilirubin and transaminases. We saw similar elevations and, additionally elevated alkaline phosphatases. In a patient treated for more than one year, and who may have ingested overdoses of CsA, it was shown that the liver was the organ containing the highest concentration of CsA, more than twofold the level found in circulation.[7] Consequently, we suspect that hepatotoxicity in our patient was probably the result, initially, of paraquat poisoning, compounded later by CsA accumulation and/or injury induced by some of the other drugs used in this case.

Peak and trough level monitoring was improved when samples were drawn at frequent intervals, but it was not possible to use the information in a meaningful way in this case, because the serum levels did not correlate with the dose administered. This phenomenon does not seem to be unique to our patient; it has been reported to occur in renal allograft recipients as well.[7]

In summary, we feel that blood levels of CsA cannot be used to indicate subsequent CsA dosage. However, peak to trough ratios may be helpful in indicating drug accumulation.

SUMMARY

Cyclosporine was administered orally every 24 hr to a paraquat poisoning victim who had a unilateral lung transplant. In the first week, blood samples were obtained 2–5 hr (peak) and 20–22 hr (trough) after administration. Daily CsA dosage was based on serum creatinine, the last CsA dose, and peak and trough serum CsA levels (RIA). However, on several days, the peak and trough values were not spread apart as expected, but they approached each other closely and even inverted. Periods of intestinal dysfunction correlated with these unusual characteristics in peak and trough levels. The 2–5-hr samples were not always at the peak but rather on the upswing of the peak, and the 20–22-hr samples were at points located at various places on the downswing, sometimes higher, other times lower, than the 5-hr values. These findings indicate that CsA absorption rates can vary significantly from day to day in sick patients during the critical time of the immediate postoperative period.

ACKNOWLEDGMENT

The authors thank Martin Lesser, Tonida Lindsay, and Abe Edelman for their expert assistance in computer programming, radioimmunoassay, and statistical analysis.

REFERENCES

1. Borel JF: In White DJG (ed): Cyclosporin A. Amsterdam, Elsevier Biomedical, 1982, pp 5–17

2. Beveridge T: In White DJG (ed): Cyclosporin A. Amsterdam, Elsevier Biomedical, 1982, pp 61–64

3. Veith FJ, Norin AJ, Montefusco CM, et al: Transplantation 32:474, 1981

4. Ryffel B: In White DJG (ed): Cyclosporin A. Amsterdam, Elsevier Biomedical, 1982, pp 45–75

5. Kamholz SL, Veith FJ, Mollenkopf F, et al: NY State J Med (in press)

6. Finney DJ: Statistical Methods in Biological Assay. London, Griffin, 1971

7. Kahan BD, van Buren CT, Lin SN, et al: Transplantation 34:36, 1982

8. Johnson EE, Hedley-Whyte J: J Appl Physiol 39:937, 1975

9. Beveridge T: In White DJG (ed): Cyclosporin A. Amsterdam, Elsevier Biomedical, 1982, pp 33–44

CLINICAL TRANSPLANTATION

KIDNEY TRANSPLANTATION

The Colorado-Pittsburgh Cadaveric Renal Transplantation Study with Cyclosporine

T. E. Starzl, T. R. Hakala, J. T. Rosenthal, S. Iwatsuki, and B. W. Shaw, Jr.

OUR EXPERIENCE with cyclosporine for cadaveric renal transplantation began in late 1979. An article by Calne et al.[1] had just been published that gave critics of our trial a lot of ammunition. Although the pathfinding report by Calne and his associates contained the good news that rejection of some cadaveric kidneys had been avoided with no drug other than cyclosporine, the bad news was that there had been a high patient mortality in these Cambridge trials, that none of the kidneys was providing normal function, and that nearly 10% of the recipients had developed lymphomas.[1]

MATERIALS AND METHODS

In spite of these warning signs, a large-scale clinical trial of cadaveric renal transplantation was mounted; this is now 3½ years old (Table 1). Sixty-six patients were treated at the University of Colorado in a non-randomized trial between December 1979 and September 1980. This was a learning period in which it was realized that cyclosporine should be used with steroids for optimum efficiency.[2] However the exact formula for the prednisone interaction with cyclosporine had not yet been worked out. In addition, the dose manipulation of cyclosporine that was frequently necessitated by the nephrotoxicity of this drug had not yet been clarified. These subtleties of management were described later[3,4] and were applied in the Pittsburgh series.

RESULTS

Phase I (1979–1980)

The results in the Colorado trials were surprisingly good in spite of a learning curve effect (Table 2). Almost 80% of the primary cadaveric grafts were still functioning at the end of 1 year, as well as 60% of the cadaveric kidneys used for retransplantation.

The 1-year results have held up well. Now, with a median follow-up of about 3 years, 68.4% of the primary grafts and half of the grafts used for retransplantation are still providing satisfactory function. The 3-year patient mortality in the trial has been 21.2%.

Phase II (1981)

The most important part of the study encompassed the calendar year 1981, during which, at the University of Pittsburgh, 65 cadaveric kidneys were transplanted to 64 patients (Table 3). Thirty-eight of the patients were primary graft recipients under cyclosporine-steroid therapy. The other 26 were undergoing retransplantation after one

---

From the Department of Surgery, University of Pittsburgh, Pittsburgh, PA.

Supported by research grants from the Veterans Administration, by Project Grant AM 29961 from the National Institutes of Health, and by Grant RR 00084 from the General Clinical Research Centers Program of the Division of Research Resources, National Institutes of Health.

Reprint requests should be addressed to T. E. Starzl, 3601 Fifth Avenue, Room 103, Falk Clinic, Pittsburgh, PA 15213.

0041-1345/83/1505-0049$01.00/0

The specter of lymphoma production with cyclosporine has been all but replaced with a comfortable understanding that most of the lesions grouped under this frightening classification are not true lymphomas as Rosenthal and others describe. The term *pseudo lymphoma* used by Iwatsuki et al. for such lymphoproliferative lesions may be an appropriate one.[7]

The good results obtained both in Denver and in Pittsburgh were without the kind of systematic recipient transfusion that has become so popular among nephrologists and without the kind of good tissue matching that at one time was envisioned as an important condition for successful cadaveric transplantation. The ways in which all of the observations made over the last several years could alter the so-called strategy of transplantation has been speculated upon elsewhere.[5] Because of the outstanding results obtained with cadaveric transplantation, the use of living donors has lost much of its attractiveness. The importance of tissue matching at the A, B, and D loci will be reduced. Since cyclosporine cannot prevent hyperacute rejection, the importance of accurately identifying preformed antidonor T-warm antibodies will be increased. As a corollary, it will become increasingly important to avoid sensitization of potential kidney recipients by deliberate transfusion. Because it has been so much easier to treat diabetics with the low steroid doses that are needed with cyclosporine, these patients have become more attractive candidates for cadaveric organs. Other patients of marginal candidacy will be more freely admitted to transplant waiting lists. The fact that the organ supply will become critical is quite obvious.

SUMMARY

The immunosuppression provided with cyclosporine and steroids has greatly increased the effectiveness of cadaveric kidney transplantation both in patients receiving their first kidneys and in those undergoing retransplantation.

REFERENCES

1. Calne RY, Rolles K, White DJG, et al: Lancet 2:1033, 1979
2. Starzl TE, Weil R III, Iwatsuki S, et al: Surg Gynecol Obstet 151:17, 1980
3. Starzl TE, Klintmalm GBG, Iwatsuki S, et al: Surg Gynecol Obstet 153:486, 1981
4. Starzl TE, Hakala TR, Rosenthal JT, et al: Surg Gynecol Obstet 154:819, 1982
5. Rosenthal JT, Hakala TR, Iwatsuki S, et al: Surg Gynecol Obstet 157:309, 1983
6. Calne RY, White DJG, Evans DB, et al: Br Med J 282:934, 1981
7. Iwatsuki S, Geis WP, Molnar Z, et al: J Surg Res 24:428, 1978

Comparison of Cyclosporine Versus Azathioprine-Antilymphocyte Globulin in Renal Transplantation

J. S. Najarian, M. Strand, D. S. Fryd, R. M. Ferguson, R. L. Simmons, N. L. Ascher, and D. E. R. Sutherland

ADULT SPLENECTOMIZED, transfused, uremic recipients of renal allografts, from cadaver or HLA-nonidentical related donors, have been randomized to one of two immunosuppressive regimens at the University of Minnesota since September 1980.[1] One group of patients received cyclosporine (CsA) and a relatively low dose of prednisone, while the other group received azathioprine (Aza) and a relatively high dose of prednisone plus antilymphocyte globulin (ALG) in the immediate post-transplant period. The preliminary results obtained in the patients entered into the trial as of April 1, 1983, are summarized here.

MATERIALS AND METHODS

Patient Population

Between September 1, 1980, and April 1, 1983, 182 patients were randomized. Prior to randomization, the patients were stratified according to donor source (cadaver or relative), presence or absence of diabetes, and number of previous transplants (in the retransplant group, only patients whose previous grafts had functioned over 1 year were included in the trial). All patients had been splenectomized and had received transfusions from up to five unrelated donors at least 1 month prior to transplantation. Ninety-two patients were randomized to the CsA group (53 cadaver, 39 related donors; 52 diabetic, 40 nondiabetic recipients, 84 primary and 8 retransplants), and 90 to the Aza group (57 cadaver, 33 related; 49 diabetic, 41 nondiabetic; 83 primary and 7 retransplants). At the time of the analysis, the mean follow-up in patients with functioning grafts was 14.6 ± 8.8 months in the CsA group and 16.7 ± 10.0 months in the Aza group.

Cyclosporine Treatment

CsA was given orally in a dose of 14 mg/kg prior to transplantation and daily for the first post-transplant week. Thereafter the dose was adjusted to ≤ 12 mg/kg/day according to trough blood levels determined by high-pressure liquid chromatography[2] and serum creatinine levels. We attempted to keep CsA levels between 100–200 ng/ml and serum creatinine < 2 mg/dl, but this objective was not always achieved. Mean (± SD) CsA dose in the recipients with functioning grafts at 1 year after transplantation was 6.3 ± 3.6 mg/kg/day. Prednisone was tapered from an initial dose of 2 mg/kg to 0.2 mg/kg/day by 1 year. Patients with elevations in serum creatinine interpreted as rejection, on the basis of biopsy or clinical course, were treated with 500 mg of methylprednisolone intravenously for 3 days or with an increase in prednisone to 2 mg/kg followed by a rapid taper to their maintenance dose.

Azathioprine Treatment

Aza was given in a dose of 5 mg/kg preoperatively and tapered to ≤ 2.5 mg/kg/day by 1 week. Prednisone dose was 2 mg/kg/day for 3 days, tapered to 0.3 mg/kg/day by 1 year. ALG (30 mg/kg/day) was administered intravenously for a total of 14 doses during the immediate posttransplant period.

Analysis of Results

Patient and graft survival rates were calculated by actuarial techniques. Graft loss was defined as either return to dialysis or death with a functioning graft. All causes of graft loss were included in the analysis, as were all deaths, even those that occurred years after graft loss and return to dialysis. Two grafts in the CsA group and 5 grafts in the Aza group failed for technical reasons, but they were not excluded from the analysis. Seventeen of the recipients in the CsA group were switched to treatment with Aza between 1 and 25 months (mean 7.5 ± 6.1 months) after transplantation (12 for nephrotoxicity, 3 for severe rejection, 1 for prolonged acute tubular necrosis, and 1 for severe thrombocytosis); these patients were included in the CsA group for statistical analysis, and 13 had functioning grafts at the time of the analysis. In the Aza group, 1 patient was switched to cyclophosphamide because of liver dysfunction (graft functioning), and 2 were switched to CsA (1 to reduce the prednisone dose

---

From the Department of Surgery, University of Minnesota Health Sciences Center, Minneapolis, MN.

Supported by NIH Grant AM 13083.

Reprint requests should be addressed to D. E. R. Sutherland, Box 280, Mayo Memorial Building, University of Minnesota, Minneapolis, MN 55455.

0041–1345/83/1505–0050$01.00/0

because of a myocardial infarct and the other because of an allergy to ALG); these patients remained in the Aza group for statistical analysis (1 has since lost graft function). Besides patient and graft survival rates, the incidence of rejection episodes, acute tubular necrosis, infections, adverse drug reactions, and hospital readmissions were determined in the CsA and Aza groups. Mean values are given with standard deviations.

RESULTS

Patient and Graft Survival Rates

The actuarial patient and renal allograft functional survival rates up to 26 months after transplantation in all CsA- and Aza-treated recipients are given in Fig. 1. At 1 year, 92% of the CsA patients and 95% of the Aza patients were alive, and 87% of the CsA patients and 80% of the Aza patients had functioning grafts. The actuarial patient survival and renal allograft functional survival rates at 1 year in the subgroups of diabetic and nondiabetic recipients of grafts from a cadaver or related donors are summarized in Table 1. None of the differences between the CsA- or Aza-treated recipients, overall or in the subgroups, is statistically significant (all p values > 0.1).

Incidence of Acute Tubular Necrosis (ATN)

In recipients of technically successful cadaveric grafts, 13 of 51 treated with CsA (25%) and 12 of 54 treated with Aza (22%) required dialysis for uremia in the immediate posttransplant period (2 CsA- and 3 Aza-treated patients lost cadaveric grafts for technical reasons and are not included in these calculations). The mean number of dialyses required before satisfactory renal function began was 7.3 ± 9.4 in the CsA group and 3.8 ± 1.4 in the Aza group ($p > 0.05$). The mean number of days from transplant to the last dialysis were 19.9 ± 24.1 days in the CsA group and 10.7 ± 3.3 in the Aza group ($p < 0.05$). Mean serum creatinine (mg/dl) at discharge was 3.1 ± 2.2 in the CsA group and 2.8 ± 1.9 in the Aza group. Two cadaveric grafts in the Aza group (3.8%) never functioned (rejected before ATN resolved), while all cadaveric grafts undergoing ATN in the CsA group eventually functioned.

Two of 39 CsA-treated (5.1%) and 1 of 31 Aza-treated recipients (3.2%) of technically successful grafts from living related donors (two related grafts in the Aza group were lost for technical reasons) required dialysis in the immediate posttransplant period. The Aza-treated recipient required only one dialysis. One of the CsA-treated recipients required seven dialyses; the graft in the other CsA-treated patient never functioned and was removed 1 month after transplantation.

Incidence of Rejection Episodes

The cumulative percentage of renal allograft recipients treated for rejection in the CsA and the Aza groups are shown in Fig. 2. Rejection was diagnosed when there was an increase in the serum creatinine (that did not decline following reduction of CsA dose in the

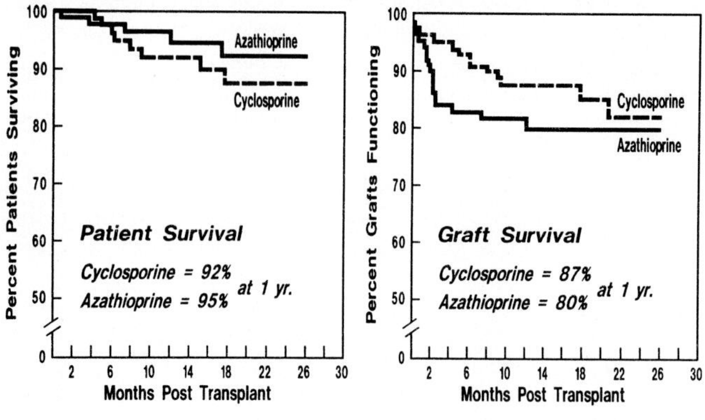

Fig. 1. Patient survival and renal allograft functional survival rates in all cycloporine- ($N = 92$) and azathioprine- ($N = 90$) treated recipients in the Minnesota randomized trial.

Table 1. Actuarial Analysis of Results of Renal Transplantation in Subgroups Randomized to Cyclosporine (CsA) of Azathioprine (Aza) at the University of Minnesota Between September 1, 1980, and April 1, 1983.

Donor	1-Year Survival Rates					
	Diabetic (*N*)		Nondiabetic (*N*)		All Recipients (*N*)	
Source	CsA	Aza	CsA	Aza	CsA	Aza
Graft						
Cadaveric	84% (30)	67% (30)	81% (23)	85% (27)	83% (53)	76% (57)
Relative	88% (22)	94% (19)	100% (17)	77% (14)	94% (39)	87% (33)
All sources	86% (52)	77% (49)	89% (40)	82% (41)	87% (92)	80% (90)
Patient						
Cadaveric	84% (30)	91% (30)	95% (23)	96% (27)	89% (53)	94% (57)
Relative	92% (22)	94% (19)	100% (17)	100% (14)	96% (39)	97% (33)
All sources	87% (52)	92% (49)	97% (40)	97% (41)	92% (92)	95% (90)

CsA group) and was usually confirmed by biopsy, using the histologic criteria of Sibley et al.[3] to differentiate rejection from CsA toxicity in the CsA group. During a follow-up period of 1–32 months, 28 of 92 CsA patients (31%) and 51 of 190 Aza patients (58%) were treated for rejection. The mean interval between transplantation and the first treatment for rejection was 94 ± 141 days for the CsA group of patients and 62 ± 70 days for the Aza group. Of the patients treated for a first rejection episode, 6 of 28 in the CsA group (21%) and 13 of 51 Aza group (25%) were treated a second time. No CsA patients have been treated for more than two rejection episodes, but 3 of the 13 Aza patients treated for a second rejection were treated for a third, and in turn, 1 of the 3 treated for a third rejection episode was treated for a fourth. Chronic or irreversible rejection has occurred in 9 of 92 CsA patients (10%) and 11 of 98 Aza patients (12%) during the 1–32 months they have been at risk.

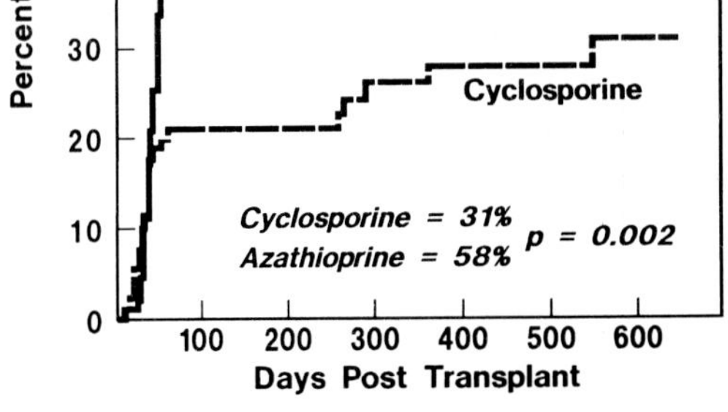

Fig. 2. Cumulative percentage of renal allograft recipients undergoing treatment for a first rejection episode in Minnesota randomized trial of cyclosporine ($N = 92$) vs. azathioprine ($N = 90$) for immunosuppression.

Comparison of Renal Function

The mean serum creatinine levels (mg/dl) at 3, 6, 12, and 24 months were 2.0 ± 0.6 ($N = 78$), 2.0 ± 0.7 ($N = 69$), 2.2 ± 0.8 ($N = 47$) and 2.0 ± 0.6 ($N = 16$) in the CsA group and 1.5 ± 0.4 ($N = 69$), 1.7 ± 0.8 ($N = 66$), 1.5 ± 0.4 ($N = 49$), and 1.4 ± 0.4 ($N = 13$) in the Aza group ($p < 0.05$ at all time points for CsA vs. Aza).

Table 2. Incidence of All Infections in Renal Allograft Recipients Randomized to Cyclosporine ($N = 92$) vs. Azathioprine ($N = 90$) in the Minnesota Randomized Trial

	No. Patients*		No. Infections	
Type	CsA	Aza	CsA	Aza
Viral	16	50	22	57
Bacterial	15	22	22	30
Fungal	11	7	16	10
Mycoplasma	1	4	1	4
Total	43 (47%)	54 (60%)	60	101

*Two patients in each group died from infections, one from CMV and one from aspergillus in the CsA group, and both from CMV in the Aza group.

Incidence of Infections

The incidence of all types of infections in the CsA and Aza groups during the 1–32 months of follow-up are summarized in Table 2. There were significantly more viral infections in the Aza group ($p < 0.05$), primarily cytomegalovirus (CMV) (Table 3), but other viral infections occurred in 12/92 (13%) CsA-treated patients (7 H. simplex, 2 H. zoster, 1 hepatitis B, 2 hepatitis non-A, non-B) and 26/90 (29%) Aza-treated patients (16 H. simplex, 9 H. zoster, 1 EBV). Fifteen of 90 (16%) CsA patients developed bacterial infections (4 respiratory, 5 urinary, 1 wound, 12 miscellaneous), not significantly different from the 22/92 (24%) Aza patients who had bacterial infections (10 respiratory, 7 urinary, 3 blood, 1 wound, 9 miscellaneous). Positive cultures from at least one site were obtained in 5 CsA- and 19 Aza-treated patients during episodes of clinical infection. There also was not a significant difference in the overall incidence of fungal infections between the CsA (11 candida, 1 aspergillosis, 3 other) and Aza (7 candida, 2 aspergillosis, 3 other) groups, although *Candida esophagitis* was seen in 4 Aza- and no CsA-treated patients.

Adverse Reactions Possibly Attributable to Cyclosporine

Of the 92 CsA-treated patients followed 1–32 months, 26 had hypertension (28%), 24 had hyperuricemia (26%); and 23 had hyperkalemia (25%). Fifteen CsA-treated patients (16%) have had neurologic symptoms (5 with tremors, 3 with paresthesias, 3 with muscle weakness, 2 with temperature sensitivity, and 2 with seizures). An increase in serum bilirubin or glutamic oxaloacetic transaminase, indicating possible hepatic toxicity, occurred in seven patients (8%), and all improved after the dose of CsA was reduced. Five patients (5%) have complained of mild hirsutism. One patient (1%) was diagnosed to have a lymphoma at 17 months after transplantation; immunosuppression was stopped, acyclovir was administered, and all evidence of lymphoma has disappeared. The patient rejected the kidney 2 months after cessation of immunosuppression and is now on chronic maintenance hemodialysis, 2.7 years after the transplant and 15 months after the diagnosis of lymphoma.

Table 3. Incidence of CMV Infections and Syndromes in Minnesota Patients Randomized to Cyclosporine ($N = 92$) or Azathioprine ($N = 90$) for Immunosuppression

Site	No. Patients with Positive Culture*		No. Patients with Syndrome	
	CsA	Aza	CsA	Aza
Urine	5	10	2	7
Blood	6	14	5	11
Throat	2	5	1	5
Bronchial	0	4	0	4
Retinitis	0	2	0	0
Ulcer	1	0	1	0
None†	–	–	1	4
Total	9 (9.8%)	18 (20.0%)	5 (5.4%)	24 (26.7%)

*Some patients had positive culture from more than one site.

†Syndrome only (seroconversion in one CsA and one Aza patient each).

Cyclosporine Nephrotoxicity

Of 92 CsA-treated patients, 68 (74%), followed for 1–32 months, have had creatinine levels > 2 mg/dl or acute elevations of serum creatinine levels that decreased when the CsA dose was reduced. Kidney biopsies were done in 28 instances, and histological features consistent with CsA nephrotoxicity without rejection were present in 26 of the specimens. Twelve patients were switched to Aza because serum creatinine remained elevated even after reduction of the CsA dose.

Conversion from Cyclosporine to Azathioprine

Of the 17 patients in the randomized trial who, for various reasons, were switched from CsA to Aza, 13 currently have functioning grafts, while 2 rejected the grafts (1 subsequently died) and 2 died with functioning grafts. The mean serum creatinine at the time of conversion was 4.8 ± 2.3 mg/dl; the most recent creatinine in the 13 patients with functioning grafts is 3.4 ± 2.4 mg/dl (mean of 6.8 ± 7.0 months after conversion).

Hospitalization

The mean number of days the patients were initially hospitalized following transplantation was 15.3 ± 8.1 in the CsA group and 19.9 ± 10.6 days in the Aza group. During the 1–32-month period of follow-up, 85/92 (71%) CsA and 71/90 (79%) Aza patients have been readmitted (137 readmissions in the CsA group, 2.1/patient; 154 readmissions in the Aza group, 2.2/patient). The mean total hospitalization time for patients requiring readmission has been 21.0 ± 17.5 days in the CsA group and 31.1 ± 38.3 days in the Aza group. None of the differences is statistically significant.

DISCUSSION

This interim analysis of a randomized trial of CsA vs. Aza shows that the renal allograft survival rates are only slightly better (by 7% at 1 year) in CsA-prednisone- than in Aza-prednisone-ALG-treated renal allograft recipients ($p > 0.1$). Apart from patient and graft survival rates, three advantages and three disadvantages are associated with the use of CsA as opposed to Aza. The disadvantages include a longer duration of ATN if it occurs in CsA-treated patients (the incidence is similar in Aza-treated patients), higher creatinine levels at all times after transplantation, and more difficulty in managing hypertension and hyperkalemia. The advantages to the use of CsA include fewer viral and bacterial infections, shorter hospitalization times, and fewer rejection episodes than in Aza-treated patients.

Some groups have stated that the availability of CsA has diminished the advantage of using related donors for kidney transplantation.[4] We disagree. We included kidneys from both related and cadaver donors in our trial, and, in the CsA group, related donor kidneys had a better survival rate than cadaveric grafts (94% vs. 83% functioning at 1 year), the same relative difference that occurred in the Aza group (87% vs. 76%).

Table 4. Comparison of Graft Survival Rates in Two Prospective Randomized Trials of Cyclosporine vs. Azathioprine in Recipients of Renal Allografts from Cadaveric Donors

	1-Yr Graft Survival Rates	
	European*	Minnesota†
Azathioprine	53%	76%
Cyclosporine	73%	83%

*European trial: Prednisone added only for rejections in CsA patients; no Aza patients were splenectomized or received ALG.

†Minnesota trial: Used prednisone prophylactically in CsA patients, added splenectomy and ALG in Aza patients.

Our results also show that graft survival rates in patients treated with Aza are as good as those treated with CsA. In fact, our results with Aza-prednisone-ALG are equivalent to those achieved with CsA in the ongoing European randomized trial of CsA vs. conventional immunosuppression (Table 4). The fact that we are unable to show a significant difference in graft survival rates between the CsA and Aza groups, while there was a significant difference in the European trial,[5] probably reflects a difference in the adjunctive measures applied by our group, as opposed to the European groups, in Aza-treated recipients. Our Aza-treated patients were heavily transfused and splenectomized and received ALG, while such was not the case in the European trial. Thus, it was possible for the European trial to show an advantage for CsA because the conventional immunosuppressive regimen did not incorporate certain features that can maximize graft survival rates.

In conclusion, good patient and graft survival rates can be obtained by immunosuppression with either CsA-prednisone or Aza-prednisone-ALG in renal allograft recipients. The advantages and disadvantages of the regimens are different, but the therapeutic ratio is nearly the same. Further analysis will be necessary to determine which regimen is the most cost-effective and which is superior for long-term maintenance of renal allograft function.

REFERENCES

1. Ferguson RM, Rynasiewicz JJ, Sutherland DER, et al: Surgery 92:176, 1982

2. Sawchuk RJ, Cartier LO: Clin Chem 27:1368, 1981

3. Sibley RK, Ferguson RM, Sutherland DER, et al: Transplant Proc (this issue)

4. Starzl TE, Hakala TR, Iwatsuki S, et al: Surg Gynecol Obstet 154:819, 1982

5. Report on the European Multicentre Trial: Lancet 2:57, 1982

Cyclosporine Immunosuppression Mitigates Immunologic Risk Factors in Renal Allotransplantation

B. D. Kahan, C. T. Van Buren, S. M. Flechner, W. D. Payne, M. Boileau, and R. H. Kerman

EVALUATION OF A new pharmacologic agent demands trials in a setting wherein established clinical practice has yielded unsatisfactory results. Some renal allograft patients display poor graft survival apparently as a result of adverse immunologic factors, including (1) lack of previous blood transfusions,[1] (2) receipt of a totally DR-mismatched cadaveric (CAD)[2,3] or highly mixed lymphocyte culture (MLC)–stimulatory living related donor (LRD) allograft,[4] and (3) strong immune responsiveness as evidenced by performances in pretransplant in vitro and in vivo cellular assays.[5] Therefore, the studies presented here compared the outcome of allografts in recipients at immunologically high risk, who were immunosuppressed with either cyclosporine (CsA) or with azathioprine (Aza), combined with initial equal amounts of prednisone. The improved graft survival in the CsA therapy group appeared to be independent of the risk factors of immune responsiveness, prior blood transfusions, splenectomy, and/or HLA matching.

MATERIALS AND METHODS

Recipients

All patients referred for renal transplantation were subjected to a 5-day hospital evaluation searching for conditions posing absolute and/or relative contraindications to the procedure.[6] After referral, no patient was transfused with blood for the purpose of immunologic conditioning. The prior transfusion history of each recipient was verified by formal inquiry to the referral dialysis unit and to previous hospital sites of admissions, as well as their servicing blood banks. Generally, packed red blood cells without leukocyte depletion by washing or freezing were used for transfusions; rarely had patients received whole blood. Of the patient population treated with CsA, 27% were not transfused and 60% received less than 5 units.

Determination of immune responder status was performed as previously described.[5] A "strong responder" end-stage renal-failure patient displayed at least two of the properties: > 33% active T cells enumerated by rosette formation with sheep erythrocytes, > 12,500 counts per min ^{3}H-thymidine (cpm-^{3}H) uptake of whole blood in the spontaneous blastogenesis assay, > 10-fold proliferation index (cpm-^{3}H) when confronted with a panel of five unrelated donors' lymphocytes compared to his own cells as stimulators, and cutaneous delayed-type hypersensitivity responses to more than one of the recall antigens—purified protein derivative of *Mycobacterium tuberculosis*, trichophytin O, trichophytin M, and/or mumps. The immune responsiveness status correlated with OKT4/OKT8 (Ortho-mune Reagents, Ortho Diagnostics Inc., Raritan, NJ) ratios measured on the Spectrum III flow cytometer. Normal individuals displayed 42 ± 8% OKT4$^+$ and 26 ± 7% OKT8$^+$ for a ratio of 1.9 ± 0.5 (mean ± 1 SD). The lower value of the 95% confidence limits spanning 2 SD was 26% OKT4$^+$, 12% OKT8$^+$, and T4/T8 = 0.9. Of the patients partitioned as strong responders and examined pretransplant with OKT reagents, 42/44 (96%) displayed T4:T8 ratios greater than 2 SD above normal (> 1.9) compared to 18% of weak responders ($p < 0.01$). On the other hand, 7/11 (64%) of patients profiled as weak responders had OKT8$^+$ cells > 12% and T4:T8 ratios < 0.9 ($p < 0.05$). Immune responder status did not correlate with cytotoxic panel reactive antibody, probably because most patients had received fewer than five transfusions and had not therefore been adequately stimulated to produce antibody.

Patients were not routinely splenectomized: 22% of the CsA group had had their spleen removed either in the distant past or because of white blood cell counts less than 3000/mm^3 at the time of evaluation. Patients were not routinely nephrectomized; 34% of the CsA group had undergone either unilateral or bilateral nephrectomy. While most patients had been nephrectomized in the distant past, a few underwent the procedure at the time of transplant evaluation, because of renin-dependent hypertension or recurrent, chronic pyelonephritis.

Cadaveric Donor (CAD) Transplantation

The procurement of cadaveric renal allografts by the en bloc technique, preservation methods, and renal trans-

---

From the Division of Immunology and Organ Transplantation, Department of Surgery, The University of Texas Medical School, Houston, TX.

Reprint requests should be addressed to B. D. Kahan, Ph.D., M.D., Division of Organ Transplantation, Department of Surgery, 6431 Fannin Street, Houston, TX 77030.

0041–1345/83/1505–0051$02.00/0

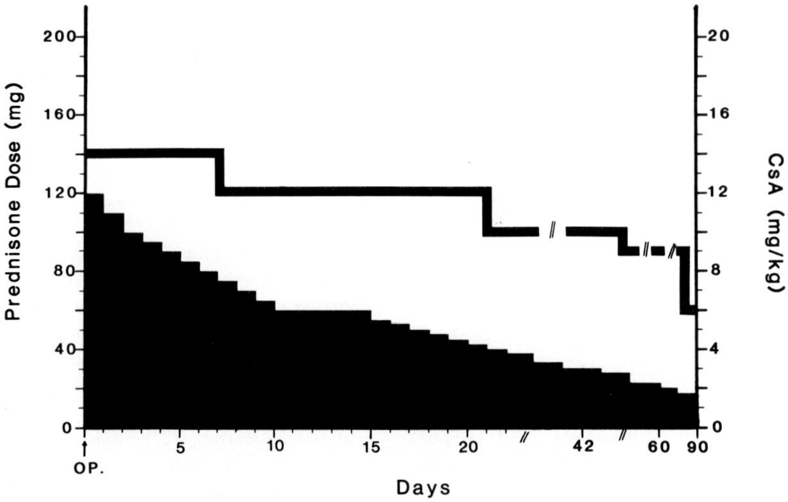

Fig. 1. The dosage taper regimen for CsA from 14 mg/kg to 6 mg/kg and prednisone from 120 mg to 25 mg in a 70-kg adult during the first 90 days after transplantation.

plant procedure have been presented previously.[6] HLA matching was used as a guide, but not a requisite, to transplantation. The only contraindication save for blood group incompatibility was a positive visual crossmatch.[7] The present report includes 100 CsA-treated cadaveric renal allografts in patients from age 8 to age 63 years, with a mean age of 37 years. The mean follow-up is 12 months. A randomized trial of the two immunosuppressive regimens for CAD transplantation was abandoned after 22 patients were accrued in the CsA arm and 19 in the Aza arm, because of the highly significant difference in outcome. There were no grafts lost to rejection in the former group. For the purposes of the data analysis herein, the 19 patients in the Aza arm were combined with the previous 92 consecutive patients treated with Aza-prednisone (Aza-P) using the same steroid regimen. This Aza-P group was compared with 100 consecutive CsA-treated cadaveric graft recipients. Although the study represents primarily a historical comparison of the outcome of the highest-risk patients between Aza and CsA groups, a common protocol was used longitudinally, and the last 25 Aza recipients overlapped the first 75 CsA patients. Graft survival was determined by the actuarial method. Since the mean follow-up (MFU) was at least 1 year, this time point was utilized for comparisons. Statistical significance was assessed by the Wilcoxon signed-rank sum test.

Living Related Donor (LRD) Transplantation

All living related potential donors underwent a 3-day evaluation[6] that included history, physical examination, psychosocial evaluation, laboratory studies, crossmatching, and digital subtraction angiography for vascular anatomy. Haploidentical LRDs were partitioned on the basis of the result of a pretransplant MLC reaction.[5] Donors whose irradiated lymphocytes evoked > 6.5-fold greater stimulation than the recipients' own cells were considered incompatible. The present report includes 50 living related renal allografts in patients from age 3 to age 56 years, with a mean age of 40 years and a mean followup of 12 months. The CsA group included 40 donors whose stimulation ratios ranged from 8–65. In addition, CsA was administered to another 10 recipients displaying stimulation ratios from 1.0–6.0 against their donors, who were considered compatible.

Treatment Regimen

The trial was performed substituting CsA for Aza. The CsA was furnished (Sandoz, Inc., East Hanover, NJ, through Dr. D. Winter) as an oral (100 mg/cc) suspension in castor oil, which, when administered, was diluted in either chocolate milk or fruit juice. The administered oral dose was 14 mg/kg preoperatively and for the first 7 days, 12 mg/kg for 14 days, then reduced to 10 mg/kg (Fig. 1). In addition, living related renal allograft recipients received oral CsA for at least 5 days preoperatively. Patients reached the maintenance dose of 6.0 ± 1.2 mg CsA daily by 90 days after transplant (Fig. 2). In addition, on the evening of and the morning after transplantation, CsA 2.5 mg/kg was infused intravenously slowly over 6 hr. CsA was otherwise used by the oral route only, except in cases of gastrointestinal catastrophies or documented poor gastrointestinal absorption.[8] Precise oral dosages were adjusted to fasting serum trough levels, as determined by the radioimmunoassay method,[9] using samples obtained 18 hr after drug administration. The presence of trough levels > 200 ng/ml or of nephrotoxic-

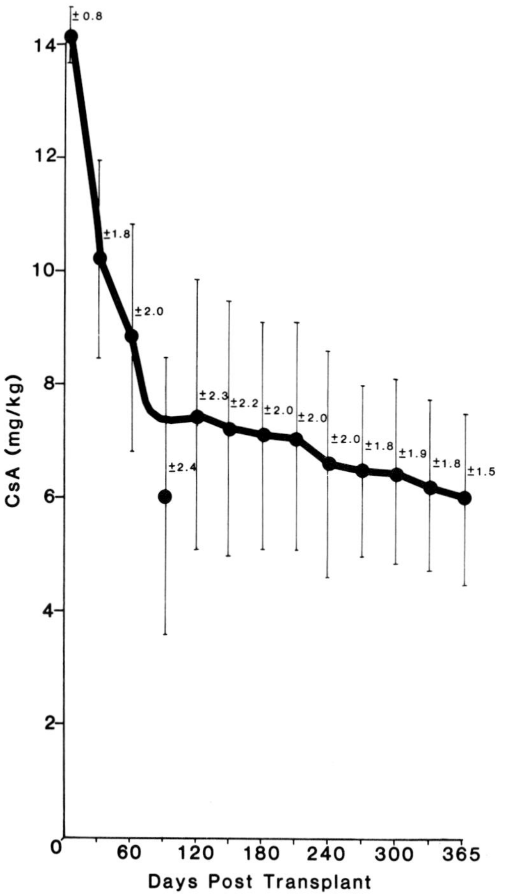

Fig. 2. Average observed CsA dose (with standard error of the mean) in 150 renal allograft recipients at serial times after transplantation.

ity demanded progressive dose reduction, which in some instances reached 3 mg/kg.

The Aza regimen has been previously reported:[6] After a loading dose of 5 mg/kg, the oral dosage is tapered to 2.5 mg/kg as tolerated, in order to avert severe myelosuppression. Antilymphocyte serum (ATGAM, Upjohn, Kalamazoo, MI) was not used in combination with Aza because at the inception of this study it was also an investigational drug.

The prednisone regimen was uniform for both groups: beginning at 120 mg/kg on the day of transplantation, tapering to 60 mg by day 10, 40 mg by day 21, 30 mg by day 42, and 25 mg by day 60 (Fig. 1). Although this regimen uses higher prednisone dosages in combination with CsA than other centers,[10,11] it not only allowed direct comparison between the immunosuppressive effects of Aza and CsA per se but also may have facilitated the use of lower CsA doses than in the other studies and thereby reduced drug-induced complications.

Rejection episodes were treated by three 8-hourly intravenous doses of 500 mg methylprednisolone, followed by increasing the oral prednisone to 3 mg/kg (usually 200 mg) for 1 day. The corticosteroids were promptly tapered to 1.5 mg/kg (100 mg) by day 5 and to 0.57 g/kg (40 mg) by day 11. The CsA dose was increased only during a rejection episode, if the trough serum level was below 100 ng/ml. Because only few patients experienced allograft rejection, the total cumulative steroid dose in the CsA group was less than half that required in the Aza group, in spite of the equal initial prednisone doses.

RESULTS

Overall Cadaveric Allograft Survival

The administration of CsA improved cadaveric graft survival from 51% in the Aza-P group to 81% in the CsA-prednisone (CsA-P) group ($p < 0.05$; Table 1). The mortality rate of 4% in the CsA group appeared to be improved, compared to 11% in the Aza group.

Outcome in Cadaveric Allograft Recipients Stratified by Immune Responder Status

Among the 111 patients treated with Aza, 75 recipients were strong and 36 weak immune responders. Figure 3 reveals that the immune responder status provided a significant index ($p < 0.001$) to predict graft outcome: Weak immune responders displayed 72% graft survival (MFU = 18.2 months), while strong responders displayed 39% function (MFU = 20 months). The mortality rate in both groups was 11%–12%.

The 100 recipients treated with CsA-P were partitioned as 75 strong and 25 weak immune responders. CsA conferred a definite advantage to the strong-responder recipients (Table 2), who displayed 80% 1-year graft survival ($p < 0.05$ versus the strong-responder Aza-P group). On the other hand, the weak-responder group experienced only slight

Table 1. Outcome of Cadaveric Renal Allografts in the Entire Group of Recipients Receiving Aza-P vs. CsA-P

Treatment	*N*	% Function*	% Mortality
Aza-P	111	51.0	11.0
CsA-P	100	81.0	4.0

*Actuarial 1-year graft survival.

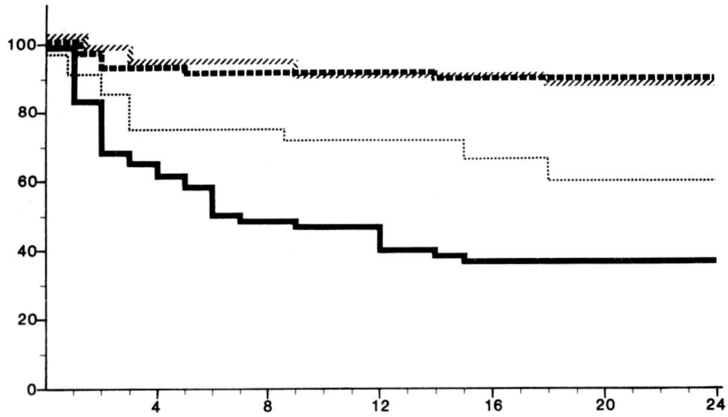

Fig. 3. Actuarial survival of grafts and patients who were partitioned as strong and weak responders before transplant.

benefit with 84% function (p = NS versus weak Aza group). The improved graft survival that presumably reflected more potent immunosuppression was not associated with an increased mortality rate. Both strong and weak immune responders in the CsA-P group (Table 2) suffered a 4% mortality.

Influence of Blood Transfusions on Allograft Outcome

When examining the impact of prior blood transfusions on allograft survival, there appeared to be a slight improvement in the 1-year graft survival in the overall CsA-P group receiving > 1 transfusion ($N = 77$, 83%) compared to the untransfused group ($N = 23$, 70%; $p < 0.05$). However, the overall group includes 25 transfused weak immune responders, who displayed good graft survival whether treated with CsA or Aza. Therefore, the role of blood transfusions as a risk factor for allograft outcome is more appropriately examined in strong-responder recipients. The 75 strong-responder recipients treated with Aza demonstrated a beneficial effect of blood transfusions: Patients who received 0, 1–4, or ≥ 5 units displayed 26%, 30%, and 52% 1-year graft survivals, respectively (Fig. 4). On the other hand, the benefit of CsA was evident even in the untransfused group. While Aza recipients displayed 26% ($N = 17$), CsA patients enjoyed 70% ($N = 20$) 1-year graft survival ($p > 0.01$). Greater than 5 pretransplant transfusions appeared to convey a slight benefit over untransfused CsA patients, namely 83% 1-year graft survival versus 70% ($p = 0.05$). However, there was no significant difference between the 70% graft survival in nontransfused versus 76% in the 1–4 unit group, just as there was no difference in survival between similar Aza groups. These findings suggest that pretransplant blood transfusions are not necessary for, but in large numbers may slightly improve, allograft survival in CsA-treated patients.

The Role of Splenectomy

Pretransplant splenectomy had been performed in 22% of the CAD recipients. There was no difference in the incidence of splenectomy in weak or strong responders. Splenectomized patients treated with Aza displayed

Table 2. Outcome of Cadaveric Renal Allografts in Recipients Stratified by Immune Responder Status

		Strong		Weak	
Treatment	N	Function	Mortality	Function	Mortality
Aza-P	111	29/75 (39%)	9/75% (12%)	26/36 (72%)	4/36 (11%)
CsA-P	100	60/75 (80%)*	1/75% (4%)†	21/25 (84%)†	1/25 (4%)†

*$p < 0.05$: strong responder CsA-P vs. Aza-P.

†p = No significant difference between CsA-P vs. Aza-P groups.

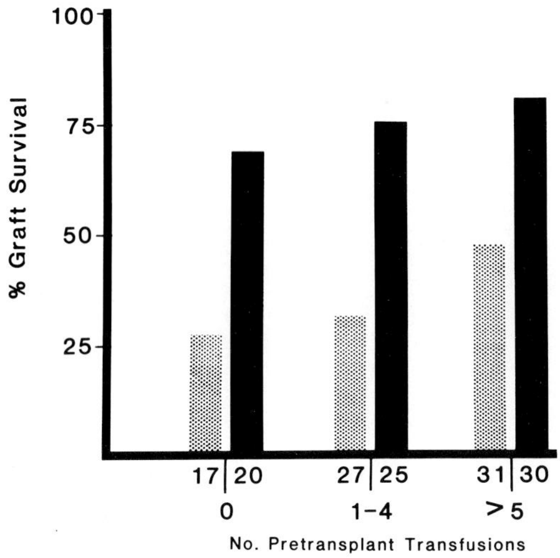

Fig. 4. Effect of administered pretransplant blood transfusions on the outcome of cadaveric renal allografts in strong immune responders treated with Aza and with CsA.

better graft survival than non-splenectomized patients (60 versus 42%, $p < .05$). Under CsA-P immunosuppression, renal allografts did not show improved survival in splenectomized compared to nonsplenectomized patients, whether they were strong or weak immune responders (Table 3).

The Role of HLA-A,B and HLA-DR Tissue Matching

Figure 5 demonstrates the outcome of renal transplantation across HLA incompatibilities in CsA- and Aza-treated recipients. In our center, HLA-A,B matching slightly improved graft survival in the overall group of Aza-treated recipients. There was 44% 1-year graft function in the 55 recipients of transplants bearing more than two HLA-A,B incompatibilities, compared to the 59% 1-year graft survival in 56 recipients with fewer incompatibilities ($p = 0.05$). HLA-DR matching, however, had a more dominant role. There was only 31% graft survival in 32 recipients with two HLA-DR mismatches, compared to 59% survival in 79 recipients with only 1–2 mismatches ($p = 0.05$). When incompatibilities at all loci were combined and analyzed, the most compatible group with $\leq$ 2 HLA-A,B and 0–1 HLA-DR incompatibilities showed 70% (28/40) compared to 38%, 46%, and 31% graft survival with greater degrees of incompatibility ($p = 0.01$). On the other hand, there was no significant difference among the graft outcomes of CsA-treated patients receiving grafts matched or mismatched at the HLA-A,B and/or HLA-DR loci. Although there was no significant difference between the outcome of well-matched grafts in recipients treated with Aza (70%) or CsA (80%), mismatched grafts clearly displayed improved survival in CsA-treated compared to Aza-treated patients (83 vs. 38, 83 vs. 46, 71 vs. 31; all $p = 0.01$) (see Fig. 5).

Outcome of Living Related Haploidentical Renal Allografts Across Stimulatory MLC Reactions

Cochrum et al.[4] demonstrated that the level of pretransplant MLC reactivity between living related donor and recipient pairs predicts the outcome of haploidentical grafts, presumably by virtue of this in vitro reaction to quantitate the potency of the haplodisparity to provoke in vivo graft rejection. The series of patients treated with Aza confirmed the results of Cochrum et al. There was 85% actual 1-year graft survival ($N = 20$, mean follow-up 27.2 months) in recipients of allografts from donors eliciting stimulation index (S.I.) < 6.5 vs. 57% ($N = 20$, MFU = 29.5 months) for S.I. > 6.5. Because of the adverse

Table 3. Influence of Pretransplant Splenectomy on the Survival of Cadaveric Donor Renal Allografts

Splenectomy	Immune Responder Status* Strong	Weak	Total
Yes	12/15 (80%)†	6/7 (86%)	18/22 (82%)
No	48/60 (80%)‡	15/18 (83%)‡	63/78 (81%)
Total	60/75 (80%)	21/25 (84%)	81/100 (81%)

*Recipients were stratified as strong and weak immune responders as described in Materials and Methods.

†Actuarial 1-year graft survival with percentage in parentheses.

‡Comparisons of splenectomy vs. no splenectomy in both strong and weak responder groups separately and combined failed to reveal statistical significance.

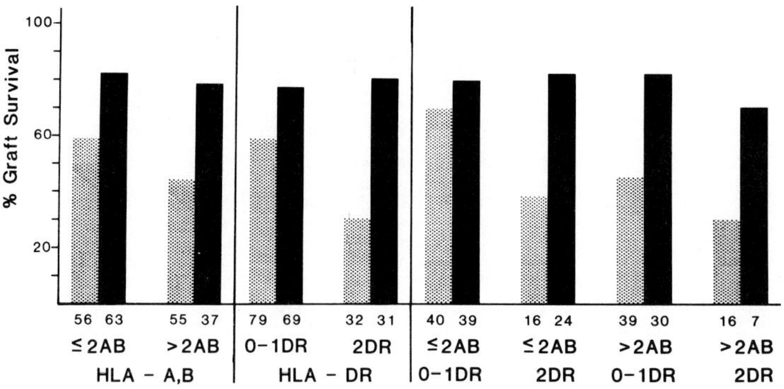

Fig. 5. The effect of HLA-A mismatches on the outcome of renal allografts in the 100 recipients of cadaveric organs treated with Aza and with CsA.

result with Aza-P, our program had excluded donors who provoked stimulation ratios > 6.5. Forty recipients of grafts from stimulatory living related donors were treated substitutively with CsA, according to the same protocol as cadaveric kidney recipients. The actuarial graft survival of 92% was markedly improved over the 57% and 51% function observed at 12 months and at 18 months, respectively, in Aza-treated patients (Fig. 6; $p < 0.01$).

Causes of Graft Loss in the 150 CsA Recipients

Table 4 summarizes all causes of graft loss in recipients of 100 CAD and 50 LRD grafts. Rejection was an infrequent cause of graft loss. Arterial thrombosis occurred in four CAD cases. Three thromboses occurred at day 7 and one at day 18. The etiology of this event is uncertain. No changes in intrinsic coagulation factors were observed. Cases of increased erythrocyte sedimentation rate were observed, but not always associated with thrombosis. There was no thrombocytosis (data not presented). One patient who lost her first graft to thrombosis at day 7 was retransplanted, and although she thrombosed her arteriovenous polytetrafluorethylene (PTFE) arteriovenous fistula graft at 5 days and was heparinized for 2 days thereafter, her kidney has functioned well for over 1 year.

Six grafts were abandoned due to sepsis in the recipient. The one cadaveric graft abandoned because of severe hypertension might have been salvaged by conversion of the immunosuppressive regimen to Aza. This possibility probably also applies to the two cases of primary-graft nonfunction, since two of our other cases were converted to Aza with acquisition of good renal function, as described in detail elsewhere.[12] One pediatric cadaveric recipient lost her graft due to recurrent oxalosis.

There were four deaths in the CAD group: one at 4 months due to viral sepsis following

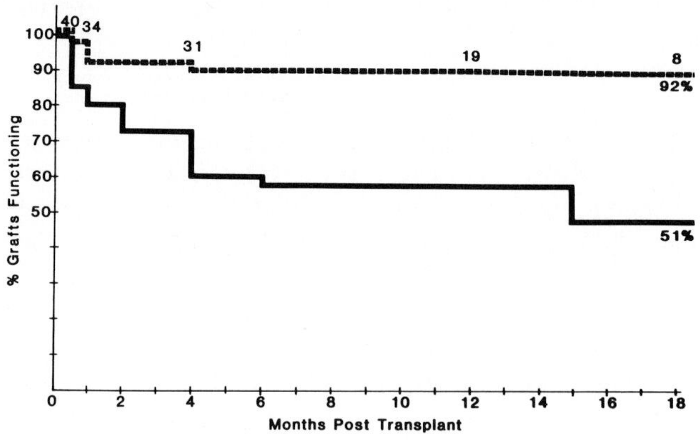

Fig. 6. Actuarial survival of renal allografts from LRD causing > 6.5 stimulation ratio in pretransplant mixed lymphocyte culture reactions in recipients treated with CsA-P and with Aza-P.

Table 4. Causes of Graft Loss in 24 of 150 CsA-Treated Recipients

Cause	CAD (100)	LRD (50)
Rejection	3	1
Thrombosis	4	0
Abandoned		
Sepsis	4	2
HTN	1	0
Primary nonfunctioning	2	0
Recurrent disease (oxalosis)	1	0
Death with functioning graft	4	2
Total loss (percent)	19 (19%)	5 (10%)

hemigastrectomy and vagotomy for exsanguinating pyloric channel ulcer, one at 2 weeks due to pulmonary sepsis in a 56-year-old weak immune responder, one at 2 months due to myocardial infarction in a 52-year-old man, and the fourth due to disseminated herpes and staphylococcal infection. The deaths in the LRD group were due to aspergillosis in a 45-year-old diabetic man and to *Serratia marcescens* septicemia emanating from an infected PTFE vascular access graft that caused septic arthritis and meningitis.

Incidence and Severity of Rejection in CsA Recipients

Table 5 summarizes the rejection episodes in 100 CAD and 50 LRD renal recipients. Although 30% of LRD and 25% of CAD recipients received increased steroids for suspected allograft rejection, retrospective review of patient records revealed that 20% and 16%, respectively, of these episodes were insensitive to prednisone therapy but reversed after reduction of the CsA dose, suggesting that they represented nephrotoxicity. Thus, 10% of LRD and 9% of CAD graft recipients suffered "true" rejection episodes, and only 2% of LRD and 3% of CAD grafts were lost due to this cause. There was no significant difference between the incidence of treated, of actual, or of irreversible rejection episodes leading to graft loss between recipients of living related donor and cadaveric grafts. The low incidence of rejection probably reflects the potent immunosuppressive properties of CsA.

Table 5. Rejection Episodes in CsA-Treated Recipients

	LRD (50)	CAD (100)
Treated rejection episodes	30%	25%
Confirmed rejection episodes	10%	9%
Grafts lost to rejection	2%	3%

Risk of Serious Infection with CsA-P Therapy

Because the CsA-P combination potently suppressed allograft rejection, the incidence of serious infection requiring readmission or prolonged hospitalization was examined in these 150 patients. Among the 100 CAD recipients, 25 patients displayed serious infections. There was no significant difference in the incidence of infections between strong and weak immune responders. Of the 25 weak-responder recipients treated with CsA, 8 (32%) suffered infections necessitating admission or prolonging primary hospitalization: namely, three bacterial pneumonias, of which one was fatal; three severe viral syndromes; one peritonitis due to perforated sigmoid diverticulitis; and one nocardial, followed by cryptococcal, fungal infection. Of the 75 strong responder cadaveric graft recipients treated with CsA, 18 (24%) suffered a similar array of infections: nine viral sepsis leading to death in two patients and abandonment of the graft in three; one *Staphylococcus aureus* septicemia; four Nocardia or streptomyces infections; two peritonitis due to perforated sigmoid diverticulae, leading in one case to abandoning the allograft; one *Listeria* meningitis; and one pneumocystis pneumonia. The incidence of infection was similar in 10 living related allograft recipients of low MLC-stimulation ratio donors (30%) and 40 recipients of high MLC-stimulation ratio donors (22%). In the entire LRD group there were five significant bacterial infections, of which two involved PTFE arteriovenous fistulas (one fatal), one pneumonia, one perforated gastric ulcer, and one perinephric abscess. One *Listeria* meningitis responded promptly to ampicillin therapy. Three serious CMV infections were conservatively managed without sacrificing the transplants. One case of aspergillosis pneumonia was fatal.

Therefore, 38/150 (25%) of the entire group of consecutive CsA-treated patients experienced infections that prolonged their hospital course or required readmission. Of this group, 11/38 (29%) infections occurred after increased steroid therapy for putative rejection. In 10/11 (91%) instances, retrospective analysis of available data including renal biopsy did not confirm the initial impression of allograft rejection. Therefore, increased steroid therapy in patients undergoing the potent CsA-P immunosuppressive regimen described here may trigger serious infection and should only be initiated in the presence of unequivocal evidence of rejection. If these cases of unnecessary antirejection therapy are excluded from the analysis, 27/150 (18%) of patients treated with this CsA-P regimen developed serious infections, and only three patients succumbed to sepsis.

DISCUSSION

An improved outcome of renal transplantation has been achieved by the use of CsA rather than Aza in combination with prednisone.[9–11] The present study assessed the significance of known risk factors on the outcome of cadaveric and living related donor grafts in CsA-treated patients. Improved graft survival was achieved without concern for the lack of favorable prognostic indicators: preconditioning by donor-specific or third-party blood transfusions, nephrectomy or splenectomy, tissue matching, or modulation to a weak immune responder status. For example, in the highest-risk, nontransfused, cadaveric allograft, strong-responder recipients, there was only 26% graft survival using Aza, but 70% using CsA.

The freedom from preconditioning by blood transfusions has two potential advantages. First, it may reduce the waiting time for transplantation, not only by obviating the 2–3 month period for blood administration, but also by reducing the hazard of evoking cytotoxic antibodies that produce positive crossmatches. Second, it may avert the risks of transfusion-acquired infections, including hepatitis or immunodeficiency syndromes. While transfusions are not critical to the CsA effect, they may afford synergistic immunosuppression. The effect of blood transfusions to activate T suppressor cells[13] may be synergistic with the capacity of CsA to spare suppressor cells, as reported by Leapman et al.[14] and by Hess et al.[15] To wit, a modest improvement to 83% allograft survival was observed in strong-responder CsA cadaver graft patients who had received > 5 transfusions prior to transplant evaluation. However, this additional boost in allograft survival above the 70% observed in untransfused CsA patients is much less important than in the comparable, untransfused Aza group.

Pretransplant splenectomy appears to improve allograft survival in Aza-treated patients.[16,17] However, this procedure poses a surgical hurdle. Some patients decline the transplant procedure when confronted with mandatory splenectomy, particularly in the few centers where nephrectomy is also a prerequisite. Furthermore, HLA mismatching does not appear to obviate the benefit of CsA therapy. The independence of graft outcome from the stricture of HLA matching may reflect a unique sensitivity of HLA-DR activation to CsA treatment. While this initial analysis suggests that CsA mitigates the need for pretransplant transfusions, for splenectomy, and for HLA matching, controlled trials of these variables will be essential to assess their potential individual and aggregate benefit. By virtue of its apparent independence from these strictures, CsA affords the opportunity to expeditiously transplant end-stage renal-disease patients, as illustrated by the fact that 12 LRD and 5 CAD recipients in this series were transplanted without dialysis therapy. Therefore, under the umbrella of CsA therapy, transplantation appears to be an excellent mode of primary therapy for end-stage renal disease. CsA may thus reduce end-stage renal-disease costs by removing the hurdles of splenectomy and blood transfusion, which usually demand hemodialysis as well as the need for HLA compatibility that prolongs waiting time and escalates organ procurement costs by organ shipment solely for better HLA compatibility. Furthermore, expeditious primary transplantation of suitable candidates has the possibility to relieve the psychologic dependency of the patient that occurs with chronic dialysis and therefore maintain vocational activity.

The most encouraging result of this clinical series is the apparent immunologic selectivity of CsA. Few grafts were lost due to rejection, and only 10% of patients actually suffered rejection episodes. One cannot exclude the possibility that the four grafts lost to arterial thrombosis actually represent a new, distinct form of rejection. However, the pathologic specimens that showed glomerular capillary thrombosis failed to reveal immunoglobulin deposition. Of interest is the observation that 7 of 116 grafts in the Canadian multicenter trial were also lost to thrombosis.[18] The major obstacle to identifying rejection was the more frequent occurrence of nephrotoxic CsA side effects. Because of the high price in terms of increased infection rate when nephrotoxicity was inadvertently treated with increased steroids and because of the infrequency of alloimmunity under CsA therapy, extreme caution must be exerted in establishing this diagnosis. Furthermore, the potent antirejection effects of CsA were not accompanied by a similar degree of suppression of nonspecific immunity: The incidence and mortality rate due to sepsis was not increased over comparable Aza-treated patients, even among the weak-responder group.

While the present studies suggest that the CsA-P combination provides potent induction of immunosuppression, it may be possible to maintain the unresponsiveness with less immunosuppression.[19] For example, none of eight patients induced with CsA-P and later converted to Aza-P has experienced rejection episodes. Furthermore, prednisone has been withdrawn from six haploidentical LRD recipients without adverse effects, in a fashion akin to that described by First et al.[20] for HLA-identical LRD transplants under Aza therapy. These findings augur for the development of indices reflecting the onset of unresponsiveness, thereafter permitting manipulation of the immunosuppressive regimen to achieve the minimal immunosuppression consistent with continued graft function.

SUMMARY

A group of 150 CsA-treated recipients of 100 CAD donor and 50 LRD kidney allografts was analyzed for the impact of immunologic risk factors determining transplant survival with Aza immunosuppressive therapy. One-year cadaveric graft function in CsA-treated recipients was independent of blood transfusion history, of HLA-A,B and/or HLA-DR mismatches, of prior splenectomy, and of strong vs. weak pretransplant immune status. Of the 10% of patients who suffered a rejection episode, only 3% lost their grafts for this cause. A 4% patient mortality rate was observed in both the LRD and CAD groups. Therefore, the combination of CsA and prednisone provides potent immunoprophylaxis of allograft rejection without increased patient mortality. This selective potency vitiates the need not only for pretransplant immune conditioning by transfusions or splenectomy but also for HLA matching, thereby offering the prospect of expeditious transplantation as a primary mode of end-stage renal-disease therapy.

REFERENCES

1. Opelz G, Terasaki PI: N Engl J Med 299:799, 1978

2. Ting A, Morris PJ: Lancet 1:1047, 1978

3. Moen T, Albrechtsen D, Flatmark A, et al: N Engl J Med 303:850, 1980

4. Cochrum KC, Perkins H, Payne R, et al: Transplant Proc 5:391, 1973

5. Kerman R, Kahan BD: Ann Clin Res 13:244, 1981

6. Kahan BD, Conner WT: In American College of

Surgeons, *Manual of Preoperative and Postoperative Care*. Philadelphia, Saunders, 1983, p 182

7. Kissmeyer-Nielsen F, Olsen S, Posborg-Peterson V, et al: Lancet 2:662, 1966

8. Kahan BD, Ried M, Newburger J: Transplant Proc 15:446, 1983

9. Kahan BD, Van Buren CT, Lin S, et al: Transplantation 34:36, 1982

10. Starzl T, Weil R, Iwatsuki S, et al: Surg Gynecol Obstet 151:17, 1980

11. Ferguson RM, Rynasiewicz J, Sutherland DER, et al: Surgery 92:176, 1982

12. Flechner SM, Van Buren CT, Kahan BD: Transplant Proc (in press)

13. Kerman R, Flechner SM, Van Buren, et al: Transplant Proc (in press)

14. Leapman SB, Filo RS, Smith EJ, et al: Transplantation 30:404, 1980

15. Hess AD, Tutschka PJ, Santos G: J Immunol 128:360, 1982

16. Stuart FP, Reckard CR, Ketel BL, et al: Ann Surg 192:553, 1980

17. Fryd DS, Sutherland DER, Simmons RL, et al: Transplant Proc 13:48, 1981

18. Stiller CR, Keown P, Laupacis A, et al: Transplant Proc (in press)

19. Calne RY, White D, Thiru S, et al: Lancet 2:1323, 1978

20. First MR, Munda R, Fidler JP, et al: Transplant Proc 13:319, 1981

The Canadian Trial of Cyclosporine: Cyclosporine Therapy Compared to Standard Immunosuppression in Renal Transplants: An Exploration of Nephrotoxicity

C. Stiller, London, Canada, for The Canadian Transplant Study Group

THE CANADIAN TRANSPLANT Study Group (CTSG) is conducting a multicenter randomized study of cyclosporine and prednisone (CsA-P) vs. azathioprine and prednisone (standard therapy: STD) in recipients of cadaveric renal transplants. The initial analysis in June 1982 involving the first 210 patients has been reported elsewhere.[1] Entry into the trial has been closed, and there are now 291 patients (142 CsA-P, 149 STD) in the study, with a follow-up of 4–28 months (mean, 19 months).

In this paper we briefly review the actuarial graft and patient survival obtained in June 1982 and then examine cyclosporine nephrotoxicity in more detail. For all analyses except the actuarial graft and patient survival, data on all 142 CsA-P patients have been used. Other complications are dealt with in detail elsewhere in this volume.[2]

MATERIALS AND METHODS

The protocol and initial results of the CTSG trial have been described previously.[1] An initial oral loading dose of 20 mg/kg/day of cyclosporine was given within 12 hr prior to surgery, and the patients then received 10 mg/kg every 12 hr. Cyclosporine serum levels were measured frequently by radioimmunoassay at the participating centers' laboratories (usually 2–3 times a week, and often daily), and the cyclosporine dose was adjusted to achieve trough cyclosporine serum levels of 100–400 ng/ml. If the patient was unable to take the drug by mouth, it was given by intravenous infusion. Cyclosporine could be discontinued and patients switched to alternate immunosuppressive therapy, but a concerted attempt was made to keep these switches to a minimum. There was no common protocol for switching patients.

On day 14, patients were started on prednisone 1 mg/kg body weight on alternate days, which was reduced by 5 mg every other day, clinical conditions allowing, to a level of 0.3 mg/kg body weight on alternate days. This dosage was maintained until 3 months, when it was lowered to 0.25 mg/kg on alternate days if there was no evidence of rejection. At 6 months, the prednisone was further reduced to 12.5 mg every other day, clinical conditions allowing. Acute rejection was treated with steroids to a maximum of 4.5 g of methylprednisolone (or its equivalent) over 7 days. If an acute rejection occurred prior to 14 days after transplantation, maintenance prednisone therapy could be started immediately after high-dose steroid therapy was discontinued. Cytotoxic agents or antilymphocytic globulin were not used in cyclosporine-treated patients.

Initial nonfunction was defined as a requirement for dialysis immediately after transplant, or a serum creatinine greater than 10 mg/dl, in the absence of hyperacute or accelerated rejection, renal artery thrombosis, or post-renal obstruction.

The effect of treatment and predetermined prognostic factors on patient and graft survival were analyzed using product limit estimate survival curves. Significance was tested by both the log rank and the Mantel-Haenszel methods. All mean values cited in the text are followed by the standard deviation (SD). Significance over contingency tables was determined by the Mantel-Haenszel test.

RESULTS

Patient and Graft Survival

On June 1, 1982, 103 CsA-P and 107 STD patients had been followed for at least 1 month after transplantation, with a mean follow-up of 8 months. Overall average patient survival was significantly greater in CsA-treated patients (97.1% vs. 89.6%; $p = 0.03$), and the product limit estimate of the 1-year survival was 96.6% in the CsA-P group and 86.4% in the STD group.

CsA-P treated patients had a significantly greater overall average graft survival than patients on STD therapy (83.5% vs. 67.0%; $p = 0.003$). The product limit estimate of the

From the Canadian Transplant Study Group, University Hospital, London, Ontario, Canada.

Reprint requests should be addressed to Dr. C. R. Stiller, Centre for Transplant Studies, University Hospital, London, Ontario, Canada.

0041-1345/83/1505-0052$01.00/0

Table 3. Effect of Initial Cyclosporine Levels

Initial Cyclosporine Level* (ng/ml)	No. of Patients	Rejections in First 7 Days (%)	Patients with No Rejections During First 100 Days (%)	Graft Losses (%)
100	25	28	40	16
100–199	44	25	36	25
200–400	31	55	23	19
> 400	30	30	13	20

*Mean trough cyclosporine level during first 3 days after transplantation.

deteriorating renal function. The patients in this group all lost their grafts more than 200 days post-transplant, with no evidence of acute rejection. It was not clear whether this was caused by chronic rejection or cyclosporine nephrotoxicity. Of patients with initial nonfunction, 33% (21/64) lost their grafts in the first 100 days, compared to 14% (10/63) of patients whose kidneys functioned immediately.

Long-Term Graft Function

Forty-one patients in the CsA-P group and 30 in the STD group still had functioning grafts 500 days after transplantation and had not been switched to alternate immunosuppression. The serum creatinine level (mmole/liter) in the CsA-P patients rose from 108 ± 82 on day 90, to 176 ± 77 on day 180, to 195 ± 83 on day 360, to 213 ± 99 on day 500. In the patients in the STD group, the levels were 146 ± 61 on day 90, 150 ± 61 on day 180, 149 ± 51 on day 360, and 150 ± 63 on day 500. The cyclosporine dose (mg/kg/day) was 9.5 ± 4.3 on day 90 and 8.3 ± 4.5 on day 500. The corresponding CsA serum levels (ng/ml) were 262 ± 312 and 148 ± 87.

Switches

Twenty-two patients were switched from CsA-P to STD therapy 2–465 days after transplantation. Seven patients received azathioprine and steroids immediately following cessation of cyclosporine, 3 patients received ALG and steroids followed by azathioprine, and 12 patients received steroids alone for 1–33 days and then were placed on azathioprine. In one patient each, ALG or azathioprine was started on the last day of cyclosporine therapy. Otherwise, there was no overlap of cyclosporine with cytotoxic agents. Two patients developed easily reversible leukopenia, and no acute rejections were seen at the time of switching. The reasons for and outcomes of switching are shown in Table 5. Of the 7 patients switched for nonfunction, 3 had improved graft survival after switching. All 11 patients switched because of impaired function had a decrease in their serum creatinine levels, but this was transient in 3 patients, who subsequently required nephrectomy. One patient later died of cardiac arrest. All 3 patients who were switched for reasons unrelated to renal function had a decrease in serum creatinine after switching.

Table 4. Causes of Graft Loss

	Cyclosporine	Standard
Renal artery thrombosis	3	1
Initial nonfunction	10	4
Accelerated or hyperacute rejection	2	3
Acute rejection	7	29
Deteriorating renal function	7	1
Infection	1	4
Deaths with functioning kidneys	6	7
Total	36	49

DISCUSSION

Cyclosporine is an immunosuppressive agent with which one can achieve a 1-year renal graft survival of approximately 80%, with acceptable infectious complications. Its most troublesome side effect is nephrotoxicity, manifested by a detrimental effect of long rewarm and perfusion time on graft survival, a high incidence of initial nonfunction, a rela-

Table 5. Switches from Cyclosporine

Reason	No.	Days After Transplantation	Creatinine at Switch	No. Presently Functioning	Present Creatinine	Days Since Switch
Nonfunction	7	26–106 (59)*	923 ± 87	3	181 ± 92	65–475 (268)*
Impaired function	11	87–465 (235)*	436 ± 241	7	165 ± 44	373–587 (501)*
Hyperacute rejection	1	2	681	1	212	477
Lymphoma	1	127	89	—	—	—
Lymphomatous change	1	192	159	1	97	201
Vomiting	1	399	324	1	192	165
Total	22		578 ± 335	13		169 ± 55

*Number in parentheses is the mean.

tively high mean serum creatinine in functioning grafts, and possibly a predisposition to hypertension.[2] Unfortunately, CsA-induced nephrotoxicity may be very difficult to differentiate from chronic rejection. This problem needs to be addressed by careful and systematic review of a large number of renal biopsies in patients whose clinical courses have been well studied.

Long perfusion time is associated not only with an increased incidence of graft loss but also with a high incidence of initial nonfunction. Both the magnitude of the CsA serum trough levels achieved at the time of transplantation and the length of machine perfusion had separately definable effects on the incidence of initial nonfunction. The CsA serum levels achieved in the first 3 days after transplantation vary considerably in patients given the same loading dose of 20 mg/kg/day; the measurement of CsA levels in the early post-transplant period is therefore important and allows rapid adjustment of the dose to achieve target CsA serum levels. It is not known whether the trough or peak CsA serum level is more important in causing nephrotoxicity. It may be that continuous intravenous infusion of CsA during the first few days after transplant avoids high peaks of CsA and allows better titration of the dose. The patients in this study were given a loading dose of 20 mg/kg before transplantation, and that may have predisposed to the high incidence of initial nonfunction. There was no correlation between the length of rewarm time and the incidence of initial nonfunction. It is unclear why long perfusion time should have more of an effect on initial nonfunction than long rewarm time.

Cyclosporine-treated patients with initial nonfunction have an increased incidence of early graft loss (especially primary nonfunction), a longer initial hospitalization, and a higher serum creatinine level during the first 180 days after transplantation than their counterparts without initial nonfunction. They are also treated for more rejection episodes than patients whose kidneys function immediately. The diagnosis of rejection is difficult in a patient whose kidney is not functioning, and some of the episodes treated as rejections in these patients may not have been true rejections. As more experience has been gained with the use of cyclosporine, many rises in serum creatinine levels that would previously have been treated with high-dose steroids are now being managed by decreasing the dose of CsA.

Patients with initial CsA levels of < 100 ng/ml have a relatively low incidence of initial nonfunction and also do not experience more rejection episodes in the first 7 days than patients with higher initial CsA levels. In fact, patients with lower serum CsA levels experienced fewer rejections in the first 100 days than patients with higher levels. This significant trend may reflect the higher incidence of initial nonfunction in the patients with relatively high initial CsA levels, which were mistakenly treated as rejection episodes. It is highly unlikely that a high CsA level itself predisposes to rejection.

In the CsA-P group there was a gradual upward drift in serum creatinine between day

90 and day 500. Seven CsA-P–treated patients lost their grafts more than 200 days after transplantation because of gradually deteriorating renal function (compared to one in the STD group). It is uncertain whether these patients were experiencing cyclosporine-induced nephrotoxicity or chronic rejection.

Twenty-two patients were switched from CsA-P to STD therapy, and many had significant and maintained decreases in serum creatinine levels. Long-term function and survival of these grafts is unknown. None had acute rejections at the time of switching, despite the fact that many were maintained on steroids alone for a number of days after cyclosporine was discontinued. However, severe leukopenia, infections, and acute rejections at the time of switching have been reported.[3] This warrants a policy of aggressively lowering the dose and level of CsA before switching patients to azathioprine.

ACKNOWLEDGMENTS

We acknowledge the support of the Medical Research Council of Canada, Richard and Jean Ivey Fund, London, Ontario; Sandoz Ltd., Basel; the Michael Fung Endowment Fund, London, Ontario; and the University Hospital Transplant Research Fund, London, Ontario.

Centers involved in this study were Vancouver General Hospital (C. E. Reeve), University of Alberta Hospital, Edmonton (F. Harley), Calgary Foothills Hospital (J. Klassen), Health Sciences Centre, Winnipeg (J. Jeffery), Toronto General Hospital (P. Halloran), Toronto St. Michael's Hospital (R. Bear), St. Joseph's Hospital, Hamilton (D. Ludwin), Montreal General Hospital (M. Mangel), Notre Dame Hospital (P. Daloze), Maisonneuve-Rosemont Hospital (R. Dandavino), Victoria General Hospital, Halifax (P. Belitsky), and University Hospital, London (P. Keown).

Executive Committee: G. Arbus, R. Bear, R. Dandavino, J. B. Dossetor, J. Jeffery, A. S. MacDonald (Chairman), M. Robinette, C. R. Stiller.

Management Committee, Centre for Transplant Studies and Statistical Consultants: H. Cheung, M. Gent, M. Grace, W. Howson, P. A. Keown, J. Koval, A. Laupacis, B. Lockwood, I. MacNeill, L. Moist, N. R. Sinclair, C. R. Stiller, G. Wells.

REFERENCES

1. Canadian Transplant Study Group. N Engl J Med (in press)

2. Canadian Transplant Study Group: Transplant Proc (this issue)

3. Canafax D, Sutherland DER, Simmons R, et al: Transplant Proc (this issue)

Australian Trial of Cyclosporine (CsA) in Cadaveric Donor Renal Transplantation

A. G. R. Sheil, B. M. Hall, D. J. Tiller, M. S. Stephen, J. P. Harris, G. G. Duggin, J. S. Horvath, J. R. Johnson, J. R. Rogers, and J. Boulas

THE INCIDENCE OF failure due to rejection in cadaveric donor renal (CAD) transplantation has fallen recently as a result of advances in tissue matching and the recognition of the importance of preoperative blood transfusions. However, many grafts are still lost to rejection, and in the others, reversible rejection occurs with high frequency. Repetitive high-dose corticosteroid therapy is often required, and those patients who retain functioning grafts must be treated indefinitely with corticosteroids and antimetabolites. In the early postoperative months, complications of therapy are frequent and severe. Bone marrow depression, infections, pancreatitis, and gastrointestinal hemorrhage may all be life-threatening, while the development of Cushingoid features is distressing for most patients. In the long term, bone necrosis, lens cataract formation, infections, vascular degeneration, and cancer all occur in significant proportions of patients.[1] While reduction of rejection is a prime aim of a new immunosuppressive agent, we nevertheless would accept gladly an equivalent failure rate to rejection if these currently inescapable complications were to disappear.

We report here the results of prospective controlled trials of the use of CsA for first and second CAD transplants compared with azathioprine (Aza), prednisone (P), and antithymocyte globulin (ATG). We followed the pioneering experience of the Cambridge group, using their recommended CsA dose and administration as sole maintenance therapy.[2] However, unlike them, in an effort to achieve optimal immunosuppression and to determine practicability of use of CsA for all patients in a cadaveric donor transplant program, we elected to administer the agent preoperatively to all patients and to continue therapy in full dosage irrespective of early graft function.

MATERIALS AND METHODS

Sequential patients receiving first and second CAD allografts who had previously received at least 5 units of blood transfusion were randomly allocated either to a CsA-treated group or a control group receiving conventional therapy (Aza group). Diabetics and those with a history of malignancy other than localized skin malignancy were excluded. Kidney grafts were obtained from a sharing program in which grafts were allocated on the basis of HLA matching and negative direct T-cell crossmatch after storage by machine perfusion.

CsA (Sandoz Ltd., Basel, and Sandoz Pty. Ltd., Australia) was given in the dose 17 mg/kg p.o. preoperatively, and half this dosage was given twice daily for 28 days. The dose was then gradually reduced to 10 mg/kg by day 50 after transplantation. The Aza group was given Aza (3 mg/kg p.o.) and methyl prednisolone (MP), Ig intravenously (IVI) preoperatively. Aza was continued in the same daily dosage postoperatively, with reduction or cessation of therapy if toxicity occurred. MP was continued in the dosages of 500 mg and 250 mg IVI on the first and second postoperative days before change to oral P (100 mg/day). P dosage was gradually reduced to a daily maintenance dose of 10–15 mg by 6 weeks. ATG (15 mg/kg) was given IVI on alternate days from the time of operation for 7 doses.

Rejection was diagnosed clinically and confirmed whenever possible by examination of percutaneous biopsy specimens. Oliguric postoperative biopsies were performed each 7–10 days if not contraindicated by coagulopathy or wound complications. Rejection was treated in both groups by pulse MP therapy over 3 days (Ig, 500 mg, 250 mg). CsA patients then stopped corticosteroid therapy, while Aza patients continued with oral P in gradually decreasing doses.

From the Renal and Transplantation Units, Royal Prince Alfred Hospital and the Department of Surgery, University of Sydney, New South Wales, Australia.

Reprint requests should be addressed to Professor A. G. R. Sheil, Department of Surgery, New South Wales, 2006 Australia.

0041-1345/83/1505-0053$01.00/0

RESULTS

Primary Grafts

After 30 months there are 30 patients in each arm of the trial. Of the entire 60 patients, 3 (5%) died. One CsA patient died of viral pneumonia soon after change to Aza-P therapy. A second CsA patient drowned accidentally. One Aza patient died of herpes simplex viral infection. In the CsA group, 1-year and 2-year graft survivals were both 70%. In the control group, the respective survivals were 80% and 70%. However, five CsA patients required change from CsA to Aza-P therapy. In one patient, this was because of mood depression 11 months after transplantation. In the other four, it was because of primary nonfunction of renal grafts for periods from 5 weeks to 3 months after transplantation; all four grafts began to function 3–14 days after changing to standard therapy, and good function continued in three, the fourth patient dying of pneumonia. When the four patients with functioning grafts after change to Aza-P therapy are considered CsA treatment failures, 1- and 2-year graft survivals in continuously CsA-treated patients are both 56%.

Tissue matching based on the presence or absence of 2B and 2DR antigens for CsA patients showed 12 with no or one antigen shared with donors, 10 with two antigens shared, and 8 with three or four antigens shared. Respective patient numbers for control patients were 10, 15, and 5. Patients with serum antibodies against lymphocytes from a panel of blood donors numbered 9 (30%) in the CsA group and 16 (56%) in the control group. Highly sensitized patients (>80% antibodies) numbered 3 in both the CsA and control groups.

The causes of 9 (30%) graft failures in the CsA group were rejection (5; 17%), death of patient (2), bleeding following biopsy (1), and technical failure (TF, 1). Of the 5 grafts lost to rejection, 2 were because of hyperacute rejection (HAR), 2 acute rejection (AR), and 1 chronic rejection (CR). In the standard therapy group, 8 (27%) grafts failed, 7 (23%) because of rejection (1 HAR, 3 AR, 3 CR), and 1 was TF.

If the grafts lost to rejection and TF are excluded, reversible rejection episodes in the first 3 postoperative months occurred in 19 (63%) CsA patients, who required 1–8 (mean, 3) treatments for rejection. Five (17%) CsA patients had no rejection episodes. In the Aza group, 21 (70%) patients received 1–6 (mean, 3.6) treatments for rejection. Only 1 (3%) patient had no rejection episode.

In the CsA patients, 3 grafts were nonfunctional because of rejection or TF. Immediate good function (GF) occurred after operation in 5 (17%), while persisting nonfunction requiring change to standard therapy occurred in 4 (13%). The remaining 18 patients achieved GF 4–38 (mean, 23) days after transplantation, while full CsA treatment continued. Lowest levels of serum creatinine achieved were 90–410 (mean, 180) μmole/liter. In the Aza group, 3 grafts were nonfunctional because of rejection or TF. Immediate GF occurred in 12 (40%). The remaining 15 patients diuresed 2–32 (mean, 13) days after transplantation. Lowest levels of serum creatinine were 65–185 (mean, 119) μmole/liter.

In the CsA group, excluding 6 patients who lost grafts within the first 2 weeks, there were no patients without complications of therapy. Nine developed coagulopathy. Of these, 2 required operation for bleeding. Four patients became thrombocytopenic, but bleeding did not occur. Seventeen (57%) developed infections. Most were bacterial, affecting the urinary tract (11 patients), operation site (3), shunt sites (3), chest (4), and peritoneal cavity (1). However, 5 patients developed one or more viral infections [herpes zoster (1), herpes simplex (4), cytomegalovirus (CMV) (2)], 1 of which (CMV pneumonia) was fatal. A further 2 patients developed pyrexia of unknown origin. Three patients developed peptic ulceration, 1 requiring operation because of bleeding from a duodenal ulcer. Mild abnormalities of tests of liver function (LFT) were detected in most patients, but only 1 became jaundiced. In all patients, liver function returned to normal spontaneously or with minor reduction in CsA dosage. Most patients developed a mild increase in body hair, and in 2 this complication was considered serious. One patient changed to Aza-P subsequently developed squamous cell carcinoma of the skin (SCC).

In the Aza-P group, 14 (47%) patients developed coagulopathy, 2 requiring operation for hemorrhage. Seventeen (57%) became thrombocytopenic, but hemorrhage did not occur. Nine (30%) developed severe bone marrow depression requiring modification of therapy. There were 30 episodes of bacterial infection and 17 of viral infections, and 4 patients had pyrexia of unknown origin. One patient developed peptic ulceration but did not require operation. Mild abnormalities of LFT were common postoperatively, but only one patient became jaundiced, and this was resolved with a decrease in Aza dosage. Five (17%) patients developed SCC, 1 diabetes, and 4 transplant renal artery stenosis.

Secondary Grafts

Of 6 CsA-treated patients to receive secondary grafts, 4 (67%) survive, 2 (33%) with FG. Causes of deaths were bacterial pneumonia in 1 patient and ischemic enteritis following return to dialysis after graft removal in a second. Causes of graft failure were HAR (1), AR (1), TF (1), and patient death (1).

Of 8 Aza-P patients, 5 (62%) survive, 3 (37%) with FG. However, 1 of these is considered a treatment failure because of severe bone marrow depression requiring change to CsA. Causes of deaths were bacterial pneumonia (2) and ruptured sigmoid colonic diverticulum (1). Reasons for graft failures were AR (2) and patient deaths (3).

DISCUSSION

The relatively good results with primary grafts in the control patients (97% patient survival, 1- and 2-year graft survivals of 80% and 70%) reflect results that can be achieved in CAD transplantation with conventional immunosuppressive agents and selection criteria including multiple blood transfusions before operation and exclusion of diabetic patients. Even so, it may be expected that after a further 10 years, ½ of the patients treated successfully so far will have died or lost grafts, and most of the remainder will have suffered from one or more disorders such as serious infections, vascular degeneration, lens cataract development, bone necrosis, and cancer.[1]

That the results in the CsA-treated group were equivalent (93% patient survival, 1- and 2-year graft survivals both of 70%) is encouraging. Even though it was necessary to suspend CsA treatment in some patients and complications were many, most difficulties were overcome, and surviving patients are in excellent health and spirits. It remains to be seen if renal function will continue over the long term in most patients or if unexpected complications will occur.

The encouraging results in both arms of the trial could not be explained by tissue matching. In the CsA group, well-matched patients were only 26% of the total, and in the Aza-P group 17%. Patients previously sensitized as shown by the presence of serum antibodies before transplantation were unevenly distributed, forming 30% of CsA patients and 56% of Aza-P patients. However, highly sensitized patients (>80% antibodies) were evenly distributed, there being 3 in each group. While the presence of antibodies in general did not appear to affect adversely the results in either group, 2 of 3 highly sensitized patients in the CsA group rejected grafts, and the other highly sensitized patient required repeated therapy for rejection. In the Aza-P group, 1 of 3 highly sensitized patients rejected the graft. It remains to be seen if oral CsA may be inadequate to control rejection in highly sensitized patients.

In this trial, CsA proved to be at least as immunosuppressive as our best standard therapy, and possibly a little more so. Grafts lost to rejection were fewer in the CsA group (17% vs. 23%), there were fewer rejection episodes (mean, 3 vs. 3.6), and patients with no rejection episodes were more numerous (17% vs. 3%). Even so, significant rejection did occur in the CsA group. Of particular concern is the incidence of hyperacute and acute rejection in both the primary-graft and secondary-graft trials, where the proportions of grafts lost to these causes were 13% and 33%, respectively. We are concerned that, because CsA was administered by mouth before the operation, blood levels may not have been effective at the time of operation because of delayed absorption of the agent in patients prepared for operation, a factor that may be of increased importance in highly sensitized patients. We hope to decrease HAR and AR by administering the preoperative dose of CsA IVI to ensure adequate blood levels at the time of graft revascularization. It may also prove necessary to add other immunosuppressants such as corticosteroids or ATG in the perioperative period with the hope that improved immunosuppression will not be offset by increased complications of therapy.

Of all the complications suffered by patients in the CsA group, nephrotoxicity was of most concern. With the circumstances in Australia of organ procurement, preservation, and the need for HLA-DR tissue matching performed after donor death, most grafts are implanted 24–40 hr after harvesting. Immediate function occurs in approximately 50% of grafts, and postoperative diuresis in the rest within 1 month, facts attested to in the control arm of this trial. Nephrotoxicity was demonstrated in the CsA group in all parameters studied. Immediate function occurred in only 17% of patients, while persisting nonfunction occurred in 13%. Postoperative diuresis was delayed by a mean of more than a week, compared to Aza-P patients. The adequacy of renal function achieved by the CsA group was less than that of the Aza-P group, as indicated by comparative mean levels of serum creatinine of 180 and 119 mm/liter, respectively. Furthermore, we have reported that in some grafts there is histologic evidence of graft damage that may be attributable to CsA or the combined effects of CsA and graft ischemia.[3] It appears to us that the dosage of CsA used must be close to the maximum dictated by nephrotoxicity in this cadaveric donor program. Clearly, it is important that we work toward improved methods of organ procurement, tissue matching, and preservation to decrease the extent of ischemic damage to grafts used.

The five patients in the CsA group who required change to Aza-P must be considered CsA treatment failures. However, it should be noted that failure was not due to rejection, and 4 of the 5 grafts still function. In the evaluation of an immunosuppressive agent, these patients are difficult to classify, as effective immunosuppression was achieved in the important first weeks after transplantation. Even so, the option of early effective immunosuppression with reversible renal failure due to nephrotoxicity is not attractive as a form of management because of the long period of uncertainty as to outcome following operation for both patients and clinicians, the need for repeated investigations—some invasive—to analyze progress, and histologic evidence or renal parenchymal damage in these patients.[3] We now plan to change therapy routinely after 1 month in patients receiving CsA who remain oliguric following renal transplantation.

While complications were numerous in both CsA-treated and control patients, those in the CsA group tended to be much less threatening and more easily managed. Most encouraging was the virtual absence of severe bone marrow depression, a complication that occurred in 30% of control patients. Viral infections were also notably fewer in CsA patients. A particular benefit to the morale of CsA patients was the absence of the feared Cushingoid physical features notable in standard therapy patients. Of potential importance is the virtual absence of SCC in CsA patients; this complication occurred with usual frequency in the control group. We also note that renal artery stenosis, which is thought to have an immunological component, has occurred in the standard therapy group but not so far in the CsA group.

Despite nephrotoxicity, it is clear that good results can be achieved by administering CsA preoperatively to all patients in a CAD transplantation program and continuing it in full dosage irrespective of early graft function. With these methods, most grafts diuresed while full therapy continued, and in the others, effective immunosuppression was achieved and good function followed cessation of CsA therapy. Thus, for best immunosuppression, the requirement of CsA administration at the time of or before transplantation[4] can be met and the need to restrict CsA therapy to patients with diuresing grafts[2] avoided.

REFERENCES

1. Mahony JF, Sheil AGR, Etheredge SB, et al: Med J Aust 2:426, 1982

2. Calne RY, Rolles K, White DJG, et al: Lancet 2:1033, 1979

3. Farnsworth A, Hall B, Bishop A, et al: Transplant Proc (in press)

4. Borel JF, Feurer C, Magnee C, et al: Immunology 32:1017, 1977

The Requirements for Maintenance Steroids in Cyclosporine-Treated Renal Transplant Recipients

C. Stiller, London, Canada, for The Canadian Transplant Study Group

CYCLOSPORINE (CsA) is an effective immunosuppressant in renal transplantation that has been used with and without maintenance steroid therapy. The Canadian Transplant Study Group (CTSG) has reported an 80.4% 1-year actuarial cadaveric renal graft survival in 103 patients treated with CsA and alternate-day prednisone started on day 14.[1] A European multicenter study in which patients were treated with CsA alone achieved an estimated graft survival at 6 months of 73%.[2] Although 82% of the CsA group with functioning grafts were receiving CsA alone at the time of reporting, only 27% of the patients never received steroids.

To determine if maintenance steroids improve graft survival and function in CsA-treated patients, the CTSG is conducting a double-blind study in which patients receive CsA and alternate-day prednisone for the first 90 days following transplantation and then are randomized into receiving either prednisone or placebo. Prior to commencing this study, 69 renal transplant patients were entered into a non-blind "interim study" comparing CsA and prednisone with CsA alone. The early results of this study are reported here.

MATERIALS AND METHODS

Seven Canadian transplant centers participated in the study, with patient entry occurring between August 1982 and January 1983. Patients were not eligible for entry if they had (1) evidence of acute or progressive liver disease, (2) a previous generalized or metastatic malignancy or a localized malignancy within the previous year, (3) a positive Terasaki T-cell crossmatch between either current or noncurrent sera and donor T lymphocytes, (4) a disease requiring maintenance steroid therapy, or (5) previously been included in this trial. There were no transfusion requirements for entry, and both living related and cadaveric donors were accepted.

A balanced, restricted randomization by center was used. A computer-derived randomized block of varying size was generated and noted in a series of opaque envelopes held by the research pharmacist at each participating center. When the decision for transplantation was made, the patient signed the final consent and the envelope was opened (admission before allocation). The study was not blinded.

The intraoperative protocol in use at each participating center was applied to both groups. An attempt was made to keep the length of machine perfusion (perfusion time) and surgical anastomosis time (rewarm time) as short as possible.

Cyclosporine was given as a loading dose of 15 mg/kg orally within 12 hr prior to surgery, and the patients then received 7.5 mg/kg every 12 hr. Trough CsA serum levels were determined frequently by radioimmunoassay, and the oral dose was adjusted to achieve trough levels of 100–300 ng/ml during the first 60 days after transplantation. After 60 days, centers attempted to achieve trough CsA serum levels of 50–200 ng/ml.

Acute rejection episodes in either group were treated with oral or intravenous steroids to a maximum of 4.5 g of methylprednisolone or its equivalent over 7 days. High-dose steroids were continued for a maximum of 14 days. No cytotoxic drugs or antilymphocytic products were used in patients receiving CsA. If necessary, CsA could be discontinued and the patients switched to alternate therapy (azathioprine and prednisone), but an attempt was made to keep these switches to a minimum. Patients in the no-prednisone group could be given maintenance steroids if clinical conditions required.

The effects of treatment and predetermined prognostic factors on patient and graft survival were analyzed using product limit estimate survival curves. Significance was tested by the Mantel-Haenszel method. The prognostic factors that were tested in univariate analyses were type of transplant (living related or cadaveric), number of transfusions prior to surgery, number of previous kidney transplants, length of rewarm time, and presence or absence of machine perfusion.

RESULTS

Patient Entry

Sixty-nine patients were entered; 36 received prednisone and 33 no prednisone. Of

---

From the Canadian Transplant Study Group, University Hospital, London, Ontario, Canada.

Reprint requests should be addressed to Dr. C. Stiller, Centre for Transplant Studies, University Hospital, London, Ontario, Canada.

0041-1345/83/1505-0054$01.00/0

Table 1. Entry Characteristics

	No Prednisone	Prednisone
Age	35	35
Males	25	20
Females	11	13
Living related	6	13
Machine-perfused	7	8
Perfusion time >24 hr	2	2
Rewarm time >45 min	2	2
Previous transplant	6	7

the patients receiving prednisone, 29 received alternate-day and 1 received daily prednisone, starting on the day of transplant. Six patients received alternate-day prednisone starting on day 14. Post-transplant follow-up ranged from 5–173 days, and the median length of follow-up was 5.5 months. No patients were excluded after entry. The number of patients entered per center varied from 2–15. The two treatment groups were balanced for all entry characteristics examined except for the type of transplant (Table 1). Twelve recipients of grafts from related donors were in the prednisone group, and six in the no-prednisone group.

Patient and Graft Survival

Actual patient and graft survival of all 69 patients was 95.6% and 86.9%, respectively. There was no difference in graft survival between patients receiving prednisone (86.1%) and patients not receiving prednisone (87.9%) (Table 2).

The effect of risk factors in all 69 patients was examined. The 18 patients who received kidneys from a living related donor had a superior overall graft survival (94.4%), compared to patients receiving a cadaveric kidney (84.3%), but this was not statistically significant. The overall cadaveric graft survival in patients receiving prednisone was 79.2%, compared with 85.2% in patients receiving no prednisone. Thirteen patients received grafts from one-haplotype-identical related donors, and one graft was lost. Patients receiving their first kidney transplant had a significantly better graft survival than patients who had been previously transplanted (91.1% vs. 69.2%; $p = 0.03$). All living related transplants were done in patients who had not had a previous transplant. The graft survival of patients who received a cadaveric kidney and had never been previously transplanted was 89.5%.

There was no difference in graft survival in patients who received 0–4 transfusions (87.9%) and those who received more than 4 transfusions (85.7%). Five patients received no transfusions prior to surgery, and all have functioning grafts. The method of kidney preservation (machine perfusion or cold storage) and the length of rewarm time (≥35 min) had no significant effect on graft survival. Only four patients received kidneys that had been perfused for longer than 24 hr, and 2 lost their grafts. None of the 4 patients who had a

Table 2. Graft Survival by Prognostic Factor

Prognostic Factor	No. of Patients	Graft Survival Rate	Cumulative Graft Survival*	Significance
Prednisone	36	86.1	83.8	0.82
No prednisone	33	87.9	87.8	
Living related	18	94.4	94.1	0.32
Cadaveric	51	84.3	83.0	
First transplant, cadaveric kidney	38	89.5	—	
No previous kidney	56	91.1	89.8	0.03
Previous kidney	13	69.2	68.4	
0–4 transfusions	33	87.9	87.5	0.75
>4 transfusions	35	85.7	83.5	
Perfused	15	87.0	85.8	0.91
Not perfused	54	86.7	86.7	
Rewarm ≤35 min	38	89.5	87.8	0.46
Rewarm >35 min	22	81.8	81.8	

*Product limit estimates of cumulative survival at 1 year.

rewarm time greater than 45 min lost the graft.

The deaths were due to septicemia and candidal peritonitis, severe metabolic encephalopathy, and hemorrhage after renal biopsy. The other six graft losses were due to renal artery thrombosis (1), accelerated rejection (1), acute rejection (3), and initial nonfunction and rejection (1).

Switches from Cyclosporine and Between Treatment Groups

Nine patients were switched to azathioprine and prednisone 2–51 days after transplant. Six were in the no-prednisone and 3 in the prednisone group. The reasons for switching were initial nonfunction (5), nephrotoxicity (2), inability to achieve adequate CsA levels (1), and hemolytic anemia (1). All grafts are still functioning with a serum creatinine level of 2.0 ± 0.8 mg/dl, except for 1 patient who was switched because of initial nonfunction.

Twelve patients in the no-prednisone group are on maintenance prednisone because of recurring rejection. Twelve (41%) of the 29 no-prednisone patients with functioning grafts are still receiving CsA alone. Eight patients have required no steroids.

Graft Function and Rejections

There were 33 rejection episodes treated in the no-prednisone and 30 in the prednisone group. Eight patients in the no-prednisone and 12 in the prednisone group had no rejection episodes.

The incidence of initial nonfunction was 36%; 11% in patients receiving kidneys from related donors and 45% in patients receiving cadaveric kidneys.

Table 4. Infectious Complications

	No Prednisone	Prednisone
Septicemia	1	2
Abscess	0	2 (lung, perinephric)
Systemic fungal	0	1* (candida peritonitis)
Cytomegalovirus	1 (mild)	0
Other viral†	2	6
UTI		
Simple	8	6
Recurrent	0	2
Skin and wound	3	5
Pneumonia	3	0

*This patient also had septicemia.

†Herpes zoster, herpes simplex, veruceae vulgaris, infectious mononucleosis.

The serum creatinine level of all patients 90 days after transplantation was 2.1 ± 0.7 mg/dl (Table 3). Although the serum creatinine level was higher in the no-prednisone group compared with the prednisone group on day 30, the levels in both groups were similar on day 90. Serum creatinine level at day 90 of recipients of living related grafts was 2.2 ± 0.7 mg/dl. The mean CsA level 60 days after transplantation was 209 ± 164 ng/ml, and the mean CsA dose was 9.3 ± 4.1 mg/kg/day.

Complications

The infectious complications in both groups are listed in Table 4. There are too few infections to comment on the relative incidence in the two groups. There were no neoplasms. Urologic complications were ureteric fistulae (2), a large hydrocele (2), and a necrotic ureter (1). One patient required nephrectomy 2 days after transplantation because of a renal artery thrombosis due to a kinked renal artery. Other vascular complications were deep venous thromboses (2), pul-

Table 3. Serum Creatinine Levels

Group	30 days	60 days	90 days
Total	3.7 ± 3.2 (60)*	2.1 ± 1.0 (51)	2.1 ± 0.7 (47)
Prednisone	3.1 ± 3.1 (31)	2.0 ± 1.0 (27)	2.1 ± 0.7 (24)
No prednisone	4.2 ± 3.4 (29)	2.3 ± 0.9 (24)	2.1 ± 0.7 (23)
Living related	2.1 ± 0.8 (17)	2.0 ± 0.8 (14)	2.2 ± 0.7 (13)

*Number in parentheses is number of patients.

monary embolus, and thrombophlebitis of the iliac vein. Sixteen patients in the prednisone and 10 in the no-prednisone group had hypertension. Thirteen patients had white cell counts of <3500/cc. All but 1 patient were on CsA at the time of leukopenia. Six patients had WBC counts of 2500/cc or less. They occurred 5–86 days after transplantation, and none was associated with clinical CMV infections. Leukopenia resolved in 2 patients on CsA alone immediately after they were given prednisone. Three patients (all in one center) had a Coombs-positive hemolytic anemia (mean hemoglobin level, 3.6 g/dl). One patient was switched to azathioprine and prednisone, and the hemolysis spontaneously resolved in the other 2 patients. Two episodes of hepatotoxicity (increased bilirubin and SGOT) were both associated with CsA serum trough levels greater than 700 ng/ml and resolved when the CsA dose and serum level were decreased. Other complications included the onset of seizures (2), gastritis (2), and acute pancreatitis (1). Cyclosporine-induced hirsutism, gingival hyperplasia, tremor, and parathesia occurred as previously reported, but these were not a major clinical problem.

DISCUSSION

The CTSG has reported a 1-year actuarial graft survival of 80.4% in 103 cadaveric renal transplant recipients treated with cyclosporine and prednisone.[1] The event causing graft loss occurred prior to 32 days in 15/17 patients. Although the follow-up in the current study is relatively short, the overall graft survival (86.9%) is consistent with the previous study.

Six prognostic factors were examined for their effect on graft survival, and only the presence or absence of a previous transplant had a significant effect (69.2% vs. 91.1%; $p = 0.03$). Patients who received a cadaveric kidney and who had not had previous transplant had a graft survival similar to patients who received a kidney from a related donor. No effect of transfusion on graft survival was seen. Because long perfusion time and rewarm time were detrimental to graft survival in our previous study, an attempt was made to keep these to a minimum. Only 4 patients had a perfusion time greater than 24 hr, and 4 had a rewarm time greater than 45 min; 2 of the former and none of the latter patients lost their grafts.

Maintenance steroids are used in CsA-treated patients in an attempt to achieve a graft survival and function rate superior to that achieved with CsA alone. However, the requirement for steroids has not been established. In this study, the relatively small number of patients in each group does not allow a definitive statement, but patients randomized into the no-prednisone group had a graft survival and function similar to the patients in the prednisone group. Although there was no difference in the number of rejection episodes in the two groups, 33% of the no-prednisone patients were placed on maintenance steroids because of rejection. It may be possible to wean some of these patients off steroids with time.

In our previous study, the serum creatinine level 90 days after transplantation was 2.6 ± 1.8 mg/dl, compared to 2.0 ± 1.5 mg/dl in patients treated with azathioprine and prednisone.[1] In an attempt to decrease the amount of cyclosporine nephrotoxicity, the initial CsA dose in this study was 15 mg/kg/day (compared to 20 mg/kg/day in the previous trial), and a trough CsA level of 50–300 ng/ml was aimed for. The serum creatinine level of all patients who reached 90 days after transplantation was 2.0 ± 0.7 mg/dl. There was no difference in the serum creatinine level between the prednisone and no-prednisone groups at day 90. Patients in the no-prednisone group had a higher incidence of initial nonfunction, were switched to azathioprine more frequently, and had a higher serum creatinine level at day 30 than patients on prednisone. Although none of these differences was statistically significant, they suggest that graft function during the first 30 days may be better in the prednisone than the no-prednisone group. Recipients of grafts from related donors had fewer problems with initial nonfunction than patients who received cadaveric grafts, but their serum creatinine level at 90 days (2.3 ± 0.7 mg/dl) was disappointingly high (the equivalent level in living related patients treated with azathioprine and prednisone, and excluded from the previous CTSG study, was 1.6 mg/dl).

Leukopenia has rarely been reported in CsA-treated patients. However, in this study, 19% of patients had a white blood cell count of <3500/cc, and 6 had counts of 2500/cc or less. Cytomegalovirus infection can cause leukopenia. None of these patients had clinical CMV infections, but subclinical CMV infections cannot be excluded. Because leukopenia is not as severe as that seen with azathioprine therapy, it may have been missed in the past. The previously reported trend toward an increased incidence of vascular complications (especially renal artery stenosis and thrombosis)[1] in CsA-treated patients was not seen in this study.

This study confirms that cyclosporine is an effective immunosuppressant in renal transplantation during the first few months following transplantation and that acceptable graft survival can be achieved with CsA alone. However, graft survival in patients who have had a previous failed transplant continues to be disappointing. Although not optimal, graft function as reflected by the serum creatinine level has improved compared to a previous study conducted by our group. This may be due to shorter rewarm and perfusion times, a lower CsA dose, or more experience with the drug, but this has not been established. To determine if maintenance steroids are needed in CsA-treated patients, a large double-blind study of maintenance prednisone vs. placebo is required.

ACKNOWLEDGMENTS

We acknowledge the support of the Medical Research Council of Canada, Richard and Jean Ivey Fund, London, Ontario; Sandoz Ltd., Basel; the Michael Fung Endowment Fund, London, Ontario; and the University Hospital Transplant Research Fund, London, Ontario. Centers involved in this study were Vancouver General Hospital (C. E. Reeve), University of Alberta Hospital, Edmonton (F. Harley), Calgary Foothills Hospital (J. Klassen), Health Sciences Centre, Winnipeg (J. Jeffery), Toronto General Hospital (P. Halloran), Toronto St. Michael's Hospital (R. Bear), St. Joseph's Hospital, Hamilton (D. Ludwin), Montreal General Hospital (M. Mangel), Notre Dame Hospital (P. Daloze), Maisonneuve-Rosemont Hospital (R. Dandavino), Victoria General Hospital, Halifax (P. Belitsky), and University Hospital, London (P. Keown). Executive Committee: G. Arbus, R. Bear, R. Dandavino, J. B. Dossetor, J. Jeffery, A. S. MacDonald (Chairman), M. Robinette, C. R. Stiller. Management Committee, Centre for Transplant Studies and Statistical Consultants: H. Cheung, M. Gent, M. Grace, W. Howson, P. A. Keown, J. Koval, A. Laupacis, B. Lockwood, I. MacNeill, L. Moist, N. R. Sinclair, C. R. Stiller, G. Wells.

REFERENCES

1. Canadian Transplant Study Group: A Randomized Clinical Trial of Cyclosporine in Cadaveric Renal Transplants (in press)

2. Report on the European Multicentre Trial: Lancet 2:57, 1982

A Prospective Randomized Substitutive Trial of Cyclosporine as a Prophylactic Agent in Human Renal Transplant Rejection

Presented by R. A. Sells

ALTHOUGH the fungal cyclicpeptide cyclosporine A (CsA) (Sandimmun) is known to be a potent immunosuppressive in reducing graft rejection in humans, early trials indicated that high doses of the drug combined with concurrent steroids were associated with severe infection and an unacceptably high incidence of tumors.[1] For this reason, and because CsA presented the first opportunity for steroid-free immunosuppression in human transplant recipients, Calne and his colleagues developed the first extensively applied CsA regime[2] and demonstrated successful suppression in diuresing cadaveric transplant recipients. Because of these encouraging results and the desire to explore long-term CsA prophylaxis *without* steroids, a prospective randomized trial was set up to compare CsA alone with azathioprine (Aza) and prednisolone (P) in recipients of immediately functioning first and second cadaveric renal transplants. The preliminary results have been published,[3] and this report gives the results updated to a minimum patient follow-up of 1 year.

MATERIALS AND METHODS

Patients in each participating center who were admitted for cadaveric renal transplantation between January 1 and December 31, 1981, were considered eligible for the trial. The criteria for entering patients into the trial were as follows: recipients of immediately functioning first and second cadaveric renal grafts who showed no evidence of chronic liver disease or antibodies against hepatitis B surface antigen, who were not insulin-dependent diabetics, and who had not received immunosuppressive agents during the previous 3 months. Informed consent was obtained from these patients after an explanation of the purpose of the trial and the method of allocation to it. Pretransplant dialysis and transfusion, cadaveric renal transplantation, and HLA-A,B and HLA-DR matching of donor and recipient were carried out according to the policy of each individual unit. Patients who were not electively transfused before transplantation received 2 units of whole blood during the operation. All patients were given 500 mg methylprednisolone intravenously before the vascular clamps were released from the graft. Early diuresis was encouraged by ensuring adequate hydration during anesthesia (usually with maintenance of a central venous pressure around 11 cm H_2O) together with the elective administration of 30–40 g mannitol intravenously or, if heart failure was present, up to 250 mg furosemide. In some centers, dopamine 1–3 μg/kg/min was administered intravenously for 5 days. The urine volume was observed postoperatively for 6 hr, and if the flow from the graft exceeded a mean value of 50 ml/hr, the patient was declared eligible for the trial. Randomization was then carried out using sealed envelopes, and each patient was allocated to receive Aza and P (control group) or CsA (experimental group).

In the control group, conventional prophylactic antirejection therapy was prescribed in accordance with each unit's usual policy, which consisted of azathioprine 1–2 mg/kg orally (with or without a single loading dose of 5 mg/kg given intravenously), rising to a maintenance dose of 2.5–3 mg/kg, or less if bone marrow suppression occurred, and prednisolone 20 mg/day orally. Rejection was treated in this group according to each center's practice, either by giving repeated daily injections of 0.5 g or 1 g methylprednisolone intravenously or by increasing the dose of oral prednisolone to 3 mg/kg/day, with 25 mg/day decrements every 3 days eventually reverting to 20 mg/day maintenance; after 6 months, this dose was reduced by 1 mg/day each month.

Patients in the experimental group were given CsA prophylaxis alone: For the first 14 days, a maintenance dose of 17 mg/kg/day was given in divided doses every 12 hr, initially by intramuscular injection (up to four doses) and then orally. The dose was reduced at day 15 to 15 mg/kg/day and at monthly intervals thereafter by 2 mg/kg/day to a maintenance dosage of 6 mg/kg/day. This regimen was modified in the event of acute systemic side effects (such as jaundice, vomiting, or severe tremor), evidence of nephrotoxicity, or a predose plasma CsA concentration exceeding the recommended level of 400 μg/ml as indicated by serial determination using a

---

From eight European Centers (see Acknowledgments).

Reprint requests should be addressed to R. A. Sells, Royal Liverpool Hospital, Prescot Street, Liverpool L78XP, UK.

0041-1345/83/1505-0055$01.00/0

this CsA-treated group (86.7%) is significantly superior to the survival rate in CsA patients who received 3 or more prior transfusions (68.9%; $p < 0.005$).

Long-Term Graft Function

The previously noted nephrotoxic effect of CsA[4] was studied by measuring serial serum creatinine levels in control patients and in CsA patients who remained on their original treatment for 1 year. The results are plotted in Fig. 2, from which it may be seen that there is a consistently higher mean serum creatinine in the CsA group than among the controls. No significant deterioration in renal function was seen in either group between 4 months and 1 year after transplantation.

Side Effects

In the CsA group, the most common problem, hirsutism, occurred in 37% of cases and varied in severity from a minimal increase in facial hair to considerable hairiness of trunk or limbs. The problems causing most concern in the CsA-treated patients were anorexia, nausea, and tremor, which caused conversion to conventional treatment in 6 cases. Gingival hypertrophy, seen in 32 patients, ranged from mild (in 19 cases) to severe enough to require formal dental hygiene (in 5). Two benign breast lumps have been removed from 2 CsA patients (one fibroadenoma, one gynecomastia). Transient hyperbilirubinemia (serum bilirubin exceeding 30 μmole/liter on at least one occasion) was seen in 23 CsA patients.

In the control patients, the dominant side effect has been the development of a Cushingoid appearance in 54%, and 14 patients developed bone marrow depression, requiring cessation of azathioprine therapy. There were three cases of peptic ulceration, two requiring surgery, and one (gastric) ulcer contributed to the patient's death.

Infections were observed with equal frequency and proportion in each group: CsA-treated patients suffered 84 bacterial, 17 viral, and 3 fungal infections, and in the control group, 93 bacterial, 19 viral, and 1 fungal infections occurred.

Excluded Patients

During the period of the trial, 99 patients received grafts with early postoperative oliguria and were thus excluded from the trial and were given azathioprine and prednisolone postoperatively. The graft survival probability estimate in this group is 53%, the same as in the trial control group.

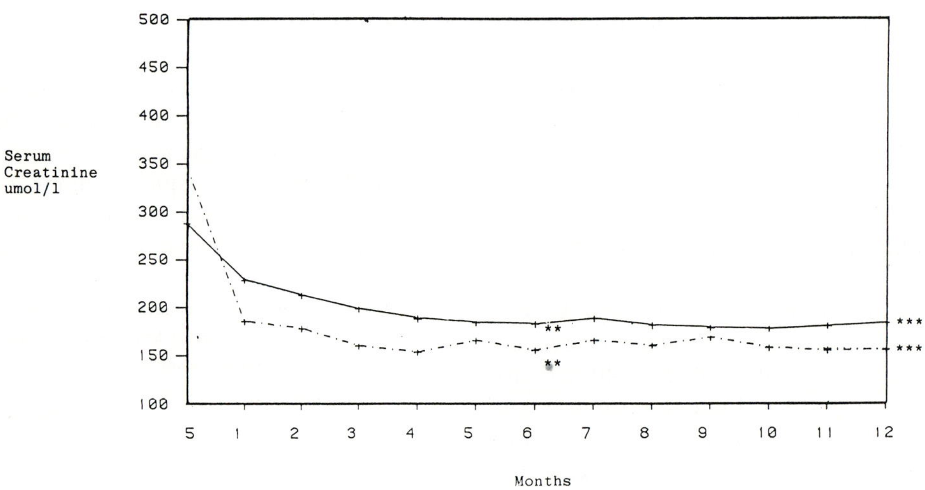

Fig. 2. **Mean creatinine levels of patients with graft functioning at 1 year ($p = 0.003$ at 6 months, <0.001 at 1 year).**

DISCUSSION

The 1-year follow-up in both groups of patients presented here confirms our first cautiously expressed view that renal transplant survival is superior in patients treated with CsA as a first-line immunosuppressive compared with azathioprine and steroid prophylaxis.[3] There does not seem to be any difference in patient survival between the two groups, and the incidence of infections appears equal. The precise diagnosis of CsA nephrotoxicity is difficult to achieve in all cases and may only be recognized retrospectively after the drug has been stopped. Routine blood level estimations,[6] when more widely available, will undoubtedly enable improved titration of dosage against function, with, hopefully, a reduction in toxicity, but recent observations indicate that histologic appearances of CsA-induced renal injury may look very similar to those of immune rejection (Mihatsch, unpublished data). Despite these diagnostic difficulties, 84 patients (72%) of the CsA group had functioning grafts at 1 year—60 (51%) of whom were maintained on CsA alone—compared with 51% in the control group.

For the first time we report here a demonstrable difference in graft survival in CsA-treated patients who have or have not received blood transfusions. The marked difference in 1-year survival (86.7% in untransfused vs. 68.9% in multiply transfused recipients) appeared despite transfusion of 2 units into all previously untransfused patients at the operation. The control patients exhibited the "transfusion effect,"[7] with a 10% improvement in graft survival after multiple transfusions.

The possible interaction between blood transfusions and CsA in transplantation has recently been investigated in experimental animals: The pretransplant administration of donor-specific blood together with CsA induced considerable heart-graft prolongation in Lewis recipients of AC1 and BUF hearts;[8] Homans et al. described similar results using spleen cells and CsA;[9] and Dumble et al. have shown that skin-graft survival was prolonged in rabbits treated with CsA and donor blood before grafting.[10] Divergent results, however, were obtained by Marquet et al., who, using BN hearts transplanted into Wag recipients, indicated that CsA given postoperatively abrogated the immunosuppressive effect of adoptively transferred, blood transfusion–induced isogeneic suppressor cells, with consequent loss of graft protection. This last experiment seems to mimic more closely the clinical situation reported in this trial concerning blood transfusion and CsA. However, the explanation for our observation must await further studies, in particular, assays for peripheral blood suppressor cells in humans. But the prospect of abandoning preemptive transfusion, with its risk of sensitization, in favor of postoperative CsA therapy alone is an attractive one, although more data on graft survival in untransfused CsA-treated recipients is needed before transfusions are abandoned. Meanwhile, the results of this trial indicate a superior outcome in patients treated with CsA alone, and its adoption as a first-line immunosuppressive drug in clinical renal transplantation seems justified.

ACKNOWLEDGMENTS

The following centers participated in this study: Basle (F. Harder, R. Loertscher); Cambridge (R. Y. Calne, D. J. G. White); Hannover (R. Pichlmayr, J. Klempnauer); Innsbruck (R. Margreiter, M. Spielberger); Liverpool (R. A. Sells, J. W. Colbert); Manchester (R. W. G. Johnson, M. Wise); Munich (W. Land, H. Lutjens); Portsmouth (M. Slapak, H. A. Lee). Trial coordination and data analysis: Sandoz Ltd., Feltham, UK, and Basle, Switzerland (T. Beveridge, W. Maurer, T. W. Poole, E. Wiskott, A. J. Wood).

REFERENCES

1. Beveridge T: Transplant Proc 15:433, 1983
2. Calne RY, White DJG, Evans DB, et al: Br Med J 282:934, 1981
3. Report on the European Multicentre Trial: Lancet 2:57, 1982
4. Donatsch P, Abisch E, Homberger M: J Immunoassay 2:19, 1981

5. Kaplan EL, Meier P: J Am Statist Assoc 53:457, 1958

6. White DJG, McNaughton D, Calne RY: Transplant Proc 15:454, 1983

7. Opelz G, Sengar DPS, Terasaki PI: Transplant Proc 5:253, 1973

8. Miller CM, Martinelli GP, Racelis D, et al: Transplantation 33:335, 1982

9. Homans WP, Williams KA, Millard PR, et al: Transplantation 31:423, 1981

10. Dumble LJ, King HP, Clunie GJA, et al: Transplant Proc 15:1000, 1983

Living Related Kidney Transplants Treated with Cyclosporine

T. Oka, Y. Ohmori, I. Aikawa, J. Ioka, Y. Kadotani, H. Nomura, S. Suzuki, and I. Hashimoto

CYCLOSPORINE (CsA), a powerful new immunosuppressant, has improved the 1-year graft survival from a previous 50%–55% to nearly 80% in recipients of kidney grafts from cadaveric donors.[1,2]

There are, however, fewer reports on its clinical use in living related kidney transplants where the matching levels of histocompatibility is uniform, and primarily better graft survivals have been achieved with conventional immunosuppressive therapy consisting of azathioprine and steroids. The question is whether it is justifiable to apply CsA to these recipients, running the risk of nephrotoxicity.

We started clinical trials of CsA in parent-to-child kidney transplants in April 1982. The present report describes our initial experiences in these patients treated with CsA, especially in regard to their graft function and the association between CsA plasma levels and the occurrence of side effects.

MATERIALS AND METHODS

Patients

Twenty patients, including 3 children under the age of 12 years, received kidney transplants from their parents between April 1982 and April 1983. The age of the recipients ranged from 8 to 40 years. The follow-up period was 3–55 weeks, with a mean of 30 weeks.

Immunosuppression

CsA was administered orally in a dose of 10 mg/kg for 5 days before transplantation, expecting a sufficient state of immunosuppression to be achieved at the time of operation. Postoperatively, CsA was given in a single daily dose of 14 mg/kg, tapering by 2 mg/kg each month until a maintenance dose of 8 mg/kg was reached. The dose of CsA was reduced at the time when plasma levels were high or when major side effects appeared.

When CsA was used in combination with steroids, the steroid dose was half that used in our conventional immunosuppressive regimen. Prednisolone (50 mg/day) was administered on the day of transplantation, supplemented by 1 g of intravenous methylprednisolone during operation, and tapered to a maintenance dose of 10 mg/day at 3 months. Acute rejection crises were treated with bolus doses of methylprednisolone.

Plasma Levels of Cyclosporine

CsA plasma levels were measured using a radioimmunoassay kit (supplied by Sandoz Ltd., Basel). Twenty-four-hour pharmacokinetic activity was determined in the patients on two occasions: when they were on hemodialysis before transplantation and when the grafts were functioning well. For posttransplant monitoring, CsA trough and peak levels were determined just prior to and 2–4 hr after oral administration of the drug at intervals of a few days.

RESULTS

Graft Outcome

All the grafts showed good diuresis soon after revascularization, and serum creatinine (S-Cr) levels fell to normal range within a week after transplantation. To date, all the patients have functioning grafts, except one who died of acute pancreatitis at 3 months after transplantation. In 2 of these patients, CsA was converted to bredinin and then to azathioprine at 1 month because of leukocytopenia, probably induced by latent cytomegalovirus infections, evidenced by inclusion bodies discovered in incidental biopsy specimens of gastric mucosa. S-Cr levels began to rise in five patients to over 2.0 mg/dl at 1–6 months after transplantation, although the rate subsequently stabilized (see Fig. 1).

Rejection Episodes

The patients treated with CsA had a significantly lower incidence of acute rejection epi-

From the Department of Surgery, Kyoto Prefectural University of Medicine, Kyoto, Japan.

Reprint requests should be addressed to Dr. T. Oka, Department of Surgery, Kyoto Prefectural University of Medicine, Hirokoji, Kawaramachi, Kamikyoku, Kyoto 602, Japan.

0041-1345/83/1505-0056$01.00/0

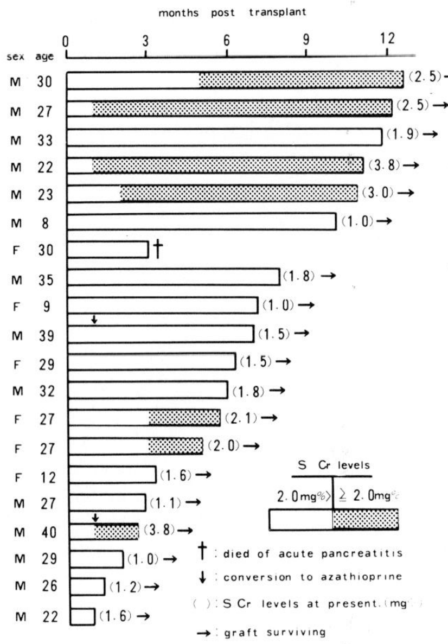

Fig. 1. Graft survival in 20 living related kidney transplant recipients treated with cyclosporine. Horizontal arrows indicate that patients are surviving with functioning grafts and a cross means death of a patient. Vertical arrows show the time when cyclosporine was changed to conventional immunosuppressive therapy. Shaded areas represent serum creatinine levels of more than 2.0 mg/dl. Serum creatinine levels at present are shown in parentheses.

sodes, even though the steroids had been reduced by half the level used in conventional immunosuppression ($P < 0.05$) (Table 1). Patients experiencing these episodes with CsA immunosuppression were often afebrile and had no graft swelling. In the later stages, there was a slow and slight rise of S-Cr levels, but patients never required hemodialysis. To date, no graft has been lost due to rejection.

Side Effects and Complications

The side effects of CsA did not cause great morbidity in our patients (Table 2). Hirsutism was most common and seen in almost all. This was especially prominent in two 9- and 12-year-old girls, although this subsided with a reduction of the CsA dose. Tremor and gingival hypertrophy were less common. No serious systemic infection was encountered. Acute pancreatitis, the only cause of death in one patient, was not considered to be related to CsA therapy.

Table 1. Frequency of Acute Rejection

Immunosuppression	Cases	Crises	Frequency
Conventional	151	79	52%
Cyclosporine	20	6	30%*

*$p < 0.05$.

Table 2. Complications and Side Effects of Cyclosporine in 20 Living Related Kidney Transplants

Complication or Side Effect	No. of Cases	Percentage
Hirsutism	15	75%
Hypertension	14	70%
Nephrotoxicity	7	35%
Hepatotoxicity	7	35%
Tremor	6	30%
Infection		
Cystitis	3	15%
CMV infection	2	10%
Leukocytopenia	2	10%
Acute pancreatitis	1	5%
Gum hypertrophy	1	5%

Frequent and important side effects of CsA were hepatotoxicity and nephrotoxicity. Hepatotoxicity, defined as a higher serum concentration of more than 100 Karmen units of transaminases, were observed in 7/20 (35%) patients. Two of these patients also had hyperbilirubinemia. These episodes were resolved with a reduction of CsA or with conversion from a single to a divided administration of the same daily CsA dose. Acute nephrotoxicity, which was diagnosed by increased S-Cr levels of more than 30% of baseline, an improvement of impaired renal function with a reduction of CsA dose, and/or the absence of diffuse interstitial-cell infiltration in histology, was experienced in 7 (35%) cases. These acute nephrotoxicity episodes responded well to a reduction of the CsA dose, but a slightly deteriorated renal function at a later stage was a matter of some concern. The mean S-Cr level in the CsA-treated patients, except for 3 pediatric patients, was significantly higher at 3 months ($p < 0.001$) and 6 months ($p < 0.001$) after transplantation, compared with that of the patients treated with conventional immunosuppression, suggesting chronic nephrotoxicity caused by CsA (see Fig. 2).

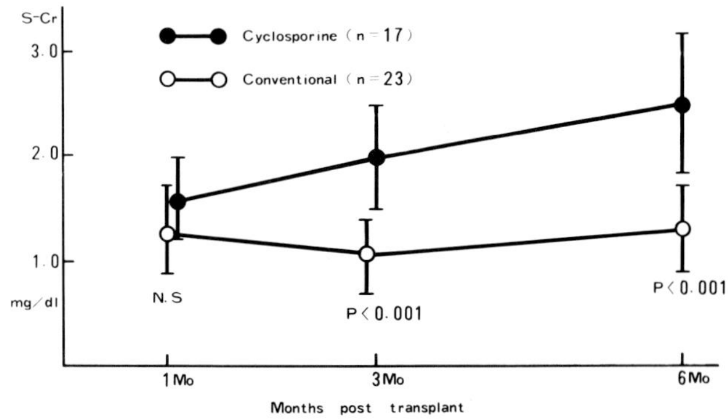

Fig. 2. Posttransplant changes of serum creatinine levels (mean ± S.E.). Serum creatinine levels in 17 patients treated with cyclosporine are significantly higher than those in 23 patients with conventional immunosuppressive therapy at 3 and 6 posttransplant months ($p <$ 0.001).

Cyclosporine Plasma Levels

In 24-hr pharmacokinetic studies of CsA in nine patients with functioning grafts, given an oral dose of 14 mg/kg, plasma levels reached a peak, ranging from 600 to 2000 ng/ml at 2–4 hr after administration, and tapered to trough levels of 100–400 ng/ml (Fig. 3). Thus, a marked difference in the ability to absorb and to eliminate CsA was found among individuals.

CsA plasma levels in nine patients on hemodialysis, given in oral dose of 10 g/kg, are shown in Fig. 4. Five of nine patients showed almost the same pattern of absorption and elimination as those with functioning grafts. In the remaining four, the peak time was delayed showing a bipolar pattern. In any case, trough levels of CsA in patients requiring hemodialysis were low. These results indicate that in patients suffering from acute tubular necrosis following cadaveric kidney transplant, CsA can be safely given without apprehension for its accumulation in the body.

Cyclosporine Plasma Levels and Toxicity

Peak and trough levels of CsA in plasma were compared between patients with nephro- and/or hepatotoxicity and those without them during the first and the second months after transplantation. In patients with toxicity, a mean ± SE of all values assayed during 10 days before and after its onset were evaluated for comparison.

The episodes of hepatoxicity were concentrated during the first month, while those of nephrotoxicity were distributed over 2 months.

The incidence of nephrotoxic episodes was significantly dependent on the CsA trough

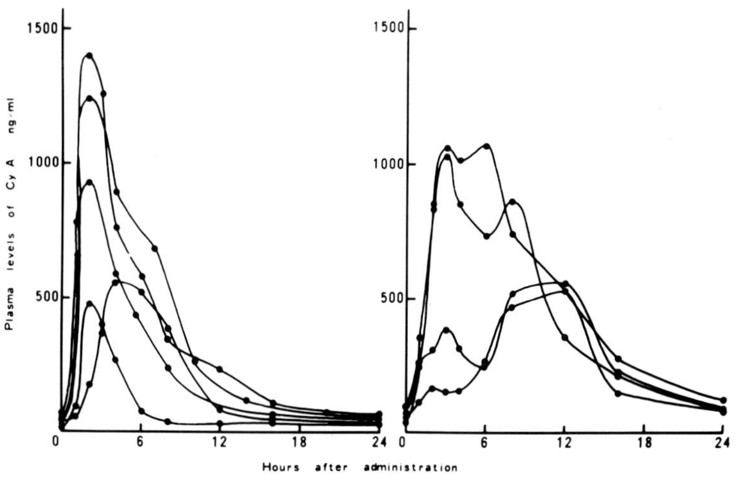

Fig. 3. Twenty-four-hour pharmacokinetic studies of cyclosporine plasma levels in 9 patients with well functioning grafts at a single oral dose of 14 mg/kg.

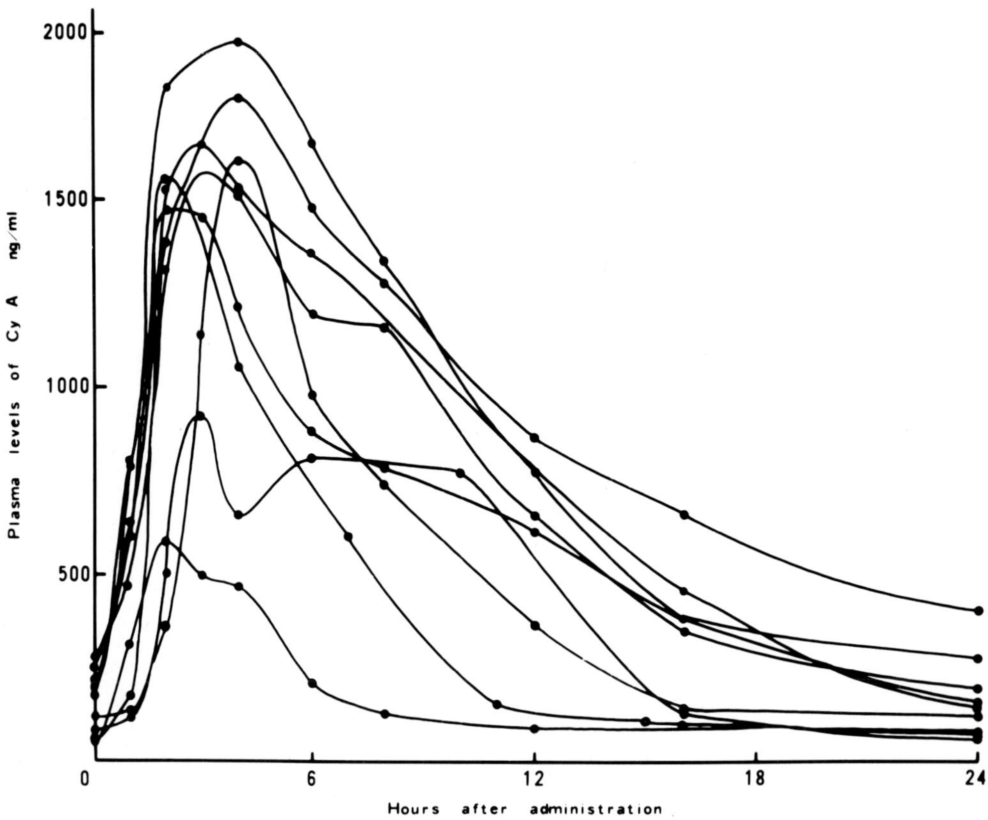

Fig. 4. Twenty-four-hour pharmacokinetic studies of cyclosporine plasma levels in 9 patients on hemodialysis before transplantation at a single oral dose of 10 mg/kg. Two different patterns are observed; five patients show almost the same pattern as those with functioning grafts (left), and in the remaining 4, the peak time is delayed, showing a biopolar pattern (right).

levels during the first month ($p < 0.01$) and on the peak levels during the second month ($p < 0.05$). The trough levels in the patients with hepatotoxicity were also significantly higher than those in the quiescent patients ($p < 0.05$), whereas there was no difference in peak levels among the patient groups during the first month (Table 3).

Mean Daily Dose of Cyclosporine and Serum Creatinine Levels

The association between a mean daily dose of CsA/kg during each month of post-transplantation and S-Cr levels at the end of the month were assessed retrospectively, in an attempt to search for an optimal CsA dose in living related kidney transplants (Fig. 5).

Table 3. Association Between CsA Plasma Levels and Side Effects

	1–30 Days After Transplantation			31–60 Days After Transplantation		
	No. of Patients	Trough (ng/ml)	Peak (ng/ml)	No. of Patients	Trough (ng/ml)	Peak (ng/ml)
Quiescence*	5	109 ± 11	1088 ± 64	6	114 ± 17	674 ± 61
Hepatotoxicity†	7	209 ± 32‡	1209 ± 146	—	—	—
Nephrotoxicity†	4	222 ± 26§	1125 ± 135	3	185 ± 24	1001 ± 102‡

*Mean ± SE of values assayed during 30 days.

†Mean ± SE of values assayed during 10 days before and after onset.

‡$p < 0.01$.

§$p < 0.05$.

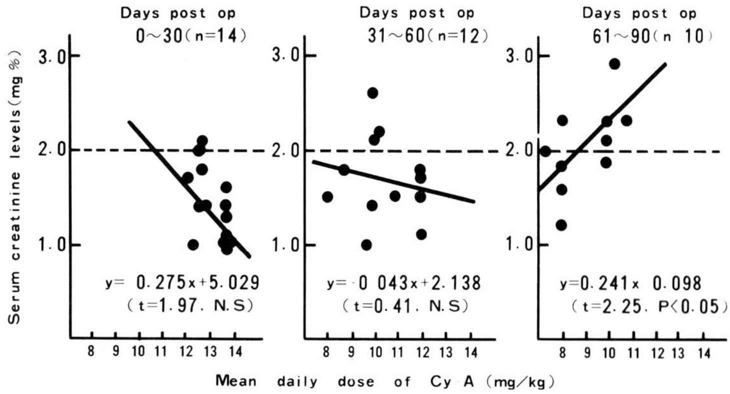

Fig. 5. Mean daily dose of cyclosporine (mg/kg) during each posttransplant month and serum creatinine level (mg/dl) at the end of each month. Significant correlation is found between daily dose of cyclosporine and serum creatinine level during the third posttransplant month.

During the first month, a mean daily dose of 14 mg/kg was efficiently and safely administered for a maintenance of S-Cr levels below 2 mg/dl. During the second month, no association was found between S-Cr levels and a mean CsA dose. On the other hand, during the third month, a significant correlation was found ($p < 0.05$): The larger the daily dose, the higher the S-Cr levels. As a result, it is likely that an optimal CsA dose is 14 mg/kg/day during the first month and below 8 mg/kg/day during the third month in living related kidney transplants.

DISCUSSION

The graft survival rate in our 170 consecutive living related kidney transplants treated with conventional immunosuppression was 84% at 1 year and 67% at 5 years. However, there were considerable complications, including fatal infections (6%) and aseptic necrosis of femoral heads (28%). Expecting CsA to achieve better graft survival and less morbidity, we started clinical application in living related kidney transplants. Although a long-term prognosis cannot be made, since the number of patients is too small and the follow-up period too short, it has been encouraging that to date no graft has been lost due to rejection and there have been no life-threatening complications. Not only were acute rejection episodes significantly less frequent, but they also were easily reversed in the CsA-treated patients, compared with those under conventional immunosuppression. These results show the potent immunosuppressive activity of CsA, especially in the early stage of post-transplantation.

However, episodes of nephrotoxicity were not infrequent in this series. Peak CsA plasma levels during the first month were almost the same in all patients, ranging from 1000 to 1200 ng/ml, whereas trough levels were significantly higher in the patients with toxicity. This suggests that our starting dose of 14 mg/kg can be safely administered, unless patients have decreased ability to eliminate the drug, causing high trough levels. On the other hand, nephrotoxicity during the second month is thought to be caused by an overdose of CsA, since peak levels were significantly lower in the quiescent patients.

S-Cr levels at a later stage of post-transplantation were higher in the CsA-treated patients, although not progressive, in accordance with the findings reported by Ferguson et al., who supposed it to be due to mild chronic nephrotoxicity of the drug.[3]

Our retrospective analysis of an association between a mean of daily dose CsA during each posttransplant month and S-Cr levels reveals that initially too much CsA was used in our trials. Immunosuppression with a reduced dose of CsA as well as the routine monitoring of peak and trough levels will hereafter hopefully decrease the incidence of toxicity in living related kidney transplants; otherwise, some new trials, such as a conversion from CsA to azathioprine at a certain stage of posttransplantation[4] or an alternate-day administration of CsA,[5] may be feasible.

REFERENCES

1. Calne RY, White DJG, Evans DB, et al: Br Med J 282:934, 1981

2. Starzl TE, Weil R, Iwatsuki S, et al: Surg Gynecol Obstet 151:17, 1981

3. Ferguson RM, Rynasiewicz JJ, Sutherland DER, et al: Surgery 92:175, 1982

4. Morris PJ, French ME, Ting A, et al: In White DJG (ed): Cyclosporin A, Amsterdam, Elsevier Biomedical, 1982, p 355

5. Ferguson RM, Rynasiewicz JJ, Najarian JS, et al: Transplant Proc 15:480, 1983

Improved Outcome in Renal Transplant Recipients Above 55 Years of Age Treated with Cyclosporine and Low Doses of Steroids

O. Ringdén, L. Öst, G. Klintmalm, A. Tillegård, I. Fehrman, H. Wilczek, and C. G. Groth

IN MANY CENTERS, uremic patients of advanced age have not been considered for renal transplantation. During the last 10 years, we have accepted an increasing number of patients up to 70 years of age. In these elderly patients, graft rejection was less common than in younger renal transplant recipients.[1,2] Nevertheless, graft and patient survival was poorer in the older patients. This was due to high morbidity and mortality consequent to infections and cardiovascular, cerebrovascular, and gastrointestinal complications. Furthermore, the elderly patients had a higher incidence of steroid diabetes and osteonecrosis, complications that could be attributed to steroid therapy. Because of the poor outcome following renal transplantation when using conventional immunosuppression in patients of advanced age, these patients were selected for a trial with the new immunosuppressive agent, cyclosporine A (CsA).[3,4] In this trial, we also included some other high-risk patients, namely, those who had diabetic nephropathy, those who did not tolerate azathioprine, and children. CsA is a powerful inhibitor of T cell–dependent immune reactions;[5] in renal transplantation, the drug has been given either alone[6] or together with low doses of steroids.[3,4,7] We report here our experience of using CsA in these special-category patients. Special emphasis is on the results in the patients above 55 years of age.

MATERIALS AND METHODS

Between January 1980 and February 1983, 57 renal transplant recipients were treated with CsA. Thirty-one nondiabetic patients were 55 years of age or older. The mean age of these patients was 60 years, with a range from 55 to 71 years. All 31 patients received cadaveric kidneys. Twenty-four of the patients received their first graft, 5 their second graft, and 2 their third. Nine diabetic patients (age range, 37–60 years) received a cadaveric kidney, 8 of them for the first time and 1 for the second time. Seven other recipients of cadaveric kidneys (age range, 28–53 years) were treated with CsA because of assumed or proven azathioprine intolerance, 5 of them receiving their second renal graft. First kidney grafts from living related donors were given to 10 recipients (age range, 2–40 years). Two of these were children, 2 and 13 years of age, respectively, and 1 of them was a diabetic; the remaining 7 patients were assumed to have a reduced tolerance to azathioprine.

When the trial was started, the CsA treatment was begun at 17 mg/kg/day.[3] The dose was then reduced by 2 mg/kg every month until it reached 9 mg/kg. Approximately halfway through the study, the protocol was changed. The initial dose was reduced to 15 mg/kg/day, and the first reduction was carried out at 2 weeks. Two months after transplantation, the dose had been dropped to 9 mg/kg/day. If side effects occurred, the dose was reduced at a faster rate.

On the day of operation, 0.5 g of i.v. hydrocortisone was given. Early on, prednisolone was started at 60 mg/day; later in the study, the initial dose was 100 mg/day. The dose was tapered to reach 15 mg/day after 1 month and 10 mg/day after 3 months. With both protocols, the accumulated steroid dose during the first 6 months was 2.7 g. Rejection episodes were treated with i.v. methylprednisolone, 1.5–1.75 g given over a 5-to-9-day period.[4]

The outcomes for the nondiabetic patients 55 years of age or older who were treated with CsA were compared to those for 92 grafts in 83 patients above 55 years of age who were treated with conventional immunosuppression and received their transplants between 1973 and 1980. These patients were given azathioprine in a standard dose (1–3 mg/day). Early on, prednisolone was started at a dose of 200 or 120 mg/day. The dose was then tapered to 30–40 mg/day at 1 month and 10 mg/day at 1 year. The accumulated steroid dose for the first 6 months was 6.8 or 6.2 g. Many of these patients were given horse antilymphocyte globulin during the first 2 weeks (Behringwerke, Germany).[8] In 1979–80, prednisolone therapy was begun at a dose of 40 or 30 mg/day (accumulated dose, 5.3 or

---

From the Department of Transplantation Surgery, Huddinge Hospital, Karolinska Institute, Stockholm, Sweden.

Reprint requests should be addressed to Dr. O. Ringdén, Department of Transplantation Surgery, Huddinge Hospital, S-141 86 Huddinge, Sweden.

0041–1345/83/1505–0057$01.00/0

4.5 g). Many of these patients were given high-potency rabbit antithymocyte globulin for 2 weeks.[9] Among these patients, the treatment of rejection varied from a total of 1.75–5.0 g of i.v. methylprednisolone given over a period of 5 to 9 days.

The statistical analysis of the actuarial survival curves was made with Student's t test. In the analysis of absolute numbers, Fisher's exact probability test and/or X^2 analysis with Yates' correction were used.

RESULTS

Side Effects

Among our 57 patients treated with CsA, the following side effects could be attributed to CsA treatment: nephrotoxicity in 36 (63%), tremor in 16 (28%), hepatotoxicity in 11 (19%), hirsutism in 16 (28%), and gingival hyperplasia in 13 (23%). Hirsutism occurred in 13/24 of the younger patients and in 3/33 of the patients above 55 years of age ($p < 0.01$).

Most side effects could be reversed by reducing the dose of CsA. The most disturbing of these side effects was nephrotoxicity: This occurred once in 17 patients, twice in 9 patients, three times in 2 patients, and four times in 3 patients. Because of nephrotoxicity, 8 patients were switched to therapy with azathioprine.

Infections

Infections were common. Six patients had serious cytomegalovirus (CMV) infections. Three older patients died of CMV interstitial pneumonitis, in spite of discontinuation of CsA. Oral herpes simplex infections were seen in six patients, and one patient had keratitis caused by this virus. Four patients developed septicemia and three patients had bronchopneumonia; one diabetic patient died of bronchopneumonia. Two patients developed Legionnaires' disease; both survived. A 63-year-old woman with a Bricker bladder was given a third cadaveric kidney graft; she developed an intraabdominal abscess and septicemia and died of bronchopneumonia. Wound infections occurred in two patients and pyelitis or pyelonephritis in three.

Rejections

Twenty-five patients (44%) never had a rejection episode, 24 patients had one, 4 had two, and 3 had three. The rejections could easily be reversed by the use of i.v. steroids. Only two grafts were lost because of rejection while on therapy. One irreversible rejection occurred 2 weeks after transplantation; the other occurred in a patient who had been switched to azathioprine because of nephrotoxicity.

Patient and Graft Survival

Six of the 9 diabetic patients receiving cadaveric grafts have functioning kidneys 7–37 months after transplantation. Thrombosis occurred in one kidney 7 months after transplantation, and the patient died 2 months later on dialysis. Another diabetic patient died of bronchopneumonia and septicemia 9 months after transplantation. In a 57-year-old diabetic patient who developed Legionnaires' disease, CsA was discontinued and the graft was rejected; the patient is now back on dialysis.

Among the seven patients with azathioprine intolerance who received cadaveric kidneys, one lost his graft due to early rejection; the other six grafts are functioning 3–19 months after transplantation.

All of the 10 kidneys obtained from relatives are functioning 3–37 months after transplantation.

Patients above 55 years of age. Among the CsA-treated patients over 55 years of age, four died of infections and one graft was rejected after the patient had been switched to azathioprine. Four more grafts were lost. A 55-year-old man with glomerulonephritis received a third graft, which never functioned. This graft, as well as the two earlier ones, showed signs of glomerulonephritis. Two further kidney grafts never functioned, one probably because of preservation damage and another because of vascular thrombosis. One renal graft was lost because of thrombosis 2 weeks after transplantation. One of the patients with a nonfunctioning graft died later of an arrhythmia during dialysis. Thus, 9/31 grafts were lost among these patients.

Among the 29 patients above 55 years of age who were treated with CsA and received their first or second cadaveric kidney, the actuarial 2-year graft survival rate was 73% (Fig. 1). The corresponding figure in 83 patients 55 years of age or older and treated with conventional immunosuppression during the preceding 7-year period was 41% ($p < 0.01$) (Fig. 1). The actuarial patient-survival rate at 2 years was 85% among the CsA patients compared with 59% among the controls ($p < 0.01$) (Fig. 2).

The two groups of patients above 55 years of age were compared for a number of factors that may have influenced the graft and patient survival rates, such as age, number of second grafts, pretransplant dialysis,[10] pretransplant blood transfusions,[10] and HLA-A,B[11] and HLA-DR match grade[12] (Table 1). There was a significantly higher proportion of patients in the CsA group who had received pretransplant blood transfusions (93%) than in the group of patients treated with conventional immunosuppression (77%) ($p < 0.05$).

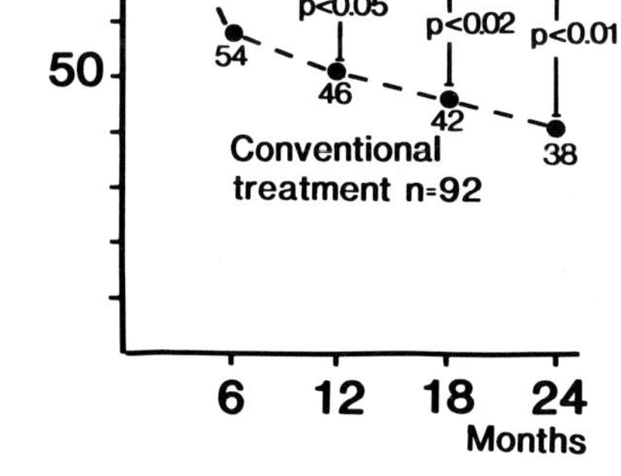

Fig. 1. Actuarial kidney graft survival in patients 55 years of age or older treated with cyclosporine A and in patients receiving conventional immunosuppressive treatment (first and second grafts only).

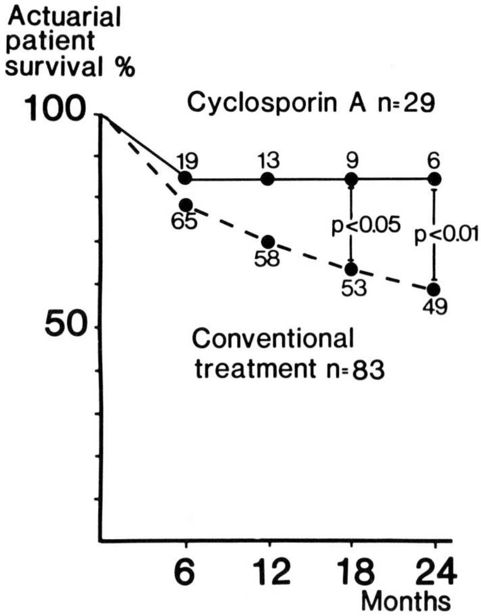

Fig. 2. Actuarial patient survival in patients 55 years of age or older treated with cyclosporine A and in patients receiving conventional immunosuppressive treatment (first and second grafts only).

Otherwise there was no difference between the two groups regarding the various prognostic factors.

The frequencies of a number of complications occurring within 6 months after transplantation that could be attributed to the immunosuppressive treatment in general or the steroid therapy in particular were compared among the 92 controls and the 22 patients treated with CsA that had a follow-up time of at least 6 months. There were no significant differences between the two groups (Table 2).

DISCUSSION

Several of the well-known side effects of CsA treatment were seen among our patients. Hepatotoxicity, tremor, and hirsutism disappeared or improved when the dose of CsA was reduced. Interestingly, hirsutism was more common among the younger patients. The incidence of gingival hyperplasia in this series is probably underestimated: In a smaller group of the patients examined by a dentist,

Table 1. Factors Possibly Affecting First- and Second-Graft Survival Rates Among Renal Transplant Recipients Above 55 Years of Age

Period	Treatment	No. of Patients	Patient Age (mean ± SE)	2nd Graft	Pretransplant		No. of HLA-A,B Incompatible		No. of HLA-DR Incompatible	
					Dialysis	Transfusions	< 2	> 2	0	1–2
1980–82	Cyclosporine A & prednisolone	29	60.0 ± 0.7	17%	86%	93%*	72%	28%	43%	57%
1973–80	Azathioprine & prednisolone	92	61.0 ± 0.4	15%	72%	77%*	68%	32%	27%†	73%†

*Statistically significant difference: Fisher's exact test $p < 0.05$.

†Retrospective analysis in 49 patients.

Table 2. Complications Occurring During the First 6 Months after Transplantation in Renal Transplant Patients Above 55 Years of Age

	Azathioprine ($N = 92$)		Cyclosporine A ($N = 22$)	
Treatment	No.	%	No.	%
Steroid side effects				
Steroid diabetes	25	27%	4	18%
Psychosis	5	5%	1	5%
Gastrointestinal complications				
Colon perforation	5	5%	0	
Pancreatitis	1	1%	1	5%
GI bleeding	1	1%	1	5%
Serious infections				
Pneumonia	26	28%	2	9%
Bacteremia	8	9%	2	9%
Meningoencephalitis	0		1	5%
Infections classified by agent				
Bacteria	18	20%	4	18%
Virus	35	38%	8	36%
Protozoa	2	2%	1	5%

all were found to have gingival hyperplasia, although most of the patients were asymptomatic. A major problem in the clinical use of CsA is nephrotoxicity.[3,4,9,13,14,15] Fourteen percent of the patients were switched to conventional treatment because of nephrotoxicity. Many of these patients belonged, however, to the first patients treated with CsA at our center, and drug serum-level determinations were not available at that time. In retrospect, it seems likely that some switches may have been unnecessary.

In all patient groups treated with CsA, the patient and graft survival rate was very satisfactory. We are especially encouraged by the results in the elderly patients: These are far superior to those achieved at our center previously with conventional immunosuppression. It should be noted, however, that in 1980 when CsA was introduced at our center, we also began to give pretransplant blood transfusions to all patients. As a consequence, significantly more patients in the CsA group had received pretransplant blood transfusions. Since in previous series at our institution even patients given blood transfusions have had a 2-year graft survival rate of only 50%, the present results could not be ascribed to a transfusion effect.[10] Also in 1980, we introduced donor-recipient selection based on DR matching. As a consequence, the number of patients receiving kidneys with 0 DR incompatibility was somewhat higher in the CsA group. This difference, however, did not reach statistical significance.

According to the protocol, the CsA patients received approximately 2–4 g less prednisolone during the first 6 months after transplantation than the patients given conventional immunosuppression. In spite of this, there was no difference in the frequency of hyperglycemia and psychosis, both side effects that may be attributed to steroid therapy. It is too early to say whether the reduced steroid regimen will have any effect on the incidence of osteonecrosis, as this complication appears much later after transplantation.[16] Gastrointestinal complications, as well as infections, were equally common whether the patients were treated with CsA or with azathioprine. It must be noted, however, that the analysis concerning complications covered only events during the first 6 months after transplantation: The differences in patient survival rate did not reach significance until 18 months. That the patient survival was superior, at this later stage, must have its explanation in that the various complications were more amenable to treatment in the CsA patients.

SUMMARY

Fifty-seven "special category" renal transplant recipients were given CsA and low-dose prednisolone. In patients above 55 years of age, the 2-year-graft and patient survival rate was 73% and 85%, respectively, as compared with 41% and 59% among patients in the same age groups treated with conventional immunosuppressive therapy during a preceding 7-year period ($p < 0.01$). In diabetics and patients with azathioprine intolerance, 12/16 cadaveric grafts and 10/10 related grafts are functioning 3–37 months after transplantation.

REFERENCES

1. Öst L, Groth CC, Lindholm B, et al: Transplantation 30:339, 1980

2. Lundgren G, Fehrman I, Gunnarsson R, et al: Transplant Proc 15:601, 1983

3. Ringdén O, Bergstrand A, Collste H, et al: Scand J Urol Nephrol (Suppl) 64:220, 1981

4. Ringdén O, Collste H, Klintmalm G, et al: Transplant Proc 14:100, 1982

5. Borel JF, Feurer C, Magnee C, et al: Immunology 32:1017, 1977

6. Calne RY, Rolles K, Thiru S, et al: Lancet 2:1323, 1978

7. Starzl TE, Weil R, Iwatsuki S, et al: Surg Gynecol Obstet 151:17, 1980

8. Groth CG, Berg B, Collste H, et al: Scand J Urol Nephrol 15:295, 1981

9. Groth CG, Lundgren G, Ringdén O, et al: Scand J Urol Nephrol (Suppl) 64:200, 1981

10. Fehrman I, Groth CG, Lundgren G, et al: Transplantation 30:324, 1980

11. Berg B: Tissue Antigens 18:306, 1981

12. Berg B, Möller E: Tissue Antigens 18:316, 1981

13. Klintmalm G, Bergstrand A, Ringdén O, et al: Transplant Proc 15:493, 1983

14. Klintmalm G, Ringdén O, Groth CG: Transplant Proc (this issue)

15. Calne RY, White DJG, Evans DB, et al: Br Med J 282:934, 1981

16. Svahn T, Elmstedt E, Lewander R, et al: Scand J Urol Nephrol (Suppl) 29:135, 1975

Randomized Comparison Between Cyclosporine and Conventional Therapy Plus Minnesota Antilymphocyte Globulin in Cadaveric Renal Transplantation

P. Halloran, D. Ludwin, M. Aprile, J. Lien, N. White, and the Canadian Transplant Study Group

CYCLOSPORINE (CsA) is a major development in clinical modulation of immune responsiveness and appears to be of proven benefit in management of renal allograft recipients, compared to azathioprine.[1–4] However, it is not yet clear whether CsA is superior to antilymphocyte antibodies.[5,6] In an earlier publication, we reported on our preliminary results (first 45 patients) of a randomized trial comparing cyclosporine plus prednisone to a protocol of azathioprine, prednisone, and intravenous Minnesota (horse) antilymphoblast globulin (MALG), given both prophylactically and therapeutically.[5] The purpose of the present report is to update our experience in this trial, which now includes 68 patients.

MATERIALS AND METHODS

This experience is part of the Canadian Multicentre Cyclosporine Trial and represents the combined experience of the two centers that opted to treat all of their "standard" therapy recipients with MALG as well as azathioprine and prednisone. MALG was provided through the courtesy of Dr. Richard Condie, University of Minnesota; CsA was provided through the generosity of Sandoz Pharmaceuticals.

The criteria for eligibility and exclusion have been outlined elsewhere.[2,3] In brief, all patients receiving cadaveric grafts, regardless of number of previous grafts, were eligible, providing they gave informed consent prior to randomization, had received at least 2 units of blood, and did not have a positive T-cell crossmatch, abnormal liver function, or a history of malignancy or previous treatment with cytotoxic drugs. After randomization, patients received either the MALG-standard therapy protocol or the CsA protocol. The former consisted of MALG 20 mg/kg preoperatively and daily postoperatively, administered over 8–24 hr into a large central vein, and prednisone (usually 0.5 mg/kg/day for 6 weeks, followed by a gradual reduction to approximately 15 mg/day). MALG therapy was continued for 14–21 days (mean, 18.5 ± 3) and was reinitiated for severe rejection episodes thereafter. Azathioprine was usually given 3 mg/kg preoperatively i.v., then not restarted until the MALG dose began to be tapered at 2–3 weeks. Cyclosporine was given in a loading dose of 10 mg/kg, then daily p.o. in divided doses to maintain 12-hr trough levels of 50–300 ng/ml (followed by RIA). Prednisone was started on alternate days from day 14 and rapidly tapered. Rejections were treated with Solumedrol.

RESULTS

The characteristics of these patients (Table 1) were similar in the two randomized groups. The MALG had a slight excess of males, diabetics, second transplants, and older patients, and both groups received kidneys that were predominantly (94%) machine-perfused, usually for greater than 24 hr, as is standard practice in the MORE kidney distribution system. The median follow-up time was 9 months in both groups. Four patients in the CsA group were switched to standard therapy for poor function on cyclosporine; for analysis they are retained in the CsA group. Three of these 5 kidneys are functioning on standard therapy.

Patient survival has been excellent, with only one death (in the MALG group, from CMV infection), for an overall patient survival of 96% for the MALG group and 100% for the CsA group (Table 2). Graft survival in the two groups was not significantly different, although the survival was better in the MALG group. Actual graft survival is 27/31 (87%) in the MALG group and 27/37 (73%) in the

From the Trihospital Nephrology Service, Toronto General Hospital, Toronto, and the Division of Nephrology, St. Joseph's Hospital, Hamilton, Ontario, Canada.

Supported by a grant from the Medical Research Council of Canada.

Reprint requests should be addressed to Dr. P. F. Halloran, Mount Sinai Hospital, Suite 435, 600 University Ave., Toronto, Ontario, Canada M5G 1X5.

0041-1345/83/1505-0058$01.00/0

Table 1. Characteristics of the Randomized Patients and Their Grafts

Variable	MALG-Standard Therapy Group	Cyclosporine Therapy Group
Number	31	37
Age (mean)	41	39
Male sex	23 (74%)	22 (59%)
Previous transplants	7 (23%)	6 (16%)
Diabetes	8 (26%)	5 (14%)
Perfusion time		
0 hr	2	2
0–24 hr	9	9
> 24 hr	20	26
Switched from CsA to standard therapy	0	5*
Median follow-up time (months), with range	9 (1–19)	9 (1–23)

*Switch was made at week 1, 3, 5, 11, and 26, respectively.

Table 2. Graft Survival*

Variable	MALG-Standard Therapy Group	Cyclosporine Therapy Group
No. of grafts lost	4	10
Immediate loss (vascular occlusion)	0	3
Primary nonfunction	1	3
Uncontrolled rejection	2	4
Death	1	0
Actual no. of grafts surviving	27 (87%)	27 (73%)
Actuarial 1-year graft survival	92%	74%

*There were no significant differences between the two groups.

CsA group. Actuarial 1-year graft survival is 92% for MALG and 74% for CsA.

Causes of the 4 graft losses in the MALG group were patient death (1 case), rejection (2 cases), and prolonged primary nonfunction with later rejection (1 case). Causes of the 10 graft losses in the CsA group were early vascular occlusion (3 cases), rejection (4 cases), and prolonged primary nonfunction, with or without later rejection (3 cases). Thus, in 61 patients whose grafts achieved function, rejection was responsible for only 6 graft losses, reflecting the increasing rarity of this cause of graft loss.

Renal function in the MALG group was superior to that in the CsA group, both early and late (Table 3). In the early period, the incidence of nonfunction in the CsA group was significantly greater than in the MALG group and tended to last longer, as reflected by the "turn-on time" (days to urine output greater than 1 liter) and by number of patients requiring dialysis. In the latest follow-up results, serum creatinine was significantly higher in the CsA group (2.5 vs. 1.7), which represents a 32% decline in renal function. The incidence of rejection episodes was higher on CsA than on MALG in the initial

Table 3. Early and Late Renal Function

	MALG-Standard Therapy Group	Cyclosporine Therapy Group	Significance
Turn-on time* (± SD) (days to urine output > 1 liter)	1.6 ± 3	7.1 ± 11	$p < 0.02$
Proportion of patients dialyzed†	8/31 (26%)	22/34 (65%)	$p < 0.005$
Renal function at last follow-up visit	27	27	
Excellent (creatinine ≤ 1.5)	13 (48%)	3 (11%)	
Good (creatinine 1.6–2.0)	9 (33%)	8 (30%)	
Fair (creatinine 2.1–3.0)	3 (11%)	10 (37%)	
Poor (creatinine > 3.0)	2 (7%)	6 (22%)	$p < 0.025$
Mean serum creatinine	1.7 ± 0.7	2.5 ± 1.0	$p < 0.005$
Cumulative rejection episodes			
Up to day 30	0.5 ± 0.6 (N = 29)	1.4 ± 0.9 (N = 34)	$p < 0.001$
Up to day 90	1.0 ± 1.3 (N = 26)	1.9 ± 1.1 (N = 30)	$p < 0.02$
Up to 1 year	2.0 ± 2.2 (N = 12)	2.1 ± 1.2 (N = 16)	NS

*Excluding patients who never achieved function.
†Excluding 3 technical failures.

period, although differences disappear by 1 year.

DISCUSSION

Experience with CsA has indicated that this agent is capable of inducing approximately 80% graft survival in unmatched cadaveric transplants, 1-year actuarial survival being 73%,[3] 80%,[4] and 84%[5] in controlled studies and approximately 80% in each of two uncontrolled studies.[1,2] In the European controlled study, the patients were not treated with antilymphocyte antibodies, and the 1-year graft survival was 53%, compared to 82% in the Minnesota study in which control patients received MALG. In the Canadian trial, a similar dichotomy appeared: Patients receiving standard therapy who did not receive antilymphocyte globulin had a graft survival of 50%, compared to the present results for those who received antilymphocyte antibodies. Although graft survival was lower in the CsA group in the present study, this may have been due to the fortuitous occurrence of three early vascular thromboses in the CsA group, without such accidents, the actual graft survival approaches 80% in this group. Whether these losses were indeed fortuitous or were due in part to some property of CsA is not possible to determine at present. However, other large experiences with CsA to date have not detected a striking incidence of renal vascular occlusion.

When the present results are seen in conjunction with those reported elsewhere, we can conclude that both antilymphocyte antibodies (plus azathioprine) and CsA can induce graft survival of 80% or more, with excellent patient survival. The results in terms of renal function are not comparable: Renal function in patients treated with antilymphocyte globulin plus azathioprine is superior to that in cyclosporine-treated patients. The follow-up creatinine values suggest that the CsA patients have about 32% less renal function than the MALG patients, on average. Which therapy should one choose? In favor of cyclosporine are its ease of administration, lack of requirement for central venous lines, lower potential for anaphylactic reactions, susceptibility to monitoring, chemical purity, and lower tendency toward CMV infections.[7] Also, as a newer agent, it may be that results with this agent or a nonnephrotoxic successor will improve with use, whereas the results with heterologous antilymphocyte antibodies may be at the peak of their development. In favor of antilymphocyte antibodies are the superior early and late renal function, the short term of therapy, the possible use of human and murine monoclonal antibodies in the future, the low cost, and the absence of nephrotoxicity, giving superior renal function. Unknown, and currently unknowable, in this complex comparison are the long-term survival figures and complication rates in both groups, especially the important question of the long-term consequences of CsA nephrotoxicity. For example, will the 32% decrease in renal function in patients on CsA decrease their ultimate graft survival and increase their vascular complications?

Our experience with CsA, which was not as favorable as that reported in some centers, may be colored by some interaction between this drug and a local variable, such as mode of kidney preservation. In our area, most kidneys are preserved by pulsatile perfusion, usually for greater than 24 hr. The Canadian multicenter trial has suggested that this variable is associated with poorer graft survival and function.[4] Whether the results with CsA can be improved with a change in renal preservation will be determined by a prospective trial that we are undertaking at present.

Given the facts cited here, we believe that CsA and antilymphocyte antibodies will both find their place in the armamentarium of renal transplantation units. The fact that only 6/61 grafts that achieved function have been lost due to uncontrolled rejection points out the declining incidence of this event. Indeed, it is conceivable that appropriate combinations of CsA and MALG may be able to abolish graft loss due to acute rejection without impairing patient well-being. The task of evaluating the relative role of each of these agents will occupy us for some time. We believe that future immunosuppression in transplantation is likely to be intermodal, utilizing the beneficial properties of a variety of immunosuppressives as the situation warrants. At present, we must conclude that exclusive reliance on CsA, to the exclusion of antilymphocyte antibodies in most renal transplant units, is not justified on the basis of our results.

REFERENCES

1. Calne RY, White DJG, Evans EB, et al: Br Med J 282:934, 1981
2. Starzl TE, Klintmalm GBF, Weil R, et al: Surg Gynecol Obstet 153:486, 1981
3. Report on the European Multicentre Trial: Lancet 2:57, 1982
4. Canadian Multicentre Cyclosporine Trial: N Engl J Med (in press)
5. Najarian JS, Ferguson RM, Sutherland DER, et al: Transplant Proc 15:438, 1983
6. Halloran PF, Lien J, Aprile M, et al: Transplant Proc 15:627, 1983
7. Peterson PK, Rynasiewicz JJ, Simmons RL, et al: Transplant Proc 15:457, 1983

Cadaveric Renal Transplantation with Cyclosporine: Experiences in 148 Patients at a Single Institution

W. Land, L. A. Castro, K. Günther, C. Hammer, C. Hillebrand, W.-D. Illner, N. Schmeller, B. Schneider, W. Siebert, R. A. Zink, and H. Zöttlein

SINCE NOVEMBER 1980, 195 renal transplantations have been performed at our center using cyclosporine as a new immunosuppressive agent. Twenty-five patients were treated with cyclosporine as the sole immunosuppressive agent in the European Multicentre Trial.[1] Outside a control study, cyclosporine, in combination with small doses of methylprednisolone, was used in 157 cadaveric renal transplantations as well as in 5 living related donor transplantations. Cyclosporine, in combination with steroids, was used in 8 combined renal and pancreatic transplantations. This article reports our experiences with 148 cadaveric renal transplantations performed by March 1983, using cyclosporine in combination with steroids as basic immunosuppressive therapy.

MATERIALS AND METHODS

Patient Population

This study includes 140 consecutive transplants of cadaveric renal allografts performed between March 1982 and March 1983 on recipients aged 9–61 years. No patients were excluded from cyclosporine treatment, neither patients with known liver disease nor patients with primarily nonfunctioning kidneys without immediate diuresis. Of the 140 patients, 115 got a primary renal allograft and 25 received a secondary or tertiary allograft. All recipients had received at least 3 random type-specific blood transfusions prior to transplant. Eight patients (aged 25–49 years) suffering from Type I diabetes mellitus and end-stage renal disease received combined renal and pancreatic allografts.

Immunosuppressive Protocol

Basic immunosuppression. Cyclosporine was administered intravenously before the operation and on day 1 postoperatively in a dose of 4 mg/kg of body weight and continued by oral administration in a dose of 15 mg/kg for 1 month after transplantation, when it was decreased by 2 mg/kg monthly to a maintenance level of 6–7 mg/kg. Methylprednisolone was begun at 8 mg daily immediately after the operation and maintained at that level.

Antirejection treatments. Antirejection treatment consisted of 3 i.v. bolus injections of 500 mg methylprednisolone during the first rejection episode. The second and third rejection episodes were treated by administration of ALG/ATG over a period of 7 days, in combination with methylprednisolone in a dose of 125 mg i.v. daily until reversal.

"Triple" immunosuppressive therapy. In recipients of a secondary or tertiary renal allograft and in patients with preformed antibodies higher than 50%, cyclosporine, azathioprine, and methylprednisolone were administered during the first week posttransplant as follows: cyclosporine was given as described above; azathioprine in a dose of 2 mg/kg initially, then decreased to 1 mg/kg; methylprednisolone (i.v.) in a dose of 500 mg daily, tapering to 30 mg daily.

From the second week after transplantation, the original basic immunosuppressive treatment was continued. Antirejection treatment was applied as described above.

Combined Renal and Pancreatic Transplantation

Pancreas transplantation was performed using the technique of segmental pancreatic allografting by occluding the duct system with Ethibloc. Postoperative management consisted of cyclosporine administration in combination with steroids; in addition, administration of heparine, antibiotics, and Somatostatine.

Incidence of Infections Under Cyclosporine Therapy

The incidence of infections described in this report concerns only the manifestation of severe infections requiring hospitalization of the transplant patient. In addition to careful clinical assessment and appropriate

From the Transplantation Center, Klinikum Grosshadern (Departments of Surgery, Internal Medicine I and Urology), University of Munich, Munich, Germany.

Supported in part by the Kuratorium für Heimdialyse e. V. Neu-Isenburg, Arbeitsgemeinschaft der Bayerischen Krankenkassenverbände, Germany, and Sandoz Ltd., Basel, Switzerland.

Reprint requests should be addressed to Prof. Dr. W. Land, Dept. of Surgery, Klinikum Grosshadern, Marchioninistr. 15, D-8000 München 70, Germany.

0041-1345/83/1505-0059$01.00/0

microbiologic tests for evidence of infectious diseases, detailed laboratory investigations were carried out whenever an overt virus disease was suspected.

Fine-Needle Aspiration Cytology

The methodology used has been described elsewhere.[2] In brief, fine-needle aspiration has to be done under sterile conditions by placing a spinal needle into the cortex of the graft. The aspirated material was dispersed into a centrifuge vial by means of 5 ml RPMI medium held in the suction syringe.

The mouse monoclonal antibodies used were directed against pan-T lymphocytes (OKT3), helper-inducer T lymphocytes (OKT4), and cytotoxic/suppressor T lymphocytes (OKT8).

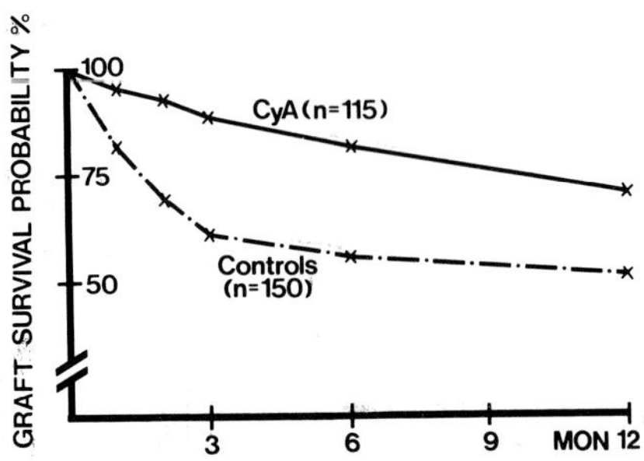

Fig. 1. Graft survival rates in primary renal transplantation, comparing cyclosporine-methylprednisolone treatment (CsA) vs. historical controls (azathioprine-steroids treatment).

RESULTS

Cadaveric Renal Transplantation

The overall graft survival rate (graft survival probability as calculated by the Cutler-Ederer test) after primary cadaveric renal transplantations in 115 consecutively treated patients under cyclosporine-methylprednisolone therapy is depicted in Fig. 1; the result in the historical control group (steroids + azathioprine; $N = 150$) is shown for comparison. At 1 year, the graft survival probability is 70% in the cyclosporine group compared to 50% in the control group. The difference of 20% is statistically significant. The overall graft survival rate after secondary or tertiary cadaveric renal transplantation in 25 patients under cyclosporine-methylprednisolone therapy is depicted in Fig. 2. The 1-year graft survival probability of 70% is identical to that obtained in the primary renal allograft group, although during the first 6 months after transplantation there was a slightly higher incidence of graft losses. Of these 25 patients, 18 were treated during the first week following transplantation by using the "triple" immunosuppressive protocol (see below).

Of the original 115 patients treated with cyclosporine after primary renal transplantation, 111 are currently alive. Of the 4 patients who died, 2 did so with functioning grafts, 1 from spontaneous intracerebral hemorrhage at 1 month and the other from acute cardiac failure at 6 months. One patient with a primary nonfunctioning kidney (ATN) died from acute cardiac failure at 1 week, another patient from sepsis at 6 months. There was an immunologic cause of graft loss only in 14 patients, and a nonimmunologic cause of graft loss in 3. All the original 25 patients treated with cyclosporine after retransplantation are alive. There was an immunologic cause of graft loss in 6 patients and a nonimmunologic cause of graft loss in 1.

"Triple" Immunosuppression in Immunologically High-Risk Patients

As described in Materials and Methods, 26 immunologically high-risk patients (18 retransplantations and 8 recipients with preformed antibodies > 50%) were treated with cyclosporine, azathioprine, and steroids during the first week after transplantation. The result of this pilot study is depicted in Fig. 3. We observed a 1-year graft survival probability of 70%. Remarkably, all irreversible graft rejections occurred during the first 3 months after transplantation. In none of these 26 patients treated initially with the "triple" immunosuppressive regimen has either severe infection or malignancy been seen so far.

Combined Renal and Segmental Pancreatic Transplantation

The results obtained with this kind of surgical treatment in Type I diabetics with end-stage renal disease are listed in Table 1. Although our experience with cyclosporine therapy in combined renal and pancreatic transplantation is limited to 8 cases, the

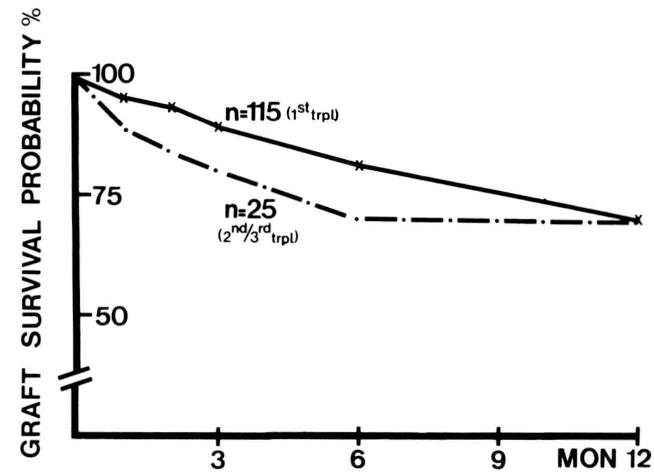

Fig. 2. Graft survival rates in primary renal transplantation ($N = 115$) compared to retransplantation ($N = 25$).

results obtained with this new immunosuppressive agent are encouraging and promising.

Incidence of Infectious Diseases Under Cyclosporine Treatment

The incidence of clinically manifested severe infections that required hospitalization is listed in Table 2. Of the original 140 patients treated with cyclosporine after cadaveric renal transplantation, only 13 (9%) were hospitalized with a bacterial infection (1 death due to sepsis), 9 (6%) with a viral infection, and 2 (1.3%) with a fungal infection.

Immunologic Monitoring: Fine-Needle Aspiration Cytology

Due to the difficulty in detecting acute rejections in patients treated with cyclosporine, recourse was made to fine-needle aspiration cytology. The method allows not only estimation of onset, severity, and course of rejection but also measurement of the impact of treatment and differentiation between cyclosporine side effects, acute tubular necrosis, and acute cellular rejection. Differentiation of the inflammatory cell populations by monoclonal antibodies has proved that with increasing severity of rejection, high numbers of lymphocytes of the cytotoxic/suppressor cell compartment invade the graft. Helper cells therefore decrease relatively in terms of percent (Fig. 4).

This observation of a high influx of cytotoxic cells into the graft during rejection was not changed after introduction of cyclosporine as the immunosuppressant. Despite its powerful effect on graft rejection, no change in lymphocyte numbers in the peripheral blood could be seen. During rejection under cyclo-

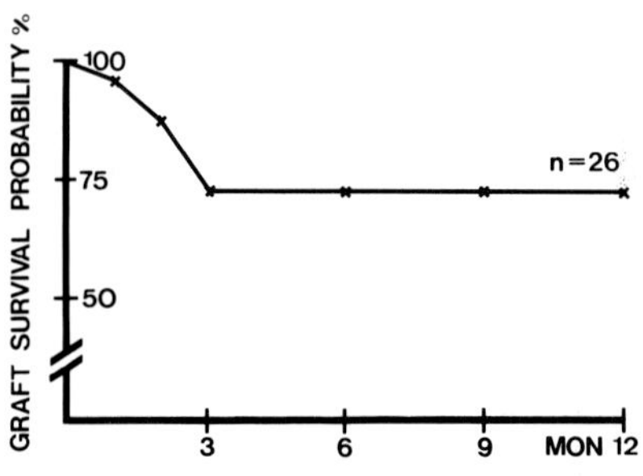

Fig. 3. Graft survival rate in immunologically high-risk patients treated with cyclosporine, azathioprine, and methylprednisolone during the first week following transplantation.

Table 1. Results of Combined Pancreatic and Renal Transplantation in 8 Patients Treated with Cyclosporine and Steroids*

Patients alive	7
Function of both grafts	5†
Function of the renal graft (2 years)	1
Rejection of both grafts (1 month)	1
Death (acute liver failure)	1

*At the Transplantation Center, Munich, 1979–1983; $N = 12/11$.

†2 years, 1 year, 5 months, 4 months, and 3 months, respectively.

Table 2. Incidence of Infectious Diseases in 140 Cyclosporine-Methylprednisolone–Treated Patients

No. of Patients (*N* = 13/140)	Bacterial Infections: Manifestation	Associated with ART*	Outcome
9	UTI, prostatitis, pyelonephritis	No	Recovery
1	Graft infection at biopsy	Yes	Transplantectomy
1	Otitis media	No	Recovery
1	Endocarditis	No	Recovery
1	Pneumonia, sepsis	No	Death

No. of Patients (*N* = 9/140)	Viral Infections: Manifestation	Pathogen	ART	Outcome
5	Interstitial pneumonia: cerebral signs, general symptoms	CMV	Yes (3) No (2)	Recovery
2	Herpes genitalis, Herpes simplex (generalized)	Herpes virus	Yes (1) No (1)	Recovery
2	Fever, pneumonia	Unknown	No	Recovery

No. of Patients (*N* = 2/140)	Fungal Infections: Manifestation	Pathogen	ART	Outcome
1	Tracheitis	*Candida albicans*	No	Recovery
1	Sepsis, UTI	*Candida albicans*	Yes	Recovery with graft loss

*ART: Antirejection therapy.

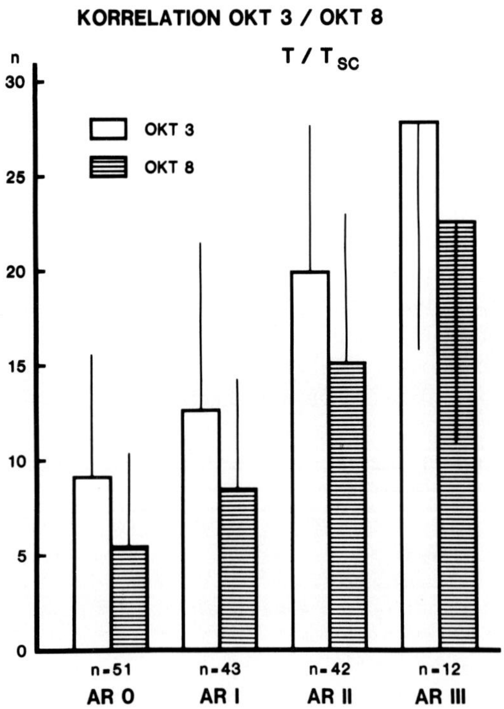

Fig. 4. OKT8^{+} cells increase in the graft with increasing severity of the rejection reaction.

sporine therapy, lymphocyte numbers increased in the graft, but less than with conventional therapy. Surprisingly enough, no impact on helper cells was seen under cyclosporine therapy. A new aspect was analyzed (Table 3) when conversion of numbers of helper and cytotoxic suppressor cells was measured in the peripheral blood and in the graft. High numbers of lymphocytes in the periphery and the graft, preferably belonging to the

Table 3. Behavior of Peripheral Granular Lymphocytes and T4/T8† Cells in Rejection Episodes vs. Viral Infections

	Rejection Episode 0	Rejection Episode 2	Virus Infection
Lymphocytes in fine-needle biopsy	8.5	23.9	31.7
Lymphocytes in peripheral blood	7.7	6.3	18.3
OKT3	9.8	18.3	29.2
OKT4	4.8	8.2	4.5
OKT8	4.9	13.3	25.6
OKT4/OKT8 ratio	1.2	0.7	0.2
In peripheral blood	2.6	2.4	0.45

T8 compartment, heralded in virus infection. The ratio of T4 to $T8^+$ cells was below 0.5 in aspirate and peripheral blood.

A further sign distinguishing virus infection from acute rejection seems to be the number of large granular lymphocytes—supposedly responsible for the natural killer activity. During acute rejection, peripheral blood lacks large granular lymphocytes. In the graft, large granular lymphocytes reach up to 12% of the inflammatory cell compartment. During virus infection, however, large granular lymphocytes increase in the peripheral blood and the graft to values up to 25%, with the mean of 14, i.e., 10%.

DISCUSSION

The results reported confirm the potential usefulness of cyclosporine in combination with low doses of steroids to improve the graft survival in cadaveric renal transplantation with an extremely low incidence of morbidity and mortality. Compared with the historical controls treated with conventional therapy at our center, a 20% difference in the results obtained with the use of cyclosporine was observed. Interestingly enough, the 70% 1-year graft survival probability under cyclosporine-methylprednisolone therapy was observed in primary renal transplantation as well as in retransplantation. By using a short-term "triple" immunosuppressive regimen (cyclosporine, azathioprine, methylprednisolone) immediately after surgery, a 70% 1-year graft survival rate of cadaveric renal allografts could also be achieved in immunologically high-risk patients. Although these results are similar to those reported by others,[3-6] one has to be careful in interpreting the current improved graft survival rates as definite long-term results. Thus, within ½ year the 6-month graft survival rate of 90% came down to the 12-month graft survival rate of 70% at our own institution. Nevertheless, when evaluating the results at our institution, one has to take into account that no exclusion criteria for the use of cyclosporine were applied, as had been done in the European Multicentre Trial. This circumstance represents one of several difficulties in comparing the efficacy of the combined cyclosporine treatment with that of cyclosporine monotherapy.

As far as the results in immunologically high-risk patients are concerned, a valid conclusion cannot be drawn from the data obtained at the present time. Nevertheless, two aspects seem worthwhile to discuss: (1) Our first clinical impression of a strong immunosuppressive potency of the "triple" regimen used is confirmed by experimental studies showing a synergistic immunosuppressive effect of cyclosporine and azathioprine in three different animal allograft models.[7] (2) According to our observations (no incidence of severe infection or malignancy), such a combined immunosuppressive therapy seems to be safe for the patient, provided all three drugs are administered only for a short period of time.

Apart from the improved results in graft survival rates, the decreased morbidity, particularly in terms of decreased infectious diseases, is one of the remarkable advantages of cyclosporine treatment. Infections remain an important and typical complication of renal transplantation, which often has led to graft loss or patient death. Therefore, the decreased incidence of severe infectious diseases (of bacterial, viral, or fungal origin) as observed by us and others[3,8] is tremendously encouraging. In this context, it remains to be studied in the future why particularly the incidence of viral infections is lower than expected in light of the mode of action of cyclosporine. Despite all the advantages, there is, however, one serious disadvantage in the use of cyclosporine: It makes the early detection of rejection episodes a difficult procedure, especially in patients with primarily nonfunctioning kidneys. A lot of "classical" rejection symptoms have completely (or partially) disappeared and are no longer seen by clinicians. This obvious difficulty with cyclosporine use has given rise to a search for new and better methods for immunologic monitoring. One of us (C. H.) tried to use P. Häyry's fine-needle aspiration cytology as a method helpful for the accurate detection of rejection episodes. Although this method is not fully convincing from the practical point of view at the present time, some conclusions can be drawn: Fine-needle biopsy, in combination with highly specific monoclonal antibodies, provides some important new information about the background of high-lymphocytic inflammation. Clinical statements like onset, severity, and progress of an acute rejection given by the aspiration cytology can be confirmed and precised with this method in certain circumstances. A possible new prominent example is to differentiate between acute rejection and virus infection with the help of monoclonal antibodies and by differentiating large granular lymphocytes from other cell populations. With this information, unnecessary and dangerous immunosuppressive therapy in cases of nondiagnosed viral infections might be avoided.

Parallel to the improvement of the results in cadaveric renal transplantation under cyclosporine therapy, the results of combined renal and pancreatic transplantation have improved, although the number of patients treated with this surgical method at our institution is too small to draw any valid conclusion. Nevertheless, in view of the current uncertain state of the art relating to the technique of pancreatic grafting, the introduction of cyclosporine in the clinical pancreatic allografting program seems to improve the results in this field of organ transplantation slightly but steadily.

REFERENCES

1. Report on the European Multicentre Trial: Lancet 2:57, 1982
2. Hammer C, Land W, Stadler J, et al: Transplant Proc 15:356, 1983
3. Hakala TR, Starzl TE, Rosenthal JT, et al: Transplant Proc 15:465, 1983
4. Calne RY, White DJG, Evans DB, et al: Br Med J 282:934, 1981
5. Calne RY, Rolles K, White DJG, et al: Lancet 2:1033, 1979
6. Najarian JS, Ferguson RM, Sutherland DER, et al: Transplant Proc 15:438, 1983
7. Squifflet JP, Sutherland DER, Field J, et al: Transplant Proc 15:520, 1983
8. Peterson PK, Rynasiewicz JJ, Simmons RL, et al: Transplant Proc 15:457, 1983

Cyclosporine in Cadaveric Renal Transplantation: A Prospective Randomized Trial

P. McMaster, I. G. Haynes, J. Michael, D. Adu, T. Vlassis, S. Roger, J. Turney, S. Stock, J. Buckels, P. Mackintosh, and M. Ezzibdeh

AZATHIOPRINE AND steroids have formed the basis of nonspecific immunosuppression in cadaveric renal transplantation since the early 1960s.[1] While modifications in immunosuppression protocols have occurred over the years, leading to a reduction in steroid dosage[2] and in some units the use of antilymphocytic globulin,[3] no major new therapeutic agent has proved its clinical value. Thus, the early in vitro demonstration of the immunosuppressive properties of cyclosporine A (CsA) by Borel[4] and the initial animal studies in organ transplantation aroused great interest.[5] It seemed clear that cyclosporine A, a fermentation of the fungus *Trichoderma-polysporum,* had significant immunosuppressive properties and, by a more selective action, apparently produced little myelosuppression. The success of these experimental organ transplant studies led Calne et al. to initiate an early evaluation of cyclosporine A in organ transplantation in humans.[6] These clinical studies confirmed the marked immunosuppressive activity of cyclosporine A, but the development of nephrotoxicity made management difficult.[7] In addition, CsA in conjunction with other immunosuppressive agents gave a high incidence of infection. These problems have led to different clinical protocols of management being developed in cadaveric renal transplantation. The European Multicentre Trial, using CsA alone, clearly demonstrated good early graft survival,[8] although some centers have since added steroids to their CsA protocol. In North America, CsA has been routinely used in conjunction with steroids without the development of major systemic infection.[9] However, some units have found clinical management difficult, and their early experience with CsA has been less encouraging.[10]

As yet, there is no universally agreed protocol for the use of CsA in clinical cadaveric transplantation, and the need for steroids in conjunction with CsA has been debated. Our earlier experience suggested that CsA alone from the time of transplantation was associated with a high incidence of early acute rejection requiring steroid boluses in the crucial early postoperative phase, yet we were reluctant to adopt the protocol of continuous steroid administration, as it seemed likely from the European study that we would "condemn" many of our patients to continuous long-term steroids unnecessarily.

There have been few single-center randomized prospective studies of CsA in cadaveric grafting,[11,12] and this paper represents our assessment of the early results of CsA in conjunction with short-term steroids (STS) in cadaveric transplantation in a single-center randomized study.

MATERIALS AND METHODS

Our clinical trial began in May 1981, and all patients who were to receive a cadaveric renal graft were considered for entry into the trial. Patients prior to entry onto the transplant waiting list received 2 units of whole blood. Patients were excluded from consideration of the trial if they were insulin-dependent diabetics, aged less than 10 years, or had evidence of hepatic dysfunction. In addition, patients were entered into the trial only after a full explanation to each individual had been given and informed consent had been obtained.

Patients received a cadaveric graft with a negative crossmatch on the basis of the best available HLA-A, B match; prospective HLA-DR matching was not used in patient selection.

Prior to transplantation, each patient received 1 g of Solumedrone intravenously and 5 mg/kg of body weight of azathioprine as an intravenous bolus in addition to

From the Queen Elizabeth Hospital, Birmingham, England.

Reprint requests should be addressed to Dr. McMaster.

0041-1345/83/1505-0060$01.00/0

perioperative ampicillin and flucloxicillin. During and immediately following transplantation, patients were transfused to maintain their intravascular volume using central venous pressure monitoring, and mannitol 20 g was given intravenously and, when necessary, a Lasix infusion. Only those patients who put out >400 ml of urine from their grafted kidney—via a Tizzard bladder-ureteric catheter—in the first 8 hr were entered into the study. Patients were randomly allocated to Group I (CsA and STS) or Group II (prednisolone and azathioprine).

By April 1983, 68 patients had entered the study and had been followed up for at least 6 months. Thirty-five patients had received CsA and STS (Group I), and 33 patients conventional treatment (Group II).

Group I Patients

Patients in Group I received during the first postoperative month 15 mg/kg CsA in divided morning and evening doses, reducing on day 28 to 12 mg/kg. By the end of the second month, a further dose reduction to 10 mg/kg was made, and at 3 months a variable reduction to 6–10 mg/kg, depending on clinical function. In addition, Group I patients received 10 mg of oral prednisolone twice a day for the first 14 days postoperatively.

Acute rejection episodes confirmed by renal biopsy were treated with 1 g of Solumedrone i.v. on 3 consecutive days. Unless renal function then returned to prerejection levels, prednisolone 20 mg/day was reintroduced.

The CsA regime was modified if function deteriorated without clinical features of rejection and biopsy failed to confirm evidence of allograft rejection. The CsA dose was intially reduced by 25%, and, if within 7 days improvement in function did not occur, a further reduction was made.

Group II Patients

Conventionally treated patients in Group II received azathioprine 2.5 mg/kg/day postoperatively in a single evening dose and prednisolone 10 mg twice a day. Azathioprine dosage was not reduced unless leukopenia developed (WBC count < 4000); steroids were reduced to 17.5 mg/day at 3 months.

Comparison of Groups I and II

Both groups of patients were compared for factors that might influence patient and graft survival. These features are summarized in Table 1.

The success of the two immunosuppressive protocols was determined on the basis of patient and renal graft survival; the incidence, timing, and severity of renal rejection episodes; and the total steroids administered to patients in each group. In addition, renal and hepatic function was monitored and an evaluation made of the early morbidity of each regime.

Patients in Group I have been followed up for a mean of 14.8 ± 4.7 months and those in Group II for a mean of 15.0 ± 4.4 months.

Table 1. Factors That Might Influence Patients and Graft Survival

	Group I (CsA + STS) (N = 35)	Group II (Aza + P) (N = 33)
Age (mean + range)	36 (10–64)	34 (15–53)
Sex		
Male	22 (63%)	21 (64%)
Female	13 (37%)	12 (36%)
Blood group		
O	11 (31%)	11 (33%)
A	18 (51%)	19 (57%)
B	5 (14%)	2 (6%)
AB	1 (3%)	1 (3%)
Pretransplant transfusions		
2 units	28 (80%)	30 (91%)
2–5 units	4 (11%)	3 (9%)
> 5 units	3 (8%)	0
Primary renal disease		
Chronic pyelonephritis	5 (14%)	2 (6%)
Glomerula nephritis	16 (45%)	11 (33%)
Polycystic kidney	0	5
Hypertension	5 (14%)	6 (18%)
Other	9 (28%)	9 (27%)
Previous graft	5 (14%)	1 (3%)
HLA-A,B mismatches		
0	4 (11%)	2 (6%)
1	7 (20%)	11 (33%)
2	22 (63%)	19 (57%)
3 or 4	2 (6%)	1 (3%)
Mean	1.6	1.5
HLA-DR mismatch	1.4	1.0

RESULTS

There was no significant difference between the two random patient populations, and the degree of HLA-A,B mismatching was the same as was the retrospective HLA-DR matching.

Patient and Graft Survival

In Group I, two patients died with a functioning renal transplant, one of CMV viremia and the other of a myocardial infarction at 1 month. In Group II, one patient died with a functioning graft due to bacterial infection and heart failure. In addition, one patient from each group has died since returning to dialysis, one of an overwhelming infection and the other of acute pancreatitis on dialysis.

In Group I, eight grafts (22.8%) have been lost from allograft rejection at 4, 4, and 6 weeks and 7, 9, 9, 15, and 19 months, and an

Table 2. Rejection Episodes

Number of Rejection Episodes	Group I	Group II
0	13	12*
1	14	11
2	4	8
> 2	4	2
Mean	0.8	0.9*
Time of onset of rejection (days)	13.3 ± 15.4	6.4 ± 2.5†

*NS, Mann-Whitney U test.
†$p < 0.05$, Kolmogorov-Smipnov test.

additional graft has been lost because of technical complications. In Group II, rejection resulting in the loss of kidneys in five patients (15%), two within 4 weeks of transplantation and one each at 3, 5, and 7 months. However, four other kidneys in Group II have been lost, due in three cases to recurrence of the original pathology (focal segmental sclerosis and Type I mesangial capillary disease), and in one other case, graft loss was related to perfusion and technical complications.

In Group I, 37% of the patients had no evidence of rejection episodes, while in Group II it was 36%, and the total number of rejection episodes was the same in each group. However, the clinical pattern of rejection and the time of onset of rejection was significantly different between the two groups (see Table 2).

First acute rejection episodes were evident in Group II at a mean of 6.4 ± 2.5 days, while in Group I acute rejection occurred in a mean of 13.3 ± 15.4 days. This difference is statistically significant ($p < 0.05$), and the clinical pattern of rejection was different. Acute rejection in Group II was almost invariably associated with a high temperature, leukocytosis, graft tenderness, and a sharp fall in urine output and rise in chemistry, whereas in Group I obvious clinical signs of rejection were rarely present and graft tenderness or leukocytosis were rare. The clinical management within the first 2 weeks of transplantation in Group I was relatively uneventful, while in Group II patients, acute severe clinical features of rejection were frequently apparent.

Table 3 shows the mean total steroids administered in each patient group within 3 months and 6 months of transplantation. Oral prednisolone was discontinued at 14 days in Group I and reintroduced only if progressive deterioration in function was seen in patients whose biopsies confirmed features of definite cellular rejection. When no improvement was seen, the dose of CsA was reduced, and if function then improved, a component of nephrotoxicity was considered to be present. However, in some patients no clear distinction could be made, and it seems likely that both mild rejection and nephrotoxicity were present concomitantly in some patients.

Of the 35 patients in Group I, 10 have been converted from CsA to prednisolone and azathioprine. Two patients were converted in less than 3 months, 1 because of severe nephrotoxicity and the other because of a distal colitis after having been previously treated for ulcerative colitis. In 5 patients in whom rejection persisted after two episodes of rejection treatment, conversion was made to prednisolone and azathioprine, but all grafts were ultimately lost due to rejection. Two additional patients have been converted from CsA to prednisolone and azathioprine because of nephrotoxicity. One of these grafts was subsequently lost because of rejection; the other continued to function 10 months after

Table 3. Steroids Administered During Acute Rejection and During the First 6 Months of Cyclosporine Treatment

	Group I	Group II	Significance
Total steroids (i.v.) during rejection	4171 ± 386	4181 ± 291	NS
Oral prednisolone			
3 months	754 ± 46	1800 ± 89	< 0.05
6 months			
CsA alone	754 ± 46		
CsA + prednisolone	2554 ± 241	3156 ± 181	< 0.05

improvement in function following conversion from CsA to prednisolone and azathioprine. One further patient was converted at 12 months because of tremor and gingivitis. At 6 months, of the 29 functioning grafts in Group I, 26 are on CsA and 16 require steroids.

Renal Function

Immediate graft function obviating the need for dialysis occurred in 23/35 patients in Group I and in 20/33 in Group II. The mean number of dialyses required was 2.0 in Group I and 2.6 in Group II. Six patients in Group I required >10 dialyses, whereas only 2 in Group II required that many.

While graft survival was satisfactory in Group I, renal function in patients treated with CsA was inferior to Group II, prednisolone and azathioprine at 3 months, and then at each 3-monthly interval after 12 months. At 1 year, the mean urea was 14.7 ± .05 for Group I and 6.5 ± 1.9 for Group II. Creatinines were 227 ± 90 mmole/liter for Group I and 121 ± 40.7 mmole/liter for Group II ($p < 0.02$). This disparity remained constant throughout the study period, although fewer patients remained in the cyclosporine group, having been converted to prednisolone and azathioprine over this period.

Complications

Hypertension was present in the majority of patients in both groups: 75% of the patients in Group I and 69% of those in Group II were receiving antihypertensive treatment.

Persistent hyperkalemia was observed in four of the CsA-treated patients (serum K 6-7.1 mmole/liter) inappropriate to their renal function. This was associated with a hyperkalemia metabolic acidosis.[13]

Infection remains the major life-threatening complication within the first year after transplantation. Clinically significant and potentially hazardous infection was common in both groups, with 48% of patients in Group I and 72% of patients in Group II experiencing significant infection episodes. Minor viral herpetic infections were particularly common in both groups of patients. Minor signs of CsA toxicity were seen in all patients, with an increase in hair growth and gum hypertrophy, but in only three patients did gum hypertrophy prove slow to resolve with reduced CsA doses and dental hygiene. Table 4 summarizes the main clinical complications. It is of interest that the only patient who showed evidence of avascular necrosis of the head of the femur was in Group I. Moderate Cushingoid features appeared in the majority of prednisolone and azathioprine patients, and there was a significant increase in the incidence of "indigestion" in Group II, although no proven case of peptic ulceration was found.

DISCUSSION

This study again demonstrates the impressive immunosuppressive properties of cyclosporine A in clinical cadaveric transplantation. It seems clear also that not all patients on CsA require continuing steroids after transplantation to prevent rejection. However, in many patients, after cessation of steroids there was a progressive deterioration in function that was halted only by reintroducing steroids. In this protocol, steroids were given only during the early postoperative period in an endeavor to prevent severe acute rejection episodes requiring high doses of steroids in the immediate postoperative period. Although the same

Table 4. Complications

	Group I	Group II
Infective complications		
Bacterial	12 (33%)	15 (45%)
Fungal	1 (3%)	1 (3%)
Viral	6 (17%)	5 (15%)
Wound	1 (3%)	2 (6%)
UTI	6 (17%)	8 (24%)
Chest infection	10 (28%)	14 (42%)
Noninfective complications		
"Indigestion"	1 (3%)	6 (17%)
Proven DU	1 (3%)	0
Diabetes	2 (6%)	1 (3%)
Avascular necrosis	1 (3%)	0
DVT	0	1 (3%)
Cushingoid features	2 (6%)	14 (42%)
Hypertension	26 (75%)	23 (69%)

number of rejection episodes were recorded in each group, the delay in onset of rejection in patients on CsA and steroids is apparent. By stopping the steroids after the immediate postoperative period, that is, at 14 days, it may then be possible to identify CsA-treated patients in whom continued steroids is unnecessary; if function deteriorates, steroids may again be introduced.

The overall renal function in patients on CsA as measured by urea and creatinine at 3, 6, and 12 months, is inferior to that of conventionally treated patients and must give rise to concern about the long-term kidney function.

Also of concern is the difficulty in clinical practice of managing CsA patients whose function deteriorates. Once the early postoperative period has passed, repeated renal biopsies are both inconvenient and potentially hazardous as a means of assessing the reason for deterioration in function. The current measurement of CsA levels now seems of more value than it did in earlier studies and may well be of help. We have adopted the approach of reducing CsA dosage in the face of deterioration of function occurring late after transplantation. However, this has rather assumed that nephrotoxicity and rejection do not occur concomitantly. This may be an unwarranted assumption, and although we found it difficult to prove in several of our patients, it seemed likely that both were present. Also, we have been loath to attribute significant cellular infiltrate to a drug-induced "cellular nephritis," as has been suggested by others.[14] We suggest that until biopsies from patients not receiving cadaveric grafting (heart and liver transplantation) are available, this question will prove difficult to resolve.

In the European Multicentre Trial, an impressive reduction in allograft loss due to rejection was found when compared to conventional treatment.[8] However, in our own study of cadaveric grafting in tranfused patients, no significant difference in the incidence of graft loss due to rejection has been found.

With the exception of nephrotoxicity, patients on cyclosporine A have faired well, and the main difference between this study and previous ones in failing to demonstrate significant difference is probably accounted for by the relatively satisfactory conventional results achieved on prednisolone and azathioprine. The difference in morbidity in the two groups is little, with the exception of Cushingoid faces, and this probably related to the low level of steroids administered in our conventionally treated group. Previous studies have shown that high-dose steroid regimes achieve no improvement in graft survival when compared to low-steroid regimens and at a higher mortality.[2] Although the number of patients who have had to be converted from cyclosporine A to conventional treatment has been disappointing, a relatively higher number of CsA (6/12, 52%) patients remain steroid-free than could ever have been achieved in conjunction with azathioprine.

REFERENCES

1. Starzl TE: Renal Transplantation, Earlbourne, England, Saunders, 1964, p 171

2. McGeown MG, Kennedy JA, Loughridge WGC: Lancet 2:648, 1977

3. Ferguson RM, Rynasiewicz JJ, Sutherland DER: Surgery 92:176, 1982

4. Borel JF, Feurer C, Gubler HU, et al: Agents and Actions 6:468, 1976

5. Calne RY, White DJG: IRCS Med Sci 5:595, 1977

6. Calne RY, White DJG, Thiru S, et al: Lancet 1:1323, 1978

7. Calne RY, Rolles K, White DJG, et al: Lancet 2:1033, 1979

8. Report on the Multicentre Trial: Lancet 2:57, 1982

9. Starzl TE, Hakala TR, Rosenthal JT, et al: Surg Gynecol Obstet 154:819, 1982

10. Sweny P, Farrington K, Younis F, et al: Transplant Proc 13:1981

11. Ferguson RM, Rynasiewicz JJ, Sutherland DER, et al: Surgery 92:175, 1982

12. Hakala TR, Starzl TE, Rosenthal JT, et al: Transplant Proc 15:465, 1983

13. Adu D, Turney JH, Collier I, et al: (in press)

14. Najarian JS, Ferguson RM, Sutherland DER, et al: Transplant Proc 15:438, 1983

Renal Transplantation Using Cyclosporine in Pediatric Patients 3 to 17 Years Old

S. B. Conley, E. D. Brewer, S. M. Flechner, C. T. Van Buren, and B. D. Kahan

CYCLOSPORINE (CsA) is a powerful immunosuppressant drug, biochemically unrelated to existing drugs that modify the immune response. It inhibits many T-cell functions and alters the T-cell helper-cell-to-suppressor-cell ratio. Its use was first reported in the United States by Starzl in 1980,[1] after having been used in Europe since 1978.[2] There has now been significant experience with this drug in renal transplantation in adult patients,[1–4] but the experience reported in childhood transplant recipients is limited. Starzl and colleagues have reported the use of CsA in three pediatric renal transplant recipients and eight pediatric liver transplant recipients.[5] All three renal transplant recipients tolerated the drug well and had functioning grafts 4–6 months after transplantation. We report here our experience with cyclosporine in 15 pediatric renal transplant recipients, after 1–20 months of follow-up.

MATERIALS AND METHODS

Fifteen children, ages 3–17 years, have received renal allografts with cyclosporine and prednisone immunosuppression. Time elapsed since transplantation has been 1–20 months. Seven patients received grafts from living related donors (LRD), for a total experience using CsA of 44 patient months. Five of these seven patients who received LRD grafts are prepubertal or in early puberty. Eight patients received grafts from cadaver donors (CAD), for a total experience using CsA of 42 patient months. Five of these eight patients who received CAD grafts are prepubertal or in early puberty (Table 1).

The CsA dosages used are given in Table 2. Initial dosage was 14 mg/kg of body weight daily p.o., tapering to a mean of 10 mg/kg daily at 1 month after transplantation and to a mean of 7 mg/kg daily at 4 months after transplantation. Trough serum levels (≥18 hr after the dose) were used to regulate the dosage during the first month after transplantation, with the goal of maintaining the trough serum level at 100–200 ng/ml. Levels were measured by radioimmunoassay.[6] Prednisone had been given initially in four divided doses of 2–3 mg/kg of body weight daily, tapering as given in Table 3. Seven children who had received azathioprine just prior to our conversion to the use of CsA and who had continued function of their transplants were analyzed for prednisone dosage given. These seven patients ranged in age from 12 to 16 years. One received a CAD transplant; six received LRD transplants.

RESULTS

Of the 15 patients, 13 have functioning grafts 1–20 months after transplantation. Seven of eight CAD grafts are functioning; six of seven LRD grafts are functioning. Serum creatinine levels range from 0.6 to 2.3 mg/dl, with 12/13 patients having serum creatinine

Table 1. CsA Therapy for Pediatric Renal Transplant Recipients

Patient	Age	Sex	Months Since Transplant	Serum Creatinine (mg/dl)
Living related Donor				
M. N.	3*	M	5	0.6
Y. G.	9*	F	1	0.9
T. H.	15*	M	2	1.0
M. M.	15*	M	(Immediate loss)	(Dialysis)
P. L.	15*	M	1	1.7
R. S.	15	M	14	2.3
A. G.	16	F	20	1.4
Cadaver				
M. P.	9*	F	4	1.0
K. T.	9*	F	(Loss at 4 months)	(Dialysis)
J. C.	11*	M	4	1.3
S. S.	13*	F	11	0.9
K. H.	14*	M	10	1.4
S. D.	15	M	4	1.5
A. T.	15	M	1	1.3
H. W.	17	F	4	1.1

*Prepubertal children.

From the Department of Pediatrics and the Department of Surgery, Division of Organ Transplantation, The University of Texas Medical School, Houston, TX.

Reprint requests should be addressed to Dr. Susan B. Conley, Department of Pediatrics, The University of Texas Medical School, 6431 Fannin, Houston, TX 77030.

0041–1345/83/1505–0061$01.00/0

Table 2. Daily Oral CsA Dosage

Initial	14 mg/kg
1 month	10 mg/kg (range, 7–13 mg/kg)
4 months	7 mg/kg (range, 6–12 mg/kg)
12 months	7 mg/kg (range, 6–8 mg/kg)

levels of $\leq$1.7 mg/dl. The loss of the CAD (patient K.T.) was caused by the recurrence of oxalosis. The loss of the LRD graft (patient M.M.) was caused by cortical necrosis secondary to vascular insufficiency in the immediate postoperative period. No grafts have been lost to rejection.

Three patients have had rejection episodes, 6 days, 24 days, and 5 months after transplantation, respectively. All patients had CsA serum trough levels of <60 ng/ml at the time of the rejection episode. All recovered after high-dose prednisone therapy. Two patients required hemodialysis during the rejection episodes.

Hirsutism has been the most frequent side effect of the drug, being present in all 14 patients who have received the drug for >1 month. Mild nephrotoxicity, marked by rises in serum creatinine of >25%, has occurred in 5 patients. In each instance, the serum creatinine has returned to its previous level with reduction of the CsA dosage. In addition, 1 patient had a doubling of the serum creatinine related to trimethoprim-sulfamethoxisole therapy. Five children have had tremor, which resolved spontaneously. Hypertension occurred universally in the 14 patients but has been difficult to control in only 2 patients. Possible hepatotoxicity, marked by a rise in levels of serum liver enzymes but not a rise in the serum bilirubin level, has been noted in 1 patient. Hyperkalemia, a serum potassium of >5.5 meq/liter, has been noted in 2 patients. Neither serious infection nor gingival hyperplasia has been noted.

Table 4. CsA Toxicity (*N* = 14)

	No. of Patients	Percentage
Hirsutism	14	100
Nephrotoxicity	5	36
Tremor	5	36
Hypertension (difficult to control)	2	14
Possible hepatotoxicity	1	7
Hyperkalemia	1	7
Serious infection	0	—
Gingival hyperplasia	0	—

The prednisone dosages used have been significantly lower than dosages given to the previous seven patients, whom we had transplanted using azathioprine (Table 3). One patient has been off prednisone for 5 months, since 15 months after transplantation.

DISCUSSION

Cyclosporine appears to have significant potential as an immunosuppressant agent in pediatric renal allograft recipients. The most serious question that has been posed about the use of CsA in a patient of any age has been whether it is unacceptably nephrotoxic.[7–9] In our series of patients, nephrotoxicity appears to be a minor problem, although it is possible that undetected chronic nephrotoxicity is present in these patients. Levels of serum creatinine are elevated above normal for patient size in all the children, even though they are <2 mg/dl in all but one patient. Further experience will demonstrate whether renal function in patients receiving CsA is sufficient to allow growth.

Other drug-related side effects have also been of minor consequence. Hirsutism has been a universal side effect; tremor has been frequent. Neither has been an indication to stop using the drug. Serious infections have not occurred in these children. (See Table 4.)

Table 3. Prednisone Dosage (mg/kg of body weight daily)

	Initial	At 1 Month	At 4 Months
Azathioprine	0.95 (range, 0.70–1.2) (*N* = 7)	0.61 (range, 0.42–1.0) (*N* = 7)	0.48 (range, 0.38–0.74) (*N* = 6)
Cyclosporine	0.74 (range, 0.42–2.0) (*N* = 14)	0.35 (range, 0.31–0.41) (*N* = 8)	0.22 (range, 0.17–0.26) (*N* = 3)

Growth may be enhanced because the use of CsA appears to allow for the use of less prednisone. This reduction in the prednisone dosage can often be attributed to the fact that patients treated with CsA have fewer rejection episodes than do patients treated with azathioprine. They are therefore recycled back to higher doses of prednisone less often than are patients on azathioprine. Our experience currently is not long enough to assess growth. Our longest-term CsA renal transplant recipients have had bone ages of >12 years, so we have not expected to see much growth in them. We are encouraged that growth may occur, since our youngest patient, at 3 years old, has grown at a rate of 2 cm/month in the 5 months since he received his transplant.

The major advantage of the drug has been that rejection has been prevented in most patients, occurring in only 3/14 patients and responding to high-dose prednisone therapy in all 3 patients. No grafts have been lost to rejection; the only two graft losses were secondary to recurrent disease and to vascular insufficiency.

More extensive experience is needed with the use of cyclosporine in children, but this preliminary experience indicates the drug holds promise as an effective agent for preventing rejection and has an acceptable level of toxicity.

REFERENCES

1. Starzl TE, Weil R, Iwatsuki S, et al: Surg Gynecol Obstet 151:17, 1980
2. Calne RY, White DJG, Thiru S, et al: Lancet 2:1323, 1978
3. Report on the European Multicentre Trial: Lancet 2:59, 1982
4. Kahan BD, Van Buren CT, Lin SN: Transplantation 34:36, 1982
5. Starzl TE, Iwatsuki S, Malatack JJ, et al: J Pediatr 100:681 1982
6. Donatsch P, Abisch E, Homberger M, et al: J Immunoassay 2:19, 1981
7. Klintmalm GBG, Iwatsuki S, Starzl TE: Lancet 1:470, 1981
8. Trompeter RS, Chantler C, Haycock GB: Lancet 1:1218, 1981
9. Thomson AW, Cameron ID: Scot Med J 26:139, 1981

Cyclosporine and Steroids: Effects on the Clinical Course After Renal Allotransplantation

H. Bunzendahl, K. Wonigeit, J. Klempnauer, C. Brölsch, and R. Pichlmayr

CYCLOSPORINE (CsA) monotherapy has proved to be an effective immunosuppressive regimen in the European Multicentre Trial.[1] However, rejection crises demanding high doses of steroids for treatment have been frequent, and the number of steroid-free patients has remained small. The concept of combining CsA with steroids in low doses proposed by Starzl[2] and Najarian[3] tries to increase efficacy and to decrease toxicity and side effects of CsA therapy. After participation in the European Multicentre Trial, we continued the use of CsA in kidney and liver transplantation. A combination of CsA and prednisolone was chosen. Results of renal transplantation with special emphasis on rejection episodes are reported here.

MATERIALS AND METHODS

In 1982, 104 kidney transplants from cadaveric donors and 9 from living related donors have been performed at our institution. The combination protocol with CsA and prednisolone was used in 75 of them. Early in 1982, only high-risk patients were selected because of limited supply of CsA. Later it became the standard protocol for immunosuppression. This explains a high ratio of patients with special risk factors within this group (Table 1).

Of 75 patients, 33 had one or more risk factors (age over 50, diabetes, or multiple transplants), and 8/17 patients with second and third grafts had lost a previous graft from early acute rejection. CsA therapy was started with an oral dose 6 hr before transplantation and continued irrespective of graft function. The dosage protocol was as follows: Cyclosporine, preoperatively through week 1, 14 mg/kg of body weight p.o.; through week 2, 11 mg/kg; and thereafter, 8 mg/kg. Prednisolone, weeks 1–4, 2.0–0.3 mg/kg; weeks 4–8, 0.3–0.15 mg/kg; and thereafter, 0.15 mg/kg. Cyclosporine was given in divided doses.

Rejection episodes were treated with methylprednisolone 500-mg boluses for 1–5 days maximum. Diagnosis of rejection was based on clinical signs, laboratory, nuclear medicine, and biopsy (74 biopsies in 45 patients). In addition, the subcapsular hydrostatic pressure (SHP) was measured in 30 patients over a period of 15–20 days; this facilitated the diagnosis of rejection.[4]

The daily dosage of CsA was reduced beneath the protocol if signs of CsA toxicity (nephrotoxicity, hepatotoxicity, tremor) were present or if measured CsA levels were unacceptably high. CsA levels were determined by RIA from plasma, and later during the year from whole blood.[5] Patients remained in the hospital routinely for about 4 weeks; outpatients were controlled regularly.

RESULTS

Patient and Graft Survival

The actuarial graft survival of all patients at 3, 6, and 12 months is 81%, 76%, and 73%, respectively (Fig. 1). Of 75 patients, 73 are alive. A 57-year-old female with preexisting aortic valvular disease succumbed after 4 months to bacterial endocarditis with a functioning graft. A 29-year-old female with a second transplant died suddenly at home 6 weeks after transplantation. Autopsy findings were compatible with sepsis. The graft had never functioned. In 16 patients grafts were lost for reasons specified in Table 2.

Acute Tubular Necrosis (ATN)

The time of cold storage was 37.7 ± 7.6 hr (range, 18–54 hr). No machine perfusion was used. Postoperative dialysis was necessary in 53.3% of the patients. The average length of dialysis in patients whose grafts finally functioned was 15.9 ± 1.4 days. In this group with ATN, eight grafts were lost with signs of rejection; only two grafts were rejected after primary function.

Rejection Episodes

Of 75 patients, 38 were never treated for rejection. Nine additional patients were

From the Klinik für Abdominal- und Transplantationschirurgie, Medizinische Hochschule, Hannover, Germany.

Reprint requests should be addressed to Dr. Bunzendahl, Klinik für Abdominal- und Transplantationschirurgie, Medizinische Hochschule, Hannover, Konstanty Gutschow Straße 8, D-3000 Hannover 61, Germany.

0041-1345/83/1505-0062$01.00/0

Table 1. The 75 Patients in the Study

Transplants	
First graft	58 (77.3%)
Second graft	11 (14.7%)
Third graft	6 (8.0%)
Sex	
Male	48 (64.0%)
Female	27 (36.0%)
Age	38.7 ± 11.3 years
Risk factors	
Age > 50 years	13 (17.3%)
Diabetes mellitus	5 (6.7%)

treated for rejection because of clinical suspicion; during their treatment, objective findings, such as biopsy or CsA levels, led to correction of the rejection diagnosis and therapy. A total of 47 patients, therefore, did not have rejection episodes at all. In 16 patients, rejection could be confirmed by clinical signs, response to steroids, or biopsy. The remaining 12 patients are classified as questionable rejections. Their biopsies show slight interstitial infiltrates. Although this suggests primarily nephrotoxicity, rejection cannot be ruled out with certainty in these cases.

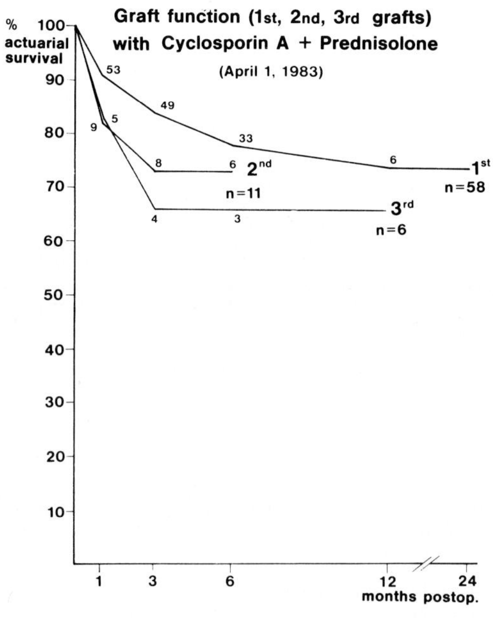

Fig. 1. Actuarial graft survival of 75 patients with first (1), second (2), and third (3) transplants (no exclusions; minimum follow-up, 5 months).

Table 2. Causes of Graft Loss in 16 Patients

Diagnosis	Period of Function (days)
Immunologic failures	
Acute rejection with ATN	0
Acute rejection with ATN	0
Acute rejection and urinary tract obstruction	22–52
Acute rejection after withdrawal of immunosuppression	10–27
Steroid-resistant rejection after positive crossmatch*	1–36
Low CsA levels with phenytoin	0
Low CsA levels with phenytoin	27–37
Late rejection with low CsA levels after erroneously long CsA reduction	16–111
Chronic rejection	1–312
Nonimmunologic failures	
Arterial thrombosis on day 6	0
Arterial thrombosis on day 14	0
Hemorrhage after biopsy	10–81
Infection of arterial anastomosis	1–23
Interstitial graft infection after urinary tract obstruction	12–63
Cortical necrosis	0
Unknown	1–68

*Crossmatch negative in donor center, retrospective test positive in our center.

The majority of confirmed rejection episodes (9/16) responded well to steroid bolus treatment and have stable graft function at the present time.

Toxicity and Side Effects

Transient increases in serum creatinine not related to rejection but accompanied by high levels of CsA occurred in 30% of all patients. Since these episodes responded well to CsA dose reduction, they had to be regarded as drug-induced nephrotoxicity. Mean creatinine values at 3 and 6 months were 160 ± 57 and 157 ± 48, respectively. At 3 months, 23.5% of all patients had a serum creatinine below 120 μmole/liter. Hirsutism was frequently observed, but very few patients complained of it. Gingival hyperplasia and tremor were rare. Steroid side effects were mild. Although a Cushingoid appearance developed in about 25% of the patients, this was usually mild or absent after 3 months. Steroid diabetes and steroid-induced bone complications have not been seen to date.

Infections

Bacterial and viral infections were observed at about the frequency previously seen with conventional immunosuppression (Table 3). They contributed to the two deaths. Pneumonia in a smoker led us to withdraw immunosuppression; the graft was subsequently rejected within 1 week. Because of prolonged CMV disease with moderate severity in one patient, immunosuppression was stopped for 6 weeks without signs of rejection. All other virus infections were of low severity and short duration.

Table 3. Infections in 75 Patients

Bacterial	
Lethal sepsis (endocarditis)	1
Suspected sepsis	1
Bacteremia	4
Pneumonia (smoker)	1
Graft infection	4
Symptomatic urinary tract infection	6
Asymptomatic urinary tract infection	30
Viral	
CMV syndrome	9
CMV seroconversion without clinical disease	6
Herpes labialis	35
Herpes simplex Type I in genital region	1

DISCUSSION

CsA differs in its chemical structure and pharmacologic properties from other immunosuppressive agents used at present. Its effects on the immune system as well as its side effects are unique. Therefore, it is not surprising that CsA changes in many ways the post-transplant course of allograft recipients. Because the results reported were not obtained in a controlled trial, they do not allow conclusions about possible superiority of this immunosuppressive regimen. But they clearly demonstrate a remarkable change in the postoperative course when compared to conventional therapy.

The frequency of rejection episodes is decreased; so is graft loss due to irreversible rejection. Classical clinical signs of rejection, such as graft tenderness and swelling, fever, and illness, are quite infrequent. Only about 20% of all patients developed clear-cut rejection episodes with typical biopsy findings. On the other hand, 60% of the patients did not show any signs of rejection at all. This is in contrast to previous experience with conventional immunosuppression and also with CsA monotherapy. This change in frequency of acute rejection was unexpected. Anticipation of rejection may have influenced the decision to treat questionable rejection episodes in some instances. In patients with otherwise uncomplicated courses, only two grafts were lost from rejection. In eight patients, however, rejection may have contributed to graft loss. Factors such as infection and prolonged ATN were involved. This reflects difficulties in differential diagnosis and adequate handling of immunosuppression in patients with complicated postoperative courses. The incidence of ATN in this study was unexpectedly high and exceeds that previously seen with conventional immunosuppression. The question arises whether this might have its cause in the combined effects of ischemic injury and acute CsA toxicity. This hypothesis is supported by findings of Devineni et al.,[6] who showed an exacerbation of CsA toxicity after ischemic renal injury in a dog model. This has prompted a change in our policy to limit the time of cold storage to 24 hr whenever possible.

Nephrotoxicity has been the most frequent side effect of CsA therapy. Although the relatively low CsA dosage has resulted in less frequent and less severe signs of toxicity, it still remains a problem in patient management. Differentiation from rejection is facilitated when plasma or blood levels are determined. Deterioration of graft function in the presence of plasma levels above 500 ng/ml or whole blood levels above 1000 ng/ml is most likely due to drug toxicity. We feel that the incidence of nephrotoxicity can be markedly reduced by avoiding levels in this range.[7] Marked nephrotoxicity, however, can also occur at lower CsA levels. Differentiation from rejection may require graft biopsy. In this situation, the measurement of the subcapsular renal hydrostatic pressure (SHP) has also proved to be of value for this purpose.[4,8] Whereas rejection is accompanied by an increase in the SHP, it remains low during CsA nephrotoxicity.

Infections, both bacterial and viral, with CsA seem to occur at similar frequency as with conventional immunosuppression. They continue to be a challenge in prevention, detection, and treatment.

SUMMARY

CsA used with steroids in 75 renal allograft recipients has shown to be very effective in reducing rejection episodes and ultimate graft loss. ATN and CsA nephrotoxicity have complicated patient management; their prevention seems to be possible. Infections have remained an important cause of morbidity and mortality. For the majority of patients, this immunosuppressive regimen results in a smooth post-transplant course.

REFERENCES

1. Report on the European Multicentre Trial: Lancet 2:57, 1982
2. Starzl TE, Weil R III, Iwatsuki S, et al: Surg Gynecol Obstet 151:17, 1980
3. Najarian JS, Ferguson RM, Sutherland DER, et al: Transplant Proc 15:438, 1983
4. Wagner E, Pichlmayr R, Wonigeit K, et al: Transplant Proc 15:489, 1983
5. Donatsch P, Abisch E, Homberger E, et al: Immunoassay 2:19, 1981
6. Devineni R, Keown P, Stiller C, et al: Transplant Proc (this issue)
7. Wonigeit K, et al: (submitted for publication)
8. Wagner E, Pichlmayr R, Wonigeit K, et al: Transplant Proc (in press)

Cyclosporine for Steroid-Resistant Rejection in Azathioprine-Treated Renal Graft Recipients

A. S. MacDonald, P. Belitsky, A. Cohen, J. Crocker, R. Gupta, S. G. Lannon, and J. White

THE PRESUMED MECHANISM of action of cyclosporine (CsA) is such that its most appropriate use should be to prevent rather than treat established graft rejection.[1] The drug has been shown to be unable to reverse established skin-graft rejection in mice.[2] On the other hand, it can reverse graft-vs.-host disease in marrow recipients.[3] We report here our experience with the use of CsA in the treatment of steroid-resistant renal allograft rejection in a group of patients previously maintained on azathioprine and prednisone.

MATERIALS AND METHODS

Twelve patients, five males and seven females, aged 8–40, were entered into the study between March and November 1982. There were three living related donor (LRD) and nine cadaveric (CAD) graft recipients. One of the latter had been treated initially with cyclosporine but was switched to conventional therapy at 105 days. All the others were on maintenance azathioprine and prednisone from the time of their transplants, 16 days to 10 years previously. One patient had two separate rejection crises treated.

Rejection was diagnosed on clinical grounds and confirmed by needle biopsy in all but one patient. Rejection was defined as acute if it occurred in a patient with previously stable function and resulted in rises in serum creatinine of at least 100 mmole/liter/day on 3 consecutive days, accompanied by the usual morphologic changes of inflammatory cell infiltration. Rejection was considered to be chronic if the rise in serum creatinine took place slowly over a period of weeks to months and was accompanied by biopsy changes of fibrosis, loss of glomeruli, obliterative arteritis, and minimal inflammatory cell infiltrate, or if multiple acute episodes occurred with persistence of renal dysfunction. Steroid resistance was considered to be present if the patients failed to respond to two 5-day courses of high-dose prednisone therapy (10 mg/kg of body weight on days 1 and 2, 5 mg/kg on day 3, 3 mg/kg on day 4, and 2 mg/kg on day 5) and in the absence of biopsy evidence of acute tubular necrosis. There were six patients each with chronic and acute rejection in the study.

Informed consent was obtained. The patients discontinued azathioprine and began cyclosporine, 20 mg/kg in divided dosage, with subsequent doses adjusted to maintain serum trough levels of 100–400 ng/ml. The drug was given for at least 10 days in conjunction with low-dose steroids and then discontinued, and the patients restarted on azathioprine, with the exception of two patients who remained on CsA.

RESULTS

The results are summarized in Table 1; the acute cases, in Fig. 1. Six CAD kidney recipients had seven rejection episodes within 3 months of transplantation. All seven rejection episodes were reversed by CsA. In six of the episodes, the serum creatinine began to fall within the 10-day treatment period, and in the other, diuresis was evident within 17 days of starting CsA. In four patients, including the three children (ages 4, 8, and 12 years), the creatinines have normalized and remained so for the follow-up period of 8–12 months without further rejection episodes. Two children had two rejection episodes prior to the institution of CsA for steroid insensitivity; the other had one. One of the adult patients had had a previous severe steroid-resistant rejection in the first month after grafting that responded to antithymocyte globulin (ATG) despite biopsy evidence of extensive fibrinoid necrosis. Thirty days later, he developed an equally severe rejection, which on biopsy was characterized by extensive fibrinoid necrosis but only moderate cellular infiltrate. Much to our surprise, he had a delayed but gratifying response to cyclosporine. This drug was continued thereafter. The initial improvement has not been sustained, and over the succeeding 6 months, the creatinine has slowly risen. Another patient has had a similar course, with

From the Transplant Service, Dalhousie University, Halifax, Nova Scotia, Canada.

Reprint requests should be addressed to Dr. A. S. MacDonald, Department of Surgery, Victoria General Hospital, Halifax, Nova Scotia B3H 2Y9, Canada.

0041-1345/83/1505-0063$01.00/0

Table 1. Results of Treatment with Cyclosporine

Months from Transplant to Resistant Rejection	No. of Patients	No. of Rejection Episodes	Immediate Results			Ultimate Results			
			Reversed	Stable	Failed	Normal	Stable	Worse	Lost
0–6	6	7	6	1	0	4	0	1	1
6–18	3	3	0	0	0	0	0	1	2
60–120	2	2	0	0	2	0	0	0	2

two rejections reversed by CsA, and now has stable good function on azathioprine and prednisone. The last patient in the group had an excellent response to CsA with normal creatinine in the next 12 months of follow-up, but ultimately his graft function slowly deteriorated on maintenance steroids and azathioprine, and he is now dialysis dependent.

In contrast, the fate of patients with chronic rejection was less salutary. Two patients with slowly deteriorating LRD grafts 60 and 120 months after transplantation showed no improvement after 10 days of CsA. Both were ultimately regrafted. Three other patients, at 14, 16, and 17 months, respectively, with more rapid deterioration, all with multiple previous steroid-responsive rejections, had finally become unresponsive to high-dose prednisone. Unfortunately, the loss of function continued unabated despite at least 10 days of CsA therapy. Only one patient in the group responded. She had originally been treated with CsA with only one mild rejection, easily reversed with prednisone at 10 days. She was switched to azathioprine at 90 days, and 5 months later had a severe rejection episode. Steroids were not helpful, and she was put back on CsA. She had a prompt response, but it has not been sustained. Over the past 12 months, the creatinine has slowly but steadily risen, and biopsies confirm chronic rejection.

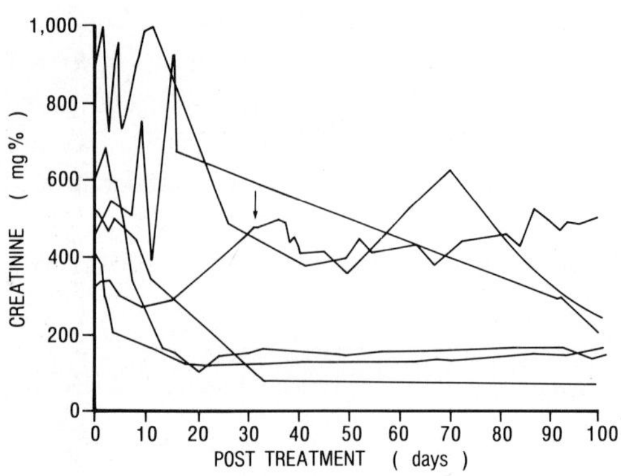

Fig. 1. Serum creatinine curves for acute rejections in 6 patients treated with 10 days of oral cyclosporine. The "↓" indicates a second episode in one patient.

DISCUSSION

Calne and his colleagues had reported that cyclosporine was not particularly effective in reversing rejection crises in kidney transplant recipients. However, at that time, the nephrotoxicity of the drug and the hazards of combining it with other immunosuppressives were not fully appreciated. The experimental evidence is conflicting. Leapman et al.[4] suggested the CsA could inhibit secondary responses of primed T cells in mixed lymphocyte cultures. This was at odds with the results of Lindsey et al.,[5] who could not show any effect for CsA in preventing secondary antibody responses to bovine serum albumin (BSA) in BSA-immunized rabbits. Furthermore, Borel was unable to reverse established skin-graft rejection in mice.[2] However, the drug is clearly effective in reversing established graft-vs.-host disease.[3] In this study, we have found that CsA can reverse severe rejections, but only within the first few post-transplant months. Rejection occurring in the second year, whether of rapid onset and progression, as in 4 of our patients, or of the slow, chronic type, is unaffected, at least by a short course (1–3 weeks) of CsA.

If CsA affects only T cells and then only during the early stages of antigen sensitization, one must postulate that early rejection episodes within the first few months are still largely or wholly T-cell dependent. Presumably, conventional therapy with azathioprine and prednisone, while unable to suppress the immune response completely, is adequate to control B-cell activation. Thus, the repeated rejections are not antibody-mediated and are, therefore, still reversible by a T-cell active agent. Delayed use of CsA as described by Borel is ineffective because B-cell activation has already taken place by the time the drug has been given, and, as has been mentioned, neither primary antibody production, once started, nor secondary antibody responses are affected by CsA.

We certainly favor this explanation, as it fits our clinical experience with the use of CsA in presensitized renal graft recipients in a study not yet published. The drug cannot prevent hyperacute or accelerated rejections in this type of patient, although it is effective in this hyper-responsive group if kidneys, bearing antigens to which the recipient is sensitized, can be avoided.

The uniform success of CsA in reversing early severe rejections in kidney transplantation is encouraging, as it provides an alternative to antilymphocyte serum. In view of the expected costs of CsA, its use for continuous maintenance therapy may be prohibitively expensive. Its use for short-term therapy of rejection may be a suitable option.

ACKNOWLEDGMENT

We wish to thank Miss Alice Whelan, R.N., and Miss Pat Miller, R.N., for help with both the care of the patients and data retrieval and analysis.

REFERENCES

1. Wagner H: Transplant Proc 15:523, 1983
2. Borel JF: Transplant Proc 13:344, 1981
3. Powles RL, Clink HM, Spence D: Lancet 1:327, 1980
4. Leapman SB, Filo RS, Smith EJ, et al: Transplant Proc 12:246, 1980
5. Lindsey NJ, Harris KR, Norman HB, et al: Transplant Proc 12:252, 1980

A Critical Look at Renal Allografts That Failed in Patients Receiving Cyclosporine

T. Kovithavongs, W. H. Lakey, R. Boake, K. B. Bettcher, P. McCormick, and J. B. Dossetor

THERE HAS BEEN overwhelming evidence in recent literature supporting the notion that cyclosporine (CsA) is a superior immunosuppressive drug compared with azathioprine and prednisone in organ transplantation.[1] In this report, we examine why some renal allografts failed in patients who received CsA with the aim of identifying factors that might be avoided so that graft survival could be further improved. The analysis is made on 37 kidneys transplanted since January 1981, when this center entered the CsA trial of the Canadian Multicentre Transplant Study Group. Details of the 16 patients who received CsA and the other 21 patients treated with conventional or standard medications are listed in Table 1. All patients had a negative crossmatch by standard complement-dependent cytotoxicity. In the standard treatment group, patients received azathioprine (Aza) at a dose of 2.5 mg/kg/day plus prednisone (P) 1.5 mg/kg/day on the day of transplantation. Subsequently, Aza was given at a dose that maintained WBC counts of not less than $4000/mm^3$, and P was gradually tapered to a maintenance dose of 15–20 mg on alternate days by about 6 weeks. In CsA-treated patients, a loading dose of 20 mg/kg was given orally several hours prior to surgery, followed by a twice daily dose to maintain trough blood levels of 100–400 ng/ml, as measured by radioimmunoassay with kits provided by Sandoz Ltd. As oral administration proved unsatisfactory in some patients (see below), those entered later into the trial were given CsA intravenously, using a loading dose that was ¼ the oral loading dose. In addition, this later group of patients also received alternate-day P starting on day 14 at 1 mg/kg, which was rapidly reduced by 5 mg to 0.3 mg/kg until 3 months, at which time it was maintained at 0.25 mg/kg. In both groups of patients, each rejection episode was treated by i.v. methylprednisolone (MP), 1 g/day for 3–4 days, with a total of 15–16 g allowed per patient in 4–5 courses. Local irradiation, 150 rad on four occasions, was included in the treatment protocol, should the patient prove resistant to i.v. MP therapy.

From the Departments of Medicine, Laboratory Medicine, and Surgery, University of Alberta, Edmonton, Alberta, Canada.

Supported by the Medical Research Council of Canada (Grant MT 6011) and the Canadian Multicentre Transplant Study Group, CMTSG, London, Ontario, Canada.

Reprint requests should be addressed to Dr. T. Kovithavongs, Room 1046, University Hospital, Edmonton, Alberta, Canada.

0041-1345/83/1505-0064$01.00/0

STANDARD TREATMENT GROUP

Of the 21 kidneys followed for a period of 6–26 months, 7 were lost, 6 of them by rejection. Three were rejected in 3 weeks. One was rejected at 40 days, possibly aggravated by the use of lithium for the treatment of Aza-induced neutropenia.[2] Two remaining grafts were lost by chronic rejection at 140 days and 14 months, respectively. One graft had a persistent urinary leak from a ureteropelvic rupture that was unable to heal and was removed after 310 days. At the time of nephrectomy, the kidney was functioning reasonably well and was maintaining a serum creatinine of 240 μmole/liter. Of the 14 functioning grafts, 2 never had a rejection episode. The serum creatinine of these graft recipients when last seen ranged from 106–548 μmole/liter.

There were no instances of persistent nonfunction in the group.

CSA-TREATED GROUP

Six kidneys were lost in this small group of 16, seemingly making CsA treatment no dif-

Table 1. Clinical Data

Patient	Age	Sex	Original Renal Disease*	Blood Transfusion	Clinical Course†
Standard treatment group					
A. S. (1)	51	F	Polycystic	Yes	Rejected in 3 weeks
T. T.	25	F	Trauma	Yes	Rejection +, Cr 170 (3 mo), 143 (24 mo)
V. A.	40	M	MGN	Yes	No rejection, Cr 110 (3 mo), 125 (26 mo)
S. C.	54	F	CPN	Yes	Rejection +, Cr 100 (3 mo), 153 (25 mo)
J. T.	34	F	CGN	No	Cr 80 (3 mo), 240 (310 days); urinary leak from ureteropelvic rupture led to graft removal
W. B.	40	M	Alport's	Yes	Rejected day 40
J. A.	30	M	CGN	Yes	Rejection +, Cr 180 (3 mo), 126 (21 mo)
J. H.	40	F	CPN	Yes	Rejection +, Cr 140 (3 mo), 440 (21 mo)
J. K.	58	M	Nephrosclerosis	Yes	Rejection +, Cr 130 (3 mo), 106 (6 mo); moved
P. H. (2)	38	M	DM	Yes	Cr 160 (3 mo), rejected 14 mo; deceased
R. C.	27	M	MGN	Yes	Rejection + + +, Cr 460 (3 mo), 195 (17 mo)
R. J.	41	M	DM	Yes	Rejection +, Cr 115 (3 mo), 138 (15 mo)
A. P. (3)	46	F	CPN	Yes	Rejection + + +, Cr 85 (3 mo), 548 (15 mo)
R. M.	25	M	CGN	Yes	Initial nonfunction, Cr 130 (3 mo), 116 (6 mo); moved
M. S.	44	F	DM	Yes	Rejected in 3 weeks
L. C. (2)	50	M	Nephrosclerosis	Yes	Rejection +, Cr 135 (3 mo), 154 (12 mo)
M. D.	26	M	CPN	Yes	Rejection + + + +, Cr 145 (3 mo), 279 (12 mo)
S. K.	25	F	CGN	No	Chronic rejection, Cr 595 (3 mo) led to CAPD 140 days
A. S. (2)	51	F	Polycystic	Yes	Rejection +, Cr 105 (3 mo), 183 (10 mo)
R. H.	40	M	HSP	Yes	Rejected in 3 weeks; deceased
F. P.	41	F	DM	Yes	Rejection +, Cr 115 (3 mo), 152 (9 mo)
Cyclosporine-treated group					
P. H. (1)	37	M	DM	Yes	LMC +; rejected day 9
R. B.	46	F	CGN	Yes	Rejection +, Cr 130 (3 mo), 149 (25 mo)
R. L.	45	M	CGN	Yes	No rejection, Cr 170 (3 mo), 195 (23 mo)
R. M.	56	M	Alport's	Yes	No rejection, Cr 150 (3 mo), 170 (20 mo)
P. E.	40	M	CPN	Yes	Essentially never functioned
W. H. B.	64	M	CGN	Yes	Kidney never functioned; deceased
E. E.	52	F	IgA Nephropathy	Yes	Rejection + + +, Cr 235 (3 mo), 268 (15 mo)
L. C. (1)	50	M	Nephrosclerosis	Yes	Kidney never functioned
E. B.	39	M	CGN	Yes	Kidney never functioned; LMC +
L. M.	63	F	Polycystic	Yes	No rejection, Cr 105 (3 mo), 120 (9 mo)
L. S.	39	M	CGN	Yes	No rejection, Cr 150 (3 mo), 153 (8 mo)
B. K.	42	F	CGN	Yes	Rejection +, Cr 105 (3 mo), 131 (8 mo)
A. W.	53	F	CGN	Yes	No rejection, Cr 245 (3 mo), 181 (8 mo)
L. B.	25	F	DDD	Yes	Rejection +, Cr 95 (3 mo), 118 (7 mo)
P. L.	64	M	CGN	Yes	No rejection, Cr 280 (3 mo), 180 (6 mo)
D. O.	28	F	DM	Yes	Rejected day 15

*CPN = Chronic pyelonephritis
CGN = Chronic glomerulonephritis
DDD = Dense deposit disease or MPGN Type II
DM = Diabetes mellitus
HSP = Henoch-Schonlein purpura
MGN = Membranous glomerulonephritis
†Creatinine (Cr) levels in μmole/liter.

ferent from standard therapy. However, four grafts never functioned from the time they were implanted. These four recipients never put out urine and required regular hemodialysis treatment; the kidneys had poor function on serial renal scanning from the beginning. Three of these are illustrated in Figs. 1–3. Patient E.B. had a positive lymphocyte-mediated cytotoxic (LMC) crossmatch (Fig. 3). He also had subtherapeutic CsA blood levels in the first 2 weeks despite initial i.v. CsA administration and supposedly adequate oral dosage. The course of the fourth patient (Fig. 4) is more difficult to interpret because (1) the initial isotope flow scan was acceptable, (2) there was some residual renal function prior to transplant, (3) multiple antibiotics were given that might have been synergistic with CsA nephrotoxicity, and (4) he needed continuous ambulatory peritoneal dialysis (CAPD), which might have influenced CsA blood levels and made their regulation more difficult. All four kidneys had been subjected to machine perfusion times of longer than 30 hr, a risk factor for CsA recently identified in the Canadian Multicentre Trial[3] and probably responsible for graft loss in these four patients.

The remaining two failed kidneys functioned after implantation despite similarly long perfusion times. Both were grafted into Type I diabetics (both of whom had visceral neuropathic symptoms). In neither of them were therapeutic CsA blood levels achieved in the first 3–7 days (Figs. 5 and 6). The kidneys were rejected on days 9 and 15, respectively. The LMC crossmatch was positive in patient P.H. (Fig. 5) and remained so throughout the course, whereas in patient D.O. (Fig. 6) it was negative initially but turned positive on day 3.

Of the 10 functioning grafts, 6 never suffered a rejection episode. Mean serum creatinine at 3 months was 166 μmole/liter (vs. 164 in the standard treatment group), and when last seen, it ranged from 118–268 in these patients.

INFLUENCE OF MACHINE PERFUSION TIME

Long reanastomosis time (<45 min) and long machine perfusion time (>24 hr) have been implicated as risk factors in patients receiving CsA in the recent Canadian CsA trial.[3] Long perfusion time is also associated with a high incidence of initial nonfunction regardless of the initial (mean first 3 days)

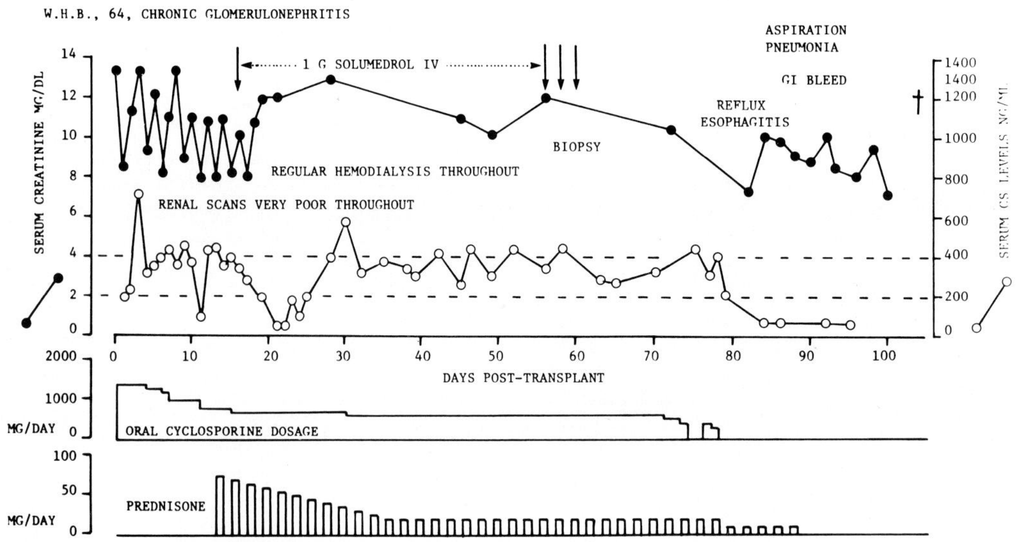

Fig. 1. Clinical course of patient W.H.B., who received a kidney with a warm ischemic time of 21 min and a machine perfusion time of 40 hr.

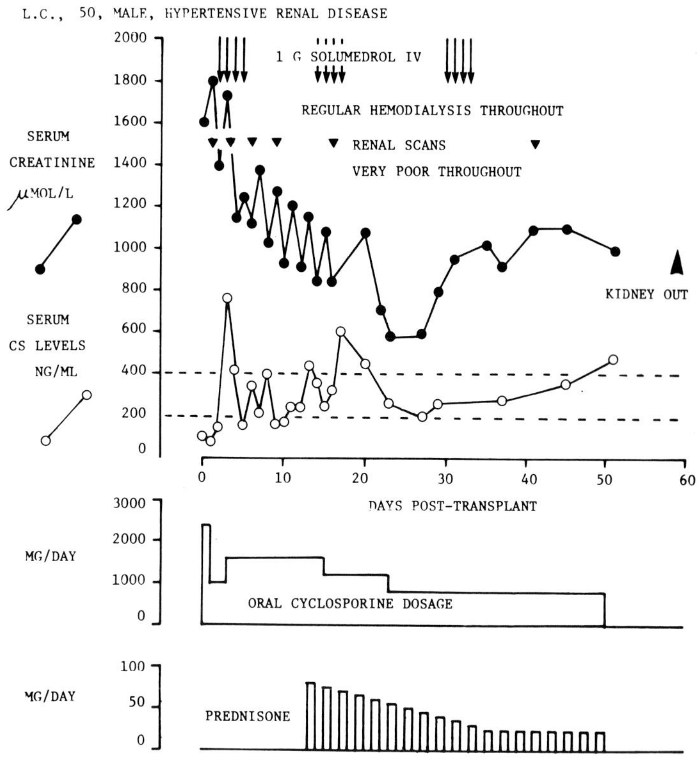

Fig. 2. Clinical course of patient L.C., who received a kidney with a machine perfusion time of 43.5 hr.

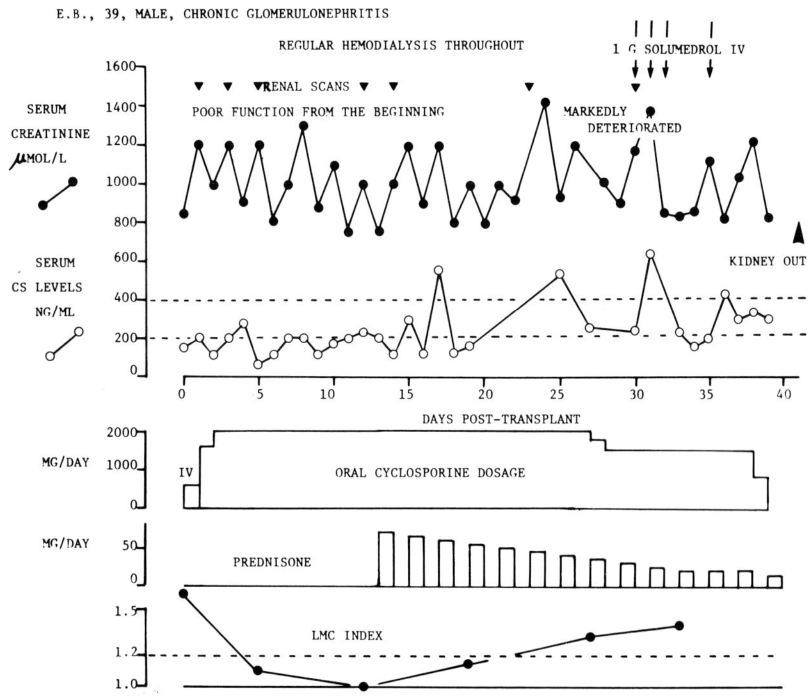

Fig. 3. Clinical course of patient E.B., who received a kidney with a reanastomosis time of 76 min and a machine perfusion time of 40.5 hr.

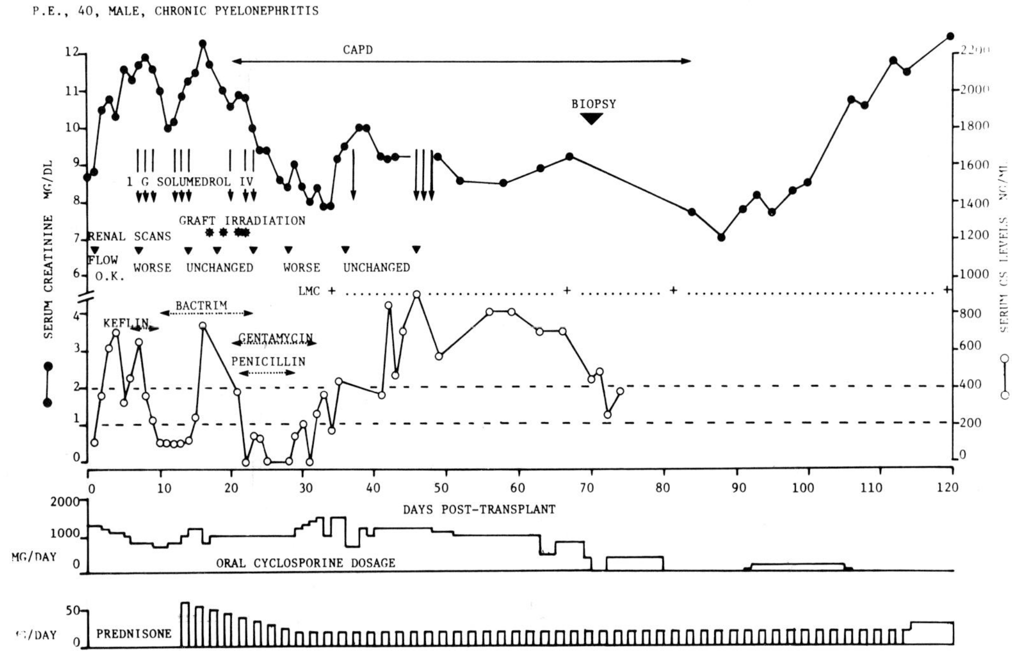

Fig. 4. Clinical course of patient P.E., who received a kidney with a machine perfusion time of 34.3 hr. (See text for discussion.)

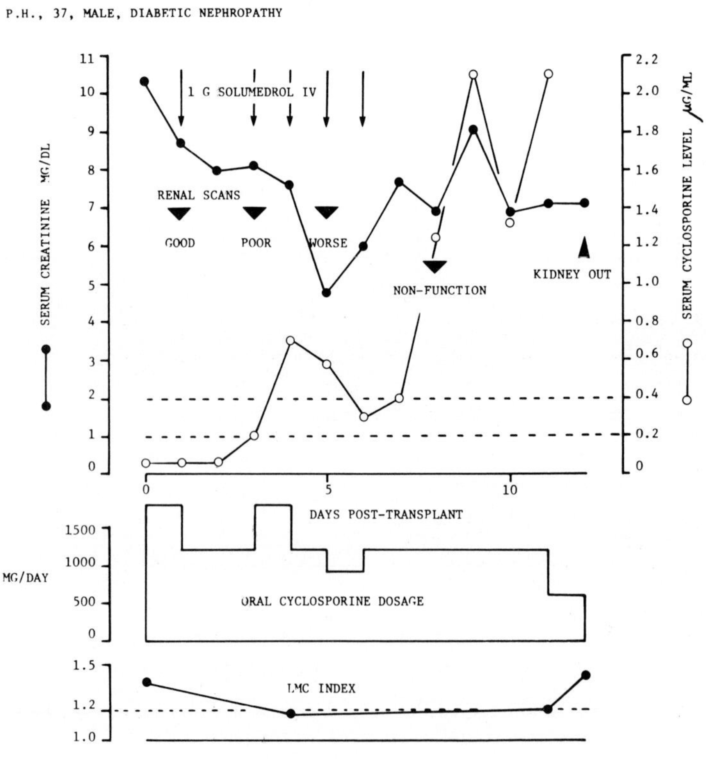

Fig. 5. Clinical course of patient P.H., who received a kidney with a machine perfusion time of 42.6 hr. Note the positive LMC throughout the course, initial subtherapeutic CsA blood levels, and very high levels later on.

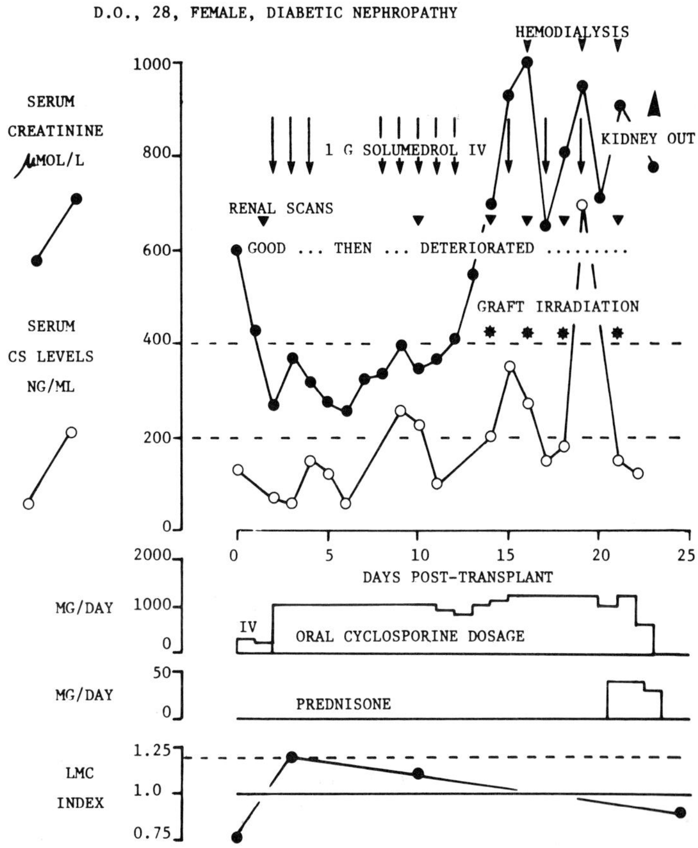

Fig. 6. Clinical course of patient D.O., who received a kidney with a machine perfusion time of 34.5 hr. Note initial subtherapeutic CsA blood levels.

CsA trough levels.[4] Initial nonfunction is characterized by lack of significant urine output, delay in fall of serum creatinine to less than 50% of pretransplant value in 3 days (in the absence of rejection), and need for dialysis. Our analysis (Fig. 7) shows no significant influence of warm ischemic time or reanastomosis time on graft failure, but initial nonfunction occurred in 7/16 kidneys that had been cold-perfused for longer than 30 hr [Fig. 4 (C)]. All three kidneys with initial nonfunction in the standard treatment group regained function in 6–11 days, and two (J.K. and R.M., Table 1) had normal renal function when followed up to 6–10 months. The third patient (J.T.), also with normal renal function, had a persistent urinary leak, which led to graft nephrectomy on day 310.

In contrast, in CsA-treated patients, four kidneys with initial nonfunction regained function. This accounts for 4/6 graft losses in this group; all four had perfusion times longer than 30 hr. In one instance (E.B., Table 1), revision of an anastomosis lengthened the reanastomosis time to 76 min. Before implantation of another kidney (into W.H.B.), it was necessary to join double renal arteries, prior to cooling, prolonging the warm ischemic time to 21 min. None of these had a mean blood CsA trough level of >400 ng/ml in the first 3 days, a level thought to be associated with high incidence of initial nonfunction despite a short perfusion time.[4]

DISCUSSION

At first glance, CsA did not seem to be superior to standard therapy in improving graft survival in kidney transplantation, as comparable numbers of grafts were lost in both groups over the same period of time (37% in the CsA-treated group vs. 33% in the standard treatment group). On close exami-

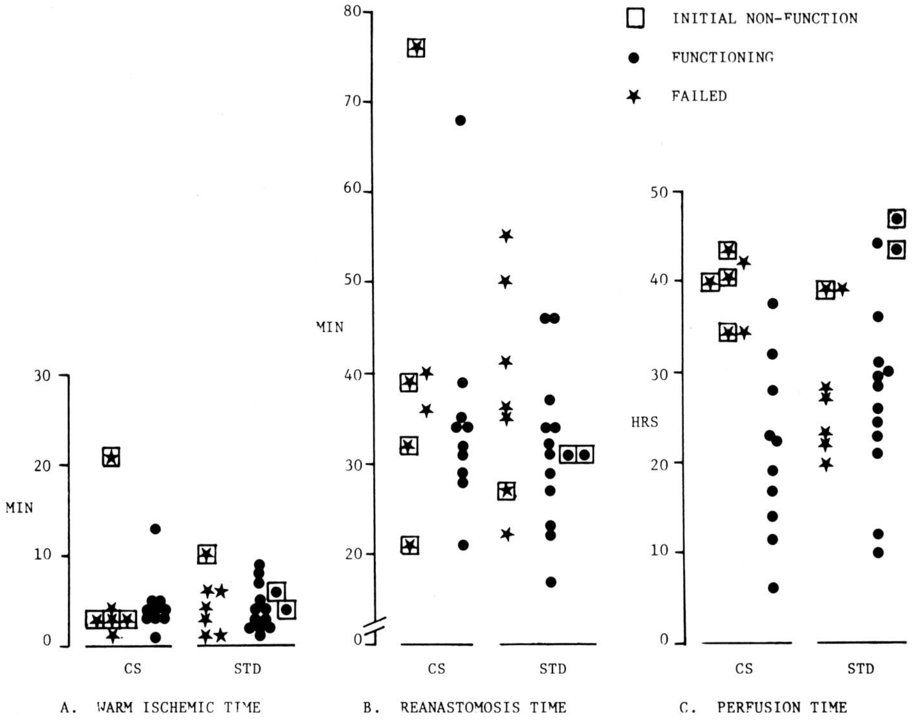

Fig. 7. Influences of (A) warm ischemic time, (B) reanastomosis time, and (C) machine perfusion time on initial graft function, graft success, and graft failure.

nation, however, CsA is superior in preventing graft rejection, as only 2/6 kidneys lost in CsA patients was caused by that mechanism (and in neither were adequate early CsA levels achieved), compared with 6/7 in the other group. In addition, 6/10 functioning grafts in CsA-treated patients suffered no rejection, compared with 2/14 in the other group ($p < 0.02$). As rejection is the most important mechanism for graft loss, CsA is a superior drug compared with azathioprine and prednisone.

CsA is a highly nephrotoxic agent. This has been amply demonstrated in transplantation of organs other than the kidney.[5,6] It is therefore not unexpected that CsA might have a detrimental effect on renal allografts that have been damaged by other nephrotoxic agents[7,8] or by mechanical injury such as prolonged perfusion of the renal vasculature by machine.[3] Whereas all three kidneys that had been perfused for more than 30 hr and developed initial nonfunction recovered their function in the standard treatment group, none of the four initially nonfunctioning kidneys in CsA-treated patients regained function [Fig. 7 (C)].

In a recent experience (not included in this analysis), we observed the immediate failure of a pair of kidneys, obtained from a 16-year-old boy who shot himself in the head, following implantation into patients loaded with CsA. We speculate that the kidneys may have suffered ischemic injury from disseminated intravascular coagulation triggered by the release of thromboplastin from the damaged brain into the circulation, despite the lack of proper documentation beyond a mildly elevated serum creatinine (155 μmole/liter) in the donor prior to bilateral nephrectomy. Alternatively, CsA may enhance the tendency to clot in microcirculations, as has been suggested by the recurrence of hemolytic uremic syndrome in a renal transplant.[9] Whatever the mechanism, it is very probable that we are just beginning to recognize factors that might be synergistic to the nephrotoxic effect of CsA. Prolonged perfusion is one that can be avoided.

Equally important is the observation in the two CsA-treated patients who failed to achieve a therapeutic blood level in the first 3–7 days (Figs. 1 and 2) and who subsequently rejected their grafts. This points out the importance of measuring CsA blood levels at frequent intervals after transplantation and the need to regulate the dose more quickly. As i.v. CsA preparations are now available, it should be possible in the future to give it as a constant i.v. infusion for the first 5–7 days to ensure a certain blood level that is therapeutic and yet minimally nephrotoxic. By avoiding factors that could contribute to undue renal injury on the one hand and eliminating nephrotoxic as well as subtherapeutic blood levels on the other, it should be possible to further enhance renal allograft survival in patients on CsA.

ACKNOWLEDGMENT

We thank our medical, surgical, and nursing colleagues for their care of these patients, Maureen Coulson for excellent record keeping, and Joan Clark for her excellent secretarial assistance.

REFERENCES

1. Beveridge T: Transplant Proc 15:433, 1983

2. Kovithavongs T, Marchuk L, Schlaut J, et al: Transplant Proc (in press)

3. Stiller CR: New Engl J Med (in press)

4. Laupacis A: (personal communication, April 1983)

5. Klintmalm GBG, Iwatsuki S, Starzl TE: Lancet 1:470, 1981

6. Kennedy MS, Deeg HJ, Storb R, et al: Clin Res 30:69, 1982

7. Hows JM, Palmer S, Gordon-Smith EC: Transplantation 33:382, 1982

8. Kennedy MS, Deeg HJ, Siegel M, et al: Transplantation 35:211, 1983

9. Leithner C, Sinzinger H, Pohanka E, et al: Lancet 1:1470, 1982

HEART AND LUNG TRANSPLANTATION

Cyclosporine in Cardiac Transplantation: A 2½ Year Follow-Up

P. E. Oyer, E. B. Stinson, S. W. Jamieson, S. A. Hunt, M. Perlroth, M. Billingham, and N. E. Shumway

CYCLOSPORINE A (CsA) was obtained in the Stanford Cardiovascular Laboratories for experimental studies in 1978. During the ensuing 2 years, its immunosuppressive properties and general lack of toxic side effects were confirmed in several cardiac allograft systems. On the basis of these observations and preliminary clinical trials of the drug in renal transplantation at other institutions, CsA was introduced into the clinical transplant program at Stanford in December 1980. Since that time, all patients undergoing cardiac transplantation have received CsA for postoperative immunosuppression. Reported here is a summary of the updated results of this experience[1,2] and a comparison of selected aspects of such with previous experience using conventional immunosuppression in cardiac recipients.[3-5] Important changes in the techniques of postoperative management of such patients mandated by use of this new immunosuppressant are also discussed.

From the Departments of Cardiovascular Surgery, Cardiology, and Pathology, Stanford University School of Medicine, Stanford, CA.

Reprint requests should be addressed to Dr. P. E. Oyer.

0041-1345/83/1505-0065$01.00/0

MATERIALS AND METHODS

A total of 68 cardiac transplants were performed in 66 patients between December 1980 and May 1983. Several characteristics of this patient group, including their preoperative diagnoses, are outlined in Table 1. The cumulative follow-up duration was 60.3 patient-years, with a maximum follow-up of 2.5 years. All patients except one received orthotopic allografts; one received a heterotopic graft because the only available donor heart was judged too small to fully support his circulation. Two patients, whose initial immunosuppression included CsA, underwent retransplantation, one because of acute graft failure (not due to rejection) and another because of hemodynamically significant constrictive pericardial disease that developed several months after initial transplantation. Three additional patients in the series, who had received cardiac allografts 5–8 years earlier, underwent retransplantation because of coronary atherosclerosis in their previous cardiac allografts.

CsA was administered in concert with relatively low-dose corticosteroid therapy, as outlined in Table 2. During the initial experience (patients 1–28), CsA was given according to a fixed tapering protocol as shown, with minor adjustment of dosages based primarily on evidence of renal function abnormality. In addition, rabbit antithymocyte globulin (RATG) was given as an initial 2–4-dose course, sufficient to lower the fraction of circulating T cells (rosette method) to <2%. Although CsA serum levels were measured in all of the first 28 patients, dosages of the drug were only rarely adjusted on the basis of these data.

The occurrence of four lymphoid malignancies in this initial group of patients prompted a reduction in the overall level of immunosuppression, as outlined in the lower panel of Table 2. This reduction was achieved by omitting use of RATG, except for the treatment of

Table 1. Cyclosporine Patient Summary

Total number of patients	66
Total number of transplants	68
Male/female	52/14
Age range (years)	13–52 (mean, 36.9)
Retransplants	5
Preoperative diagnoses	
Coronary artery disease	
Native heart	21
Transplant heart	3
Cardiomyopathy	38
Viral myocarditis	1
Acute graft failure	1
Coronary embolus (pregnancy)	1
Congenital heart disease	1
Constrictive disease (transplant heart)	1
Valve disease with myopathy	1
Follow-up periods	
Range (months)	0.06–28.5
Average (months)	10.9
Cumulative duration	724 patient-months (60.3 patient-years)

rejection episodes not controllable with corticosteroid therapy alone. In addition, CsA dosages were adjusted more closely on the basis of serum levels to achieve a targeted trough level in the range of 100–300 ng/ml. This modification has resulted generally in more rapid reduction of administered CsA, as compared to the initial patient group. Follow-up is currently too short to determine whether these modifications in the immunosuppressive protocol have reduced significantly the incidence of lymphoproliferative disease in cardiac recipients.

Table 2. Cyclosporine Maintenance Immunosuppression

Initial protocol	(N = 28 patients; Dec. 1980–Jan. 1982)
Cyclosporine	18 mg/kg/day (starting dose); dosage reduced by 2 mg/kg/day at monthly intervals
Prednisone	1 mg/kg/day (initial dose); decreased to 0.2 mg/kg/day by end of 2 months
RATG	2–4-dose initial course
Modified protocol	(N = 38 patients; Jan. 1982–present)
Cyclosporine	18 mg/kg/day (starting dose)*; dosage adjusted to maintain serum levels at 100–300 ng/ml
Prednisone	1 mg/kg/day (starting dose); decreased to 0.2 mg/kg/day by end of 2 months

*Cyclosporine starting dose attenuated in severely debilitated patients with compromised renal and hepatic function.

The diagnosis of acute graft rejection, as previously reported, can be reliably confirmed only by endomyocardial biopsy. As yet, neither the electrocardiogram nor other noninvasive techniques have demonstrated suitable sensitivity and specificity to establish the diagnosis of rejection in patients treated with CsA. It has therefore been necessary to biopsy all patients more frequently, even during the late postoperative period, than was formerly the case in patients treated with azathioprine.

The histologic findings associated with rejection in patients receiving CsA differ somewhat from those occurring during rejection among conventionally treated patients, particularly in terms of myocardial edema. Thus, although interstitial edema was formerly an early hallmark of rejection in patients maintained on azathioprine, this finding is usually minimal or absent during rejection in patients treated with CsA, even in the presence of severe cellular infiltrates and myocardial cell necrosis. The criteria for diagnosis of acute rejection during CsA treatment have become slightly more stringent than previously; thus, patients with mild myocardial infiltrates alone, a finding previously considered indicative of rejection and treated as such, were not judged to be rejecting. Rather, such patients were evaluated by more frequent biopsies and treated for rejection only if histologic changes progressed in severity to include evidence of myocyte necrosis or more severe cellular infiltration. Often, mild lymphocytic infiltrates were documented to resolve spontaneously during such observation periods, although in most instances, progressive changes occurred requiring augmented immunosuppression.

Rejection episodes were usually treated either with pulsed methylprednisolone therapy (1000 mg daily intravenously for 3 days), holding constant the oral corticosteroid dosage, or with augmentation of oral prednisone dose to 100 mg/day, followed by tapering to near previous maintenance levels during the subsequent 2 weeks. RATG has been reserved only for those episodes that remained uncontrolled after at least two courses of pulse therapy with methylprednisolone or when histologic changes were observed to be rapidly progressive or unusually severe.

CsA levels were measured twice weekly during the first 1–3 months after transplantation and at least monthly thereafter. Measurements were performed in serum separated from whole blood at room temperature using reagents supplied by Sandoz Ltd., Basel. Measured levels were not normalized to hematocrit values or to lipid levels.

A group of 99 consecutive patients who underwent cardiac transplantation between 1976 and 1980 and received azathioprine immunosuppression were compared to those who received cyclosporine in order to assess the potential advantages and disadvantages of the latter agent. The use of historical controls to evaluate current therapy is recognized to provide data of limited statistical validity; however, this method does serve to provide baseline data against which reasonable conclusions can be drawn.

RESULTS

Rejection

Although the incidence of rejection among patients maintained on CsA was slightly lower than in those treated with conventional agents, this difference was not significant statistically. The incidence of rejection observed in the two groups during the first 60 postoperative days is shown in Fig. 1. It is important to note that, although the use of CsA has not appreciably reduced the frequency of rejection of cardiac allografts, mortality resulting from this complication has been reduced to near zero in this series. The number of deaths due to acute rejection among CsA patients and azathioprine patients are given in Table 3. It is also noteworthy that this reduction in mortality occurred despite the inability to detect rejection onset in CsA patients by noninvasive methods, as previously mentioned.

Infection

The overall incidence of infection among CsA patients was slightly lower than that previously observed in the azathioprine group.

Table 3. Causes of Death

	Azathioprine Patients ($N = 99$)	Cyclosporine Patients ($N = 66$)
Infection	40	5
Rejection	10	1
Malignancy	3	2
Graft atherosclerosis	1	2
Pulmonary hypertension	2	1
Sudden death	3	0
Pulmonary embolus	1	0
Cardiomyopathy	1	0
Acute graft failure	0	1
CVA	0	1
Cerebral edema	0	1
Total	61	14

Four categories of infection—bacterial, viral, fungal, and nocardial—have been observed in patients receiving CsA. No infections due to *Pneumocystis carinii* have yet occurred in this series. The incidence of infection of all types, calculated actuarially, is shown in Fig. 2 for the two groups of patients.

As in the case of rejection, the *incidence* of infection was only modestly reduced in comparison to patients treated with azathioprine; however, the *mortality* observed among those receiving CsA was substantially lower. Table 3 summarizes the number of deaths in each group resulting from infection. Among the CsA patients who died of infection, two deaths resulted from bacterial infection, two from fungal infection, and one from viral (cyto-

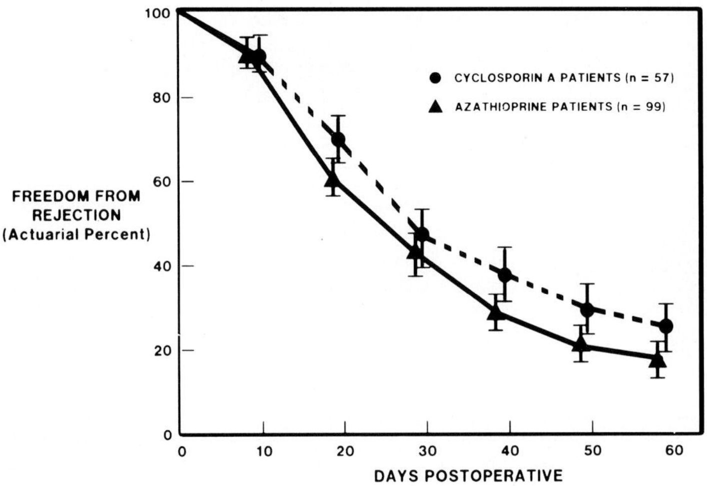

Fig. 1. Actuarial incidence of rejection among patients maintained on CsA compared to the control group of patients maintained on azathioprine. The incidence of rejection was not statistically different in the two groups. Brackets denote 1 SEM.

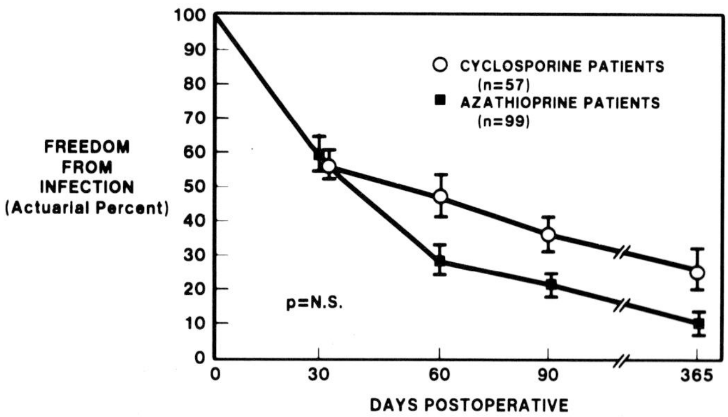

Fig. 2. Actuarial incidence of infection of all types among patients taking CsA compared to the azathioprine control group. The *incidence* of infection was not significantly different in the two groups. Brackets denote 1 SEM.

megalovirus) pneumonia. It is notable that three additional fungal infections occurred in the CsA group; these were successfully treated with amphotericin-D, confirming that this nephrotoxic drug can be used safely in conjunction with CsA. Careful monitoring of renal function and prompt modification of drug dosages if renal compromise occurs are mandatory during such treatment, however. Similarly, use of other nephrotoxic antibiotics, most notably those of the aminoglycoside group, have been used safely in patients receiving CsA with close surveillance of dosages, serum levels, and renal function.

Other Observations

The rate of recuperation of cardiac allograft recipients after operation appears to have improved in a subjective sense since the introduction of cyclosporine. This undoubtedly has resulted partially from the substantial "steroid-sparing" effect of the drug. In addition, the apparent improved "treatability" of rejection and infection episodes and the consequent reduction of the morbidity associated with these complications have allowed substantial reduction in the time required in the intensive care unit and in the overall hospitalization period after transplantation (43 hospital days for CsA patients vs. 72 days for azathioprine patients). The overall mean cost of the transplant hospitalization has, as a consequence, been substantially reduced, from \$100,000 ± \$47,000 for patients treated with azathioprine to \$72,000 ± \$38,100 for those who received CsA (and for whom such cost data are currently available, $N = 48$).

Side Effects and Complications

Several adverse or potentially adverse consequences of CsA administration have been observed. First, most patients have exhibited mild degradation of renal function, with serum creatinine ranging from 1.5–2.5 mg/dl. Such renal dysfunction appears to persist chronically, but with no evidence of progression during the late follow-up period. This CsA-induced dysfunction has not been clinically important, except when concomitant therapy with other nephrotoxic drugs has been necessary, as discussed previously. Four patients, all of whom exhibited severe cardiogenic renal and hepatic dysfunction preoperatively, required hemodialysis during the first 2 weeks after surgery; all recovered adequate renal function thereafter. It would appear, therefore, that such patients with compromised metabolic status preoperatively might benefit from attenuated initial cyclosporine dosages.

A second and possibly related side effect of CsA administration is the development of hypertension in most patients in this series, often within 1 month postoperatively. Adequate control of blood pressure has been difficult to achieve in some cases, even with intensive combination antihypertensive therapy. This observation is in distinct contrast to that in patients maintained on azathioprine, among whom approximately 20% developed hypertension, presumably resulting from corticosteroid-induced salt retention; in these cases, diuretic therapy alone was usually sufficient for adequate control.

A third apparent effect of CsA that could potentially influence negatively the late outcomes of cardiac recipients receiving this agent is the development of a characteristic form of myocardial fibrosis that may appear on biopsy specimens as early as 2–4 weeks after transplantation. This fibrotic pattern, not observed in conventionally immunosuppressed patients, has occurred in nearly all patients receiving CsA. On the basis of postmortem examination of the hearts of two patients in the series who died more than 1 year after transplantation, it would appear that the fibrosis is not progressive. Moreover, cardiac catheterization with volume-loading studies performed in several patients at 2 years after surgery has demonstrated no evidence of restrictive myocardial dysfunction. Thus, the long-term importance of the myocardial fibrosis observed in CsA-treated cardiac recipients remains undefined.

Finally, lymphoproliferative disease (LPD) has occurred in six patients in this series. All cases occurred within 6 months after transplantation. Two resulted in death, and one was an incidental autopsy finding in a patient who died of a subphrenic abscess following surgery to repair a ruptured splenic artery aneurysm. A fourth patient died of graft atherosclerosis 1 year after diagnosis of LPD, which was localized to unilateral inguinal nodes and was treated with local irradiation and the antiviral agent acycloguanosine; no evidence of LPD was observed at postmortem examination of this patient. The remaining two patients are currently receiving irradiation therapy in combination with acycloguanosine.

Although the etiology of the lymphoid proliferation in these patients remains unclear, several lines of circumstantial evidence suggest an association with Epstein-Barr virus (EBV). First, EBV antibody titers were elevated at the time of diagnosis in four of the five patients for whom such data were available. Second, the EBV genome was incorporated into the tumor-cell DNA of all four patients in whom the assay was performed. Finally, lymphocytes from the tumor of one patient were easily grown in tissue culture, suggesting that the cells were infected with virus. Further studies of lymphoid tissue from these tumors are in progress.

Notwithstanding the real and potential side effects and complications associated with CsA noted, survival among the group of cardiac recipients that has received the drug has clearly been improved substantially, within the constraints of the current follow-up period. The actuarial survival of these patients is compared to that observed among two groups of azathioprine-treated patients in Fig. 3, stratified as outlined. The survival statistics for patients selected for transplantation but for whom no suitable donor could be readily identified are also shown. The causes of death for all patients who received CsA and for the 99 patients in the azathioprine control group are given in Table 3.

DISCUSSION

Experience with cyclosporine immunosuppression in clinical cardiac transplantation now spans nearly 2.5 years. During this time, CsA has clearly contributed to improved survival rates for cardiac recipients. Moreover, because it has allowed substantial reduction in corticosteroid dosages and their associated side effects, compared to previous patients treated with azathioprine, the overall quality of life among CsA patients has been improved. The superior survival statistics among these patients has not been accounted for by an important reduction in the incidence of rejection and infection, but rather by more successful treatment of these two complications and a consequent reduction in mortality. Inasmuch as rejection and infection continue to occur, however, prompt diagnosis and treatment thereof remain important to the successful long-term management of CsA-treated cardiac allograft recipients.

The high incidence of hypertension among

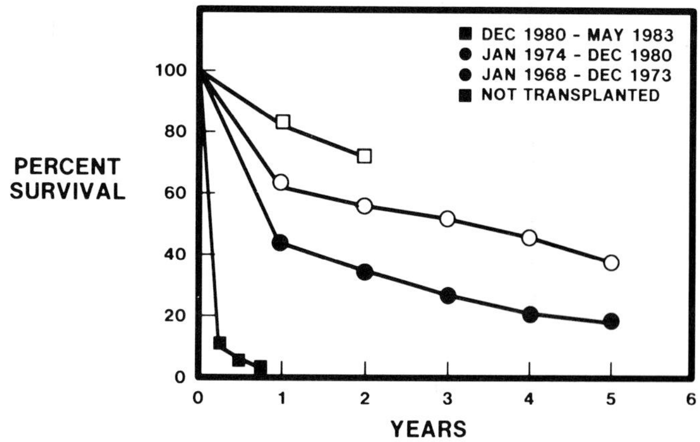

Fig. 3. Actuarial survival probabilities of cardiac allograft recipients, stratified according to date of transplantation. The upper curve depicts the survival of patients treated with cyclosporine. The lower curve reflects the survival of patients selected for transplantation but for whom no suitable donor could be readily identified.

patients treated with CsA is clearly of concern in regard to the potential adverse late sequelae. Although blood pressure has been controlled reasonably well in most patients, some continue to exhibit mild to moderate elevation of arterial diastolic pressure. Detailed studies of these patients are currently in progress to determine the mechanism by which hypertension occurs. Information gained in these studies may provide the basis for more specific and effective therapy.

The frequency at which lymphoproliferative disorders were observed in this series is also of substantial concern. The apparent higher prevalence of these disorders in the cardiac allograft population, compared to CsA-treated renal allograft recipients at other centers, remains unclear. Compared to renal recipients, the higher overall level of immunosuppression, particularly in those patients receiving the initial dosage protocol (Fig. 2), may have contributed to this higher incidence. The likelihood that these tumors may be viral-induced suggests the possibility that early intervention with antiviral agents, or conceivably even their prophylactic use in selected patients, may permit control of these disorders in some cases.

The occurrence of accelerated allograft coronary atherosclerosis, a well-recognized complication in patients treated with azathioprine, has recently been observed in two patients in the cyclosporine series; death has resulted in both, in one case suddenly and in the other within 2 months following an acute myocardial infarction. This form of atherosclerosis has been presumed due to incomplete control of the immune response, leading to chronic coronary endothelial damage. Physiologic processes to repair this damage then result in progressive endothelial hyperplasia, culminating in obstructive atherosclerotic lesions. Although it was initially hoped that CsA might afford sufficient control of this low-grade immune-mediated coronary endothelial damage to eliminate this form of atherosclerosis, such does not appear to be the case. Follow-up is currently too short to determine the rate at which this complication will occur among CsA-treated patients.

SUMMARY

Immunosuppression of cardiac allograft recipients with CsA has afforded distinct improvement in terms of survival, rehabilitation, and hospitalization costs. Several alterations in the management of these patients have been necessary, however, and certain complications of this form of immune therapy have been observed that did not occur in previous experience with azathioprine immunosuppression. Although the long-term consequences of cyclosporine treatment of cardiac recipients remain to be fully defined, current data analysis supports the contention that this form of therapy indeed represents an important advance in clinical transplant immunology.

REFERENCES

1. Oyer PE, Stinson EB, Jamieson SW, et al: Heart Transplant 1:284, 1982

2. Oyer PE, Stinson EB, Jamieson SW, et al: Transplant Proc 15:1247, 1983

3. Cabrol C, Gandjbakhch I, Guiraudon G, et al: Heart Transplant 1:120, 1982

4. English TA, Cory-Pearce R, McGregor C: Heart Transplant 1:112, 1982

5. Baumgartner WA, Reitz BA, Oyer PE, et al: Curr Prob Surg 16:1, 1979

Experience with Cyclosporine in Cardiac Transplantation

R. L. Hardesty, B. P. Griffith, R. F. Debski, and H. T. Bahnson

AT THE UNIVERSITY of Pittsburgh in March 1981, cyclosporine A (CsA), with the addition only of steroids, was adopted as the immunosuppressive agent for cardiac transplantation, which had been resumed at the health center 9 months previously. The regimen used was similar to that employed for transplantation of kidneys and livers, all based on previous work of Starzl (who had recently joined our staff) and his associates.[1,2] Believing that CsA was a better drug, we elected and attempted to avoid other agents and to use smaller doses of steroids in order to reduce the morbidity associated with steroids.

After 23 patients had been treated solely with CsA and steroids,[3] the number of deaths due to chronic rejection prompted a change in the immunosuppressive regimen. Rabbit antithymocyte globulin (RATG) was added if myocyte necrosis could not be eliminated by pulses of steroids. An additional 19 patients received cardiac allografts between July 1982, when the immunosuppressive regimen was changed, and April 1983.

MATERIALS AND METHODS

Patient Selection

All 42 patients were NYHA class IV and met the criteria described by Baumgartner et al.[2] Ages ranged from 8–54 years (median, 40 years). Twenty-four patients were suffering from idiopathic cardiomyopathy and 18 from ischemic heart disease. ABO blood type was compatible in all cases, and compatibility of donor lymphocytes with recipient serum was desired and evaluated.

A mismatch against donor lymphocytes (trypan blue) was known after implantation of the donor heart in 4 of the initial 23 cases and in 1 of the last 19. Two mismatches, done retrospectively, occurred with a preoperative percentage of reactive antibodies of zero (O PRA).

Immunosuppression

In our initial experience, a loading dose of CsA of 17.5 mg/kg was given prior to transplantation, but oliguria, which appeared soon after surgery and did not seem to be related to the operation, prompted a reduction of the loading dose to 10 mg/kg. Following transplantation, the maximal tolerated dose was given in two equally divided portions at 12-hr intervals. The dose was often limited by renal toxicity, less commonly by hepatic toxicity. Recipients of a cardiac transplant seemed more sensitive to the toxic effects of CsA than did recipients of other organs, for unknown reasons. The maintenance dose was usually adjusted so that the creatinine was 2 mg/dl or less, and rarely was a maximal dose of 17.5 mg/kg/day achieved. Whole blood levels of CsA (measured by high-performance liquid chromatography) have been monitored recently to achieve trough levels of 250–500 ng/ml. Appropriate approval of the Institutional Review Board (IRB) for the use of CsA was obtained.

Large initial doses of steroids were rapidly tapered to low maintenance levels. Methylprednisolone (1 g) was given as circulation was restored to the donor heart during transplantation. Prednisone (200 mg/day), in two divided doses, was started after operation, and the daily dose was reduced by 20 mg each day to a maintenance dose of 20 mg daily by the tenth day. If oral medication was not tolerated, an equivalent dose of methylprednisolone was given intravenously.

To treat rejection, hydrocortisone (1 g i.v.) was given, usually without alteration of the dose of prednisone. The number and frequency of pulses varied, depending on the degree of rejection as determined by endomyocardial biopsy. Severe rejection was treated with three daily doses of hydrocortisone; less severe rejection was treated with pulsed doses at 3-, 5-, or 7-day intervals.

RATG was not used in the initial 23 patients. In the few instances when toxicity precluded use of CsA, azathioprine was used temporarily. The immunosuppressive regimen changed in July 1982, and 19 patients received transplants between then and April 1983. Myocyte necrosis was initially treated with three daily pulses of hydrocortisone (1 g), but if evidence of rejection did not resolve after two or three courses of this pulse therapy, 1 g of antithymocyte globulin (Stanford) was given daily for 3 days until improvement occurred.

Operative Technique and Donor Procurement

Orthotopic cardiac transplantation was performed using the conventional operative technique. The method

---

From the Department of Surgery, University of Pittsburgh School of Medicine, Pittsburgh, PA.

Reprint requests should be addressed to Dr. R. L. Hardesty, Department of Surgery, University of Pittsburgh, School of Medicine, 1084 Scaife Hall, Pittsburgh, PA 15261.

0041-1345/83/1505-0066$01.00/0

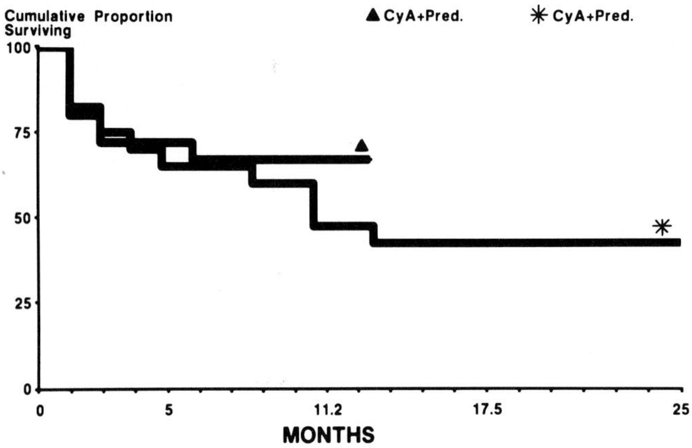

Fig. 1. Cumulative survival of the initial 23 patients at 1 year and at 2 years.

of preservation of the donor heart varied with respect to the use of cardioplegia. All donor hearts after excision were immediately immersed and transported in a 4°C solution of electrolytes. Most donor hearts were perfused with 1000 ml of clear cardioplegic solution (4°C) before cardiectomy, and recently, additional doses of blood cardioplegia have been given during implantation. The latter method has been associated with a reduced need for postoperative inotropic support.[5]

RESULTS

Mortality

The cumulative actuarial survival of the initial 23 patients at 1 year was 61%, and at 2 years 41%, (Fig. 1), whereas for the 19 patients in whom rescue therapy with RATG was used for myocyte necrosis not responsive to pulse therapy with steroids, the cumulative survival was 79% at 9 months (Fig. 2). Three deaths resulted from acute rejection within the first 3 months in the first group; one occurred in the second group (described below). The initial series contained four deaths at 8–13 months due to chronic rejection and obliterative coronary artery disease; this time period has not yet elapsed in the second group.

Infection contributed significantly but not greatly to mortality, as only two patients in each group (4/42) died with infection. Two other factors, neurological complications and selection of patients, were responsible for the remaining deaths, and these factors were related in that neurologic complications occurred primarily in the patients who were most severely ill prior to operation.

Rejection

Endomyocardial biopsies, obtained with the Caves-Schultz bioptome, provided a morphologic index of rejection;[6] and concomitant right heart catheterization with cardiac output by

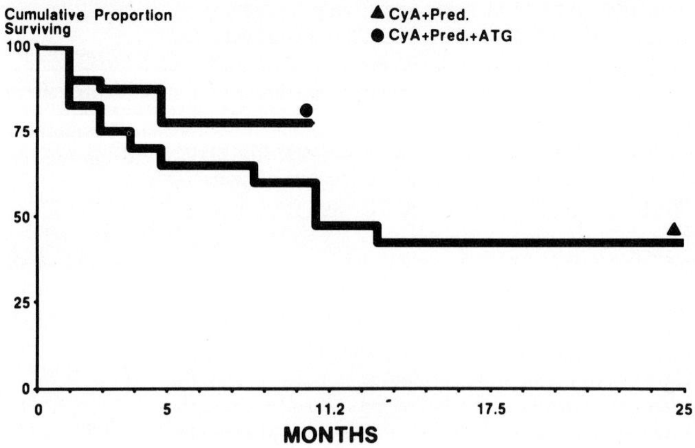

Fig. 2. Cumulative survival of the last 19 patients (upper line), who received ATG, compared with the first 23 patients (lower line), who did not receive ATG. Rescue therapy with RATG was used for myocyte necrosis not responsive to pulse therapy with steroids.

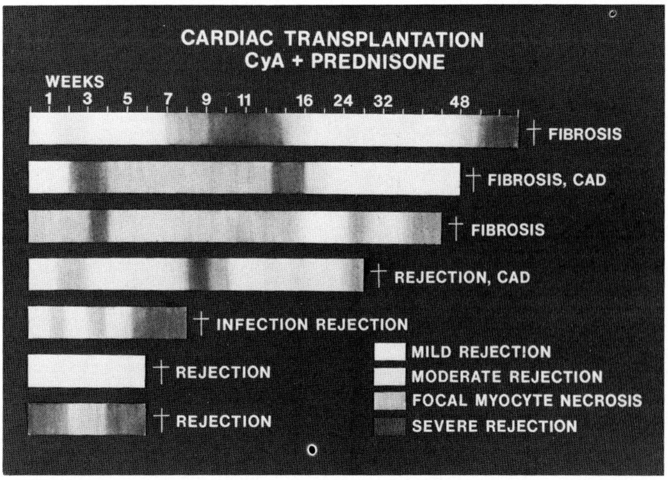

Fig. 3. Persistent histologic rejection not reversed with pulse therapy or increased maintenance of steroids leading to death in the first group of 23 patients. Evidence at autopsy of rejection or of severe fibrosis, rejection's late result, indicated the need for additional immunosuppression.

thermodilution, pulmonary and systemic arterial, and right atrial pressures provided hemodynamic confirmation of the morphologic criteria for the degree of rejection. Electrocardiographic voltage, arrhythmia, clinical criteria of low cardiac output, and ventricular diastolic gallop were of only limited usefulness in the detection of early rejection.

An important lesson from our initial experience was the fact that persistent histologic rejection, as reflected in focal myocyte necrosis,[6] was not always reversed with pulse therapy of hydrocortisone, nor with an increased maintenance dose of prednisone (30–40 mg/day). As a consequence, three patients with acute rejection died within 3 months of transplantation, and four died of chronic rejection and restrictive cardiomyopathy at 8–13 months. Two of the latter died unexpectedly with an acute myocardial infarction (Fig. 3).

This observation prompted the addition of RATG if myocyte necrosis could not be eliminated by pulses of steroids without an increase in the maintenance dose of prednisone. The cumulative actuarial survival of 19 patients at 9 months is 79% (Fig. 2), and chronic rejection, by histologic criteria, is not persisting in the 6 patients receiving rescue therapy with RATG (Fig. 4). Since compiling these data, 1 patient has died of acute rejection on her sixth postoperative day; the severity of her rejection was not recognized, and she had received

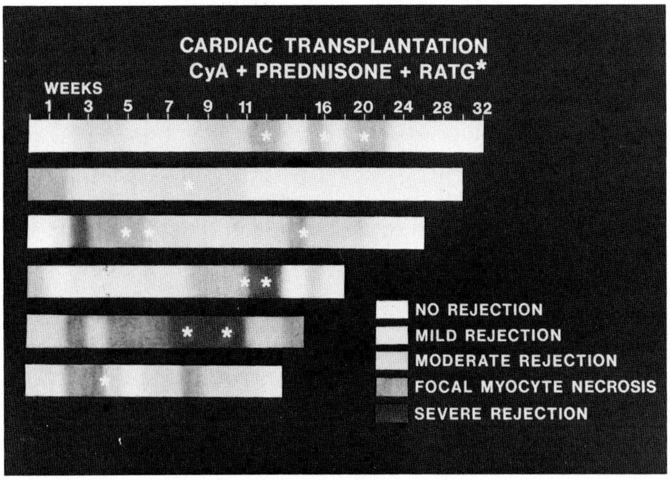

Fig. 4. Histologic rejection initially not reversed with pulse steroid therapy but reversed with rescue therapy of RATG in 6 of the last 19 patients. Stars indicate a 3-day course of RATG.

neither pulsed steroids nor RATG. Her CsA dosage had been lowered on the first postoperative day because of renal toxicity but had been raised incremently to 10 mg/kg/day until death. CsA level on the fourth postoperative day was 234 ng/ml.

Compatibility of donor lymphocytes with recipient serum was desired, but a mismatch against donor lymphocytes was known after implantation of the donor heart in 4 of the initial 23 patients and 1 of the last 19. None died of hyperacute rejection. Two of the 4, not treated with RATG, survived and are free of chronic rejection, and 2 died of rejection within 2 months. The one patient among the last 19 whose lymphocytotoxic crossmatch was incompatible is alive and free of chronic rejection without treatment with RATG.

Infection

Infectious episodes in 33 patients were monitored by the Division of Infectious Diseases for a mean period of 9 months, a minimum of 3 months. The rate of infection decreased in time (Table 1). Herpes viral infections, bacterial pneumonia, and other intrathoracic infections (empyema, mediastinitis) account for the majority of infections and infection-related deaths (Table 2).

Infectious episodes occurred in 79% of the 33 patients followed, with an average of 1.54 episodes per patient. Nine infections were associated with death, and infection was thought to be the cause of death in four of these.

Lymphoma

A monoclonal mixed histiocytic-lymphocytic lymphoma occurred in one patient, ultimately resulting in his death. The lymphoma was first evident at 3 months and at autopsy was present in cervical nodes, nasopharynx, and both lungs. Studies indicated a new infection with Epstein-Barr virus, as immunoglobulins to viral capsid antigen (IgG and IgM) were detected concomitantly with the lymphoma. IgG remained elevated until death, and Epstein-Barr nuclear antigen (EBNA) was later identified in the nuclei of the lymphoma cells. This patient had not received RATG.

Table 1. Infection Rates per Quarter

Quarter	Episodes per Patient	No. of Patients
1	0.82	33
2	0.58	26
3	0.17	26
4	0.31	16
>4	0.10	10

Table 2. Symptomatic Infections

	Episodes	No. of Patients	Death
Epstein-Barr cytomegalic virus	11	10	4
Bacterial pneumonia	10	9	2
Herpes simplex virus	8	8	0
Intraabdominal	5	4	1
Herpes zoster	3	3	0
Other intrathoracic	3	3	1
Mediastinal	3	3	0
Urinary tract	2	2	0
Central nervous system	1	1	0
Disseminated toxoplasmosis	1	1	1
Pneumocystis	1	1	0
Otitis	1	1	0
Primary bacteremia	2	1	0

Adverse Reactions to CsA

Hypertension tended to begin in the first postoperative week, developed irrespective of preoperative historical hypertension or measurable postoperative CsA renal toxicity, and was difficult to control with diuretics and peripheral vasodilators. It appeared atypical in that the usual sleep-related fall in diastolic pressure was not observed. It was associated with a slightly elevated peripheral vascular resistance and generally with normal blood renins.

Other troublesome adverse reactions included hirsutism, a fine tremor of the upper extremities, nasal congestion, hyperplasia of the gums, and transient gastrointestinal ileus.

Convulsions occurred in 11/43 patients. The time of occurrence relative to the operation, the absence of localizing signs on examination, the absence of focal abnormalities on sequential contrast-enhanced computerized tomographic scanning of the brain, and normal spinal fluid pressures and analyses made air emboli, systemic arterial emboli, and infection unlikely causes of the seizures. These observations may implicate CsA as a contributing cause.

DISCUSSION

Cyclosporine A for cardiac transplantation has provided powerful immunosuppression and allowed lower doses of steroids and thus fewer of the morbid effects from steroids. In our initial experience with 23 patients treated with CsA and steroids alone, rejection occurred with an intolerable frequency, and it appeared that optimal survival required the addition of antithymocyte globulin to the immunosuppressive regimen. The continued absence of rejection following rescue therapy with RATG in 6 of the last 19 patients (Fig. 4) is responsible for an improved 79% cumulative survival at 9 months compared to the 61% cumulative survival at 1 year for the initial 23 patients. It appears significant that among the initially treated group, 7 patients had histologic evidence of moderate rejection (focal myocyte necrosis), which was not reversed with pulsed therapy of steroids nor by an increased dose of maintenance prednisone (30–40 mg/day). Three of these 7 patients died of acute rejection within 3 months, and 4 died of chronic active rejection at 8–13 months. As a consequence, the cumulative survival of these 23 patients at 2 years was 41% (Fig. 1). The projected 2-year cumulative survival of the last 19 patients should not decrease greatly, because new episodes of rejection have not occurred after 3 months in either group. The anticipation of continued long-term survival is further justified by the experience that the rate of infection has decreased in time (Table 1) and has accounted for a small number of deaths (Table 2).

Because two patients had incompatible lymphocytotoxic crossmatches in spite of preoperative PRA screens of zero, the lymphocyte panel has been expanded from 18 to 36 donors. All major A and B loci will be represented at least three times in the expanded donor panel, and results can still be obtained within 4 hr.

The addition of antithymocyte globulin raises a concern about the possibility of causing an increased incidence of lymphoma. The association of a new Epstein-Barr viral infection and the subsequent identification of EBNA in the lymphoma of the single patient who died from a lymphoma have led to a prospective trial of treatment with acyclovir for those patients who develop a new infection or have a reactivation of Epstein-Barr virus. Three patients have received acyclovir for this reason up to the present.

We continue committed to avoiding the morbid side effects of steroids if possible and use large initial doses that are rapidly tapered to low maintenance levels. Increasing the maintenance dose of prednisone from 20 mg/day to 30–40 mg/day did not reverse the chronic rejection, myocyte necrosis, and resultant fibrosis among the patients who did not receive RATG. Low doses of short-acting pulsed steroid therapy with hydrocortisone (1 g) were used to treat myocyte necrosis as opposed to high doses of longer-acting methylprednisolone.

The initial desire not to use antithymocyte globulin was based on the impression that CsA, when combined with low-dose prednisone, would improve survival over the previously used immunosuppression with azathioprine, steroids, and antithymocyte globulin.[1,2,7,8] We were concerned about the potentially increased mortality and morbidity associated with the use of multiple immunosuppressive drugs. The low incidence of severe, persisting, or potentially fatal rejection had RATG not been used (7 instances in the first 23 cases and 6 in the second 19) supports a directed and selective use of RATG for rescue rather than for routine prophylaxis.

Proper evaluation of these conclusions may require correlation of evidence of rejection with blood levels of cyclosporine, a measurement now available to us. The child who died with rejection and coronary artery disease at 7 months may have been on a subtherapeutic dose of CsA; she was receiving Dilantin and phenobarbital, which are known to lower strikingly the blood level of CsA. A child who is currently being treated with the same medications for control of seizures requires 30 mg/kg/day of CsA to maintain a whole-blood trough level of 200–500 ng/ml.

SUMMARY

CsA has provided powerful immunosuppression for cardiac transplantation and allowed lower doses of steroids, with lessening of morbidity from the steroids. In our initial experience with these two agents alone, the significance of rejection in morbidity and mortality resulted in the addition of rabbit antithymocyte globulin. More recent experiences suggest that optimal long-term survival requires rescue therapy with antithymocyte globulin when myocyte necrosis persists in spite of pulsed steroids.

REFERENCES

1. Starzl TE, Weil R III, Iwatsuki S, et al: Surg Gynecol Obstet 151:17, 1980
2. Starzl TE, Klintmalm GBG, Porter KA, et al: N Engl J Med 305:266, 1981
3. Griffith BP, Hardesty RL, Deeb GM, et al: Ann Surg 196:324, 1982
4. Baumgartner WA, Reitz BA, Oyer PE, et al: Curr Prob Surg 16:51, 1979
5. Hardesty RL, Griffith BP, Deeb GM, et al: Transplant Proc 15:1253, 1983
6. Griffith BP, Hardesty RL, Bahnson HT, et al: Transplant Proc 15:1241, 1983
7. Pennock JL, Oyer PE, Reitz BA, et al: J Thorac Cardiovasc Surg 83:168, 1982
8. Calne RY, Rolles K, White DJG, et al: Lancet 2:1033, 1979

Cyclosporine for Cardiac Transplantation: U.K. Trial

J. Wallwork, R. Cory-Pearce, and T. A. H. English

CYCLOSPORINE (CsA) was first introduced as part of the immunosuppressive regimen for patients undergoing cardiac transplantation in December 1980.[1] The potential advantages of the use of cyclosporine are considerable and include improved immunosuppression with fewer rejection episodes, reduction in corticosteroid requirements, reduced incidence of serious infection, and elimination of the need for azathioprine. Cyclosporine in combination with other immunosuppressive agents has been used at Papworth Hospital since March 1982, and reported here are the results of the clinical trial until May 1983. In light of the results, the advantages and disadvantages of cyclosporine are discussed, as well as the choice of protocol and subsequent changes against the background of continuing development to determine optimal regimens at this and other centers.

MATERIALS AND METHODS

Between March 1982 and May 1983, 21 patients underwent orthotopic cardiac transplantation. Patient data and preexisting diagnosis are given in Table 1. Patients were selected for transplantation according to previously established criteria. Data from an historical group of 29 patients transplanted between 1979 and 1982 who received azathioprine, prednisolone, and horse ATG (HATG) immunosuppression have been used for comparative purposes.

Initially, CsA (Sandoz Ltd., Basel) was administered with low-dose steroids (protocol I in Table 2) in the belief that there was evidence of overimmunosuppression in previous CsA-based regimens.[2] In particular, the appearance of several lymphomas was of concern. CsA dose in our early experience was adjusted from the fixed-dose regimen of the protocol according to the patient's renal function. Because of the occurrence of early moderate and severe rejection episodes, in one case fatal, the protocol was modified as shown in Table 2. These modifications will be discussed further, the major change being to introduce a course of intravenous HATG (Upjohn, Kalamazoo, MI) for a 10-day period. The daily dose of HATG was adjusted according to daily T-cell counts by the rosette method to maintain circulating T cells at 10% total lymphocytes or 100 cells/mm^3 absolute.

Serum trough CsA levels have been measured three times weekly by radioimmunoassay developed by Sandoz Ltd., and, more recently, CsA dose has been adjusted to maintain trough levels in the range 200–500 ng/ml instead of using the stepwise reduction called for in the original fixed-dose regimen.

Endomyocardial biopsy was performed at weekly intervals, or on suspicion of rejection, and histologic features graded as shown in Table 3. Therapy was instituted for rejection episodes that showed evidence of myocyte necrosis. Persistent mild infiltrates seen on two or more subsequent biopsies were also treated as rejection episodes.

Rejection episodes were treated according to the protocol outlined in Table 4, and since the introduction of protocol II, additional courses of HATG for moderate or severe rejection have not been used.

RESULTS

Rejection

The occurrence of rejection episodes is outlined in Table 5. Twenty-one patients have been at risk in the predischarge period, 14 patients postdischarge. Five of 8 rejection episodes prior to discharge occurred in the first 6 patients receiving CsA and steroids alone. Four of these rejection episodes occurred within the first 2 weeks of transplantation, and all were moderate or severe. Contrary to other reports,[3] severe rejection was not indolent in nature but caused hemodynamic changes and death of one patient at 10 days. Since the introduction of additional ATG in June 1982, there have been three mild rejection episodes in the early postoperative period. The one severe rejection episode occurred late in the only patient receiving CsA and steroids alone who did not reject in the early postoperative period. He received intravenous sulphadimidine and trimethoprim therapy for a late pneumocystis infection, and

---

From Papworth Hospital, Papworth Everard, Cambridge, England.

Reprint requests should be addressed to J. Wallwork, Papworth Hospital, Papworth Everard, Cambridge CB3 8RE, England.

0041-1345/83/1505-0067$01.00/0

Table 1. Patient Summary

Patients	21
Age	19–52 (mean, 39 years)
Sex	18 males, 3 females
Diagnosis	
Ischemic heart disease	14
Cardiomyopathy	7
Follow-up	
Range	14 days–14 months (mean, 7 months)
Status	
Alive	16
Discharged	14
Died	5 (4 early, 1 late)
Hospitalized	3

CsA levels were low in spite of increased oral CsA dose. This rejection episode was aborted with a course of intravenous methylprednisolone and HATG. This case has been previously reported.[4]

The previously described pattern of fine interstitial fibrosis in endomyocardial biopsy specimens of patients receiving CsA[5,6] has not been a feature in our experience.

Infection

Infective complications of the whole group are outlined in Table 6. Not included are secondary bacterial infections that occurred in both patients who died, one as a result of primary CMV infection, and the other, systemic toxoplasmosis. All other infection episodes of clinical significance—or requiring antibiotic therapy, in the case of bacterial infection—have been included. One patient who suffered primary CMV infection also developed a severe candida esophagitis requiring treatment with intravenous amphotericin B.

Table 3. Definition of Rejection and Treatment of Rejection Episodes

Histologic Grade	Cellular Focal	Infiltrate General	Myocyte Necrosis	Erythrocyte/ Polymorphonuclear Infiltrate
Minimal	+	–	–	–
Mild	+	+	–	–
Moderate	+	+	+	–
Severe	+	+	+	+

Table 4. Protocol for Rejection Episodes

Rejection	Cyclosporine	Prednisolone	HATG
Early	No change	1g i.v. × 3	3–5 days if resistant or severe
Late	No change	↑1 mg/kg/day Reduce to maintenance over 10 days	—

Table 5. Rejection Episodes, March 1982–May 1983

	Early (Predischarge)	Late
Mild	3	7
Moderate	3	0
Severe	2*	1
Total	8	8

*Including 1 resulting in death.

It is of note that in spite of the reintroduction of HATG into the immunosuppressive regimen, no herpetic infections have occurred.

Antibiotic usage, compared with the previous group of patients treated with conventional immunosuppression, has been reduced, as has the workload on the bacteriological laboratory (Table 7). The incidence of biopsy procedures requiring prophylactic antibiotic

Table 2. Maintenance Immunosuppressive Protocols

	Protocol I (Patients 1–6)			Protocol II (Patients 7–21)		
	Cyclosporine	Prednisolone	ATG	Cyclosporine*	Prednisolone	ATG
Initial	18 mg/kg/day	500 mg i.v. 125 mg i.v. × 3 0.3 mg/kg/day	—	18 mg/kg/day p.o.	500 mg i.v. 125 mg i.v. × 3 1 mg/kg/day	Horse i.v., 10 days (T cells = 10%)
Maintenance	Reduce weekly by 2 mg/kg/day to 10 mg/kg/day	0.3 mg/kg/day	—	Reduce weekly by 2 mg/kg/day to 10 mg/kg/day	1 mg/kg/day to 0.3 mg/kg/day at 2 weeks	—

*Cyclosporine dose adjusted according to renal function and trough serum level (200–500 ng/ml)

Table 6. Infection Episodes, March 1982–May 1983

Infection	Early (1-3 months)	Late
Bacterial		
Coliform pneumonia	1	0
Septicemia	1	0
Pneumocystis	0	2
Viral		
CMV	3*†	0
Fungal		
Candida esophagitis	1*	0
Parasitic		
Toxoplasmosis	1†	0
Total	7	2

*Same patient included in both categories.
†Including 1 patient who died.

cover is the same in both groups. Some reduction in the investigating workload results from a shorter in-hospital stay, but nevertheless both these differences reflect the diminution of infective problems in CsA-treated patients.

Deaths

Causes of death in the five patients who have died in this series are outlined in Table 8. Four of the deaths occurred during the initial in-hospital period following transplantation. The first two patients to die received CsA and prednisolone alone, and the first patient died of severe acute rejection associated with, retrospectively, low CsA levels, having received 18 mg/kg/day. Endomyocardial biopsy 48 hr prior to death was normal. Previous reports had described rejection in CsA-treated patients as being indolent in nature, but this is obviously not the case in this patient. The second death occurred in a

Table 7. Antibiotic Usage and Change in Bacteriologic Workload

	Conventional Immuno-suppression	Cyclosporine
Antibiotic usage, 90 days (mean g/patient)		
Benzyl penicillin	12.5	7.1
Flucloxacillin	43.0	18.0
Gentamycin	1.1	0.1
Others	79.3	12.5
Bacteriologic investigative workload (6-month survivors) (mean tests/patient)		
	363.0	192.0

Table 8. Causes of Death

Patient No.	Cause	Days After Transplant
3	Rejection	10
4	Toxoplasmosis	36
12	Graft failure	24
14	Multisystem failure, cerebral hemorrhage	11
15	CMV	80

patient who was toxoplasma sero-negative who received a heart from a toxoplasma sero-positive donor and developed primary systemic toxoplasmosis. The third patient to die exhibited sudden cardiac dysfunction while receiving prophylactic HATG, CsA, and steroids, and repeated endomyocardial biopsy showed no evidence of cellular infiltration. Full supportive care including balloon counterpulsation was instituted, but the patient died some 2 weeks later in what appeared to be an unconfirmed humoral-mediated rejection episode. Donor-specific antibodies were absent, and direct crossmatch against the donor was negative. Neither repeated endomyocardial biopsy through his terminal illness or postmortem histology showed any lymphocytic cellular infiltrate characterizing cell-mediated rejection. For this reason, it has been difficult to classify the cause of graft failure in this patient. The fourth patient to die was in gross cardiac failure, requiring dopamine support preoperatively, and developed diffuse cerebral hemorrhage postoperatively and subsequent multisystem failure without evidence of rejection. The fifth patient to die had an uncomplicated postoperative course and was discharged 5 weeks following transplantation. He subsequently developed clinical signs and symptoms of primary CMV infection, which was confirmed by transbronchial biopsy. Bone marrow suppression and resulting neutropenia led to the development of secondary bacterial pulmonary and systemic infection, and he died 80 days after transplantation. He is the only patient to have died after discharge from the hospital.

Survival and Hospital Stay

Sixteen of 21 patients survived (Table 1), and currently 80% of patients have been discharged from the hospital. In-hospital stay has been reduced, compared with azathioprine-based immunosuppressive therapy (Table 9), and within this overall reduction of in-hospital stay, the average time spent barrier-nursed in intensive care has been reduced from 28 to 10 days. The low incidence of infective complications in the patients discharged from the hospital may be a result of the steroid-sparing effect of CsA-based immunosuppression. This has enabled mean steroid usage compared with conventionally treated patients to be halved during the first 90 days following transplantation (Table 10). Daily steroid dose is reduced to 0.2 mg/kg/day by 1 month after transplantation. Although long-term survival has probably been improved, our follow-up period is yet too short for valid statistical analysis.

Cyclosporine-Related Toxicity

Side effects attributable to CsA have been noticed in all patients. Mild tremor in the early postoperative period has been common, as has hirsutism. Some patients have exhibited postural-dependent edema, which has been attributed to "capillary leak" as a result of CsA therapy. Hepatic toxicity attributable to CsA therapy has not been identified.

The most important toxic effect of cyclosporine has, as in other series, been nephrotoxicity.[3,7] All patients have had a degree of nephrotoxicity, exhibited in the early postoperative period by decreased creatinine clearance, rising urea, and absence of the usual diuretic response following cardiac transplantation. Subsequent renal function in the later postoperative period has also been impaired. Although this would not appear to have a clinical disadvantage to the patient, the degree of impairment nevertheless reflects the loss of $\frac{1}{3}$–$\frac{2}{3}$ of renal reserve and must therefore be regarded as significant. Figure 1 shows a comparison between the creatinine clearance of patients previously undergoing cardiac transplantation and receiving conventional immunosuppression with our current group of patients. There is a statistically significant difference from day 4 onwards ($p <$ 0.05). Nephrotoxicity becomes particularly important when it is necessary to administer other potentially nephrotoxic agents. However, close monitoring of the CsA levels, renal function, and, when appropriate, drug levels of other agents enables such drug combinations to be administered safely.

Table 9. Length of Hospital Stay (Days)

	Mean	Median
Conventional immunosuppression	81	75
Cyclosporine	51	44

Table 10. Steroid Usage to 90 Days

	Conventional Immunosuppression	Cyclosporine
Mean (g)	12.05	4.85

Probably associated with nephrotoxicity, CsA therapy has resulted in a significant increase in the presence of diastolic hypertension following cardiac transplantation. Nine of 10 patients who have survived longer than 90 days have required antihypertensive therapy. In the early postoperative period, alpha blockers have been found to be effective but rapidly become less effective, and currently our outpatients receive Nifedipine for blood pressure control. The precise mechanism of this hypertensive action of CsA and its long-term significance are unknown.

Lymphoma and other lymphoproliferative disorders have not occurred in our series to date. It is too early to attach any firm conclusions to this observation.

DISCUSSION

The actual and putative advantages of cyclosporine as the main immunosuppressive agent following cardiac transplantation have been, and are increasingly being, reported.[2,3,7] Our experience is similar to that of others in that the choice of protocols and drug combinations associated with CsA-based immunosuppressive regimens is still in a state of flux. Before introducing CsA following cardiac

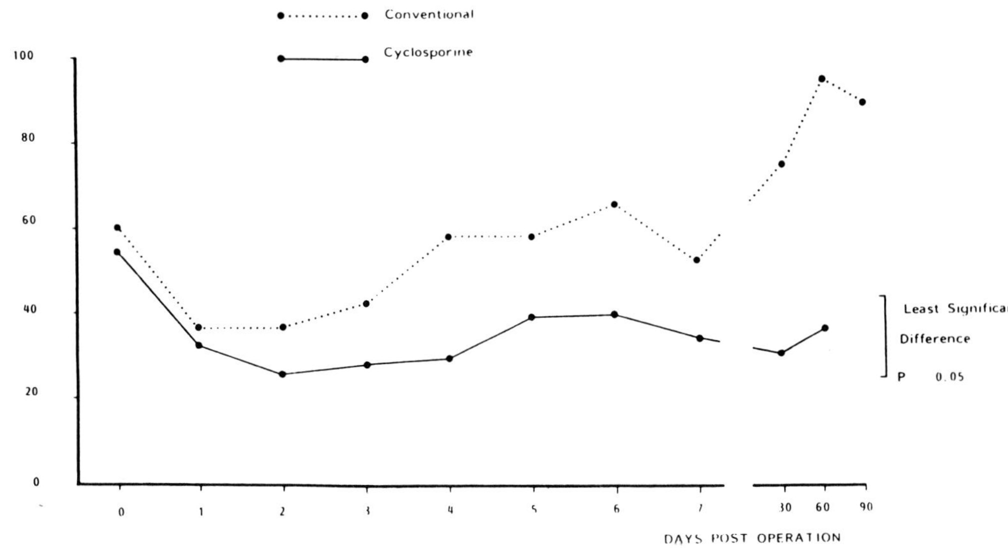

Fig. 1. Creatinine clearance.

transplantation here, particular note was taken of the early experience at Stanford. Using cyclosporine, prednisolone, and an attenuated course of RATG, there was evidence that the patients were being overimmunosuppressed. Such evidence included the low incidence of rejection, a high incidence of viral infection (particularly herpetic), and of most concern, the early occurrence of a significant number of lymphomas. It was also the impression that rejection in these patients, when it did occur, appeared to be a more indolent process giving rise to few clinical sequelae and histologically having more focal changes seen on endomyocardial biopsy. Because of these early reports, and in particular because of the high incidence of lymphoma, we decided to discontinue prophylactic use of ATG and to combine CsA in a similar fixed-dose regimen with low-dose oral steroids. However, our initial experience with the first six patients, all but one of whom had a moderate or severe rejection episode within the first 2 weeks following transplantation, requiring ATG therapy, suggested to us that in an attempt to prevent overimmunosuppressing our patients, we had indeed to some degree been giving inadequate immunosuppression in the early postoperative period. This caused us to modify our immunosuppressive regimen. We did not wish greatly to increase the steroid component, as steroid sparing seemed to us to be a major advantage of CsA immunosuppressive therapy. Others, using higher steroid dosage, have reported the early occurrence of rejection of moderate or severe nature requiring further increased steroid therapy.[7] Mindful of the potential increased risk of lymphoma, we nevertheless introduced an initial short course of intravenous horse ATG into the immunosuppressive regimen. The degree of immunosuppression attained was attenuated from conventional therapy. We aimed to reduce the T-cell fraction of the total lymphocyte count to approximately 10%, compared with the reduction to 1% called for in the original Stanford experience. Although this modification in our immunosuppressive regimen has reduced the incidence of early rejection to approximately 27%, which may again suggest overimmunosuppression, we have not encountered any increased incidence of viral, particularly herpetic, infections and have to date had no case of lymphoma or lymphoproliferative disease. Furthermore, because of the mild nature of the rejection episodes, massive additional immunosuppressive therapy in the early postoperative period has been unnecessary. It may well be that, in the light of subsequent experience, the 10-day course of ATG may be reduced, but we have so far seen no evidence of morbidity or mortality associated with this regimen. It is of interest—and demonstrates the uncertainty that is currently present in the choice of CsA-based protocols—that at the time we reintroduced ATG, others had abandoned its use.[3]

Although in common with others we have found a reduced incidence of rejection episodes, the definition of what constitutes a rejection episode has become more blurred, and detection by noninvasive means has become less reliable. We believe the so-called cyclosporine effect seen on biopsies, implying a benign cellular infiltrate, is not proven and that all cellular infiltrates should be regarded with suspicion. We consider that they represent an immunologic, active process, whether advantageous or detrimental. To reserve treatment for rejection and until myocyte necrosis occurs on biopsy, already implying a certain degree of graft damage, appears to us to go against the philosophy of detecting rejection early and avoiding cumulative myocyte damage. We therefore would regard the occurrence of a static mild cellular infiltrate as evidence of a rejection episode until future developments can define those infiltrates that are benign. We have seen no reports of cellular infiltrates in the myocardium of hearts taken from patients receiving CsA for other organ transplants and have seen no cellular infiltrates at necropsy in the kidneys of CsA-treated patients who have died following cardiac transplantation.

One of the disadvantages of CsA therapy with respect to rejection has been the absence of reliable indicators of rejection, in particular the relative insensitivity of summated ECG voltages previously regarded as a good indicator of impending rejection episodes.[8] This has been attributed to the relative lack of edema seen in the heart during rejection episodes with CsA. Nevertheless, we still feel it is important to monitor ECG voltages regularly. More frequent biopsies have been performed in the early follow-up period, at 2-weekly intervals for the first 2 months and then monthly until 6 months and 3-monthly after that.

Other disadvantages of CsA therapy include adverse drug reactions. Minor problems such as fine tremor, hirsutism, and postural edema have been noted in many patients. More important, and in keeping with others' experience, has been the almost universal occurrence of some degree of nephrotoxicity. Although this has had little effect on the patients' well-being, the degree of renal dysfunction assessed by serum creatinine and creatinine clearance tests represents a significant impairment of renal function. Certainly, in the first few days following transplantation, the normally expected diuretic phase is inhibited, and serum creatinine and urea rise markedly. As experience is gained in the practical use of CsA, these effects can be anticipated and attenuated; nevertheless, in the late postoperative period, renal dysfunction is impaired. The long-term consequence of such renal dysfunction has yet to be determined. Similarly, hypertension has occurred following cardiac transplantation in the majority of patients, and this is a change from the experience of patients not receiving CsA. Again, the mechanism by which hypertension occurs and its late consequences are the subject of current investigation both here and elsewhere[3] in an attempt both to define the pathophysiology and to predict future adverse consequences. Hypertension with CsA therapy following renal transplantation was not a particularly noted feature, perhaps because hypertension is common in these patients.

In spite of these disadvantages, there are several benefits that have accrued since introducing cyclosporine. It is undoubtedly steroid-sparing, and it appears reasonable to assume that by reducing the side effects of corticosteroids, considerable morbidity in the late follow-up period may be avoided. In particular, this may enable the somewhat rigid criteria

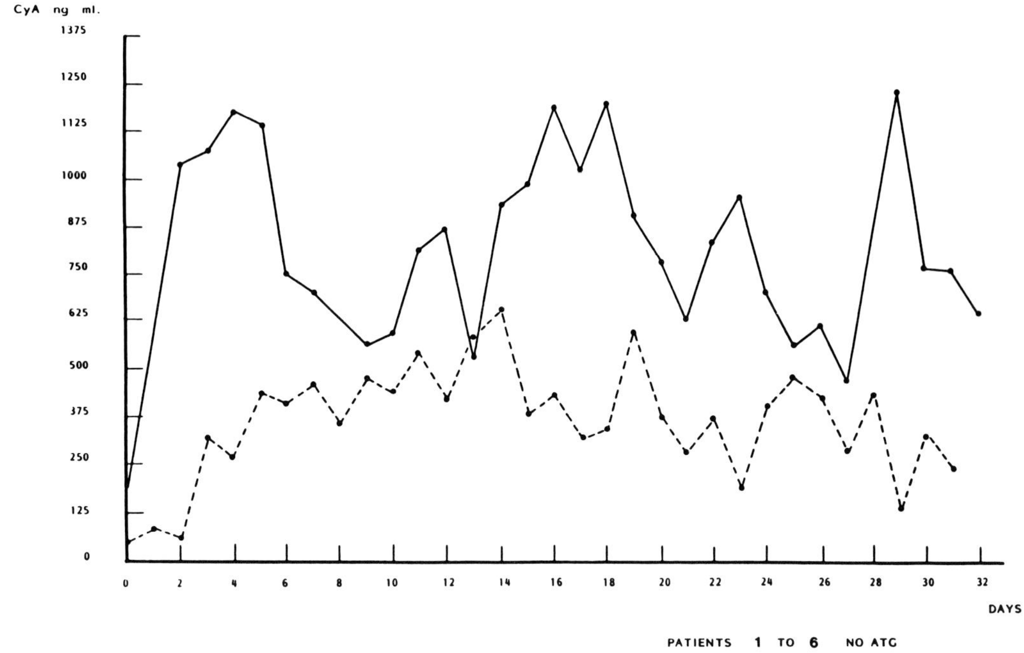

Fig. 2. Cyclosporine for cardiac transplantation. Mean CsA serum levels of 17 heart transplant patients for the first 32 days posttransplant. ●—●, Patients 1–6, no ATG given; ●----●, Patients 7–17, ATG given.

for cardiac transplantation to be relaxed and thus widen its application. We have observed a low incidence of rejection with few infective problems on our current regimen, and this has led to considerably reduced intensive care and initial hospital stays, which has beneficial resource and cost implications.

There are, however, important developments for the future that we hope will lead to further improvements using cyclosporine. There is great variability in absorption between individuals, and in the same patient at different times of recovery following transplantation, and as yet no method is available to assess the degree of immunosuppression achieved by any particular drug dose or indeed circulating serum drug level. However, as more data become available, it appears, certainly within the first month following transplantation, that a serum trough level of 200–500 ng/ml gives adequate clinical immunosuppression without producing clinically significant nephrotoxicity. Figure 2 demonstrates that as our experience improved, mean CsA trough levels were lower and less erratic from day to day. This also demonstrates an important aspect of additional prophylactic ATG therapy, which has enabled us to build up CsA levels slowly. This minimizes early nephrotoxicity without risk of underimmunosuppression and allows us to tailor the initial CsA dose to preexisting hepatic and renal dysfunction in particularly sick recipients. From a practical point of view, this enables us to dramatically reduce or even temporarily cease CsA therapy if clinically indicated, without risk of rejection. During the early recovery phase following cardiac transplantation, absorption and excretion of CsA may vary as hepatic function improves, and we now adjust the CsA dose according to the serum levels.

The advent of cyclosporine has had a major impact in cardiac transplantation as in other forms of organ transplantation. It is a drug that has clear advantages but can have considerable adverse effects and must be used with caution. Future development of less toxic analogs and greater experience in its use will further enhance the outlook for patients requiring cardiac transplantation.

ACKNOWLEDGMENTS

Cyclosporine was supplied by Sandoz Products Ltd. Cyclosporine levels were kindly performed by Dr. David White, Department of Clinical Surgery at Addenbrooke's Hospital, Cambridge. Equine ATG (Atgam) was supplied by Upjohn, Kalamazoo, MI.

REFERENCES

1. Oyer PE, Stinson EB, Jaimeson SW, et al: Heart Transplantation 1:285, 1982

2. Oyer PE, Stinson EB, Reitz BA, et al: In White DJG (ed): Cyclosporin A. New York, Elsevier Biomedical, 1982

3. Oyer PE, Stinson EB, Jaimeson SW, et al: Transplant Proc 15:1247, 1983

4. Wallwork J, McGregor CM, Cory-Pearce R, et al: Lancet 1:366, 1983

5. Billingham ME: Heart Transplantation 1:25, 1981

6. Griffith BP, Hardesty RL, Bahnson HT, et al: Transplant Proc 15:1241, 1983

7. Griffith BP, Hardesty RL, Deeb GM, et al: Ann Surg 196:324, 1982

8. Baumgartner WA, Reitz BA, Oyer PE, et al: Curr Prog Surg 16, 1979

Cardiac and Cardiopulmonary Transplantation Using Cyclosporine For Immunosuppression: Recent Texas Heart Institute Experience

D. A. Cooley, O. H. Frazier, G. A. Painvin, L. Boldt, and B. D. Kahan

SIX MONTHS AFTER the cardiac transplantation performed by Christiaan Barnard in Cape Town,[1] the first successful cardiac transplantation at the Texas Heart Institute was performed on May 2, 1968.[2] During the ensuing 18-month period, 19 patients underwent elective cardiac transplantation. Because problems of infection and rejection were encountered in these early attempts, the program was virtually abandoned. Only Shumway and colleagues at Stanford University maintained a sustained interest in cardiac transplantation.

During the past decade, however, advances have been made in the clinical application of cardiac transplantation for patients with end-stage myocardial disease.[3] At present, we estimate approximately 10,000 end-stage cardiac patients in the United States could benefit from transplantation. Improvements in patient selection, graft preservation, and immunosuppression have increased survival for heart transplant recipients. The recent addition of cyclosporine as an adjunct to the immunosuppression necessary in the transplant patient has caused renewed interest in this method.[4,5] Cyclosporine (CsA), an endecapeptide extracted from fungi, appears to induce potent reversible preferential suppression of T lymphocytes while sparing the nonspecific immune system.

Review of the world experience has shown that between 1972 and 1982, 346 patients underwent heart transplantation; 51 of these were treated with cyclosporine. With a cumulative follow-up of 1200 patient-years (mean, 3.4 years), the survival rate is 57%. During this 10-year period, 43% of the recipients died: 20% from rejection, 14% from infection, 3% from accelerated atherosclerosis, 3% from acute graft failure in the operating room, 2% from malignancy, and 1% from other causes. The probability of survival has been 82%, 70%, and 52% at 1 year, 3 years, and 5 years, respectively. Since the introduction of cyclosporine, there has been a 50% decrease in the incidence and mortality of the major complications (rejection and infection).

A new program of cardiac (Table 1) and cardiopulmonary transplantation using cyclosporine has been initiated recently at the Texas Heart Institute. This report summarizes this recent experience. Surgical techniques have been described previously.[6,7]

MATERIALS AND METHODS

Patient Selection

Heart transplantation. Most patients referred for cardiac transplantation have end-stage heart disease due to coronary artery disease with global left ventricular dysfunction, idiopathic cardiomyopathy, or previously treated valvular heart disease associated with cardiomyopathy. They are generally in NYHA Functional Class IV, with a prognosis limited to weeks or months. Upon examination, candidates are screened for contraindications to transplantation, including age greater than 50 years, elevated pulmonary vascular resistance above 8 Woods units, active infection, recent pulmonary infarction, diabetes mellitus requiring insulin, marked obesity, severe peripheral vascular disease, significant renal disease greater than can be attributed to prerenal azotemia or hepatic congestion, unrelenting life-limiting conditions (malignant neoplasm), and psychosocial abnormalities that would prohibit post-transplantation rehabilitation.

Candidates are subjected to an in-depth evaluation

From the Division of Surgery, Texas Heart Institute of St. Luke's Episcopal and Texas Children's Hospitals; and the Division of Immunology and Organ Transplantation, Department of Surgery, The University of Texas Medical School, Houston, TX.

Presented at the First International Congress on Cyclosporine, May 16–19, 1983, Houston, TX.

Reprint requests should be addressed to Denton A. Cooley, M.D., Texas Heart Institute, P.O. Box 20345, Houston, TX 77225.

0041-1345/83/1505-0068$01.00/0

Table 1. Cardiac Transplantation at the Texas Heart Institute

Referred for evaluation	49 patients
Rejected for transplantation	40 (81%)
Accepted for transplantation	9 (19%)
Died waiting for transplant	2
Transplanted	7
Ischemic heart disease	3
Idiopathic cardiomyopathy	3
Rheumatic heart disease	1
Cumulative follow-up	830 patient-days
Early death	1
Rejection episodes	9%/patient-month
Fatal rejection	0%/patient-month
Infection episodes	30%/patient-month
Fatal infection	0%/patient-month

during admission to the Texas Heart Institute, including a complete medical history, physical examination, and laboratory studies (biochemical, microbiologic, hematologic, radiologic, and immunologic). Cardiac catheterization is performed to define precisely cardiac abnormalities and measure pulmonary vascular resistance. Assessment of the patient's psychosocial status is then undertaken. A supportive social structure with a history of medical compliance is necessary.

After the patient has been accepted as a suitable candidate by the Medical Review Board, informed consent is obtained with a full discussion of current risks, complications, and expected survival of cardiac transplant recipients. Patients are then placed on a heart transplant waiting list.

Cardiopulmonary transplantation. The resurgence of interest in organ transplantation includes the combined replacement of the heart and lungs. Candidates for cardiopulmonary transplantation include patients with cardiogenic pulmonary hypertension, either acquired or congenital (Eisenmenger's syndrome), primary pulmonary hypertension, end-stage chronic obstructive pulmonary disease, interstitial pulmonary fibrosis, cystic fibrosis, pulmonary atresia, and pulmonary AV fistula.

Donor Selection

Heart transplantation. Potential donors are evaluated as thoroughly as possible. Donors must be 15–40 years of age with normal heart function as defined by electrocardiogram, physiologic performance, physical examination, and history. Also included in the evaluation protocol are an SMA, chest roentgenogram, coronary angiography for men over 35 years and women over 40 years of age, blood and urine cultures, and erythrocyte typing. Contraindications include obvious sepsis, malignancy, primary heart disease, tuberculosis, systemic disease involving the heart, chronic hypertension, and high-dose inotropic support. Brain edema <48 hr and ventilatory support <100 hr with normal gas exchange are required.

After brain death has been established, appropriate studies of tissue compatibility are completed. The donor and recipient must be ABO compatible and reasonably comparable in terms of body weight, with a negative crossmatch by the visual eosin-exclusion lymphocytotoxicity method. The microlymphocytotoxicity technique is used to detect HLA-A, HLA-B, HLA-C, and HLA-DR determinants. Cadaveric hearts can be used even if donor-recipient antigenic differences are found, except for a donor incompatibility of HLA-A2. Recipients bearing three or four antigen identities or cross-reactivities with the cadaveric donor are accorded first preference.

Cardiopulmonary transplantation. Potential donors are evaluated using the same criteria used for heart transplantation. More importance is placed, however, on matching the donor organs for size and fit. According to statistics published by Stanford, only 25% of potential cadaveric donors have suitable lungs for transplantation due to complications of brain death.[8]

Immunosuppressive Monitoring

Early diagnosis of graft rejection is essential. Cyclosporine is started 6 hr before the procedure and is then administered daily in doses to maintain therapeutic plasma trough levels of 100–200 ng/ml. Prednisone is begun during the procedure and is continued thereafter in divided doses of 120 mg, tapering to 20 mg on the 120th post-transplant day. Transvenous endomyocardial biopsies are performed, beginning on the second postoperative day and continued weekly if rejection is not noted and twice weekly if rejection occurs. After the first postoperative month, biopsies are done twice monthly, then monthly. The endocardial biopsy technique can be performed percutaneously, rapidly, and safely. Routine biopsy specimens may reveal evidence of mild rejection prior to clinical symptoms. Features include myocardial interstitial edema, myocardial mononuclear cell infiltrates, endocardial mononuclear pyroninophilic cell infiltrates, perivascular cuffing, and myocytolysis in even mild rejection (Fig. 1). Steroids are given if rejection is encountered, beginning with Solu-Medrol, 1500 mg/day, then prednisone, 200 mg/day tapering to 20 mg on day 120. Myocytolysin seems to be the only significant pathologic finding of rejection with cyclosporine.

Routine postoperative monitoring for the first 3 weeks includes daily chest roentgenograms and lab work including SMA-6, CBC, and trough levels for CsA. Immunomonitoring includes spontaneous blastogenesis, LMC, pan-T cells, T_h/T_s ratio, and CDC. Following hospital discharge, patients are initially seen weekly in the clinic for routine lab work.

CASE REPORTS*

Case 1

A 43-year-old man was first admitted to the Texas Heart Institute on May 26, 1982, with

*As of May 1, 1983.

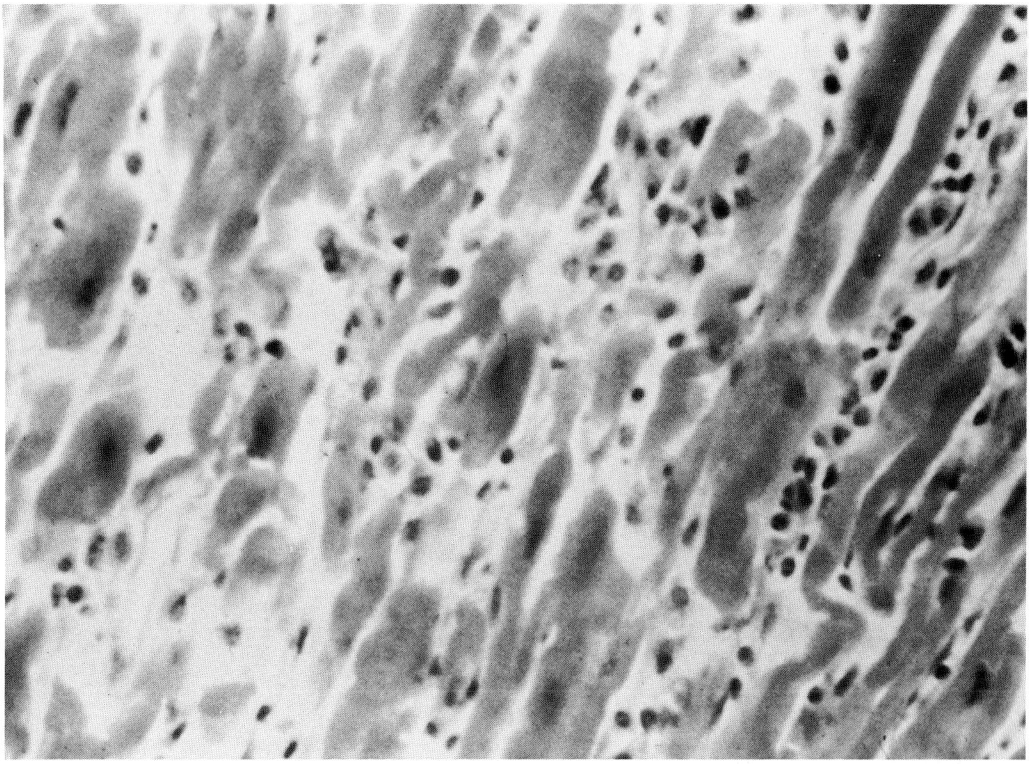

Fig. 1. Endomyocardial biopsy specimen showing representative histopathologic findings during an episode of rejection. Note the interstitial mononuclear infiltrate and perivascular inflammatory infiltrates.

a diagnosis of ischemic heart disease. He had a history of two myocardial infarctions, in 1975 and 1978, and had undergone single vessel bypass and resection of a left ventricular aneurysm in Cleveland, OH, in 1978. He did well until March 1982, when he sustained a subendocardial myocardial infarction, which precipitated congestive heart failure. He was referred to the Transplant Service on June 8, 1982. At this time, he was essentially bedridden, with an ejection fraction of 8%.

Surgery on both the donor and recipient began simultaneously at 11:30 p.m. on July 4, 1982, and was completed uneventfully approximately 2 hr later, as the transplanted heart began to beat spontaneously. Cold ischemic time for the allograft was 48 min.

The early postoperative clinical course was unremarkable. No cardiac support drugs were necessary, and the patient was extubated after 8 hr in the recovery room. Strict handwashing and sterile dressing changes were the only isolation techniques observed. Prednisone was given orally on a tapering basis in conjunction with CsA throughout the postoperative period. On the 26th post-transplant day, an endomyocardial biopsy specimen was abnormal, and the patient was pulsed for rejection. Additionally, he developed acute cholecystitis requiring cholecystectomy and a lung abscess requiring right pulmonary lobectomy. Subsequently, an empyema was drained. His recovery from infectious complications was complete, and he has been discharged from the hospital for outpatient care. A recent heart catheterization showed no abnormalities. All pressures were normal.

Case 2

A 45-year-old woman in NYHA Functional Class IV with progressively worsening cardiomyopathy of unknown origin was admitted for consideration for transplantation. She was accepted into the program, and transplantation was performed on August 5, 1982.

Routine postoperative immunosuppression was begun. Her postoperative course was complicated by an episode of rejection on August 31, 1982 (27th postoperative day). At that time, she was pulsed for rejection with Solu-Medrol/prednisone standard taper. Two weeks after transplantation, she developed disseminated pulmonary tuberculosis. This had appeared despite a preoperative negative PPD skin test. The pulmonary infection responded promptly to antituberculous therapy, and she was discharged after 6 weeks of

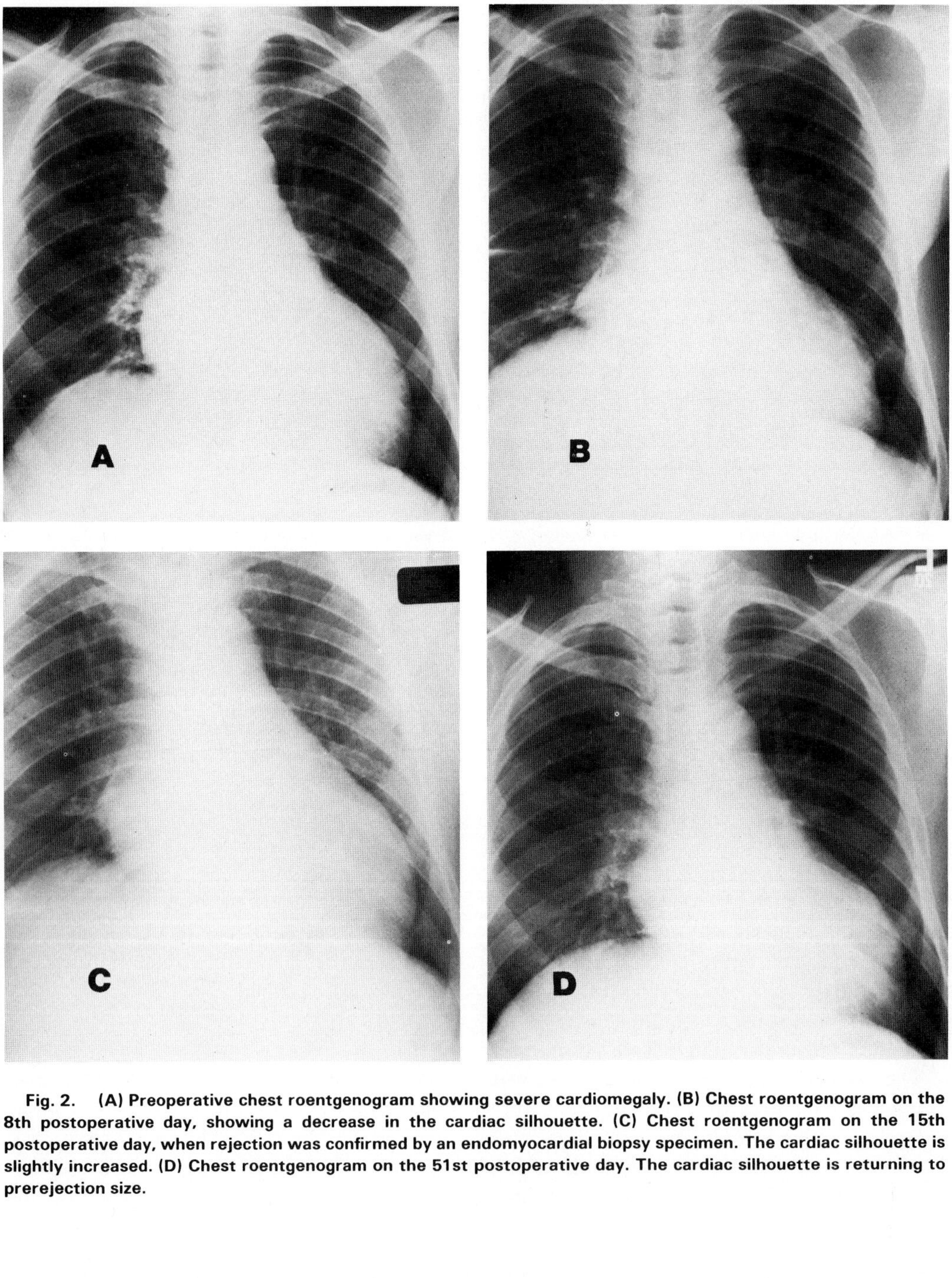

Fig. 2. (A) Preoperative chest roentgenogram showing severe cardiomegaly. (B) Chest roentgenogram on the 8th postoperative day, showing a decrease in the cardiac silhouette. (C) Chest roentgenogram on the 15th postoperative day, when rejection was confirmed by an endomyocardial biopsy specimen. The cardiac silhouette is slightly increased. (D) Chest roentgenogram on the 51st postoperative day. The cardiac silhouette is returning to prerejection size.

hospitalization. She is presently totally rehabilitated, works part-time, and is a housewife and mother.

Case 3

The third transplantation in this series was performed on a 50-year-old man on December 28, 1982. He was admitted with a diagnosis of idiopathic cardiomyopathy. Cardiac symptoms had first occurred in 1974. Ischemic time was 35 min during the transplantation.

The patient's postoperative course was routine until January 12, 1983 (15th post-transplant day), when rejection was diagnosed by endomyocardial biopsy. He was pulsed for rejection starting with 1500 mg Solu-Medrol, followed by 200 mg of prednisone tapered. A biopsy specimen on January 17 was still abnormal but returned to normal by January 21. In this patient, a chest roentgenogram taken at the time of rejection showed cardiac enlargement. Although roentgenograms are not definitive in the diagnosis of rejection, cardiomegaly may, in some patients, be associated with an episode of rejection, and routine chest films can aid in the diagnosis (Fig. 2).[9] No other postoperative complications occurred. A mild case of herpes simplex was cultured but disappeared without treatment. The patient is now totally rehabilitated.

Case 4

The next patient in this series was admitted with a diagnosis of cardiomyopathy secondary to aortic valve disease. This 52-year-old man underwent transplantation on January 13, 1983. He had undergone aortic valve replacement in 1979.

Immunosuppression consisted of the standard CsA and steroid tapers. There were no postoperative complications, and he was discharged from the hospital 3 weeks after transplantation. He is following a normal course of rehabilitation.

Case 5

This 28-year-old man was admitted with a diagnosis of idiopathic cardiomyopathy. At that time, he was bedridden and had an ejection fraction of 5%. A liver biopsy, which was done to clarify an elevated bilirubin of 4.2, was normal, and showed only passive congestion related to this cardiomyopathy. He was accepted into the program, and transplantation was performed on February 28, 1983. He developed renal failure in the postoperative period, and died suddenly on day 23 of cardiac arrest. The postmortem examination did not reveal the cause of death. The heart showed some hypertrophy but was otherwise unremarkable.

Case 6

The sixth patient was a 48-year-old male who was admitted with end-stage ischemic heart disease. He had undergone aortocoronary artery bypassing (×7) in January 1983 at another hospital. On March 27, 1983, he underwent cardiac transplantation. He was discharged 4 weeks later without any complications.

Case 7

A 40-year-old male was admitted to the Texas Heart Institute with a diagnosis of severe emphysema secondary to alpha-1 antitrypsin deficiency and cor pulmonale with tricuspid insufficiency and compensated right heart failure. He had become totally disabled in April 1982 because of progressive cardiorespiratory failure. On admission, he was bedridden, severely dyspneic at rest, and cyanotic with oxygen. On November 23, 1982, he underwent cardiopulmonary transplantation. He received cyclosporine both p.o. and i.v.

His postoperative course was complicated by persistent bilateral pleural effusion necessitating repeated thoracentesis, progressive respiratory distress with subsequent reintubation, and chronic malnutrition. A positive culture for Legionnaire's disease was obtained. On December 15, he was returned to the operating room following dehiscence of the tracheal anastomosis. Within hours, he again showed signs of an air leak and was pronounced dead that evening, 3 weeks after transplantation. Autopsy confirmed tracheal disruption and severe bilateral pneumonia. There was no evidence of rejection.

DISCUSSION

At present and for the foreseeable future, cardiac transplantation is the most effective and practical means for salvage of patients with terminal heart disease. Transplantation now promises the recipient a substantial prolongation of life. The procurement of suitable donors, however, remains a continuing obstacle. Many qualified recipients die awaiting the arrival of a donor. Efforts to prolong the period that an allograft may be safely preserved outside the body should help alleviate some of the logistic problems that now exist.

The use of cyclosporine has given the recipient a considerably better chance to survive and avoid allograft rejection. In a Stanford study, rehabilitation rates were found to be 90%, compared to 70% previously.[10] A decrease in the incidence of rejection episodes in the postoperative period, particularly when prednisone had been combined with CsA, was also noted. In more than 50 heart transplant patients treated with CsA, only 0.89 episodes of rejection per patient during the initial 60 postoperative days were noted, versus 1.22 episodes with conventional treatment. The incidence of infection was also decreased by approximately 50%, and mortality associated with infection decreased from 31% to 11%. These effects also extend to earlier hospital discharge (42 vs. 72 days) and, thus, a decrease in the overall costs associated with transplantation ($51,000 vs. $90,700). The routine use of transvenous endomyocardial biopsy for the diagnosis of early rejection has also improved survival rates, which are now 82% at 1 year and 50% at 5 years. With the decreased threat of rejection and reduced costs associated with shorter hospitalizations, cardiac transplantation should become a more widely accepted procedure.

REFERENCES

1. Barnard CN: Capetown S Afr Med J 41:1271, 1967

2. Cooley DA, Bloodwell RD, Hallman GL: J Cardiovasc Surg 9:403, 1968

3. Jamieson SW, Oyer PE, Reitz BA, et al: Heart Transplantation 1(1):86, 1982

4. Calne RY, White DJG, Thiru S: Lancet 2:1323, 1978

5. Kahan BD: Texas Heart Inst J 9(3):253, 1982

6. Cooley DA, Frazier OH, Kahan BD: Texas Heart Inst J 9(3):247, 1982

7. Cooley DA: Techniques in Cardiac Surgery. Philadelphia, Saunders, 1983

8. Reitz BA: Heart Transplantation 1(4):291, 1982

9. Baumgartner WA, Reitz BA, Oyer PE, et al: Cardiac Homotransplantation. Chicago, Yearbook Medical Publishers, 1979

10. Oyer PE, Stinson EB, Jamieson S, et al: Heart Transplantation 1(4):285, 1982

New Onset of Hypertension Following Cardiac Transplantation: A Preliminary Report and Analysis

M. E. Thompson, A. P. Shapiro, A. M. Johnsen, R. Reeves, J. Itzkoff, E. Ginchereau, R. L. Hardesty, B. L. Griffith, H. T. Bahnson, and R. McDonald, Jr.

CARDIAC transplantation has been used with increasing success over the past 15 years for the treatment of patients with intractable congestive heart failure. During this period, refinements in imunosuppressive management have resulted in a 1-year survival of 63% and a 5-year survival of 39% for patients operated on between 1974 and 1981 receiving azathioprine and prednisone.[1] For the past 2 years, a new immunosuppressive agent, cyclosporine A (CsA), has been used with equally good success.[2] One of the most notable and unexpected findings in patients receiving CsA is the almost universal development of systemic arterial hypertension. This observation is in sharp contrast to that in patients receiving azathioprine and prednisone, in whom postoperative hypertension developed in less than 20%.[3] This paper reports observations made in 18 long-term survivors of cardiac transplantation in whom postoperative hypertension developed in association with the use of CsA for immunosuppression.

MATERIALS AND METHODS

This group of 18 long-term survivors of cardiac transplantation was gleaned from a total of 33 adults undergoing transplantation at the University of Pittsburgh from March 1981 through December 1982. In this group, 28 patients survived 1 or more months following cardiac transplantation, and of these, 26 ultimately developed hypertension. The 2 patients who did not develop hypertension died of a combination of infection and rejection within 2–3 months following surgery. The 18 individuals constituting this report are those in whom adequate follow-up data have been obtained to date and are representative of the larger group of hypertensive cardiac transplant patients.

Demographic information was collected by interview with respect to patient age, sex, weight, previous personal history of hypertension, family history of hypertension, and reason for cardiac transplantation. Hypertension was defined as being present if three separate measurements of systolic and/or diastolic blood pressure exceeded 140 mmHg and 90 mmHg, respectively. Complete right heart catheterization was performed pre- and postoperatively. Arterial pressure was measured either directly with an intraarterial catheter or indirectly with a sphygmomanometer. Mean arterial pressure was calculated as ⅓ the pulse pressure plus the diastolic pressure. Cardiac output was determined using the indocyanine green technique, the Fick cardiac output method, or the thermodilution method.[4-6] Systemic vascular resistance was calculated using the formula

$$\text{SVR (dynes/sec/cm}^{-5}) = \frac{\text{mean arterial pressure}}{\text{cardiac output}} \times 80$$

All hemodynamic measurements were obtained while the patients were receiving their usual medical therapy. In the preoperative patients, for example, some were receiving inotropic agents, diuretics, and vasodilators. Postoperatively, the right heart catheterization was performed in conjunction with routine endomyocardial biopsy. Consequently, some patients were started on antihypertensive agents prior to the initial postoperative observations. In all instances, representative postoperative values are reported. The paired two-tailed Student's t test was used for statistical analysis.[7] The mean maintenance dose of prednisone and CsA was 18 mg/day and 6 mg/kg/day, respectively.

Pre- and postoperative renal function was assessed using the serum creatinine value.[8] Values for supine and erect circulating peripheral renin activity and 24-hour urinary excretion of catecholamines were determined.[9,10] In addition, 17/18 patients underwent postoperative 24-hr ambulatory blood pressure monitoring using an Avionics recorder (Del Mar Avionics, Irvine, CA).[11]

Long-term treatment of hypertension was instituted in a stepwise manner. Treatment consisted of a diuretic (hydrochlorothiazide or furosemide) to control intravascular volume; vasodilator therapy (hydralazine or prasozin); sympatholytic therapy (beta blockers and/or the

From the Department of Medicine, Divisions of Cardiology and Clinical Pharmacology/Hypertension, and the Department of Surgery, University of Pittsburgh School of Medicine, Pittsburgh, PA.

Reprint requests should be addressed to Mark E. Thompson, M.D., Division of Cardiology, 789 Scaife Hall, University of Pittsburgh, Pittsburgh, PA 15261.

0041–1345/83/1505–0069$01.00/0

alpha-blocking agent clonidine); and, finally, a more potent vasodilator (minoxidil).

Of the 18 patients, only 1 was receiving no treatment at the time of this report, 1 was being treated with furosemide alone, and 1 was taking hydralazine alone. Four patients received furosemide and a vasodilator, 3 were receiving a diuretic and a beta blocker, and 1 was receiving a vasodilator and a beta blocker. Six patients were treated with a diuretic, vasodilator, and sympatholytic agent, while another patient received minoxidil in addition to the three aforementioned drugs.

RESULTS

The 18 patients with hypertension (17 males, 1 female) ranged in age from 25–54 years. The mean follow-up time from transplantation was 11.8 months (5–24 months). Arterial hypertension was first noted on an average of 50 days following transplantation (median, 42 days; range, 6–139 days). Only 2 patients had a prior personal history of hypertension; a family history of hypertension was obtained in 10. The development of hypertension appeared to be independent of patient age, sex, weight, or reason for transplantation. Postoperative blood pressure measurements obtained in conjunction with cardiac output and used to calculate systemic vascular resistance were as follows: average systolic pressure, 154 ± 14 mmHg; average diastolic pressure, 95 ± 13 mmHg; average mean arterial pressure, 116 ± 13 mmHg. The average preoperative cardiac output was 3.7 ± 1.2 liters/min; the postoperative value was 4.9 ± 0.9 liters/min ($p < 0.01$). The average systemic vascular resistance preoperatively was 1707 ± 595 dyne/sec/cm^{-5}, and the postoperative peripheral vascular resistance was 1941 ± 418 dyne/sec/cm^{-5} ($p > 0.2$). The preoperative serum creatinine was 1.2 ± 0.3 mg/dl, and the postoperative value was 2.2 ± 0.8 mg/dl ($p < 0.001$). The postoperative mean values for supine and erect peripheral renin activity were 4.8 ± 3.2 ng/ml/3-hr incubation and 9.6 ± 7.8 ng/ml/3-hr incubation, respectively (normals: supine, 1.5–5 ng/ml/3-hr incubation; erect, 5–15 ng/ml/3-hr incubation). The postoperative mean values for 24-hr urinary catecholamine excretion were: norepinephrine, 11.7 ± 8.5 m*M*; epinephrine, 2.1 ± 2.8 m*M*; dopamine, 55 ± 40.8 m*M* (the upper limit of normal: norepinephrine, 40 m*M*; epinephrine, 10 m*M*; dopamine, 200 m*M*).

Twenty-four-hour ambulatory blood pressure monitoring was accomplished in 17/18 patients. The average 24-hr systolic and diastolic blood pressures were 135 mmHg and 91 mmHg, respectively; the average daytime pressures were 136 mmH and 91 mmHg, respectively; the average nighttime sleeping pressures were 133 mmHg and 90 mmHg, respectively. The average nighttime fall in blood pressure levels in these patients was 1.6% and 0.3%, respectively, and the average fall in pulse rate, 10%, which is in sharp contrast to the 10%–15% fall in systolic and diastolic blood pressure and 15%–20% fall in pulse rate observed by us in patients with essential hypertension and in normotensive individuals.[11] Only 3/17 patients showed a fall of 10% or more in systolic and diastolic blood pressures, while 8 demonstrated an actual rise in these pressures, ranging from 1.5%–18%. A representative example of a 24-hr ambulatory blood pressure record showing a rise in systolic and diastolic blood pressures during sleep is illustrated in Fig. 1.

Eleven patients have been closely followed

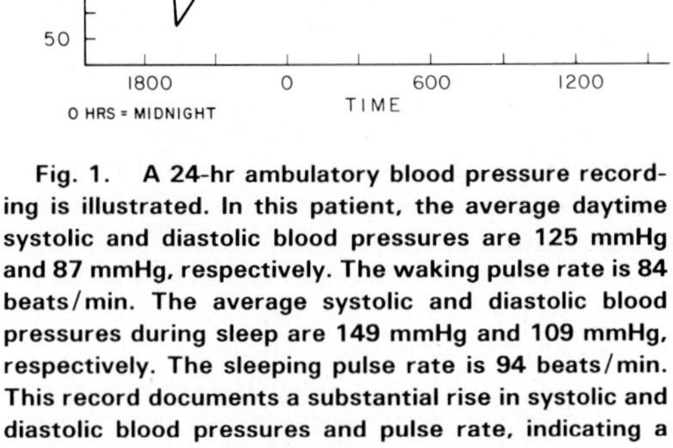

Fig. 1. A 24-hr ambulatory blood pressure recording is illustrated. In this patient, the average daytime systolic and diastolic blood pressures are 125 mmHg and 87 mmHg, respectively. The waking pulse rate is 84 beats/min. The average systolic and diastolic blood pressures during sleep are 149 mmHg and 109 mmHg, respectively. The sleeping pulse rate is 94 beats/min. This record documents a substantial rise in systolic and diastolic blood pressures and pulse rate, indicating a disturbance in neurogenic blood pressure control.

in the Hypertension Clinic. In these 11, treatment of hypertension was similar to that of the overall group and was initiated in the hospital in most instances. In only 6/11 patients did the sequential addition of drugs in a stepwise fashion result in a significantly lower blood pressure: (1) beta blocker added to diuretic and hydralazine in 3 patients; (2) clonidine added to hydralazine and a diuretic in 1 patient; (3) minoxidil added to a diuretic, hydralazine, and beta blocker in 1 patient; and (4) a diuretic and hydralazine following no therapy in 1 patient. In this group, the average of the highest systolic and diastolic blood pressures were 167 mmHg and 108 mmHg, respectively. The average pulse rate associated with the highest blood pressures was 100 beats/min, and the average serum creatinine was 2.0 mg/dl. The average lowest systolic and diastolic pressures were 144 mmHg and 93 mmHg, respectively. The average pulse rate associated with the lowest blood pressures was 97 beats/min, and the average serum creatinine was 1.7 mg/dl. The failure to achieve ready lowering of systolic and diastolic blood pressures in the patients followed in the Hypertension Clinic indicate the relative difficulty encountered in treating this group of patients.

DISCUSSION

The predictable development of systemic hypertension following cardiac transplantation in patients receiving prednisone and CsA as immunosuppressants represents a unique problem. The circumstances surrounding the development of hypertension are unusual in that the characteristic demographic factors associated with hypertension (age, race, sex, body weight) and family history did not seem to influence the development of postoperative hypertension.[12] Rather, the hypertension seen following cardiac transplantation seems to be related partially to the hemodynamic and neurogenic changes associated with the received heart, but at least as important a factor seems to be the use of CsA. This latter association is further strengthened by noting the infrequent report of hypertension when prednisone and azathioprine have been used as immunosuppressants following cardiac transplantation.[3]

The mechanism responsible for the development of this "new" hypertension following cardiac transplantation when CsA is used remains to be determined. Multiple factors obviously determine the level of systemic blood pressure. These may be divided into two groups: group A, short-term modulation of blood pressure, which depends on the central nervous system and is mediated through baroreceptors and chemoreceptor reflexes, and group B, long-term maintenance of blood pressure, which depends on the renin-angiotensin system, aldosterone production, vascular tone, and intravascular volume.[13]

Evidence of an aberration in the central nervous system's control of blood pressure has been demonstrated by 24-hr ambulatory blood pressure monitoring. In the patient undergoing cardiac transplantation, 14/17 showed only a modest fall or actual rise in the diastolic blood pressure during sleep, compared to the ambulatory state. The failure of the blood pressure to fall with sleep contrasts sharply with the response noted in patients with essential hypertension and even renal hypertension, in which we have noted a fall in blood pressure during sleep.[11] This finding is indicative of an abnormal response of the baroreceptors to a rise in blood pressure. Usually, a rise in blood pressure results in a decrease in sympathetic tone and reflex vasodilatation, which would be expected to return the blood pressure to the baseline state.[13] In normal circumstances, one would also expect a slowing of the pulse rate, but this response is blunted in post-transplant patients because the heart is denervated. An average fall in pulse rate of only 10% was noted in the transplant patients, compared to a 15%–20% fall in other hypertensive patients.[11] The absence of change in the resting pulse rate when the patient changes from the supine to the erect position and the minimal slowing of the heart rate following administration of the beta blocking agents provide additional evidence of altered neural response in patients following cardiac transplantation. Altered responsiveness of the denervated heart to pharmacologic manipulation has also been documented by Shaver et al.[14]

The long-term mechanisms that influence the level of systemic blood pressure are also modified in patients undergoing cardiac transplantation. While the relationship between mean arterial blood pressure and cardiac output may be expressed in terms of mean arterial pressure equals cardiac output times systemic vascular resistance, the factors that determine systemic arterial pressure and cardiac output are regulated in a mutually independent manner.[13] Following cardiac transplantation, the received heart provides a statistically significant increase in cardiac output from 3.7 liters/min to 4.9 liters/min ($p < 0.01$). At the same time cardiac output increases, the total peripheral vascular resistance in the "old vascular tree" remains unchanged postoperatively, compared with preoperative values (1941 dynes/sec/cm^{-5} vs. 1707 dynes/sec/cm^{-5}, respectively; $p > 0.2$). Failure of the appropriate preoperative elevated systemic vascular resistance to return to the normal range following an increase in cardiac output to normal postoperatively was associated with a sustained elevation of blood pressure (preoperative average blood pressure, 80 mmHg, vs. 116 mmHg postoperative; $p < 0.001$).

Altered vascular compliance may contribute to the sustained increase in total peripheral vascular resistance observed in these patients. This abnormality may be a consequence of the sustained increase in peripheral vascular resistance that is characteristic of patients with intractable congestive heart failure.[15] This vasoconstrictive response to congestive heart failure over a prolonged period of time, which is mediated neurogenically and hormonally, may result in permanent changes in the arteriolar resistance vessels, much as has been noted in patients with essential hypertension.[16]

Alternative explanations for the sustained elevation of systemic vascular resistance were investigated in several ways. First, a determination of 24-hr urinary catecholamine excretion was made. No increase in the production of catecholamines was detected to explain the sustained elevation of blood pressure. Second, supine and upright peripheral renin activity (PRA) was measured. While PRA is at the upper limit of the normal range, it must be remembered that sodium restriction and diuretic therapy were imposed on most of these patients. These observations serve to exclude excessive renin production by the kidneys as an explanation for the sustained level of systemic hypertension observed. Accordingly, the role of the kidneys in contributing to the development of hypertension following cardiac transplantation using CsA for immunosuppression requires an explanation other than one related to excess renin production.

CsA has been clearly demonstrated to be nephrotoxic.[17] In the present group of patients, the creatinine level preoperatively was 1.1 mg/dl, and the postoperative level was 2.2 mg/dl ($p < 0.001$). Even this modest degree of renal impairment may indicate that the development of hypertension is the result of salt and water retention, perhaps through an effect on tubular function. An association between CsA administration, altered renal function, and the development of hypertension has also been reported by Joss et al.[18] Twenty-five of 29 patients less than 17 years of age without preexisting cardiovascular or renal disease developed hypertension while receiving CsA following bone marrow transplantation. A rise in BUN, creatinine, and associated fluid retention preceded a rapid rise in diastolic blood pressure. Convulsions occurred in 6/7 patients with diastolic blood pressures in excess of 120 mmHg. Treatment in the form of diazoxide and diuresis with mannitol and furosemide was required. These workers also suspected that impairment of renal function contributed to the development of hypertension, although the precise mechanism remains to be elucidated. Further support for this concept is provided by the observations made in the long-term following of 11 patients seen in the Hypertension Clinic. The highest mean systolic and diastolic blood pressures were associated with mean serum creatinine levels of 2.0 mg/dl, while the lowest pressures were associated with a mean serum creatinine level of 1.7 mg/dl. The necessity for maintenance doses of steroids may also have contributed to some extent to the development of hypertension in this group of patients.[19] However, in patients undergoing cardiac transplantation who received a combination of prednisone and azathioprine for immunosuppression, a sustained elevation of blood pressure is unusual, as is an elevation of the serum creatinine during long-term follow-up.

SUMMARY

New onset hypertension has been observed to develop in a group of patients undergoing cardiac transplantation while receiving CsA for immunosuppression. The hypertension develops independently of known risk factors. The cause of hypertension is unknown, but it is associated with normalization of the cardiac output, maintenance of an abnormally elevated systemic vascular resistance, a distortion of neurogenic control, and a modest impairment of renal function, which may result in an increase in intravascular volume as a result of an impairment in sodium excretory function. No abnormalities have been demonstrated in peripheral renin activity nor in urinary catecholamine levels. A systematic approach to the treatment of hypertension used diuretics to reduce excess intravascular volume, vasodilators to reduce vascular tone, and sympatholytic drugs to attenuate the effects of circulating catecholamines and the sympathetic nervous sytem. In spite of this multifaceted approach, the hypertension has been relatively resistant to treatment. Further studies will be required to define the mechanisms of this new form of hypertension and to establish an effective and rational mode of therapy.

REFERENCES

1. Pennock JL, Oyer PE, Reitz BA, et al: J Thorac Cardiovasc Surg 83:168, 1982
2. Griffith BP, Hardesty RL, Deeb GM, et al: Ann Surg 196:324, 1982
3. Oyer PE, Stinson EB, Jamieson SW, et al: Transplant Proc 15:1247, 1983
4. Hamilton WF, Moore JW, Kinsman JM, et al: Am J Physiol 99:534, 1932
5. Selzer A, Sudrann RB: Circ Res 6:485, 1958
6. Ganz W, Swan HJC: Am J Cardiol 29:241, 1972
7. Snedecor GW, Cochran WG: In Statistical Methods (6th ed). Ames, IA: Iowa State University Press, 1967, pp 59–60
8. Tietz H (ed): Fundamentals of Clinical Chemistry. Philadelphia: Saunders, 1976, p 986
9. Haber EJ, Koerner T, Page LB, et al: J Clin Endocrin and Metab 29:1349, 1963
10. Laverty R, Taylor KM: Analyt Biochem 22:269, 1968
11. Reeves RA, Shapiro AP, McDonald RH Jr, et al: Environ Health Perspect (in press)
12. Gifford RW, Cooper ES, Hill M, et al: Circulation 64:1079A, 1981
13. Guyton AC: Circulation 64:1079, 1981
14. Shaver JA, Leon DF, Gray S, et al: N Engl J Med 281:822, 1969
15. Zelis R, Flaim SF: Mod Con Cardiovasc Dis 51:79, 1982
16. Klintmalm GBG, Iwatsuki S, Starzl TE: Lancet 2:470, 1981
17. Folkow B, Hallbäck M, Lundgren Y, et al: Circ Res 32 (Suppl 1):2, 1973
18. Joss DV, Barrett AJ, Kendra JR, et al: Lancet 1:906, 1982
19. Popovtzer MM, Pinnggera W, Katz FH, et al: Circulation 47:1297, 1973

Single Lung Transplantation with Cyclosporine Immunosuppression

S. L. Kamholz, F. J. Veith, C. M. Montefusco, K. L. Pinsker, F. P. Mollenkopf, R. Kaleya, J. Goldsmith, A. J. Norin, E. E. Emeson, S. N. Cannarella, and M. L. Gliedman

INCREASED SUCCESS in experimental lung and heart-lung transplantation has been achieved with use of cyclosporine (CsA) immunosuppression.[1–4] In previous studies using standard therapy—prednisone (P), azathioprine (Aza), and/or antilymphocyte globulin (ALG)—the mean survival of canine single lung allograft (SLA) recipients was only 2–3 weeks, with rejection being the major cause of death.[5] We have noted a marked improvement in the mean survival (≧5 months) with good allograft function of canine SLA recipients treated with CsA. In the current report, results in 28 canine and 2 human CsA-treated SLA recipients are analyzed.

MATERIALS AND METHODS

Canine Recipients

Left lung allotransplantation was performed in 28 dogs, using previously described surgical techniques.[6] Donor and recipient animals were unmatched male mongrels, each weighing 20–25 kg. CsA dissolved in corn oil was administered to all canine SLA recipients. The inital oral dose was 17 mg/kg/day. This was tapered by 4 mg/kg/day decrements, commencing 5–6 weeks after transplantation. In 5 dogs (Nos. 1, 8, 15, 19, 23), CsA was discontinued after 75–399 days of therapy.

Additional immunosuppressive agents were administered as follows:

Group 1. Eight dogs (Nos. 1–5, 21–23) received Aza, 2 mg/kg/day p.o. for the first 2 weeks after transplantation only.

Group 2. Eight dogs (Nos. 6–10, 24–26) received P, 2 mg/kg/day p.o., which was tapered by 0.5 mg/kg every 7–10 days until a maintenance dose of 0.5 mg/kg/day was achieved.

Group 3. Four dogs (Nos. 11–14) received Aza and P on the same schedule as in groups 1 and 2. In addition, intravenous methylprednisolone (MP), 750–1000 mg, and rabbit antidog ALG, 3.5 ml intramuscularly, were administered daily for 1–3 days following transplantation.

Group 4. Eight dogs (Nos. 15–20, 27, 28) received CsA only.

All canine SLA recipients were evaluated with weekly chest roentgenograms (CXR), periodic ventilation/perfusion ($\dot{V}/\dot{Q}$) lung scans, bronchoalveolar lavage (BAL) with analysis of cell content and cytotoxic T-cell activity, and, when indicated, open lung biopsy. Details of the interpretation of lung scans[1,7] and evaluation of the results of BAL[8,9] have been previously published. A diagnosis of allograft rejection was established by one or more of the following: presence of infiltrate in the SLA on CXR; decreased perfusion to the SLA on $\dot{V}/\dot{Q}$ scan, increase in cytotoxic T-cell activity on BAL; or histologic findings of allograft rejection[2,5] on open lung biopsy. Upon diagnosis, treatment was instituted with MP, 50 mg/kg/day i.v. for 3 days, followed by P in tapering doses, as previously reported.[1,2]

Human Recipients

Patient 1. Left lung allotransplantation was performed in a 68-year-old white male because of chronic severe respiratory failure due to idiopathic pulmonary fibrosis. The donor organ was obtained from a brain-dead 17-year-old white male with compatible blood group and appropriate hilar dimensions. Immunosuppressive therapy was identical to that employed in canine group 1 recipients, with the addition of varying doses of corticosteroids (because the patient had been treated with long-term P preoperatively).

Patient 2. Left lung allotransplantation was performed in a 25-year-old white male because of terminal acute respiratory failure due to accidental paraquat poisoning. The lung donor was a brain-dead 19-year-old ABO- and hilar-size-compatible white male. Immunosuppressive treatment was similar to that employed in patient 1. The surgical techniques used in human allotransplantation have been previously reported.[7]

Human SLA recipients were monitored with daily CXR, serial arterial blood gases (ABG) and pulmonary hemodynamic measurements, and daily microscopic and bacteriologic examination of sputum. Bronchial anastomotic healing was assessed by repetitive bronchofiber-

---

From the Departments of Surgery, Medicine, and Pathology, Montefiore Medical Center, and the Albert Einstein College of Medicine, New York, NY.

Supported by NIH-NHLBI Program Project Grant HL 17417 and by the Manning Foundation.

Reprint requests should be addressed to Dr. S. L. Kamholz, Pulmonary Division, Montefiore Medical Center, 111 East 210th Street, New York, NY 10467.

0041-1345/83/1505-0070$01.00/0

scopic examination in patient 2. At postmortem examination, multiple sections of the SLAs and of the transplant bronchial anastomoses were obtained and subsequently analyzed.

RESULTS

Canine Recipients

Mean survival of the 28 canine SLA recipients exceeded 5 months, with 10/28 dogs surviving >150 days and 4/28 dogs surviving >350 days (Table 1). Roentgenographic and scintigraphic assessment of the SLA function revealed clear CXR and ≧30% of total blood flow to the transplanted lung on $\dot{V}/\dot{Q}$ scan in 9/10 long-surviving SLA recipients.

Nine of 10 canine SLA recipients with ≧5 months survival were in group 1 (CsA + Aza) or group 4 (CsA alone). None of the dogs treated with the multiagent regimen (group 3) survived more than 9 weeks, and only 1 dog (No. 8) in the CsA + P treatment group (group 2) had prolonged survival (9 months).

Manifestations of allograft rejection were noted in 22/28 (79%) of the canine SLA recipients (Table 1). An earlier median date of onset of recognizable rejection phenomena was noted in treatment groups 2 and 3 and similar, later date of onset in groups 1 and 4. Reversibility of manifestations of SLA rejection was noted in 28/38 (74%) episodes (Table 1), as documented by clearing of infiltrates on CXR, improvement in perfusion to the SLA on $\dot{V}/\dot{Q}$ scan, and/or resolution of histologic features of rejection when open lung biopsy was repeated.

Of the six dogs that never demonstrated rejection, dog 1 survived almost 3 years (1053 days) with excellent SLA function and entirely normal histology at postmortem examination. Dog 6 died of infection without rejection 68 days after transplantation. The remaining four dogs (Nos. 7, 12, 14, 25) died within 4–8 days of transplantation. However, when previous canine SLA recipients treated with standard immunosuppression died 4–8 days postoperatively, histologic findings of allograft rejection were characteristically present at postmortem examination.[5]

CsA therapy was discontinued in 5 animals (Table 2), despite the fact that 3/5 (Nos. 8, 19, 23) had prior episodes of allograft rejection that had been successfully treated. These dogs were receiving maintenance P when CsA was stopped. Four of these 5 survived >100 days after discontinuation of CsA. Rejection occurring in these animals after cessation of CsA was reversible with MP or P therapy.

Human Recipients

Patient 1. As a result of perioperative cardiopulmonary arrest, the patient developed

Table 1. Survival and Rejection Episodes in Canine Lung Allograft Recipients

Group	No. of Dogs	No. Surviving >150 days	Survival (days) Median (range)	Survival (days) Mean ± SE	Rejection No. with Episodes* (median date of onset)†	Rejection Treatment Responses Total Episodes‡
1	8	6	185 (21–1053)	279 ± 116§	7 (day 44)	10/13
2	8	1	45 (6–282)	69 ± 32	5 (day 27)	6/10
3	4	0	13 (4–65)	24 ± 14	2 (day 13)	1/2
4	8	3	107 (7–522)‖	183 ± 65	8 (day 41)	11/13
All	28	10	75 (4–1053)	155 ± 42	22 (day 40)	28/38

*Difference among groups in frequency of rejection episodes not significantly different by chi-squared method.
†22/28 dogs (79%) had at least one episode of rejection.
‡Treatment response: improved CXR, $\dot{V}/\dot{Q}$ scan, lavage or biopsy after MP therapy, which occurred in 74% of episodes.
§Survival in group 1 significantly greater than in group 2; t test, $p = 0.10$.
‖Dog 19 is still alive.

Table 2. Discontinuation of Cyclosporine

Dog (Group)	Day of Discontinuation	Rejection Before Discontinuation	Rejection After Discontinuation	Treatment of Rejection	Survival After Discontinuation (days)
1 (1)	399	No	No	None	654
8 (2)	258	Yes	Yes	Prednisone	24
15 (4)	205	No	Yes*	Methylprednisolone/prednisone	210
19 (4)	144	Yes	No	Prednisone	378†
23 (1)	75	Yes	Yes	Prednisone	115

*Dog 15: first rejection 111 days after discontinuation.
†Dog 19 is still alive.

severe oliguric renal failure and recurrent pulmonary edema. Despite intensive therapy, including repetitive peritoneal dialysis, the patient died 17 days after surgery. At postmortem examination, intraalveolar edema, septal fibrosis, and hyaline membrane formation were noted in the SLA.

Patient 2. The postoperative course was complicated by four episodes of allograft rejection and by persistent *Pseudomonas aeruginosa* infection in the remaining paraquat-damaged right lung. The episodes of rejection were successfully reversed with MP (and, on two occasions, equine antihuman ALG). In addition to specific therapy for pseudomonas infection, a right pneumonectomy was performed 16 days after left lung transplantation. Thus, the left SLA provided all respiratory gas exchange for this patient for more than 1 month after right pneumonectomy. The patient died of respiratory failure 7 weeks after transplantation due to a recurrent bronchopleural fistula at the right pneumonectomy stump. At postmortem examination, the transplant bronchial anastomosis was well healed; there was no evidence of rejection in the SLA.

DISCUSSION

The utilization of CsA immunosuppression in canine SLA recipients has resulted in a dramatic improvement in allograft survival with function, as compared to previous results achieved with standard immunosuppressive therapy. The 185-day median survival of group 1 recipients, and the fact that 6 of these 8 dogs survived >5 months, are highly suggestive that CsA and initial Aza is the best immunosuppressive regimen for canine single lung transplantation, although statistical significance (mean survival) was only demonstrated for the superiority of CsA + Aza (group 1) over CsA + P (group 2).

Although nearly 4/5 of the canine SLA recipients did have evidence of rejection, this was reversible more frequently (74% of episodes) and more completely than was observed when rejection occurred in canine SLA recipients treated with standard immunosuppression.[10] We have also observed that CsA therapy may be discontinued in some animals without the subsequent onset of progressive rejection (Table 2). Even when manifestations of rejection have been present prior to cessation of CsA (dogs 8, 19, 23), subsequent rejection phenomena that occur following discontinuation of CsA are usually reversible with increased doses of P. Four of 5 dogs in which CsA was stopped survived >100 days (range, 115–654) thereafter, suggesting the presence of immunologic unresponsiveness to the SLA, the mechanism of which is not yet known.[11]

Two human SLA recipients have been treated with CsA + Aza. The efficacy of CsA could not be evaluated in patient 1. In patient 2, episodes of rejection were fully reversible, and the allograft provided total pulmonary function for this patient for >1 month after contralateral pneumonectomy. The SLA did not reveal any evidence of rejection at postmortem, and the transplant bronchial anastomosis was well healed.

SUMMARY

We have shown that CsA therapy markedly enhances the survival of canine SLA recipients. In patient 2, we were encouraged by the absence of rejection and the presence of a well healed bronchial anastomosis at autopsy. Although optimal utilization of CsA in experimental and clinical lung transplantation remains to be defined, we believe that this experience supports the feasibility of the SLA as a therapeutic option for patients with end-stage lung disease.

ACKNOWLEDGMENT

The expert technical assistance of Israel Colon and Michael Torres is greatly appreciated. Our sincere thanks to Steven Levine and Louisa Greco for efforts in manuscript preparation.

REFERENCES

1. Veith FJ, Norin AJ, Montefusco CM, et al: Transplantation 32:474, 1981
2. Norin AJ, Emeson EE, Kamholz SL, et al: Transplantation 34:372, 1982
3. Reitz BA, Burton NA, Jamieson SW, et al: J Thorac Cardiovasc Surg 80:360, 1980
4. Reitz BA, Wallwork JL, Hunt SA, et al: N Engl J Med 306:557, 1982
5. Veith FJ, Sinha SBP, Blumcke S, et al: J Thorac Cardiovasc Surg 63:509, 1972
6. Veith FJ, Richards K: Ann Surg 171:553, 1970
7. Veith FJ, Koerner SK, Siegelman SS, et al: Ann Surg 178:463, 1973
8. Pinsker KL, Norin AJ, Kamholz SL, et al: Acta Cytol 24:558, 1980
9. Emeson EE, Norin AJ, Kamholz SL, et al: Transplant Proc 15:550, 1983
10. Veith FJ, Koerner SK, Siegelman SS, et al: Ann Thorac Surg 16:172, 1973
11. Norin AJ, Emeson EE, Veith FJ: Transplant Proc 15:508, 1983

LIVER AND PANCREAS TRANSPLANTATION

Report of Colorado-Pittsburgh Liver Transplantation Studies

T. E. Starzl, S. Iwatsuki, D. H. Van Thiel, J. C. Gartner, B. J. Zitelli, J. J. Malatack, R. R. Schade, B. W. Shaw, Jr., T. R. Hakala, and J. T. Rosenthal

THE PURGATORY in which liver transplantation was mired has ended in the cyclosporine era. Long-term survival after liver replacement was achieved in 1964 with dogs[1] and in humans[2] beginning in 1967. The longest surviving patient is now in her 14th postoperative year.

In spite of such tantalizing successes, the operation was unpredictable and unreliable, with 1-year survival rates that did not improve with increased experience over a 16-year period.[3] Of the first 111 patients, less than 1/3 lived for 1 year. The 1-year survival rose to 50% in a second but small series of 30 patients, but in a third series, the survival sank again, almost to the original level. The overall 1-year survival rate for 170 patients was 33%.

From the Departments of Surgery, Medicine, and Pediatrics, University of Pittsburgh Health Center, University of Pittsburgh, Pittsburgh, PA.

Supported by research grants from the Veterans Administration, by Project Grant AM 29961 from the National Institutes of Health, and by Grant RR 00084 from the General Clinical Research Centers Program of the Division of Research Resources, National Institutes of Health.

Reprint requests should be addressed to Dr. Starzl, 3601 Fifth Avenue, Room 103, Falk Clinic, Pittsburgh, PA 15213.

0041-1345/83/1505-0071$01.00/0

MATERIALS AND METHODS

We have used cyclosporine (CsA) with prednisone in all liver transplantations since early 1980.[3] The standard therapy begins with a 5-day burst of steroids, leveling off at about 20 mg/day in adults after a few days. The dose of CsA is 6 mg/kg i.v. or 17 mg/kg orally. When nephrotoxicity of CsA is suspected, the CsA dose is reduced; in a few instances it has been replaced temporarily with azathioprine.

RESULTS

The survival in the first 67 consecutive recipients in the cyclosporine era is summarized in Fig. 1 and contrasted with the pooled previous experience. All of the CsA patients in Fig. 1 had their operations before May 1, 1982, and thus have minimum 1-year follow-ups. The 1-year and subsequent survival was doubled overnight compared to past expectations.

Of the first 67 recipients in the CsA series treated over a period of <2 years, 42 passed the 1-year mark. This was almost as many survivors as had been acquired in the nearly 17 preceding years. Six of the 42 one-year survivors subsequently died. In four, the cause of the late failure was recurrence of the original disease (two hepatic malignancies, one example each of Budd-Chiari syndrome and B-virus chronic hepatitis) (Table 1). The other late deaths were caused by an airway obstruction secondary to an upper respiratory infection in one patient and by complications

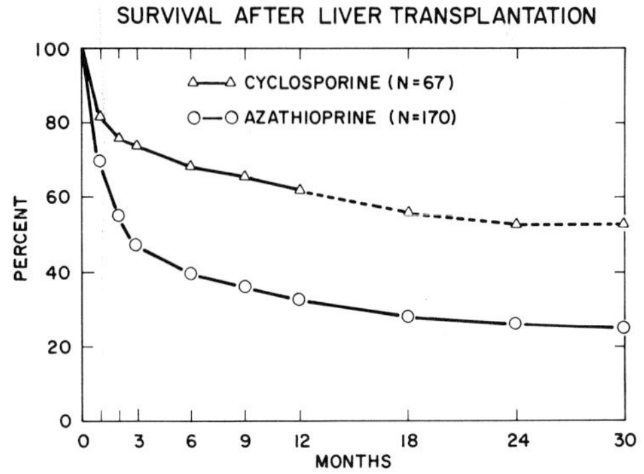

Fig. 1. Life survival curves of patients under conventional immunosuppression vs. CsA-steroid therapy. In the latter group, note that survival after 1 year is actuarial.

Table 1. Late Deaths Under Cyclosporine-Steroid Therapy

Original Diagnosis	Cause of Death	Time (Months)
Chronic active hepatitis	Airway obstruction, tonsillitis	12
Cholangiocarcinoma	Recurrent cancer	13
Budd-Chiari syndrome	Recurrent Budd-Chiari syndrome	15
Chronic active hepatitis	Recurrent chronic active hepatitis (B virus)	15
Budd-Chiari syndrome	After retransplantation (for chronic rejection)	20
Hepatoma (fibrolamellar)	Recurrent cancer	33

after retransplantation in a patient whose first graft was chronically rejected (Table 1). In spite of these six deaths after 1 year, the late decline of the life-survival curve has been slower than in past patients who entered the second postoperative year under azathioprine and prednisone (Fig. 1).

A natural question would be whether these results could be explained by a sudden change in candidacy criteria or by a difference in the diseases for which transplantation was performed. Analysis according to the recipient diseases showed that this was not the case. Instead, the results with almost all of the diseases were improved (Table 2). This was obvious with all the diagnoses that contributed heavily to the case material before and after the introduction of cyclosporine, such as biliary atresia, nonalcoholic cirrhosis, primary hepatic malignancy, primary biliary cirrhosis, and the heterogenous group of inborn errors of metabolism.

With these improved results, the pace of liver transplantation has quickened. Between 1963 and the end of 1979, the average yearly caseload was not much over a dozen. The number of transplantations rose to 30 in 1981 and to 80 in 1982 (Table 3). In the first 4 months of 1983, 34 liver replacements were

Table 2. Influence of Disease on 1-Year Survival in 237 Patients*

	Conventional Therapy		Cyclosporine + Steroids	
	No.	After 1 Year†	No.	After 1 Year‡
Biliary atresia	51	14 (27.0%)	11	6 (54.5%)
Nonalcoholic cirrhosis	46	16 (34.8%)	16	9 (56.3%)
Primary liver malignancy	18	5 (27.8%)	9	6 (66.7%)
Inborn errors§	15	8 (53.3%)	10	7 (70.0%)
Alcoholic cirrhosis	15	4 (26.7%)	0	—
Primary biliary cirrhosis	6	1 (16.7%)	6	5 (83.3%)
Sclerosing cholangitis	7	2 (28.6%)	3	2 (66.7%)
Secondary biliary cirrhosis	4	3 (75.0%)	5	1 (20.0%)
Budd-Chiari syndrome	1	1 (100.0%)	3	3 (100.0%)
Miscellaneous‖	7	2 (28.6%)	4	3 (75.0%)

*The same case material was analyzed in detail elsewhere,[3] but with shorter follow-ups.

†32 of these 52 patients are still alive with follow-ups of 3½–13½ years.

‡36 of these 42 patients are still alive with follow-ups of 1–3¼ years.

§Alpha-1-antitrypsin deficiency (17 examples), Wilson's disease (3), tyrosinemia (2), glycogen storage disease (2), sea blue histiocyte syndrome (1).

‖Neonatal hepatitis (3 examples), congenital hepatic fibrosis (2), Byler's disease (2), adenomatosis (1), hemachromatosis (1), protoporphyria (1), acute hepatitis B (1).

Table 3. Yearly Total of Orthotopic Liver Transplantations

Year	No. of New Patients	Retransplantation	Total
1963	5	0	5
1966	1	0	1
1967	6	0	6
1968	12	2	14
1969	6	1	7
1970	10	1	11
1971	11	0	11
1972	11	1	12
1973	13	4	17
1974	20	1	21
1975	9	4	13
1976	14	3	17
1977	21	2	23
1978	19	2	21
1979	11	0	11
1980	15	0	15
1981	26	4	30
1982	62	18	80
1983*	24	10	34
Total	296	53	349

*January–April, 1983.

done, a rate that extrapolates to 100 for this year.

To be a service, a new surgical procedure must be within the capability of more than the occasional surgeon. Until 1982, virtually all our liver transplantation procedures over a span of 19 years were performed by a single surgeon. During 1982, 40% of the procedures were performed by another young faculty member or by the fellows, and this year this figure has been 70% (Table 3).

In 1983, most of the adult patients have had pump-driven nonheparin venovenous bypasses during the anhepatic phase, when the portal vein and vena caval systems must be obstructed. This simple technique has removed the urgency of the implantation and should place the operation of liver replacement within the grasp of a much greater number of surgeons.

We have had one example of multiple intestinal "lymphomatosis" in a liver recipient 6 months postoperatively. His cyclosporine dose was dropped from 20 mg/kg/day to 1.4 mg/kg/day, and the steroid dose was reduced from 25 mg/day to 10 mg/day. After several months on these almost homeopathic drug doses, he began to reject his liver, necessitating resumption of more standard immunosuppressive therapy (Fig. 2). The rejection was easily controlled, and this boy has returned to his university studies; he has no evidence of lymphoma. At autopsy, one other liver recipient had similar lymphoproliferative lesions as an incidental finding.

DISCUSSION

Most of the mortality that remains with liver transplantation is perioperative and is

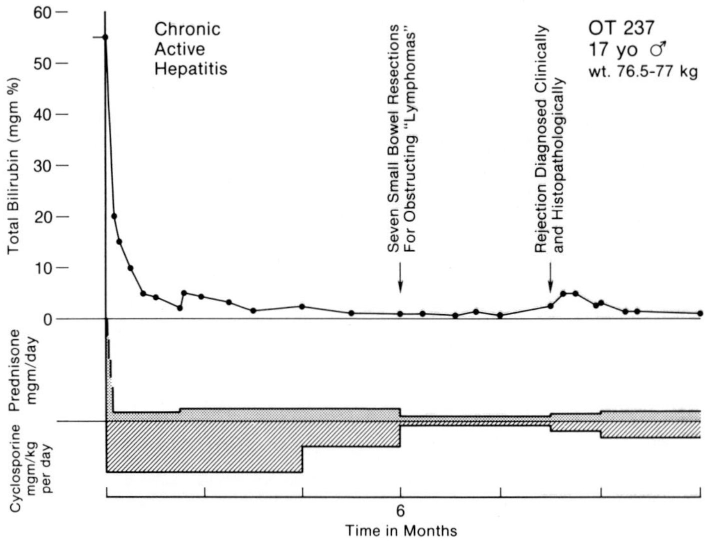

Fig. 2. Course of a 17-year-old boy with chronic active hepatitis, who developed "pseudo lymphomas" of the small intestine. Note that immunosuppression was drastically reduced, followed by evidence of rejection, which was easily reversed. The patient is now well and without evidence of malignant disease.

Table 4. Change in Pattern of Surgeons Performing Liver Transplantation Since Introduction of Cyclosporine

	1963–1979	1980–1981	1982	1983 (4 months)
New patients	170	40	62	24
Total transplantations	191	45	80	34
Transplantations by single surgeon (T. E. Starzl)	187 (97.9%)	45 (100%)	48 (60%)	10 (29.4%)

related to technical surgical errors, to inadvertent use of damaged homografts, and to continuing acceptance into candidacy of patients who are moribund and with irreversible pathophysiology of other organ systems.

One of the recent developments that may further reduce perioperative mortality is the nonheparin venovenous bypass system now being used for almost all adult recipients. Aside from reducing the stresses to the operating surgeon, an extra incentive to use the bypass is the protection to the recipient kidneys offered by avoidance of inferior vena caval occlusion. This will be important because it may be that a physiologic or mechanical renal injury could amplify the potential nephrotoxicity of cyclosporine. In liver recipients, the necessity to juggle the CsA doses in the face of renal failure may force a decision to switch temporarily to azathioprine.[3] Starting the postoperative period with good renal function is one of the premonitors of success.

When CsA was first used clinically, the appearance of lymphomas in an alarming number of patients cast a shadow over the fate of this new drug. As it has turned out, the mere chronicling of these so-called lymphomas is a relatively meaningless exercise. The lesions are almost always a manifestation of Epstein-Barr virus infection,[4] and thus they imply overimmunosuppression. More important, virtually all the lymphoproliferative lesions (Iwatsuki has appropriately called them pseudolymphomas[5]) can be expected to involute spontaneously providing immunosuppression is stopped or reduced and if the temptation is resisted to use the toxic (and immunosuppressive) chemotherapeutic regimens that are customarily recommended by hemotologic oncologists. Lightening of immunosuppression apparently led to disappearance of the intestinal lesions in one of our liver recipients. The story of the appropriate treatment of these pseudolymphomas has been most completely worked out in renal recipients and is discussed by Dr. Tom Rosenthal elsewhere in this volume.

SUMMARY

Immunosuppression with cyclosporine and prednisone has transformed liver transplantation from an agonizingly difficult and highly unpredictable experimental undertaking to one that can be defended as a bona fide service.

REFERENCES

1. Starzl TE, Marchioro TL, Porter KA, et al: Surgery 58:131, 1965

2. Starzl TE, Groth CT, Brettschneider L, et al: Ann Surg 168:392, 1968

3. Starzl TE, Iwatsuki S, Van Thiel DH, et al: Hepatology 2:614, 1982

4. Bird AG: In White DJG (ed): Cyclosporin A. Amsterdam, Elsevier Biomedical, 1982, p 307

5. Iwatsuki S, Geis WP, Molnar Z, et al: J Surg Res 24:428, 1978

Special Aspects of Immunosuppression with Cyclosporine in Liver Transplantation

K. Wonigeit, C. Brölsch, P. Neuhaus, M. Burdelski, E. Schmidt, W. Lang, and R. Pichlmayr

IN LIVER transplantation, there is a particular need for a potent but highly selective method of immunosuppression. Since no artificial support for reversible episodes of hepatic dysfunction is available, acute rejection means a much higher risk to the patient than in renal transplantation. On the other hand the liver recipient is particularly compromised with regard to infection because of the extent of the surgical procedure and the poor preoperative condition resulting from terminal liver insufficiency. This makes it highly desirable to limit the amount of nonspecific immunosuppression as far as possible.

Cyclosporine (CsA) meets several of the particular requirements for immunosuppression in liver transplantation. The absence or low degree of bone marrow toxicity leaves phagocyte function, the most important line of defense against bacterial infection, intact. Furthermore, it has a remarkable degree of selectivity in its action on T cells, with little effect on B cells. These advantages of CsA immunosuppression have already been shown to improve the results of clinical liver transplantation.[1,2] In the first liver recipients treated with CsA in our center, we have found a marked reduction in the incidence of acute rejection episodes when compared to conventional immunosuppression.[3] In this report, results obtained with a subsequent series of patients who were treated with two different cyclosporine regimens are described. The great potential of this drug is confirmed; however, its use in liver transplantation was found to be associated with problems rarely seen in other allograft recipients. These problems can be overcome by prolonged intravenous treatment in the early post-transplant course and by intravenous monitoring of CsA blood levels.

MATERIALS AND METHODS

Patients

Sixteen consecutive liver transplantations performed in 15 patients between July 1982 and February 1983 are reported. Six recipients suffered from hepatocellular or cholangiocellular tumors, and one patient from liver metastases of a carcinoid tumor; seven recipients had liver cirrhosis, one a Budd-Chiari syndrome (Tables 1 and 2).

Immunosuppression

Immunosuppressive treatment in all patients consisted of a combination of cyclosporine and prednisolone. The prednisolone dose was essentially according to the regimen described by Starzl, with minor modifications.[2] Two different CsA regimens were used. With regimen I, CsA was given intravenously only for 1–2 weeks after transplantation at a dosage of 5 mg/kg/day, followed by oral administration of 12 mg/kg/day. With regimen II, a dosage of 5–10 mg/kg/day was given intravenously over a period of 4 weeks, followed by oral treatment with 14 mg/kg/day. The exact dosage under regimen II was adjusted according to the CsA blood level and clinical status. Intravenous CsA was generally given as a 4–6-hr infusion, oral CsA in two daily doses. Treatment of rejection episodes consisted of bolus injections of 500 mg methylprednisolone; with regimen II, the CsA dosage was also increased.

Measurement of CsA Blood Levels

In the initial period of the study, CsA levels were determined in plasma. Subsequently, measurements were made in whole blood in order to avoid problems arising from temperature-dependent variations in the cellular binding of CsA. Trough levels were determined 12 hr after oral and 20 hr after i.v. administration. All estimations were performed by radioimmunoassay (RIA) according to the procedure described by Donatsch.[4] Reagents were provided by Sandoz, Basel.

From the Klinik für Abdominal- und Transplantationschirurgie, Medizinische Hochschule, Hannover, Germany.

Supported in part by Stiftung Volkswagenwerk (AZ I/36 057).

Reprint requests should be addressed to Dr. Wonigeit.

0041-1345/83/1505-0072$01.00/0

Table 1. Patients Treated According to Regimen I

Transplant No.	Age (years)	Sex	Diagnosis	Rejection (no. of episodes)	Survival Time	Cause of Death
66	38	F	Budd-Chiari	Reversible (1)	11 months (alive)	
67	21	M	Tumor	Reversible (1)	6 weeks	Small bowel perforation
68	20	M	Tumor	Irreversible →	2½ months (alive); retransplantation (No. 71)	
69	36	F	Cirrhosis	Irreversible	24 days	Hepatic failure

Diagnosis of Rejection

The diagnosis of rejection was made using procedures described previously.[3] All rejection episodes were confirmed histologically.

RESULTS

Patients Under Short-Term Intravenous CsA Treatment (Regimen I)

Table 1 summarizes the results obtained in four patients treated with CsA according to regimen I. Patient 67 received intravenous treatment for 2 weeks, the other 3 patients for only 4–6 days before changing to oral application. All four patients developed typical acute rejection 5–15 days after transplantation, characterized by clear-cut increases in enzyme and bilirubin levels and histologically by massive lymphocytic infiltration and tissue damage in the graft. In two patients, this responded well to intravenous methylprednisolone. One recovered completely and is doing well; the other subsequently developed small bowel perforation and died. In the other two patients, rejection was irreversible. Patient 67 developed a severe rejection episode followed by severe irreversible cholestasis. The CsA plasma level determined on day 16 after transplantation was very low (<40 ng/ml trough level). Furthermore, plasma levels 2, 4, and 6 hr after oral intake on the following days failed to increase. The immunosuppression was then changed to ALG and azathioprine, which led to a decrease in the enzyme levels but did not resolve the cholestatic syndrome. This patient was retransplanted 10 weeks after the first transplantation and then treated with CsA according to regimen II (see transplant 71 in Table 2). The last patient in this group initially had an excellent postoperative course but then developed irreversible acute rejection, which proved lethal. Retrospective analysis of CsA plasma levels in this patient also revealed low or undetectable trough levels. We concluded that these two patients suffered from malabsorption of CsA and that irreversible rejection resulted from inade-

Table 2. Patients Treated According to Regimen II

Transplant No.	Age (years)	Sex	Diagnosis	Rejection (no. of episodes)	Survival Time	Cause of Death
70	41	M	Tumor	Reversible (1)	27 days	Multiple organ failure
71*	20	M	Tumor	Reversible (1)	7 months (alive)	
72	4	M	Cirrhosis	Reversible (1)	7 months (alive)	
73	48	F	Cirrhosis	None	26 days	Multiple organ failure
74	57	M	Tumor	None	6 months (alive)	
75	49	M	Cirrhosis	None	16 days	Cardiac failure
76	51	F	Tumor	None	11 days	Cardiac failure
77	21	F	Cirrhosis	None	12 days	Septicemia
78	50	M	Tumor	Reversible (1)	4 months (alive)	
79	34	F	Cirrhosis	Reversible (2)	4 months (alive)	
80	27	M	Tumor	None	3 months (alive)	
81	2	M	Cirrhosis (biliary atresia)	None	3 months (alive)	

*Retransplantation of no. 68.

quate immunosuppression. This led us to modify the immunosuppressive regimen.

Patients Under Long-Term Intravenous CsA Treatment (Regimen II)

The purpose of the modified CsA treatment according to regimen II was to ensure sufficient loading of the patient with CsA by prolonged intravenous administration and to monitor this by frequent determinations of CsA blood levels. During phases of clinical quiescence, blood levels of 500 ng/ml were aimed at, and during manifest rejection, levels of 800–1000 ng/ml. Since in kidney patients trough levels above 1000 ng/ml are frequently associated with severe toxic complications (own unpublished observation), we tried to avoid blood levels above this value. When changing from i.v. to oral administration, absorption from the intestine was tested by determining CsA blood levels 2, 4, 6, and 8 hr after administration. Effective absorption was assumed when a clear-cut peak was observed after 2–4 hr.

The results obtained in 10 patients treated with this regimen are given in Table 2. Four patients developed single rejection episodes, and 1 patient two rejection episodes, all of which resolved after increasing the intravenous dose of CsA to 10–12 mg/kg/day, accompanied by 3–5 bolus injections of 500 mg methylprednisolone on consecutive days.

Figure 1 shows the results of patient 78, who developed acute rejection on day 10 after transplantation, which fully resolved after treatment. During the third post-transplant

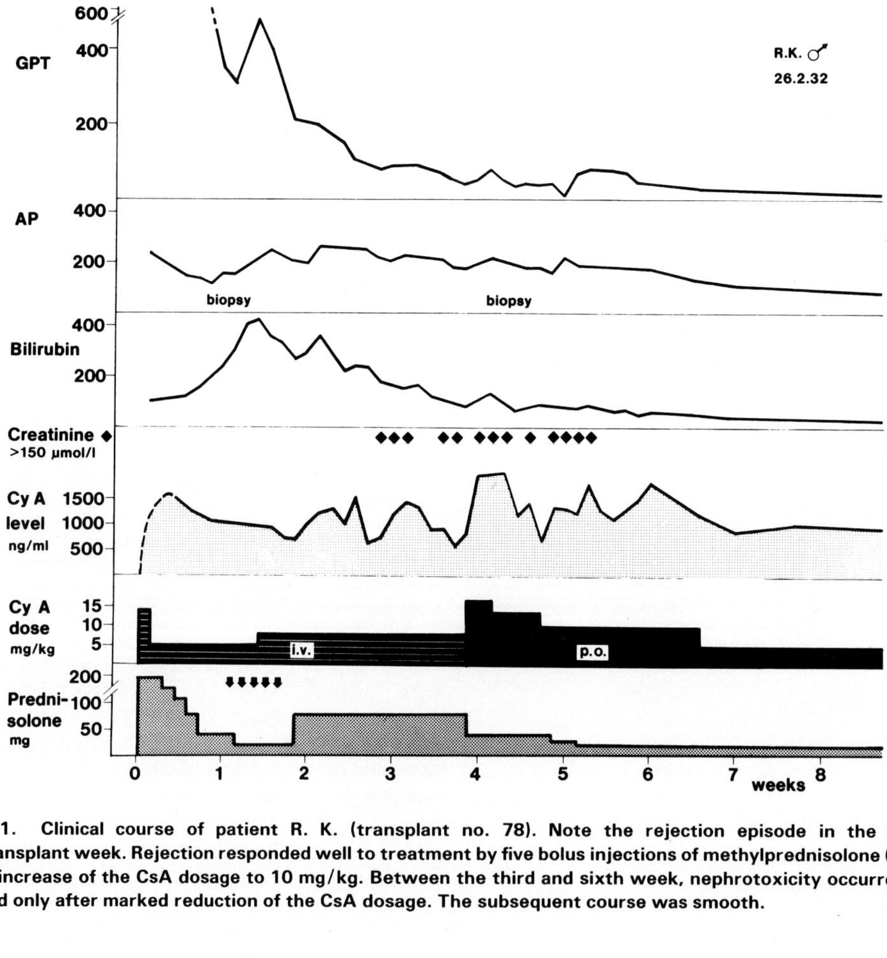

Fig. 1. Clinical course of patient R. K. (transplant no. 78). Note the rejection episode in the second post-transplant week. Rejection responded well to treatment by five bolus injections of methylprednisolone (arrow) and an increase of the CsA dosage to 10 mg/kg. Between the third and sixth week, nephrotoxicity occurred; this resolved only after marked reduction of the CsA dosage. The subsequent course was smooth.

week, the serum creatinine level increased above 150 μmole/liter, indicating that nephrotoxic concentrations of CsA had been reached. Very high CsA blood levels during weeks 5 and 6 were accompanied by slight but clear-cut increases in serum transaminases, alkaline phosphatase, and bilirubin. A needle biopsy on day 30 revealed cholestasis and some parenchymal damage without any sign of rejection.

Figure 2 shows the course of patient 80, who experienced no rejection episodes. He had already been changed to oral CsA on day 23, which was followed by a marked increase in trough levels. Despite excellent graft function, the cholinesterase levels of this patient remained depressed for about 6 weeks and recovered only when the oral CsA dosage was reduced and the CsA blood level had decreased.

Change in Dose Requirements with Increasing Time After Transplantation

It was a common observation in all patients that the dosage required to maintain blood levels around 500 ng/ml markedly decreased with time and showed great individual variability. Similar observations have also been made in kidney recipients (own unpublished observations).[5] Whereas the long-term dosage of 5–8 mg/kg/day is very similar in both groups of patients, the dosage required in the early course in liver patients usually exceeds that given to kidney recipients.

DISCUSSION

The results of this study underline the importance of potent immunosuppression in liver transplantation and reveal unexpected problems with the use of cyclosporine. CsA

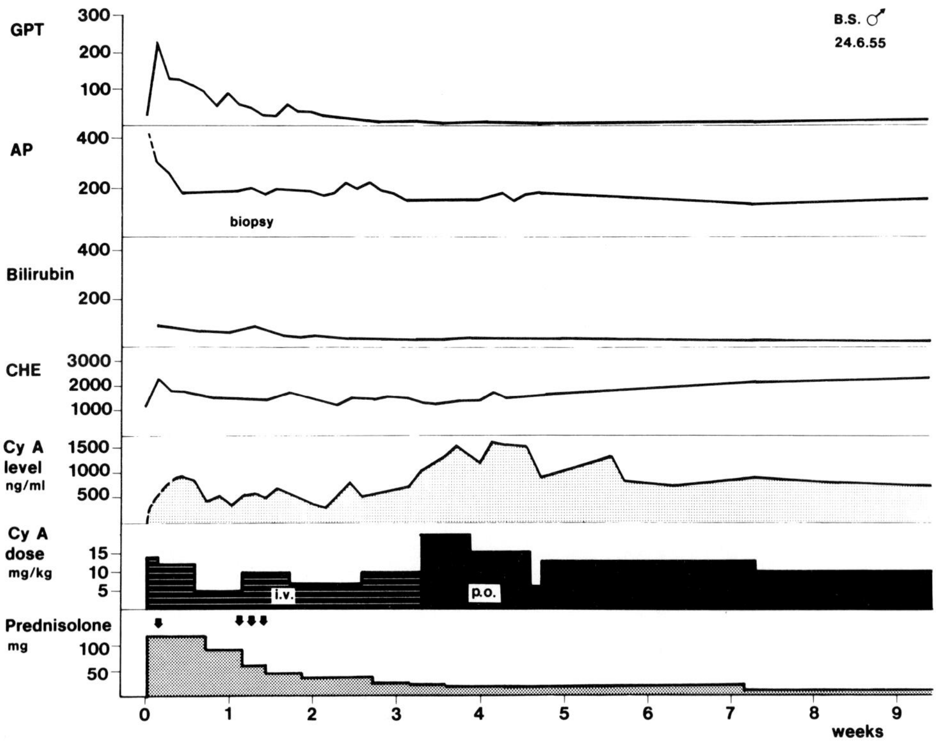

Fig. 2. Clinical course of patient B. S. (transplant no. 80) without signs of rejection or toxicity. Interestingly, cholinesterase did not reach the normal range (>1900) before CsA was reduced to 10 mg/kg p.o. This may indicate a suppression of the synthetic capacity of the liver by higher CsA dosages.

treatment according to regimen I was based on our experience in clinical kidney transplantation, where particularly low-dose cyclosporine had proved effective.[6] Therefore, the loss of two liver grafts from irreversible rejection was totally unexpected. Retrospectively, it is evident that these patients had insufficient blood levels, probably as a result of reduced absorption of the drug. The cause of the malabsorption has not been fully clarified. Important factors may be inadequate emulsification of the drug because of disturbed bile secretion and/or disturbed intestinal function. If there is enterohepatic recirculation of CsA, as recently suggested by Kahan et al.,[7] this would also be reduced by malabsorption [Fig. 3 (A and B)]. A similar effect can be expected when a major part of the bile is drained with a T tube. The obvious solution to the problem of malabsorption is the prolonged parenteral application of CsA as used in regimen II.

Figure 3 (C) shows another potential risk of CsA therapy in liver transplantation, namely, reduced metabolism and excretion during periods of disturbed liver function. Although this effect was not observed in this series of patients, it can be anticipated that it may occur during acute liver allograft rejection, in particular when the drug is given intravenously. We have occasionally seen this type of disturbed cyclosporine metabolism in renal allograft recipients with reduced liver function (K. Wonigeit, unpublished observation). This state is easily recognized by frequent monitoring of CsA blood levels, which show a rapid increase. By appropriate adjustment of the CsA dose, correction is usually possible before manifestation of overt clinical side effects. If not treated, a vicious circle will be started, with further deterioration in liver function duc to thc hcpatotoxicity of CsA.

The results obtained in patients treated according to regimen II clearly demonstrate its usefulness. None of these patients developed irreversible rejection. The rejection crises observed were generally moderate and responded promptly to treatment. A particularly important point is the enhancement of the i.v. CsA dosage to 10 or even 15 mg/kg/day during periods of rejection. This of course bears the risk of intoxication and therefore requires intensive blood-level monitoring and constant alertness for clinical signs of manifest toxicity. We feel that this immunosuppressive strategy can markedly reduce the requirement for steroids. This might be important in face of the high frequency of bacterial infections in liver allograft recipients.

The particular relevance of blood-level determinations for liver transplantation only became obvious during the course of this

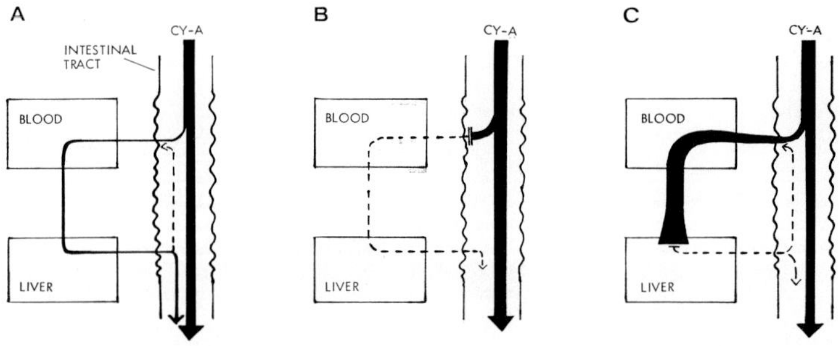

Fig. 3. Schematic representation of particular problems of CsA therapy in liver transplantation. (A) Normal absorption of drug from intestine and secretion of unchanged or biochemically modified drug by the liver. The dotted arrow indicates a possible enterohepatic recirculation of the unmodified drug. (B) Disturbances in bile production or in intestinal function can reduce the absorption rate. This can best be overcome by intravenous treatment. (C) Impaired graft function due to ischemic, toxic, or immunologic damage can reduce drug metabolism and excretion, leading to excessive drug accumulation and intoxication. Disturbances of type B and C are not mutually exclusive. Combinations or a rapid change from one to the other may render the choice of the correct CsA dosage very difficult.

study. The interpretation of the data was performed on a purely empirical basis. It is already clear that the RIA determines not only the unmodified drug but also a number of its metabolites.[8,9] It is likely that the metabolic pathway of CsA in liver allograft recipients will be affected by changes in graft function and that this can alter the proportions of unmodified drug and its metabolites in the blood. Thus, it is obvious that further refinement of CsA immunosuppression will be dependent on the clarification of its detailed pharmacodynamics.

SUMMARY

In a series of 16 consecutive orthotopic liver transplants performed in 15 patients, two different CsA immunosuppressive regimens were used. Of 4 patients treated according to regimen I with a short term i.v. course of CsA and subsequent oral administration, 2 underwent irreversible rejection due to malabsorption of the orally given CsA. In regimen II, the i.v. treatment was prolonged to 28 days and the dosage adjusted according to the blood levels. Rejection treatment consisted of bolus injections of methylprednisolone and increased CsA dosage. None of the 12 patients treated according to regimen II developed irreversible rejection. It is concluded that disturbed drug absorption and/or metabolism occur more frequently in liver allograft recipients than in other transplant patients. These problems can be overcome, however, by prolonged intravenous treatment and by intensive blood-level monitoring. Under these precautions, immunosuppression with CsA can be regarded as clearly superior to conventional treatment in liver transplantation.

REFERENCES

1. Calne RY, Williams R, Lindop M, et al: Br Med J 283:115, 1981

2. Starzl TE, Iwatsuki S, Klintmalm GP, et al: Transplant Proc 13:281, 1981

3. Pichlmayr R, Brölsch C, Neuhaus P, et al: Transplant Proc 15:1279, 1983

4. Donatsch P, Abisch E, Homberger E, et al: J Immunoassay 2:19, 1981

5. Stiller CR, Keown PA, Sinclair NR, et al: In White DJG (ed.): Cyclosporin A, Amsterdam, Elsevier Biomedical, 1982, pp 379–386

6. Bunzendahl H, Wonigeit K, Klempnauer J, et al: Transplant Proc (this issue)

7. Kahan BD, Ried M, Newburger J: Transplant Proc 15:446, 1983

8. Niederberger W, Schaub P, Beveridge T: J Chromatog 182:454, 1980

9. Carruthers SG, Freeman DJ, Koegler JC, et al: Clin Chem 29:180, 1983

Hepatic Homograft Survival in Pediatric Orthotopic Liver Transplantation with Cyclosporine and Steroids

B. J. Zitelli, J. C. Gartner, Jr., J. J. Malatack, B. W. Shaw, Jr., S. Iwatsuki, and T. E. Starzl

CYCLOSPORINE (CsA) used with steroids has been a major influence in the improved survival of patients undergoing orthotopic liver transplantation. The overall results of patient survival have been published elsewhere.[1,2] Part of the increased survival rate is dependent on retransplantation for homograft failure. We report our experience of patient and homograft survival as well as major causes for graft failure.

MATERIALS AND METHODS

From May 11, 1981, to March 7, 1983, 43 patients ranging in age from 7½ months to 18 years received 57 orthotopic liver homografts. Table 1 lists the indications for transplantation. Patients reported here have been assigned OT (orthotopic transplant) numbers, which allows one to follow and compare the course of any one patient in previous or subsequent publications. Details of patient selection and immunosuppression have been described in detail elsewhere.[1-3] Briefly, patients were given oral CsA (17.5 mg/kg) or an intravenous infusion of CsA (5 mg/kg) a few hours preoperatively. Intravenous CsA was continued at 5 mg/kg/day, divided twice daily, until oral CsA could be begun at 17.5 mg/kg/day, divided twice daily. Most pediatric patients were given a burst of steroids beginning the day of surgery (100 mg methylprednisolone) and rapidly tapered to a baseline dose (20 mg/day of prednisone) 4–5 days postoperatively. This baseline steroid dose was further decreased pending the patient's clinical course.

If clinical signs of rejection appeared, the immunosuppression regimen was modified. Initially, a single bolus of hydrocortisone (500–1000 mg) was given intravenously. If the patient showed only moderate improvement, a cycle of prednisone similar to that given immediately postoperatively was also begun. In addition, CsA doses were occasionally increased, monitoring clinical and laboratory evidence for nephrotoxicity. Whole blood CsA levels were measured by high-pressure liquid chromatography[4] in patients transplanted since January 1983, and CsA doses were adjusted to achieve trough levels of 100–400 ng/ml.

Graft failures occurred when irreversible and progressive hepatic injury was noted by increases in bilirubin and hepatocellular and canalicular enzymes as well as worsening prothrombin time.

RESULTS AND DISCUSSION

From 5/11/81 to 3/7/83, 43 pediatric patients received 57 hepatic homografts. Overall patient survival to 3/7/83 is 63% (27/43). Thirteen patients (30%) received multiple transplants; 12 patients received two homografts, and 1 patient received three homografts. The overall patient survival of retransplanted patient is 38% (5/13).

Twenty-four overt graft failures occurred in the 57 homografts (42%). Of the 16 patients who died, transplantation in 6 patients took place while the patient was moribund, and the patient expired shortly after surgery. Graft function was assessed shortly prior to death. Those six grafts are not included in graft failures.

Causes of graft failure and contributing causes of graft failure are listed in Table 2. Although the primary cause of graft failure is given, other factors often contributed to graft injury. At times it was difficult to determine which was the dominant factor responsible for graft failure. The most prominent pathological event found in the graft at retransplantation or autopsy helped determine the major factor. Infarction, rejection, vascular accidents, and infection were the major causes of graft failures (Table 3).

Infarction

Hepatic infarction accounted for the loss of eight grafts (33%). All but two of these grafts never had adequate function and were marked by an immediate and continued postoperative enzyme elevation, often in the thousands. Bili-

From the University of Pittsburgh Health Center and School of Medicine, Children's Hospital of Pittsburgh, Pittsburgh, PA.

Reprint requests should be addressed to B. J. Zitelli, Children's Hospital of Pittsburgh, 125 DeSoto Street, Pittsburgh, PA 15213.

0041-1345/83/1505-0073$01.00/0

Table 1. Indications for Pediatric Liver Transplantation

Biliary atresia	18
Metabolic	
Alpha-1-antitrypsin deficiency	7
Glycogen storage Disease I	1
Hereditary tyrosinemia	1
Wilson's disease	2
Sea blue histiocyte	1
Biliary hypoplasia	4
Chronic active hepatitis	3
Familial cholestasis	3
Neonatal hepatitis	1
Biliary obstruction	1
Benign liver tumor	1
Total	43

rubin also rose, and clotting studies worsened. Death occurred if retransplantation did not occur within 72–96 hr. Reasons for graft infarction were not clear because vessels were all patent at retransplantation or autopsy. Possible factors for infarction might include transplantation of an already injured graft or damage to the graft during harvesting, transport, or implantation. An example of the latter might be OT 279B, who suffered an intraoperative cardiac arrest. The graft never functioned well.

Two patients, OT 232 and OT 240, had a delayed onset of massive hepatic infarction. OT 232 had an absent inferior vena cava. Each had initial good function postoperatively but suffered subsequent fulminant hepatic necrosis and death at 12 and 10 days, respectively. Both grafts had patent vascular anastomoses at postmortem examination. Both patients, however, had preformed T-cell warm antibodies directed against the graft. Whether acute rejection was contributory to the infarction is purely speculative.

Table 3. Status of Surviving Grafts

Discharged survivors*	26
Bilirubin < 1.5 mg/dl	24
SGOT < 100 IU	25
Status	
Well	24
Chronic rejection	1
Mild rejection	1

*OT 246, not included, recently underwent a third transplant and is still hospitalized.

Rejection

Rejection occurred as a major cause of graft failure in 29% (7/24) of grafts. In addition, it was a contributing factor in the failure of another 4 grafts. Pathological features of rejection have been described elsewhere.[5–7] In most cases, rejection was manifested by fever, malaise, hepatomegaly with induration of the graft, ascites, and vague abdominal discomfort. Bilirubin increased and canalicular enzymes increased, usually out of proportion to the hepatocellular enzymes. Generally an ominous prognostic feature has been the disappearance of bile ducts within the portal triads.[2,7] Clinically, rejection mimicked other disorders, especially biliary tract obstruction and portal vein occlusion. If the patient did not respond to specific therapy directed toward rejection, the pathological process could be determined with certainty only with specific investigations such as cholangiography and angiography, as well as biopsy. In addition, these clinical entities may not be exclusive of each other, and it is at least theoretically possible that they may contribute to one another. Such an example might be decreased hepatic blood flow during rejection

Table 2. Causes of Graft Failure

Failure (No.) ($N = 24$)	Major Cause	Contributing Cause
Hepatic infarction (8)	OT 265, 271A, 271B, 240, 232,284A, 203A, 279B	—
Rejection (7)	OT 216, 214A, 203B, 266A, 229A, 246A, 250A	OT 232, 214B, 240, 191
Vascular accident (5)	OT 220, 259A, 273A, 267, 214B	OT 232, 259B, 266A
Infection (4)	OT 201, 191, 259B, 279A	OT 259A, 266A, 246A

causing vascular thrombosis and/or infection.[8]

OT 266A had clinical and pathological evidence for chronic rejection while on 18 mg/kg/day of CsA. Prior to retransplantation, CsA kinetics studies demonstrated poor oral absorption at that dose. Retransplantation occurred 57 days after the initial transplant. Pathology of the initial graft demonstrated severe rejection and a branch hepatic artery thrombosis. Cyclosporine was increased to 29 mg/kg/day, achieving adequate blood CsA levels, possibly preserving good function of the second graft. No nephrotoxicity was noted. This patient demonstrated the possible interplay of several pathological processes as well as the possible potential value of measuring CsA levels. In addition, this patient was representative of many of our patients who received higher than the standard CsA dose and appeared to tolerate it without overt nephrotoxicity.

Vascular Accidents

Vascular complications accounted for the loss of 5 (21%) grafts. OT 220A had no portal vein found at transplant, and the portal anastomosis was made to the recipient's vena cava. The graft failed from portoprival flow. OT 259A suffered both portal vein thrombosis and hepatic artery thrombosis; OT 267 thrombosed the hepatic artery; OT 273A had a

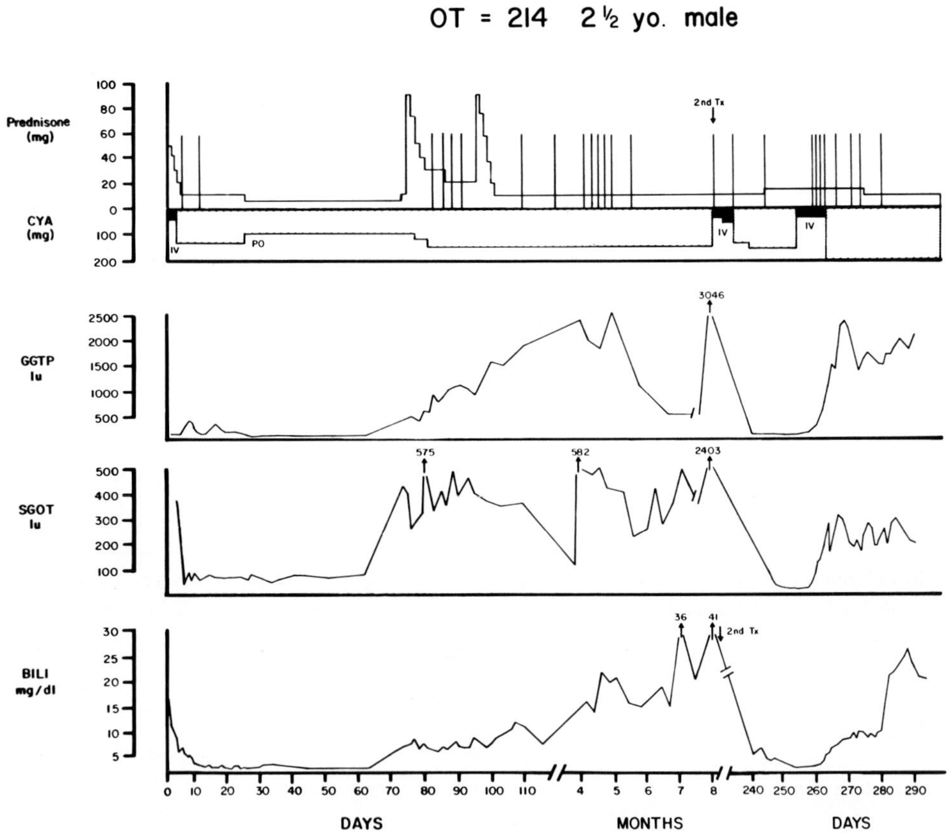

Fig. 1. Clinical course of OT 214. Note the late onset of rejection marked by rises in SGOT, GGTP, and bilirubin. Rejection persisted despite aggressive immunosuppression, culminating in retransplantation on day 241. The course of the second transplant was marked by rises in the same laboratory studies. Steroid boluses did not alter the course. Postmortem examination confirmed the premortem diagnosis of portal vein thrombosis. Vertical bars during steroid therapy indicate large boluses of i.v. steroid. The CsA graph indicates i.v. dosing by the solid bar and oral dosing by the open bar.

thrombosis of the portal vein and inferior vena cava; and OT 214B had a thrombosed portal vein. Vascular complications may have been contributory in the failure of another 3 cases.

The course of OT 214A and B is depicted in Fig. 1. The first graft was lost to rejection, and the second to a portal vein thrombosis. This patient was unusual because unrelenting rejection occurred several weeks after achieving normal liver functions—later than most patients. Despite continued high-dose steroids, the course of rejection was unaltered. The patient became increasingly debilitated with high-dose immunosuppression. The clinical course and laboratory findings of rejection and portal vein thrombosis were similar. We have since changed our approach to patients with chronic rejection. Once it is determined that rejection is irreversible through lack of response to increased immune suppression and pathological evidence, retransplantation is considered earlier. The patient's immune suppression is decreased to avoid overimmunosuppression. The surgery is often easier because vital structures already have been skeletonized and the patient is not debilitated from chronic overimmunosuppression.

Infection

Infection leading to graft failure occurred in 4 (17%) patients and was a contributing factor in another 3 losses. In patients OT 201 and OT 279A, biliary tract reconstruction may have been the initial inciting event, leading to biliary sepsis and graft failure. The second liver of OT 259B was grafted to vessels already infected with candida and *Pseudomonas aeruginosa*. OT 191 emphasized Starzl's concept of septic hepatic gangrene.[5] The patient had a large fungal abscess. The homograft injured from rejection or vascular insult is much more susceptible to infection than one not injured.

Hepatic homograft loss was a frequent complication of transplantation. Acute hepatic infarction, rejection (despite the use of CsA and steroids), vascular accidents, and infection were primary causes of graft failure. Early retransplantation may be beneficial in preventing patient death with initial graft loss.

Surviving Grafts

The current status of 27 surviving patients is listed in Table 3. One patient recently underwent a third transplant (not in the time frame discussed above) and will not be included in the following discussion. Of the 26 remaining survivors, 24 (92%) have bilirubins under 1.5 mg/dl. Of the 2 patients with elevated bilirubins, OT 206 has chronic rejection and may require retransplantation; OT 237 has mild rejection due to drastic lowering of immunosuppression because of an intestinal lymphoma. OT 206 is the only patient who has an SGOT of >100 IU. Daily prednisone dose averages 0.4 mg/kg/day, and the mean CsA dose is 15.5 mg/kg/day. Cyclosporine doses in patients transplanted prior to 9/82 average only 10 mg/kg/day. Patients transplanted subsequently, however, have an average dose of 25.6 mg/kg/day. Generally, this dose is able to be decreased to 8–10 mg/kg/day within the first postoperative year.[9] It appears, therefore, that the vast majority of surviving grafts have excellent function.

CONCLUSIONS

Hepatic homograft failures occur frequently (42%) and remain a major cause of morbidity and mortality in pediatric liver transplant patients. Graft infarction (33%), rejection despite the use of CsA and steroids (29%), vascular accidents (21%), and infection (17%) are major causes of graft failure. Attempts to control rejection may involve using higher doses of CsA than previously accepted, and children may tolerate larger oral doses with little nephrotoxicity. Despite a 30% retransplantation rate, 92% of surviving grafts are associated with bilirubins of <1.5 mg/dl, indicating excellent function of surviving grafts.

ADDENDUM

Since submission of this manuscript, OT 206 underwent successful retransplantation for chronic rejection. Her bilirubin and enzymes are within normal limits.

REFERENCES

1. Starzl TE, Iwatsuki S, Malatack JJ, et al: J Pediatr 100:681, 1982

2. Starzl TE, Iwatsuki S, Van Thiel DH, et al: Hepatology 2:614, 1982

3. Malatack JJ, Zitelli BJ, Gartner JC, et al: Transplant Proc 15:1292, 1983

4. Sawchuk RJ, Cartier LL: Clin Chem 27:1368, 1981

5. Starzl TE, Putnam CW: In Experience in Hepatic Transplantation. Philadelphia, Saunders, 1969

6. Porter KA: Transplant Rev 2:129, 1969

7. Fennell RH, Roddy HJ: Pathol Ann 14(2):155, 1979

8. Groth CG, Porter KA, Otte JB, et al: Surgery 63:658, 1968

9. Iwatsuki S, Starzl TE, Shaw BW Jr, et al: Long-Term Use of Cyclosporine in Liver Recipients: Reduction of Doses in the First Year to Avoid Nephrotoxicity (Paper presented to the American Society of Transplant Surgeons, Chicago, June 3, 1983)

Pancreas Transplantation: Overview and Current Status of Cases Reported to the Registry Through 1982

D. E. R. Sutherland

EVIDENCE THAT the complications of diabetes are secondary to disordered metabolism is very convincing, and many diabetologists are now making intense efforts to maintain euglycemia in diabetic patients.[1] Pancreas transplantation has had limited application because of technical difficulties, uncertainty of the timing of the operation relative to the development of diabetic complications, and imperfect immunosuppressive regimens. These problems are gradually being overcome, and the number of transplants performed has increased dramatically in recent years.

The Pancreas Transplant Registry has information on 264 pancreas transplants performed in 247 diabetic patients at 34 institutions between December 17, 1966, and December 31, 1982 (Fig. 1), 3 more than in a previous summary of cases reported through 1982.[2] Additions include one late report of a 1978 case that was not known at the time of the last report to the Transplantation Society,[3] plus two previously unreported cases from 1982. In addition, 53 pancreas transplants in 50 new patients performed at 21 institutions (8 new) have been reported to the Registry between January 1, 1983, and May 15, 1983, bringing the total number of known pancreas transplants at the time of the First International Congress on Cyclosporine to 317 in 297 patients; of these, 257 were performed in 243 patients (241 new) since July 1, 1977. There is insufficient follow-up time on the 1983 cases for analysis. The details on the 60 transplants performed in 56 patients before June 30, 1977 (57 cases reported to the old ACS/NIH Registry), have previously been summarized.[4] The current status of 204 pancreas transplants, performed in 193 (191 new) patients, reported to the Registry between July 1, 1977, and December 31, 1982, are summarized in this report.

Individual Institutions

The six institutions with the largest pancreas transplant experience since 1977, Minnesota,[5,6] Lyon,[7,8] Stockholm,[9,10] Cambridge,[11,12] Detroit,[13] and Zurich,[14] have published details on all except their most recent cases. Some of the other institutions have also published reports on their latest pancreas transplants, most of which are referenced in a recent comprehensive review article.[4]

As of May 1983, 34 patients have functioning grafts and are insulin-independent, 26 for more than 1 year (Table 1). Seven other grafts functioned for more than a year before the recipients either died with a functioning graft (1 Lyon patient) or the grafts failed and the patients resumed exogenous insulin (2 Cambridge, 2 Lyon, 1 Birmingham, and 1 Minnesota patient). The other 163 grafts ceased to function at <1 year because of technical complications, rejection, or death of the recipient. Of the 193 patients who received transplants between July 1, 1977, and December 31, 1982, 35 (18%) died from perioperative problems or from diabetic complications within the first 3 months after transplantation; 24 died several months or years after transplantation; and 134 (69%) of the patients are currently alive.

RESULTS

Technique

Of the 204 pancreas transplants performed between July 1, 1977, and December 31,

From the Department of Surgery, University of Minnesota, Minneapolis, MN.

Presented at the First International Congress on Cyclosporine, Houston, TX, May 16–19, 1983.

Reprint requests should be addressed to Dr. David Sutherland, Box 280, University of Minnesota Hospital, 420 Delaware Street S.E., Minneapolis, MN 55455.

0041–1345/83/1505–0074$01.00/0

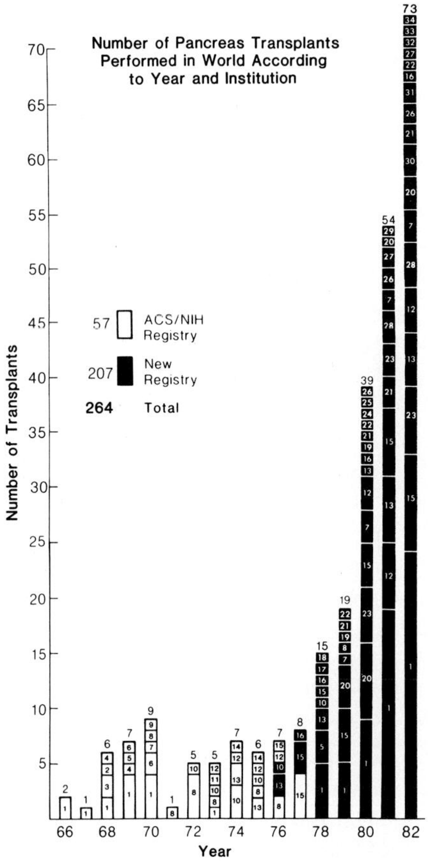

Chronological Order	Number Transplants
1. Univ. Minnesota	76
2. Univ. Rio de Janeiro	1
3. Univ. Sao Paulo	2
4. Perrando H., Resistencia	2
5. Univ. Colorado	4
6. Univ. Calif., Irvine	3
7. Univ. Cincinnati	10
8. Montefiore H., New York	11
9. N.Western Univ., Chicago	1
10. Guys H., London	8
11. Rush H., Chicago	1
12. Univ. Zurich	17
13. Huddinge H., Stockholm	20
14. Univ. Gothenberg	2
15. Herriot H., Lyon	33
16. Parkland H., Dallas	4
17. Univ. Montpellier	1
18. Dalhousie Univ., Halifax	1
19. Univ. Iowa	2
20. Univ. Cambridge	15
21. Univ. Munich	7
22. Univ. Innsbruck	3
23. Mt. Carmel H., Detroit	14
24. Univ. Erlangen, FRG	1
25. Univ. Miami	1
26. Univ. Genoa	5
27. Univ. Rome	3
28. Qu. Eliz. H., Birmingham	7
29. Univ. Helsinki	1
30. Louisiana St. Univ., Shreveport	3
31. Univ. Wisconsin	2
32. Univ. Leeds	1
33. Univ. Cardiff	1
34. Univ. St. Luc, Brussels	1

Fig. 1. The number of pancreas transplants in the world by year and institution as reported to the American College of Surgeons/National Institute of Health (ACS/NIH) Registry and the new Pancreas Transplant Registry between December 17, 1966, and December 31, 1982. Each institution is assigned a number according to the chronological number by which they did their first transplant.

1982, 1 was a pancreaticoduodenal graft (PD) (failed), 8 were whole pancreas (all silicone-rubber-injected Minnesota cases),[5,15] and 195 were segmental pancreas grafts. The current status of the whole and segmental pancreas grafts, according to the method of handling the pancreatic duct, are summarized in Table 2. The long-term function rate, so far, is approximately the same for all techniques except duct ligation, and almost all of these grafts failed early for technical reasons (not necessarily related to the method of handling the duct).

Association with Kidney Transplants

Kidney transplants were performed either before, simultaneous with, or after 153/204 (75%) of pancreas transplants reported to the Registry since July 1, 1977 (Table 3). Of those 193 patients, 49 were reported not to have end-stage diabetic nephropathy (25%), but proteinuria and other clinical manifestations of nephropathy were present in some members of this group.

Immunosuppression

Cyclosporine with or without other agents (usually prednisone) has been administered to 76 recipients of pancreas allografts, while azathioprine and prednisone (with or without antilymphocyte globulin preparations) have been administered to 125 recipients of pancreas allografts since July 1, 1977. The percentage of patients with functioning grafts in

Table 1. Pancreas Transplant Experience of Individual Institutions Reporting ≥ 7 Cases, 7/1/77–12/31/82

Institution	No. of Transplants (Patients)	Functioning as of 5/18/83 No.	Months (Technique)*
Minnesota	62 (57)	13	42, 47, 58 (open duct); 6, 8, 16, 29, 30 (silicone injection); 6, 9, 16, 19, 21 (pancreaticoenterostomy)
Lyon	28 (27)	4	6, 13, 14, 26 (neoprene injection)
Stockholm	14	3	13, 14, 19 (pancreaticoenterostomy)
Cambridge	15 (14)	1	45 (polyisoprene injection)
Detroit	14	0	—
Zurich	13	3	11, 25, 35 (prolamine injection)
Cincinnati	9 (7)	2	9 (duct-ureterostomy); 17 (neoprene injection)
Munich	7 (6)	2	13, 23 (prolamine injection)
Birmingham	7	3	14, 20, 24 (polyisoprene injection)
≤ 5 cases (17 institutions)	35 (34)	3	6 (pancreaticoenterostomy);† 12, 29 (prolamine injection)‡
Total	201 (193)	34	5–58

*All functioning pancreas grafts other than in the Minnesota and Genoa series were transplanted simultaneously with a kidney. The Minnesota open-duct and silicone-injected grafts currently functioning were all transplanted after a previous kidney graft, as was one (19 months) enterically drained graft; the other pancreaticoenterostomies were in non-kidney transplant patients.

†Brussels.

‡Genoa.

each group is summarized in Table 4. Technical as well as immunologic failures are included in the calculations.

DISCUSSION

There has been an obvious resurgence of interest in pancreas transplantation in recent years, as emphasized by the fact that more than 25% of the pancreas transplants performed since 1966 were done in 1982. The success rate, however, remains low, and only 17/73 (23%) pancreas transplants performed in 1982 are currently functioning.

In the past, pancreas grafts failed at a relatively high rate for technical reasons. Most of the recent grafts have ceased to function even when there were no apparent technical problems. Thus, it is uncertain why the graft loss rate should be so much higher for the pancreas than for the kidney or the heart. The pancreas may be more susceptible to rejection than other organs, as has been suggested in rat allograft experiments,[16] but other experiments, in dogs, have shown that pancreas allografts are rejected later than the kidney allografts.[17,18]

In most instances, biopsies have not been performed in pancreas grafts that lost function; thus, it is uncertain whether rejection or some other process has been responsible for deterioration of function. Fibrosis from duct injection has been implicated,[4] but late graft losses have been observed even when other techniques have been used. In fact, in one

Table 2. Techniques Used for 8 Whole and 195 Segmental Pancreas Transplants, 7/1/77–12/31/82

Method	No. of Cases	Functioning as of 5/18/83 No.	Percent	Duration (months)
Ducto-, cysto-, or ureterostomy	5	1	20%	8
Duct ligation	9	0	0%	—
Open-duct intraperitoneal	17	3	18%	42–58
Pancreaticoenterostomy	41	9	22%	6–21
Duct injection with polymers	131*	21	16%	5–45
Total	203	34	17%	5–58

*Neoprene in 37 (5 functioning), prolamine in 36 (7), silicone in 28 (5), polyisoprene in 21 (4), cyanoacrylate in 9 (0).

Table 3. Pancreas Transplants (1 PD, 8 Whole, 195 Segmental) in Association with Kidney Transplants, 7/1/77–12/31/82

Association	No. of Cases	Functioning as of 5/18/83 No.	Percent	Duration (months)
Pancreas before kidney	2	0	0%	—
Pancreas alone	51	6	12%	7–29
Pancreas after kidney	54	9	17%	5–58
Pancreas plus kidney	97*	19	20%	6–45
Total	204	34	17%	5–58

*Two patients had previous kidney transplants.

Table 4. Cyclosporine vs. Azathioprine for Pancreas Allografts Transplanted 7/1/77 to 12/31/82

Immunosuppression	No. of Patients	Functioning as of 5/15/83* No.	Percent
Cyclosporine	76	18	24%
Azathioprine	125	16	13%

*Does not include 3 identical-twin transplant recipients who were not immunosuppressed.

patient, a biopsy of a pancreas graft performed 6 months after transplantation, and 4 months after recurrence of hyperglycemia, showed normal islets except for the absence of beta cells.[5] It is unlikely that rejection is responsible for selective loss of beta cells, and it is possible that the factor(s) responsible for destruction of beta cells in the native pancreas are still present in the recipient—recurrence of diabetes in some cases could be akin to the recurrence of glomerular nephritides seen in some kidney transplant recipients. In some patients with simultaneous kidney and pancreas grafts from the same donor, late loss (>1 year) of pancreas graft function has occurred even while the kidney has continued to function. Again, it is unlikely that rejection would selectively destroy the pancreas and not the kidney, and recurrence of disease in the new pancreas is more likely. Nevertheless, pancreas grafts can function for prolonged periods and perhaps indefinitely, as exemplified by the number of recipients—26—whose grafts have functioned more than 1 year, including 1 patient who is nearly 5 years beyond pancreas transplant.

It remains to be seen whether the use of cyclosporine will improve the pancreas transplant survival rate. The proportion of patients with grafts currently functioning is higher for those treated with cyclosporine than for those treated with azathioprine, but the average follow-up time is also shorter in the cyclosporine group.

Ultimately, pancreas transplantation should primarily be applied to diabetic patients before the development of serious complications. Such a step will require an immunosuppressive regimen with a very high therapeutic ratio.

It may be possible, however, to identify patients who are at high risk to develop secondary complications, such as those with joint stiffness,[19] as well as those in whom intensified exogenous insulin therapy regimens may be inappropriate because their epinephrine response and other counterregulatory mechanisms are inadequate to compensate for inadvertently induced episodic hypoglycemia.[20] Current immunosuppressive protocols, particularly those that include cyclosporine, may be sufficiently effective to allow selected patients from within these subgroups to be considered for pancreas transplantation, along with the renal allograft recipients who currently constitute the majority of the pancreas transplant population.

REFERENCES

1. Unger RH: Diabetes 31:479, 1982

2. Sutherland DER: Cryobiology 20:245, 1983

3. Sutherland DER: Transplant Proc 15:1303, 1983

4. Sutherland DER, Goetz FC, Najarian JS, et al: Clin Endocrinol Metab 11:549, 1982

5. Sutherland DER, Goetz FC, Elick BA, et al: Transplantation 34:330, 1982

6. Sutherland DER, Goetz FC, Elick BA, et al: Transplant Proc 15:1322, 1983

7. Dubernard JM, Traeger J, Pozza G: Transplant Proc 15:1318, 1983

8. Traeger J, Dubernard JM, Pozza G: Transplant Proc 15:1326, 1983

9. Groth CG, Lundgren G, Ostman J, et al: Transplant Proc 12:68, 1980

limited number of cases, some aspects of our experience with CsA in clinical pancreatic transplantation can nevertheless be remarked upon.

The effect of CsA on pancreatic graft survival does not appear, at least at present, as impressive as for other transplanted organs: the rate of early failures was the same as with conventional therapy, but it could also depend on other factors, such as technical problems not yet completely solved or poor condition of the recipients. Over the long term, it seems that CsA can improve pancreatic graft survival, but this observation must be confirmed in a larger series of patients. The main disadvantage of the use of CsA from the beginning is nephrotoxicity, which is difficult to distinguish from rejection. The higher number of dialysis treatments required in the CsA-treated patients in the early posttransplant period and the more elevated plasma creatinine levels testify to the difficulties of the CsA treatment. For these reasons, we actually prefer to employ the conventional treatment at the beginning and introduce CsA some weeks later, after stabilization of renal function.

Endocrine function in the transplant patients treated with CsA alone is more satisfactory, a logical consequence of the suppression of the steroids, which are diabetogenic.

The immunoglobulin abnormalities and the lymphoproliferative syndromes that occurred in some patients receiving CsA and ALG were most likely the consequence of major immunosuppression induced by the association of the drugs, perhaps mediated by a virus or other microorganism.

SUMMARY

Cyclosporine A is a potent immunosuppressive agent, successfully employed in kidney and liver transplantation, that has potential use in pancreas transplantation.

The relatively poor results of pancreas transplantation, due to technical problems and the high frequency of complications occurring in end-stage diabetics, do not allow an accurate estimation of the real effect of CsA in preventing rejection and of eventual improvement in pancreatic graft survival. The metabolic advantages of the elimination of steroids are apparent.

Our experience indicates that the association of CsA with other immunosuppressive agents, mainly with ALG, is a real risk, and great care must be taken with combined CsA therapies.

REFERENCES

1. Calne RY, Rolles K, White DJG, et al: Transplant Proc 13:344, 1981

2. Starzl TE, Weil R, Iwatsuki S, et al: Surg Gynecol Obstet 151:17, 1980

3. Dubernard JM, Traeger J, Neyra P, et al: Surgery 84:633, 1978

4. Traeger J, Dubernard JM, Pozza G, et al: Transplant Proc 15:1326, 1983

5. Traeger J, Dubernard JM, Pozza G, et al: Horm Metab Res (Suppl) 13:63, 1983

6. Touraine JL, El Yafi S, Bosi E, et al: Transplant Proc (this issue)

Experience with Cyclosporine Versus Azathioprine for Pancreas Transplantation

D. E. R. Sutherland, P. L. Chinn, F. C. Goetz, B. A. Elick, and J. S. Najarian

ALTHOUGH PANCREAS transplantation has great potential as a treatment for diabetes mellitus, its application has been limited for a variety of reasons, partly because of technical problems with the procedure and partly because of the need for generalized immunosuppression, thus restricting the procedure to patients whose complications are considered more serious than the potential side effects of chronic immunosuppression.[1] For application to nonuremic, nonrenal allograft recipients, a generalized immunosuppressive regimen with a high therapeutic ratio is needed.

Cyclosporine (CsA) was used to treat pancreas allograft recipients shortly after its introduction into clinical practice, with the hope that the pancreas transplant success rate might increase.[2] Recent data from the Pancreas Transplant Registry show that a higher percentage of pancreas grafts are functioning in patients treated with CsA than with other immunosuppressive regimens.[3] However, other changes in patient management and in patient selection could also be responsible for the improved results. Furthermore, the results of pancreas transplantation in recipients treated with CsA at the University of Minnesota do not indicate that CsA results in higher pancreas graft survival rates.

The most recent series of pancreas transplants at the University of Minnesota began in 1978.[4] Initially, azathioprine (Aza), along with antilymphocyte globulin (ALG) and prednisone, was used for immunosuppression. In 1980, we began to treat recipients of pancreas grafts with CsA, unless they were already on Aza, to prevent rejection of a kidney graft from a related donor and were receiving a subsequent hemipancreas graft from the same donor.[5] In such cases, the recipients were simply maintained on the same immunosuppressant that had proved to be successful in preventing rejection of the kidney from the specific donor. Most of the other patients (including ones with a previous kidney graft from a cadaveric or related donor who received a cadaveric pancreas transplant or ones who had not previously been given a kidney and who received a pancreas graft from a related or cadaveric donor) were treated with CsA, either indefinitely or until the side effects of CsA prompted us to convert the recipient to immunosuppression with Aza. The results of pancreas transplants in the recent Minnesota series, according to whether the recipients received Aza or CsA for immunosuppression, are described here.

MATERIALS AND METHODS

Patient Population and Pancreas Transplant Techniques

Between July 25, 1978, and April 27, 1983, 72 pancreas transplants were performed in 65 patients (26 male, 39 female), including 7 retransplants in 6 patients. Forty patients had previously received renal transplants for treatment of end-stage diabetic nephropathy; 25 had not had previous kidney grafts and did not require dialysis treatment at the time of pancreas transplantation. Forty-two of the pancreas grafts were from cadaveric donors, and 30 were from related donors (15 HLA-identical and 5 nonidentical siblings, 5 identical twins, 4 parents, and 1 cousin). All 30 of the transplants from related donors (11 had previously given a kidney to the recipient) were of a portion of the pancreas only (segmental), as were 29 of the grafts from cadaveric donors; 13 pancreas grafts from cadaveric donors were of the whole gland.[6,7] A variety of

Presented at the First International Congress on Cyclosporine, Houston, TX, May 16–19, 1983.

From the Departments of Surgery and Medicine, University of Minnesota, Minneapolis, MN.

Supported in part by NIH Grants AM 19269 and RR 400.

Reprint requests should be addressed to Dr. David Sutherland, Box 280, University of Minnesota Hospital, 420 Delaware Street S.E., Minneapolis, MN 55455.

0041–1345/83/1505–0076$01.00/0

techniques were used to manage or suppress exocrine secretions.[6] Nineteen of the 72 transplants failed for purely technical reasons (7/42 from cadaveric and 12/30 from related donors, including 2/5 from identical twins): 2/2 duct-ligated, 8/15 open-duct, 7/21 pancreaticojejunostomies, and 2/34 duct-injected (0/4 prolamine, 2/30 silicone rubber). The recipients of pancreas grafts from identical twin donors were not immunosuppressed (3 technically successful, 2 unsuccessful) and, along with the 17 technically unsuccessful allografts, were eliminated from this analysis on the effect of immunosuppression on pancreas allograft functional survival. The follow-up period on the 50 technically successful pancreas allografts performed in 45 patients (5 had two transplants) ranges from 1–58 months (mean of 19.9 ± 15.0 months).

Immunosuppression

The basic immunosuppression protocol used in our pancreas transplant program has been described in detail previously.[6] Of 34 technically successful pancreas allografts from cadaveric donors, 9 recipients (all with previous renal allografts) were simply maintained on their current doses of Aza (≤ 2.5 mg/kg), their prednisone doses were temporarily increased to 2.0 mg/kg/day (tapered to 0.3 mg/kg/day by 1 year), and ALG 30 mg/kg/day was administered for 14 days. One of the 9 patients received CsA temporarily 2–4 weeks after pancreas transplantation but was then switched back to Aza (at a time the pancreas graft was functioning) because of CsA nephrotoxicity; this patient is tabulated in the Aza group. Eighteen of the 25 recipients treated with CsA following transplantation of a technically successful cadaveric pancreatic allograft had previously received kidney grafts (15 of the 18 were on Aza and 3 were on CsA before the pancreas transplant), while 7 had not had previous kidneys. In the first 8 CsA-treated recipients of technically successful cadaveric pancreas allografts, Aza and ALG were given for the first 1–2 weeks, and CsA was started only when oral feedings were begun. In the other 17, CsA was begun at the time of transplantation and was given intravenously in a dose of 3–5 mg/kg/day for 1–2 weeks before oral CsA (≤ 14 mg/kg/day) was begun.

Of 16 technically successful pancreas grafts from related donors, 10 recipients (9 HLA-identical, 1 cousin) were treated with CsA. None of the 10 patients had previously received renal allografts. One of the 10 was treated with Aza, prednisone, and ALG for 2 weeks before conversion to CsA; the other 9 received CsA intravenously for 1–2 weeks before conversion to oral CsA (≤ 14 mg/kg) and reduction of prednisone to ≤ 0.2 mg/kg/day. Two patients were switched from CsA to Aza at 8 and 10 months, respectively, because of CsA toxicity, but they are tabulated in the CsA category. Six recipients of technically successful pancreas grafts from related donors were treated with Aza; 5 had previously received kidneys from the same donor, and the 3 whose donors were HLA-identical simply remained on their maintenance doses of Aza and prednisone, while the 2 whose donors were HLA-nonidentical received a 10-day course of ALG 20 mg/kg/day (prophylactically in 1 and at 2 weeks for a possible rejection episode in the other). The other Aza-treated recipient of a technically successful related graft (HLA-nonidentical) received CsA 2–4 weeks after transplantation but then was switched back to Aza because of an ileus and inability to absorb CsA.

Metabolic Studies

Metabolic studies before and after transplantation included 24-hr plasma glucose profiles, oral and intravenous glucose tolerance tests, and determination of serum C-peptide concentration and 24-hr total urinary C-peptide secretion. The methods used have been described in detail previously.[8] Serum C-peptide concentrations were < 1.0 ng/ml and urinary C-peptide secretion rates were < 1 n*M*/24 hr in all except one recipient pretransplant; after transplantation, C-peptide levels were above baseline as long as the patient had a functioning graft. However, only patients who remained insulin-independent were counted as having fully functioning grafts, and even if C-peptide levels were above baseline (indicating partial graft function), the patient was not tabulated as having a functioning graft if exogenous insulin treatment was required to maintain euglycemia.

Diagnosis of Pancreas Graft Rejection

The recipients of the 50 technically successful allografts all became insulin-independent and were normoglycemic or nearly normoglycemic, at least initially, after transplantation. If hyperglycemia recurred, a presumed diagnosis of rejection was made. Two patterns were seen: In some, recurrence of hyperglycemia and the need for resumption of exogenous insulin treatment was rapid; in others, either the fasting or postprandial plasma glucose levels increased above the previously established baseline, but hyperglycemia was not severe or rapidly progressive. Hyperglycemia was usually associated with a decrease in serum C-peptide and urinary C-peptide excretion rates; in some patients, however, C-peptide levels remained elevated in association with an increase in plasma glucose. This situation was recognized retrospectively; if antirejection treatment had been instituted, it was not effective, and it was presumed that insulin resistance or an increased need for insulin secondary to steroid administration existed. A reduction of prednisone dosage was sometimes, but not always, associated with a decrease in plasma glucose levels and obviation of the need for exogenous insulin. Many patients with good graft function had chronically high serum amylase levels (particularly those with open ducts, but also some with duct injection or pancreaticojejunostomy-type grafts); in these cases, rejection was always associated with a decrease in serum amylase levels, usually to normal. We were not able to detect increases in serum amylase levels when pancreas graft endocrine dysfunction occurred.

In some cases (now a routine), when loss or decrease of graft endocrine function occurred, pancreas graft biopsies were performed; at least in one biopsy, loss of beta cells occurred without signs of rejection.[6] In the other cases where biopsies were done, histologic features consistent with rejection (diffuse mononuclear cell infiltration in the pancreatic parenchyma and acute or chronic vasculitis) were seen, but in some grafts (particularly the duct-injected ones) fibrosis was also present—a feature that could be a sequela of either duct occlusion or rejection.

Treatment of Pancreatic Allograft Rejection Episodes

Of the 50 pancreas allograft recipients, 34 had episodes or recurrence of hyperglycemia interpreted, at least initially, as rejection. In 16 instances, no antirejection measures were instituted, and, when clinically indicated, exogenous insulin treatment was permanently resumed. In the other 18 cases, antirejection treatment was administered. A variety of protocols were used.

In the Aza group, 4 recipients of cadaveric pancreas allografts (all with previous kidneys) were treated with an increase in oral prednisone only, 2.0 mg/kg/day, tapered to 0.25 mg/kg/day by 1 month. One recipient of a pancreas graft from an HLA-nonidentical sibling (donor of a previous kidney) received Aza and prednisone in maintenance doses only for the first 2 weeks after pancreas transplantation; an increase in plasma glucose and development of a swollen, tender graft then occurred, 500 mg of methylprednisolone was administered intravenously, prednisone was temporarily increased to 2 mg/kg, and ALG 20 mg/kg was administered for 10 days.

In the CsA group, two recipients of cadaveric grafts (one with and one without previous kidney transplants), one recipient of a graft from an HLA-identical sibling (no previous kidney transplant), and one recipient of a graft from a cousin (no previous kidney transplant) were treated with increased doses of oral prednisone by the protocol outlined above when hyperglycemia recurred. Seven CsA-treated recipients of cadaveric pancreas grafts (five with and two without previous kidneys) and two CsA-treated recipients of pancreas grafts from HLA-identical siblings (neither with a previous kidney transplant) were treated with methylprednisolone 500 mg i.v. for 3 days, an increase in oral prednisone, and ALG 20–30 mg/kg/day for 5–10 days (after conversion to Aza in one of the latter).

RESULTS

Overall Patient and Pancreas Graft Functional Survival

Fifty-five of the 65 pancreas graft recipients are currently (May 1983) alive (83%), including 39/45 recipients of 50 technically successful allografts (87%). Eighteen of the 72 pancreas grafts are currently functioning (25%), including 17/50 technically successful allografts (34%). Three recipients of technically successful allografts died of cardiovascular problems within the first 2 months of transplantation, while their grafts were functioning (on CsA), and 3 died after loss of graft function (2 Aza-treated patients of myocardial infarcts at 21 and 51 months, respectively, and 1 CsA-treated patient of CMV infection at 3 months after transplantation).

The duration of graft function in the 50 technically successful pancreas grafts according to immunosuppression, donor source, and pancreas transplant technique is summarized in Table 1. Currently, 8/15 Aza-treated and 9/35 CsA-treated patients have functioning graft. The overall results of Aza- and CsA-treated patients cannot be strictly compared, however, since donor source also influences the outcome: 10/16 grafts from related and 7/34 from cadaveric donors are currently functioning. Even within the donor-source subcategories, a valid comparison of the efficacy of azathioprine and cyclosporine cannot be made if all the recipients are included, since 5 of the 6 Aza-treated recipients in the related group had had previous kidney grafts from the same donor as the pancreas and had demonstrated that Aza was effective in preventing rejection of an organ from the particular donor in question.

Outcome According to Immunosuppression in Nonrenal Allograft Recipients of Pancreas Grafts from Related Donors

There were 11 patients in this category, of whom 10 (all with pancreaticojejunostomies) were treated with CsA and prednisone and the other (silicone-injected graft) with Aza for maintenance immunotherapy. The Aza-treated recipient received CsA 2–4 weeks after transplantation, but when an operation to drain a pseudocyst was required, Aza was started in place of CsA, and the graft lost function 2 months after transplantation. Of the 10 recipients treated with CsA, 5 currently have functioning grafts (all from HLA-

Table 1. Results According to Immunosuppression in 50 Technically Successful Pancreas Allografts at the University of Minnesota

	No. of Grafts	No. Functioning as of 5/15/83	Duration of Function (months)	No. Not Functioning	Time of Loss of Function (months)
Azathioprine	15	8		7	
Related	6	5		1	
Open duct	1	1	46		
Silicone	3	2	5, 29	1	2*
Pancreaticojejunostomy	2	2	2, 18		
Cadaveric	9	3		6	
Open duct	6	2	41, 57	4	2, 2, 3, 4
Prolamine	1			1	2
Silicone	2	1	1	1	2
Cyclosporine	35	9		26	
Related†	10	5		5	
Pancreaticojejunostomy	10	5	1, 6, 9, 16‡, 20	5	1§, 1‖, 2¶, 9‖, 9‡
Cadaveric	25	4		21	
Prolamine	2	0		2	2, 3
Silicone	23	4	1, 8, 15, 28	19	1§, 1**, 1(×3), 2§, 2(×8), 3(×3), 7, 12

*The only Aza-treated recipient of a related-donor pancreas graft who lost graft function had not had a previous kidney from the same donor and was HLA-mismatched with the donor. The other 5 had previously received kidneys from the same donor (3 HLA-identical, 2 nonidentical), and all have retained graft function during the period of follow-up.

†None had previously received kidney grafts.

‖Related grafts from HLA-nonidentical donors. All other related donors of grafts to CsA-treated recipients were HLA-identical.

¶Recurrent disease, not rejection.

‡Switched to Aza at 8 months.

**Patient rejected after stopping CsA.

§Died with functioning graft.

identical siblings) at 1, 6, 9, 16, and 20 months, respectively (the one with the functioning graft at 16 months was switched to Aza at 10 months; the others have remained on CsA). Of the 5 recipients who eventually lost graft function, 1 died at 1 month of cardiovascular disease; 2 rejected the grafts from HLA-mismatched donors at 1 month (cousin, no biopsy) and at 9 months (father, rejection biopsy confirmed); 1 rejected an HLA-identical graft at 9 months (biopsy confirmed), 1 month after conversion to CsA for nephrotoxicity; and 1 recipient of an HLA-identical graft became hyperglycemic at 2 months: biopsy of the graft at 6 months showed no evidence of rejection and beta cells were absent in otherwise normal islets, so recurrent disease rather than rejection was implicated.[6] Thus, no recipients of grafts from HLA-identical siblings who have received cyclosporine continuously for maintenance immunosuppression have lost graft function, and the only losses of technically successful grafts from related donors in CsA-treated recipients have been in those who were HLA-mismatched, were converted to Aza, or, in one case, were presumed a victim of recurrent disease.

Outcome According to Immunosuppression in Recipients of Pancreas Grafts from Cadaveric Donors

The results of transplantation of cadaveric pancreas grafts in recipients given CsA or Aza for immunosuppression can be compared without the influence of donor selection, because the degree of mismatching for HLA antigens was similar in both groups. The results obtained in recipients of technically successful cadaveric pancreas allografts ac-

Table 2. Results According to Immunosuppression in Recipients of Pancreas Grafts From Cadaveric Donors at the University of Minnesota

	Grafts Functioning as of 5/15/83		Grafts that Lost Function	
Immunosuppression (*N*)	No.	Months	No.	Time of Loss (months)
Azathioprine (9)*	3 (33%)	1, 41, 57	6	2(×4), 3, 4
Cyclosporine (25)	4 (16%)			
Previous kidney (18)†	3			
Aza (15)	2	8, 28	13	1‡, 1, 2(×6), 3(×3), 7, 12
CsA (3)	1	15	2	2, 2‡
No previous kidney (7)	1	1	6	1(×3), 1‡, 2, 2

*All had previous renal allografts.

†Of the 18 with previous kidney allografts, 15 were switched from Aza to CsA, and 3 were already on CsA at the time of pancreas transplantation.

‡Died with functioning grafts.

cording to immunosuppression are summarized in Table 2. The overall graft survival rate is slightly higher in Aza-treated recipients but the CsA group was weighted by inclusion of patients with no previous transplants, and it is possible that chronic immunosuppression or uremia prior to pancreas transplantation could have influenced the results.

Treatment of Rejection Episodes in Recipients on Cyclosporine or Azathioprine for Maintenance Immunosuppression

Five patients in the Aza group received antirejection therapy when hyperglycemia recurred subsequent to sustained periods of normoglycemia after pancreas transplantation. Three recipients of cadaveric grafts had sudden and severe hyperglycemia occur 2–3 months after transplantation, and none responded to treatment with an increase in oral prednisone alone. One recipient of a cadaveric graft had a less rapidly progressive elevation of plasma glucose levels, and C-peptide levels never fell entirely below baseline levels. An increase in prednisone dosage was instituted, with no immediate improvement, and the patient remained on exogenous insulin for 4 months, at which time insulin was withdrawn, C-peptide levels returned to normal, and the patient remained normoglycemic with no need for exogenous insulin (Fig. 1). This patient is now insulin-independent 42 months after pancreas transplantation but does have episodes of postprandial hyperglycemia. The one recipient of a pancreas graft from an HLA-nonidentical sibling donor of a previous kidney who became hyperglycemic at 2 weeks had not had immunosuppression increased initially but responded to treatment with methylprednisolone and ALG, became normoglycemic within 1 week of treatment, and has remained euglycemic during a 6-month follow-up period. It appears that an increase in immunosuppression may be necessary when a pancreas graft is transplanted from an HLA-nonidentical donor even when a previous kidney graft from that donor is functioning, but such an increase is unnecessary when the donor is an HLA-identical sibling (3/3 cases so handled have had continuous pancreas graft function without rejection episodes).

Thirteen recipients on CsA for maintenance immunosuppression were treated for rejection at the time of recurrence of hyperglycemia. There was no response to an increase in oral prednisone alone in two recipients of cadaveric grafts (both with rejection confirmed by biopsy). The one recipient of an HLA-identical sibling graft treated with an increase in oral prednisone alone also did not respond, but this was the one with recurrent disease rather than rejection, as documented by biopsy.[6] Recurrence of hyperglycemia at 2 weeks in the recipient of the graft from a cousin (not documented by biopsy) had a transient improvement after receiving oral prednisone but lost graft function by 1 month.

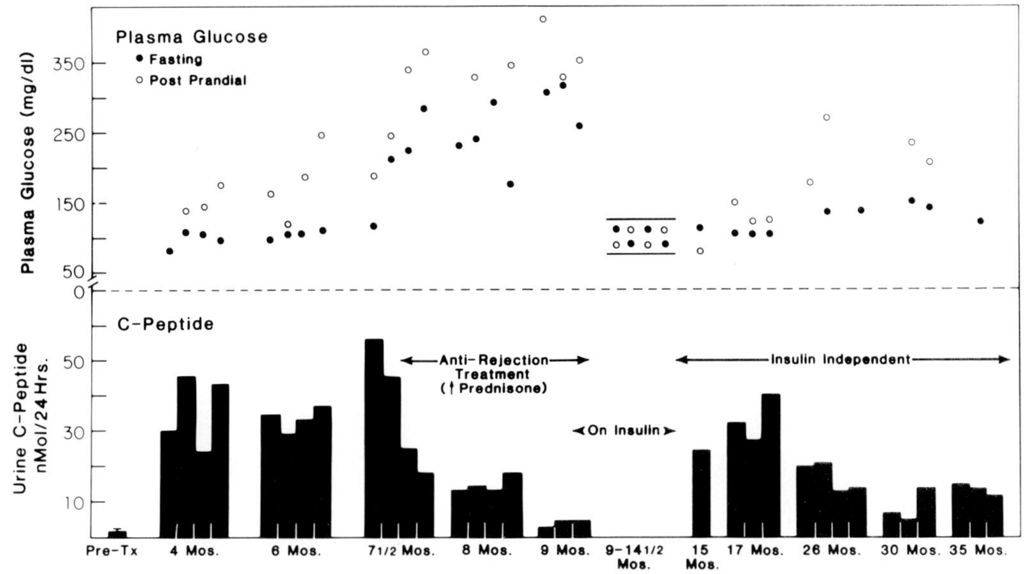

Fig. 1. Urine C-peptide excretion and plasma glucose levels before, during, and after antirejection treatment with prednisone in a renal allograft recipient of a cadaveric segmental pancreas transplant on azathioprine for maintenance immunosuppression. Prednisone dosage was temporarily increased and exogenous insulin resumed following diagnosis of rejection. Exogenous insulin was stopped 4 months later, and the patient is currently insulin-independent at 42 months after transplantation.

Two of the nine recipients treated for rejection with ALG were recipients of related grafts; one improved and was able to become insulin-independent (the one who did not was the one who had been switched to Aza a month previously) and has remained so over the entire period of follow-up (20 months), but glucose tolerance tests are abnormal. Of the seven recipients of cadaveric grafts treated for rejection episodes with ALG, four improved and were able to become insulin-independent following the treatment, but only one has maintained this state (now 7 months after transplantation). Rejection was confirmed by biopsy in all nine ALG-treated patients.

Two patients treated with ALG developed cytomegalovirus infections. Both had received Aza prior to pancreas transplantation because of previously placed renal allograft rejections. One received high-dose ALG (30 mg/kg/day for 10 days, in contrast to a dose of 20 mg/kg/day for 5–10 days in the other recipients) and died of CMV, while the other recovered from the CMV infection but lost graft function.

DISCUSSION

The patient survival rate following pancreas transplantation has improved in recent years and is now nearly equivalent to that achieved in renal allograft recipients. The pancreas graft survival rate, however, remains much lower than that of renal allografts, even when technically unsuccessful grafts are eliminated from analysis. Data from the Pancreas Transplant Registry show that a higher percentage of pancreas grafts are functioning in CsA- than in Aza-treated recipients,[3] but in our own personal experience at Minnesota, the pancreas graft functional survival rate is at least as high, if not higher, in Aza- than in CsA-treated recipients.

If all technically successful pancreas transplants (cadaveric and related donors), including patients who previously received a kidney from the same donor as the pancreas, are included in the analysis, 53% of Aza- and 26% of CsA-treated recipients currently have functioning grafts. If patients with previous kidneys from the same donor are eliminated, no recipients (one Aza- and three CsA-treated) of pancreas grafts from HLA-nonidentical related donors have functioning grafts, but 5/7 grafts from HLA-identical siblings are functioning (71%) in CsA-treated recipients. Of the two failed HLA-identical grafts, one was from recurrence of diabetes (not rejection), and one was after switching to Aza because of CsA toxicity.

The function rate of pancreas grafts from cadaveric donors is slightly higher in Aza- than in CsA-treated recipients. The discordance between the results in Minnesota and those in the Registry for CsA-treated recipients of cadaveric pancreas allografts might possibly be explained by patient selection. Most of our Aza-treated patients had previously received renal allografts and were chronically immunosuppressed. Nearly ⅓ of CsA-treated recipients of cadaveric allografts in our series were nonuremic, nonrenal allograft recipients. Other institutions using CsA perform pancreas transplants simultaneously with kidney allografts, and the uremic condition may potentiate the immunosuppressive effect of CsA. The diagnosis of rejection of a synchronously placed pancreas allograft might also be facilitated by monitoring renal allograft function from the same donor. Nevertheless, even with the theoretical advantages of simultaneous kidney and pancreas transplantation, it appears that immunosuppressive regimens tested so far are less effective in maintaining long-term function of pancreatic than of renal allografts. The ultimate future of pancreas transplantation lies in performing the procedure before secondary complications reach end stage. An immunosuppressive regimen applicable to these patients must be found. The only subcategories of diabetic pancreas allograft recipients in whom high success rates have been achieved are (1) those who have previously received renal allografts from the same related donor as the pancreas (in which case azathioprine is adequate if already used) or (2) in nonrenal allograft recipients of pancreases from HLA-identical siblings. In the latter subcategory, no patients given CsA continuously for maintenance immunosuppression have rejected pancreas grafts.

SUMMARY

Graft survival rates following transplantation of pancreases from cadaveric donors continue to be low in both CsA- and Aza-treated recipients. Although the long-term prognosis is relatively poor, rejection episodes in CsA-treated pancreas recipients can be reversed by ALG. Good graft survival rates can be achieved by transplantation of hemipancreases from HLA-identical siblings to CsA-treated recipients. The greatest benefit in our program has been achieved in this category of patients. A cyclosporine protocol that will consistently prevent rejection of cadaveric pancreatic allografts in nonuremic, nonrenal allograft diabetic patients needs to be developed.

REFERENCES

1. Sutherland DER: Transplantation 15:1303, 1983
2. Calne RY, Rolles K, White DJG, et al: Lancet 2:1033, 1979
3. Sutherland DER: Transplant Proc (this issue)
4. Sutherland DER, Goetz FC, Najarian JS: Transplantation 28:485, 1979
5. Sutherland DER, Goetz FC, Rynasiewicz JJ, et al: Surgery 90:159, 1981
6. Sutherland DER, Goetz FC, Elick BA, et al: Transplantation 34:330, 1982
7. Sutherland DER, Chinn PL, Elick BA, et al: Transplant Proc (in press)
8. Sutherland DER, Najarian JS, Greenberg B, et al: Ann Intern Med 95:537, 1981
9. Dubernard JM, Traeger J, Touraine JL, et al: Transplant Proc 13:305, 1981

BONE MARROW TRANSPLANTATION

Cyclosporine in Clinical Marrow Transplantation: The Baltimore Experience

P. J. Tutschka, A. D. Hess, W. E. Beschorner, E. R. Farmer, R. Saral, R. Brookmeyer, and G. W. Santos

IN A NUMBER OF preclinical studies in a rat bone marrow transplant model, it was shown that the then novel immunosuppressive agent cyclosporine A (CsA) had a remarkable potential for allogeneic bone marrow transplantation.[1–3] It was highly immunosuppressive, yet not toxic to marrow or stem cells; it prevented acute graft-vs.-host disease (GVHD) when given to recipients of allogeneic, MHC-mismatched marrow grafts; it accelerated the development of immunocompetence after grafting; and it rapidly led to the establishment of specific transplantation tolerance.[4,5]

Based on the rather successful preclinical animal studies and preliminary clinical transplant studies,[6] we started in 1980 to use cyclosporine clinically in patients who were grafted with allogeneic bone marrow. So far, the patients have been entered into three studies, two of which are still ongoing. Those three clinical trials form the basis of the present report.

CYCLOSPORINE TO PREVENT GRAFT-VS.-HOST DISEASE: A PILOT STUDY IN PATIENTS RECEIVING ALLOGENEIC MARROW TRANSPLANTS

Between 9/2/80 and 12/9/81, cyclosporine was administered to 22 consecutively entered patients, who were transplanted with genotypically HLA-identical bone marrow as therapy for a variety of lymphohematopoietic malignancies or aplastic anemia. Eleven patients had acute nonlymphocytic leukemia, six patients acute lymphocytic leukemia, one patient chronic myelogenous leukemia, one acute myelofibrosis, two aplastic anemia, and one patient therapy-refractory non-Hodgkin's lymphoma. As conditioning, the patients received either a combination of Busulfan and cyclophosphamide (patients with nonlymphocytic leukemia and chronic myelogenous leukemia), a combination of cyclophosphamide and fractionated total body irradiation (lymphocytic leukemias, non-Hodgkin's lymphoma), or cyclophosphamide and single-exposure total-body irradiation (aplastic anemia). The recipients had a median age of 20.5 years (range, 12–43) and were sex-matched with their respective donors in 13 cases.

From the Bone Marrow Transplant Program, Oncology Center, The Johns Hopkins University School of Medicine, Baltimore, MD.

Supported by NIH-NCI Grants CA 15396 and NIH-NIADD 1R01 AM 25602.

A. D. H. is a scholar of the Leukemia Society of America.

Reprint requests should be addressed to Dr. P. J. Tutschka, The Ohio State University Hospitals, 410 W. 10th Avenue, Room N-1027, Columbus, OH 43210-1228.

0041-1345/83/1505-0077$01.00/0

All patients were given cyclosporine orally, unless the oral preparation had to be substituted for a period of time with an intramuscular preparation due to a gastrointestinal intolerance. The patients received 20 mg/kg on days 0–3 (first dose given 12 hr before the marrow infusion), 50 mg/kg on days 4–28, and 12.5 mg/kg on days 29–180.

The aim of this pilot study was to evaluate if cyclosporine was stem cell–toxic, could prevent the development of acute graft-vs.-host disease, and at the same time accelerate the development of immune competence and tolerance. Furthermore, the incidence and severity of any toxic side effects of therapy with cyclosporine were to be identified.

Of the 22 patients entered into the study, 1 died at day 10 after transplantation, too early to evaluate for engraftment, but was found at autopsy to show islands of recovering marrow activity. The remaining 21 patients engrafted promptly and showed early recovery of peripheral counts 14–19 days after transplantation (median) without any evidence for stem cell impairment by cyclosporine.

The main objective, to attempt to prevent the development of graft-vs.-host disease, was not achieved in this pilot study. Of the 22 patients, 1 patient developed severe gastric intolerance to CsA, requiring discontinuation of the agent. Within a week after stopping CsA, the patient developed severe GVHD and died later with interstitial pneumonia. Of the remaining 21 patients, 11 showed no evidence of GVHD. However, 7 patients died before they reached day 70 after transplantation, at a time when they were still at risk for developing GVHD. If these patients are excluded, the observed absence of graft-vs.-host disease was 4/14 patients, or 28.5%. Cutaneous GVHD was seen in 5 patients, and systemic GVHD, which affected in no case more than two organ systems, was present in another 5 patients.

Three of the 5 patients that showed cutaneous GVHD were given steroid therapy, and all patients responded and became long-term survivors. Of the 5 patients with systemic GVHD, all were treated with methylprednisolone. Four of those 5 patients responded and had complete resolution of the GVHD; 2 of those 5 patients survived, but 3 patients died, of interstitial pneumonia in one case and sepsis in two cases. Interstitial pneumonia was seen in 6 patients and was fatal in all of them. Sixteen patients did not show any interstitial pneumonia; however, 9 of those patients survived for less than 100 days, while still at risk for developing interstitial pneumonia. Therefore, the observed incidence was 6/13 patients, or 46%. The median day of onset was 12 days, with a range of 9–60 days.

Liver function abnormalities were seen in the majority of patients. Fourteen patients showed a bilirubin of > 2 mg/dl, 7 patients showed an SGOT of > 100 IU/liter, and 8 an SGPT of > 100 IU/liter. Seven patients showed an elevation of all three parameters. In all patients who showed liver abnormalities, these were associated with either GVHD or veno-occlusive disease, and no correlation could be established between cyclosporine and liver function abnormalities.

Renal function abnormalities were seen in a majority of patients as well. Seventeen patients showed a creatinine of > 2 mg/dl, and 6 patients an elevation of > 4 mg/dl. Nine patients had sustained elevated creatinine levels of > 2.5 mg/dl for more than a week. Three of these patients required dialysis. All of these patients ultimately recovered their renal function, but the duration of renal failure was quite long, showing a median duration of 18 days, with a range of 6–29 days.

A strong association with renal function abnormalities and Amphotericin B therapy could be established. Of the 12 patients treated with Amphotericin B, 11 showed creatinine levels of > 2.5 mg/dl, and in only 1 patient was renal failure encountered without concomitant therapy with Amphotericin B. This highly significant association of renal failure with concomitant administration of Amphotericin B and cyclosporine could not be established with the administration of antibacterial antibiotics including aminoglycocides.

Attempts were made to correlate cyclosporine serum levels, as measured by radioimmunoassay (RIA),[7] and the observed side effects. In all patients, cyclosporine serum levels were determined twice daily, one being a trough level determined immediately prior to such cyclosporine administration and the other a peak level determined 8 hr after each cyclosporine administration. No correlation could be observed between trough levels and presence or absence of GVHD, nor could any correlation be established between peak levels of cyclosporine and liver or renal function abnormalities.

The pilot study, conducted with these 22 patients, indicated several points.[8] It seemed possible that cyclosporine indeed reduced the incidence and severity of GVHD. Renal failure was encountered as a most prominent side effect, suggesting that the therapeutic range was operationally quite narrow. Serum levels, as measured by RIA, were probably not predicting for or correlating with toxicity or biological activity. The study suggested that randomized trials needed to be conducted to establish if there was a true value of cyclosporine for clinical marrow transplantation.

RANDOMIZED DOUBLE-BLIND STUDY COMPARING THE EFFECTS OF CYCLOSPORINE-METHYLPREDNISOLONE TO CYCLOPHOSPHAMIDE-METHYLPREDNISOLONE FOR THE PREVENTION OF GRAFT-VS.-HOST DISEASE

Based on animal studies and some preliminary clinical data from a number of institutions, it was suggested that methylprednisolone was an agent that could be beneficially used in the prevention of graft-vs.-host disease.[9,10] Furthermore, studies with solid organ transplants had indicated that methylprednisolone acted synergistically with cyclosporine in preventing rejection of organ allografts.[11,12] Therefore, a combination of cyclophosphamide and methylprednisolone was used in one arm of the study and compared to a combination of methylprednisolone and cyclosporine. The aim of this study was severalfold. First, the question was asked if a combination of cyclosporine and methylprednisolone increased the therapeutic range of cyclosporine, permitting lower doses of cyclosporine yet at the same time increasing its GVHD-preventing potential. Second, it was asked if cyclosporine was a better agent than cyclophosphamide to prevent GVHD, and, third, if patients receiving a combination of cyclosporine and methylprednisolone showed an improved survival compared to patients receiving cyclophosphamide and methylprednisolone. To circumvent investigator-related bias, the study was designed as a double-blind randomized trial. Cyclosporine was given at a daily dose of 5 mg/kg on days 0–3, starting 8 hr prior to the infusion of bone marrow, followed on days 4–14 by a dose of 3.5 mg/kg/day given intravenously. If the patients had a functioning gastrointestinal system and tolerated oral cyclosporine, on day 15 the patients received oral cyclosporine at a dose of 10 mg/kg/day until day 42, at which time the dose was reduced to 7.5 mg/kg/day until day 180. Methylprednisolone administration started at day 8 with 0.5 mg/kg/day and advanced to 1 mg/kg/day on days 15–28. From then on, the steroids were tapered until day 72, with a reduction of the dose every 2 weeks. Cyclophosphamide was given at a dose of 7.5 mg/kg on days 1, 3, 7, 9, 21, and then weekly until day 100.

So far, 34 patients have been entered into this study, 17 patients on each arm. Eight patients developed clinically significant GVHD, 4 patients in each arm. Of those 8 patients, 4 have died from complications of GVHD. Overall, a total of 14 patients have died from a variety of causes. The actuarial survival curve constructed to date does not show any difference between the arms of the study, suggesting that so far a combination of cyclosporine and methylprednisolone does not appear to be superior to a combination of cyclosphamide and methylprednisolone.

THERAPY OF ESTABLISHED ACUTE GRAFT-VS.-HOST DISEASE

It had been shown previously by Powles et al. that cyclosporine might be effective in counteracting established acute graft-vs.-host disease.[6] Based on this study, we tried to ascertain if a combination of cyclosporine and methylprednisolone was beneficial in counteracting acute, clinically significant GVHD. Patients who showed GVHD of stage II received methylprednisolone at a daily dose of 2.5 mg/kg for 4 days. If they showed improvement, the steroids were tapered; if they did not show improvement, the prophylactic immunosuppression was discontinued and the patients were started on cyclosporine at a dose of 5 mg/kg/day i.v., combined with methylprednisolone at a dose of 5 mg/kg/day. So far, 15 patients have been entered into this study (10 with a diagnosis of acute nonlymphocytic leukemia, 3 with acute lymphocytic leukemia, 1 with chronic myelogenous leukemia, and 1 with aplastic anemia). The patients had a median age of 27 years and were sex-matched with their respective donors in 8 cases. Seven of those patients had received cyclophosphamide only as post-transplant GVHD prophylaxis, 4 a combination of cyclophosphamide and methylprednisolone at low doses and 4 a combination of cyclosporine and methylprednisolone. One of those patients had stage II disease, 8 showed stage III, and 6 stage IV disease. Day of onset of the disease was a median of 17, with a range of 10–28 days. Thirteen of the 15 patients (86.6%) showed complete resolution of the GVHD with a histologic improvement to grade 0 or 1. Five of the 15 patients have become long-term survivors, with a median survival of > 276 days (range, 184–482 days). Ten patients died, 1 with GVHD and viral gastroenteritis, 1 with GVHD and interstitial pneumonia, 1 from sepsis, 1 from interstitial pneumonia, and 1 from interstitial pneumonia and viral gastroenteritis; in 5 patients only viral gastroenteritis could be documented. This study suggested that cyclosporine, in combination with methylprednisolone, was a most effective agent in treating established acute GVHD but that this combination regimen was associated with a high complication rate, whereby in particular a high degree of fatal hemorrhagic gastroenteritis was observed.

These rather preliminary data indicate that the true efficacy of cyclosporine as a prophylactic agent for GVHD cannot yet be established. These data are in agreement with the results of other bone marrow transplant groups, in particular the studies reported by the Seattle group, where in randomized studies no clear cut advantages of cyclosporine over methotrexate could be established.[13] The preliminary data indicating that cyclosporine in combination with methylprednisolone is an effective agent to counteract ongoing GVHD have to be treated with caution, as only historical controls are available. Furthermore, the relatively low overall salvage rate of 33% indicates that the combination regimen is associated with a number of complications, possibly correlated to a high degree of immunosuppression afforded by cyclosporine and methylprednisolone. Clearly, further controlled studies are needed, in particular those using different drug regimens, to establish the true value of cyclosporine for prevention and treatment of acute graft-vs.-host disease.

REFERENCES

1. Borel JF, Feurer C, Magnee C, et al: Immunology 32:1017, 1977

2. Tutschka PJ: Blut 39:81, 1979

3. Tutschka PJ, Beschorner WE, Hess AD: Blut (Suppl) 25:241, 1980

4. Tutschka PJ, Beschorner WE, Allison AC, et al: Nature 280:148, 1979

5. Van Bekkum DW, Knoon S, Zurcher C: Transplant Proc 12:278, 1980

6. Powles RL, Barrett AZ: Lancet 1:327, 1980

7. Donatsch P, Abish E, Hamberger M, et al: J Immunoassay 2:19, 1981

8. Tutschka PJ, Beschorner WE, Hess AD, et al: Blood 61:318 1983

9. Blume KG, Beutler E, Bross DJ, et al: N Engl J Med 302:1041, 1980

10. Kersey JH, Ramsay NKC, Kim T, et al: Blood 60:400, 1982

11. Starzl TE, Neil R, Iwatsuki S, et al: Surgery 151:17, 1980

12. Starzl TE, Klintmalm GBG, Parker KA, et al: N Engl J Med 305:266, 1981

13. Deeg HJ, Storb R, Thomas ED, et al: Transplant Proc 15:1385, 1983

Allogeneic Bone Marrow Transplantation: The Basel Trial with Cyclosporine

B. Speck, A. Gratwohl, B. Osterwalder, E. Signer, C. Nissen, M. Corneo, and M. Jeannet

IN JULY 1979, we initiated a prospective study using cyclosporine A (CsA) instead of methotrexate (MTX) in allogeneic bone marrow transplantation (BMT) for leukemia and severe aplastic anemia (SAA). The purpose was to document the value of CsA in clinical bone marrow transplantation, in particular its influence on engraftment, graft-vs.-host-disease (GVHD), interstitial pneumonia (IP), and survival.

MATERIALS AND METHODS

Patients between the ages of 3–42 years with acute leukemia (AL), chronic myelogenous leukemia (CML), and SAA were entered into this study. Between July 1979 and March 1983, 71 allogeneic grafts were performed; 67 had HLA-identical sibling donors (Table 1). Median age was 28 years (range, 3–42). The median observation period was 20 months (range 3–45). Four patients were grafted with HLA-one-haplotype-identical marrow from a family member. The 57 patients with leukemia were conditioned with 2 × 60 mg/kg cyclophosphamide and 1000 rad total-body irradiation (TBI) midline tissue dose from a linear accelerator at a dose rate of 7.5 rad/min. In the initial 15 patients, the lungs were shielded to receive 800 rad, but this was discontinued in the subsequent patients.

HLA-Identical Sibling Transplants in Leukemia (N = 53)

Nineteen patients had acute myelogenous leukemia (AML); 14 were in first complete remission, 5 in second. Another 19 patients had acute lymphoblastic leukemia (ALL); 8 were in first complete remission, 5 in second. Another 19 patients had acute lymphoblastic leukemia (ALL); 8 were in first complete remission, 5 in second, 3 in third, and 3 in relapse or never reached remission. Fifteen had CML. All were splenectomized before BMT. Thirteen were in chronic phase, 2 had accelerated disease with increased blast counts, severe basophilia, anemia, and thrombocytopenia.

HLA-One-Haplotype-Identical Transplants From Family Members in Leukemia (N = 4)

Three patients had ALL; 2 were in first complete remission, 1 in second relapse. One patient had AML; he never reached remission on chemotherapy.

HLA-Identical Sibling Transplants in SAA (N = 14)

All patients were conditioned with 4 × 50 mg/kg cyclophosphamide. In addition to the marrow, they were given donor buffy coat from 4 units of blood on each of 5 successive days, directly after marrow transplantation.

All patients were nursed in ultrasterile laminar air-flow rooms with gastrointestinal decontamination, skin cleansing, and sterile food for 21–45 days (median, 28 days).

CsA was given intramuscularly 20 mg/kg/day in a single dose, starting 24 hr before the infusion of the marrow, and was continued for 7 days in the initial 20 patients. The next 11 patients were given the same dose of CsA as a continuous i.v. infusion starting 24 hr before marrow transplantation and continuing for 5 days. The last 40 patients all had CsA as a continuous i.v. infusion, 20 mg/kg on the day before marrow transplantation, then 10 mg/kg for 5 days and afterwards 5 mg/kg/day for 5 more days as a continuous i.v. infusion. All patients then received the drug orally in a single daily dose of 12.5 mg/kg. This dose was maintained for 6 months, then slowly reduced, and stopped at 12 months.[1,2]

RESULTS

HLA-Identical Sibling Transplants in Leukemia (N = 53)

Results are summarized in Fig. 1. Of the 14 patients with AML in first remission, 8 (57%) survive without evidence of leukemia and without chronic problems. Six patients died: 4 of relapse, 1 of GVHD, and 1 of interstitial pneumonia. Of the 5 in second remission, 2 survive. All 3 deaths were due to leukemic relapse. Of the 8 patients with ALL in first

From the Division of Hematology, Department of Internal Medicine, Kantonsspital Basel, Basel, the Kinderspital Basel (E.S.), and the Hôpital Cantonal Geneva, Switzerland (M.J.).

Supported by Grants of the Swiss Science Foundation (3.846.0.79), the Swiss Cancer League (FOR.141.LR 79–3), and the Swiss Public Health Service.

Reprint requests should be addresssed to Dr. B. Speck, Kantonsspital, 4031 Basel, Switzerland.

0041-1345/83/1505-0078$01.00/0

Preliminary Results of Prospective Randomized Trials Comparing Methotrexate and Cyclosporine for Prophylaxis of Graft-vs.-Host-Disease After HLA-Identical Marrow Transplantations

R. Storb, H. J. Deeg, E. D. Thomas, C. D. Buckner, R. A. Clift, N. Flournoy, M. S. Kennedy, K. Doney, F. R. Appelbaum, J. E. Sanders, P. Stewart, H. Shulman, K. M. Sullivan, and R. P. Witherspoon

METHOTREXATE (MTX) and cyclosporine (CsA) have been used in uncontrolled clinical trials to prevent acute graft-vs.-host disease (GVHD) after marrow transplantation.[1-10] The rationale for their use in humans is supported by controlled studies in experimental animals that have demonstrated the effectiveness of both drugs in obviating GVHD.[11-14] In autumn 1980, two randomized prospective trials were begun in Seattle comparing the usefulness of MTX to that of CsA in patients given HLA-identical sibling marrow grafts for the treatment of acute nonlymphoblastic leukemia (ANLL) in first remission and chronic myelogenous leukemia (CML) in chronic phase. Preliminary results in patients with ANLL have been reported.[15] This report updates those results and presents new preliminary data on patients with CML in chronic phase.

MATERIALS AND METHODS

From October 20, 1980, to February 24, 1983, 78 patients with ANLL in first remission and 36 patients with CML in chronic phase were entered into the study. Patient characteristics are shown in Tables 1 and 2. Patients were referred after detailed consultation with their physicians and an interview in which advantages and disadvantages of the transplantation procedure were emphasized. Protocols and consent forms were approved by the Human Subjects Review Committee of the Fred Hutchinson Cancer Research Center.

The transplantation regimen and the randomization are outlined in Table 3. Total body irradiation was delivered from two opposing cobalt-60 sources at a dose rate of 6.5 rad/min. Details on the conditioning regimen have been reported.[16,17] The marrow was infused within 4 hr of the last dose of irradiation. All patients were given 12 mg of intrathecal MTX on alternate weeks beginning on day 32 in an effort to prevent central nervous system relapse. Patients receiving CsA were given citrovorum factor rescue.

The grading system and the treatment of acute and chronic GVHD have been discussed elsewhere.[18-20] Treatment of established GVHD consisted of prednisone, 2 mg/kg/day p.o., in patients receiving CsA prophylaxis or randomization to either prednisone or CsA 12.5 mg/kg/day orally in patients on MTX prophylaxis. The supportive care after transplantation has also been described.[16,17]

RESULTS

The results on the 78 patients with ANLL engrafted in first remission are summarized in Table 1. Thirty-six of the patients received prophylactic CsA and 42 MTX. The projected survival is 71% for patients given CsA and 55% for those given MTX (Fig. 1). This difference is not statistically significant ($p = 0.26$ by log rank test). Patients given CsA showed significantly faster engraftment as measured by recovery of granulocytes and a lesser requirement for platelet transfusions. Patients treated with CsA required red blood cell transfusions for a longer period of time than those given MTX. There was no significant difference in hospital stay between the

From the Fred Hutchinson Cancer Research Center and the University of Washington School of Medicine, Seattle, WA.

Supported by Grants CA 18029, CA 15704, CA 18221, and CA 09319, awarded by the National Cancer Institute, DHHS. E.D.T. is the recipient of Research Career Award AI 02425 from the National Institute of Allergy and Infectious Diseases. F.R.A. and P.S. are supported in part by Junior Faculty Clinical Fellowships from the American Cancer Society.

Reprint requests should be addressed to Dr. R. Storb, Fred Hutchinson Cancer Research Center, 1124 Columbia Street, Seattle, WA 98104.

0041-1345/83/1505-0079$01.00/0

Table 1. Data on 78 Patients with Acute Nonlymphoblastic Leukemia Given Marrow Grafts from HLA-Identical Siblings During First Remission

Data	GVHD Prophylaxis	
	Cyclosporine	Methotrexate
No. of patients studied	36	42
Median age in years (range)	25 (13–49)	27 (13–46)
Male/female (no. of patients)	21/15	22/20
Median months from diagnosis to transplant (range)	3 (2–8)	3 (2–10)
Post-transplant data		
Median day (range) of granulocytes $\geq 1000/mm^3$	18 (12–32)	25 (18–46)
Grade II–IV acute GVHD (% of patients)	36%	67%
Median day (range) of onset of acute GVHD	14 (10–66)	17 (7–66)
No. of patients with chronic GVHD/No. of patients at risk	20/33*	17/32
Relapse (No. of patients)	3	5
Surviving (No. of patients)	26	25
Dead (No. of patients)	10	17
Causes of death (No. of patients)		
Relapse	1	4
Interstitial pneumonia	4	5
Bacterial or fungal infections	3	3
Viral infections	1	4
Other	1	1

*Excludes patients still receiving cyclosporine <180 days after transplantation.

two groups of patients. The range of hospital days was 18–105 days (median, 32 days) for CsA-treated patients and 23–136 days (median, 40 days) for those treated with MTX.

The overall incidence of acute grades II–IV GVHD was less in patients given CsA than in those given MTX ($p = 0.04$). The rate at which acute GVHD developed was comparable in both groups of patients, as was the incidence of chronic GVHD.

Three patients in the CsA group and five in the MTX group have relapsed. Three of these patients (one in the MTX and two in the CsA group) are still alive.

Causes of death included relapse, interstitial pneumonia, and bacterial, fungal, and

Table 2. Data on 36 Patients with Chronic Myelogenous Leukemia Given Marrow Grafts From HLA-Identical Siblings During the Chronic Phase of the Disease

Data	GVHD Prophylaxis	
	Cyclosporine	Methotrexate
No. of patients studied	18	18
Median age in years (range)	30 (15–39)	26 (11–42)
Male/female (No. of patients)	12/6	12/6
Post-transplant data		
Grades II–IV acute GVHD (% of patients)	43%	37%
No. of patients with chronic GVHD/No. of patients at risk	5/9*	9/16
Relapse (No. of patients)	3†	2†
Surviving (No. of patients)	12	15
Dead (No. of patients)	6	3
Causes of death (No. of patients)		
Interstitial pneumonia	5	2
Other	1	1

*Excludes patients still receiving cyclosporine <180 days after transplantation.

†Return of cells with Philadelphia chromosome. Patients are alive.

Table 3. Transplantation Regimen

Cyclophosphamide 60 mg/kg/day × 2 days
↓
Total body irradiation 200 rad/day × 6 days
↓
Marrow graft
↓
Randomize

Cyclosporine	Methotrexate
12.5 mg/kg/day p.o. day −1 to day 50, then taper by 5%/week until day 180	15 mg/m² i.v. day 1, 10 mg/m² days 1, 3, 6, 11, and weekly until day 102

viral infections. The incidence of these complications was similar in both groups of patients studied.

Table 2 shows the data on patients with CML, 18 of whom received CsA and 18 MTX prophylaxis. Projected long-term survival is 67% for patients treated with CsA and 83% for those treated with MTX (Fig. 2). This difference is not significant ($p = 0.26$). As did patients with ANLL, CsA-treated patients with CML showed faster hemopoietic engraftment. There was no significant difference in the incidence of acute GVHD among patients treated with CsA compared to those given MTX ($p = 0.47$). Also, there were no differences in the rate of acquisition of acute GVHD nor in the overall incidence of chronic GVHD. Five patients, three in the CsA group and two in the MTX group, showed reemergence of cells with the Philadelphia chromosome. All five are alive and, upon repeated testing, the Philadelphia chromosome could not be found in two of them. The dominating cause of death in both groups was interstitial pneumonia, mostly related to cytomegalovirus.

The most significant adverse side effect of CsA was renal function impairment, a complication that has been reviewed in detail elsewhere.[21] Also, mild liver abnormalities were seen in many patients. Overall, patients given CsA received approximately 75% of their calculated drug dose during the first 100 days after transplantation, compared to 82% for patients given MTX.

DISCUSSION

The current study set out to compare the usefulness of cyclosporine to that of methotrexate for preventing acute and chronic GVHD and to evaluate the resulting effect on long-term survival in patients with ANLL in first remission and CML in the chronic phase.

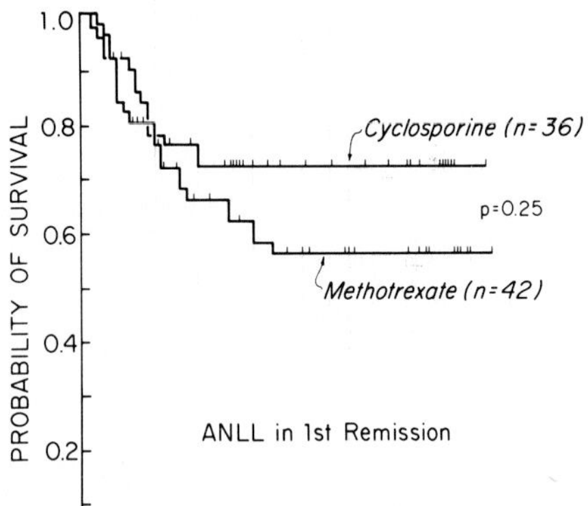

Fig. 1. Probability of survival in 78 patients with ANLL in first remission given marrow grafts from HLA-identical siblings and either methotrexate or cyclosporine after transplantation (Kaplan-Meier product limit estimates). Tick marks represent surviving patients. Survival as of May 1, 1983.

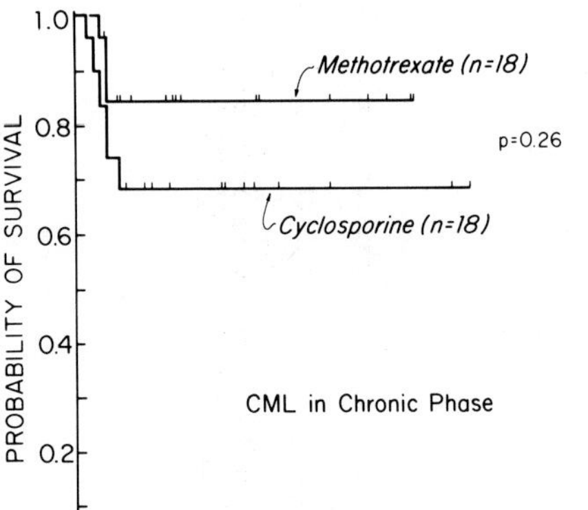

Fig. 2. Probability of survival in 36 patients with CML in chronic phase given marrow grafts from HLA-identical siblings and either methotrexate or cyclosporine after transplantation (Kaplan-Meier product limit estimates). Tick marks represent surviving patients. Survival as of May 1, 1983.

The preliminary results reported here suggest that the two drugs are equivalent. Although the incidence of grades II–IV acute GVHD was significantly decreased among CsA-treated patients with ANLL in first remission, there was only a marginal improvement in overall survival. It should be noted that the 67% incidence of acute GVHD seen in the MTX-treated patients was higher than the 40%–50% incidence customarily seen among patients transplanted for leukemia with that regimen.[22] Somewhat in contrast to results in patients with ANLL, there was no difference in the incidence of acute GVHD between CsA-treated and MTX-treated patients with CML, and survival was marginally better among patients treated with MTX. Overall, the survival seen in the present study agrees with data previously reported from this and other transplant centers for patients with ANLL and CML. The incidences of chronic GVHD and of infectious complications were comparable among both groups of patients. Consistent findings were a faster rate of granulocyte and platelet recovery after transplantation, greater requirements for red blood cell transfusions, and a higher incidence of renal function impairment in patients treated with CsA. Despite a faster rate of hemopoietic engraftment, the overall length of hospital stay was only marginally shorter in patients treated with CsA, owing to a higher incidence of complications from nonhemopoietic toxicity.

A question raised by an analysis of the European Bone Marrow Transplant Group has been the possibility of a higher incidence of leukemic recurrence among patients given CsA.[23] The current preliminary findings do not concur with that suggestion.

Our results allow the conclusion that cyclosporine is a powerful immunosuppressive agent that is equivalent to methotrexate after HLA-identical marrow transplantation for patients with ANLL in first remission and CML in chronic phase. This conclusion, however, is tentative, as the longest follow-up is only 2.5 years, and many patients are still at risk of developing chronic GVHD and recurrent leukemia.

REFERENCES

1. Storb R, Thomas ED, Buckner CD, et al: Blood 43:157, 1974
2. Thomas ED, Buckner CD, Banaji M, et al: Blood 49:511, 1977
3. Storb R, Prentice RL, Buckner CD, et al: N Engl J Med 308:302, 1983
4. Thomas ED, Sanders JE, Flournoy N, et al: Blood 54:468, 1979
5. Thomas ED, Buckner CD, Clift RA, et al: N Engl J Med 301:597, 1979
6. Powles RL, Barrett AJ, Clink H, et al: Lancet 2:1327, 1978
7. Powles RL, Clink HM, Spence D, et al: Lancet 1:327, 1980
8. Hows JM, Palmer S, Gordon-Smith EC: Transplantation 33:382, 1982
9. Tutschka PJ, Beschorner EW, Hess AD, et al: Blood 61:318, 1983
10. Speck B, Gratwohl A, Nissen C, et al: In Baum SJ, Ledney GD, Khan A (eds): Experimental Hematology Today 1981. New York, Springer-Verlag, 1981
11. Tutschka PJ, Beschorner WE, Allison AC, et al: Nature 280:148, 1979
12. Deeg HJ, Storb R, Weiden PL, et al: Transplant Proc 13:402, 1981
13. Deeg HJ, Storb R, Weiden PL, et al: Transplantation 34:30, 1982
14. Storb R, Epstein RB, Graham TC, et al: Transplantation 9:240, 1970
15. Deeg HJ, Storb R, Thomas ED, et al: Transplant Proc 15:1358, 1983
16. Clift RA, Buckner CD, Thomas ED, et al: Lancet 2:621, 1982
17. Thomas ED, Appelbaum FR, Buckner CD, et al: In Recent Advances in Bone Marrow Transplantation. New York, Alan R. Liss (in press)
18. Thomas ED, Storb R, Clift RA, et al: N Engl J Med 292:832/895 1975
19. Doney KC, Weiden PL, Storb R, et al: Am J Hematol 11:1, 1981
20. Sullivan KM, Shulman HM, Storb R, et al: Blood 57:267, 1981
21. Kennedy MS, Deeg HJ, Storb R, et al: Transplant Proc 15:471, 1983
22. Weiden PL, Seattle Marrow Transplant Team: In Gale RP, Fox CS (eds): Biology of Bone Marrow Transplantation. New York, Academic Press, 1980, p 37
23. Zwaan FE, Hermans J: Exp Hematol 10:64, 1982

Cyclosporine for the Prevention of Graft-vs.-Host Disease in 72 Patients with Acute Myeloblastic Leukemia in First Remission Receiving Matched Sibling Bone Marrow Transplants

R. L. Powles, B. Evans, C. Poole, A. Pedrazzini, M. Crofts, C. Pollard, and G. Hughes

CYCLOSPORINE (CsA) was introduced into clinical practice in August 1978[1,2] and was shown 2 years later to be useful for preventing fatal graft-vs.-host disease (GVHD) following bone marrow transplantation (BMT).[3] In this initial series of patients, it was difficult to define clearly the impact of CsA on BMT because a controlled trial was not possible comparing CsA with no treatment. In addition, the patients treated were not a homogenous group, in that they had different varieties of leukemia in either remission or relapse.

Now sufficient patients have accrued to examine a single group with acute myeloblastic leukemia (AML) in first remission receiving matched sibling transplants given only CsA to prevent GVHD, and a statement can be made about the efficacy of this form of treatment for these patients and the toxicity encountered.

MATERIALS AND METHODS

Seventy-two patients with AML received BMT during first remission at the Royal Marsden Hospital between August 1978 and May 1983. The age range was 4–46 years, with a median of 37 years.

Conditioning Regimen

Fifty-six patients received cyclophosphamide 60 mg/kg i.v. daily for 2 days, followed after 36 hr by total body irradiation (TBI) of 10 Gray given as a single dose at a dose rate of approximately 1.5 Gray/hr. An additional 11 patients were conditioned with a priming i.v. dose of cyclophosphamide 300 mg/m^2, followed 7 days later by a single i.v. dose of melphalan (85–100 mg/m^2) and 12 hr later TBI at a dose of 10 Gray. Both these groups of patients received the marrow transplant the day after the TBI. A third group of 5 patients received the same priming dose of cyclophosphamide, followed 7 days later by a single dose of melphalan 240 mg/m^2 (and no TBI) and 4 days later they received their transplants.

Bone Marrow Transplant

Approximately 2.0–3.5 × 10^8/kg nucleated bone marrow cells were given from HLA-DR matched sibling donors. The marrow was not subjected to any separation procedures prior to infusion.

Cyclosporine

Five different regimens were used: Between August 1978 and September 1982, 38 patients received intramuscular CsA 25 mg/kg, from the day prior to transplant for 5 days, followed by oral CsA 12.5 mg/kg for 175 days. During the same period, an additional three groups of patients received oral instead of intramuscular regimens as follows: from the day prior to transplant, CsA was given for 5 days at a daily dose of either 8 mg/kg (7 patients), 12.5 mg/kg (15 patients), or 35.5 mg/kg (8 patients), followed by a maintenance dose of 8–12.5 mg/kg for 175 days. In all studies the maintenance dose of CsA was titrated against toxicity, the dose being reduced by 33% if the creatinine rose above 250 μmole/liter or the BUN above 20 mmole/liter. For ~70% of the patients, the radioimmunoassay of CsA was available, and serum levels were monitored and kept within a "therapeutic" range of 500–1000 ng/ml. Since September 1982, when i.m. CsA was no longer available, 4 patients had received 12.5–25 mg/kg/day infused over 12 hr for the first 5 days after transplantation.

Forty of the 72 patients in the series have stopped taking CsA at 180 days after transplantation.

Graft-vs.-Host Disease

Initially all patients developing skin rashes had a biopsy taken, but no change was made in management, and in all but one instance there was complete resolution of the skin problem. After our first fatality with GVHD, all patients with skin GVHD received as treatment 3 days of i.v. methylprednisolone 700 mg/m^2. Recently, skin biopsies have no longer been performed.

From the Royal Marsden Hospital and Institute of Cancer Research, Sutton, Surrey, England.

Reprint requests should be addressed to Dr. R. L. Powles, R. M. H., Downs Road, Sutton, Surrey, England.

0041-1345/83/1505-0080$01.00/0

RESULTS

Graft-vs.-Host Disease

Of the 38 patients receiving i.m. CsA, 26 (68%) are alive; 71% either had proven or suspected GVHD, and 1 (3%) died of the syndrome. There was no significant difference in the results obtained for the 30 patients treated only with oral CsA; 56% are alive, 66% developed suspected or proven GVHD, and 1 (3%) died from it.

Survival

Forty-seven of the 72 patients remain alive, with a projected actuarial plateau between 26–56 months at 54%. Of the 25 deaths, 8 (11%) were due to recurrent leukemia (day 92–393; median, 189), 6 due to pulmonary edema (day 30–513; median, 92), 4 due to renal failure (day 27–84), 3 of pneumonia (day 41–65), 2 GVHD (day 49 and day 77), 1 of CNS (day 20), and 1 of carcinoma of the rectum (day 698). There were thus 23% transplant-related deaths, Four of the 8 patients receiving high initial CsA doses (35.5 mg/kg/day) died of pulmonary edema, whereas there were only 2 deaths from this cause in the whole of the rest of the series. Otherwise the causes of death could not be related to CsA administration. Although renal dysfunction occurred in over 70% of patients on CsA, death due to renal failure was not directly attributable to CsA (or serum levels). However, a correlation was found between the conditioning regimen and severe renal failure; only 1 patient died of renal failure of 56 conditioned with cyclophosphamide and TBI, whereas 3/16 patients who received melphalan (with or without TBI) died of the problem.

Age was the most important factor associated with survival; of 23 patients under 20 years of age, 78% remain alive; of 18 patients 21–30 years, 67% are alive; of 24 patients 31–40 years, 59% are alive, and only 43% are alive of 7 patients over 40 years of age.

The serum bilirubin was also a prognostic significance; 59 patients had bilirubin levels remaining <100 μmole/liter (normal <17 μmole/liter) during the first 12 weeks after transplantation and 43 (73%) are alive, whereas only 3/13 (24%) of patients are alive whose bilirubin rose about 100 μmole/liter. The cause of death of the 10 severely jaundiced (conjugated) patients was not liver failure; 3 died of pulmonary edema, 3 of infection, 2 of renal failure, 1 of GVHD, and 1 of carcinoma of the rectum.

Stopping CsA

Forty patients stopped taking CsA after 180 days, and 12 required reinstitution of the drug within 60 days due to the development of acute GVHD in either skin or liver (based on liver function tests). All had resolution of their GVHD.

DISCUSSION

It was a pity that we could not conduct a controlled trial of CsA versus nothing, but it was ethically difficult to have an untreated group of patients following transplantation. Such a study could have determined the exact contribution that CsA makes in preventing serious GVHD and also would have given a clearer picture of the toxicity of this drug in the context of patients who have other problems consequent to such a complicated procedure as bone marrow transplantation. However, it was gratifying in this present series to find that only 3% of patients died as a direct consequence of GVHD. Although GVHD occurred in some patients when, after 6 months, the drug was stopped, this was not a serious problem and readily responded to treatment. Of more concern was the still relatively high proportion (23%) of transplant-related deaths in this series of patients, and the long-term place of BMT in leukemia stands or falls upon reducing these complications. Fatal pulmonary edema (a problem that has dominated our mismatched transplant program[4]) was the most common serious occurrence, and although there was a hint it might be related to high initial doses of oral CsA, other important factors, such as the TBI, cannot be excluded. The essential lesion that appears to be central to this problem is in the vascular endothelium. Renal failure leading to death, the next most common serious complication, seemed to have a separate pathogenesis from the mild renal toxicity seen in most patients on CsA[1,5] and almost certainly was related to a drug interaction between melphalan and CsA.[6] Recently we have given the melphalan in our conditioning programs 5 days prior to receiving CsA (and the transplant), and severe renal failure is now rare. We also see intravascular hemolysis associated with hemolytic uremic syndrome occurring in about 10% of our patients on CsA following BMT,[7] and further studies are required to determine its pathogenesis.

The relationship between a raised serum bilirubin (due to liver dysfunction[8]) during the 3 months after BMT and subsequent death is curious and unexplained, particularly as the cause of death in these patients is not liver failure.

One of the more worrying potential side effects of CsA (and other powerful immunosuppressants) is the possibility that relapse of leukemia may occur more commonly in patients treated with this drug after transplantation due to a suppression of an antileukemic action of the allogeneic transplant. The low relapse rate (11%) in this series does not indicate that this occurs.

The development of new cancers in BMT patients on CsA is a possibility that we have been aware of for some time. Two young patients out of a total of 180 receiving CsA developed a new cancer (one a high grade astrocytoma, the other carcinoma of the rectum), but there is no indication that this was due to a carcinogenic effect of CsA and almost certainly was a consequence of the conditioning regimens. More patients with much longer follow-up will clarify this point.

No patients in this series developed a lymphoma, unlike some patients receiving CsA immunosuppression for other organ transplants.[9] This is probably because our patients develop excellent T-lymphocyte surveillance of EB virus-infected B-lymphocyte proliferation within a few weeks of transplant in spite of being on CsA.[10] Such T-cell surveillance is defective in other organ transplant recipients on CsA[11] and results in the rare but significant occurrence in these patients of lymphomas of B-cell origin.[12]

We have not included data in this report on serum levels of CsA in our patients in spite of having conducted over 3000 assays. The reason is that we have found the assay of very little clinical use, and although many groups refer to a "therapeutic range," no hard data at present exist for such statements, certainly in relation to GVHD. The relationship of serum levels with toxicity is more definite but has not been useful clinically because it has proved easier to use the toxic side effects themselves for determining the dose of the drug. These observations on blood level determinations of the drug are not grounds for pessimism—within the pharmacopeia, no useful drug exists that relies for its administration on determination of blood levels. Obviously it is vital to understand the pharmacodynamics of CsA, but the long-term prospects of CsA's becoming a standard drug in medical practice depends much more on learning, as with all new drugs, how its administration may be correctly judged by clinical methods alone.

ACKNOWLEDGMENT

R.P. would like to thank Peter Alexander in this project for enthusiasm, intellectual drive, and regular use of punitive discipline.

REFERENCES

1. Powles RL, Barrett AJ, Clink H, et al: Lancet 3:1327, 1978

2. Calne RY, White DJG, Thiru S, et al: Lancet 2:1323, 1978

3. Powles RL, Clink HM, Spence D, et al: Lancet 1:327, 1980

4. Powles RL, Morgenstern GR, Kay HEM, et al: Lancet 1:612, 1983

5. Hedley D, Powles RL, Morgenstern GR: In White DJG (ed): Cyclosporin A. Amsterdam, Elsevier Biomedical, 1982, pp 545–551

6. Morgenstern GR, Powles RL, Robinson B., et al: Lancet 2:1342, 1982
7. Mackenzie JC, Lumley HS, Hughes RG, et al: Exp Haematol 11 (Suppl. 13):18, 1983
8. Farthing JJG, Clark ML, Sloane JP, et al: Gut 23:465, 1982
9. Calne RY, Rolles K, White DJG, et al: Lancet 2:1033, 1979
10. Crawford DH, Powles RL, Iliescu V, et al: Exp Haematol 11 (Suppl. 13):113, 1983
11. Crawford DH, Sweny P, Edwards JMB, et al: Lancet 1:10, 1981
12. Crawford DH, Thomas JA, Janossy G, et al: Lancet 1:1355, 1980

Use of Cyclosporine as Prophylaxis of Graft-vs.-Host Disease After Human Allogeneic Bone Marrow Transplantation: Report of 38 Patients

E. Gluckman, A. Devergie, O. Poirier, and F. Lokiec

CYCLOSPORINE A (CsA) is a potent immunosuppressive drug that has little or no marrow toxicity.[1] It inhibits the first step of T-cell activation by inhibition of T helper cells for antibody production to T-dependent antigens.[2] It inhibits the generation of cytotoxic T cells induced in allogeneic mixed lymphocyte reaction and abrogates the concanavalin A–induced suppressor-cell function.[3,4] CsA has been shown to render T cells unresponsive to IL-1 and IL-2 and to inhibit the synthesis of these growth factors.[5]

The efficacy of CsA has been well established in human kidney, liver, and heart transplants.[6–8] In bone marrow transplantation (BMT), its efficacy has been questioned because its use has been limited by its nephrotoxicity.[9,10] In a preliminary report, we described the high indicence of nephrotoxicity observed in 13 patients.[11] We described the influence of the addition of other nephrotoxic drugs such as amphotericin B or aminoglycosides and non-nephrotoxic drugs such as ketoconazole as factors that increased the risk of renal failure.[12] We therefore performed pharmacokinetic studies using a radioimmunoassay (RIA) that showed the individual variability of the metabolism of the drug.[13] A test-dose method was investigated to predict the dose necessary to obtain a given plateau concentration of CsA.[14] A series of 38 consecutive patients was treated with cyclosporine A given in continuous i.v. infusion, then orally for at least 6 months. The initial i.v. dose was calculated individually according to a preliminary pharmacokinetic study. Results are reported in this article.

From the Bone Marrow Transplant Unit (E.G., A.D.) and the Department of Nuclear Medicine (O.P.), Centre Hayem, Hospital Saint-Louis, Paris, and the Centre René Huguénin, Saint-Cloud (F.L.), France.

Reprint requests should be addressed to E. Gluckman, Bone Marrow Transplant Unit, Centre Hayem, Hospital Saint-Louis, 2 place du Dr. A. Fournier, F-75475 Paris CEDEX 10, France.

0041–1345/83/0081$01.00/0

MATERIALS AND METHODS

Patients

The trial was performed from September 1981 to December 1982. Thirty-eight consecutive patients received an allogeneic BMT from an HLA-identical sibling donor and were treated for prevention of graft-versus-host disease (GVHD) by CsA. There were 14 patients with severe aplastic anemia (SAA), 6 with Fanconi anemia (FA), 12 with chronic granulocytic leukemia (CGL) (4 in accelerated phase), and 6 with acute myelogenous leukemia (AML) in first complete remission. The ages ranged from 2–37 years (median, 16). There were 23 male and 15 female patients.

Bone Marrow Transplant Procedure

Conditioning. Patients with SAA were conditioned with cyclophosphamide 150 mg/kg followed by a 6-Gray thoracoabdominal irradiation.[15] Patients with FA were conditioned with cyclophosphamide 20 mg/kg and 5-Gray thoracoabdominal irradiation,[16] and patients with leukemia with cyclophosphamide 120 mg/kg and 10-Gray total-body irradiation; the lungs were shielded to receive a maximum dose of 8 Gray. The patients received 2–7.8 $\times$ 10^8 cells/kg from an HLA-identical sibling on day 0 of transplant.

Supportive care. All patients were isolated in laminar air-flow rooms from day -8 to at least 35 days after BMT. On day -8, they were started on Ketoconazole 400 mg p.o. per day for prophylaxis of fungal infections. Oral nonabsorbable antibiotics—Cephalosporin, Bacitracin, and Gentamicin—were given for total gut decontamination as long as the patients were isolated. Oral acyclovir (800 mg/day) was given to half the patients in a double-blind placebo-controlled study for prophylaxis of herpes infection from day -8 to day 35.[17] Fever above 38°C was treated with broad-spectrum antibiotics, usually Vancomycin, Latamoxef, and Amikacin, or according to the results of bacterial isolation. Persisting fever of unknown origin was treated with Amphotericin B 0.1–0.2 mg/kg/day. All blood products were irradiated at 25 Gray.

Evaluation criteria. Engraftment was documented through marrow cellularity, blood counts, and study of genetic markers. GVHD was classified according to the Seattle criteria and proved by skin and/or gut biopsies.[18] All patients were monitored as to daily blood counts, urea, creatinine, electrolytes in blood and urine, twice weekly liver function tests, coagulation tests, weekly chest roentgenogram, viral serology, and CMV viremia.

Administration of CsA

In a preliminary study, 13 patients received from day −1 to day 5 a daily i.m. dose of 20 mg/kg, followed by 12.5 mg/kg/day p.o. divided in three doses. This study was interrupted because of the high incidence of nephrotoxicity observed in 7/13 patients; 3 patients with anuria required dialysis.[19] For this reason, pharmacokinetic studies, using RIA, were performed in a series of 15 patients comparing plasma levels observed after a single dose of CsA administered i.v. or p.o. This study showed a large variability of maximum plasma concentration and clearance of CsA from patient to patient. Furthermore, there was no correlation between the maximum CsA concentration obtained by i.v. or p.o. routes when they were studied in the same patient. Ketoconazole significantly increased the maximum concentration of CsA.[12] There was no correlation between plasma levels and nephrotoxicity. In the face of such individual variability of plasma CsA concentration, we designed a prospective study using a test-dose method with the aim of calculating the dose necessary to obtain a given plasma level of CsA. In this study all patients had a preliminary pharmacokinetic study performed before conditioning. They were given 4 mg/kg i.v. over a 2-hr period, and plasma levels were measured at 10 and 30 min and 1, 2, 4, 6, and 12 hr after the infusion. The dose was calculated according to the following formula: $Q = Cl \times C \times t$ (Q = dose of CsA to administer to the patient, Cl = plasma CsA clearance, C = desired plasmatic concentration, t = duration of the course).

CsA was given as a continuous i.v. infusion from day −1 to day 15. After day 15, it was given p.o.; the oral dose was twice the last i.v. dose, assuming that gut absorption was 50%. The dose was modified according to urea, creatinine, and plasma CsA levels. It was given for at least 3 months and then decreased slowly acccrding to GVHD symptoms and tolerance. Ten patients received an i.v. dose calculated to obtain a plateau at 700 ng/ml (Group 1), 21 patients a dose calculated to obtain a plateau at 200 ng/ml (Group 2), and 7 patients a dose calculated to obtain a plateau at 100 ng/ml (Group 3), When GVHD was observed, the dose of CsA was doubled if possible, and methylprednisolone was added at the dose of 2–5 mg/kg for a week and then tapered off. If GVHD progressed despite this treatment, it was treated either with antithymocyte globulin (ATG; Mérieux, France) or a monoclonal pan-T antibody (OKT3; Ortho). This protocol has been approved by the ethics committee of our institution.

RESULTS

Overall Results

Overall results are summarized in Table 1. All patients had a prompt marrow engraftment; 30 survived more than 100 days, with a follow-up ranging from 130–555 days (median follow-up time, 240 days). Eight patients died: 4 from acute GVHD (associated with interstitial pnemonitis in 3 cases); 1 from liver veno-occlusive disease, renal failure, and cerebral hemorrhage; 1 from leukemic relapse; 1 from pulmonary infection; and 1 from hepatic necrosis related to HbS Ag hepatitis. GVHD was observed in 32 cases (84%), grade I-II in 22 cases (57.8%) and grade III–IV in 10 cases (26.3%). It was treated with methylprednisolone and resolved in 22 cases without additional immunosuppression. In 10 cases, ATG or OKT3 was given, with a good result in 6 cases. Ultimately, the mortality related to GVHD was 10% (4/38 patients). Chronic GVHD was observed in 8/30 patients at risk who survived more than 100 days (26%). It was usually mild, limited to localized lichen planus like eruption of skin or mucosae,

Table 1. Overall Results

				Graft-vs.-Host Disease				
	No. of Patients	Renal Toxicity	Hypertension	Grade 0	Grade I–II	Grade III–IV	Chronic	Survivors > 100 Days
Group 1	10	9 (90%)	6	3	5	2	3/7	7 (70%)
Group 2	21	17 (80%)	11	2	12	7	4/16	16 (76%)
Group 3	7	4 (57%)	5	1	5	1	1/7	7 (100%)
Total	38	30 (79%)	22 (57.8%)	6 (15%)	22 (57.8%)	10 (26.3%)	8/30 (26%)	30 (79%)

centrations, of the drug are modified by liver dysfunction and drug interactions.[20] Several drugs, such as Ketoconazole[12,21] and Dilantin, increase the CsA levels; other drugs, such as phenytoin, phenobarbital, and Cimetidine, seem to decrease the CsA levels. Some drugs, such as aminoglycosides, Amphotericin B, and Cotrimoxazole,[22] seem to induce a synergistic nephrotoxicity. The distribution and binding of CsA has been well studied,[23,24] and the plasma concentration assay measures only a small fraction of CsA that is preferentially bound to membrane lipoproteins.

Our pharmacokinetic study had shown the large variability of absorption and clearance of CsA and the interaction with Ketoconazole. For this reason, we used the i.v. form given in continuous infusion in order to avoid the variability related to intestinal absorption and to obtain a constant level of CsA. The optimal plasma concentration for adequate immunosuppression is not known. It seems that complete suppression of lymphocyte proliferation was observed with sera containing >300 ng/ml of CsA as measured by RIA, with abrogation of CTL generation above 400 ng/ml.[20] We first tried to obtain a plateau at 700 ng/ml, and because of the high incidence of nephrotoxicity, the dose was decreased to 200 ng/ml and to 100 ng/ml because it is generally accepted that a plasma level of 100–200 ng/ml is satisfactory. This approach was not fully successful because nephrotoxicity was still observed, but it was not as severe as described by other authors, and none of the patients required dialysis for CsA-induced renal toxicity. It seemed that the cumulative dose of CsA during the first 15 days was not correlated with the nephrotoxicity, although it correlated with GVHD. The mean dose of 2 mg/kg we used is inferior to the dose used by others teams.[25–27] The diminution of the dose did not modify our results, as compared to the others. This was perhaps due to the fact that all our patients were on Ketoconazole. The monitoring of the plasma level of CsA did not correlate with nephrotoxicity or with GVHD. This could be due to technical problems because recently it has been demonstrated that plasma levels could be modified by temperature, CsA concentrations, hematocrit, and composition as well as concentration of lipoproteins.[28] Other methods using high-pressure liquid chromatography (HPLC) or measurement of whole blood CsA using RIA may be helpful.[29]

The mechanism of renal toxicity is unknown, and there are few data on histopathological examination. It seems that renal failure was due to acute tubular necrosis. There was no indication of immune complex damage, nor evidence of acute glomerulonephritis.[9] Some authors reported the presence of thrombosis in the capillary tufts and the arterioles of the hilum of glomeruli,[30] and others described giant mitochondria. In our autopsy material, we found changes compatible with tubulopathy. The mechanism of hemolytic and uremic syndrome[31] and hypertension is also very poorly understood. It seems to interfere with the renin-angiotensin-aldosterone system.[32] The efficacy of cyclosporine A on the prevention and treatment of GVHD has been questioned. Nevertheless, some reports seem very encouraging. It decreases the rate of rejection in SAA.[33] For prevention of GVHD, it seems that the total incidence of acute GVHD was not modified when it was compared to a MTX-treated group.[10] In our own experience, the severity of GVHD was decreased and was more easily controlled by the addition of methylprednisolone. The incidence and severity of chronic GVHD was decreased, and the quality of long-term survival was improved, in the group of patients treated with CsA.

In conclusion, there are still many questions to be answered concerning the optimal use of cyclosporine A, such as the dose and way of administration, pharmacokinetic monitoring, and mechanism of toxicity. In our hands, its utilization led to a real improvement related to a diminution of early complications of aplasia, diminution of length of hospitalization, and decrease in the severity of both acute and chronic GVHD.

REFERENCES

1. Gordon MY, Singer JW: Nature 279:433, 1979
2. Ryffel B, Götz U, Heuberger B: J Immunol 129:1978, 1982
3. Hess AD, Donnenberg AD, Tutschka PJ: J Immunol 130:717, 1983
4. Hess AD, Tutschka PJ: J Immunol 124:2601, 1980
5. Bunjes D, Harot C, Röllinghoff M, et al: Eur J Immunol 11:657, 1981
6. Calne RY, Rolles K, White DJG, et al: Lancet 2:1033, 1979
7. Calne RY, White DJG, Evans DB, et al: Br Med J 282:934, 1981
8. Reitz BA, Wallwork JL, Hunt SA, et al: In White DJG (ed): Cyclosporin A. Amsterdam, Elsevier Biomedical, 1982, p 473
9. Tutschka PJ, Beschorner WE, Hess AD, et al: Blood 61:318, 1983
10. Barrett AJ, Kendra JR, Lucas CF: Br Med J 285:162, 1982
11. Gluckman E, Arcese W, Devergie A, et al: Transplant Proc 13:368, 1981
12. Lokiec F, Poirier O, Gluckman E: In Touraine JL, Gluckman E, Griscelli C (eds): Symposia Foundation Mérieux 6. Amsterdam, Excerpta Medica, 1981, p 160
13. Lokiec F, Poirier O, Gluckman E, et al: In White DJG (ed): Cyclosporin A. Amsterdam, Elsevier Biomedical, 1982, p 497
14. Lokiec F, Poirier O, Devergie A, et al: Exp Hematol 11 (Suppl. 13):40, 1983
15. Devergie A,Gluckman E: Exp Hematol 10 (Suppl. 10):17, 1982
16. Gluckman E. Devergie A, Dutreix J: Br J Haematol 54:431, 1983
17. Gluckman E, Lotsberg J, Devergie A: J Antimicrob Chemotherapy (in press)
18. Glucksberg H, Storb R, Fefer A: Transplantation 18:295, 1974
19. Gluckman E, Devergie A, Lokiec F: Lancet 2:144, 1981
20. Keown PA, Stiller CR, Laupacis AL: Transplant Proc 14:659, 1982
21. Diererink H, Möller J: Lancet 2:1218, 1982 (letter)
22. Kennedy MS, Deeg HJ, Siegel M, et al: Transplantation 35:211, 1983
23. Beveridge T, Gratwohl A, Michot F: Curr Therapeut Res 30:5, 1981
24. Hows JM, Palmer S, Want S: Lancet 2:145, 1981
25. Powles RI, Clink HM, Spence D, et al: Lancet 2:327, 1980
26. Speck B, Gratwohl A, Nissen C: In Baum SJ, Ledney CD, Kahn A (eds): Exp Hematol Today. Basel, S Karger, 1981, p 117
27. Atkinson K, Biggs JC, Ting A: Br J Haematol 53:265, 1983
28. Nussbaumer K, Niederberger W, Keller HP: J HRC and CL 5:424, 1982
29. Abisch E, Beveridge T, Gratwohl A: Pharmaceutical Weekblad (Scientific Edition) 4:84, 1982
30. Shulman H, Striker G, Deeg HJ: N Engl J Med 305:1392, 1981
31. Hamilton DV, Calne RY, Evans DB: Lancet 2:151, 1982
32. Siegl H, Ryffel B: Lancet 2:1274, 1982
33. Hows J, Harris R, Palmer S: Br J Haematol 48:227, 1981

Postgraft Immunosuppression with Cyclosporine in Allogeneic Bone Marrow Transplantation for Severe Aplastic Anemia

J. M. Hows, J. L. Yin, P. M. Chipping, S. M. Fairhead, S. Palmer, and E. C. Gordon-Smith

ALLOGENEIC bone marrow transplantation remains the first choice of therapy for patients with severe aplastic anemia (SAA) who have a histocompatible family donor. Since the mid 1970s, improved immunosuppressive regimens have reduced the incidence of bone marrow graft failure in aplastic transplant patients. Modified total body irradiation[1] and total lymphoid irradiation[2] are both effective in reducing graft failure. In Seattle, the use of buffy coat infusions from the bone marrow donor in the postgraft period has also been successful.[3]

Modified total body irradiation[1] and the use of buffy coat infusions[3] are both associated with an increased incidence of graft-vs.-host disease. The use of irradiation may have long-term consequences such as sterility and malignancy.[4] In addition, patients irradiated in childhood may fail to grow normally. To avoid the complications of irradiation and buffy coat infusions, we have studied the effect of cyclosporine A (CsA) on graft failure and graft-vs.-host disease in a series of multiply transfused patients transplanted for SAA.

MATERIALS AND METHODS

Patients

Thirty-five patients aged 3–43 years (median, 20 years) were studied. All received marrow from mixed lymphocyte reaction-negative family donors. Thirty-three patients had human leukocyte antigen (HLA)-A, B, and DR–identical sibling donors. Patients 16 and 35 were transplanted from HLA-identical parents, and patient 22 received marrow from her mother, who was mismatched at the A locus. All 35 patients fulfilled the criteria for SAA,[5] and all had received blood transfusions prior to transplantation. Thirty-three patients had received more than 10 units of blood before admission to the hospital for bone marrow transplantation. The length of time between diagnosis and transplantation was 3–208 weeks (median, 16 weeks).

From Department of Hematology, Royal Postgraduate Medical School, Du Cane Road, London W12.

Reprint requests should be addressed to Dr. J. M. Hows.

0041–1345/83/1505–0082$01.00/0

Pregraft Conditioning Chemotherapy

Cyclophosphamide 50 mg/kg/day was given on days −5 to −2 inclusive. Patients 15, 16, and 22 received procarbazine 12.5 mg/kg on days −6, −4, and −2 and antilymphocyte globulin (Mérieux) 12.5 mg/kg on days −7, −5, and −3.

Cyclosporine A

A loading dose was commenced on day −1, 12.5 mg/kg twice daily. On day 3, maintenance treatment was started with 6.25 mg/kg twice daily. Maintenance treatment was continued for 6 months, then tapered off over the subsequent 2–3 months.

Pharmacological Monitoring

Trough (12-hr) serum CsA levels were measured three times weekly by radioimmunoassay[6] while patients were in the hospital and once weekly thereafter.

Isolation and Decontamination

Isolation and decontamination procedures were carried out as previously described.[7]

RESULTS

Marrow Cell Dose

A total of 1.5–5.1 × 10^9/kg (median, 3.1 × 10^9/kg) nucleated marrow cells were infused.

Survival

Twenty-six of 35 patients survive (74%) 7–42 months after transplantation (median survival, 18 months). The actuarial survival of this group of patients is shown in Fig. 1 and is compared with the survival of 14 similar aplastic patients transplanted at the Hammersmith Hospital in 1975 and 1979.[8] The retrospective group of aplastic patients were

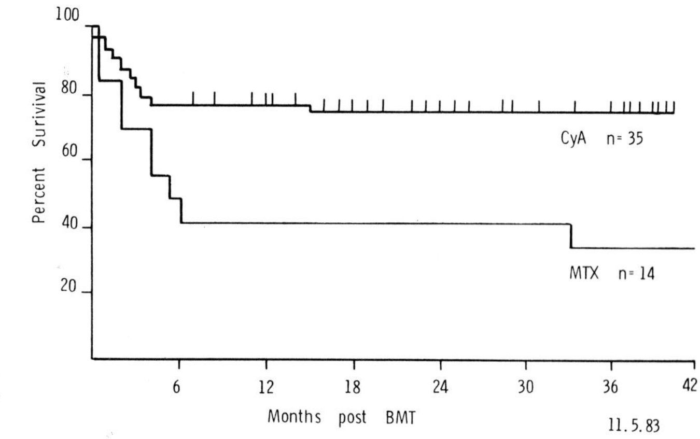

Fig. 1. Bone marrow transplantation for severe aplastic anemia. (Actuarial survival.)

treated with methotrexate in the postgraft period.

Cause of Death

Four patients died from acute graft-vs.-host disease (GVHD) and two from infection following primary graft failure. Three additional patients died from infection.

Graft-vs.-Host Disease

Thirty-two of 35 patients achieved stable engraftment. Of these, 21 (66%) developed acute GVHD. Severe disease (grade III–IV)[9] occurred in 11 patients (34%). In all patients who developed acute GVHD, CsA was continued. If severe gastrointestinal GVHD occurred, CsA was administered intravenously. The dose range was 2–5 mg/kg/day. Fifteen patients required additional immunosuppression for acute GVHD. High-dose methylprednisolone (HDMP) 20 mg/kg/day was given by i.v. bolus injection. The indication for commencing HDMP was progressive acute GVHD of grade II or more. Chronic GVHD occurred in 9 out of the 28 patients who survived >100 days after transplantation. Four patients required short courses of low-dose prednisolone (20–40 mg/day) and azathioprine for chronic GVHD. Without exception, chronic GVHD was mild and usually confined to the skin and mucous membranes.

Graft Failure

Three patients failed to engraft (primary graft failure). Two died from infection after failed retransplantation. The third patient was successfully retransplanted from the same donor. In all three cases, the nucleated bone marrow cell dose was suboptimal (2.0, 2.1, and 2.6 × 10^9/kg).

Six patients developed late graft failure 3–7 months after transplantation, following a period of established engraftment without blood-product support (Table 1). In 5 out of 6 cases, late graft failure was associated with withdrawal of CsA maintenance therapy.

CsA Toxicity

The toxic side effects attributed to CsA and the relationship of toxicity to trough serum levels of the drug are shown in Table 2.

DISCUSSION

The actuarial survival of 35 aplastic patients transplanted using CsA for postgraft immunosuppression was 74%, 7–42 months after transplantation. This result compared favorably with recently reported series where total lymphoid irradiation[2] and postgraft buffy coat infusions[3] were used to improve engraftment. Despite multiple-transfusion therapy before transplantation in 33/35 patients, only three primary graft failures occurred (9%). The higher incidence of late graft failure was closely associated with withdrawal of CsA therapy. This is an indication that maintenance therapy should be continued for longer than 6 months after transplantation in aplastic patients. In a small series of

Table 1. Late Graft Failure

Patient No.	Sex of Donor and Recipient	Duration of Graft (months)	CsA Status	Additional Factors	Treatment	Outcome
2	F → M	7	Off CsA for 4/52 weeks	None	CsA → HDMP*	Graft recovered xy → xx alive >3 years
7	M → F	5	Off CsA (noncompliance)	None	CsA HDMP	Autologous recovery xx → xy → xx alive >3 years
22	F → F	6	Reducing CsA trough serum level <60 ng/ml	Viral infection, positive direct antiglobulin test	CsA HDMP	Graft recovered (HLA marker) alive >1.5 years
25	F → M	7.5	Off CsA for 5/52 weeks	None	CyA, HDMP ATG + marrow	Poor autologous recovery xy → xx → xy alive >1 year
26	F → M	4	On CsA trough serum level 350 ng/ml	None	CsA ATG + marrow	Partial autologous recovery, good marrow function alive >1 year
27	M → M	7	Off CsA for 4/52 weeks	None	CsA Prednisolone 1 mg/kg	Autologous recovery (red cell marker) alive >1 year

*High-dose methylprednisolone 20 mg/kg by i.v. bolus.

patients transplanted for SAA in whom CsA was continued for 1 year, late graft failure after withdrawal of the drug was not seen.[10] The incidence of acute GVHD was high (66%). Although 4 patients (11%) died from acute GVHD, progression to chronic GVHD was uncommon, and long-term disability from chronic GVHD did not occur.

The most serious side effect of CsA seen was nephrotoxicity, often associated with

Table 2. Toxic Side Effects of CsA in 35 Bone Marrow Transplant Patients

Side Effect	No. of Patients Affected	Relationship to Serum Levels	Reversibility	Contributing Factors/Drugs
Nephrotoxicity* 0–4 weeks	5	Yes +++	Yes	Aminoglycosides, Vancomycin, Ketoconazole, Amphotericin B (both nephrotoxicity rows)
4–36 weeks	3	Yes ++	Yes	
Fluid retention	15	No	Yes	Methylprednisolone (fluid retention, hypertension, convulsions)
Hypertension	12	Yes	Yes	
Convulsions	4	No	Yes	
Tremor	6	Yes	Yes	? Lithium
Hyperbilirubinemia		Yes	Yes	Erythromycin, Ketoconazole, Androgens, GVHD
Hirsutism	Most	No	Yes	Minoxidal
Gastrointestinal	Most (mild)	No	Yes	GVHD, Cyclophosphamide

*Plasma creatinine >200 μmole/liter for >48 hr.

hypertension (Table 2). Nephrotoxicity correlated with high trough CsA serum levels.[10] With careful monitoring of serum CsA levels and renal function, the incidence of clinically severe nephrotoxicity was acceptable.

SUMMARY

Cyclosporine A is a useful postgraft immunosuppressive agent in bone marrow transplantation for SAA. Its use is associated with a low incidence of primary graft failure. Late graft failure was associated with withdrawal of CsA therapy. CsA does not prevent acute GVHD in aplastic transplant patients; however, morbidity and mortality from progressive chronic GVHD was not seen in this group of patients.

REFERENCES

1. Ramsay NKC, Trewan K, Nesbit ME, et al: Blood 55:344, 1980

2. UCLA Bone Marrow Transplant Team: Blood 57:9, 1981

3. Storb R, Doney KC, Thomas ED, et al: Blood 59:236, 1982

4. Barrett A: Clin Radiol 33:131, 1982

5. Camitta BM, Thomas ED, Nathan DG, et al: Blood 48:63, 1976

6. Donatsch P, Abisch E, Homberger M, et al: J Immunoassay 2:19, 1981

7. Hows JM, Palmer S, Gordon-Smith EC: Transplantation 33:382, 1982

8. Hows JM, Harris R, Palmer S, et al: Br J Haematol 48:22, 1981

9. Glucksberg H, Storb R, Fefer A, et al: Transplantation 18:295, 1974

10. Speck B, Gratwohl A, Nissen C, et al: In White DJG (ed): Cyclosporin A. Amsterdam, Elsevier Biomedical, 1982, p 491

11. Hows JM, Chipping PM, Fairhead S, et al: Br J Haematol 54: 1983

CLINICAL CASE PRESENTATIONS

The Management of Kidney Transplant Recipients Treated With Cyclosporine

B. D. Kahan

CASE NO. 1

THIS 50-year-old white male with a history of nephrolithiasis, renal hypoplasia, and hypertension leading to end-stage renal disease had been on hemodialysis since August 1980. The patient's illness began in 1953, when he developed recurrent nephrolithiasis, which was attributed to idiopathic hypercalcuria. In 1964, a left ureteral calculus was removed by a basket procedure. In 1970, he experienced severe hypertension with blood pressures as high as 285/185. Medical evaluation revealed a nonfunctioning, hypoplastic left kidney, and a 7-cm right kidney with a small right ureteral calculus. At the time of left nephrectomy, the 40-g kidney showed chronic glomerulonephritis with signs of superimposed pyelonephritis. Thereafter, renal insufficiency was documented with a blood urea nitrogen (BUN) of 32 mg/dl. Over the next 10 years, he had mild proteinuria, and his blood pressure was poorly controlled, with diastolic readings usually greater than 130. Finally, his blood pressure stabilized at 160/90 on a regimen of Aldomet, Guanethidine, Regitine, and Hydralazine. In June 1980, he developed anorexia, nausea, vomiting, malaise, fatigue, and lower extremity edema, and was begun on hemodialysis in August 1980. The patient's early course on dialysis was complicated by pericarditis, not requiring surgical intervention. His later course was complicated by severe neuropathy. He voids approximately 8 oz of urine a day and gains 5–11 pounds interdialytically. Dialyses proceed smoothly and are uncomplicated, except for lower extremity cramping during maximal ultrafiltration, and one episode of pulmonary edema in December 1980, because of dietary noncompliance. The patient's past history included: (1) glucose intolerance beginning in 1963, controlled with diet and hypoglycemic agents; (2) congestive heart failure in December 1979, treated with Digoxin; and (3) vascular calcifications in the vessels of the hands and lower extremities. Blood pressure was controlled at the time of transplant evaluation on Aldomet, 1 g/per day. Other medications included: Digoxin (0.125 mg qod), Diabinese, (100 mg tid), and Basalgel (2 tabs). The patient was maintained on a 1,800 calorie diabetic diet with sodium, potassium, cholesterol, and fluid restrictions.

On physical examination, positive findings included a moderately obese patient with a blood pressure of 170/100. There were pustules on his back, comedoes, and several de Morgan spots on his chest. Funduscopic examination revealed grade III Keith Wagner changes, copperwiring, nicking, and multiple hard exudates. Neurologic examination revealed loss of position sense in his distal lower extremities. Laboratory data included white blood cell count 14,000/mm^3, hemoglobin 10.4 g/dl, triglycerides 690 mg/dl, serum calcium 11 mg/dl, BUN 65 mg/dl, creatinine clearance 1 ml/min, and cytomegalovirus (CMV) titer positive 1:256. Urine cultures $\times 3$ showed no growth, but urinalysis showed marked pyuria. Voiding cystourethrogram was normal with no reflux. Echocardiogram showed concentric left ventricular hypertrophy and T-wave changes, suggesting lateral wall ischemia. Chest roentgenogram indicated ectasia of the aorta with prominence of

From the Division of Immunology and Organ Transplantation, Department of Surgery, University of Texas Medical School, Houston, TX.

Address reprint requests to Dr. B. D. Kahan, Division of Immunology and Organ Transplantation, Department of Surgery, University of Texas Medical School, Houston, TX 77030.

0041-1345/83/1504-0083$01.00/0

the ascending portion. Bone survey showed findings compatible with renal osteodystrophy.

The patient was accepted as a transplant candidate following right nephrectomy, which was advised due to the history of chronic infection, and following subtotal parathyroidectomy, which was advised due to the constellation of hypercalcemia, nephrolithiasis, metastatic calcification, and osteodystrophy. In February 1982, he underwent cadaveric renal transplantation and was randomized to receive azathioprine. His tissue typing was blood group A+ and HLA-A2,30; B13,27; Cw1,-; Dr1,7. He suffered an acute rejection episode that partially responded to steroid therapy. He then displayed progressive, irreversible chronic rejection associated with a severe steroid myopathy after two recyclings with prednisone that demanded withdrawal of

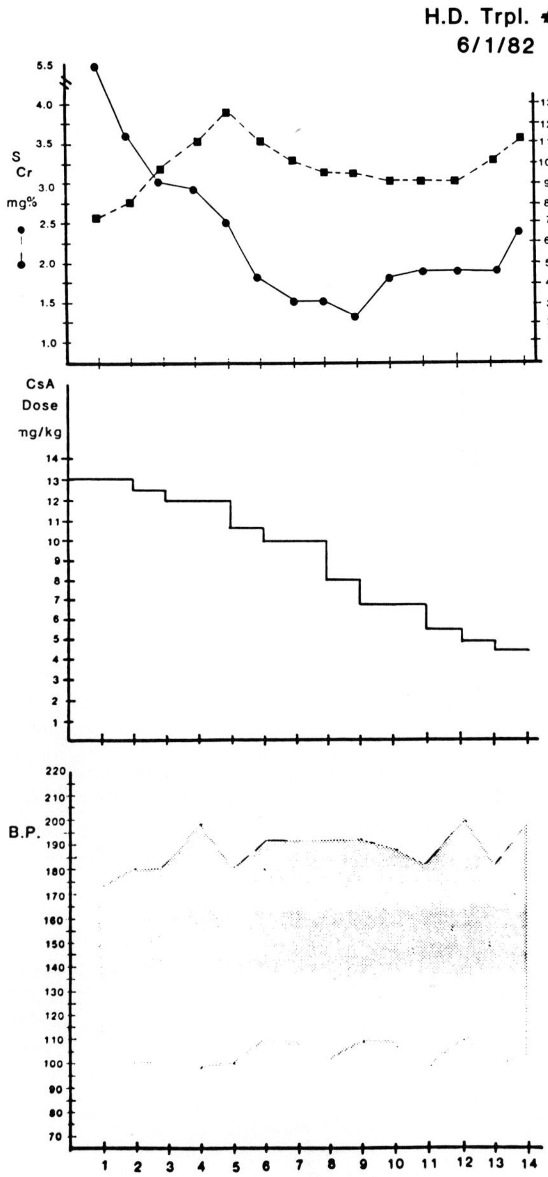

Fig. 1. Clinical course of the patient days 1–14 showing serum creatinine (mg/dl, —) and blood urea nitrogen (mg/dl, ---) in the upper panel, CsA dose (mg/kg) in the middle panel, and blood pressure shaded between systolic and diastolic readings (mm Hg) in the lower panel.

immunosuppression, transplant nephrectomy, and reinstitution of dialysis within three months.

One year later, on June 2, 1983, he underwent living-related donor transplantation from his son after being pretreated with oral cyclosporine (CsA) for three days. His immediate postoperative course revealed improvement of his serum creatinine to 1.4 mg/dl by day 9. However, on day 12 his creatinine rose to 2.1 mg/dl (Fig. 1). You will note that he had undergone a rapid CsA dose taper based on elevated serum levels. Figure 2 shows the profile of blood levels during the first 14 days. Beginning at day 4, the serum level rose and only by day 11 did it return to a lower level. A renal biopsy reported by Dr. Verani showed the picture of acute cellular rejection (Fig. 3). At this time, the urine protein was 0.30 g/24 hr, the maximum blood pressure (BP) 180/110 and stable, the urine volume approximately 1,000 cc (whereas before it was 1,800 cc), the liver function tests were normal with bilirubin 0.6 mg/dl, serum glutamic-oxalic transaminase 25 U, serum glutamic-pyruvic transaminase 93 U, alkaline phosphatase 154 U, WBC 30,000/cu mm, serum potassium 5.1 meq/liter, CO_2 28 meq/liter, and BUN 125 mg/dl. By day 15, the serum creatinine rose to 3.0. Noted was an elevated serum level of 324 ng/ml at the start of treatment.

Based on the biopsy, steroid therapy was begun, although there was little response to treatment. Indeed, several complications occurred. (1) On the 27th postoperative day, an urinary tract infection due to *Escherichia coli* was diagnosed and managed with tetracycline therapy because we wished to avoid Bactrim in order to avert synergistic nephrotoxicity. (2) There was marrow toxicity with WBC 23,000/mm^3 and 30 percent nucleated red cells on peripheral blood smear, then with the WBC falling to 7,000/mm^3. The platelets at this time fell to 22,000/mm^3. The patient was not febrile. Acyclovir was given for a suspected viral infection. Repeat renal biopsy on day 37 posttransplant showed persistent cellular changes with a diffuse mononuclear cell infiltrate extending into the tubular epithelium and endothelial hyperplasia with foamy cells and mononuclear cells. At this time, the CsA levels were low, therefore we tried to increase the drug dose to see if it helped, which it did not.

On day 93, the patient underwent conversion to azathioprine (AZA) by continuing

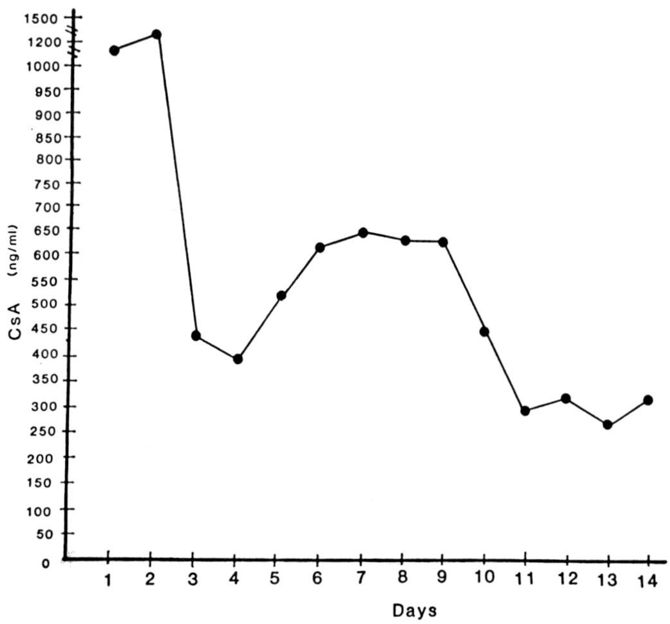

Fig. 2. The trough serum CsA levels (ng/ml) during the first 14 postoperative days.

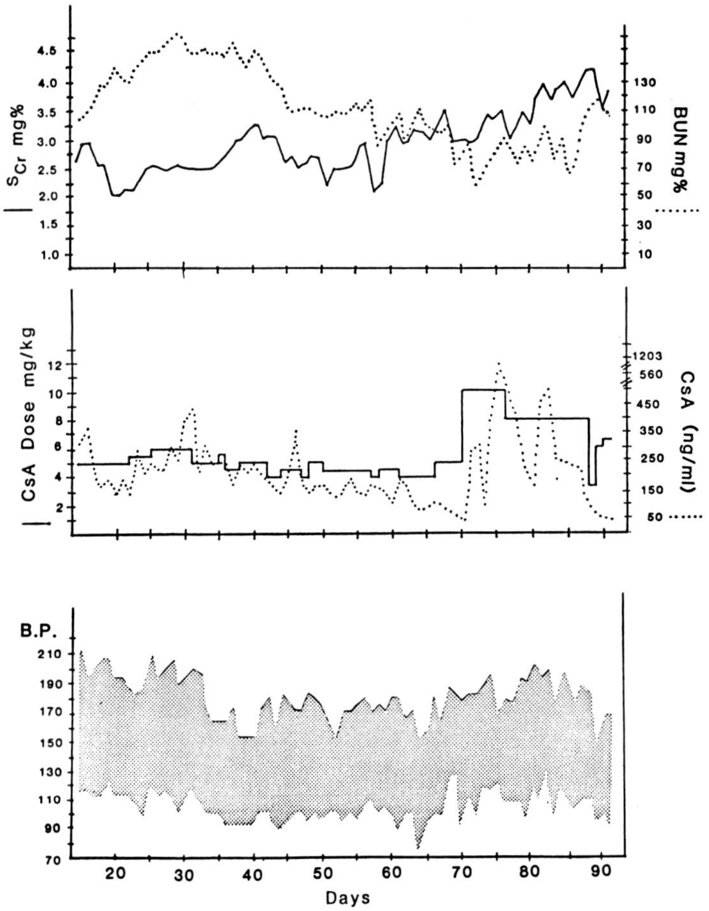

Fig. 3. The clinical course from day 15 to 90, continuing from Fig. 1, with the CsA trough serum level indicated in the middle panel (· · ·).

CsA at a 6-mg/kg dose and adding AZA at 2 mg/kg (Fig. 4). After five days, the CsA was tapered for two more days, then stopped; the AZA dose was readjusted to the tolerable level of about 2.5 mg/kg. The serum creatinine fell from 4.0 to 2.3 at 21 days after the beginning of conversion and 14 days after discontinuing CsA. Three months later, the serum creatinine was 1.6 and seven months later, namely 10 months postoperatively, it was 1.4, which has been stable.

The panelists all agreed that they would have treated the episode at day 12 as allograft rejection. They felt that the conversion from CsA to azathioprine was somewhat delayed. The case underscores the difficulty of diagnosing nephrotoxicity, particularly when serum levels are low, as well as the delayed response of improved renal function after conversion to azathioprine.

CASE NO. 2

A 29-year-old auto mechanic with known renal failure since 1978, secondary to chronic glomerulonephritis, experienced recent exacerbation of hypertension, and in January 1982, was found to be uremic. On physical examination he appeared fit. He had not been dialyzed and adamantly refused to undergo hemo- or peritoneal dialysis. His blood pressure at this time was 150/90. Laboratory data indicated white blood cell count 7,100/cu mm, hemoglobin 11.2 g/dl, hematocrit 33.0%, creatinine 8.8 mg/dl, BUN 114 mg/dl, urinary protein 0.78 g/24 hr, and creatinine clearance of 6.5 ml/min. CMV titer was

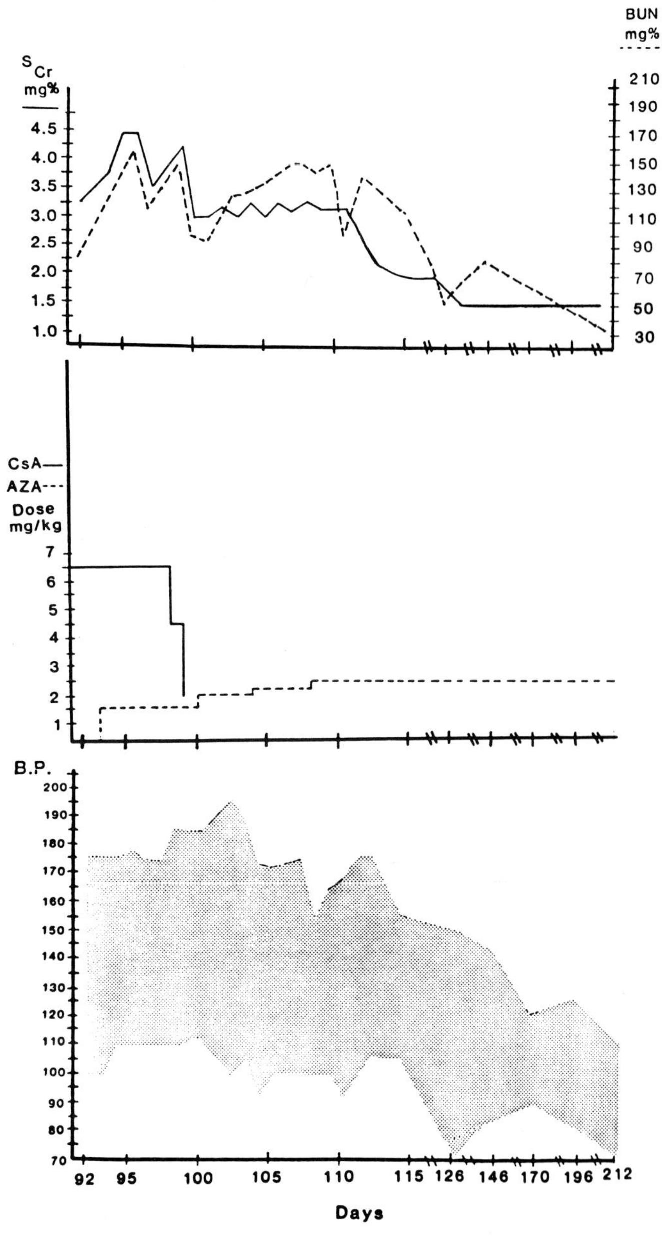

Fig. 4. The clinical course of the patient from day 92 to 212, continuing from Fig. 4. The middle panel shows the inception of azathioprine therapy at day 93.

1:512. Voiding cystourethrogram showed a small, left-sided bladder diverticulum; otherwise, the voiding cystourethrogram was normal. Two urine cultures showed no growth. Kidney tomogram showed no evidence of calcification. Bone survey and hand films were normal; there were findings equivocal for hyperparathyroidism in the distal clavicles. Tissue typing revealed ABO type B+ and HLA A23,-; B7,Bw50; Cw2,-; DR7,-. His brother's phenotype was ABO type B+ and HLA A26,A29; B52,B38; C-,-; DRw6Y,-. Donor-specific mixed lymphocyte culture (MLC) showed a stimulatory index of 65.0. Visual crossmatch using the patient's serum against the brother's peripheral blood lymphocytes (PBL) was negative at short (45 min) and long (90 min) incubation times. Reactivity of patient sera against separated donor PBL populations was negative against T cells at 37°C, B cells at 37°C, and B cells at 5°C. Comprehensive immune analysis utilizing ^{51}Cr-labeled donor PBL demonstrated the absence of donor-specific, lymphocyte-dependent antibody (LDA), complement-dependent antibody (CDA), and lymphocyte-mediated cytolysis (LMC). Similar tests against separated ^{51}Cr-labeled B-cell targets showed the LDA to be 0.5% and the CDA 3.8%; against separated ^{51}Cr-labeled T-cell targets, the LDA was 0.6% and the CDA 3.5%. Because these extensive crossmatch tests were entirely negative, suggesting the absence of presensitization in spite of high immunologic incompatibility, he underwent transplantation from the living-related donor.

In the postoperative period, his renal function slowly improved, with a fall in serum creatinine to 3.2 mg/dl and BUN 60 mg/dl at day 5 (Fig. 5). Because his tuberculin skin test was positive and there was an additional family history of the disease, he was placed on isoniazide and Rifampin postoperatively. On day 3 *Serratia marcescens* was cultured from his urine and he was treated with Bactrim. Over the succeeding days his serum creatinine rose to 5.9 mg/dl and BUN to 93 mg/dl. He was febrile once to 101.6°F on day 8 and he was persistently hypertensive, with a blood pressure of 200/100 postoperatively. There was 1.2 g/24 hr urinary protein. His liver function tests were unremarkable: bilirubin 0.1, serum glutamic-oxalic transferase 24, serum glutamic-pyruvic transferase 9, alkaline phosphatase 72. The white blood cell

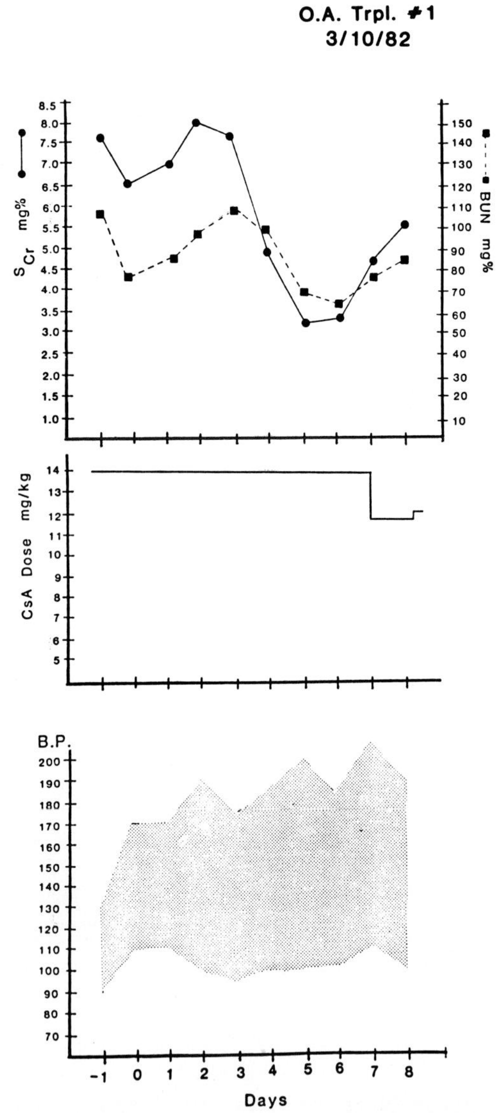

Fig. 5. The clinical course of the patient during the first eight days: upper panel shows serum creatinine (mg/dl, —) and blood urea nitrogen (mg/dl, ---); the middle panel shows the CsA dose (mg/kg); and the lower panel, the shaded area of blood pressure between systolic and diastolic (mm Hg).

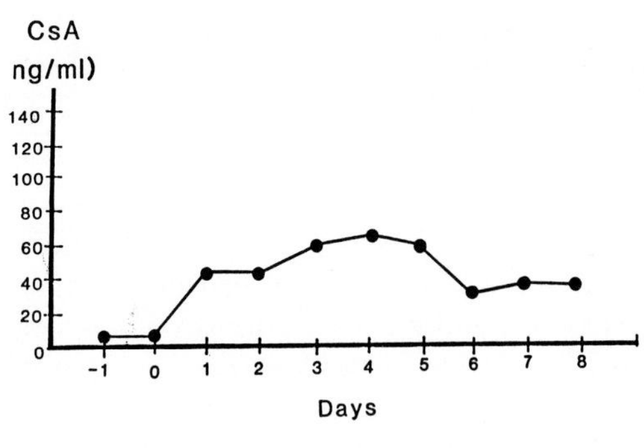

Fig. 6. Serial CsA serum trough levels (ng/ml) from the day prior to transplantation to eight days thereafter.

count remained 9,800/mm^3. Percutaneous renal biopsy showed acute cellular rejection. Analysis of CsA levels revealed that, in spite of the 14 mg/kg CsA orally, his trough level had remained low (Fig. 6). A full pharmacokinetic profile performed on day 5 showed inferior absorption, with a peak-to-trough ratio of 4.5, namely, it was inferred from these results that he had poor gastrointestinal absorption.

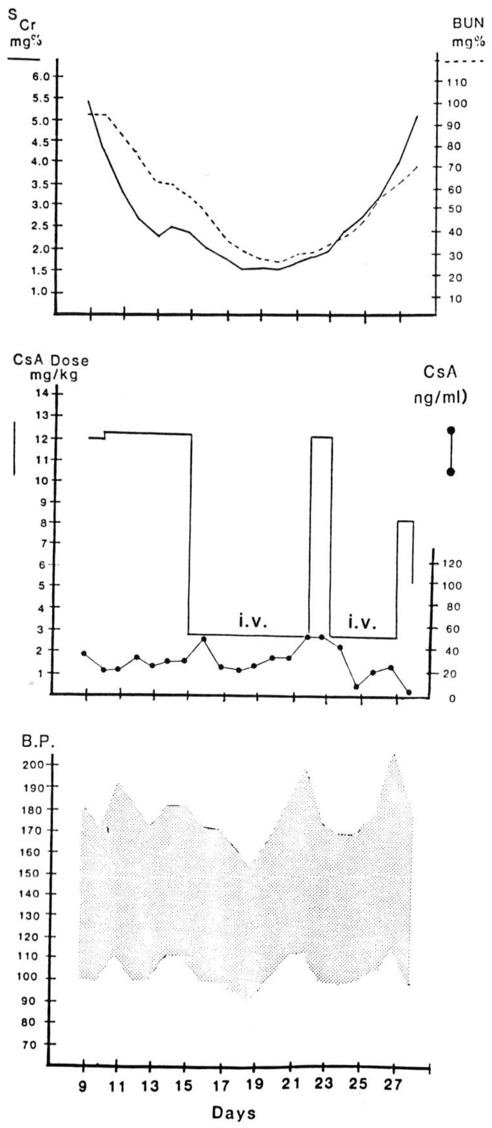

Fig. 7. The clinical course from day 9 to 28, continuing from Fig. 5.

Intravenous CsA was begun at 2.5 mg/kg/of body weight per day on day 16 (Fig. 7). The response to therapy was excellent, and the serum creatinine fell to 1.5 with BUN 30 by day 19. When the pharmacokinetic data showing poor absorption became available, they were repeated on day 14. When the data became available five days later, they demonstrated that the CsA absorption had improved: from a trough level of 36 the drug level increased to a peak of 695 ng/ml at 3 hr. Thus, on day 22, oral CsA therapy was reinsti-

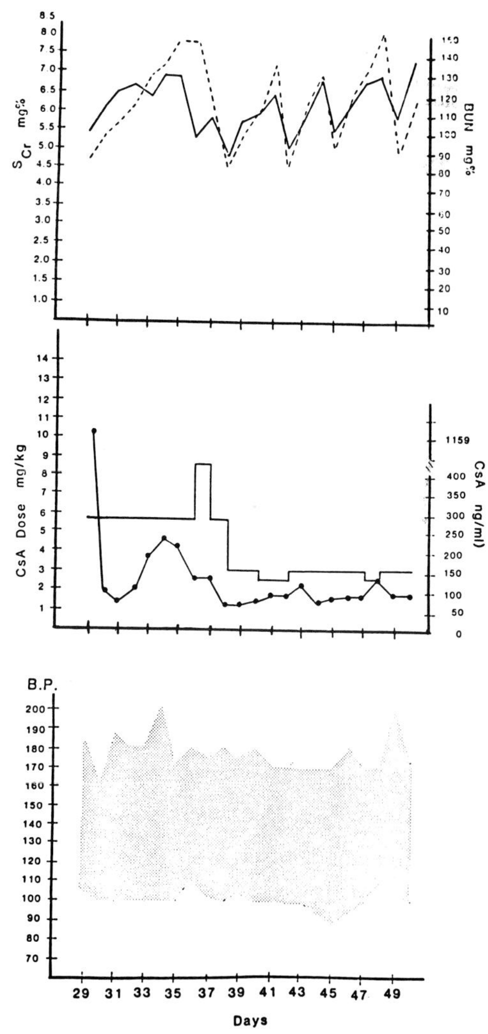

Fig. 8. The clinical course from day 29 to 50, continuing from Fig. 7.

tuted. However, the creatinine began to rise again at day 24, after just two days of oral therapy at 14 mg/kg. When the patient's serum creatinine rose to 3.2 mg/dl and BUN to 62 mg/dl, a renal biopsy was performed on day 28. There was a severe mononuclear infiltrate with hemorrhage into the interstitium; fibrin was deposited in glomeruli. Antirejection therapy was administered without benefit (Fig. 8). The graft, which was removed on day 60, showed parenchymal hemorrhage, infarction, and endothelial changes.

The panel believed that this patient had disturbed CsA absorption and probable rapid excretion due to the isoniazide and Rifampin and suggested conversion to azathioprine with possible adjunctive antilymphocyte serum therapy.

The Management of Heart Transplant Recipients Treated With Cyclosporine

B. D. Kahan

PATIENT NO. 1

THIS 49-year-old woman presented with a history of congestive heart failure that was heralded by the sudden onset of exertional dyspnea about two years prior to admission. In spite of treatment with cardiac glycosides, diuretic therapy, and afterload reduction, she progressively became worse. Over the last six months, her condition steadily deteriorated. At the time of presentation, she was New York Heart Association Functional class IV, complaining of dyspnea at rest and exertional dyspnea upon walking 30 feet. Prior to this time, she was active with a good marriage and satisfied with her life. As she now saw herself, she was unable to carry out her usual activities and faced fears of having to live a bedridden existence. This loss of control was depressing to her.

The patient's past medical history included a total abdominal hysterectomy five years prior, and plastic surgery of the left thumb. She admitted smoking two packs per day for the past 20 years, and weight loss from 150 to 110 pounds over the past 3 to 4 months. Her medications at the time of evaluation included Prazosin (1 mg t.i.d.), Lasix (40 mg q.d.), Aldactone (25 mg q.i.d.), Zaroxolyn (5 mg p.d.), and Digoxin (0.125 mg q.d.).

The blood pressure was 90/60, respirations 20, pulse 118, and weight 125 lbs. On physical examination, she presented with stigmata of right-sided heart failure: jugular venous distention; right-sided S3; right atrial pressure 13 cm H_2O; grade III/VI decrescendo murmur that increased with inspiration, best heard at the left lateral sternal margin; grade II/VI decrescendo systolic murmur best heard at the apex; and a pericardial friction rub. The liver span was 15 cm. In addition to hepatomegaly, there was 2+ pitting edema in the lower extremities.

The laboratory findings included WBC 7,800/mm^3, hematocrit (Hct) 41.6%, blood urea nitrogen (BUN) 32 mg/dl, total bilirubin 0.9 mg/dl, albumin 3.4 g/dl, serum creatinine 0.6 mg/dl, and creatinine clearance 60.9 ml/min. Electrocardiogram showed sinus tachycardia with left bundle branch block. A transvenous right endomyocardial biopsy showed focal myocardial fibrosis, lipomatosis, resolving nonspecific pericarditis, with no active inflammatory process. Chest roentgenogram showed parenchymal and hilar calcifications with an enlarged, calcified right paratracheal node. Echocardiogram in M-mode showed mild biatrial and right ventricular enlargement. Left ventricular performance study showed an ejection fraction of 12% with marked hypokinesis of both ventricles. On cardiac catheterization, there was moderate to marked left ventricular dilatation. The left and right atria were moderately dilated; there was mild pulmonary hypertension and global left ventricular dysfunction. The coronary arteries appeared normal. Upper gastrointestinal series showed calcified densities in the left lower quadrant of the abdomen, probably representing calcified mesenteric lymph nodes. The oral cholecystogram was normal. Pulmonary function studies revealed mild obstruction. All of the skin tests, including purified protein derivative (PPD), were negative. Preoperative immune assessment revealed 17.5% active T cells, spontaneous blastogenesis 11,685 cpm, panel mixed lymphocyte culture (MLC) stimulation index

From the Division of Immunology and Organ Transplantation, Department of Surgery, University of Texas Medical School, Houston, TX.

Address reprint requests to Dr. B. D. Kahan, Division of Immunology and Organ Transplantation, Department of Surgery, University of Texas Medical School, Houston, TX 77030.

0041-1345/83/1505-0084$2.00/0

25. The overall profile appeared to be that of a weak responder.

The initial impression was (1) idiopathic cardiomyopathy functional class IV with electrocardiogram stigmata of left bundle branch block; (2) a 30-pound weight loss without significant malnutrition; (3) elevated liver function tests, probably secondary to congestive liver dysfunction; (4) hyperuricemia; (5) status posthysterectomy, bilateral salpingo-oophorectomy; (6) no previous blood transfusions; (7) weak immune responder; (8) presence of autoantibodies, namely Coombs', anti-smooth muscle, and high titer positive antinuclear antibody, presumed to be secondary to hydralazine.

The patient was transplanted and came to the recovery room off pressors with a blood pressure of 150/85. Her initial course was relatively uneventful. She had endomyocardial biopsies at days 7 and 14 that were normal (Fig. 1). She was discharged on day 16 with an ejection fraction of 79% on Minipres 1 tab every 6 hr for mild hypertension, Lasix 40 mg/day for fluid retention, prednisone 50 mg daily, and cyclosporine 11 mg/kg of body weight with a serum trough level of 217 (Figs. 2 and 3). She reentered the hospital on day 24 due to a fever of 102.3°F, weight gain, and a right lower lobe infiltrate (Fig. 3). Bronchoscopy showed 4+ acid-fast bacilli. She was started on rifampin and isoniazid. It was noted that her trough serum cyclosporine value fell from 200 ng/ml to 33 ng/ml on this regimen (Fig. 4), a finding attributed to P450 induction. Because she was still febrile 72 hr later, she underwent endomyocardial biopsy (Fig. 5). We elected to treat the rejection, diagnosed on biopsy, with increased steroids (Fig. 6) and to add ethambutal to cover the infection due to *Mycobacterium tuberculosis*. In addition, the cyclosporine dose was increased. For example, on day 46, the level was 172 ng/ml, and on day 47 it was 390 ng/ml. The

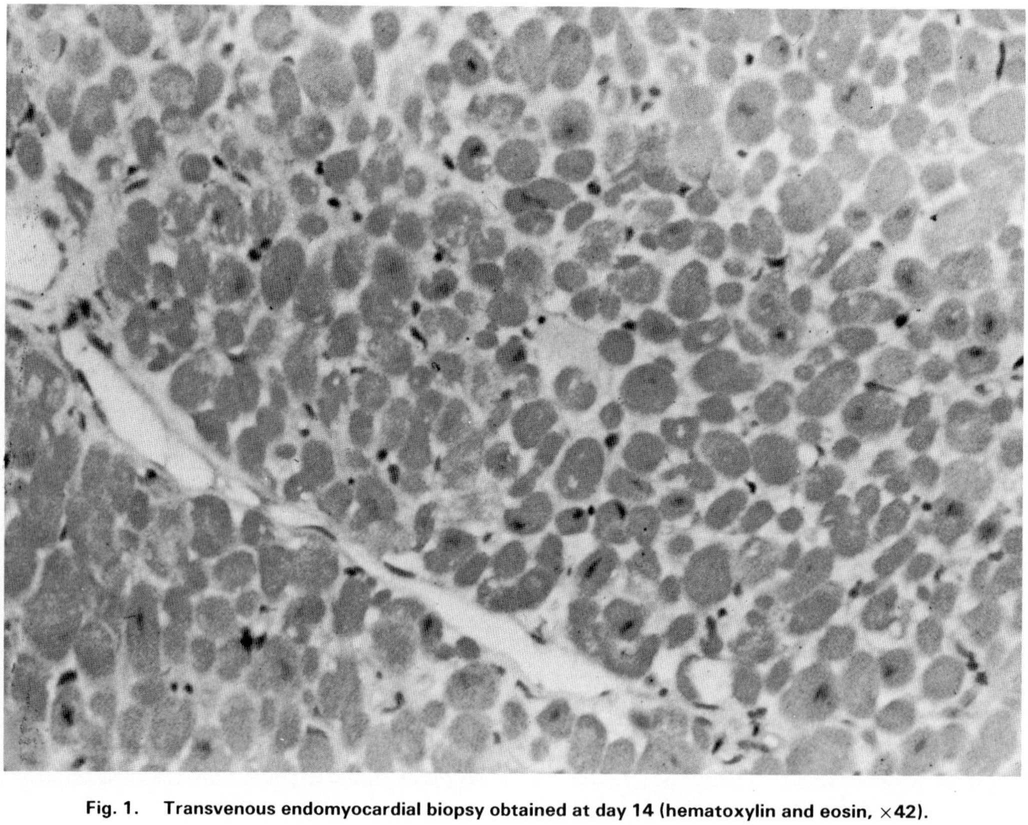

Fig. 1. Transvenous endomyocardial biopsy obtained at day 14 (hematoxylin and eosin, ×42).

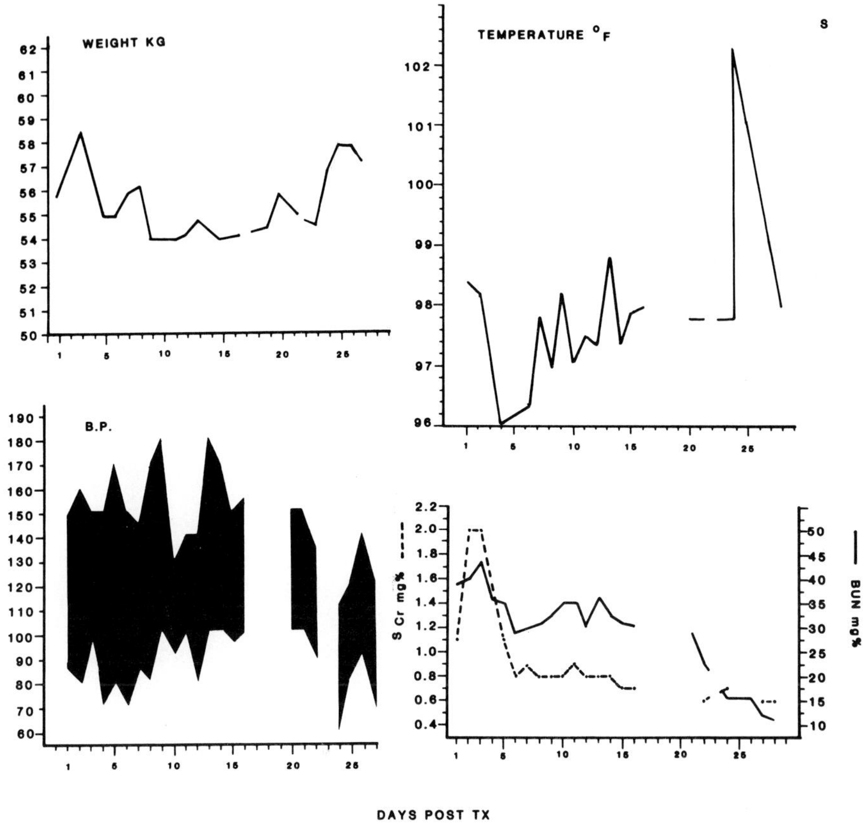

Fig. 2. Initial clinical course from days 1 to 27, showing upper left: weight (kg), upper right: temperature (°F), lower left: blood pressure shaded between systolic and diastolic (mm Hg), and lower right: serum creatinine (— — —) and blood urea nitrogen (—).

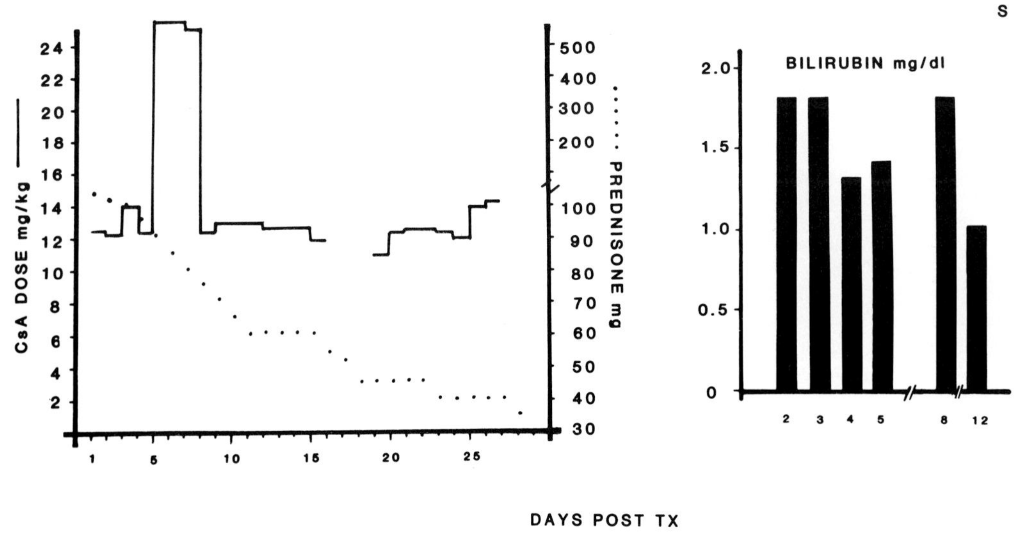

Fig. 3. (Left panel) Immunosuppressive regimen (cyclosporine —, prednisone — — —). (Right panel) Serum bilirubin values (mg/dl).

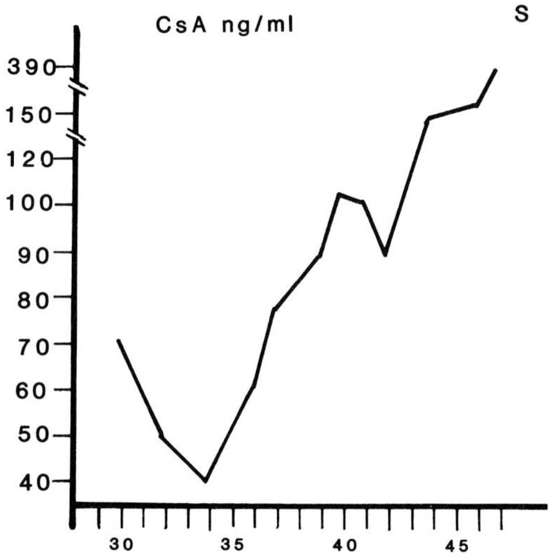

Fig. 4. Trough serum cyclosporine values (ng/ml) determined by radioimmunoassay.

patient did well; the biopsy cleared. The clinical course was benign; she was discharged on day 47 (Fig. 7). She continued well until April 29, 1983, when she was admitted due to tibia-fibular fracture from a motorcycle accident in which she struck a tree. She has convalesced without difficulty.

The discussants noted particularly the importance of other medications to alter cyclosporine pharmacokinetics and thereby reduce the immunosuppressive effect. The patient illustrates the need for cyclosporine level monitoring, as well as the potential to treat a serious infection due to *Mycobacterium tuberculosis* while continuing the immunosuppression.

PATIENT NO. 2

This 43-year-old male, electronic equipment repairman recently became totally disabled due to end-stage cardiac disease. The

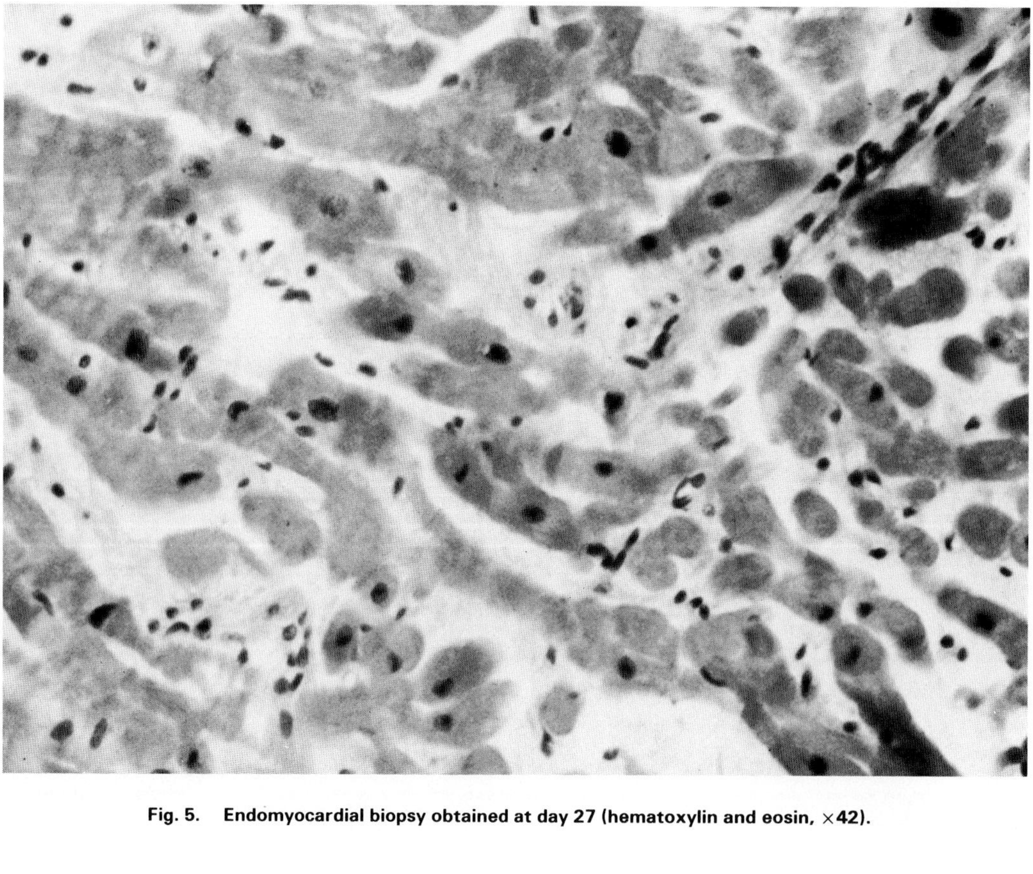

Fig. 5. Endomyocardial biopsy obtained at day 27 (hematoxylin and eosin, ×42).

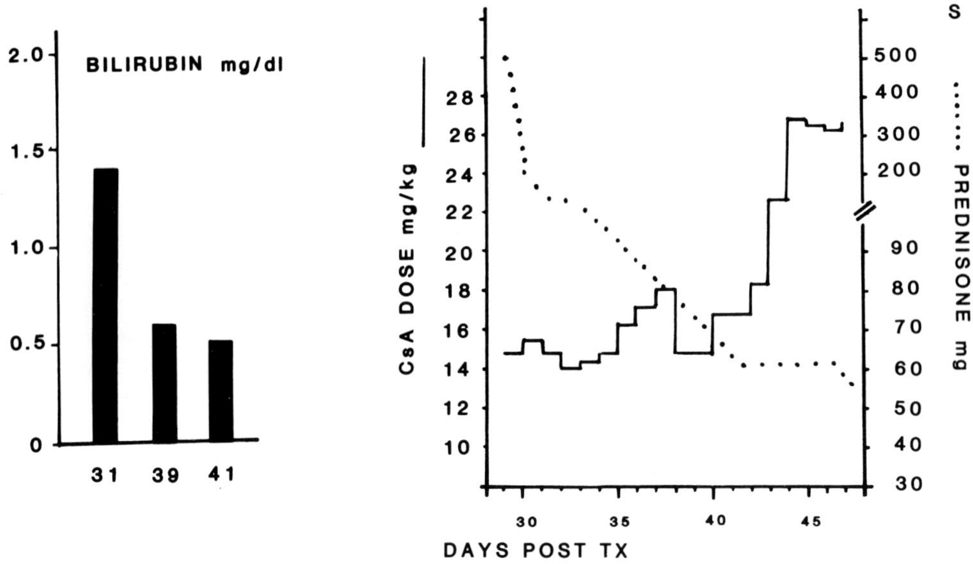

Fig. 6. Immunosuppressive regimen from days 29 to 48, continuing from Fig. 3.

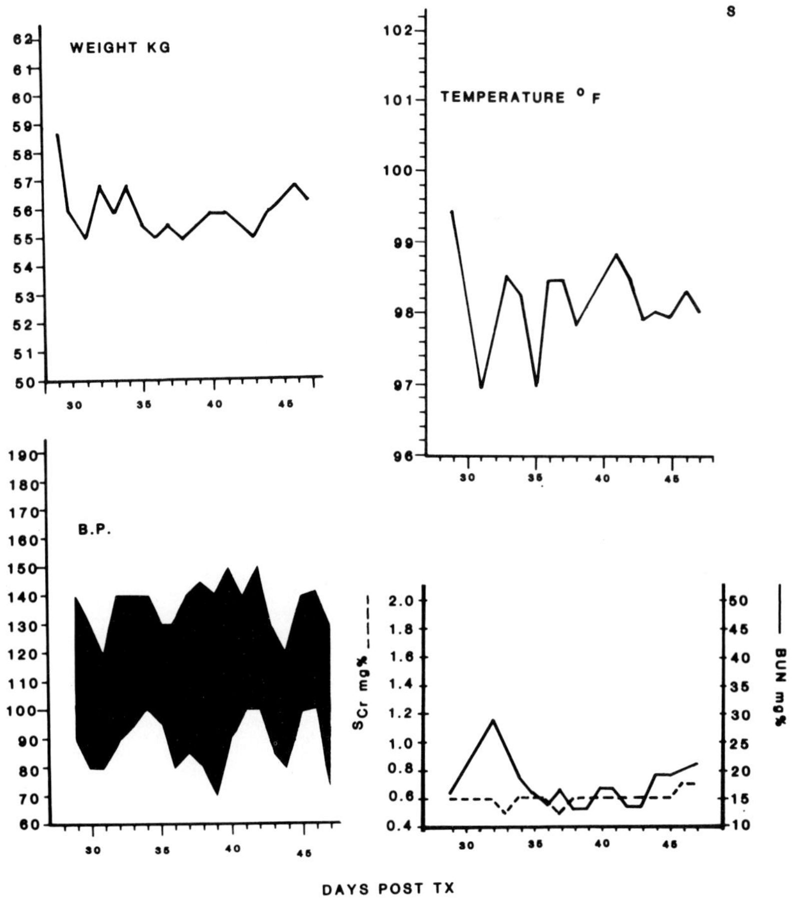

Fig. 7. Clinical course from days 28 to 47, continuing from Fig. 2.

patient had sustained a myocardial infarction in 1975, at the time of his second marriage. The patient enjoyed a full recovery from his illness except for demurring from go-cart racing. He describes an extremely stressful period of long hours and traveling on his job prior to 1978, the year he suffered a second myocardial infarction and underwent a left ventricular aneurysm resection and single-vessel coronary bypass. The patient's major risk factor for cardiovascular disease is hypertension. He also has been a smoker, but quit 15 years ago. In March 1982, he sustained a subendocardial myocardial infarction. On May 31, 1982, he came to the emergency room with congestive heart failure and was given afterload reduction, digitalis, and diuretics. He complained of being short of breath when walking around on the floor in the hospital. On nutritional assessment he admitted losing 15 pounds in the previous three months, and by objective criteria, his somatic protein stores showed a marginal deficit.

Medications at the time of evaluation included Digoxin (0.25 mg daily), Lasix (120 mg daily), Hydralazine (10 mg b.i.d.), nitroglycerine tablets (1–2 every 6 hr), Isordil (10 mg po t.i.d.), and Dilantin (100 mg 4 times a day), because he suffered from ventricular arrhythmias, which appeared to respond reasonably well to Dilantin. The laboratory findings at this time included white blood cell count 10,500/mm^3, hematocrit (Hct) 40.4%, serum creatinine 1.3 mg/dl, creatinine clearance 42 ml/min, cytomegalovirus titer IgG positive 1:1,024, BUN 21 mg/dl, total bilirubin 0.9 mg/dl, alkaline phosphatase 118 U, albumin 4.3 g/dl, serum glutamic-oxalic acid transaminase 43, and absent CPK-MB bands. The lungs were clear on chest roentgenogram, except for a calcified granuloma in the anterior

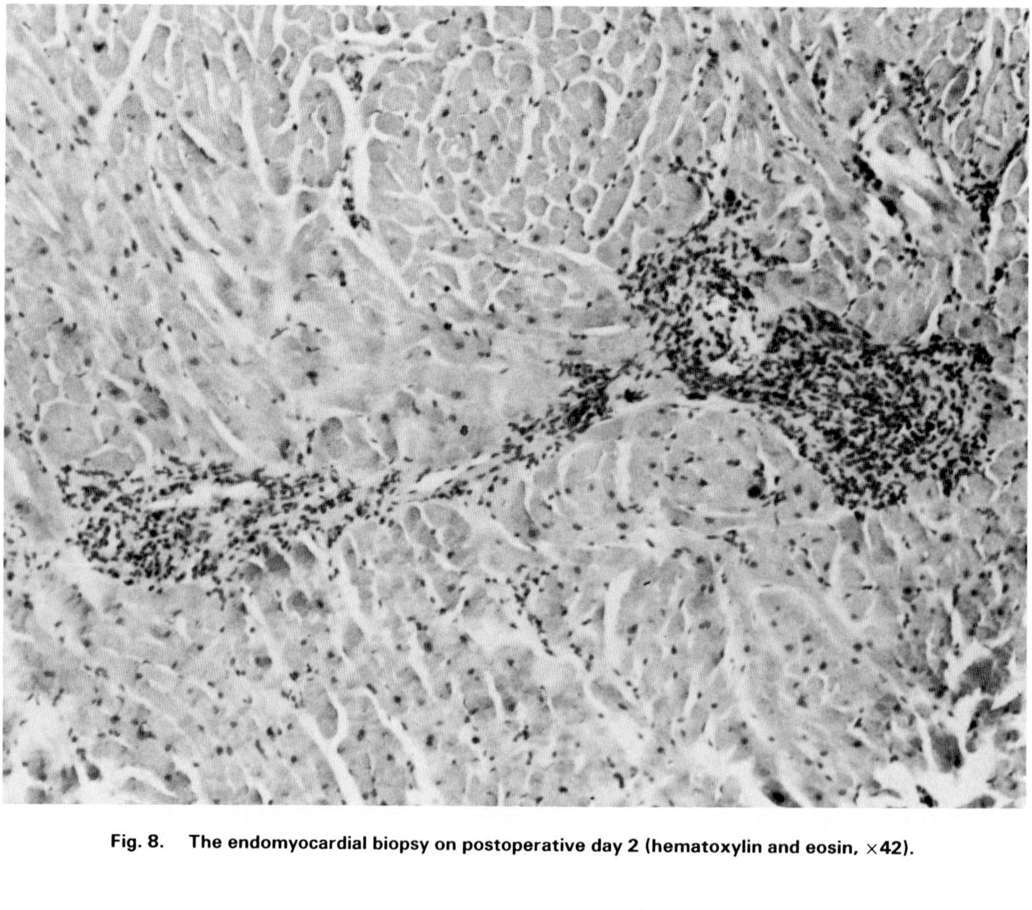

Fig. 8. The endomyocardial biopsy on postoperative day 2 (hematoxylin and eosin, ×42).

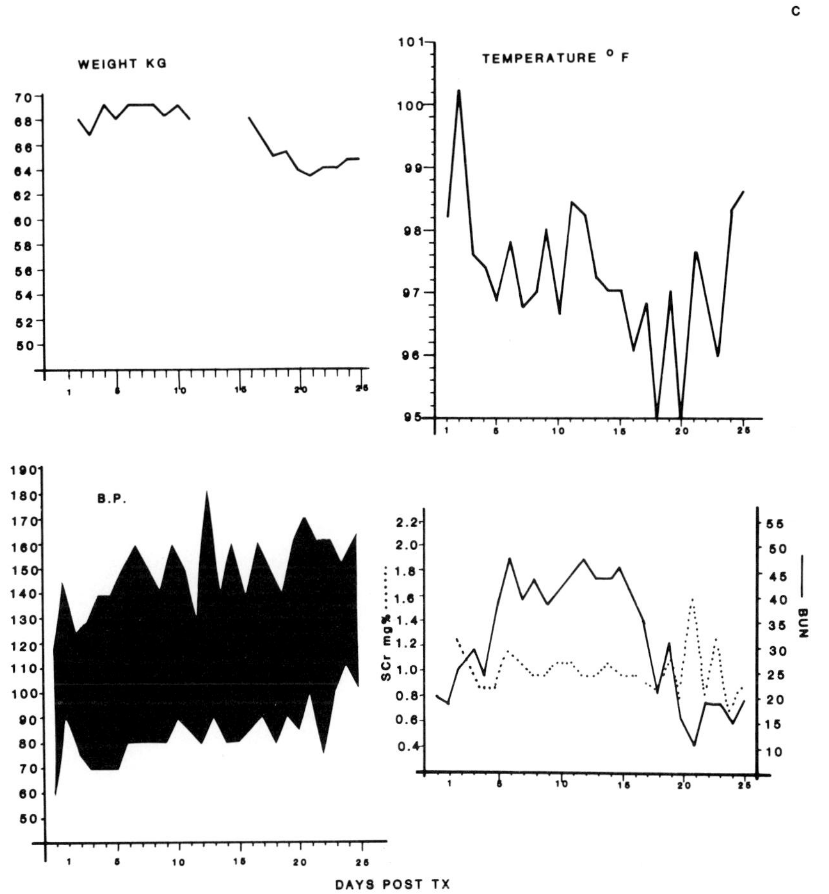

Fig. 9. The initial clinical course of the patient from days 1 to 25, including in upper left panel: weight (kg); upper right: temperature (°F); lower left: systolic/diastolic blood pressure shaded (mm Hg); and lower right: the serum creatinine (— — —) and the blood urea nitrogen (—).

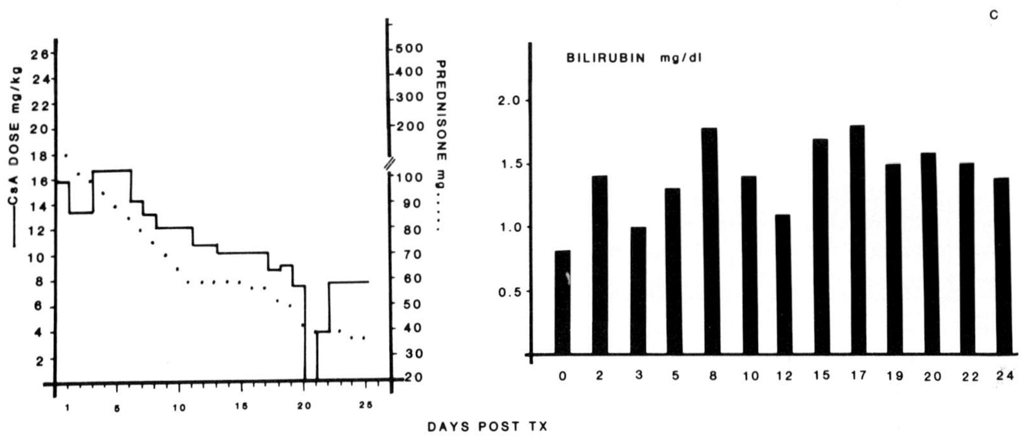

Fig. 10. (Left panel) Initial immunosuppressive regimen from days 1 to 25: cyclosporine (—), prednisone (— — —). (Right panel) Serum bilirubin values.

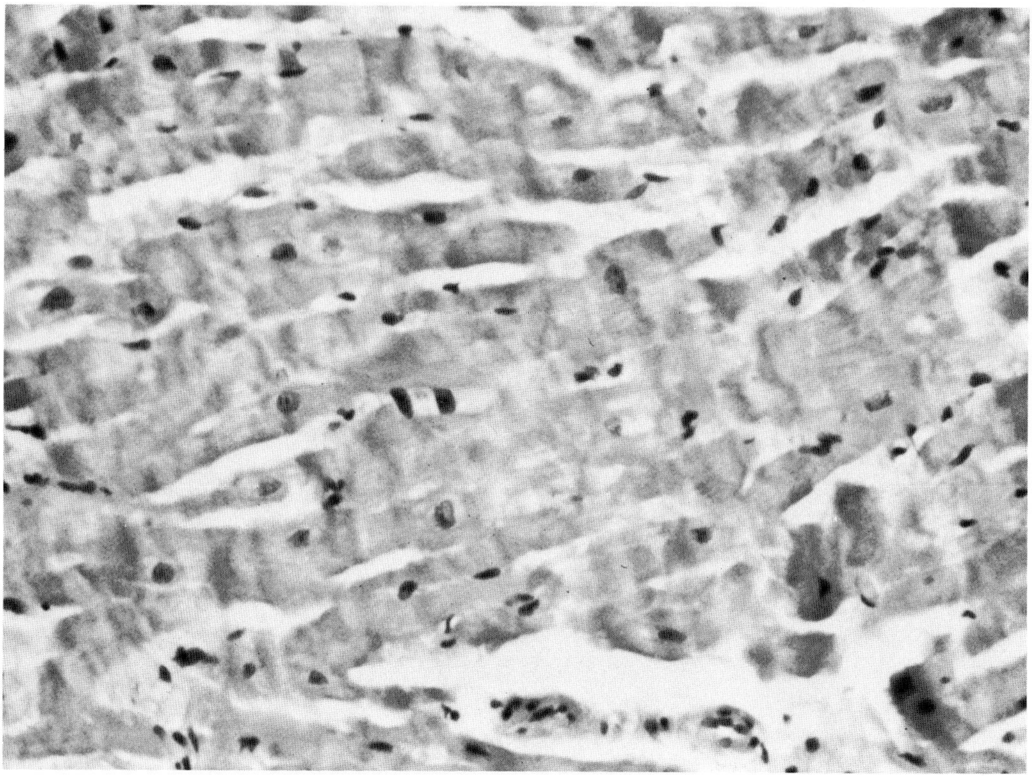

Fig. 11. Endomyocardial biopsy at day 26 (hematoxylin and eosin ×42).

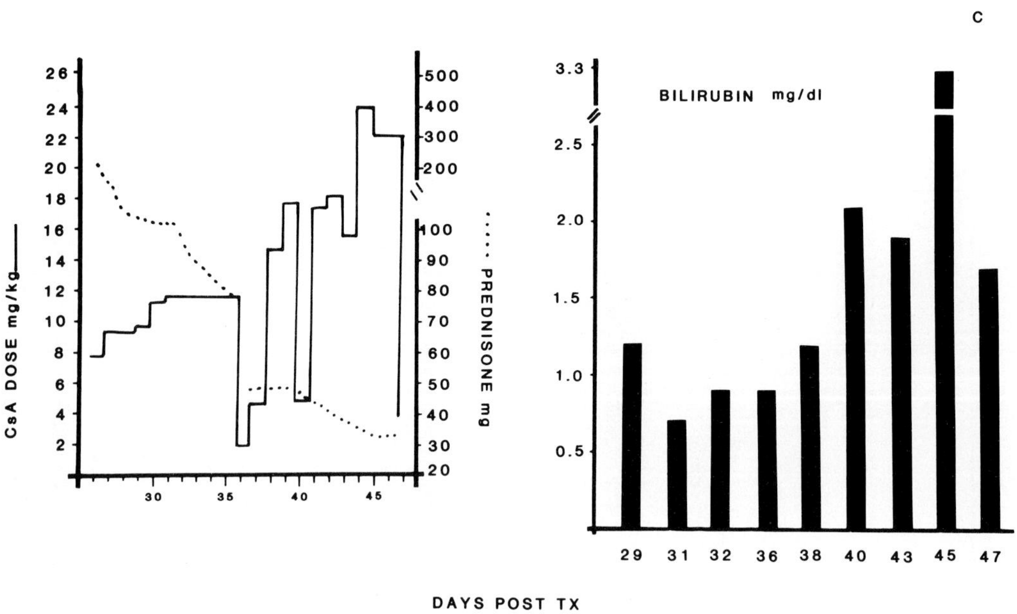

Fig. 12. (Left panel) Immunosuppressive regimen for antirejection therapy (cyclosporine —, prednisone — — —). (Right panel) Serum bilirubin values.

segment of the left upper lobe. The cardiac silhouette was enlarged. The electrocardiogram showed a sinus tachycardia with frequent premature ventricular contractions (PVCs). There were stigmata of inferior and apical myocardial infarctions. Two-dimensional echocardiogram showed left ventricular enlargement with severe regional wall motion abnormalities, including apical dyskinesis and posterior dyskinesis. Left ventricular performance study revealed generalized marked hypokinesis, as well as right ventricular and marked left ventricular dilatation. The left ventricular ejection fraction was 8%. The gallbladder was normally opacified without stones. Nuclear scan revealed a dilated, enlarged ventricle on both left and right sides. Preoperative cellular immune assessment revealed 32% total T cells, 4% active T cells, spontaneous blastogenesis 11,045 cpm, and panel MLC stimulation index 40. The overall profile suggested a weak immune responder.

The patient underwent cardiac transplantation on July 4, 1982. He returned to the recovery room with a blood pressure of 100/60 on no vasopressors, showing on electrocardiogram AV dissociation. On day 2 he displayed a fever to 101°F and underwent endomyocardial biopsy (Fig. 8). His chest roentgenogram showed a right middle lobe interstitial infiltrate with a small pleural effusion. The ejection fraction was 59%. It was elected to observe the

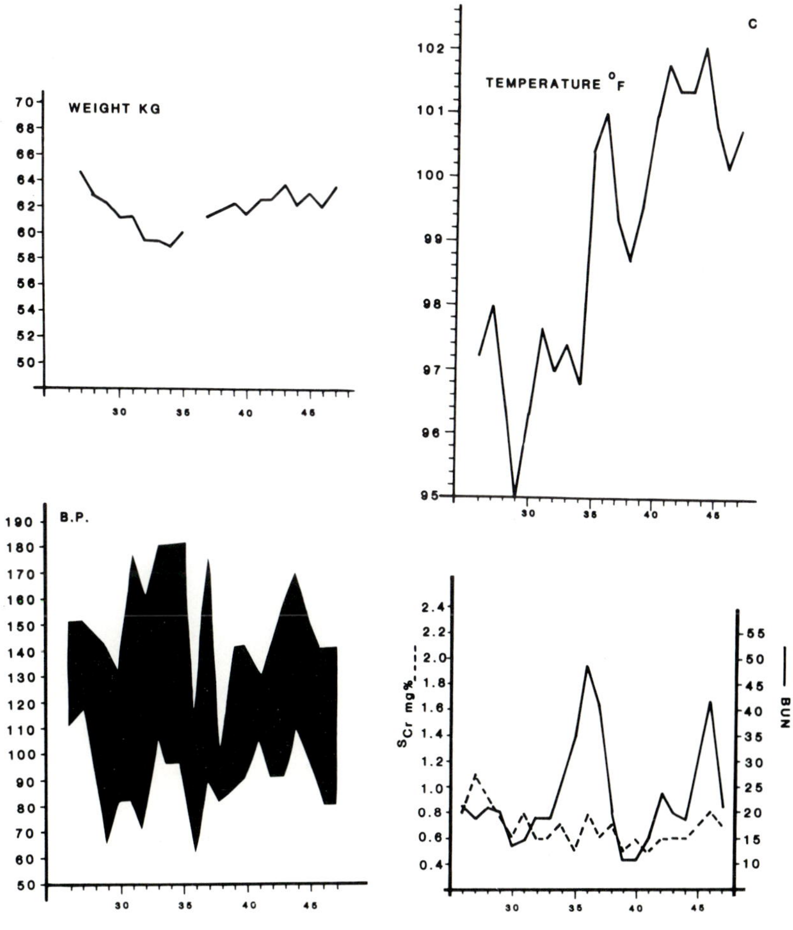

Fig. 13. The clinical course of the patient from days 26 to 47, continuing from Fig. 9.

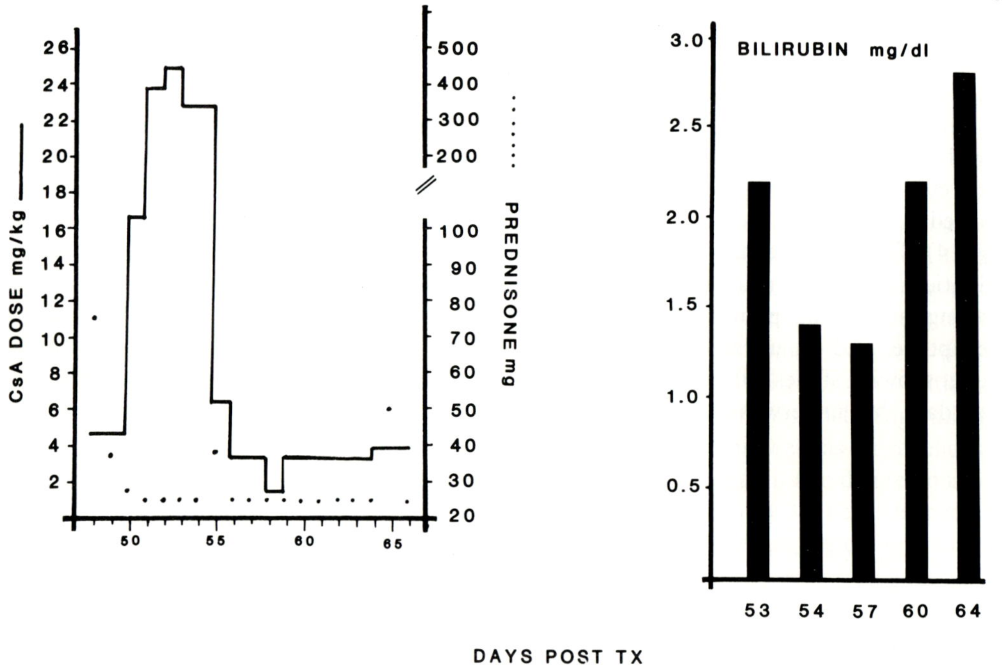

Fig. 16. Immunosuppressive regimen and serum bilirubin values, continuing from Fig. 12.

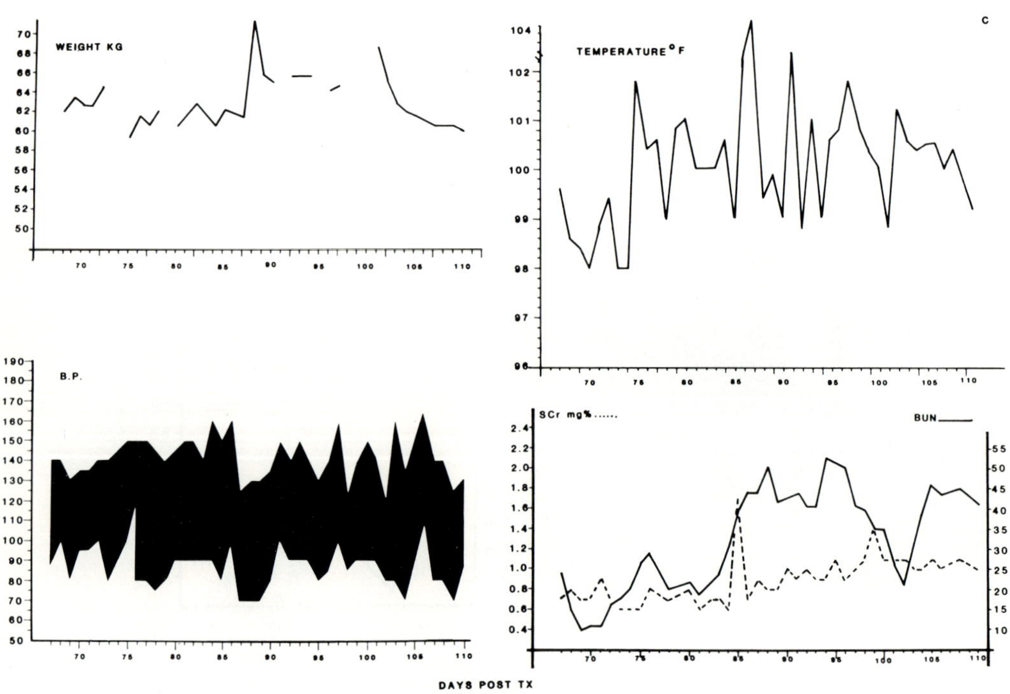

Fig. 17. Clinical course of the patient from days 67 to 110, continuing from Fig. 15.

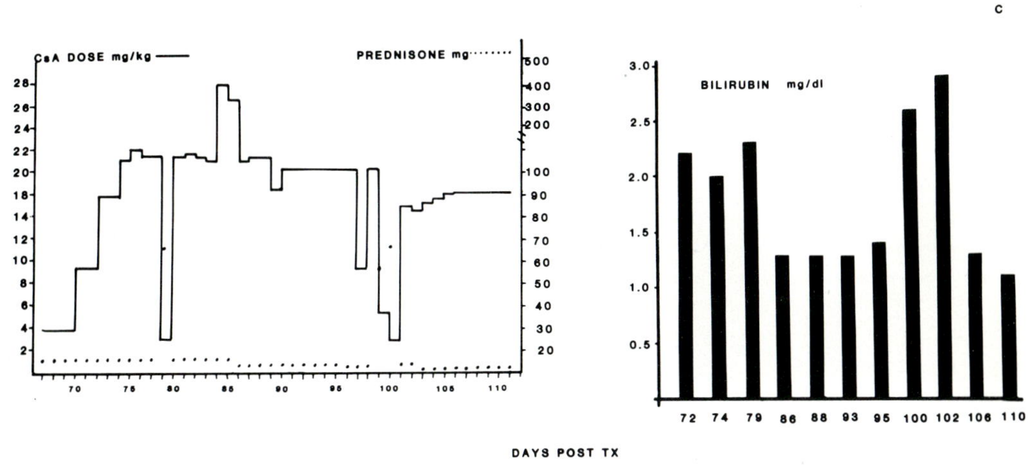

Fig. 18. **Immunosuppressive regimen and serum bilirubin values, continuing from Fig. 16.**

recurred on day 74, on day 76, and again on day 98, at which time right lung decortications were performed (Figs. 17 and 18). By day 110, the patient was afebrile. During this period, the CsA was switched to the oral route of administration, except at the time of lung operations. He was discharged on day 141.

The discussants concluded that the major impact of this patient's case was to demonstrate the severe penalty for misdiagnosing rejection (which the speaker in retrospect and the panel in prospect agreed had happened), and initiating increased steroid therapy. The patient survived only because cyclosporine did not interfere with effective treatment of bacterial infection that was exacerbated by the steroid therapy for rejection.

WORKSHOPS ON PATIENT MANAGEMENT

Practical Aspects of Renal Transplant Patient Management

B. D. Kahan

THE WORKSHOP participants were invited to pose questions to a group of panelists including Dr. Richard Wood (Oxford, UK), Dr. Paul Keown (London, Ont.), Dr. Stuart Flechner (Houston, TX), and Dr. Nicholas Tilney (Boston, MA).

Dr. Hart (Philadelphia): We are noting a lot of controversy about whether intravenous CsA should be given on the first several days after a transplant. I would like to ask the consensus about saturating the tissue stores.

Dr. Wood: Our experience was that patients treated with intramuscular CsA even after several days did not achieve optimal blood levels. Therefore, we use oral CsA as a single initial dose at the time of transplant. We give 10 mg/kg i.v., usually over 2–3 hr, starting just before the operation and running it while the patient is on the way to the operating room.

Dr. Kahan: Paul, how about the Canadian study and in your own experience?

Dr. Keown: We had traditionally only used intravenous drug when we felt that in the first 48 hr the serum levels would be low. But, as has been pointed out several times, we had a high incidence of acute tubular necrosis (ATN) and we wondered if we could get around this by a continuous intravenous infusion for the first 5 days, because what usually happens when you give the drug orally is that it does not tend to be well absorbed for the first several days. At first this looked to be the answer.

The patients received two doses of 2 mg/kg over 12 hr given continuously over a 24-hr period by Harvard pump. The patients do extremely well initially. The creatinines fall, but we have had rejection episodes in all of the last seven, although mild rejections. So I think that it may be a good way to approach the problem, but we do not have the right answer on the dosage. We are presently continuously infusing a dose that achieves a serum level of around 150 ng/ml, which is roughly the trough level we have aimed for. I think what we probably need is a serum level which is equivalent to the mean serum concentration.

Dr. Flechner: As you well know, Barry, we start our cadaveric recipients on 14 mg/kg orally when they arrive at the hospital. On the first night and second morning after the transplant, we give intravenous doses of 6 mg/kg over 6 hr and on postoperative day 1 continue on with 14 mg/kg orally. However, we have seen a few patients where levels have been very low during the first week, namely 40 ng/ml. Those patients are given an intravenous 3-mg/kg dose that day. The recipients of living related donor kidneys are given oral doses 48 hr pretransplant, other than a few patients in whom we were looking at decay curves and were treated with intravenous infusions. Obviously there will be a subset of patients with poor absorption initially, who will probably require intravenous supplements.

Dr. Hart: I have one more question. Given the state of the art of living related transplantation, namely donor-specific transfusion achieving generally good results, what does the panel feel about using CsA in living related grafts, as opposed to standard therapy, which gives excellent results?

Dr. Flechner: In Houston we have done about 40 renal transplants of high MLC-stimulatory LRD grafts with over 90% graft survival. These patients did not receive donor transfusions. There were roughly 25 patients that had third-party blood transfusions prior to the institution of the protocol or afterwards. The results are no different for the transfused versus the nontransfused groups. Our feeling

0041–1345/83/1505–0085$02.00/0

is that one does not have to administer either third-party or donor-specific blood transfusions. The second half of the coin that we are looking at now is the possibility of identifying with in vitro tests those patients in whom steroids may be withdrawn with excellent graft survival on CsA alone.

Dr. Keown: We have relatively limited experience in Canada in terms of donor-specific transfusions with haploidentical living related recipients, but our experience with CsA in this setting is very similar to the Houston experience with 88% graft survival.

Dr. Wood: In Britain we perform very few LRD transplants. We are using donor-specific transfusions, and we have decided to use conventional immunosuppression in that group rather than CsA, because I think we wanted to follow the established protocol.

Dr. Charles Zukoski (Tucson, AZ): Do you give it once a day, twice a day, three times a day, how do you give it?

Dr. Wood: Once a day, never twice a day.

Dr. Keown: We have always given it twice a day from the very beginning, but there is no question that it works for many people giving it once a day. We don't really know the answer. If you look at the pharmacokinetic curves and you want to achieve a serum level which is going to be relatively constant, the drug should be given at least twice a day, or perhaps more frequently. But the problem is that the pharmacokinetic curves don't always tell the full story of its true biological effects. It may well be that although it disappears from the plasma relatively quickly, it may still have a prolonged biological effect.

Dr. Flechner: We give the drug basically once a day. However, we—actually Barry has performed extensive pharmacokinetic analyses on the patients. There are patients identified that have a rapid decay curve with a short half-life under 10 hr, who need to be given drug twice a day. By the same token, a couple of patients will certainly be identified to have very prolonged half-lives and handle the drug differently. They may be amenable to taking the drug every other day. Basically, all patients were given the drug once a day, unless there is a reason to alter the regimen.

Dr. Melisatis (New York): The British crossover experience suggests that a lot of patients on maintenance CsA achieve a lower serum creatinine if the dose is reduced. Do you think your patients are on higher doses than are necessary?

Dr. Flechner: I think the universal agreement is that the drug is nephrotoxic and probably in most patients, other than those whose creatinines are under 1 [mg/dl] (and there are very few of those), that conversion improves the creatinine. However, will there be successive loss of the graft to rejection? Based on all the data obtained at these meetings, the drug is improving allograft survival. Probably we will lose grafts by decreasing CsA doses, in spite of improving the patients' renal function.

Dr. Keown: The answer to your question "Are some people on more drug than they actually need?" is unquestionably important. We can get people down to doses lower than we have them on, but you run a risk of eventually precipitating acute rejection. Our only four late rejections were all in that circumstance, namely, where we took someone who had a creatinine of 2.0–2.5 mg/dl and progressively and deliberately reduced the dose. They eventually rejected, and in spite of therapy they all had permanent serum creatinine levels in the range of about 4 mg/dl. I think the two effects of nephrotoxicity and the immunosuppressive potential of the drug are probably dissociated effects. You may have someone who is exquisitely sensitive to the nephrotoxic effects of the drug, yet still requires a certain threshold in the serum to maintain immunosuppression.

Dr. Kahan: Paul, is your opinion the same as Stuart's, that 3 months might be too early to routinely convert people? Doesn't the Canadian trial intend to study this issue?

Dr. Keown: Yes, the problems that we are undertaking at the moment demand that everybody receive CsA and prednisone for the first 90 days. Then we randomize them into two groups, one receiving continuing prednisone and the other receiving placebo. The question here is, can we withdraw prednisone first? In addition, those people who do not have satisfactory graft function, namely, a creatinine level over 2.5 mg/dl after that point, will be re-randomized to receive either continuous CsA or azathioprine/prednisone. We may well have an answer after this study.

Dr. Kahan: Richard, we can't ask you this question since you presented the data that we are all talking about.

Dr. Tilney: I think your question of whether 3 months is too early may be an important one, Barry. All the trouble with rejection that we had in three or four patients occurred upon conversion at the end of 3 months. We have now switched patients at 4–6 months, and we have had no trouble at all. I am not sure that your question is not slightly germane.

Dr. Max Sanders (Chapel Hill, NC): I would like to ask the panel what they do with cadaveric recipients that they treat early with CsA, and then are facing a 4-week period of anuria from ATN.

Dr. Kahan: All right, let's start with Nick. You were initially worried about a diuresing kidney in your patients.

Dr. Tilney: We certainly were; that is one reason [for] sticking slavishly to Roy Calne's initial data, that we either just did not use it in kidneys which did not diurese immediately or cut back considerably on the dose. What happens when you cut back on the initial dose is rejection with loss of the kidney. Now, we just close our eyes and plow ahead with full dose, and the kidneys will all come back. In our particular part of the country, about half of the grafts do not diurese initially anyway, because the kidneys are all about 37 hr old, which is considerably longer than [in] the Canadian trial.

Dr. Wood: We really do very much the same. I do not think that we have the same preservation problems that you have, because of the shorter distances to move kidneys. There are few kidneys in the U.K. that are put on the perfusion machine, and most are transplanted within 24 hr. Most of our kidneys work straight away, so we don't really have a particular problem. In cases where we have had patients on CsA, the kidneys tend to function straight away. We make sure that the scan shows perfusion and do biopsies to rule out rejection, and in all but one case the kidneys did satisfactorily.

Dr. Keown: In general, I agree. We try to get the CsA level down as low as possible. Rarely, if anuria is truly prolonged, [say, of] several weeks' duration, then we switch. In general we try to ride it out.

Dr. Kahan: So what you are saying is that during the anuric stage you watch the blood levels carefully. If the patient is toxic, you reduce the drug, and you will be more compulsive about that than you would be in the diuresing kidney. Stuart, any other thoughts? Stuart has studied immediate graft function and his article will be in *Transplantation* in a month or two.

Dr. Flechner: Our study echoes what everyone has said, simply that the incidence of ATN is 38%, no matter what kind of immunosuppression. The immediate number of dialysis treatments in ATN required using CsA was four, the same number as was required in our azathioprine group. So I am sure that there will be a couple of cases of primary nonfunction and a couple of cases of very prolonged ATN, just as with other forms of immunosuppression. I think it is mainly due to donor injury. The question of the drug level is probably more important early on in that group. One should avoid toxic levels and, as mentioned, try to keep them under 200 ng/ml, especially during the oliguric phase.

Dr. Heider (Galveston, TX): Those of us who work with children would obviously like to reduce the dose of prednisone. Listening to the papers, I have a vague feeling that prednisone may be helping [to] prevent CsA toxicity.

Dr. Flechner: Actually we do not know. The reason I say that is that most of our patients are on prednisone. We don't have a comparable control group. The only other thing I would say is, especially as far as children are concerned, I think this opens up the question of what we were talking about before, live donor transplantation. This may be the one opportunity to transplant most children with a kidney from the mother or father and eventually withdraw the steroids. Right now we have two children a year post-transplant off steroids completely. But your question is very specific, and I can't answer it because we do not have patients on CsA alone.

Dr. Kahan: Paul, do you have any definitive information?

Dr. Keown: No, but there is evidence from both Pekka Hayry's study today and from our control study that those who receive CsA alone during the first few weeks tend to have higher serum creatinines. I am not sure if there are any true data available.

Dr. Wood: I think there is some evidence that prednisolone reduces toxicity. We had a group of patients, as you may remember from the presentation, who had prednisolone added because of rejection, and their mean serum creatinine was in the region of 369. Now you normally expected that figure to come down in the group on CsA alone to a mean value of 242. But these patients in fact dropped their serum creatinine to 168, so I think there is evidence, from admittedly small numbers of patients, that it probably does reduce toxicity.

Dr. Kahan: Richard, did you have any insight into that question I posed to Dr. Pekka Hayry, which is whether prednisone is acting by virtue of increasing drug metabolism or at the level of the kidney? In other words, are we basically using steroids as P450 inducers to lower blood levels, or are we actually seeing effects of the steroid at the level of the kidney?

Dr. Wood: We don't really have any hard data on that at this time. I think that we will when we get down to analyzing the materials by peroxidase staining, for we will note fairly detailed information on infiltrates in these kidneys and how they compare to the patient on CsA alone. I hope that some day in the future we will get that information.

Could I just say one thing about CsA? I think it just requires a little bit of caution because in our series we had 4 deaths in 55 patients who received CsA and prednisone, with death in a patient on CsA alone. There were 13 patients who had prednisone added to the CsA, with 3 deaths from infection in that subgroup. We are just a little bit concerned that CsA plus prednisone may be oversuppression.

Dr. Tilney: My emotions about initial steroids are obviously colored by our first year and a half with patients who did not receive steroids. As far as nephrotoxicity is concerned, we had so much trouble with rejecting kidneys that we never had a chance to look for nephrotoxicity. I feel certain that the lower doses of prednisone that we are allowed to use now with CsA puts us all in a much greater position, as far as steroid sparing is concerned. So we have not had so much trouble with infection or death as we used to have with azathioprine and high-dose steroids.

Dr. Kahan: I think that gives you a smattering of opinion. I don't think that there are any firm conclusions; anybody can take their own stand on this one.

Dr. Rubin (Boston, MA): My question is, what is the role of blood transfusions?

Dr. Tilney: Well, I don't have any idea about this issue. All of our patients are transfused.

Dr. Wood: I don't have definitive information, but I certainly have some opinions. The information presented by Bob Sells from the European Multicentre Study suggests that CsA tends to reduce the transfusion effect. I think that is something for the future that we should study in detail. We have a number of nontransfused patients on the program. But in the long term, if it proves to be the case that CsA does reduce the transfusion effect, I think it would be a tremendous benefit. I think one of the problems we have with transplantation is that we often take a short view of our patients, thinking about a particular phase of the graft at a time. We do not take a long-term view that kidneys don't last forever. In a 20-year-old patient, we must be thinking in terms of the possibility of [their] requiring a second graft. If we can avoid a transfusion and use matched grafts, we will reduce sensitization and be able to offer better long-term service to our patients.

Dr. Keown: Yes, this is obviously a very important question. From the Canadian study, though, all people were transfused. There was a very dramatic difference in dose dependency of the number of transfusions in the conventionally treated group, but no dose dependency in the CsA group. Even the small differences shown between less than and more than 5 transfusions were totally excluded by taking into account the other risk factors. In our second study, with 17 patients, there is absolutely no effect of transfusions. My personal feeling is that the effect is minimal.

Dr. Fletchner: Basically, we have the approach of not transfusing patients. I think in the living related transplantation group, our data is a little bit more than preliminary. I get the feeling that we do not need to transfuse living related recipients. I think it needs more follow-up and a few more centers doing the studies, but my overall impression is that you don't have to give the transfusion, because you never had it. In the cadaveric group, Dr. Kahan, in his plenary talk, showed our data dividing patients based on transfusions, and all groups are within the 70%–80% range. One group with greater than 5 units in the 78%–80% range—not much of a statistically significant difference. I think again more numbers are needed, but certainly the days of untransfused recipients on Imuran and prednisone getting 30%–40% graft survival are over, and the question is, can we bump it up from 75%–80% to 85%–90% with more blood? I think we have to weigh the question that Dr. Wood posed, namely, are we depriving transplantation to more people because we are sensitizing, in order to get a 5% increase in graft survival?

Dr. Kahan: Bob Sells, we wanted to get your comment on the transfusion issue.

Dr. Sells (Liverpool, UK): Thank you. There are only two trials of CsA presented at this meeting [that] have really got a significant number of untransfused patients included in them, that is, Dr. Kahan's and the European trial. In both groups there was a fairly heavy, obvious eyeball difference in the controls, but not in the CsA group. In the case of the European trial, there was a statistically significant difference in favor of the untransfused state. Should we be not transfusing in the hope that CsA will prevent the problems already alluded to—sensitization, etc.? It seems to me that there are two points which are very germane: [First,] if we stop transfusing patients in the hope that the effect will be sustained by other groups and that you can substitute for the transfusion by giving CsA, that's fine so long as the patient remains on CsA, but of course in the nephrotoxic group, then you are perhaps unfairly laying those patients open to the vicissitudes of a post-transplant existence without the protective effect of previous transfusion. Second, I wish that somebody would do an animal experiment which precisely mirrors the clinical situation that we are discussing. Looking through the literature, I can find nobody who has done random transfusions in animals and then given them allografts of any tissue in any species followed by CsA. I think that that would be an extremely interesting experiment.

Dr. Kahan: Is anyone from the Dutch group here, because they did do the work on monkeys and blood transfusions presented at the First International Symposium on Cyclosporine. Would you like to comment?

Dr. Marquet (Rotterdam): We have done quite a lot of studies addressing this point in monkeys and beagle dogs, wherein the transfusion effect is produced very easily. CsA alone gave the same outcome as seen in animals receiving transfusions and CsA. From these studies one would conclude that there is no benefit of the transfusions.

Dr. Birtch (Springfield, IL): I have two questions. The perfusion injury that the Canadians reported I found very interesting, and I would be interested to know whether the other units have found a similar perfusion injury in their patients. This is obviously important to all of us, since we ship kidneys all over the country and all over the world. The second question is that if one of our major goals is to reduce or eliminate steroids, I find it a little surprising that there is not more clinical work using combinations of CsA and azathioprine, both obviously in somewhat reduced doses, attempting to get away from steroids altogether. I wonder whether there is such information that has not been passed out, besides the heart and lung transplant group.

Dr. Tilney: The perfusion injury thing interests me very much. In our own series of about 40 azathioprine-treated cadaveric grafts and about 40 CsA-treated grafts, the time of perfusion has been about exactly the same, that is, about 37 hr. In our small series, there is absolutely no difference in eventual renal function between quick perfusions and long perfusions.

Dr. Wood: I cannot comment on the perfusion injury since none of our kidneys are perfused, but I could comment on the question of conversion. We have in fact converted a number of patients from azathioprine to CsA and then gradually eliminated the steroids. These are patients with long-term steroid complications of various kinds, and that is a generally reasonable experience. The interesting thing about that is that many of these patients who have skin problems have actually experienced improvement in their skin following withdrawal of azathioprine and starting CsA. The steroids were not changed for many months.

Dr. Kahan: What was the skin problem?

Dr. Wood: These are patients with very thin skin from prednisone.

Dr. Kahan: I guess the question is, no steroids, just azathioprine and CsA from the beginning. Have you thought about that, Richard?

Dr. Wood: We have not, I must say.

Dr. Kahan: I guess the idea would be azathioprine and CsA for, like, 3–4 months and then maybe stop one of them and go with the other one.

Dr. Wood: I just wonder if that would not put us back into the problems that we experienced with immunosuppression in the initial experience.

Dr. Kahan: I think that has been the fear, and I am glad Richard mentioned that. Patients treated in this fashion experienced many problems, particularly the series from London that reported a tremendous incidence of sepsis and poor patient survival.

Dr. Keown: Well, first regarding the perfusion injuries, by all statistical means that we can use, we cannot explain the poor graft survival by any other factor. It is additive to the injury that is seen with the long reanastomosis time. I think this is an interaction between several factors causing damage to the kidney, including high doses of CsA that were used particularly in the early days of our experience. I think the reason, perhaps, that we are not seeing it as frequently now and that other groups may not be seeing it is that we have had a learning curve and over the last 3 or 4 years we have learned that it is much safer to give lower doses of the drug, and so I would hope that this problem will gradually disappear. In regard to the combination of drugs, I think the idea is very sound, and we have discussed it a lot. But the worry is sepsis, because animals treated with subtherapeutic amounts of the combination of drugs have had a high incidence of sepsis. It is probably not yet ready for clinical trial.

Dr. Flechner: This question of cold storage vs. pumping concerns everybody. Simply, the data from our program, where the vast majority of kidneys are preserved and transplanted in under 24 hr, is a 30% ATN rate in cold-stored kidneys and a similar rate in perfused kidneys. No other differences were ascertained; the preservation times were equal. There was no difference in the 1-year graft survival of ATN and non-ATN kidneys or perfused vs. cold-stored kidneys. The real question is what happens after extended preservation times to 36, 40, 44 hr; I do not have data on that. As far as the question of multiple immunosuppressants [is concerned], the animal experiments show a very high sepsis rate with CsA and azathioprine. Since these mechanisms of action are quite different, one on lymphocytes and the other on granulocytes, mainly, I think there will be compounded toxicity. Also, all of us using CsA have been aware of the cancer risk and have tried to minimize other forms of immunosuppression. I think when we use an agent such as this, combining other forms of immunosuppression raises these kinds of questions.

Question: Dr. Najarian compared CsA with his antilymphocyte serum in a protocol. I wonder whether CsA has been combined with the ATGAM preparation from the Upjohn Corporation?

Dr. Kahan: Why don't I just answer this quickly with a simple answer: no. As far as I know, there is no group that has used Upjohn ATGAM with CsA, so we don't have any idea about this combination. I think I stated at the time of my presentation that we had wanted to have as a control group azathioprine, prednisone, and Upjohn ATG, but at the time we started, Upjohn ATG was not yet approved, and we could not do a trial that involved two experimental drugs, so we could not do that trial.

Marty Mozcs (Chicago, IL): Is there any information coming out of the CsA trials concerning transplanting sensitized patients, specifically, those patients who have a historically positive crossmatch and currently negative [test]?

Dr. Keown: We have done, I think, a total of 13 who were specifically sensitized; . . . they had a historically positive T-cell crossmatch with a currently negative test, irrespective of the B-cell crossmatch. Of those 13, I think 9 are surviving at about 3–6 months and apparently doing well. So, the impression was that this group had the same graft survival as patients who were not previously sensitized. However, there is no comparison group, because we have never transplanted people with a historically positive crossmatch. But one group in Toronto, using a rabbit anti–T cell serum in the same situation of a historically positive crossmatch, has had similar results. So there is no question, you can transplant.

Dr. Wood: Most of our patients have positive crossmatches due to autoantibodies. Of this group, 20%–25% of patients have positive crossmatches with their donor and react with a panel of cells. On examining the antibodies, we feel the majority of them are autoreactive.

Dr. Ettenger (Los Angeles, CA): What is the relevance of DR antigen matching at this point? Is there any reason to do it anymore with CsA?

Dr. Tilney: We try to match the DR as much as possible, but in our region we only see it about twice a year, so I have no opinion.

Dr. Wood: We try very hard to match for DR, and before we started looking at CsA, we felt that DR matches were very important. Statistically speaking, we found that patients receiving completely DR-matched kidneys have an advantage over the patients who receive either completely DR-mismatched or only a one-DR match. We really have not got enough numbers to say whether the effects of CsA and DR are additive. We will have to wait and see, but I think it is very important to continue matching, in order to avert sensitization.

Dr. Kahan: What you are saying is that if you have a two-DR-matched recipient, you would not put the kidney into another patient, you would use that patient. In other words, if you have a matched patient, you would obviously use that patient, but the issue is, would you not put a kidney into a two-DR-mismatched recipient?

Dr. Wood: We have done this in cases of clinical urgency, but we usually find a well-matched patient in our national pool.

Dr. Keown: Within the Canadian population, it looks as though DR matching is a significant factor in the conventionally treated patient. But within the CsA-treated group in our study, there was no demonstrable effect. Now, only about a third of the patients were fully DR-typed.

Dr. Doherty (Belfast, N. Ire.): I think that our experience with conventional therapy to date differs from Dr. Tilney, suggesting that there is no reason to give more than 20 mg prednisone daily from day 1. I just wonder if in our trials with CsA, would they now make it reasonable to use the lowest dose of prednisone, and would it be a good idea to try to remove this variation of dosage from comparative groups?

Dr. Flechner: I think we in Houston begin with 120 mg prednisone; that may be too much prednisone. Any time you use it, you always think you are giving too much, i.e., that you can get away with using less or half, until you experience a breakthrough rejection. Anecdotally, two patients were started on low-dose prednisone, one an older patient who happened to be a retransplant, another a female who had lupus and had been on steroids for a long time before. Both of these patients had what we thought were early rejections, and we felt we really can't use low doses. I think we need to have more knowledge about the drug. From my observation, prednisone should be begun in everybody, and the question is how fast do you taper and who do you taper it from? My opinion is that I am not sure, in the North American population of patients, [if] beginning with 20 mg day of prednisone daily would be adequate for induction. I think the first time the antigen is presented is when you want to give the maximum immunosuppression, starting with 60 or 80 mg of prednisone for 1 week only.

Dr. Kahan: The question may relate to the different types of patients we are dealing with. That could be part of the problem that prevents us from generalizing. It may depend on how immunoresponsive the patient is. I think that it will be difficult to generalize. Paul, what do you think? You have a broader experience with at least induction steroids.

Dr. Keown: Well, we do, but I do not know if we can give you any firm answer. I think we are still very much in the dark. We know that we can give much less prednisone with CsA, but how much less, we just don't know. I think we will see, as we look back in retrospect, 2–3 years from now, there are different groups of people that require more or less, and we will eventually be able to pick them out. But what we have done in Canada is start with alternate-day steroids. We start with 1 mg/kg from day 1, and by the end of 3–4 weeks [increase] to 15–20 mg every other day.

Dr. Tilney: I think, emotionally, everybody agrees with you. In our unit, we have been slowly lowering the steroid dose for about 5–8 years with standard Imuran, long before CsA came along. Then, about 2 years ago, we started a trial in which about 20 azathioprine-treated patients were given low-dose, that is, 35 mg prednisone/day starting at the time of transplantation, as compared to our usual dose, namely, 75 mg down to 50 mg. Of those 20 patients who received 35 mg/day from the time of transplantation, 14 of them lost their kidneys resoundingly. We got so nervous, we went back up again; now our results on our standard therapy are back where they used to be.

Dr. M. Williams (Baltimore, MD): Can you review precise pharmacologic data related to the dosing interval?

Dr. Kahan: I think I can answer your question directly. The relative bioavailability of CsA is the same whether you give one dose a day, two doses a day, or three doses a day. By that I mean if you give a patient 900 mg and measure the area under the serum CsA curve of the absorption, it is the same as if you had given the patient two doses of 450 or three doses of 300. So the bioavailability is good. The rationale for single-day dosage is actually from Tom Beveridge's study, which suggested that there was a moiety with a half-life of about 24 hr. There were some animal studies from Sandoz, also, that suggested that there was a half-life of 24 hr. Now, the confusing [point] that has emerged at this conference in Jerry Newburger's analysis of our data is that the major moiety that we see in our patients by RIA seems to have a half-life between 10 and 14 hr. Now, generally, you dose drugs based on one half-life. So the question has resurrected itself of why aren't we administering CsA twice a day? I think the best answer

mg/kg intravenously. We, at last, by pharmacokinetic analysis, have gotten reasonable results with 2 mg/kg given intravenously.

Dr. Wallwork: There is no doubt we initially used too much CsA. We just came out and arbitrarily determined a dose, which was a little cavalier. We knew we had to cut the dose down, and I think that even anything 10 mg/kg/day is too much; 2 mg/kg/day is probably just about the level you should give. I have had to give intravenous CsA on two occasions since then to patients simply because the patient could not eat, because he had *Candida esophagitis,* so I gave him a very low dose.

Dr. MacKensie: This is a semantic problem defining really what you mean by nephrotoxicity. It is nephrotoxic in a sense that you have unwanted side effects. Cyclosporine has effects on the kidney which will result in oliguria, which will progress to anuria if you are giving too much, but I do not think you should adjust adequate CsA levels according to urine flow. It is much more comfortable to see the patients producing urine, but you know in a couple of days the patients will produce urine if you keep their CsA levels under tight control. You want your patients to be adequately immunosuppressed initially. You are not bothered about whether they produce 10 cc/hr or 50 cc/hr of urine, because you know within a couple of days' time, the renal function will improve.

Dr. Wallwork: What does your creatinine go up to?

Dr. MacKensie: The creatinine will at least double over the preoperative; it will not go sky high. It is not acute tubular necrosis that one is confronting.

Dr. Wallwork: What will it go up to?

Dr. MacKensie: An average of about 3 mg/dl.

Dr. Wallwork: I think that is the early problem. The later problem with the kidneys, if you have a creatinine of 1.5 mg/dl, you are talking about a loss of a third of your renal reserve. With a creatinine of 2 ng/dl, you are talking about loss of half of your renal reserve, and this may not exhibit any significant problems in the way that your patients walk around or behave, but nevertheless [it] is a worry and a concern.

Dr. MacKensie: Now you are talking about the later effects, not about the acute effects.

Dr. Wallwork: What I am saying is that whatever you do with the drug, it will hurt the kidneys. Early in the postoperative period, you can see oliguria or anuria, although I agree that the patient will diurese later. However, that compared with the previous group of patients treated with conventional therapy. CsA cardiac allograft recipients do not have the usual spontaneous early diuresis that rid of preoperative edema. For this reason, it is a little more difficult to manage their pulmonary edema and their effusions than was previously true. Anything which will produce early diuresis is surely better for the patient.

Dr. Wallwork: Dr. Oyer, what do you have to say about that? You have the biggest experience, and you are staying very quiet.

Dr. Oyer: We do not really have the data one way or another to suggest that you should or should not give it intravenously. On a theoretical basis, Dr. MacKensie is on very firm ground that if one measures levels very closely during that period of time and they do not get much out of that target range, then it would seem the primary method by which to treat them. I do not have any strong convictions about it, basically. I think there is probably more than one way to skin a cat, and in this particular case, obviously you can get good results without terrible renal problems. I think either method is a reasonable management plan.

Question: Dr. Wallwork, why do you use ATG when from previous experience with renal transplant patients there are a number of disadvantages? Eight percent of the patients given ATG will be sensitized through it with that course, thereby at least precluding further use of the drug; reports from our center and others indicate that prophylactic ATG leads to a marked exacerbation of postoperative infections.

Dr. Wallwork: Much of the data you have referred to is historical data on the use of ATG in renal transplantation. Up until the advent of CsA, prophylactic ATG was uniformly used in cardiac transplant centers. I think the renal transplant surgeons got into trouble when they gave it initially; they daily gave a fixed dose per kilogram and didn't monitor the T cells very carefully. They probably gave too much. If you give too much immunosuppression, you get problems. I was very concerned when we started that we were giving too much immunosuppression, and I think that everybody would now agree that that was what was happening. I decided that we would go with steroids and CsA alone, and I think I was giving too little. I don't want to reverse direction and give too much again, so the amount of ATG I am giving is actually quite a small dose. The dose is determined by the T-cell count; some days I may not give any. This protocol gives me a base to build upon and change CsA dose and not worry about rejection during that time when the pharmacokinetics are changing. Liver function is getting better because of relief of passive congestion, and CsA requirements may increase. In fact, nobody knows what the ideal is, but we have not seen any great increase in infection by using this protocol. We've seen much less early rejection that needs to be treated with steroid pulse therapy, and at that point probably much more immunosuppression than at baseline. One must choose which protocol to follow: Are you going to give them all a higher dose of immunosuppressant to avoid rejection, or are you going to give them less initial therapy and end up treating more for rejection? It may very well be that if I was getting a lot of problems with infection or lymphoma, I might then reduce my immunosuppressive regimen, but I think we need to avoid marked changes.

Dr. Van Buren: Your protocol is predicated upon doing immune monitoring for rosettes on a daily basis, 7 days a week?

Dr. Wallwork: Well, for the days that you give the ATG—which is 10 days postoperatively, which was picked out of a hat; it could have been 7 days.

Question: Do you need to worry about ATG sensitivity during pulse therapy?

Dr. Wallwork: No, I haven't had to. Certainly when we used to give horse ATG prophylactically, but some patients become sensitized. Recently, sensitization with horse or rabbit ATG has not been a major problem.

Dr. Van Buren: Has hypertension been a postoperative problem? If so, how do you treat it?

Dr. Oyer: Hypertension has been a substantial problem in almost all the patients in our series, so that most of them are requiring more than simple diuretic therapy. In the past, with azathioprine treatment, about 20% of the patients were hypertensive and were relatively easily treated with this diuretic alone. That hypertension was basically based on the salt retention properties of corticosteroids is certainly a new ballgame in regard to hypertension. Obviously, one would expect that the long-term effects of hypertension are going to be the same and maybe worse in the cardiac recipient than they are in the general population with hypertension. It could be potentially worse because of strong accelerated atherosclerosis which occurs in the cardiac allograft, and the adverse effect of hypertension on that process still remains to be delineated. As far as treatment [is concerned], we have no fixed protocol, but the treatment tends to be as it is in the general essential-hypertension population. One, two, or probably in some cases, three antihypertensive agents are used until a reasonable combination can be determined. It is certainly a problem for most of the patients in our series, with the hypertension beginning as early as 2 or 3 weeks postoperatively.

Dr. MacKensie: I agree with Dr. Oyer's remarks that it is very common and most do require more than simple diuretics. We are exploring the etiology of it, but haven't found any relationship to renal function or renin level. It is unclear why so many are significantly hypertensive. We found captopril probably the best drug, but often they do require multiple pharmaceutical agents to achieve reasonably satisfactory blood pressure control.

Question: Are you all using antiplatelet drugs following cardiac transplantation?

Dr. Oyer: Yes, we are using persantine alone. A couple of patients are on aspirin, but most are on persantine alone.

Question: Is the purpose of the antiplatelet drug to prevent atherosclerosis?

Dr. Oyer: Yes. We have had very recently two patients develop that accelerated atherosclerotic process, so clearly that problem is still with us. We had originally hoped that CsA would keep under a little better control the immune response in the late period. Clearly, it hasn't completely controlled it. There are not enough data yet to consider the two groups of patients (conventional vs. CsA therapy) in terms of frequency of that problem. The upshot is that we are currently considering adding aspirin to the dipyridamole regimen.

Question: What dose are you using?

Dr. Oyer: It is variable, depending upon how much they can tolerate. Usually the maximum dose is 300 mg/day. Some patients just can't tolerate that much because of gastrointestinal problems, but we push it to the limit that they can tolerate.

Question: On those two patients, have they had any particularly prolonged rejection episode?

Dr. Oyer: No, neither one was really out of the ordinary. One thing that just came out before I came out here was that one of the patients who had preoperative triglyceride levels in the normal range over the course of the year and a little over a year that it took him to develop the advanced atherosclerosis, his triglyceride levels went up astronomically.

Question: Have you instituted dietary therapy?

Dr. Oyer: All the patients throughout the years have been instructed as far as dietary control of atherosclerosis, so they all get the routine instructions regarding that diet.

Dr. Van Buren: The marked advance of atherosclerosis may also be due to the steroid therapy. In lupus patients, progression of premature atherosclerosis seems to be related to high-dose steroids. Dr. MacKensie, do you routinely use antiplatelet drugs?

Dr. MacKensie: Yes, we use aspirin and a ratrum in more moderate doses of aspirin. We use one or at the most two a day, since its only effects are due to membrane acetylation. You can demonstrate that there is a prolonged antiplatelet effect for a long time after one dose. We don't push hard to get large doses into the patients.

Dr. Wallwork: We use half an aspirin daily combined with persantine therapy.

Dr. Van Buren: In light of the recently presented data, has any group represented here needed to convert a patient from CsA to azathioprine?

Drs. Oyer, Wallwork, MacKensie: No.

Dr. Oyer: We have switched two patients the other way, converting from conventional therapy to CsA, due to severe bone lesion because of steroids. Both cases were successful in reducing the steroid dose. One got down below 10 mg/day, and the other is now on about 6 mg of prednisone per day. In terms of reducing the steroids, conversion of the patient to CsA has been quite successful. The second patient we switched is currently doing well but is having problems because before we made the switch, he had severe osteoporosis of the spine. He was 6′4″ tall when transplanted and is now 5′10″. He is doing reasonably well after the conversion. The other person had to be converted back to azathioprine after about 4 months of gastrointestinal problems because he couldn't tolerate CsA and had uncontrollable vomiting under the most inopportune circumstances. He just couldn't tolerate CsA on the basis of gastrointestinal toxicity.

Question: Do you use reverse isolation?

Dr. MacKensie: We use it from the time the endotracheal tube is in place. The patient is kept in reverse isolation for 24 hr. This also discourages unwanted visitors.

Dr. Wallwork: I would agree. Reverse isolation may have had a greater role in the early days of transplantation with higher-dose immunosuppression. We still do it for approximately 7 days following surgery, but that is mostly to cut down traffic and keep the nosy out, I am sure.

Dr. Oyer: We still do the same thing just the way it has always been done. I would agree that the primary function is as has been described. Almost all the infections that we see are mostly nosocomial infections. Most of the organisms are ubiquitous. I don't believe that reverse isolation is particularly useful as a primary deterrent to infection.

Question: Even for a heart-lung transplant recipient?

Dr. Oyer: The same is probably true for these patients, but we still use reverse isolation. We have always done it that way and are set up to do it.

Dr. Wallwork: Probably the first patient not placed in reverse isolation will get infected!

Dr. Van Buren: How long do you keep the patient in the ICU?

Dr. Wallwork: It is a difficult concept, but our patients remain on ICU care postoperatively. Then about two or three days the patients are in the same room on what you would call ward care for maybe another 7 days, and then they are just transferred to the ward.

Question: When they go to an intermediate unit, is the unit monitored and a nurse with them in the room?

Dr. Wallwork: No, it is not a monitored unit; they just go up to the ward.

Question: Is electrophysiologic monitoring worthwhile to manage the patient?

Dr. Wallwork: We started a study to look at the electrophysiologic function of the transplanted heart. Similar work has already been done but was redone in the light of more sophisticated electrophysiologic studies. All patients have some form of dysfunction, but this isn't clinically a problem; it is only revealed on fine testing. We don't monitor the patients.

Question: Do you always put in a pacemaker following cardiac transplantation?

Dr. Wallwork: Yes, they all get a pacemaker. There are two reasons for that: (1) Historically, we had two patients drop down dead postoperatively, presumably due to an arrhythmia, and (2) we are involved in a grant to study them.

Dr. Van Buren: Do you place pacing wires for temporary use?

Dr. Wallwork: No, this is a permanent pacemaker.

Dr. Van Buren: This is for all the cardiac allograft recipients?

Dr. Oyer: We would put a temporary pacing wire on the atrium just for the insurance. Occasionally, we will pace patients during the first 24 hr. Sometimes their sinus node doesn't recover for a few hours, so we place these wires routinely, and I would say they are used in 1/20 patients. In the past, we have measured electrocardiographic voltage from that wire on a daily basis as well, but inasmuch as the voltage is no longer particularly useful for diagnosing rejection, we don't do that anymore.

Question: What about myocardial markers?

Dr. Oyer: That has been a research project at Stanford. For a number of years, at the time of transplantation, we have implanted tiny metallic screws into the myocardium along the septum so that postoperatively we could take a Cini angiogram or a Cini film 3- or 4-sec shot. A computer program is being developed to deliver the motion of those markers so you can extract a whole array of physiologic information. We are still planning those studies, although it has never been useful therapeutically. It has been basically a research project, so that in the long term one can very easily noninvasively assess what the heart is doing.

Dr. MacKensie: Could you not get the same information from an echo?

Dr. Oyer: The study was actually begun before the echo was in widespread use, and it provides in many ways very similar information, but since the markers are in a fixed location, I think it is probably a little more accurate than one can get with a 2-D.

Dr. Van Buren: Let me move into a different area. Instead of talking about the practical problems we have addressed, could you now perhaps answer a question of what will be the role of cardiac transplantation in the future, once functional centers are established. Should cardiac transplantation and/or heart-lung transplantation be used as primary therapy to treat a complex pediatric cardiac lesion? Is there any role for this in the future?

Dr. MacKensie: I think there is going to be a broadening of the scope of cardiac transplantation, that is, increased numbers of centers doing transplants. It is never going to be a common undertaking. I think the indications for transplantation may themselves broaden; for example, the non-insulin-dependent diabetic may be an acceptable cardiac transplant; in fact, we have had such a patient. Others with chronic disabling diseases which are nonfatal may become candidates. I think the rather stringent acceptance criteria which were outlined by Stanford were entirely appropriate for the original application of cardiac transplantation, but they probably can be liberalized. I never see cardiac transplantation becoming a very common undertaking. I wouldn't have thought it appropriate that huge numbers of centers began transplanting and doing occasional heart transplants. I think this is something to be done by those where there is a large team who are going to devote considerable care and attention to it. I don't think that CsA is going to revolutionize the field. It is not going to develop another outburst of activity similar to what coronary artery bypass has done. It still is going to be a rather limited undertaking, I think.

Dr. Wallwork: I would agree. One of the limitations is going to be donors, and I think that whatever you are going to do, you are only going to be able to get a certain number of adequate donors. That in the end will probably be the thing that limits cardiac transplant activity. Certainly I think that many centers may very well start in the future. I don't know.

Dr. Van Buren: What is the [greatest] number of organs you have retrieved from a specific donor? You have, I am sure, been involved with multiple organ transplantation. I know that is a logistic problem at times.

Dr. Oyer: Probably four is the most that we have done, probably if you include the cornea. We have been involved with harvesting both kidneys, the liver, and the heart on several occasions of which I am aware. Of course, it takes a little more coordination and certainly a little more effort on everybody's part. Certainly, it is easier for the people harvesting the kidneys to take the kidneys only. We certainly appreciate the extra time they spend and the extra coordination involved. But certainly it can be done when these donors provide multiple organs.

Dr. Van Buren: Are you usually contacted by individual physicians or by specific organ procurement centers?

Dr. Oyer: It happens in several different ways. We get occasional calls directly to us from hospitals in the area and sometimes a distance away from our specific area regarding a potential heart donor. In those cases, we generally contact the Northern California Transplant Bank to see if somebody needs a kidney. Most of the organs we get now come from Los Angeles or San Diego and through the renal transplant centers down there. The Southern California groups have organized things very well, and they have been very generous [in] calling us when they have a suitable donor. The Northern California Transplant Bank, which is in San Francisco, also calls us when they have a recipient who might be suitable. The network is a little complicated in how these donor calls come through. I think we have really only scratched the surface in terms of educating the public and doing all things in terms of success of heart transplantation and all forms of translantation. I might just say one other thing about your question for the future. I think certainly the future of heart-lung transplantation really revolves around the quality of the immunosuppression that becomes available. Certainly CsA is not going to be the final answer in the long term, and I fully agree with the other comments that even though CsA is certainly an advance in terms of bottom-line survival, it is not really going to allow every cardiac surgeon in the country to jump into heart transplantation. I really think that what will happen 10 or 20 years from now depends on developments of immunology. If someone does come up with a means, for example, to allow xenografting, then that is an entirely different ballgame in terms of how many patients can be provided with new organs of all kinds. Depending how good immunosuppression is, it may be [that] eventually, with limitations on donors removed, many other centers around the country can provide new hearts to a lot of people. If things progress, we will see patients that have failed to respond to conventional cardiac surgical treatment of their lesions, such as coronary artery bypass or valve replacement in patients with chronic mitrial stenosis, as candidates for cardiac transplantation. Depending on how good immunosuppression is, eventually one might even consider cardiac transplantation as primary treatment for some of the forms of heart disease [that] today one wouldn't think about. This may be overly optimistic.

Question: What role do you think the mechanical device can play in patients who obviously need transplant and for whom a donor is not immediately available?

Dr. Oyer: I would have to answer that by qualifying that it depends upon how well the mechanical devices function. This is not just merely in terms of physiologic function but also in terms of how easy they are to put in and how easy they are to take out and so forth. In principle, I think they can be useful and probably applied in a limited number of patients. First of all, the practical problem is that one obviously would not like to have to operate on a severely sick recipient when he is going downhill, put one of those devices in, and then sometime later come back and operate on him again for another major operation, the cardiac transplant procedure. One would like to avoid that. Deciding when we are going to intervene with a mechanical device is not necessarily a simple matter. One should avoid operating on a patient who is too ill to benefit, but nevertheless, deciding when to implant the device may not be straightforward. Secondly, most of the people who die waiting for transplantation die suddenly. There is no real opportunity to put a mechanical device into that sort of patient. They may be doing reasonably well and die suddenly. There are those sorts of practical problems with using mechanical devices as a bridge for cardiac transplantation. In principle, I think it depends on how well those devices develop in the future.

CYCLOSPORINE TOXICITY

The Nephrotoxicity of Cyclosporine in Renal Transplant Recipients

S. M. Flechner, C. Van Buren, R. H. Kerman, and B. D. Kahan

CYCLOSPORINE (CsA), a fungal peptide with unique immunosuppressive action, has been demonstrated to be an effective agent to prevent allograft rejection in human renal transplantation. However, its potent immunosuppressive activity has been accompanied by nephrotoxicity, which was initially observed during the first clinical trials of this drug in Cambridge, England.[1] This unfortunate side effect has complicated the management of renal transplant recipients using CsA and raises questions as to the future widespread use of this agent.

CsA-induced nephrotoxicity has been observed as early as a few days posttransplant. This led to the early recommendation that CsA be withheld until an immediate posttransplant diuresis is observed.[2] Currently, many centers begin CsA prior to transplantation.[3-5] A more perplexing problem has been the differentiation between CsA-induced nephrotoxicity and allograft rejection. This report describes the impact of nephrotoxicity on both cadaveric (CAD) and living-related (LRD) renal allograft recipients. The effect of CsA on early graft function, long-term renal function, and allograft rejection will be presented.

MATERIALS AND METHODS

Patient Population

The study population consisted of 150 recipients of renal transplants (100 CAD, 50 LRD) performed at the University of Texas Medical School at Houston between January 1981 and March 1983. These recipients were immunosuppressed with CsA and prednisone (no other agent was used in combination with CsA). A concurrent group of 47 CAD recipients immunosuppressed with azathioprine (AZA) and prednisone were used as a control population. Both inpatient and outpatient medical records were used for data analysis.

Immunosuppressive Regimen

LRD recipients received CsA (14 mg/kg of body weight orally) beginning 48 hr, and CAD recipients received 14 mg/kg of body weight beginning 6–12 hr pretransplant. Postoperatively, recipients received 14 mg/kg for week 1; 12 mg/kg weeks 2–3; 10 mg/kg weeks 4–12; and thereafter dosing was predicated on measurements of 24-hr serum trough levels of CsA, as determined by radioimmunoassay (RIA; reagents supplied by Sandoz, Ltd., Basel, Switzerland).[6] At each interval, dosage adjustments were made in an effort to keep trough levels in a range of 100–200 ng/ml. CsA (2–3 mg/kg) was given intravenously when the oral route could not be used.

Each recipient received steroids in tapering doses, beginning at 120 mg prednisone on the first postoperative day. This was tapered to 30 mg day 60, 25 mg day 90, down to 15 mg at 1 year.

Ten recipients (6.6%) were converted from CsA to AZA for presumed intractable nephrotoxicity.[7] These patients and their level of renal function are included in the data analysis.

Organ Procurement

LRD nephrectomy was done in standard fashion, and all kidneys were removed only after an in situ diuresis was demonstrated. All CAD kidneys were removed locally from heart-beating donors with warm ischemia times under 10 min. All kidneys were initially flushed with a cold (4°C) intracellular electrolyte solution (Collins-2). The majority of CsA-treated CAD kidneys (69) were preserved by simple cold storage in iced Collins-2 solution. There were 31 CsA-treated CAD kidneys preserved by pulsatile perfusion on a MOX-100 (Waters, Co.) pump. Machine-stored kidneys were preserved using plasma protein fraction (plasmanate enriched with albumin) and were used only if acceptable viability criteria were maintained.[8]

Acute Tubular Necrosis

Acute tubular necrosis (ATN) was defined as the need for supportive dialysis for any reason during the first posttransplant week. A DTPA and Hippuran radioiso-

---

From the Division of Immunology and Organ Transplantation, Department of Surgery, University of Texas Medical School, Houston, TX.

Address reprint requests to Dr. S. M. Flechner, Division of Immunology and Organ Transplantation, Department of Surgery, University of Texas School of Medicine, Houston, TX 77030.

0041–1345/83/1505–0088$01.00/0

topic renal scan was obtained on each recipient the first 24 hr posttransplant. The diagnosis of ATN was established by the typical scan findings of decreased tubular excretion of Hippuran with preserved renal perfusion.[9] Immunosuppressive drugs were administered at the same doseage schedules for patients with or without ATN.

Renal Dysfunction

Episodes of renal dysfunction were categorized as to the incremental rise in creatinine, either greater than or less than 25% of baseline values. Serum CsA trough levels, daily doses of CsA (mg/kg), clinical signs of rejection (fever, graft enlargement, oliguria, hypertension, proteinuria), and renal biopsies were compared during these events. Episodes of renal dysfunction associated with <25% increases in creatinine or trough levels >200 ng/ml were treated by reducing the CsA dose 50–100 mg. Renal dysfunction with larger increases in creatinine, clinical signs of rejection, and diffuse cellular infiltrates on renal biopsy were treated with steroid pulse therapy.

Data Analysis

Data analysis was done using the chi-square statistic, Student's t test, and actuarial life table methods. Significance was set at the 95% confidence limit for each test. There were no patients excluded from the analysis for any reason. Graft loss was recorded on the date of transplant nephrectomy, return to chronic dialysis, or patient mortality.

RESULTS

Early Graft Function

The 150 CsA-treated and 47 AZA-treated kidneys were transplanted without hyperacute rejection. Only one LRD recipient (2%) experienced ATN (due to a technical problem). The incidence of ATN in CsA-treated CAD kidneys (38%) was not statistically different from that of AZA-treated (45%) kidneys (Table 1). A significant difference ($p < 0.01$) did emerge in the incidence of ATN between those 69 CsA-treated CAD kidneys preserved by cold storage (30.4%) and those 31 preserved by pulsatile perfusion (54.8%). However, no significant difference in mean preservation time between the two methods of preservation was observed to account for these results (Table 2).

Table 1. Incidence of ATN in 150 CsA-Treated and 47 AZA-Treated Renal Transplant Recipients

	Cyclosporine Treated		Azathioprine Treated
	LRD (%)	CAD (%)	CAD (%)
Immediate function	50	62	25
ATN	1(2)	38(38)	22(45)
Total	50	100	47

CAD: CsA versus AZA, p = NS.

Table 2. Mean Preservation Times (hr) of 100 CsA-Treated Cadaver Kidneys

	Cold Storage	Pulsatile Perfusion
Immediate function	18.3 ± 4.1 (48)	22.5 ± 5.1 (14)
ATN	20.4 ± 5.6 (21)	20.7 ± 4.6 (17)

NOTE. The number of kidneys is given in parentheses. There were no significant differences in preservation times.

The fate of the 150 CsA-treated allografts during the first 30 days revealed that 89 (59%) of 150 experienced a progressive improvement in renal function, with a creatinine level of ≤1.5 mg/dl by day 14. In 46 (31%) of 150, the fall in creatinine was more protracted, reaching 2–3 mg/dl by day 30. Graft loss during the first month occurred in 15 (10%) of 150: primary nonfunction in 2, arterial thrombosis in 4, sepsis in 5, and rejection in 4.

Eventual Graft Function

The one-year actuarial patient and graft survival for these CsA- and prednisone-treated recipients is reported in another article in this issue.[10] The occurrence of ATN did not appear to cause a significant deleterious effect on cadaveric allograft survival (Fig. 1), although two cases of primary nonfunction did occur.

The longitudinal analysis of CAD recipients (Table 3) revealed a continuous decrease in the administered daily dose of CsA, from a mean of 7.11 mg/kg at six months to 4.52 mg/kg at two years posttransplant. The group mean creatinines (mg/dl) remained relatively stable at each interval, from 1.87 at six months to 2.00 at two years posttransplant. However, the distribution of creatinine values demonstrated a decreasing frequency in the percentage of recipients at each interval with a creatinine <2 mg/dl. While 66% of CAD recipients had a creatinine <2 mg/dl at six

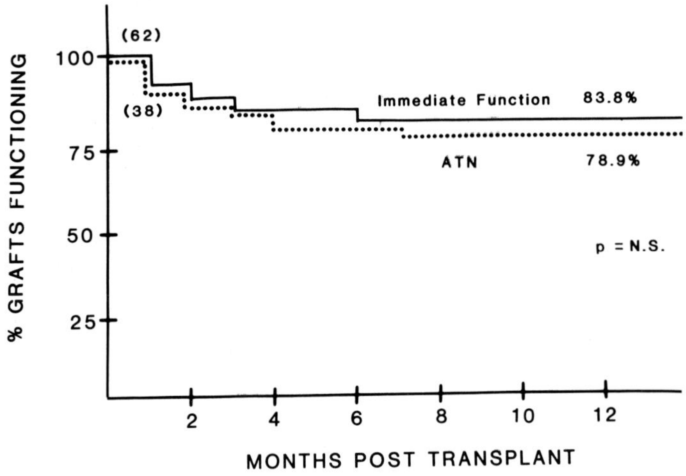

Fig. 1. Actuarial cadaveric renal allograft survival in kidneys with immediate function or posttransplant acute tubular necrosis. There was no statistically significant difference in graft survival between the two groups. Included in the ATN group are two cases of primary nonfunction.

months, only 42% had a creatinine <2 mg/dl at two years.

The longitudinal analysis of LRD recipients (Table 4) also revealed a continuous decrease in the mean daily doses of CsA, from 7.17 mg/kg at six months to 6.18 mg/kg at 18 months posttransplant. However, the LRD recipients were receiving about 1 mg/kg more CsA daily than their CAD counterparts at each follow-up interval. The group mean creatinine values remained stable during the follow-up, from 1.60 at six months to 1.59 at 18 months. The distribution of creatinine values also appeared to be stable, as 70% or more of LRD recipients maintained creatinines <2 mg/dl up to 18 months posttransplant.

Posttransplant Renal Dysfunction

The impact of CsA nephrotoxicity was felt by most recipients in that 138 (92%) of 150 required an increased rate of taper of CsA from the original protocol (see Materials and Methods) due to presumed nephrotoxicity or increased CsA levels. At present, the mean follow-up for the group is 11 ± 5 months. During this period, 812 episodes (5.4 ± 2.1/patient) of creatinine elevations <25% of baseline were observed. These were treated by a 50–100 mg reduction in the daily CsA dose, with resolution of most events.

There were 61 episodes (55 patients) of renal dysfunction associated with creatinine elevations of >25% of baseline. Retrospectively, 19 episodes (17 patients) were due to acute rejection based on the presence of clinical signs of rejection, diffuse mononuclear cell infiltrates on renal biopsy, and either a response to steroid pulse therapy or progression to graft loss due to rejection. The response to steroid pulse therapy was varied, in that five (26%) of 19 of episodes progressed to graft loss, and in only five (26%) of 19 did renal function return to normal (creatinine <2 mg/dl). In nine (47%) of 19, residual renal

Table 3. Renal Function in CsA-Treated Cadaveric Recipients (Mean ± SD)

	Months Posttransplant			
	6	12	18	24
n	60	34	17	7
CSA (mg/kg)	7.11 ± 1.94	5.88 ± 1.71	5.09 ± 1.47	4.52 ± 0.58
Creatinine (mg/dl)	1.87 ± 0.69	2.12 ± 0.80	2.06 ± 0.52	2.00 ± 0.33
Distribution				
<2	66%	53%	53%	42%
2–3	26%	32%	41%	58%
>3	08%	15%	06%	0%

Table 4. Renal Function in CsA-Treated Living-Related Recipients (Mean ± SD)

	Months Posttransplant		
	6	12	18
n	33	21	10
CSA (mg/kg)	7.17 ± 1.42	6.82 ± 1.51	6.18 ± 1.76
Creatinine (mg/dl)	1.60 ± 0.57	1.68 ± 0.65	1.59 ± 0.39
Distribution			
<2	78%	76%	70%
2–3	19%	14%	30%
>3	03%	10%	0%

impairment occurred, with creatinine values remaining 2–3 mg/dl. Fifteen (78%) of the 19 episodes occurred during the first 30 days posttransplant. The mean CsA trough levels were 186 ± 86 ng/ml during these rejection episodes.

The remaining 42 episodes (38 patients) were due to CsA nephrotoxicity. These were not accompanied by clinical signs of rejection, and no diffuse mononuclear cell infiltrates were present on renal biopsies. All episodes responded either to a reduction in the CsA dose or conversion (10 patients) to AZA and CsA withdrawal.[7] However, in only 14 (33%) of 42 of episodes did creatinine values return to within 10% of baseline, and 16 (42%) of 38 of patients were left with permanent renal impairment (creatinine 2–3 mg/dl). Only eight of these episodes occurred during the first 30 days posttransplant, and seven (87%) of these eight were associated with CsA trough levels >200 ng/ml. The other 34 episodes occurred after the first month, the majority between days 60 and 100. CsA levels were not helpful in delayed nephrotoxic events, in that 20 (59%) of 34 were associated with trough levels <200 ng/ml.

Nephrotoxicity Versus Rejection

The differentiation between nephrotoxicity and rejection was often difficult, and no single clinical or laboratory parameter appeared to be pathognomonic for either event. However, a pattern consistent with rejection did emerge (Table 5). Nearly 90% of rejection episodes occurred by day 45, most by day 30. Rejection episodes were usually associated with rapid rise in creatinine over two to four days, with elevations >25% of baseline in all patients. Clinical signs were not common (fever >100°F, proteinuria, graft enlargement, hypertension in only one-third of patients), except for diminished urine volumes. In 15 (78%) of 19 of rejection episodes, urine output dropped by 25%, and in 12 (63%) of 19, by 50% of previous volumes. During these events, renal biopsies have diffuse cellular infiltrates.

Significant nephrotoxic events (creatinine >25% baseline) generally occurred between days 60 and 100. Those few that occurred the first 30 days were usually associated with elevated (>200 ng/ml) CsA trough levels. The increase in creatinine level was more insidious and urine outputs are maintained. Renal biopsies may have patchy, focal mononuclear cell infiltrates, but marked edema and necrosis are absent. These differences were not initially evident, and 16 episodes of nephrotoxicity (eventually responsive to CsA dose reduction or conversion) were first treated with steroid pulse therapy (unsuccessfully).

DISCUSSION

CsA has been demonstrated to act early and reversibly on the triggering mechanisms

Table 5. Nephrotoxicity Versus Rejection

Parameter	Favors Rejection	Favors Nephrotoxicity
Rate of Cr rise	3–4 Days	5–7 Days
Creatinine increase	>25%	≤25%
Occurrence	<Day 30	>Day 30
CsA levels	<200 ng/ml	>200 ng/ml
Biopsy	Heavy cellular infiltrate	Negative
Clinical signs	Decreased volume 25%	No change

controlling T-cell activation and clonal expansion.[11] Therefore, adequate drug levels to prevent T-cell proliferation should be present at the time of alloantigen presentation. An unacceptably high rate of CsA nephrotoxicity, which caused a delay in drug administration, could therefore impair initial immunologic induction. LRD recipients treated with CsA for 48 hr pretransplant did not experience posttransplant ATN. CAD recipients treated with pretransplant CsA did not have an increased ATN rate compared with AZA controls. In addition, those CsA kidneys with ATN did not suffer diminished graft survival. Therefore, CsA can be safely administered prior to alloantigen presentation.

However, a significant difference in the ATN rate between the two methods of preservation used in our program was observed. Kidneys preserved by cold storage had a lower rate of ATN (30.4% versus 54.8%) than those preserved by pulsatile perfusion. Preservation times were similar in both groups, and in most cases were less than 24 hr. While there were no CsA-treated kidneys with extended preservation times (>40 hr), data from the Canadian Transplant Study Group describes a deleterious effect on graft survival from prolonged perfusion preservation.[12] Kidneys in which revascularization can be predicted to occur within 24 hr are thus more likely to have immediate function if preserved by simple cold storage.

The effect of CsA on long-term allograft function was evaluated. The present series confirms earlier reports of mild renal dysfunction in allograft recipients treated with CsA, which does not appear to be progressive up to two years posttransplant. However, a clear difference did emerge between the LRD and the CAD recipients. The mean creatinines were 0.5 mg/dl lower at each interval in the LRD group, and about 25% more LRD recipients had creatinine levels <2 mg/dl at each interval. In addition, the LRD recipients were receiving about 1 mg/kg more CsA daily than the CAD recipients.

These differences may imply that progressive long-term deterioration in renal function in CsA-treated CAD recipients is due to ongoing immunologic damage rather than drug-induced nephrotoxicity. If true, this would question the appropriateness of routine conversion to alternative (less potent) forms of immunosuppression for all recipients. An alternative explanation may be a permanent injury incurred during cadaver organ recovery and preservation. In either case, longer follow-up is needed to assess the rate of progression of changes in renal function and the long-term stability of those grafts with impaired function.

Renal dysfunction posttransplant associated with small creatinine elevations of ≤25% of baseline are due to CsA nephrotoxicity and usually respond to a decrease in the CsA dose of 50–100 mg. CsA trough levels are helpful if elevated (>200 ng/ml). Creatinine elevations >25% are very significant and lead to permanent renal impairment in two-thirds of patients. About 30% of these episodes are due to acute rejection, which usually occurs during the first 30 days posttransplant (Table 5). Acute rejection is not common in CsA-treated patients overall (17 of 150, 11%), especially after the first 2 months posttransplant. Patients with low CsA levels (<100 ng/ml), negative renal biopsies, and continued creatinine elevations are candidates for conversion to AZA.[7]

In summary, CsA nephrotoxicity is the most common cause of posttransplant renal dysfunction, but excellent allograft survival can be achieved with careful monitoring of patients. Currently, most patients are dosed to their tolerance of renal toxicity. Future investigations are needed to disclose the minimum dose required for each individual patient to ensure adequate immunosuppression with minimal nephrotoxicity. This will require further understanding of the mechanism of action, absorption, metabolism, and elimination of the drug.

REFERENCES

1. Calne RY, Thiru S, McMaster P, et al: Lancet 2:1323, 1978

2. Calne RY, Rolles K, Thiru S, et al: Lancet 1:1033, 1979

3. Starzl TE, Klintmalm GB, Weil R, et al: Surg Gynecol Obstet 153:486, 1981

4. Ferguson RM, Rynasiewicz J, Sutherland DR, et al: Surgery 92:175, 1982

5. Flechner SM, Payne WD, Van Buren CT, et al: Transplantation 36:268, 1983

6. Kahan BD, Van Buren CT, Lin SN, et al: Transplantation 34:36, 1982

7. Flechner SM, Van Buren C, Kerman R, et al: Transplant Proc (in press)

8. Magnusson M, Stowe NT: Urol Clin North Am 3:491, 1976

9. Shanahan WS, Klingensmith WC, Weil R: Am J Radiol 136:249, 1981

10. Kahan BD, Van Buren C, Flechner SM, et al: Transplant Proc (this issue)

11. Weisinger D, Borel JF: Immunology 156:454, 1980

12. Stiller CR, et al: Transplant Proc (this issue)

13. Hamilton DV, Calne RY, Evans DB, et al: Lancet 1:1218, 1981

Renal Effects of Cyclosporine: Clinical and Experimental Observations

R. Devineni, N. McKenzie, J. Duplan, P. Keown, C. Stiller, and A. C. Wallace

CYCLOSPORINE (CsA) has been shown to be an effective immunosuppressive agent in experimental and clinical organ transplantation.[1-5] We had not found significant nephrotoxicity in a canine cardiac transplant model during acute or chronic CsA administration despite wide fluctuations in serum CsA level.[5] In humans, however, significant nephrotoxicity has been common.

A more specific examination of the renal effects of CsA was therefore undertaken on the dog.

MATERIALS AND METHODS

Healthy adult male mongrel dogs weighing between 20 and 25 kg were used. Group A ($n = 4$) served as controls. Groups B, C, and D ($n = 5$) received 15, 10, and 5 mg/kg of body weight CsA, respectively.

The dogs were premedicated with Xylazine (5 mg/kg i.m.) and atropine (0.04 mg/kg i.m.). Anesthesia was induced with thiopental sodium (8 mg/kg i.v.) and maintained with halothane 1.5% and room air/O_2. Normal saline was infused to induce a brisk diuresis. A midline laparotomy was performed and both ureters exposed. They were ligated distally and the proximal ends cannulated with polyethelene tubing draining into measuring flasks (Fig. 1). The left renal artery was isolated at its origin and controlled with a rubber snare. Samples of blood and urine were taken (T_0). Biopsies were taken from both kidneys using a no. 10 Tru-Cut bioptome (Travenol Laboratories Inc., Deerfield, IL).

Heparin (1,000 units) was given i.v. and the left renal artery occluded. At the end of 1 hr, urine volumes were measured, urine and blood samples obtained (T_1), and blood flow to the left kidney was restored. CsA in 50 ml of D5W was infused over the next hour in groups B, C, and D in doses of 15, 10, and 5 mg/kg, respectively. Urine volumes were measured and blood and urine samples obtained over the next two hr (T_2 and T_3). Finally, biopsies were taken from both kidneys before the animal was killed.

Biochemical measurements included blood urea nitrogen (BUN), creatinine, electrolytes, bilirubin, and liver enzymes in the serum and N-acetyl-B-glucose aminidase (NAG), gamma-glutamyl transferase (γ-GT), and creatinine in the urine. Serum CsA was determined at T_2 and T_3 in groups B, C, and D.

Tissue samples from both kidneys were subjected to light and electron microscopic examination.

RESULTS

Urine Flow (Fig. 2)

In control animals, there was a significant reduction in the urine output from the left kidney after 1 hr of ischemia, with gradual recovery over the next 2 hr ($p < 0.05$). In groups B and C, the reduction in urine output is more pronounced in the left kidney than the right ($p < 0.01$). In group D, the smaller dose of CsA (5 mg/kg) is better tolerated by both kidneys. With the exception of animals in group B (CsA 15 mg/kg), all the other groups show an improvement in urine output with time.

Renal Tubular Enzyme Release

The changes in urinary NAG and γ-GT excretion are shown in Figs. 3–6. In group A, the increase in left kidney urinary NAG was significant ($p < 0.05$), while the γ-GT remained unchanged. In groups B, C, and D, urinary NAG and γ-GT levels are significantly increased and more so from the left kidney than the right ($p < 0.05$ to $p < 0.0001$).

Urinary and serum creatinine, BUN, serum lactate dehydrogenase (LDH), alkaline phosphatase, bilirubin, and electrolytes did not change significantly at any time.

Histologic Findings

Light microscopic abnormalities were most prominent in group B left kidney biopsies following ischemia and high-dose CsA infu-

From the Divisions of Cardiovascular and Thoracic Surgery, and Nephrology, and the Department of Pathology, University Hospital, London, Canada.

Address reprint requests to Dr. N. McKenzie, University Hospital, P.O. Box 5339, Postal Station A, London, Ontario, Canada N6A 5A5.

0041-1345/83/1505-0089$01.00/0

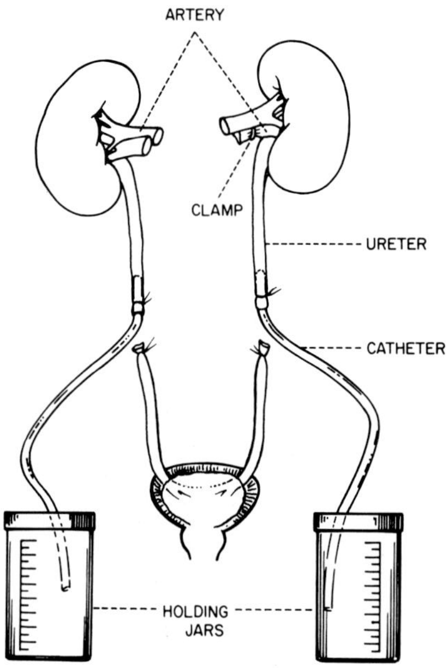

Fig. 1. Drawing showing cannulation of both ureters and temporary occlusion of the left renal artery.

sion. These comprised predominantly proximal convoluted tubule (PCT), epithelial cellular swelling, hydropic degeneration, and necrosis. The glomerulus was not overtly affected.

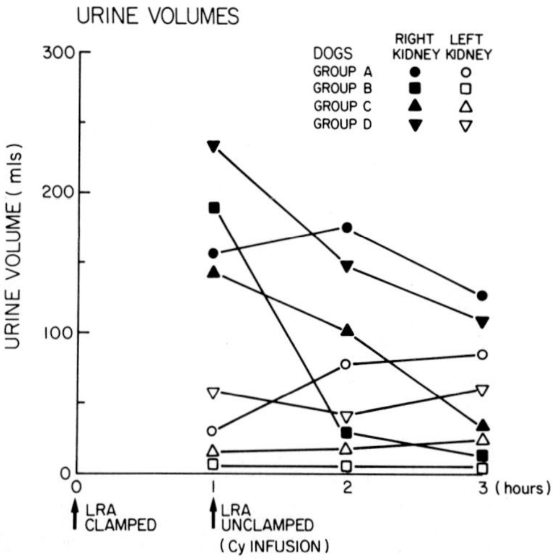

Fig. 2. Urine flows at intervals after cyclosporine infusion. Each point represents the mean value of 4 experiments in group A (control) and 5 experiments in groups B, C, and D. The solid symbols show results from the nonischemic right kidney, and the open symbols results from the temporarily ischemic left kidney.

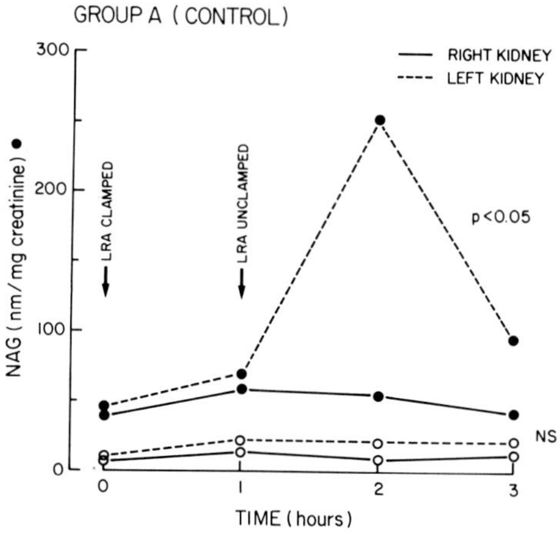

Fig. 3. Urinary gamma-GT excretion at intervals after saline infusion in group A (control) animals. Each point represents the mean value of 4 experiments.

Electron microscopy revealed cytoplasmic vacuolation, loss of brush border, increased number of lysosomes, and cellular necrosis. These changes were most prominent in the PCT cells, and to a lesser extent in the distal convoluted tubular cells. The glomeruli did not show any abnormalities. These findings

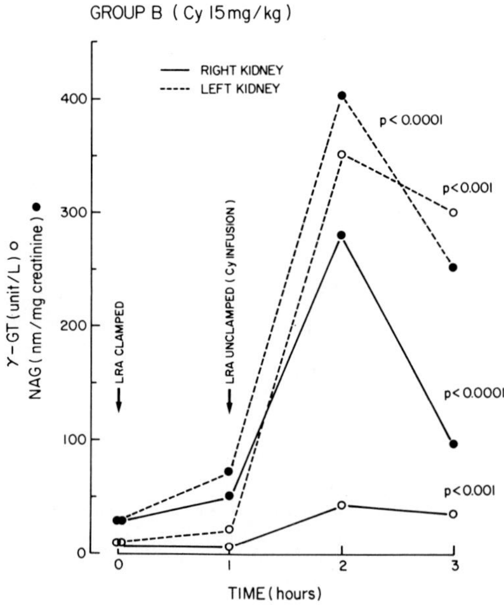

Fig. 4. Urinary gamma-GT excretion at intervals after cyclosporine infusion in group B animals (15 mg/kg body weight). Each point represents the mean value of 5 experiments.

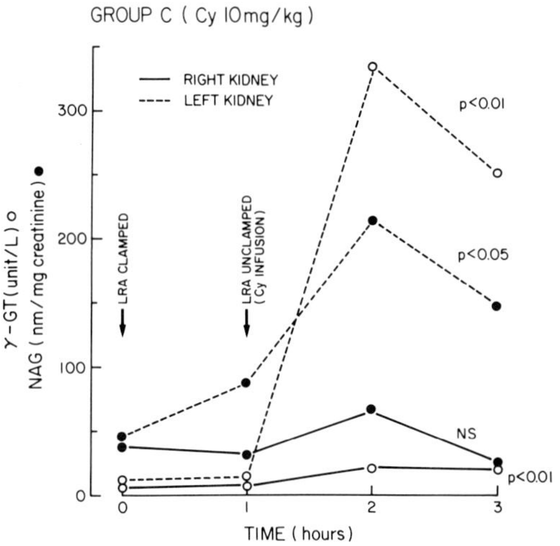

Fig. 5. Urinary gamma-GT excretion at intervals after cyclosporine infusion in group C animals (10 mg/kg body weight). Each point represents the mean value of 5 experiments.

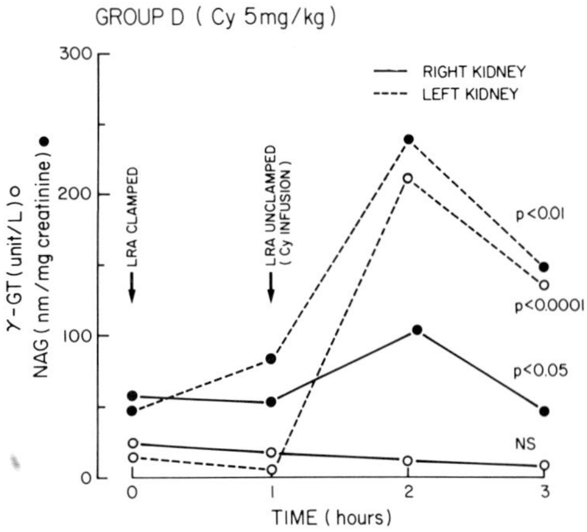

Fig. 6. Urinary gamma-GT excretion at intervals after cyclosporine infusion in group D animals (5 mg/kg body weight). Each point represents the mean value of 5 experiments.

were seen in all the CsA groups. There was no correlation between the functional status and morphologic picture of the kidneys.

DISCUSSION

The results of experimental and clinical organ transplantation using CsA as the major immunosuppressive drug have been encouraging.[2–5,8] The incidence of graft rejection and infection has been greatly reduced with a concomitant decrease in morbidity.[4,8] However, nephrotoxicity of CsA has posed a major problem.[4,9] Biochemical and structural changes in the kidneys have been reported in experimental animals treated with CsA.[6]

In this study we attempted to simulate the common clinical situation of impaired renal function by subjecting one kidney to a short period of ischemia prior to CsA administration. Each animal could thus act as its own control. An acute dose-dependent nephrotoxic effect of CsA was shown, the principal effect being on cells of the proximal convoluted tubules (PCT).

NAG is a hydrolytic enzyme present in the cells of the PCT and is released into the tubular lumen following damage to the epithelial cell brush border. γ-GT, which catalyzes the hydrolysis of gamma-glutamyl bond of reduced glutathione, is also concentrated in the brush border of the PCT epithelial cells. The urinary levels of both these enzymes are increased following nephrotoxic insult.[10,11] Ischemia alone will cause a significant elevation of NAG, but not of γ-GT (group A). After the administration of CsA, animals in groups B, C, and D show significant increase in both these urinary enzymes, with the left kidney being more profoundly affected. In groups C and D, these changes were not progressive.

The light and electron microscopic findings are similar to those noted by Whiting et al.[6] The most obvious structural damage is seen in the PCT and may explain the increase in urinary enzymes. No change, however, was seen in the endoplasmic reticulum.

In our series of clinical cardiac transplantation using CsA, renal insufficiency has been the dominant problem,[4] occurring in 10 of 14 patients. Elevated postoperative serum renin levels (18–24 ng/liter), which return to normal in 7–10 days, have been consistently found and seem unrelated to renal status. Urinary NAG, γ-GT and β_2-microglobulin are elevated in the first 3 weeks posttransplant and fluctuate with serum CsA levels. The urine output following surgery seems to follow a consistent pattern. In spite of adequate urine output during and after surgery, oliguria develops in 6–8 hr. The serum CsA levels have been between 50 and 400 ng/ml (on CsA given p.o. in a dose of 7–10 mg/kg weight 4 hr preoperatively). The oliguria fails to respond to fluids and diuretics and progresses to anuria. With expectant management, the diuretic phase begins in 48–72 hr, with a fall in BUN and serum creatinine. During the oliguric phase, the urine sodium is low (4–8 meq/liter) and the urine osmolarity is low (<350). These findings are contrary to those described by Whiting et al.[6] Though there is evidence of PCT injury, the cause of impairment of glomerular filtration has yet to be ascertained. Inadequate renal perfusion and cortical ischemia is an attractive hypothesis.[6] High serum renin levels are commonly seen following routine nonpulsatile cardiopulmonary bypass (CPB),[12] and we have confirmed this in a control clinical group of routine CPB patients. However, no significant increase in urinary NAG, γ-GT, and beta-2-microglobulin is seen in these patients, implying a different mechanism for CsA nephrotoxicity.

The acute renal effects of CsA in the clinical setting have been, fortunately, reversible and do not seem related to the peak serum CsA level. However, the kidneys may remain susceptible to high serum levels of CsA, and we strive to maintain trough levels between 150 and 250 ng/ml. At high levels, biochemical evidence of nephrotoxicity is consistently seen without any enhanced immunologic protection.

The long-term effects of CsA on renal function need to be carefully assessed. Two of our cardiac transplant recipients on CsA show biochemical evidence of renal impairment, with impaired creatinine clearance, at 18–24 months posttransplant, with adequate cardiac graft function. Renal biopsy on one of them shows moderate to severe interstitial nephritis with glomerular and PCT damage.

SUMMARY

The results of this experimental study show that there is acute renal PCT damage caused by CsA and that the magnitude of this damage is related to the dose of CsA and temporary ischemia. These changes appear to be reversible with lower CsA levels.

The occurrence of oliguria and anuria in clinical cardiac transplant patients does seem to be related to peak serum CsA levels, and its etiology remains to be ascertained.

ACKNOWLEDGMENT

We thank Sandoz of Basel, Switzerland, for supplying the cyclosporine used in these studies.

REFERENCES

1. Borel JF: Transplant Proc 13:344, 1981

2. Morris PJ: Transplantation 32:349, 1981

3. Calne RY, White DJ, Thiru S, et al: Transplant Proc 13:349, 1981

4. Devineni R, McKenzie FN, Kostuk WJ, et al: Heart Transplant 2:219, 1983

5. McKenzie FN, Stiller CR, Wall WJ, et al: Transplant Proc 15:1244, 1983

6. Whiting PH, Thomson AW, Blair JT, et al: Br J Exp Pathol 66:83, 1982

7. Sweny P, Hopper J, Gross M, et al: Lancet 1:663, 1981

8. Oyer PE, Stinson EB, Jamieson SW, et al: Heart Transplant 1:285, 1982

9. Klintmalm GBG, Iwatsuki S, Starzl TE: Lancet 1:470, 1981

10. Wellwood JM, Ellis BG, Price RG: Br Med J 3:408, 1975

11. Beck PR, Chaudhury AK: Clin Chem 22:528, 1976

12. Landymore RW, Murphy DA, Kinley CE, et al: Ann Thorac Surg 28:261, 1979

Cyclosporine in Patients With Oligoanuria After Cadaveric Kidney Transplantation

L. A. Castro, G. Hillebrand, W. Land, B. Schneider, K. Günther, and H. J. Gurland

RENAL damage due to cyclosporine is well documented.[1–3] Experience with its use after kidney transplantation is not yet sufficient to predict its potential toxicity. The nature of the clinical situation in which cyclosporine is given, especially after kidney transplantation, makes it easy to over- or underestimate the true frequency and significance of nephrotoxicity. Moreover, the kidney has limited possibilities of responses to different injuries (for example, coexisting ischemia, other drugs, or the immunologic process itself), and it is generally impossible to implicate the drug as the causative factor in primary nonfunctioning graft. Accordingly, the clinical protocol for the multicenter European study required that cyclosporine should be used only in patients having a good diuresis after transplantation.[4] This initially reasonable recommendation has been breeched by several authors[5,6] in some cases, and our group is able to review here the experiences accumulated with 164 consecutive cadaver renal graft recipients treated with cyclosporine during an oligoanuric phase after transplantation.

MATERIALS AND METHODS

During the two-year period 1981–1982, 59% of cadaver renal grafts treated with cyclosporine were accompanied by oligoanuria (urine volume under 500 ml per day) after transplantation. In all cases, serum creatinine concentrations were sufficiently elevated to require dialysis (higher than 8 mg/dl).

Levels of blood urea nitrogen (BUN), creatinine, uric acid, calcium, phosphorus, bilirubin, and transaminases were determined. Renal biopsy was performed in 52 patients. The remaining 112 were classified solely on clinical grounds as having acute renal failure or primary nonfunctioning graft.

Cyclosporine was administered intravenously prior to transplantation in a dose of 3 mg/kg of body weight and was continued orally at daily doses of 16 mg/kg for two weeks postoperation, at which time it was decreased to a maintenance level of 12 mg/kg per day.

Pharmacokinetics were studied in five patients who were anuric and compared with five nonanuric control patients having a similar range of serum levels. These studies were performed over a 12-hr period, taking blood samples every 2 hr after oral administration or hourly during hemodialysis with a 1 m^2 cuprophan dialyzer. The radioimmunoassay (RIA) for cyclosporine was performed with materials provided by the Sandoz Co., Basel, Switzerland, using methods previously described.[7,8]

The following subjects were investigated: (1) incidence and possible cause of oligoanuria after cadaveric renal transplantation, (2) mean period of time of this phase of renal failure after transplant (both incidence and duration were compared with a historical group of 100 patients treated with azathioprine), (3) graft survival in cases with primary functioning and nonfunctioning grafts, (4) pharmacokinetics of cyclosporine in renal failure with oligoanuria, and (5) clearance of cyclosporine during dialysis.

RESULTS

Posttransplant oligoanuria occurred in 59% of cyclosporine-treated patients. This rate was lower than that found in patients treated with azathioprine (74%). Thus, the use of cyclosporine did not appear to increase the incidence of oligoanuria after renal transplantation. The high incidence of primary nonfunctioning grafts in both cyclosporine- and azathioprine-treated patients was more likely due to prolonged cold ischemia time (81.8% for kidneys with over 36 hr of ice storage). The mean period of oligoanuria was 28.6 days for patients treated with cyclosporine and 22.4 days in the retrospective group of patients with primary nonfunctioning graft treated with azathioprine.

The graft survival rate at six months was

From the Department of Internal Medicine I, and Surgery and Transplantation Center, Klinikum Grosshadern, University of Munich, Munich, West Germany.

Address reprint requests to Dr. Luis A. Castro, Nephrology Department, Med. Klinik I, Klinikum Grosshadern, P.O. Box 701 260, D-8000 Muenchen 70, F.R.G.

0041–1345/83/1505–0090$01.00/0

85% in patients with primary functioning grafts and 64% in patients with oligoanuria after transplant (Fig. 1). In contrast, in patients treated with azathioprine, the difference was only 6%.

Cyclosporine was associated with hyperbilirubinemia (defined as a bilirubin increase greater than 1.0 mg/dl [17.8 μmol/liter] for periods longer than a week with no other demonstrable cause) in 48% of the anuric patients. This hyperbilirubinemia was dose-related and could usually be reduced by a dose adjustment (a decrease of 4 mg/kg) and need not contraindicate further administration.

The pharmacokinetics studies showed that the plasma peak in the anuric patients was registered between 2 and 4 hr after ingestion; this was equivalent to results in five control patients with good renal function (Fig. 2). In spite of reduced plasma protein binding in uremia, removal rate was observed to be less than 10% of the rate of presentation to the dialyzer.

During the 4-hr period of dialysis, the plasma concentration of the drug did not change significantly. However, average values for cyclosporine steady-state plasma levels were, in some cases, higher than those found in patients with functioning grafts, suggesting a cumulative increase after several days.

Histologic findings attributable to cyclosporine therapy were observed in 24 of the 52 cases studied by biopsy (Table 1).

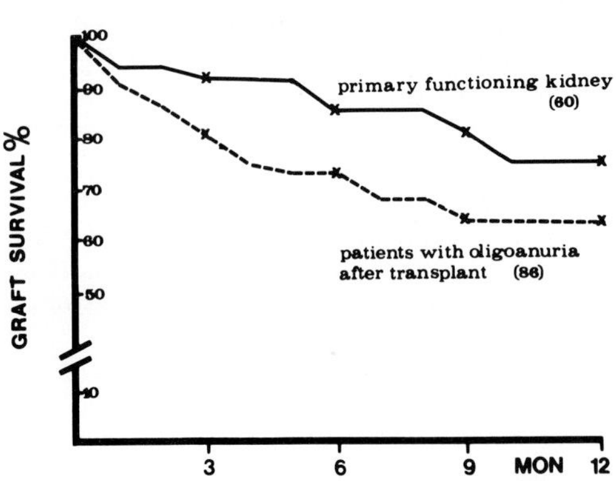

Fig. 1. Cadaveric renal transplantation.

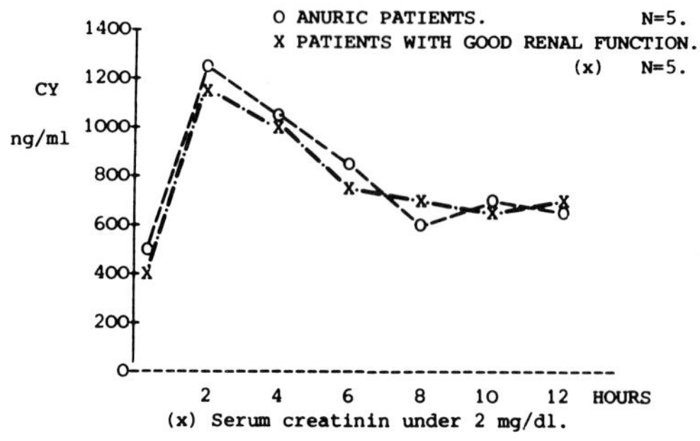

Fig. 2. Serum levels following oral dose of 17 mg/kg.

DISCUSSION

The incidence of oligoanuria (primary nonfunctioning graft) was lower in the cyclosporine group than in the retrospective group of patients treated with azathioprine and is possibly related to the cold ischemia time. However, the period of renal failure was longer in the cyclosporine patients, suggesting that the interaction of several factors, such as ischemia, concomitant drug therapy, or in some instances, rejection episodes, can hinder restitution of renal function. The results of renal graft survival were significantly poorer in patients having oligoanuria after transplantation in both groups (a 21% difference in the group treated with cyclosporine).

Hyperbilirubinemia and other side effects associated with administration of cyclosporine during the anuric phase are primarily dose-related and can usually be handled by adjustment of dosage. These complications do not prohibit further therapy.

Because of the high lipid solubility of cyclosporine, redistribution to other tissues can influence toxic side effects. With repeated

Table 1. Histologic Findings Observed in Renal Grafts From Patients Treated With Cyclosporine

Tubular changes
Diffuse vacuolization
Microcalcifications
Megamitochondria
Interstitium
Hypercellularity around groups of damaged cells
Vascular changes
Arteriole necrosis without infiltrations[9,10]

administration, redistribution can occur and the tissue concentration may not fall despite low observed serum levels. If the dosage is increased (based on the low serum levels), the toxic effect may be prolonged. The rate of tissue uptake from the blood depends on blood flow rate; therefore, it is not surprising that the liver, kidney, and brain show the highest levels and are the target organs for toxicity. The rapid development of rejection in some cases after interruption or dose reduction may also depend on a shift of cyclosporine from lymphocytes to other tissue compartments. The relation between the plasma half-life and the immunologic effect of cyclosporine or its metabolites has not been established.

Those factors that impair drug clearance will prolong the half-life and may lead to increased toxicity. Since the liver is the primary route of excretion and the role of the kidney is secondary, adjustments in dosage are indicated whenever hepatic clearance is impaired.

From the clinical point of view, episodes of rejection are difficult to detect in patients whose transplant kidney is oligoanuric, and convincing histologic patterns of cyclosporine nephrotoxicity were evident only in some cases.

It can be concluded that the incidence of oligoanuria after cadaveric renal transplantation is no higher with cyclosporine than with azathioprine therapy, but its mean duration was longer. Moreover, absorption and elimination processes after oral administration of cyclosporine were not different in patients with oligoanuria than in controls with normal kidney function. The plasma concentration with cyclosporine did not change significantly during dialysis, so no compensatory administration is required.

These results indicate that cyclosporine can be used in patients with oligoanuria after cadaveric renal transplantation without adverse consequences from overdose or excessive immunosuppression. The serum levels of cyclosporine did not rise during oliguric periods and did not show changes during dialysis, suggesting that the substance is protein-bound and not dialyzable.

REFERENCES

1. Calne RY, White DJG, Thiru S, et al: Lancet 2:1323, 1978

2. Powles RL, Barrett AJ, Clink H, et al: Lancet 2:1327, 1978

3. Klintmalm GBG, Iwatsuki S, Starzl TE, et al: Lancet 1:470, 1981

4. European Multicentre Trial: Lancet 2:57, 1982

5. Hall BM, Tiller DJ, Sheil AGR, et al: Lancet 2:876, 1981

6. Keown PA, Stiller CR, Ulan RA, et al: N Engl J Med 305:227, 1981

7. Donatsch P, Abisch E, Homberger M, et al: Immunoassay 2:19, 1981

8. Kahan BD, Van Buren CT, Lin S, et al: Transplantation 34:36, 1982

9. Mihatsch MJ, Olivieri M, Marbet U, et al: Lancet 1:1162, 1981

10. Shulman H, Striker G, Deeg HJ, et al: N Engl J Med 305:1392, 1981

Nephrotoxicity of Cyclosporine in Combination With Aminoglycoside and Cephalosporin Antibiotics

P. H. Whiting, J. G. Simpson, and A. W. Thomson

OPPORTUNISTIC infection as a consequence of immunosuppressive therapy is frequently encountered in the postoperative management of allograft recipients. This may be counteracted by the prophylactic or therapeutic administration of broad-spectrum antibiotics, such as the aminoglycoside gentamicin or "second generation" cephalosporins. Gentamicin, however, is potentially nephrotoxic,[1,2] and there is evidence that it can exacerbate renal functional impairment attributable to cyclosporine-A (CsA) in both laboratory animals[3] and bone marrow transplant patients.[4] On the other hand, cephalosporin antibiotics can be used in instances where renal function is poor, although their influence, if any, when administered together with CsA has not been ascertained. We have therefore conducted a comparative study of renal function and structure in rats given immunotherapeutic doses of CsA together with gentamicin or cephalosporin antibiotics.

MATERIALS AND METHODS

Cyclosporine-A

CsA was dissolved initially at 20°C in anhydrous ethanol. A 10% solution of the CsA-containing ethanol in olive oil, was then prepared and 25 mg/kg of body weight administered to the conscious rat by gastric intubation.

Antibiotics

Each of these was injected in aqueous solution (0.25–0.35 ml). Gentamicin sulphate (Nicholas Laboratories Ltd., Slough, U.K.) was administered intraperitoneally (50 mg/kg), while claforan (Roussel Labs. Ltd.), cefuroxime (Glaxo Labs., Greenford, Middlesex, U.K.) and cephradine (Squibb & Sons Ltd., Hounslow, Middlesex) were each given subcutaneously (100 mg/kg).

Experimental Protocol

Groups of eight Sprague-Dawley rats (mean weight 300 g) were given either CsA or one of the antibiotics daily for 14 days. An additional four groups received CsA in combination with either gentamicin, claforan, cefuroxime, or cephradine. Analyses of serum and urine were conducted immediately before the start of treatment and at seven and 14 days. On day 14, the animals were killed by terminal ether anesthesia and autopsies performed on six of each group.

Blood and Urine Sampling

Whole blood samples (1.5 ml) were collected from the cleaned tail tips of rats anesthetized with diethyl ether into plain tubes. Serum expressed from the clotted blood was stored at −20°C until assayed. Urine free of fecal contamination was collected overnight (16 hr) from animals placed in metabolic cages and starved throughout the collection period.

Biochemical Investigations

Estimations of serum urea and creatinine and urinary *N*-acetyl-β-D-glucosaminidase (NAG) levels were conducted as previously described.[5]

Preparation of Tissues for Microscopy

Kidney blocks were fixed in 10% neutral buffered formalin and processed to acrylic resin, 2-μm sections were stained with hematoxylin and eosin.

RESULTS

In this and in previous studies we have observed no significant pathologic effect attributable to the CsA vehicle (ethanol/olive oil).

Renal Function

The effects of CsA and of each antibiotic either alone or in combination with CsA are shown in Fig. 1. There were minor but significant increases in urea levels in the CsA or gentamicin groups on day 7, but only in the

---

From the Departments of Chemical Pathology and Pathology, University Medical Buildings, Foresterhill, Aberdeen, U.K.

Supported in part by a grant from the Grampian Health Board.

Address reprint requests to Dr. P.H. Whiting, Department of Chemical Pathology, University Medical Buildings, Foresterhill, Aberdeen AB9 2ZD, U.K.

0041-1345/83/1505-0091$01.00/0

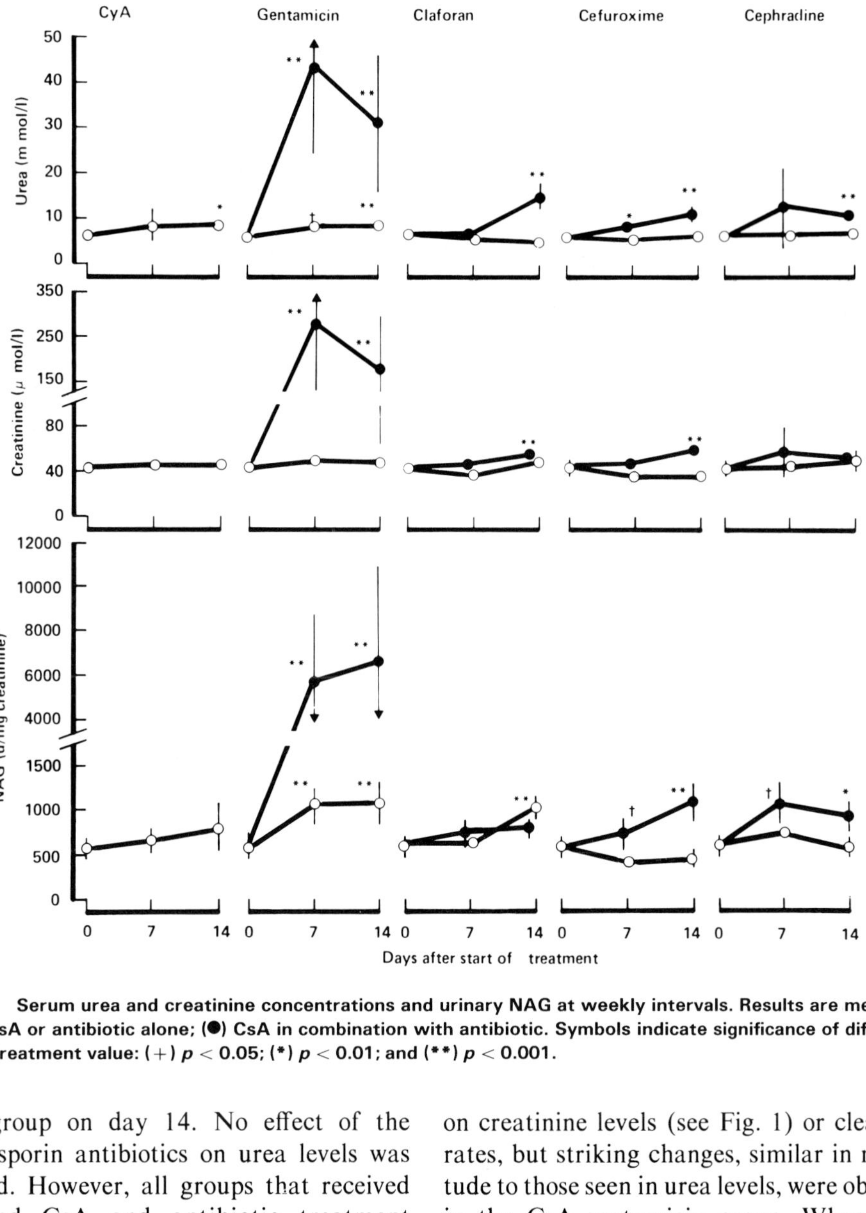

Fig. 1. Serum urea and creatinine concentrations and urinary NAG at weekly intervals. Results are means ±1 SD. (○) CsA or antibiotic alone; (●) CsA in combination with antibiotic. Symbols indicate significance of difference from pretreatment value: (+) $p < 0.05$; (*) $p < 0.01$; and (**) $p < 0.001$.

latter group on day 14. No effect of the cephalosporin antibiotics on urea levels was observed. However, all groups that received combined CsA and antibiotic treatment showed evidence of renal functional impairment within 14 days. In the case of gentamicin, the fivefold increase in serum urea was particularly marked, especially in view of the relatively minor changes in the other three groups. Concomitant decreases in urea clearance rates (data not shown) reflected the alterations in serum urea.

None of the drugs on its own had any effect on creatinine levels (see Fig. 1) or clearance rates, but striking changes, similar in magnitude to those seen in urea levels, were observed in the CsA-gentamicin group. When given with the cephalosporin antibiotics, CsA had either minor or no effect (cephradine) on serum urea and clearance rates.

The adverse effect of combined CsA and gentamicin administration is further emphasized by the six-fold elevation in urinary NAG activity. In contrast, the cephalosporins produced, at most, a twofold increase when combined with CsA.

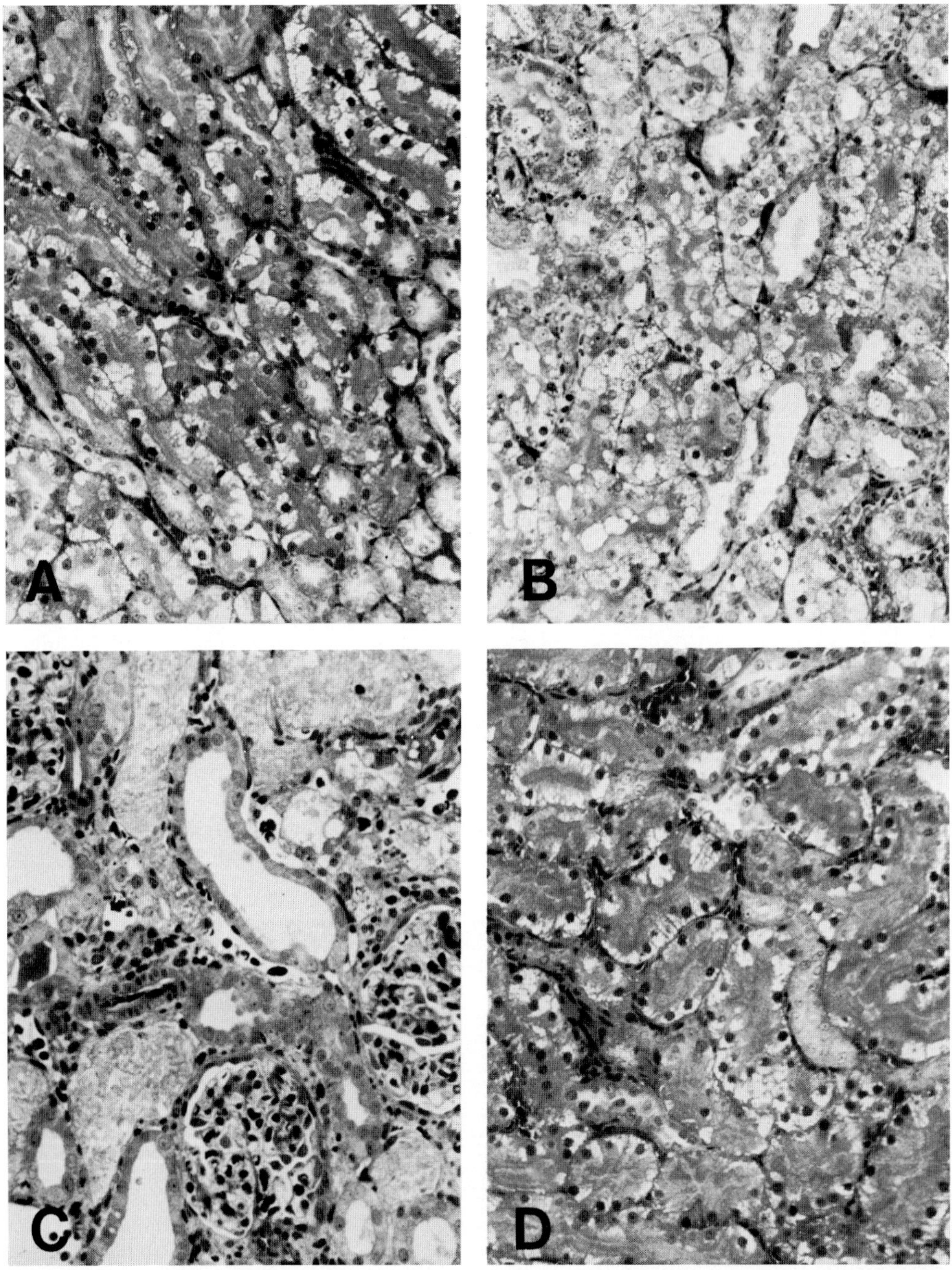

Fig. 2. Effects on renal tubules of CsA alone or in combination with antibiotics. (A) With CsA alone, only proximal straight tubular vacuolation; (B) with CsA and gentamicin, more pronounced proximal straight tubular vacuolation accompanied by (C) proximal convoluted tubular necrosis; (D) with CsA and a cephalosporin (claforan), similar proximal straight tubular changes to those seen after CsA alone (hematoxylin and eosin, × 150).

Renal Structure

None of the animals treated with any of the four antibiotics alone showed renal structural abnormalities. In the group treated only with CsA, abnormalities were restricted to the proximal straight tubule (thick descending limb of the loop of Henle); in most of the kidneys examined, a variable proportion (33%–50%) of the straight tubular profiles exhibited fine vacuolation of the cytoplasm of the epithelial cells, with no evidence of frank necrosis (Fig. 2A).

The kidneys of animals receiving both CsA and gentamicin were grossly abnormal, showing two distinct zones of renal damage. The proximal straight tubular epithelium was again vacuolated, but to a greater degree; more cells were involved and the vacuoles were larger (Fig. 2B). Some of the affected cells showed additional total necrosis. The other and more severe zone of damage involved the proximal convoluted tubule. Most convoluted tubular profiles were totally necrotic and surrounded by a mixed inflammatory cell infiltrate (Fig. 2C). Those cells still retaining recognizable nuclei showed gross coarse cytoplasmic vacuolation.

In none of the kidneys of animals treated concomitantly with CsA and any of the three cephalosporins was there tubular necrosis. The only abnormalities present in these combination groups were the same straight tubular changes as those observed in animals receiving only CsA (Fig. 2D).

DISCUSSION

In this study conducted over two weeks, we have shown that rats treated with 25 mg/kg CsA exhibit minor renal functional impairment, with attendant proximal straight tubular cell vacuolation. Our comparison of the influence of gentamicin and cephalosporin antibiotics on renal function and structure in CsA-treated animals has confirmed the potent synergistic nephrotoxicity that the aminoglycoside exerts in combination with the immunosuppressive agent. In addition to pronounced inhibition of glomerular filtration rate and striking enzymuria, administration of CsA together with gentamicin led to severe proximal straight and convoluted tubular cell damage. In the latter instance, the effect was due at least in part to gentamicin. On the other hand, administration of each of the cephalosporin antibiotics with CsA caused substantially less nephrotoxicity than in the CsA-gentamicin combination. Indeed, the only abnormalities observed were those attributable to the immune suppressant.

Both aminoglycoside and cephalosporin antibiotics are handled by the renal tubules, but they have distinctly different effects, as assessed by enzymuria, on membranes of the proximal tubule.[6] Moreover, tubulotoxic doses of cephalosporins are well in excess of those used in this investigation.[7] Since cephalosporins have a similar spectrum of antibacterial activity to gentamicin, it would seem appropriate to avoid combination of CsA and gentamicin, both of which are potentially nephrotoxic. On the basis of the present investigation, it would appear that when infection is encountered in CsA-treated patients, the use of cephalosporin antibiotics can be safely contemplated.

REFERENCES

1. Wilfert J, Burke I, Bloomer AJ, et al: J Infect Dis 124S:148, 1971
2. Mondorf AW, Breier J, Hendus J, et al: Eur J Clin Pharmacol 13:133, 1978
3. Whiting PH, Simpson JG, Davidson RJL, et al: Br J Exp Pathol 63:554, 1982
4. Hows J, Harris R, Palmer S, et al: Br J Haematol 48:227, 1981
5. Thomson AW, Whiting PH, Blair JT, et al: Transplantation 32:271, 1981
6. Mondorf AW, Hendus J, Breier J, et al: In Dubach UC, Schmidt U (eds): Current Problems in Clinical Biochemistry, vol. 9. Bern, Hans Huber, 1979, p 192
7. Sack K, et al: Med Welt 29:1233, 1978

Renal Failure in Heart Transplant Patients Receiving Cyclosporine

J. Egel, A. Greenberg, M. E. Thompson, R. L. Hardesty, B. P. Griffith, H. T. Bahnson, R. L. Bernstein, and J. B. Puschett

THE use of cyclosporine-A (CsA) for immunosuppression in human allograft recipients has resulted in prolonged graft survival, but suspected renal and hepatic toxicity have complicated administration in some patients.[1-4] Case reports have appeared suggesting that, in renal and liver transplant recipients, CsA may cause a mild azotemia reversible by a reduction in drug dosage,[1,2] but a large series has never been reported. Evaluation of nephrotoxicity in renal transplant recipients is complicated by the uncertain contribution of rejection to any renal impairment. Thus, the mechanism and clinical significance of CsA nephrotoxicity has remained unclear.

The patients reported here represent our early experience with the use of CsA and corticosteroids as immunosuppressive therapy for cardiac transplantation. There was a pronounced tendency for moderately to severely impaired renal function to develop in the first postoperative week. Although vasopressors were generally required during this period, clinically, these patients appeared to be neither in a severe low output state nor volume depleted. Urine sodium was generally quite low and the ratio of blood urea nitrogen to serum creatinine (BUN:Scr) tended to be markedly elevated early in the postoperative period. The observed renal impairment was usually of three to six days' duration, with spontaneous recovery in most cases. CsA was usually withheld or the dosage reduced if azotemia was noted.

From the Renal Electrolyte Division, University of Pittsburgh, Pittsburgh, PA 15261.

Address reprint requests to Dr. J. Egel.

0041-1345/83/1505-0092$01.00/0

There was also a marked tendency for our transplant recipients to develop renal impairment weeks to months after operation. This did not appear to be a continuation or incomplete resolution of the early azotemia described above, as frequently, late azotemia occurred in patients who maintained normal renal function in the early postoperative period. All patients were asymptomatic and urine output was maintained. In most instances, the dose of CsA was reduced when azotemia was noted. Thus far, it has not been necessary to discontinue therapy with CsA in any patient.

Disproportionate hyperkalemia was seen frequently in our group. In most cases this was not associated with conditions known to elevate serum potassium, but occasionally was associated with the use of potassium-sparing diuretics or potassium-containing salt substitutes.

The use of CsA in our cardiac transplant recipients was associated with a syndrome characterized by oliguria, a disparate increase in BUN compared to Scr concentration, and intense urinary sodium avidity. There was no evidence for decreased effective blood volume, making prerenal azotemia an unlikely possibility. As few patients required dialysis, acute tubular necrosis was also unlikely. This evidence strongly suggests that the decline in renal function was due to CsA nephrotoxicity.

Of interest regarding the mechanism of the early renal impairment seen in our CsA-treated patients are the recent reports that aspirin and other nonsteroidal antiinflammatory agents that inhibit prostaglandin synthetase can reduce renal function. Like the CsA toxicity seen early on in our patients, renal failure due to these drugs is characterized by sodium avidity and disproportionate hyperkalemia.[5] As CsA given chronically in high doses leads to tubular damage in animals,[6–9] a direct toxic effect on renal tubular cells is an alternative explanation for the renal impairment observed in our patients.

In view of this evidence, CsA was also a likely culprit for the late renal impairment noted in this series. Most of these individuals were free of acute medical illnesses and were not receiving other nephrotoxic medications when azotemia was discovered, making alternative causes of renal impairment unlikely.

Morphologic changes in renal tubules or glomeruli were not observed in necropsy specimens from patients in our series. A large series of biopsy and necropsy specimens may be necessary to establish the presence or absence of specific morphologic changes in this clinical situation.

REFERENCES

1. Powles RL, Clink H, Sloane J, et al: Lancet 2:1327, 1978

2. Klintmalm GBG, Iwatsuki S, Starzl TE: Lancet 1:470, 1981

3. Gluckman E, Devergie A, Lokiec F, et al: Lancet 2:144, 1981

4. Shulman H, Striker G, Deeg H, et al: N Engl J Med 305:1392, 1981

5. Tan SY, Shapiro R, Franco R, et al: Ann Intern Med 90:783, 1979

6. Blair JT, Thomson AW, Whiting PH, et al: J Pathol 138:163, 1983

7. Farthing MJG, Clark ML: Biochem Pharmacol 30:3311, 1981

8. Thomson AW, Whiting PH, Blair JT, et al: Transplantation 32:271, 1981

9. Whiting PH, Thomson AW, Simpson JG: Br J Exp Pathol 63:88, 1983

Nephrotoxicity in Marrow Graft Recipients Treated With Cyclosporine

J. M. Hows, J. M. Smith, A. Baughan, and E. C. Gordon-Smith

NEPHROTOXICITY in bone marrow transplant patients treated with cyclosporine-A (CsA) was first reported by the Royal Marsden Group.[1] When CsA was given prophylactically in the post graft period to prevent graft-versus-host disease, the most common nephrotoxicity seen was a mild reversible increase in the plasma creatinine.[2] As clinical experience with CsA increased, it was noted that a minority of bone marrow–transplant patients developed clinical features of renal impairment and occasionally acute renal failure.[3]

We have reviewed the clinical features of nephrotoxicity occurring in 33 bone marrow–transplant recipients treated with CsA and have attempted to identify risk factors associated with the onset of severe renal impairment.

MATERIALS AND METHODS

Patients

Thirty-three of 40 consecutive marrow transplant recipients were studied. Thirty-one received grafts from HLA-identical sibling donors, and two patients received grafts from parental donors, one HLA identical and one mismatched at the A locus. All patients received oral CsA throughout the study. Three patients who received intravenous CsA were excluded from the study, as were four patients in whom insufficient pharmacologic data were available. Relevant clinical data are shown in Table 1.

Cyclosporine-A Dose Schedule

CsA was begun on day −1 with a loading dose of 12.5 mg/kg of body weight twice daily. On day +3, the dose was reduced to an average maintenance dose of 6.25 mg/kg of body weight twice daily. Throughout the study, a dose reduction of 50% was made and/or doses were omitted if the plasma creatinine rose to 150–200 μmole/liter.

Antibiotic Therapy

Tobramycin, mezlocillin, and a cephalosporin were given intravenously to neutropenic patients developing a fever of >38°C. Ten leukemic patients received piperacillin and cefotaxime as first-line intravenous antibiotics.

Pharmacologic Monitoring

Serum CsA measurements. A radioimmunoassay was used.[4] The assay was sensitive in the range 62–4,000 ng/ml, with an interassay variation of ±5%. Trough (12-hr) venous blood samples were collected three times weekly from all hospitalized patients and once weekly after discharge from hospital.

Serum aminoglycoside measurements. A standard microbiologic plate diffusion method was used. Venous blood samples were taken immediately before dose for trough measurements and 1 hr after intravenous administration of the antibiotic for peak measurements. The dose was adjusted to keep serum levels in the therapeutic range (Tobramycin peak, 5–12 mg/liter; trough, <2 mg/liter; amikacin peak, 20–30 mg/liter; trough, <4 mg/liter).

Biochemical Monitoring. Daily estimations of renal and hepatic function were carried out on hospitalized patients by standard laboratory methods. Weekly estimations were continued after patients were discharged from hospital.

RESULTS

Early Nephrotoxicity (0–4 Weeks of CsA Therapy)

There was a close correlation between maximum plasma creatinine and maximum trough serum CsA concentration, $r = 0.93$ $p < 0.001$ (Spearman's correlation coefficient), and also between the maximum plasma urea and maximum trough serum CsA concentration ($r = 0.88$, $p < 0.001$) (Fig. 1A and Fig. 1B). Most patients developed a mild increase in plasma creatinine that was asymptomatic; however, eight patients developed clinical features of nephrotoxicity. The most frequent clinical signs were periorbital and peripheral edema with weight gain (eight patients), hypertension (three patients), and acute oliguric renal failure (two patients). Seven patients responded to dose reduction and

From the Department of Hematology and M.R.C. Leukemia Unit, Royal Postgraduate Medical School, Du Cane Road, London W12, England.

Address reprint requests to Dr. J. M. Hows.

0041-1345/83/1505-0093$01.00/0

Table 1. Clinical and Pharmacologic Data in 33 BMT Patients

	Aplastic Anemia	Leukemia
No. of patients	20	13 4 AML 9 CGL
Median age (range)	18 (3–43)	23 (7–36)
Pregraft chemotherapy	*CY 50 mg/kg × 4	CY 60 mg/kg × 2 †DN 60 mg/sq m × 1
Total body irradiation	0	5–6 × 200 cGy
Aminoglycosides post-BMT	19 Patients	4 Patients

*CY, cyclophosphamide.
†Daunorubicin, CGL patients only.

appropriate diuretic therapy, whereas one patient required hemodialysis for five weeks before her renal function improved. Risk factors identified for the development of clinically severe nephrotoxicity were trough serum CsA levels of >500 ng/ml (Fig. 1), nephrotoxic antibiotics (Fig. 2), and hyperbilirubinemia (Fig. 3).

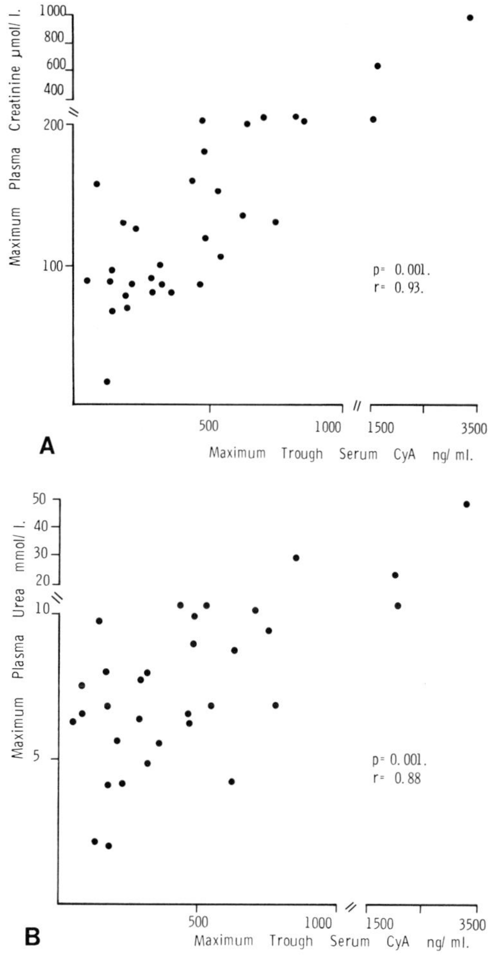

Fig. 1. (A) Correlation between maximum trough serum CsA and maximum plasma creatinine during first four weeks of CsA therapy $r = 0.93$ (Spearman's correlation coefficient), $p < 0.001$. (B) Correlation between maximum trough serum CsA and maximum plasma urea during first four weeks of CsA therapy, $r = 0.88$, $p < 0.001$.

Late Nephrotoxicity (4–36 Weeks of CsA Therapy)

Late nephrotoxicity was defined as a nephrotoxic episode occurring after more than four weeks of CsA therapy, where the plasma creatinine rose to >200 µmole/liter. Six patients developed such episodes, and in five, an increase in serum CsA concentration occurred. Other features of late CsA nephrotoxicity were hypertension (six patients), red cell fragmentation (six patients), and thrombocytopenia (three patients). The prothrombin time, partial thromboplastin time, and thrombin time remained normal. Antihypertensive therapy was necessary in five patients. One patient developed grand mal epilepsy associated with hypertension and high-dose methylprednisolone administration during the nephrotoxic episode. We have since observed grand mal attacks in three other patients treated with high-dose methylprednisolone and CsA concurrently.[5]

DISCUSSION

Nephrotoxicity during the first month of CsA therapy in the 33 bone marrow–transplant patients studied was usually confined to a mild increase in the plasma creatinine without clinical features. In a minority of patients (eight of 33), a more severe episode of nephrotoxicity occurred. Clinical features included fluid retention, hypertension, periorbital and peripheral edema, and rarely acute oliguric renal failure. Except for the patient who

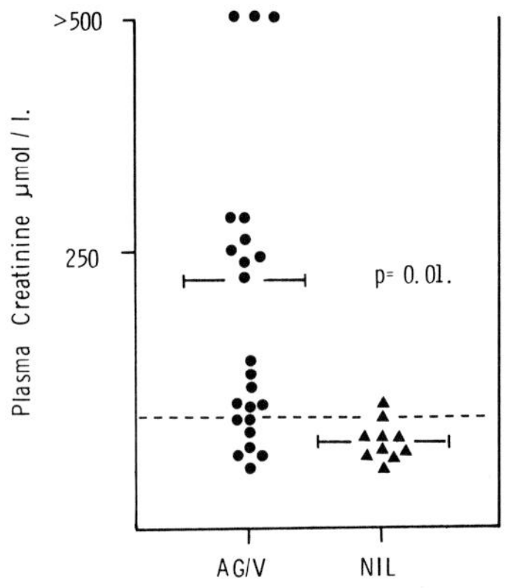

Fig. 2. Effect of nephrotoxic antibiotics on plasma creatinine in CsA-treated patients. AG/V, aminoglycosides and/or vancomycin. NIL, no nephrotoxic antibiotics.

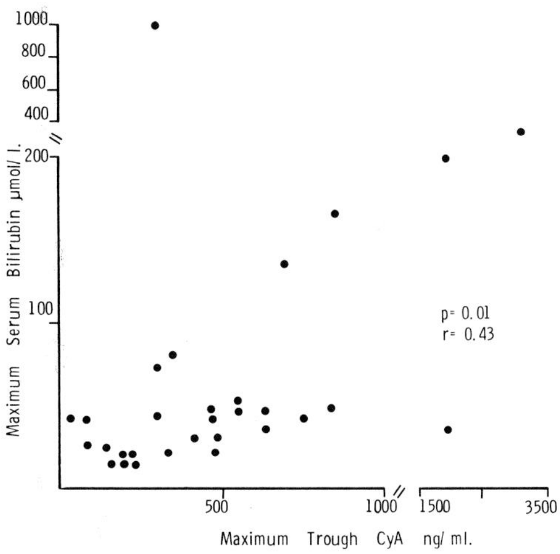

Fig. 3. Correlation between maximum trough serum CsA and maximum serum bilirubin in the first four weeks of CsA therapy ($r = 0.43$, $p < 0.01$). Preexisting hyperbilirubinemia is associated with nephrotoxic serum CsA levels (see text).

required hemodialysis, renal function improved after reduction in cyclosporine dose. Risk factors associated with serious CsA nephrotoxicity in the first four weeks of therapy were trough serum CsA levels of >500 ng/ml, use of other nephrotoxic drugs, and hyperbilirubinemia. Hyperbilirubinemia was associated with high trough serum CsA levels ($p = 0.01$) (Fig. 3). Abnormalities in hepatic function may lead to failure of metabolism of CsA and/or its excretion in the bile, resulting in nephrotoxic serum levels of the drug. Primary hepatotoxicity due to CsA may also occur. Other factors, such as infection and graft-versus-host disease, frequently cause abnormal hepatic function in the initial post-transplant period.

Nephrotoxicity occurring after four weeks or more of CsA treatment was less often associated with other nephrotoxic drugs. Although late nephrotoxicity was clinically mild in the six affected patients, the presence of hypertension and microangiopathic peripheral blood changes were similar to the hemolytic uremic syndrome (HUS). The main renal abnormality seen in HUS is glomerular capillary thrombosis, and this histologic appearance was reported recently in three bone marrow–transplant patients who died during episodes of CsA-induced nephrotoxicity.[6] It is therefore of interest that experimental work has shown that CsA inhibits prostacyclin synthesis in vascular endothelium in vitro.[7] A possible mechanism for the development of hypertension in association with CsA nephrotoxicity is an abnormality in the renin/angiotension system. Recent animal work supported this idea when it was shown that plasma renin levels in CsA-treated rats were high.[8]

In conclusion, CsA therapy in bone marrow–transplant recipients is frequently associated with mild reversible nephrotoxicity. More serious renal impairment can be reduced by appropriate dose reduction when certain risk factors are present. Major risk factors are trough serum CsA levels of >500 ng/ml, the use of other nephrotoxic drugs, and the presence of hyperbilirubinemia.

REFERENCES

1. Powles RL, Barrett AJ, Clink H, et al: Lancet 2:1327, 1978

2. Powles RL, Clink HM, Spence D, et al: Lancet 1:327, 1980

3. Hows JM, Palmer S, Want S et al: Lancet 2:145, 1981

4. Donatsch P, Abisch E, Homberger M, et al: J Immunoassay 2:19, 1981

5. Durrant S, Chipping PM, Palmer S, et al: Lancet 2:829, 1982

6. Shulman H, Striker G, Deeg HK, et al: N Engl J Med 305:1392, 1981

7. Rocchi G, Kimberti L, Fumagalli F, et al: International Conference on Prostoglandins, Florence, Italy, 1982 (abstr 59)

8. Siegal H, Rythel B: Lancet 2:1274, 1982

dosage, after which the animals were killed by cervical dislocation for removal of the liver and kidneys.

Hepatic cytochrome-P_{450} concentration and activity. The technique of Omura and Sato[8] gave a direct spectral measurement of cyt-P_{450} levels, while the level of N-demethylation of aminopyrine,[9] which is dependent on mono-oxygenase activity, gave an indirect indication of cyt-P_{450} values.

Monitoring of nephrotoxicity. Serum urea and creatinine levels were measured using a SMAC autoanalyzer (Technicon Ltd., Basingstoke, U.K.). Light microscopic sections of kidney were prepared by standard methods.

Measurement of immunosuppression. Immediately before the start of treatment, all animals received 5×10^9 sheep red blood cells intraperitoneally. Hemagglutination titers were performed on day-15 serum samples by the Takátsky microtechnique.

RESULTS

As with the untreated group, animals receiving the control vehicles showed no abnormalities in renal function and structure and no alteration in hepatic enzyme activity.

Hepatic cytochrome-P_{450} concentration and activity. Animals treated only with Aroclor showed a 240% increase in cyt-P_{450} concentration and a 100% rise in aminopyrine N-demethylase activity (Table 1). In the CsA group, there was a 30% reduction in cyt-P_{450} levels and a similar fall in the mono-oxygenase activity. When both drugs were administered together, there was a significant ($p < 0.001$) increase in cyt-P_{450} activity measured by both methods.

Renal function and structure. Aroclor alone had no effect on the kidney apart from a nonsignificant rise in serum creatinine. In the group treated with CsA, there were significant rises in serum urea and creatinine levels and these were accompanied by vacuolation and focal desquamation of the epithelium of the proximal straight segment (Fig. 1A). When CsA was administered in combination with Aroclor, these abnormalities were prevented (Fig. 1B): there was only a minor increase in serum creatinine, similar to that observed after Aroclor alone.

Immunosuppression. Animals receiving Aroclor or either of the control vehicles showed similar hemagglutination titers to the untreated group. CsA alone produced a profound immunosuppressive effect, and this was also apparent in animals receiving CsA in combination with Aroclor (Fig. 2).

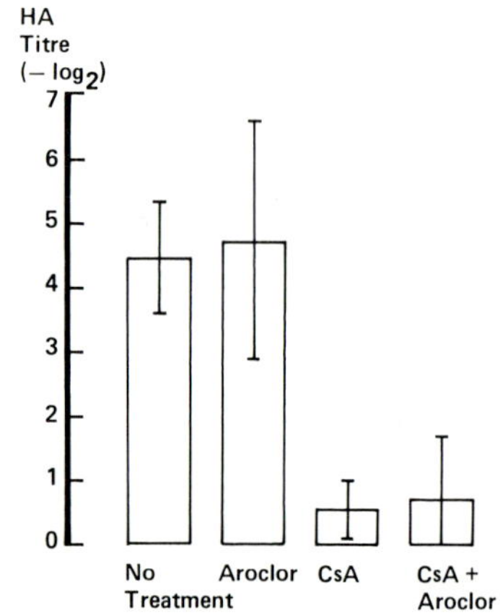

Fig. 2. Serum hemagglutination (HA) titers to sheep red blood cells after 14 days of no treatment, Aroclor, CsA, or CsA plus Aroclor. Results expressed as mean ±1 SD.

DISCUSSION

This study demonstrates that the nephrotoxicity of CsA, monitored both functionally and microscopically, is abolished by the simultaneous administration of Aroclor 1254, an inducer of hepatic drug-metabolizing enzymes, without affecting immunosuppression.

CsA is extensively metabolized in the rat, and it is probable that Aroclor, through its two- to threefold induction of cyt-P_{450}, increases the hydroxylation and N-demethylation of the immunosuppressant, thus increasing its metabolism. This is supported by our preliminary findings that animals treated with Aroclor have lower serum trough levels of CsA and implies that it is the parent CsA molecule, rather than a metabolite, that is responsible for the nephrotoxicity commonly observed with this agent.

Our demonstration that CsA itself reduces hepatic cyt-P_{450} levels by 30% has significant implications for those instances when the immunosuppressant is administered along with other pharmacologic agents metabolized in the liver, since the metabolism of these other drugs might be reduced. To our knowledge, this situation has not yet been described. The situation in which CsA is administered together with agents that inhibit its metabolism is also an important factor. Both Morgenstern et al[10] and Ferguson et al[11] have reported increased CsA toxicity associated with high serum CsA concentrations in patients treated with CsA and the antifungal agent ketoconazole; ketoconazole is a known inhibitor of cyt-P_{450}-catalyzed metabolism.

This study has shown that it is possible in the experimental animal to prevent the nephrotoxicity of CsA, while maintaining the immunosuppressive effect of the drug. Because of the proximity of the therapeutic and toxic ranges of CsA in humans, consideration might be given to a similar clinical study using an acceptable cyt-P_{450}-inducing agent, such as phenobarbitone or phenytoin.

REFERENCES

1. Powles RL, Clink HM, Spence D, et al: Lancet 1:327, 1980
2. Klintmalm GBG, Iwatsuki S, Starzl TE: Lancet 1:470, 1981
3. Calne RY, Rolles K, White DJG, et al: Lancet 2:1032, 1979
4. Blair JT, Thomson AW, Whiting PH, et al: J Pathol 138:163, 1982
5. Sandoz Ltd: Unpublished document
6. Alvares AP, Kappas A: J Biol Chem 252:6373, 1977
7. Ryan DE, Thomas PE, Korzeniowski D, et al: J Biol Chem 254:1365, 1979
8. Omura T, Sato R: J Biol Chem 239:2370, 1964
9. Burke MD, Falzon M, Milton AS: Biochem Pharmacol 32:389, 1983
10. Morgenstern GR, Powles R, Robinson B, et al: Lancet 2:1342, 1982
11. Ferguson RM, Sutherland DER, Simmons RL, et al: Lancet 2:882, 1982

Demonstration of Cyclosporine in Renal Transplants by Fine Needle Aspiration Biopsy

E. von Willebrand and P. Häyry

CYCLOSPORINE-A (CsA) has established its place as a potent immunosuppressant in organ transplantation. The most frequent side effect is nephrotoxicity.[1,2] The dose level must be adjusted for minimal nephrotoxic effect, while still giving adequate immunosuppression. However, the susceptibility of individual transplants seems to be variable. The nephrotoxic effect of CsA is reversible and dose dependent. Very high plasma levels of CsA are frequently associated with nephrotoxicity.[3] Recently, artifacts influencing serum determination of CsA have been recognized.

Fine needle aspiration biopsy (FNAB) is an atraumatic method to monitor intragraft events in renal transplantation in humans.[4,5] From the FNAB specimens, it is possible to evaluate the morphology of the transplant tubular and endothelial cells and to monitor the onset, size, and duration of the rejection episodes. Also, the effect of the immunosuppressive treatment on the inflammation can be recorded. We have previously reported that distinct, though nonspecific, changes are seen in the transplant tubular and endothelial cells in cases of CsA nephrotoxicity.[6]

In this study, we have analyzed, using indirect immunofluorescence, the presence of CsA deposits in 27 human renal allografts, correlated this to morphologic changes in the transplant parenchymal cells, to the presence of inflammation in the graft, and to the CsA serum concentrations. Finally, we have followed the effect of reduction in the drug dose.

From the Transplantation Laboratory, Fourth Department of Surgery, University of Helsinki, Helsinki, Finland.

Supported in part by Grant 1 RO1AM 26882-03 from the National Institutes of Health, Bethesda, MD, and grants from the Sigrid Juselius Foundation and the Association of Finnish Life Insurance Companies, Helsinki, Finland.

Address reprint requests to Dr. E. von Willebrand, Transplantation Laboratory, Fourth Department of Surgery, University of Helsinki, Haartmaninkatu 3, SF 00290 Helsinki 29, Finland.

0041-1345/83/1505-0095$01.00/0

MATERIALS AND METHODS

Patients and Immunosuppression

Recipients of cadaver kidney allografts receiving CsA for immunosuppression and being part of a prerandomized clinical trial (reported in another context in this meeting), were biopsied 10–360 days after the transplantation. For details of immunosuppression and patient management, see Häyry et al.[7] Serum levels of CsA were determined by radioimmunoassay.[8]

FNAB

FNABs were performed as previously described,[6] and cytocentrifuged cell smears were made from the specimens. A blood sample was obtained at the same time and processed in a similar way. Routine staining was done with May-Grünwald-Giemsa (MGG) stain.

Evaluation of the FNAB specimens has been described previously.[4,5] The intensity of morphologic changes in the renal parenchymal cells was scored from 0 to +3 from coded specimens.[6]

Demonstration of CsA deposits in the FNAB specimens was done with indirect immunofluorescence and occasionally using peroxidase anti-peroxidase (PAP) technique. Specimens were fixed with acetone (−20°C) for 10 min, treated with 1:1,000 diluted rabbit antiserum to CsA (Sandoz, Co., Basel, Switzerland), and 1:20 diluted FITC-conjugated swine antibody to rabbit IgG (Dakopatts, Copenhagen, Denmark) was used as second antibody. The rabbit antiserum to CsA has been characterized and reported to be specific for CsA (and a number of metabolites of the drug).[9] The frequency and amount of CsA in the graft parenchymal cells was evaluated from coded specimens by scoring the reaction intensity from 0 to +3. Specimens treated with normal rabbit serum were used as controls.

RESULTS

Morphologic Changes in Renal Parenchymal Cells and Localization of CsA Deposits in the Kidney

The cytologic changes in the graft parenchymal cells varied from completely normal to

Table 1. Representative Laboratory and FNAB Findings in Three Patients With CsA Toxicity and the Effect of Reduction of Cyclosporine Dose

Parameter	Prior to Reduction of CsA Dose	After Reduction of CsA Dose	
		Days 1–3	Days 5–10
Serum creatinine (μmol/liter)	391 ± 98	281 ± 18	216 ± 44
CsA dose (mg/kg/day)	10.0 ± 0.0	1.7 ± 2.3	5.0 ± 2.0
MP dose (mg/kg/day)	0.3 ± 0.0	0.3 ± 0.0	0.3 ± 0.0
Inflammation*			
Total	1.9 ± 0.5	1.7 ± 0.4	6.6 ± 2.5
Tubular cell changes†	2.8 ± 1.0	2.5 ± 0.0	2.5 ± 0.5
CsA deposits in graft†	2.0 ± 0.0	1.0 ± 0.0	0.5 ± 0.0
CsA concentration in serum (ng/ml)	231 ± 22	165 ± 0	130 ± 20

NOTE. Data are mean ± SD.
*Corrected increment units.
†Visual score from 0 to 3+.

extreme. No or only faint deposition of CsA was seen with immunofluorescence in the transplant tubular cells in cases where graft function was good and the serum creatinine level was near normal. Also in the MGG-stained smears, the tubular and endothelial cell morphology appeared normal. Prominent deposition of CsA, appearing as strongly fluorescent groups of tubular cells, was seen in cases with indisputable nephrotoxicity, poor graft function, and rising serum creatinine levels. The morphologic changes in the tubular and endothelial cells were equally prominent and appeared as strong swelling, vacuolization, and even phagocytosis.

In immunofluorescence analysis of the FNAB specimens, the antibody to CsA reacted with groups of tubular cells, and in some cases, a weak reaction with monocytes and granulocytes was also evident. The intensity of the reaction varied according to the degree of morphologic changes and to the nephrotoxicity. In immunoperoxidase analysis of the FNAB specimens, most of the positively staining tubular cells appeared to be small tubular cells, classified earlier as proximal tubular cells. In some cases, a weaker and more diffuse staining could be seen also in the distal tubular cells and in the endothelial cells.

Correlation of FNAB Findings to the Dose of the Drug and to CsA Serum Concentration

In the patients with clinical nephrotoxicity, the dose level of CsA was approximately the same, ranging from 8.5 ± 1.5 to 11.5 ± 2.0 mg/kg per day, which falls within the recommended level. The serum concentrations of CsA were not very high either, ranging from 130 ± 49 in cases with no evidence of nephrotoxicity to 195 ± 85 ng/ml in cases with nephrotoxicity. In cases of established nephrotoxicity, there were, however, prominent morphologic changes in the graft tubular cells and distinct deposition of CsA as analyzed with the immunofluorescence technique. No signs

Table 2. Differential Diagnosis of Early Renal Transplant Failure by FNAB

Serum Creatinine	FNAB: Inflammation	FNAB: Tubular Cell Changes	FNAB: CsA Deposits in Graft	Explanation
Normal	–	±	±	Well-to-do graft
Elevated	–	++	–	Acute tubular necrosis (ATN)
Elevated	–	+++	+++	CsA toxicity
Elevated	+++	+	–	Rejection
Elevated	+++	+++	+++	Rejection and CsA toxicity

of immunologic inflammation were seen in situ.

When the dose of CsA was reduced, the signs of nephrotoxicity disappeared rapidly, serum creatinine levels declined, and at the same time, the deposits of CsA diminished and disappeared in immunofluorescent staining. The morphologic changes in parenchymal cells normalized much slower. The serum CsA levels remained widely variable. On some occasions after reduction of CsA dose, a distinct inflammatory episode in situ was seen (Table 1). These inflammations, however, mostly subsided without any further immunosuppressive treatment.

Differential Diagnosis Between CsA Toxicity and Rejection Analyzed With FNAB

In the scheme of Table 2, the main alternatives are proposed for early renal transplant failure. If only CsA deposits and morphologic changes are recorded, the diagnosis of CsA nephrotoxicity emerges. If inflammation is also superimposed, rejection coexists.

DISCUSSION

Deposits of CsA are seen in parenchymal cells of a renal transplant when administration of the drug is accompanied by clinical signs of nephrotoxicity. The presence of CsA in the transplant is usually accompanied by distinct morphologic changes in the transplant tubular and endothelial cells. These changes[6] disappear when the administration of CsA is reduced or discontinued, but they seem to persist longer than the actual CsA deposits seen by immunofluorescence. Deposition of CsA in the transplants seems to have only a marginal or no correlation to the serum concentration of the drug.

Deposition of CsA in the transplant does not, as such, cause any inflammatory reaction. When a distinct inflammatory infiltrate is present in the graft, this indicates a rejection process rather than toxicity. It is more difficult to detect deposits of CsA and morphologic changes in classic histology and in frozen sections. However, some investigators have reported histologic changes that resemble those observed in our study.[10,11] With cytologic techniques, deposits of CsA and concomitant cytologic alterations in the transplant parenchymal cells seem to be easily visualized, and thus, aspiration cytology of the transplant would provide a new and more accurate method to assess CsA nephrotoxicity than the serum concentration (or whole blood) determinations.

REFERENCES

1. Calne RY, Thiru S, McMaster P, et al: Lancet 2:1323, 1978
2. Klintmalm GBG, Iwatsuki S, Starzl TE: Lancet 2:470, 1981
3. Keown PA, Stiller CR, Ulan RA, et al: Lancet 1:686, 1981
4. von Willebrand E: Clin Immunol Immunopathol 17:309, 1980
5. Häyry P, von Willebrand E: Scand J Immunol 13:87, 1981
6. Häyry P, von Willebrand E: Ann Clin Res 13:288, 1981
7. Häyry P, Ahonen J, von Willebrand E, et al: Transplant Proc (this issue)
8. Donatsch P, Abisch E, Homberger M, et al: J Immunoassay 2:19, 1981
9. Beveridge T, Grathwol A, Michot F, et al: Curr Ther Res 30:5, 1981
10. Marbet UA, Graft U, Mihatsch JM, et al: Schweiz Med Wochenschr 110:2017, 1980
11. Shulman H, Striker G, Deeg HJ, et al: N Engl J Med 305:1392, 1980

Cyclosporine, the Renin-Angiotensin-Aldosterone System, and Renal Adverse Reactions

H. Siegl, B. Ryffel, R. Petric, P. Shoemaker, A. Muller, P. Donatsch, and M. Mihatsch

MOST new compounds cause unexpected effects during their clinical testing. In the case of cyclosporine-A (CsA), which is a potent orally active immunosuppressant with an oligopeptide structure,[1] the most commonly observed adverse reactions are summarized in Table 1. However, these untoward reactions were not completely unexpected, since similar effects were observed in experimental animals administered high doses of the compound.[2]

This article is restricted to adverse renal effects, which were already reported in the first clinical trials using CsA as the sole immunosuppressant.[3] The most prominent reactions in humans are rapid, dose-dependent, but reversible, creatinine and blood urea nitrogen (BUN) increases. Histologic examination of biopsy specimens revealed tubular changes.[5,6] Glomerular thrombosis has also been reported.[7] However, the question as to whether a morphologic correlate of CsA-associated renal lesions exists is still open.

Faced with clinical reports indicating fluid retention, increased diastolic blood pressure,[8,9] and renal tubular alterations, it was decided to study the effects of CsA on the renin-angiotensin-aldosterone system (RAAS)[10] as well as on other selected endocrine parameters.

MATERIALS AND METHODS

Experiments With Spontaneous Hypertensive Rats

Male SH rats (Ivanova, Kisslegg, BRD), 8–10 weeks old and not yet hypertensively stable (blood pressure <175 mm Hg), or 12–15 weeks old with established hypertension (>180 – 250 mm Hg), were used. Each experimental group consisted of six rats.

CsA was dissolved in olive oil (5 ml/kg) and given orally by gastric tube at daily doses of 0, 20, 50, and 100 mg/kg of body weight for four weeks. The animals were weighed and observed daily. Systolic blood pressure was measured at the root of the tail, using a sphygmomanometer, twice weekly 2–3 hr after medication. The heart rate (HR) was recorded at the same times. During the measurements, the animals were kept in restraining cages at a constant temperature of 30°C.

Diuretic experiments, including clearance studies with inulin and para-aminohippuric acid (PAH), were performed weekly on all animals. Three hours after drug administration, inulin (750 mg/kg) and PAH (1,000 mg/kg) were injected subcutaneously in 10 ml distilled water. After oral administration of 50 ml/kg NaCl 0.9%, the rats were placed in metabolic cages and urine was collected after 1 and 2 hr. Urinary pH was measured immediately. Urinary Na^+ and K^+ were determined by flame photometry (Eppendorf) and Cl^- by potentiometer (EEL). Inulin and PAH were measured using standard methods.[11,12]

Blood was taken from the retroorbital plexus weekly, 4 hr after medication, to determine the plasma renin activity (PRA) and aldosterone using commercial radioimmunoassays (New England Nuclear, Boston, MA), as well as to measure the standard biochemical parameters, using an autoanalyzer (Greiner). In addition, 24-hr blood samples were taken after four weeks to determine both the CsA trough levels by radioimmunoassay[13] and the cellular electrolyte concentrations in erythrocytes.[14]

Complete necropsies were performed on all animals. Tissues from the major organs were fixed in 4% buffered formaldehyde, embedded in paraffin, cut at 3–5 μm and stained (hematoxylin and eosin, PAS, and CAB).

Experiments With Dogs

Three trained male beagle dogs about three years old and weighing between 10 and 15 kg were used. The experiment consisted of three parts, each lasting five days. The dogs were administered the solvent (olive oil) alone for five days, then the solvent and 25 mg/kg per day CsA for five days, and finally only the solvent again for five days. Blood was taken from the foreleg vein for PRA measurements twice daily, 1 hr prior to administration of either the olive oil (3 ml/kg) or the CsA and olive oil, and 5 hr after administration. A catheter was used to empty the bladder prior to the administration of 20 ml/kg NaCl 0.9%, which was carried out at the same time as the olive oil/CsA administration. The urine was then collected at

---

From Preclinical Research, Sandoz Ltd., Basel, and the Department of Pathology, University of Basel, Basel, Switzerland.

Address reprint requests to Dr. H. Siegl, Preclinical Research, Sandoz, Ltd., CH 4002 Basel, Switzerland.

0041-1345/83/1505-0096$01.00/0

Table 1. CsA Administration to Man and Animals: Major Adverse Reactions

Organ/System	Findings in Animals	Findings in Man
Kidney	Bun ↑, creatinine ↑, GFR ↓, tubular and vascular changes (rats, especially SH rats, monkeys)	+
Liver	Bilirubin and hepatic enzyme ↑, centroacinar degeneration of hepatocytes and cholostasis (rat)	+
CNS	Tremor, dysesthesia, convulsion (rat, mouse)	+
Intestine	Weight ↓, anorexia, diarrhea (rat, mouse)	+
Skin, mucosa	Hirsutism, gum hypertrophy (rat, dog)	+
Endocrine system	RAAS activated, corticosterone ↑ (dog, rat, especially SH rat, mouse)	?

1-hr intervals for 5 hr and analyzed for pH, osmolarity, Na^+, K^+, and Cl^-. The dogs were kept in restraining hangers for the daily 6-hr test period.

Calculation of the Results and Statistics

Results were expressed as means ± standard deviations. The results from the CsA-treated SH rats were compared with results from control rats obtained on the same days; results from CsA-treated dogs were compared with results obtained from the same dogs in the five-day periods before and after the CsA administration.

RESULTS

CsA possesses a high specificity for the immune system in a number of animal species without causing distinct signs of renal dysfunction at immunosuppressive doses.[15] In rats, however, dose and time-dependent functional and morphologic renal alterations did become apparent. The sensitivity of the various strains of rats tested differed as follows: SH rats (Kyoto) > normotensive Wistar > normotensive Sprague Dawley rats.

The renal functional alterations found in SH rats are summarized in Table 2. Reduced urinary volumes and electrolyte excretions were only observed in the first two weeks of drug administration, whereas in the following two weeks no significant urine volume or electrolyte excretion changes were measured. However, decreased pH was always observed. Glomerular filtration rate (GFR), measured by the elimination of inulin, and renal plasma

Table 2. Renal Functional Changes in CsA-Treated SH Rats (a 4-Week Experiment)

					URINE							
TIME IN WEEKS	CS-A DOSE MG/KG/DAY P.O.	BP	HR	PRA	H_2O	NA^+	K^+	NA^+/K^+	CL^-	PH	GFR	RPF
2	20	↑	↑	↑	(↓)	↓	↓↓	↑	↓↓	(↓)	(↓)	(↓)
	50	(↓)	↑↑	↑	Ø	↓	↓↓	(↓)	↓↓	↓	↓	↓
	100	↓↓	↑↑	(↑)	(↓)	↓↓	↓↓↓	↓	↓↓↓	↓	↓↓	↓↓
4	20	↑	↑	↑↑	Ø	(↑)	(↓)	↑	(↑)	Ø	Ø	Ø
	50	Ø	↑	(↑)	Ø	Ø	Ø	Ø	Ø	↓	(↓)	(↓)
	100	↓↓	Ø	Ø	Ø	(↓)	↓↓	↑↑	↓	↓	↓	(↓)

Ø NO EFFECT -
(↓) SLIGHT DECREASE ·
↓ DECREASE -
↓↓ DISTINCT DECREASE -
↓↓↓ SEVERE DECREASE AS COMPARED TO CONTROL

(↑) SLIGHT INCREASE -
↑ INCREASE -
↑↑ DISTINCT INCREASE IN COMPARISON TO CONTROL

Table 3. CsA Administration to Rats: Renal Morphologic Changes

Alterations	Sprague Dawley*	Wistar†	SH Rat‡
Proximal Tubule			
Isometric vacuolation	+	+	+
Inclusion bodies	+	+	+
Calcification	+	+	+
Vascular changes			
Media necrosis	−	−	+
Proliferation of myofibroblasts	−	−	+

*45 mg/kg/day given for 13 weeks.
†36 mg/kg/day given for 13 weeks.
‡20 mg/kg/day given for 4 weeks.

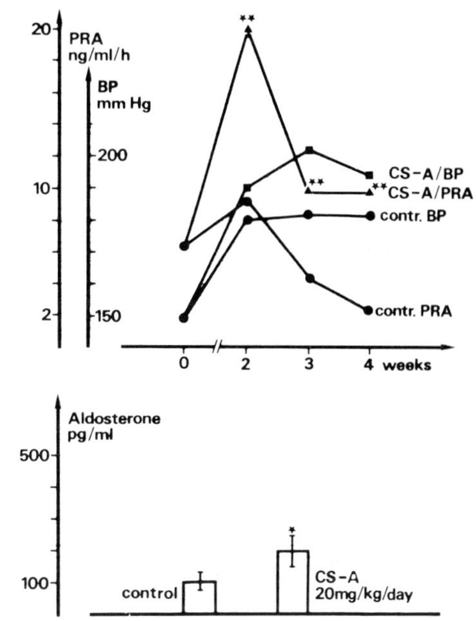

Fig. 1. CsA administration in SH rats (not yet stable hypertensive): Effects on blood pressure (BP), plasma-renin activity (PRA), and plasma aldosterone at a dose of 20 mg/kg/day.

flow (RPF), estimated by the excretion of para-aminohippuric acid, were essentially unaffected at the 20 mg/kg per day dose level. Higher doses, however, resulted in GFR and RPF reductions, as well as in increased serum BUN and creatinine concentrations. These higher doses of the compound also resulted in general toxic signs, such as anorexia and decreased body weight gain.

The morphologic alterations consisted of the following (Table 3): isometric vacuolation of proximal tubules with numerous inclusion bodies and dystrophic calcification of epithelial cells, even in young SH rats. In addition, arteriolar changes consisting of media necrosis and proliferation of myofibroblasts, similar to hypertensive vasculopathy seen typically in rats of this strain with established hypertension, were found. Thus, CsA accelerated the hypertensive vasculopathy in SH rats.

The Action on the RAAS

In beagle dogs, a significant increase of PRA with a concomitant decrease in the urinary Na^+/K^+ ratio and pH were seen after two daily doses of 25 mg/kg CsA (Table 4).

Detailed studies were performed in SH rats with emphasis on the RAAS and on cardiovascular parameters in both young SH rats with not yet stable elevated blood pressure and in older rats with established hypertension. PRA and serum aldosterone were significantly increased after CsA administration (Fig. 1). Blood pressure and HR were already increased within 10 days of drug administration. Histologic examination of the kidneys after a four week administration of 20 mg/kg revealed, besides the tubular changes, distinct vascular lesions.

Table 4. CsA Administration to Beagle Dogs: Effects on Renal Function and Plasma Renin Activity (PRA) (per Group $n = 3$)

Experiment	CsA Dose (mg/kg/day, p.o.)	Urinary Excretion 5 hr: H_2O (ml/10 kg)	Urinary Excretion 5 hr: Na^+ (meq/10 kg)	Na^+/K^+	PRA (ng/ml/hr) Mean ± SD: T_0−1 hr	PRA (ng/ml/hr) Mean ± SD: T_0 + 5 hr
Control I	—	110 ± 25	19 ± 1.8	7.66	4.6 ± 0.7	5.0 ± 0.7
CsA days 2–5	25	104 ± 9.6	14.6 ± 3.6	6.06	6.2 ± 0.1†	6.1 ± 0.8*
Control II	—	108 ± 46	17.7 ± 4.3	6.92	4.3 + 1.7	4.3 ± 1.0

Wilcoxon U test: *$2\alpha = 0.02$; †$2\alpha = 0.01$.

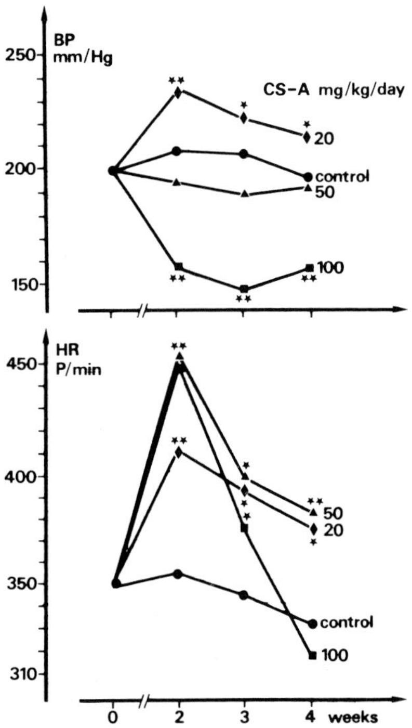

Fig. 2. CsA administration in SH rats (stable hypertensive): Effects on blood pressure (BP) and heart rate (HR).

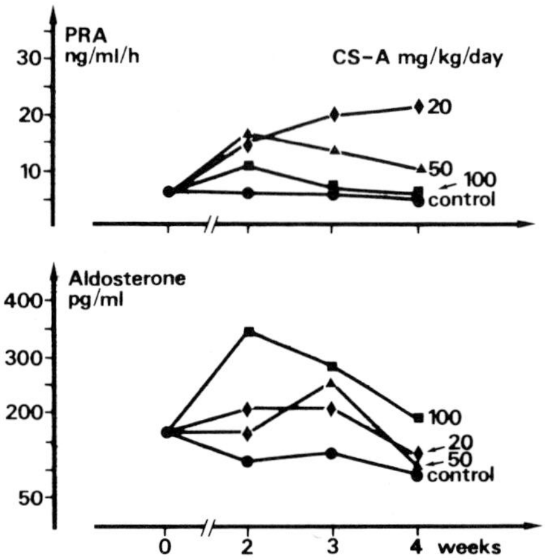

Fig. 3. CsA administration in SH rats (stable hypertensive): changes in PRA and plasma-aldosterone.

Dose Dependence

The dose dependence of CsA-associated changes was further analyzed. SH rats with stable elevated blood pressure were orally given 0, 20, 50, and 100 mg/kg CsA for four weeks. The HR was dose dependently increased for the first three weeks of the experiment, but the highly elevated values could not be fully sustained for the whole period of the study (Fig. 2). Blood pressure, on the other hand, was only increased at the 20-mg/kg dose level, whereas at the 100-mg/kg dose, significantly lower blood pressure values were recorded than in the controls.

The PRA and aldosterone findings are given in Fig. 3. Whereas a dose-dependent aldosterone increase was evident, PRA was significantly increased only at doses <50 mg/kg.

Serum Chemistry

The more important results are summarized in Table 5, and include serum BUN increases, and, to a lesser extent, creatinine increases, both indicating functional renal changes. In addition, hepatic enzymes in the serum were also increased, pointing to hepatic injury. Serum glucose values were greatly and dose-dependently increased. There were statistically significant serum Na^+ decreases and K^+ increases after four-week treatment (Table 6). Cellular K^+ concentrations, deter-

Table 5. CsA Administration in SH Rats: Changes in Clinical Chemical Parameters After 4 Weeks

CsA	Plasma Concentration (Mean)							
Dose (mg/kg/Day)	BUN (mg/dl)	Creatinine (mg/dl)	AP (IU/Liter)	Glucose (mg/dl)	Triglyceride (mg/dl)	GPT (IU/Liter)	GOT (IU/Liter)	*n*
0	16	0.45	613	108	141	72	115	6
20	23*	0.64	458	181†	301*	65	110	4
50	31*	0.87	687	220†	240	70	143*	7
100	31*	0.70	768*	259†	97*	90	151*	3

Test of variance and Student-Newman-Keuls t test.

*$2p \leq 0.05$.

†$2p \leq 0.01$.

Table 6. Electrolyte Concentration in Plasma and Erythrocytes of SH Rats After 4 Weeks CsA Administration

CsA Dose (mg/kg/day)	Plasma (Mean ± SD)		Erythrocyte (Mean ± SD)		
	Na^+ (meq/Liter)	K^+ (meq/Liter)	Na^+ (meq/Liter)	K^+ (meq/Liter)	*n*
0	140 ± 1.4	5.4 ± 0.1	21.6 ± 6.1	106.2 ± 5.1	6
20	131 ± 6†	5.7 ± 0.9	23.9 ± 10.1	99.7 ± 7.3*	4
50	133 ± 2.5†	6.8 ± 0.7†	23.2 ± 7.9	98.6 ± 4.8†	7
100	134 ± 1†	6.7 ± 0.4†	20.2 ± 7.3	102 ± 5.5	3

Test of variance and Student-Newman-Keuls t test.
*$2p \leq 0.05$.
†$2p \leq 0.01$.

mined in erythrocytes from the same animals, were decreased, whereas cellular Na^+ concentrations did not differ significantly from those of the controls.

Effects of CsA on Renal Prostaglandins

Since intrarenally produced prostaglandins play an important role in renal autoregulation and are physiologic antagonists to the vasoconstrictor effect of angiotensin-II (A-II), separate experiments were carried out in indomethacin-pretreated animals in order to study the effects of CsA under these conditions. As shown in Table 7, the CsA-induced urine retention in beagle dogs was intensified by indomethacin. Furthermore, those dogs that had not responded to CsA administration (25 mg/kg per day), showed distinct oliguria after indomethacin pretreatment.

Relation Between CsA Dose, Blood Pressure, and Vascular Changes

In order to establish the role played by the higher blood pressure in the pathogenesis of the vasculopathy, the character and severity of the arterial and arteriolar changes were analyzed in the various dose groups of SH rats given CsA for four weeks. Whereas at low doses (<50 mg/kg), an exudative type of lesion was predominant, more proliferative lesions were observed at higher doses (≥50 mg/kg). There was a dose-dependent increase of vascular changes, as shown in Table 8, but there was no relation between the vascular changes and the blood pressure after four weeks of drug administration. The proliferative lesions probably represent regenerative processes after initial injury, since animals treated with 20 mg/kg developed a proliferative change within eight weeks (data not shown). The question as to whether these vascular changes are solely caused by indirect mechanisms, such as A-II, increased sympathetic nerve activity, and transmitter-release-mediated vasoconstriction or whether CsA has a direct sensitizing effect on the vessels of SH rats is currently under investigation.

DISCUSSION

The present results indicate an intense stimulation of the RAAS in CsA-treated animals that is especially pronounced in SH rats.

Table 7. CsA Administration to Dogs: Potentiating Effects of Indomethacin ($n = 3$)

Experiment	Urinary Excretion at 5 hr (Mean ± SD)					
	CsA Dose (mg/kg/day)	H_2O (ml/10 kg)	Na^+ (meq/10 kg)	Na^+/K^+	PRA (ng/ml/hr) (Mean ± SD)	
					T_0−1 hr	T_0 + 5 hr
Control	—	110 ± 25	19 ± 1.8	7.66	4.6 ± 0.7	5.0 ± 0.7
CsA						
Day 2–5	25	104 ± 9.6	14.6 ± 3.6	6.06	6.2 ± 0.1†	6.1 ± 0.8*
Indomethacin	—	72 ± 31	14.9 ± 4.9	8.14	1.1 ± 0.4	1.6 ± 0.5
Indomethacin plus						
CsA	25	85 ± 56	7.9 ± 7.7	4.19	2.3 ± 0.6	1.8 ± 0.4

Wilcoxon U test: *$2\alpha = 0.02$; †$2\alpha = 0.01$.

Cyclosporine-Associated Hyperkalemia

R. J. Foley, C. T. Van Buren, R. Hamner, and E. J. Weinmann

CYCLOSPORINE-A (CsA) is a recently introduced immunosuppressive agent that has been used in renal,[1] cardiac,[2] liver,[3] bone marrow,[4] and pancreas[5] transplant recipients. Interestingly, CsA itself has been reported to have a nephrotoxic potential.[6] Increases in the serum concentration of creatinine and urea nitrogen have been reported after CsA administration.[7-10] Histologic studies have suggested that CsA administration may result in drug-related changes in glomeruli and tubules.[11]

Abnormalities in serum electrolytes secondary to CsA administration, on the other hand, have received relatively little notice in the published literature. Hamilton et al.[9-10] have reported their experience in renal transplant patients treated with CsA and have compared their results with patients receiving a standard immunosuppressive drug regimen. At 6 to 24 months after transplantation, the group of patients receiving CsA had a higher mean serum concentration of potassium and a lower concentration of bicarbonate.[9,10] We are unaware, however, of other studies that have systematically examined the effects of CsA on the serum electrolyte profile.

At our medical center, CsA is extensively used in renal transplant patients. We have had the impression that, in some transplant patients, there is an increase in the serum concentration of potassium that can best be ascribed to an effect of CsA on potassium metabolism. The present report documents the immediate posttransplantation course of two patients receiving CsA in whom the improvement in renal glomerular function was associated with relative hyperkalemia and in whom no other secondary causes of hyperkalemia could be discerned.

From the University of Texas Health Science Center Medical School at Houston, Divisions of Nephrology and Organ Transplantation, Houston, TX.

Address reprint requests to Dr. R. J. Foley, University of Texas Medical School, Division of Nephrology, P.O. Box 20708, Houston, TX 77025.

0041-1345/83/1505-0097$01.00/0

CASE REPORT

Patient No. 1

A 43-year-old male with end-stage renal disease secondary to glomerulonephritis underwent a living-related kidney transplant and received CsA and prednisone as the immunosuppressive agents. The living-related kidney transplant protocol includes the administration of prednisone and CsA five days prior to transplantation. Hemodialysis was initiated one week prior to transplantation, and during this period, there were no problems with management of his serum potassium. As noted in Table 1, there was a progressive fall in serum concentration of creatinine following transplantation. There was no evidence of rejection as determined by clinical examination, urinanalysis, and serial renal scans. Potassium supplements were not administered, and there was no laboratory or clinical evidence of muscle or red cell destruction. His blood pressure, which had been adequately controlled before his transplant on furosemide and metoprolol, was elevated in the posttransplantation period. Methyl-dopa, metoprolol, hydralazine, and furosemide were subsequently required to control the blood pressure. Despite the improved glomerular function, as manifested by the serum creatinine, the serum concentration of potassium increased, reaching a value of 5.6 meq/liter on postoperative day 4. The relative hyperkalemia persisted even after the administration of furosemide.

Patient No. 2

A 40-year-old female developed renal failure secondary to hereditary nephritis and was treated with chronic ambulatory peritoneal dialysis (CAPD). She had an uneventful course on CAPD and maintained a normal blood pressure and serum concentration of potassium. Six months after starting CAPD, she underwent a cadaveric kidney transplant. The serum concentration of creatinine decreased progressively in the immediate posttransplantation period. There was no clinical, laboratory, or renal scan evidence of rejection any time during her hospital course. In addition, there was no evidence of tissue destruction. Her posttransplantation course was characterized by weight gain and an increase in the blood pressure. On day 6, aldosterone and plasma renin activity were determined to be 12 ng/100 ml (normal, 4–31 ng/100 ml) and 1.6 ng/ml/hr (normal, 0.5–4.3 ng/ml/hr), respectively. Furosemide was started on day 7

Table 1. Clinical Data

Clinical Values	Pretransplant	Posttransplantation Day 1	2	3	4	5	6	7	8	9	10	11	12	13	14
Patient no. 1															
Na (meq/liter)	136.5	135	136	135	136	134	137	135	136	133	135	131	134	133	—
K (meq/liter)	4.1	3.7	4.9	4.9	5.6	5.1	5.4	5.2	5.5	4.9	5.0	4.2	4.9	5.1	—
HCO_3 (meq/liter)	24.3	25	24	24	26	26	28	27	26	27	27	27	26	27	—
Cl (meq/liter)	101	101	105	106	102	100	102	100	100	99	101	99	99	100	—
Cr (mg/dl)	7.3	2.6	1.4	1.3	1.4	1.5	1.7	1.8	1.9	1.9	1.8	2.0	1.8	1.9	—
Weight (lb)	155	151	151	151	150	150	151	151	151	151	149	151	150	150	—
BP (mm Hg)	120/84	160/105	168/110	160/110	158/100	160/106	160/108	160/102	154/100	150/100	152/108	190/116	160/108	160/100	—
Furosemide (mg/day)	160	—	—	—	40	40	40	40	40	40	40	40	40	40	—
CsA (mg/day)	—	1,000	150	1,100	1,100	1,100	1,100	1,100	850	800	800	800	750	750	—
Pred (mg/day)	—	110	105	100	95	90	85	80	75	70	65	60	60	57.5	—
Patient no. 2															
Na (meq/liter)	133	135	139	144	141	141	141	141	139	142	141	143	146	142	145
K (meq/liter)	3.9	3.7	3.5	4.3	4.1	5.0	5.4	4.9	5.0	5.4	4.9	5.4	5.5	5.4	5.4
HCO_3 (meq/liter)	22	26	26	26	28	28	28	27	26	28	27	31	31	31	30
Cl (meq/liter)	102	101	108	115	110	109	109	109	106	111	109	107	109	104	109
Cr (mg/dl)	9.6	5.5	1.7	1.3	1.2	1.3	1.3	1.4	1.4	1.2	1.4	1.4	1.2	1.4	1.0
Weight (lb)	—	110	112	111	112	112	114	114	116	114	116	116	113	113	112
BP (mm Hg)	150/84	140/80	140/90	134/96	134/86	142/80	160/90	160/96	180/90	180/94	186/100	160/100	168/94	180/102	—
Furosemide (mg/day)	—	—	—	—	—	—	—	40	80	160	160	160	80	80	80
CsA (mg/day)	—	650p.o. 100i.v.	650	650	650	700	650	650	600	600	600	600	600	600	550
Pred (mg/day)	—	110	100	95	90	85	80	75	70	65	60	60	60	60	60

posttransplantation. Despite stable serum concentration of creatinine and the subsequent administration of furosemide, the serum concentration of potassium rose to 5.0 meq/liter on posttransplant day 5 and remained elevated throughout the remainder of her hospital stay.

DISCUSSION

CsA is a cyclic endecapeptide discovered in 1972 by Borel.[11] Its effect on the immune system was first described in 1976.[12] CsA is currently being extensively evaluated in human organ transplantation.[1,2,4,5] The nephrotoxic potential of CsA, as manifested by elevations in the serum concentration of creatinine and by decreases in the creatinine clearance, was appreciated in early clinical trials.[1,5] In addition, histologic changes in the glomeruli and tubules of kidneys from patients receiving CsA have been described.[10,11] We were unaware, however, of specific reports examining the effect of CsA on potassium metabolism.

The present report details two cases in which relative hyperkalemia developed in the immediate posttransplant period and persisted for the duration of the hospital stay. In both patients, the serum concentration of potassium rose at a time the serum concentration of creatinine was decreasing and the creatinine clearance was increasing. An increase in the serum concentration of potassium in the face of an improving or a stable renal function is, in our experience, distinctly unusual in the posttransplant period in patients treated with the more usual immunosuppressive drug regimens. Particularly striking in the present patients was the development of hyperkalemia, despite the administration of prednisone and furosemide. In both patients, clinical and laboratory data failed to demonstrate evidence of endogenous potassium release from red blood cells or muscle, nor was there excessive dietary intake of potassium. No evidence of rejection was discerned in either patient during the posttransplant period, rendering it unlikely that rejection was resulting in an impairment in potassium excretion. Neither patient developed a laboratory profile consistent with type IV renal tubular acidosis, as has been reported in some transplant patients.[13,14] In addition, serum aldosterone and renin concentrations in patient no. 2 were normal at a time the extracellular fluid volume was expanded. This would suggest that aldosterone deficiency is not the proximate cause of the hyperkalemia. Neither patient was given potassium-sparing diuretics or nonsteroidal antiinflammatory agents. Patient no. 1 received a beta-blocker. Nonetheless, the beta-blocker had been administered prior to transplantation and was without any effect on the plasma potassium. Moreover, for the reasons indicated above, the electrolyte profile observed was not that of hypoaldosteronism. Finally, neither patient had clinical conditions associated with impaired tissue uptake of potassium, such as diabetes mellitus. In the aggregate, the experience noted in these two cases suggests that the hyperkalemia observed was causally related to the administration of CsA. This conclusion is supported by the temporal relationship between the administration of CsA and the rise in the serum concentration of potassium. Patient no. 1 received CsA for five days prior to transplantation and relative hyperkalemia was apparent by postoperative day 2. Patient no. 2 received CsA beginning the day of transplantation. Hyperkalemia became manifest on day 6.

The mechanism whereby CsA alters the metabolism of potassium is unknown. There are no reported data to indicate that this agent inhibits the uptake or release of potassium into tissue or inhibits the production or release of aldosterone. Preliminary studies in rats in our laboratories indicate that the acute infusion of CsA is associated with a decrease in the fractional excretion of sodium and potassium and that this effect is independent of the glomerular filtration rate and aldosterone. Unfortunately, measurements of electrolyte excretion were not obtained in the patients, but the increase in blood pressure, the weight gain in patient no. 2, and the hyperkalemia are at least consistent with the preliminary observations in rats. To the degree that the response to CsA in humans and rats is similar, the findings would suggest that, in some manner, CsA alters the tubular secretion of potassium into the urine. Hyperkalemia may then become manifest in the posttransplant period due to the catabolic effects of surgery and steroid administration.

Hamilton et al. have recently reported on the serum concentrations of potassium in renal transplant patients receiving CsA as the sole immunosuppressive agent and in patients receiving azathioprine and prednisone. The mean concentrations of potassium were significantly higher at six months posttransplantation in the CsA-treated patients as compared to those treated with a more standard immunosuppressive regimen. In a preliminary survey of 125 transplant patients at our institution, using the arbitrary criteria of a serum potassium in excess of 5 meq/liter and a creatinine clearance of 20 ml/min or greater, there was a significantly higher prevalence of hyperkalemia in patients treated with CsA and prednisone as compared to patients treated with azathioprine and prednisone. It seems reasonable to suggest, therefore, that CsA is associated with a measureable rise in the serum concentration of potassium. Neither of the two patients in the present report developed EKG or other clinical findings suggesting toxic levels of potassium. Nonetheless, the effect of CsA on the serum concentration of potassium may be of greater clinical significance in patients in whom tissue uptake of potassium is impaired, such as patients with diabetes mellitus or in patients receiving other drugs that interfere with potassium metabolism.

REFERENCES

1. Calne RY, Thiru S, McMaster P, et al: Lancet 2:1323, 1978
2. Jamieson SW, Burton NA, Bieber CP, et al: Lancet 1:545, 1979
3. Starzl TE, Klintmalm GBG, Porter KA, et al: N Engl J Med 305:266, 1981
4. Hows JM, Palmer S, Gordon-Smith EC: Transplantation 33:382, 1982
5. Calne RY, Rolles K, Thiru S, et al: Lancet 2:1033, 1979
6. Whiting PH, Thomson AW, Blair JT, et al: Br J Exp Pathol 63:88, 1982
7. Ferguson RM, Rynasiewica JJ, Sutherland DER, et al: Surgery 92:175, 1982
8. Calne RY, Rolles K, White DJG, et al: Adv Nephrol 10:335, 1981
9. Hamilton DV, Evans DB, Henderson RG, et al: Dial Transplant 11:146, 1982
10. Hamilton DV, Evans DB, Henderson RG, et al: Proc EDTA 18:400, 1981
11. Laupacis A, Keown PA, Ulan RA, et al: Can Med Assoc J 126:1041, 1982
12. Borel JF, Feurer C, Magnee C, et al: Immunology 32:1017, 1977
13. Gyory AZ, Stewart JA, George DRP: Q J Med 38:231, 1969
14. Battle DC, Mozes MF, Manaligod J, et al: Am J Med 70:786, 1981

Cyclosporine and Sodium and Potassium Excretion in the Rat

A. S. Tonnesen, R. W. Hamner, and E. J. Weinmann

CYCLOSPORINE-A (CsA) is a recently introduced immunosuppressive agent[1] that has been found to be useful in transplantation of the kidneys,[2–5] heart,[6] bone marrow,[7] and liver and pancreas.[8] A number of clinical reports have alluded to the fact that CsA is potentially nephrotoxic[3,4,8–11] and may be associated with abnormalities in urinalysis and creatinine clearance. Due to the fact that CsA is in common usage in renal transplant recipients at our institution, we have become aware that approximately 30% of patients treated with CsA develop unexplained elevations in the serum concentration of potassium. Such a finding has not been adequately documented in the existing literature, although Hamilton et al.[11] noted higher mean concentrations of potassium in renal transplant recipients receiving CsA as compared to those receiving azathioprine and corticosteroids. In the clinical context, it is often difficult to discern the significance or the mechanism of the change in potassium metabolism. Accordingly, we elected to study the effects of the acute intravenous administration of CsA to rats, with specific emphasis on the renal excretion of sodium and potassium.

MATERIALS AND METHODS

Male Sprague-Dawley rats weighing 300–400 g with free access to food and water prior to study were anesthetized with pentobarbital (50 mg/kg body weight), injected intraperitoneally and supplemented intravenously as needed. A tracheostomy was performed, and catheters were placed in the jugular veins, femoral artery, and urinary bladder. The animals were placed on a heated animal board and rectal temperature was maintained at 37°C. A volume of saline equal to 1% of body weight was administered during the surgical preparation of the animals. An intravenous infusion of 1.2 ml of normal saline, containing ^{3}H-methoxy-inulin (30 μCi/ml) (New England Nuclear Corp. Boston, MA) was given as a bolus, followed by a sustaining infusion of the same solution at a rate of 1.2 ml/hr. After a 30-min equilibration period, CsA, 20 mg/kg body weight, dissolved in cremaphor-EL in 94% ethanol and diluted 9:1 in normal saline (CEL), was infused over a 6–8-min interval. Control rats received an infusion of the diluent (CEL) or, in some experiments, normal saline alone, in a manner identical to the experimental animals. Blood and timed urine samples were obtained in three consecutive 30-min clearance periods, beginning 60 min after completion of infusion of the drug or diluent. The blood samples were replaced with equal volumes of blood from a donor rat.

Four protocols were followed. Nondiuretic rats (group I) were studied as indicated above and received only the continuous infusion of saline containing inulin at a rate of 1.2 ml/hr. A second group (group II) of rats received an infusion of normal saline equal to 10% of body weight over a 60-min interval. The infusion rate was then adjusted to match the urine flow rate. The drug or diluent was then infused, and the clearance determinations performed as already indicated. The third group of rats (group III) was studied in a manner identical to group II, except that normal saline containing 5% mannitol and potassium (5 meq/liter) was substituted for normal saline alone. The fourth group of animals (group IV) was studied under nondiuretic conditions. Prior to the infusion of CsA or CEL, a suture was placed around the aorta above the renal arteries. In the control animals, the aorta was constricted to reduce urine flow rate to a level approximately equal to or below that observed in the nondiuretic CsA animals. The CsA animals underwent the same surgical procedure, but the aorta was not constricted.

Radioactivity of blood and urine was determined in Biofluor in a liquid scintillation counter. Sodium and potassium concentrations were determined by flame photometry. Phosphate concentrations were determined in an autoanalyzer. Standard formulas were used to calculate clearance and fractional excretion rates. Clearance and excretion rates are normalized per gram of wet kidney weight (gkw). Results are expressed as the mean of means ± SEM of the three collection periods. Student's t values, regression equations, and correlation coefficients were calculated from standard formulas.

From the Division of Nephrology, Departments of Internal Medicine and Anesthesiology, University of Texas Medical School at Houston, Houston, TX.

Address reprint requests to Dr. A. S. Tonnesen, Department of Anesthesiology, University of Texas Medical School, 6431 Fannin, Houston, TX 77030.

0041–1345/83/1505–0098$01.00/0

Table 1. Effect of CsA Infusion in Nondiuretic Rats

	Controls ($N = 6$)	CsA ($N = 5$)	p
V (μl · min^{-1} · g KW^{-1})	3.9 ± 0.5	1.2 ± 0.2	<0.01
GFR (μl · min^{-1} · g KW^{-1})	926 ± 81	680 ± 67	<0.05
UNaV (neq · min^{-1} · g KW^{-1})	419 ± 102	8.3 ± 1.1	<0.01
FeNa (%)	0.30 ± 0.09	0.01 ± 0.0004	<0.02
UKV (neq · min^{-1} · g KW^{-1})	1036 ± 154	116 ± 38	<0.01
FeK (%)	27.5 ± 3.6	4.1 ± 1.8	<0.01
Serum K^+ (meq/liter)	4.55 ± 0.12	4.59 ± 0.21	NS

Values are expressed as the mean of means ± SEM. V = urine flow rate; UNaV = urinary Na^+ excretion rate; UKV = urinary K^+ excretion rate. NS = not significant.

RESULTS

Mean arterial blood pressure averaged 130 ± 19 mm Hg and increased with the onset of drug infusion to 153 ± 25 mm Hg ($p <$ 0.05). The blood pressure increase was sustained for approximately 5 min and had returned to normal in all animals before performance of the clearance measurements. The increase in blood pressure was present regardless of the state of hydration of the extracellular fluid volume. No significant changes in blood pressure were observed in animals infused with normal saline or CEL.

The animals receiving saline alone did not differ in any of the measured parameters from those receiving CEL. Accordingly, all data for nondiuretic control animals were combined. The glomerular filtration rate in nondiuretic animals receiving CsA averaged 680 ± 67 μl · min^{-1} · g KW^{-1} and was significantly lower than that of the controls, which averaged 926 ± 81 μl · min^{-1} · g KW^{-1} ($p <$ 0.01) (Table 1). Significant differences in the glomerular filtration rates were also observed in rats in which the extracellular fluid volume was expanded with either normal saline (Table 2) or normal saline plus mannitol (Table 3). In control rats in which the aorta was constricted above the renal arteries, the glomerular filtration rate was similar to CsA-infused rats that underwent the same surgical preparation (Table 4).

The absolute and fractional excretions of sodium were significantly lower in nondiuretic rats receiving CsA (8.3 ± 1.1 neq · min^{-1} · g KW^{-1} and 0.01% ± 0.0004%, respectively) as compared to the control animals (419 ± 102 neq · min^{-1} · g KW^{-1} and 0.34% ± 0.09%, $p <$ 0.02 for both). As compared to CEL controls, the absolute excretion of potassium (116 ± 38 versus 1036 ± 154 neq · min^{-1} · g KW^{-1}, $p <$ 0.01) and the fractional excretion of potassium (4.1% ± 1.8% versus 27.5% ± 3.6%, $p <$ 0.01) were significantly lower in rats infused with CsA. In addition, both the absolute (6.7 ± 3.2 versus 234 ± 25 μmole · min^{-1} · KW^{-1}) and fractional (0.43% ± 0.21% versus 8.78% ± 0.84%) rates of phosphate excretion were significantly

Table 2. Effect of CsA Infusion in Rats in Which the Extracellular Fluid Volume Was Expanded With Normal Saline

	Control ($N = 5$)	CsA ($N = 4$)	p
V (μl · min^{-1} · g KW^{-1})	46.3 ± 8.7	10.07 ± 2.0	<0.05
GFR (μl · min^{-1} · g KW^{-1})	1086 ± 33	914 ± 46	<0.01
UNaV (neq · min^{-1} · g KW^{-1})	6281 ± 860	2194 ± 608	<0.01
FeNa (%)	4.38 ± 0.53	2.78 ± 0.99	<0.02
UKV (neq · min^{-1} · g KW^{-1})	1350 ± 92	906 ± 158	<0.04
FeK (%)	33.8 ± 2.4	26.6 ± 4.3	NS
Serum K+ (meq/liter)	3.69 ± 0.08	3.82 ± 0.11	NS

Values are expressed as the mean of means ± SEM. Abbreviations as in Table 1.

Table 3. Effect of CsA Infusion in Rats in Which the Extracellular Fluid Volume Was Expanded With Saline and Mannitol

	Control ($N = 6$)	CsA ($N = 5$)	p
V (μl · min^{-1} · g KW^{-1})	154 ± 17	119 ± 14	NS
GFR (μl · min^{-1} · g KW^{-1})	957 ± 44	672 ± 69	<0.01
UNaV (neq · min^{-1} · g KW^{-1})	17732 ± 1675	13410 ± 1790	NS
FeNa (%)	13.6 ± 1.8	14.1 ± 1.7	NS
UKV (neq · min^{-1} · g KW^{-1})	1865 ± 207	1215 ± 131	<0.05
FeK (%)	56.2 ± 5.5	54.1 ± 5.3	NS
Serum K+ (meq/liter)	3.63 ± 0.13	3.38 ± 0.10	NS

Values are expressed as the mean of means ± SEM. Abbreviations as in Table 1.

lower in CsA-treated rats as compared to controls.

Expansion of the extracellular fluid with normal saline was used in an attempt to normalize the excretion of sodium. Expansion of the extracellular fluid volume with normal saline increased the rate of sodium and potassium excretion in both control and experimental animals (Table 2). Despite the significantly higher rates of sodium excretion as compared to the nondiuretic animals, the absolute and fractional excretions of sodium were still significantly lower in the experimental animals. In this group of animals, the absolute, but not the fractional, excretion of potassium was significantly lower in rats infused with CsA as compared to controls.

To further explore the relationship between sodium and potassium excretion, additional studies were performed in rats in which the extracellular fluid volume was expanded with normal saline and mannitol (Table 3). In this group of animals, both the absolute and fractional rates of sodium and potassium excretion were not different between the experimental and control animals. However, the experimental animals had a statistically significant lower absolute rate of potassium excretion.

In a further effort to equalize the rates of sodium excretion, the aorta was constricted above the renal arteries in nondiuretic rats (Table 4). The absolute as well as the fractional rates of potassium excretion were not significantly different between control and experimental animals. In the aortic-constricted control animals, the rate of Na excretion was significantly lower.

In all of the above studies, the differences in the serum concentration of potassium were not significant between groups of animals studied under the same protocol.

The relationship between the rate of potassium excretion and the logarithm of the rate of sodium excretion for all groups of animals studied is summarized in Fig. 1. In experimental animals, the correlation coefficient was 0.89 ($p < 0.01$) and the equation for the relationship was $Y = 352X - 261$, where Y is the excretion rate for potassium and X is the logarithm of the sodium excretion rate. In the

Table 4. Effect of CsA Infusion in Nondiuretic Rats With Aortic Constriction

	Control ($N = 5$)	CsA ($N = 4$)	p
V (μl · min^{-1} · g KW^{-1})	1.7 ± 0.20	1.9 ± 0.01	NS
GFR (μl · min^{-1} · g KW^{-1})	698 ± 53	837 ± 67	NS
UNaV (neq · min^{-1} · g KW^{-1})	21 ± 5	52 ± 10	<0.05
FeNa (%)	0.02 ± 0.005	.04 ± 0.008	<0.05
UKV (neq · min^{-1} · g KW^{-1})	279 ± 64	275 ± 50	NS
FeK (%)	7.8 ± 1.7	6.8 ± 1.1	NS
Serum K+ (meq/liter)	5.09 ± .22	4.86 ± .12	NS

Values are expressed as the mean of means ± SEM. Abbreviations as in Table 1.

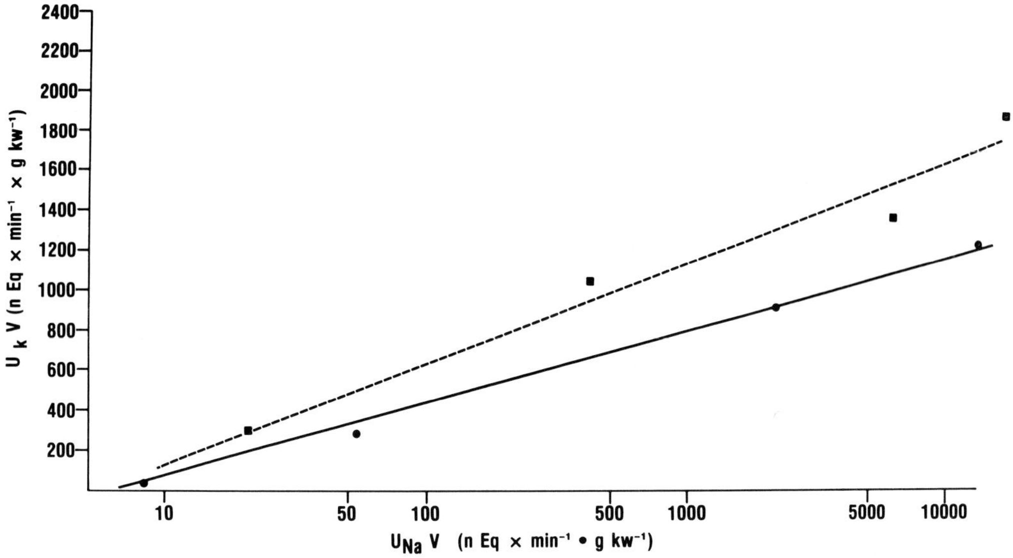

Fig. 1. Relationship between Na^+ and K^+ excretion rates in control (□——□) and CsA-treated (●——●) rats. Although the CsA-treated rats tended to excrete less K^+ at any level of Na^+ excretion, the regression lines are not significantly different.

control animals, the correlation coefficient was 0.98 ($p < 0.01$) and the equation for the relationship was $Y = 496X - 355$. There was no statistical difference between the experimental and control animals in either the slope or the intercept of the regression lines.

DISCUSSION

Although not emphasized, other investigators have reported higher mean serum concentrations of potassium in kidney transplant recipients receiving CsA as compared to patients receiving a more standard immunosuppressive regimen.[5,11] As noted in the introduction, we have observed a surprisingly high incidence of hyperkalemia in patients receiving renal transplants when CsA was used as the immunosuppressive agent. The hyperkalemia was not clearly associated with severe limitation of the creatinine clearance and did occur in patients with excellent creatinine clearances in the posttransplant period. It was not possible, given the clinical circumstances and the retrospective nature of the above observations, to study the mechanism for the hyperkalemia. It was suggested, however, that the elevation in the plasma concentration of potassium was related directly or indirectly to the administration of CsA, since a comparable group of patients treated with azathioprine instead of CsA did not manifest hyperkalemia.

The acute intravenous administration of CsA results in a transient and modest increase in blood pressure. The mechanism of this response is unknown, but it does not appear to be related to the vehicle of administration. As compared to controls, rats infused with CsA had a lower glomerular filtration rate. This finding was consistent regardless of the state of hydration of the animals. In nondiuretic animals, the infusion of CsA was associated with a lower absolute and fractional rate of sodium excretion, as well as a lower absolute and fractional rate of potassium excretion. The serum concentrations of sodium and potassium, however, were not significantly different between the groups of animals. Since potassium excretion is related to the rate of sodium delivery and/or the flow rate to the distal portion of the nephron, it was unclear from studies in the nondiuretic animals whether CsA had a direct effect on potassium excretion or whether the observed differences were related to the alteration in the renal tubular handling of sodium.

Several lines of evidence would suggest that, at least in part, the observed differences in potassium excretion in the nondiuretic animals infused with CsA were consequences of the altered renal handling of sodium. In animals in which the extracellular fluid volume was expanded and the urine flow rate increased, the urinary excretion of potassium increased, and at comparable fractional rates of sodium excretion, potassium excretion was similar in CsA rats as compared to controls. In nondiuretic control animals, constriction of the aorta above the renal arteries was employed to lower the excretion of sodium to levels comparable to those seen in the CsA-infused animals. Under such circumstances, potassium excretion was again similar between the control and experimental animals. In control animals studied under the four experimental protocols, there is a highly significant linear relationship between the rate of potassium excretion and the logarithm of the rate of sodium excretion. As summarized in Fig. 1, the relationship between these parameters in animals infused with CsA is not statistically different from controls. Taken together, the results would seem to indicate that CsA affects the renal excretion of potassium by altering the tubular reabsorption of sodium. The results also suggest that the nephron site where CsA affected sodium transport was other than the sodium potassium exchange sites in the distal tubule.

Although potassium excretion was not statistically different in CsA-infused animals as compared to controls when normalized for sodium excretion, there does appear to be a slightly lower rate of potassium excretion at any given rate of sodium excretion. Two observations might suggest that the reduced potassium excretion is not solely the result of the decrease in sodium excretion. When sodium excretions were equalized by saline loading plus mannitol, potassium excretion was still significantly lower. Secondly, when potassium excretions were equalized by aortic constriction, sodium excretion was significantly lower in control animals. It is possible, therefore, that some other factor, or factors, in addition to sodium delivery, are also operative in animals receiving CsA. Additional studies will be required to fully elucidate this issue.

We reasoned that one possible site of action of CsA was on the proximal convoluted tubule. In nondiuretic rats, we examined the renal excretion of phosphate. In the context of these studies, the excretion of phosphate was taken to reflect reabsorption in the proximal convoluted tubule. The fractional excretion of phosphate was lower in CsA-infused animals as compared to controls. The mechanism of this response is unknown at the present time, and additional studies will be required to elucidate the mechanism. We would suggest, however, that CsA directly or indirectly enhances the rate of reabsorption of filtrate in the proximal portion of the nephron and limits the distal delivery of filtrate.

Although the usual precautions in translating data from animals to humans must be considered, it is of interest that hypertension and sodium retention have also been observed in humans receiving CsA. Unlike man, however, we did not observe any alteration in the serum concentration of potassium in the rats over the time course of these studies. To the degree that the present acute infusion studies in the rat are applicable to man, CsA appears to decrease the glomerular filtration rate and the urinary excretion of sodium and potassium. If nonrenal mechanisms of potassium disposition are altered in the transplant recipient, hyperkalemia may then ensue. Clearly, specific attention must be paid to the serum concentration of potassium in patients receiving CsA, and prospective studies on sodium and potassium metabolism in such patients are indicated.

ACKNOWLEDGMENT

The authors wish to acknowledge the technical assistance of David V. Smith and the secretarial assistance of Phyllis Van Dyne.

REFERENCES

1. Borel JF, Feurer C, Gubler HU, et al: Agents Actions 6:468, 1976

2. Starzl TE, Hakala TR, Rosenthal JT, et al: Surg Gynecol Obstet 154:819, 1982

3. Starzl TE, Weil R III, Iwatsuki S, et al: Surg Gynecol Obstet 151:17, 1980

4. Calne RY, Thiru S, McMaster P, et al: Lancet 2:1323, 1978

5. Harder F, Loertscher R, Calne RY, et al: Lancet 2:57, 1982

6. Griffith BP, Hardesty RL, Deeb GM, et al: Ann Surg 196:324, 1982

7. Powles RL, Clink HM, Spence D, et al: Lancet 1:327, 1980

8. Calne RY, Rolles K, White DJG, et al: Lancet 2:1033, 1979

9. Shulman H, Striker G, Deeg HJ, et al: N Engl J Med 305:1392, 1981

10. Calne RY, White DJG: Ann Surg 196:330, 1982

11. Hamilton DV, Evans DB, Henderson RG, et al: Proc EDTA 18:400, 1981

Rat Composite Tissue Allograft Recipients Demonstrate a Dose-Related Increase in Renal Toxicity with Therapeutic Doses of Cyclosporine

C. W. Hewitt, K. S. Black, L. A. Fraser, E. B. Howard, A. Ingerman, B. Philosophe, B. M. Achauer, D. C. Martin, and D. W. Furnas

THE immunosuppressant, cyclosporine, has been used successfully to control rejection in kidney,[1,2] liver,[3] bone marrow,[4] and heart transplant patients.[5] However, it is now well established that nephrotoxic and hepatoxic side effects are associated with the administration of cyclosporine in these various transplant procedures.[1–7]

Investigations within our laboratory have centered on cyclosporine's capacity to inhibit composite tissue allograft (CTA) rejection. A CTA is made up of a composite of various tissues, which include skin, connective tissue, muscle, bone, nerve, vessels, and bone marrow. The rat hind limb has served as our CTA model in these studies.

We have previously shown that cyclosporine effectively prevents CTA rejection in the rat hind limb transplant model[8] and is superior to prior donor-specific blood transfusions, which were proven ineffective for prolonging limb allograft survival.[9]

In this article, we investigate various possible toxicities associated with composite tissue transplantation in combination with the use of cyclosporine at moderate to low levels for the inhibition of CTA rejection.

From the Reconstructive Microsurgery and Transplantation Laboratories, Division of Plastic Surgery and Division of Urology, University of California, Irvine, and the Department of Pathology, University of Southern California School of Medicine, Los Angeles, CA.

Supported in part by the American Association of Plastic Surgeons, the Smart Family Foundation, the UCI Committee on Undergraduate Scholarships, and the American Society for Surgery of the Hand.

Address reprint requests to C. W. Hewitt, Reconstructive Microsurgery and Transplantation Laboratories, Division of Plastic Surgery, University of California, Irvine, CA 92717.

0041–1345/83/15056–00100$01.00

MATERIALS AND METHODS

Lewis rats (LEW, RT1[l]) served as recipients of Lewis × Brown-Norway F_1 (LBN, $RT1^{l+n}$) allografts. LEW rats were obtained from Harlan Sprague Dawley, Inc. (Indianapolis, IN). LBN rats were obtained from Charles River Breeding Laboratories, Inc. (Wilmington, MA). The procedure for limb transplantation has been described previously in detail.[10]

Cyclosporine was solubilized in a solution of 20% Tween 80 in anhydrous ethanol at a concentration of 25 mg/ml. Cyclosporine was administered in experimental groups for 20 days as a single daily subcutaneous injection.

Five groups of LEW rats were studied: group 1—LEW limb allograft recipients received a LBN limb allograft only (controls; $n = 6$); group 2—LEW recipients received a LBN limb allograft and 2 mg/kg per day of cyclosporine ($n = 4$); group 3—LEW rats were recipients of a LBN limb transplant and received 4 mg/kg per day of cyclosporine ($n = 6$); group 4—LEW limb transplant recipients received 8 mg/kg per day of cyclosporine ($n = 6$); group 5—LEW rats received a LBN limb allograft and 25 mg/kg per day of cyclosporine ($n = 5$).

Renal function was assessed by assaying serum urea (BUN) concentrations at weekly intervals. Urea levels were determined by the Berthelot colormetric urease procedure (Sigma Technical Bulletin no. 640, Sigma Chemical Co., St. Louis, MO). Hepatic function was assessed by assaying total bilirubin levels, according to the procedure outlined in Sigma Technical Bulletin no. 605.

Hematologic analysis included white blood cell counts (WBC), total neutrophil counts, total lymphocyte counts, and total monocyte counts at weekly intervals. Cell counts were performed on a Hycell 555 blood cell counter (Hycell, Houston, TX). Differentials were carried out on Wright stained blood smears.

Regression analysis was used to determine the linear relationship of urea levels (dependent variable) with cyclosporine dose (independent variable). The completely randomized analysis of variance (ANOVA) and the Tukey multiple comparison test were used for statistical inference. Values were considered significant at $p \leq 0.05$.

RESULTS AND DISCUSSION

Figure 1 demonstrates that BUN levels rose and exhibited a significant dose-dependent

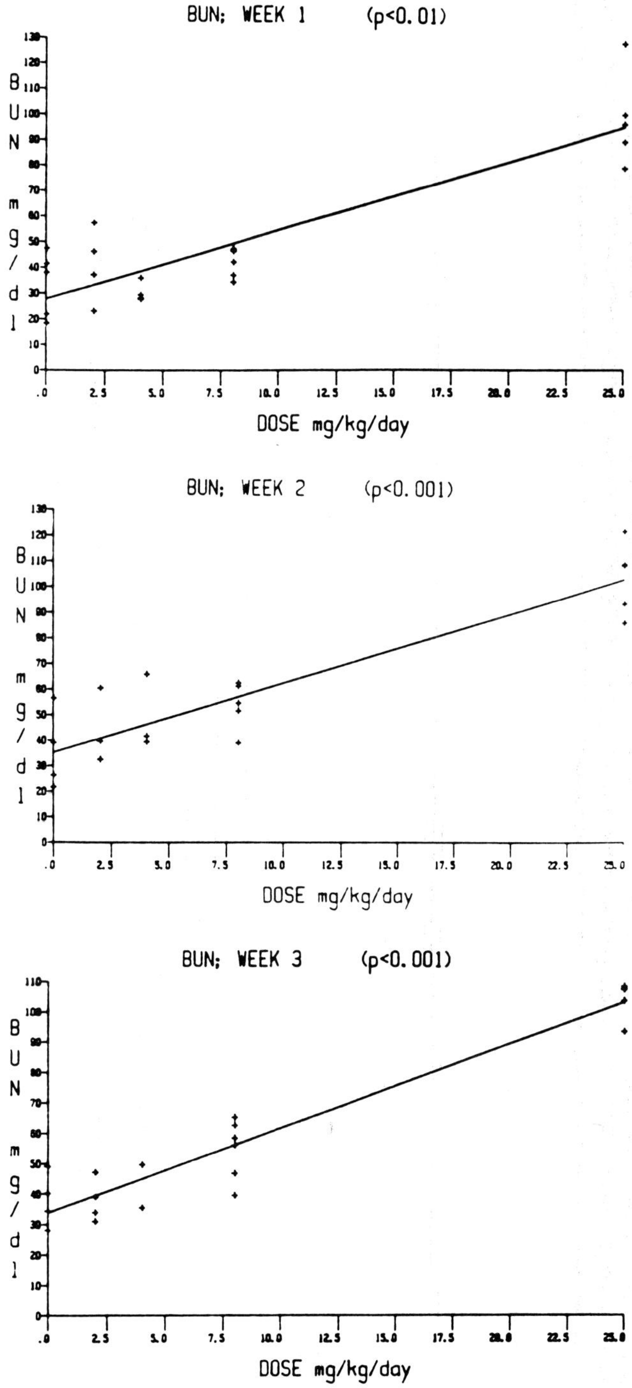

Fig. 1. Dose-dependent increase in serum urea (BUN) with increasing therapeutic doses of cyclosporine in LEW CTA recipients. *p* Values were determined by ANOVA.

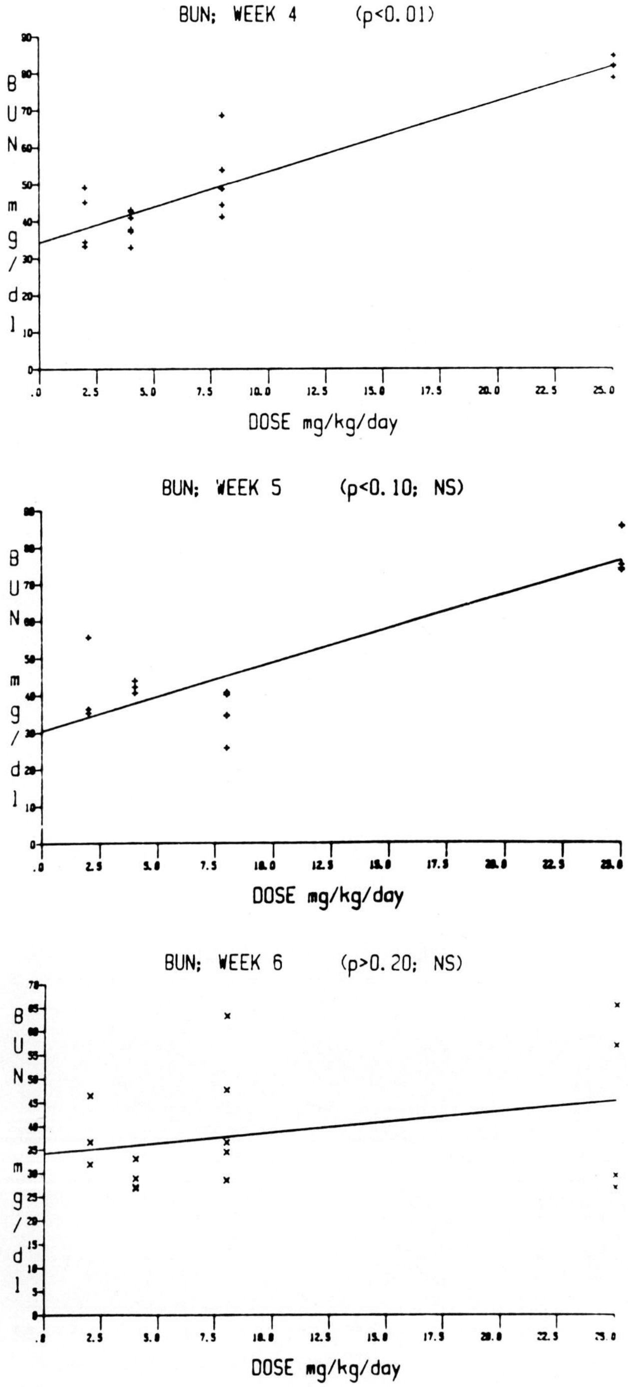

Fig. 1. Continued

linear relationship ($p < 0.05$) with the dose of cyclosporine administered. This linear relationship was observed at weeks 1 through 4 posttransplantation and corresponded to the time interval in which rats were being given cyclosporine daily (approximately three weeks posttransplantation), and an additional week that followed the completion of drug administration. However, at weeks 5 and 6 there was no evidence of renal dysfunction as determined by BUN concentration and no linear relationship to cyclosporine administration was observed ($p < 0.10$ and $p > 0.20$, respectively). The timing of these observations corresponded to two and three weeks following daily drug administration, respectively. Thus, renal function reverted to normal once the LEW CTA recipients completed their cyclosporine treatment. This is in agreement with what other investigators have observed in rats treated with a three-week course of high dosage cyclosporine.[11]

Although a dose-dependent relationship between cyclosporine and BUNs was observed in our CTA recipients at therapeutic levels, only slight increases were seen in BUNs at relatively low doses (i.e., <8 mg/kg per day). These lower doses were completely effective for preventing CTA rejection for an extended time period.

As a comparison, we have included some retrospective rat renal allograft data from LEW recipients of BN kidneys enhanced by prior blood administration and which subsequently became long-term survivors (>50 day; mean survival time was 97 days) (Table 1). As can be seen, even in this successful renal transplant group, the mean of the lowest BUN value obtained during the course of transplantation was comparable to that seen in the 8 mg/kg per day cyclosporine CTA group at week 3.

The coefficient of determination (r^2), which accounts for the proportion of the variation observed about the regression line, was determined at each week and gave the following results: 0.79, 0.83, 0.92, 0.86, 0.78, and 0.10, respectively. Thus, at week 6, the regression line accounted for very little variation in the data.

Table 1. BUN Levels in LEW Rat Transplant Recipients*

Group	Mean BUN (mg/dl ± SEM)	*n*
CTA—8 mg/kg/day cyclosporine; week 3	54 ± 4	6
LEW renal allograft recipients of BN kidneys—long-term survivors†	56 ± 5	6
CTA-controls (no cyclosporine)	38 ± 9	6

*$p < 0.05$ by ANOVA.

†Long-term survivors were induced by prior administration of donor-specific blood. The lowest BUN value during the course of the investigation for each animal was obtained retrospectively and averaged above.

Hepatotoxicity has also been associated with cyclosporine use,[12] yet, for the most part, we did not observe any significant differences ($p > 0.05$) among the various groups with respect to weekly total bilirubin analysis (Fig. 2). The exception, however, was at week 1, where the 2 mg/kg per day group exhibited a small but statistically significant elevation in total bilirubin levels. The other cyclosporine-treated groups demonstrated lower bilirubin values but were receiving higher doses. The reason for this inconsistency was not apparent.

We did not observe any significant changes in WBC, total neutrophil, and total lymphocyte counts, either during cyclosporine administration or after administration (Fig. 3). However, as other investigators reported with high-dose cyclosporine administration in rats,[11] we observed several atypical lymphocytes possessing a monocytoid appearance with increased cytoplasmic vacuolation. In addition, several lymphocytes were observed with azurophilic cytoplasmic granules. It was sometimes difficult to distinguish between these forms of lymphocytes and monocytes, which may account for the reason we observed some statistically significant ($p < 0.05$) increases in total monocyte counts, with the

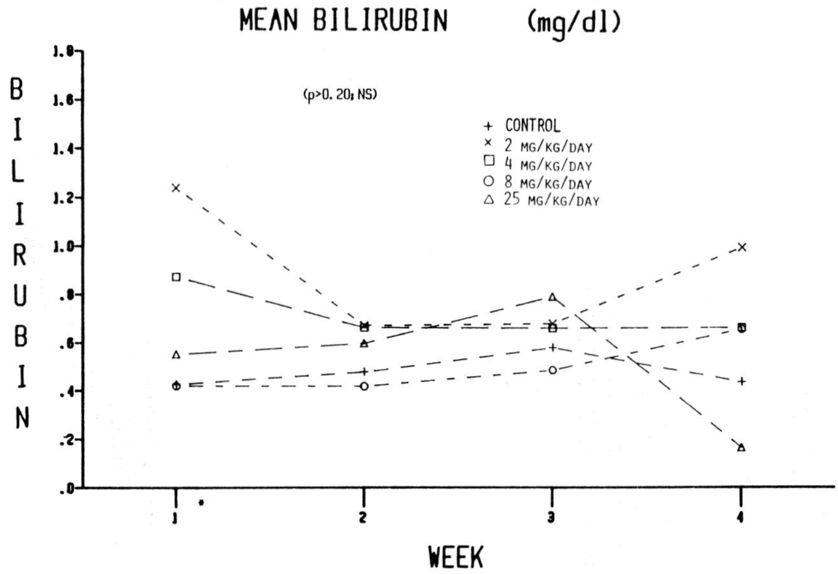

Fig. 2. Effect of cyclosporine on serum total bilirubin levels in LEW CTA recipients. *p* Values were determined by ANOVA and the Tukey multiple comparison analysis. An asterisk indicates a significant difference among groups for the week specified.

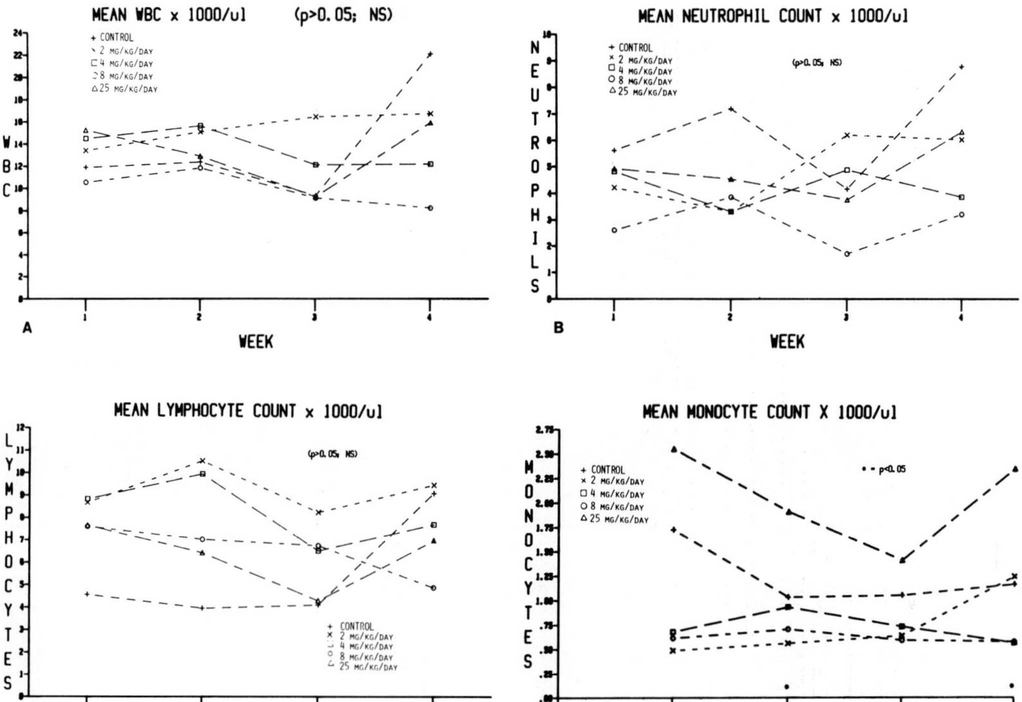

Fig. 3. Effect of cyclosporine on (A) WBC, (B) total neutrophil, (C) total lymphocyte, and (D) total monocyte counts in LEW CTA recipients. *p* Values were determined by ANOVA and the Tukey multiple comparison test. Asterisks indicate a significant difference among groups for the week specified.

highest mean values obtained in the 25 mg/kg per day group (Fig. 3).

Histologic study of kidney, liver, and spleen revealed that these tissues were essentially normal at necropsy, when the CTA rejection process appeared to be stabilized.

A review of allotransplantation of limbs has been made with the claim that limb transplants are a justifiable goal, and even at current technologic levels with respect to peripheral nerve regeneration, would be preferable to prostheses.[13] Yet, before clinical consideration could be given to such vascularized CTAs, the toxicity of the treatment regimen necessary to maintain graft acceptance would have to be minimal. The levels of cyclosporine toxicity at the lower doses in our CTA models do in fact appear to be minimal.

In this article, we have shown that there is a dose-related increase in renal toxicity in a rat CTA model as determined by BUN levels at immunotherapeutic doses of cyclosporine. However, this renal dysfunction was reversible, and low doses of cyclosporine (4–8 mg/kg per day), which are completely effective for preventing CTA rejection in this model, demonstrated only slight increases in BUN concentrations. Little, if any, other toxic effects were noted in our cyclosporine-CTA model.

ACKNOWLEDGMENT

We would like to thank Dr. David L. Winter of Sandoz, Inc., for generously supplying cyclosporine. We would also like to acknowledge the technical assistance of Brenda Mah and John Koumas, and the editorial assistance of Janet Inkster and Erin McLaren.

REFERENCES

1. Calne RY, White DJG, Thiru S, et al: Lancet 2:1323, 1978

2. Calne RY, Rolles K, White DJG, et al: Lancet 2:1033, 1979

3. Starzl TE, Klintmalm GBG, Porter KA, et al: N Engl J Med 305:267, 1981

4. Powles RL, Clink HM, Spence D, et al: Lancet 1:327, 1980

5. Oyer PE, Stinson EB, Jamieson SW, et al: Transplant Proc 15:1247, 1983

6. Klintmalm GBG, Iwatsuki S, Starzl TE: Lancet 1:470, 1981

7. Kennedy MS, Deeg HJ, Storb R, et al: Transplant Proc 15:471, 1983

8. Black KS, Hewitt CW, Fraser LA, et al: N Engl J Med 306:368, 1982

9. Hewitt CW, Black KS, Fraser LA, et al: Transplant Proc 15:514, 1983

10. Black KS, Hewitt CW, Woodard TL, et al: J Microsurg 13:162, 1982

11. Thomson AW, Whiting PH, Blair JT, et al: Transplantation 32:271, 1981

12. Klintmalm GBG, Iwatsuki S, Starzl TE: Transplantation 32:488, 1981

13. Lance EM. in Najarian JS, Simmons RL (eds): Transplantation. Philadelphia, Lea & Febiger, 1972, pp 655

Complications of Cyclosporine Therapy—A Comparison to Azathioprine

A. Laupacis, London, Canada, for Canadian Transplant Study Group

THE protocol of the randomized trial by the Canadian Transplant Study Group (CTSG) of cyclosporine and prednisone (CsA) versus azathioprine and prednisone (STD) in cadaveric renal transplantation is described elsewhere.[1,2] One hundred and forty-two patients received CsA and 149 received STD. Follow-up is from four to 28 months (mean, 19 months). Forty-one of the STD patients received three weeks of prophylactic antilymphocytic globulin (ALG) as well. This article describes the complications (other than cyclosporine nephrotoxicity) seen in both treatment groups.

MATERIALS AND METHODS

Complications were recorded on a "complication form" at least weekly during each hospitalization and at each outpatient visit. The forms were sent to the central office, where the data were checked and recorded. Any uncertainties or errors were reviewed with the clinician involved. Failure to note complications on a visit were also checked. The central office also periodically sent a summary of each patient's clinical course to the individual centers to verify the recorded data.

Cytomegalovirus (CMV) infections were diagnosed on the basis of clinical symptomatology and elevated CMV titers. Routine culturing of urine was variable by center. Urinary tract infections (UTI) were only recorded if they were treated with antibiotics. A patient with more than one treated UTI was said to have a recurrent UTI.

RESULTS

Neoplasms

Five months after transplantation, one patient in the CsA group developed a histiocytic polyclonal lymphoma of the bowel and at the base of the tongue. Cyclosporine was discontinued and the patient treated with surgery and chemotherapy. She died of hemorrhage with thrombocytopenia and a bowel perforation one month later.

One cyclosporine-treated patient had a gastric biopsy six months posttransplant, with one pathologist reporting "lymphomatous change." Repeated biopsies were negative. Cyclosporine was stopped and a gastrectomy performed, but no lesion, including the original ulcer, could be found in the surgical specimen. The patient is well nine months later.

Prior to transplant, a basal cell carcinoma of the ear and a bladder tumor were seen in two CsA patients. Both were surgically excised and have not recurred. One patient in the STD group developed actinic premalignant keratosis, which was successfully removed.

Infections

Infectious complications are listed in Table 1. Nine cases of septicemias were seen in the CsA and 11 in the STD group. In the CsA group, the septicemia was associated with a perinephric abscess (2 patients), inguinal abscess (one patient), UTI (one patient), and infected dialysis fistula (one patient). One patient developed leukopenia and septicemia after being switched to STD therapy. In the STD group, the septicemias were associated with a perinephric abscess (one patient), multiple small bowel abscesses (one patient), pseudomonas skin lesions (one patient), pneumonia (one patient), and UTI (two patients). The sources for the other septicemias were unknown.

There were nine abscesses in the CsA and seven in the STD group. In the CsA group, there were five perinephric, one lung, one

---

From the Canadian Transplant Study Group.

Supported in part by the Medical Research Council of Canada; Richard and Jean Ivey Fund, London, Ontario; Sandoz Ltd., Basel, Switzerland; Michael Fung Endowment Fund, London, Ontario; University Hospital Transplant Research Fund, London, Ontario.

Address reprint requests to Dr. C. R. Stiller, Centre for Transplant Studies, University Hospital, London, Ontario, Canada.

0041-1345/83/1505-0101$01.00/0

Table 1. Infectious Complications

Complication	Cyclosporine (142 Patients)	Standard (149 Patients)
Septicemia	9	11
Abscess	9	7
Systemic fungal	1	2
CMV	4	12
Pneumonia	11	13
Viral (non-CMV)	25	33
Oral Candidiasis	16	17
UTI (recurrent)	42 (7)	42 (18)
Wound and skin	16	19
Other major	4	5

inguinal, one recurrent skin, and one intraabdominal abscess. In the STD group there were two perinephric, one small bowel, one perianal, two skin, and one tooth abscess. When combined, the septicemia and abscess were the cause of one death and two nephrectomies in the CsA group, and three deaths and 1 one nephrectomy in the STD group.

Four CsA and 12 STD patients had CMV infections. All were mild except for two patients in the STD group in whom CMV was isolated at autopsy after death from a myocardial infarction and perforated peptic ulcer.

The incidence of other infectious complications was similar in the two groups (Table 1). The two systemic fungal infections in the STD group were due to *Candida albicans* and occurred terminally. One CsA-treated patient had peritonitis due to *C. albicans*. The other major complications were peritonitis (two patients), septic arthritis (one patient), and pyelonephritis in the untreated kidneys (one patient) in the cyclosporine group, and mycotic aneurysm, miliary tuberculosis, osteomyelitis, peritonitis, and viral ulcer of the eye in the STD group.

Surgical Complications

There were 44 clinically evident urologic complications in the study (19 in the CsA and 25 in the STD group). They were lymphocele (six patients), hydrocele (five patients), ureteric obstruction (seven patients), urinary leak (13), and postoperative or post biopsy hemorrhage (13). There was no overall difference between the two groups in the incidence of these complications.

Vascular Complications

Three patients in the CsA group had renal artery thrombosis necessitating nephrectomy, compared to one in the STD group. The latter patient developed thrombosis during emergency parathyroidectomy for hypercalcemia. Seven patients in the CsA and four patients in the STD group developed stenosis of the transplant artery. Four patients in each group suffered a myocardial infarction or sudden death.

In 18 diabetic patients treated with CsA, there were two myocardial infarctions, one below-knee amputation, two cerebrovascular accidents, and two thrombi of the internal iliac artery. In 20 diabetics on STD therapy, there was one myocardial infarction, one sudden death, one embolus to the leg, and one toe amputation.

Hepatotoxicity

There were five episodes of clinical hepatotoxicity in CsA-treated patients, all associated with trough CsA levels greater than 700 ng/ml and all resolved upon decreasing the dose. Four patients in the STD group developed clinical hepatotoxicity due to CMV infection, cholelithiasis, congestive heart failure, and hepatitis of unknown etiology. One hundred eighty days posttransplant, the mean serum glutamic oxaloacetic transaminase ± SD was 27.1 ± 20.2 U/liter in the CsA and 40.9 ± 82.6 U/liter in the STD group.

Hypertension

Hypertensive nephropathy was the primary renal disease in six cyclosporine and eight standard therapy patients. The antihypertensive regimen of all patients at their most recent clinic visit was recorded. Patients who had been switched from cyclosporine were excluded. Patients requiring any one beta-blocking agent, a vasodilator such as hydralazine or clonidine (but not minoxidil), or methyl-dopa were said to have grade 1 hypertension. Patients with grade 2 hypertension required a combination of two of the above agents, patients with grade 3 hypertension were receiving three of these agents, or minoxidil or captopril. There were 100 patients in each treatment group. Thirty-six of the patients on cyclosporine required no antihypertensive medication compared with 51 of the patients receiving standard therapy. Thirty-five cyclosporine-treated patients had grade 1 hypertension, 16 had grade 2, and 13 had grade 3 hypertension. Twenty-one of the standard therapy patients had grade 1, 20 had grade 2, and eight had grade 3 hypertension. Significantly more patients on cyclosporine had some degree of hypertension ($p = 0.03$).

Neurologic Complications

Six patients in the CsA and five in the STD group developed seizures for the first time. Transient parathesiae were common in the CsA group.

Hypertrichosis and Gingival Hyperplasia

Forty-nine patients developed hypertrichosis in the CsA group (15 moderate, one severe). Four patients in the standard group developed hypertrichosis (one severe). Twelve patients on cyclosporine had clinically evident gingival hyperplasia. None required gingivectomy. No gingival hyperplasia was seen in the standard group.

"Steroid-Related" Side Effects

One year posttransplant, the mean daily prednisone dose (±SD) in the CsA group was 9.3 ± 4.2 mg, compared with 15.2 ± 4.9 in the STD group ($p < 0.001$) (if the patient was on alternate-day prednisone, the alternate-day dose was divided by two). There was no difference in the development of cushingoid features or acne in the two groups. Aseptic necrosis of the femoral head developed in three patients in each group. Six patients in the CsA group developed hyperglycemia, requiring treatment with insulin or hypoglycemic agents, compared with 11 in the STD group. Three patients in the CsA and six in the STD group have developed cataracts.

Miscellaneous

There were five cases of gastrointestinal bleeding (one death) in the CsA and eight (two deaths) in the STD group. Hypercalcemia/hyperparathyroidism was slightly more common in the CsA (13 patients) than in the STD group (seven patients). Two patients had these disorders before transplantation. The mean serum alkaline phosphatase level 360 days posttransplant was higher in the CsA than in the STD group (193 ± 146 versus 71 ± 32, $p < 0.01$). Severe leukopenia (less than 2,000) was seen in 23 STD patients and four CsA patients. Two of the latter occurred in patients shortly after they were switched to azathioprine. One CsA patient developed hemolytic anemia on 20 mg/kg per day of CsA. This resolved when the drug was stopped, but recurred again at one-half the dose. After stopping the CsA once more, the drug was restarted at one-quarter of the original dose, with no evidence of hemolytic anemia.

One patient in the STD group delivered a healthy child. No pregnancies have occurred in the CsA group.

DISCUSSION

Although the incidence and severity of cyclosporine complications is influenced by the type of transplant and the transplant center, most clinicians have reported similar cyclosporine side effects.[2-4] Cyclosporine has been used for a relatively short time, and the true incidence of all complications (especially the uncommon ones) is unknown.

The most feared cyclosporine complication is lymphoma.[5] This occurred in one patient in this study and was fatal. Another CsA-treated patient had a gastric lesion that appeared lymphomatous on biopsy, but could not be found after CsA was stopped and gastrectomy performed. This is similar to the experience of Rosenthal et al.,[6] who reported that it may be possible to treat some cyclosporine-associated lymphomas by simply discontinuing or drastically lowering the dose of cyclosporine. The incidence of lymphoma (now approximately 0.5%) seems to be decreasing as less cyclosporine is used in each patient and concurrent therapy with cytotoxic agents is limited.

Except for a lower incidence of CMV infections in the CsA group, there was no difference in infectious complications between the two groups. One cannot separate the effects of CsA from prednisone when assessing infectious complications. Follow-up of patients treated with cyclosporine alone for autoimmune diseases will allow more accurate determination of the extent to which cyclosporine itself predisposes to infection.

The incidence of renal artery thrombosis and stenosis was higher in the CsA in the STD group. Further experience is required to determine if this difference is real. One renal artery thrombosis has occurred in the 69 subsequent patients receiving cyclosporine treated by the CTSG.[7] Cyclosporine has not decreased the incidence of vascular complications in diabetics transplanted for end-stage renal failure.

It has been suggested that cyclosporine-treated children who have received bone marrow transplants have an increased risk of seizures associated with malignant hypertension.[8] No difference in the incidence of seizures was seen in the two groups in this study.

Cyclosporine-induced hypertension is seen in cardiac transplantation.[9] In this study, hypertension was more prevalent in the cyclosporine group than in the standard group. This may reflect either cyclosporine nephrotoxicity, an effect of the drug on blood vessels, or an effect on plasma renin[10] or prostacyclin.[11] Renal biopsy may show renal microthrombi and microangiopathy.[12,13]

Cyclosporine-induced hypertrichosis is extremely common, and is manifest by increased hair growth of the whole body, especially on the arms, face, and eyebrows. It occurs in both sexes and in children (Fig. 1). Hirsutism, which is increased hair growth in the male pattern of hair distribution does not occur. Onset is usually two weeks to two months after starting cyclosporine. The amount of hair growth varies, but is usually relatively mild and cosmetically acceptable. However, it

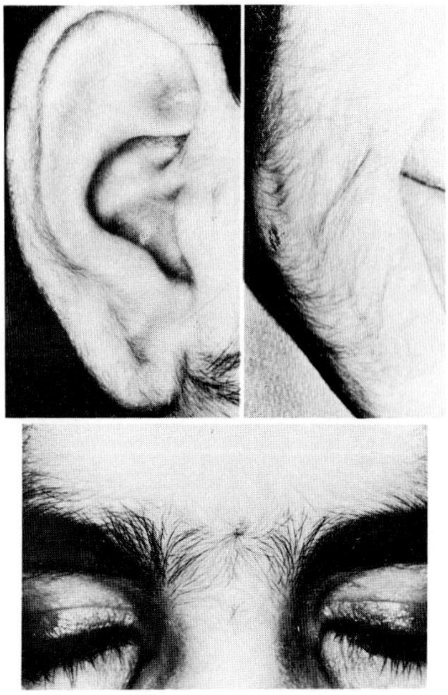

Fig. 1. Cyclosporine-induced hypertrichosis in a 10-year-old boy on cyclosporine alone after five months of therapy. Increased hair growth is seen on the arms, eyebrows, face, and ears.

may be severe enough to require discontinuation of the drug, after which it resolves in approximately two months. The severity of hypertrichosis is impossible to predict prior to therapy, although patients of Mediterranean extraction seem particularly susceptible. The cause is unknown and treatment to date has been symptomatic. Cyclosporine-induced gingival hyperplasia is clinically and pathologically similar to that seen with phenytoin[14] (Fig. 2). The time of onset and regression after discontinuation of cyclosporine is the same as with hirsutism. It appears to be more common and severe in children than adults. Factors that aggravate the hyperplasia are poor oral hygiene and dental braces. Treatment in most cases consists of good oral hygiene, but gingivectomy is occasionally required.

If further experience shows that less prednisone is required in cyclosporine-treated patients than in patients on azathioprine, this will be a major advance. Patients should be able to avoid the devastating steroid effects,

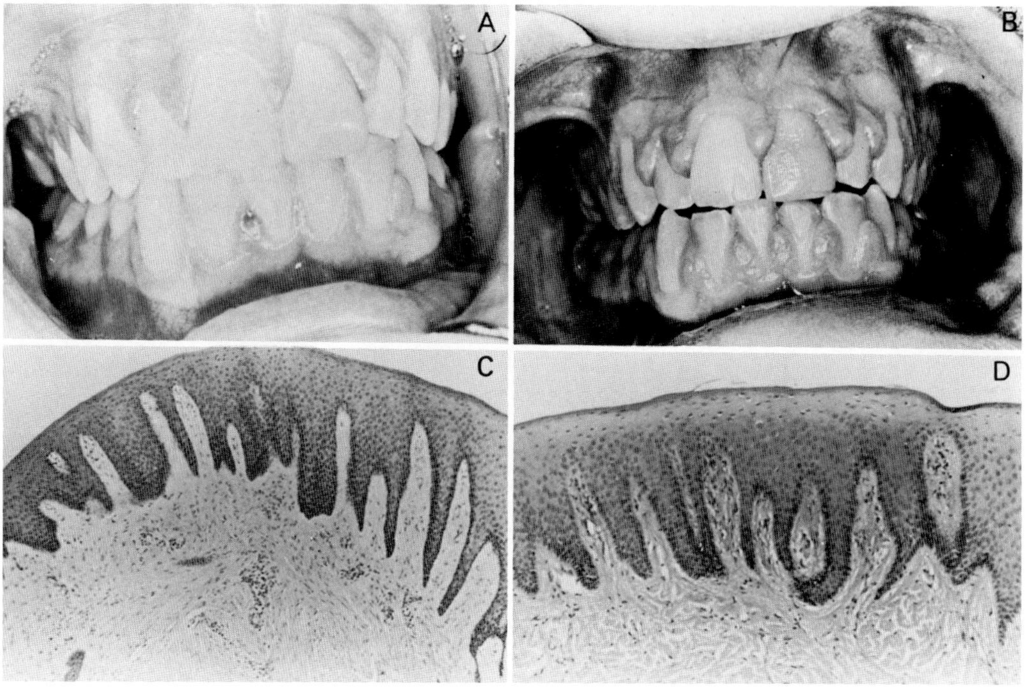

Fig. 2. Cyclosporine-induced gingival hyperplasia. A patient's gums prior to (A) and two months after cyclosporine therapy (B) demonstrate moderate gingival enlargement. Histologically, fibroplasia characterized by increased numbers of fibroblasts and an increase in the amount of collagen is seen (C). Normal gingiva is seen in D.

namely cataracts, hyperglycemia, and bone necrosis. The follow-up in this trial is too short to allow comment on the incidence of these complications.

Cyclosporine can increase bone alkaline phosphatase.[15] In this study, more patients on cyclosporine had hypercalcemia/hyperparathyroidism than patients on standard therapy. The mechanism and significance of this effect awaits further exploration.

One major advantage of cyclosporine over azathioprine is that it rarely causes severe leukopenia. The cause of the severe leukopenia in two patients on cyclosporine in this trial is unclear.

Cyclosporine is not teratogenetic in animals, even at extremely high doses.[16] It is too early to determine its effect on the human fetus, although some healthy infants have been born to mothers on cyclosporine.[17] Cyclosporine's effect on infant growth and development is not yet known, and careful documentation of growth is required in all children receiving cyclosporine.

ACKNOWLEDGMENT

We acknowledge the support of the Medical Research Council of Canada, Richard and Jean Ivey Fund, London, Ontario; Sandoz Ltd., Basel; the Michael Fung Endowment Fund, London, Ontario; the the University Hospital Transplant Research Fund, London, Ontario.

Centers involved in this study were Vancouver General Hospital (C. E. Reeve), University of Alberta Hospital, Edmonton (F. Harley), Calgary Foothills Hospital (J. Klassen), Health Sciences Centre, Winnipeg (J. Jeffery), Toronto General Hospital (P. Halloran), Toronto St. Michael's Hospital (R. Bear), St. Joseph's Hospital, Hamilton (D. Ludwin), Montreal General Hospital (M. Mangel), Notre Dame Hospital (P. Daloze), Maisonneuve-Rosemont Hospital (R. Dandavino), Victoria General Hospital, Halifax (P. Belitsky), and University Hospital, London (P. Keown).

Executive Committee: G. Arbus, R. Bear, R. Dandavino, J. B. Dossetor, J. Jeffery, A. S. MacDonald (Chairman), M. Robinette, C. R. Stiller.

Management Committee, Centre for Transplant Studies and Statistical Consultants: H. Cheung, M. Gent, M.

Grace, W. Howson, P. A. Keown, J. Koval, A. Laupacis, B. Lockwood, I. MacNeill, L. Moist, N. R. Sinclair, C. R. Stiller, G. Wells.

REFERENCES

1. Canadian Transplant Study Group: Transplant Proc (this issue)

2. Canadian Transplant Study Group: N Engl J Med (in press)

3. European Multicentre Trial: Lancet 2:57, 1982

4. Ferguson RM, Rynasiewicz J, Sutherland DER, et al: Surgery 92:175, 1982

5. Thiru S, et al: Transplant Proc 13:359, 1981

6. Rosenthal JT, Calne RY, Nagington J, et al: Transplant Proc (this issue)

7. Canadian Transplant Study Group: Transplant Proc (this issue)

8. Joss DV, et al: Lancet 1:906, 1982

9. Oyer P, et al: Transplant Proc (this issue)

10. Siegl H, et al: Transplant Proc (this issue)

11. Neild GH, et al: Transplant Proc (this issue)

12. Mihatsch MJ: Transplant Proc (this issue)

13. Shulman H, et al: N Engl J Med 305:1392, 1981

14. Wysocki GP, et al: Oral Surg 55:274, 1983

15. Rodger RSC, et al: Transplant Proc (this volume)

16. Sandoz, Ltd, Basel, Switzerland: Sandoz internal document

17. Lewis GJ: Br Med J 286:603, 1983

Cyclosporine and Liver Function in Renal Allograft Recipients

R. S. C. Rodger, J. H. Turney, I. Haines, J. Michael, D. Adu, and P. McMaster

THE usual pattern of liver function abnormalities associated with cyclosporine A (CsA) is hyperbilirubinemia, raised transaminase levels, and a normal or mildly elevated serum alkaline phosphatase.[1] It has been suggested that hyperbilirubinemia may lead to CsA accumulation because of competition for excretion via the biliary tract.[2] Hyperbilirubinemia has been reported in between 20% and 100% of renal allograft recipients receiving CsA and is thought to be dose dependent.[3–5] In studies where a lower dose of CsA has been used, the incidence of liver dysfunction is much reduced.[6,7] In this article we review the frequency and nature of liver function abnormalities in the first year after renal transplantation.

MATERIALS AND METHODS

Over an 18-month period, 66 recipients of a cadaveric renal allograft were entered in a comparative study. Patients were randomly allocated to an immunosuppressive regimen of prednisolone (20 mg per day) plus CsA or prednisolone (20 mg per day) plus azathioprine (2.5 mg/kg per day). Prior to transplantation, all patients had been transfused with at least two units of blood, and sera from all patients were negative for hepatitis-B surface antigen and antibody.

Prednisolone was discontinued in the CsA group at 14 days if there was no histologic evidence of rejection. CsA was given orally at an initial dose of 15 mg/kg per day, reducing to 12 mg/kg per day at one month. The mean dose at one year was 8.5 mg/kg per day. Hepatitis-A and -B serology and cytomegalovirus (CMV) and autoantibodies were measured in those patients with unexplained liver function abnormalities. Liver ultrasound and biopsy were performed in those patients with unexplained protracted liver dysfunction.

From the Renal and Transplantation Units, Queen Elizabeth Hospital, Edgbaston, Birmingham, U.K.

Address reprint requests to Dr. R. S. C. Rodger, Department of Medicine, The Royal Victoria Infirmary, Queen Victoria Road, Newcastle upon Tyne, U.K.

0041-1345/83/1505-0102$01.00/0

RESULTS

Thirty-five patients received prednisolone and CsA as initial immunosuppression and 31 patients received prednisolone and azathioprine. The two groups were comparable for age, sex, and primary renal disease, and actuarial graft survival at one year was 77% (CsA) and 72% (prednisolone and azathioprine). There were two deaths in each group. One patient receiving CsA died of myocardial infarction, one patient on conventional immunosuppression died of a cerebrovascular accident. The other two deaths, one from each group, were from infection.

Mean bilirubin levels were significantly higher in the CsA group in the first three months following transplantation, although hyperbilirubinemia was uncommon (Fig. 1). Aspartate aminotransferase levels were significantly higher in the CsA group in the first month only. This trend reversed, but did not reach statistical significance (Fig. 2). Alkaline phosphatase levels were significantly higher in the CsA group at all periods of comparison, with the mean levels always above the normal range (Fig. 3). However, in only one of 20 patients with an isolated elevation of alkaline phosphatase was this due to hepatic isoenzyme. In 16 patients, the increase was due predominantly to increase in the bone isoenzyme fraction. In three cases, the increase was transient and typing not performed.

Six patients (17%) in the CsA group and nine patients (29%) in the prednisolone and azathioprine group developed liver function abnormalities. In the CsA group, liver dysfunction was due to CMV infection in two cases, severe herpes simplex infection in another, and congestive cardiac failure in a fourth. The fifth case had an elevated alkaline phosphatase of hepatic origin, which rose further despite converting from CsA to conven-

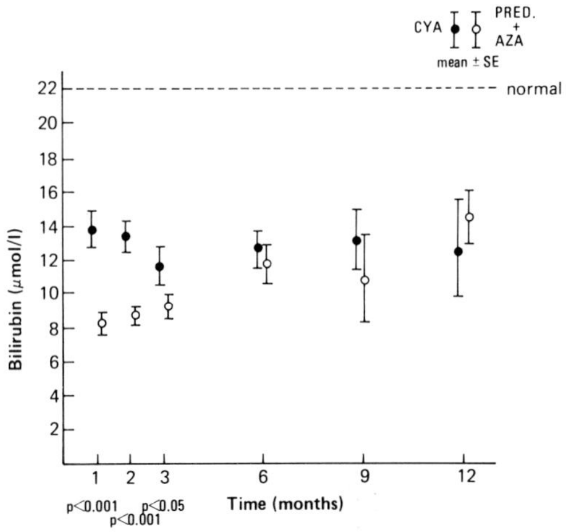

Fig. 1. Mean bilirubin levels following transplantation.

tional immunosuppression. Liver biopsy showed only minimal chronic focal inflammatory infiltrate around portal tracts. The patient also had inflammatory bowel disease, and his liver dysfunction was ultimately attributed to this. The sixth patient, who was also the oldest patient in the trial, had mild persistent hyperbilirubinemia and elevation of

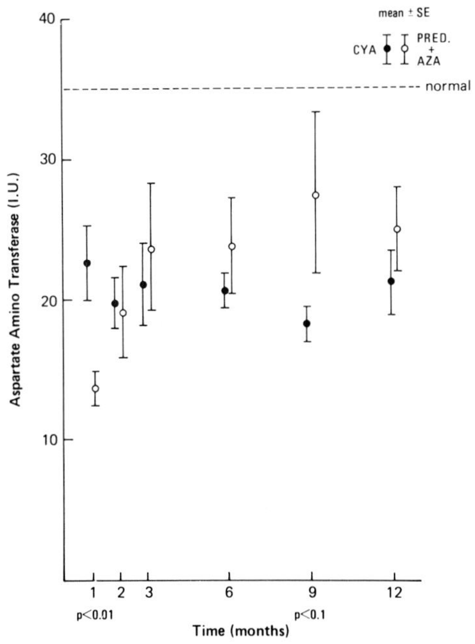

Fig. 2. Mean transaminase levels following transplantation.

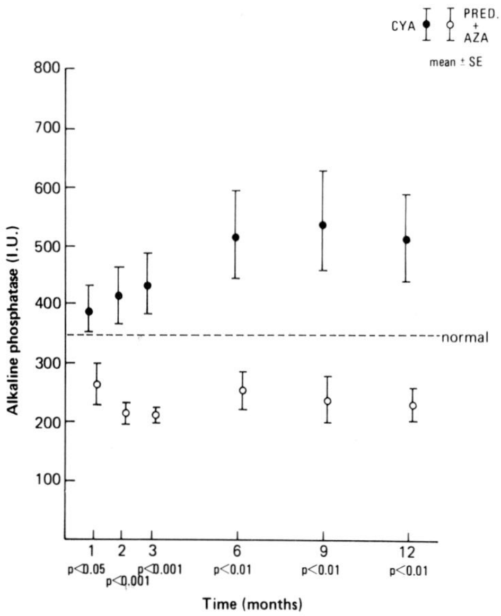

Fig. 3. Mean alkaline phosphatase levels following transplantation.

alkaline phosphatase. This was attributed to CsA, although it did not diminish on dose reduction.

In the prednisolone and azathioprine group, liver function abnormalities were due to septicemia in three cases, two of whom subsequently died, viral encephalitis in another, and hepatitis-B infection in a fifth. In four cases, liver dysfunction was unexplained, but possibly was due to azathioprine or, in two cases, isoniazid hepatotoxicity.

DISCUSSION

This study shows that at an initial dose of 15 mg/kg per day CsA provides adequate immunosuppression with no marked hepatotoxicity. Liver function abnormalities were, in fact, more common in patients receiving prednisolone and azathioprine, and CsA hepatotoxicity was seen in only one of 35 patients. In both groups, intercurrent infection was the most common cause of liver dysfunction. The fact that bilirubin levels, although in the normal range, were significantly higher in the CsA group, does, however, suggest subclinical liver dysfunction associated with the drug and is in keeping with the concept that it is dose dependent.

Loertsher[8] has also reported raised bone alkaline phosphatase levels with CsA in a third of renal allograft recipients. The long-term significance of this finding is not yet known, but alkaline phosphatase levels remained elevated a year after transplantation in some of our patients. It is an interesting speculation that some of the increase in alkaline phosphatase might occur from release from proximal tubular cells of the kidney, where the enzyme is also found, as we were unable to distinguish a renal isoenzyme from bone in our study. Although this isoenzyme is rarely found in the serum, it has been reported in cases of transplant rejection, renal failure, and acute pyelonephritis.[9-11]

ACKNOWLEDGMENT

We are grateful for the help of the Department of Clinical Chemistry, Queen Elizabeth Hospital, and the Departments of Virology and Immunology at the East Birmingham Hospital. We thank D. Cook for secretarial help.

REFERENCES

1. Klintmaln GBG, Iwatsuki S, Starzl TE, et al: Transplantation 32:488, 1981
2. Hows JM, Palmer S, Want S, et al: Lancet 2:147, 1981
3. Calne RY, White DJG, Thiru S: Lancet 2:1323, 1978
4. Starzl TE, Weil R, Iwatsuki S, et al: Surg Gynecol Obstet 151:4, 1980
5. European Multicentre Trial: Lancet 2:57, 1982
6. Ferguson RM, Rynasiewicy JJ, Sutherland DE: Surgery 92:175, 1982
7. Rodger RSC, Turney JH, Haines I, et al: Transplantation (in press)
8. Loertscher R, Mihatsch M, Harder F: Kidney Int 23:292, 1983
9. Latner AL: In Ruyssen R (ed): Enzymes in Clinical Chemistry. Amsterdam, Elsever, 1965, p 110
10. Kranc MC, Foreback CC, Curz C: Clin Chem 24:1012, 1978
11. Fontini S: Nephron 12:197, 1974

Cholestasis in Heart Transplant Recipients Treated With Cyclosporine

R. R. Schade, A. Guglielmi, D. H. Van Thiel, M. E. Thompson, V. Warty, B. Griffith, A. Sanghvi, H. Bahnson, and R. Hardesty

CYCLOSPORINE-A is being used increasingly for immunosuppression in patients undergoing organ transplantation. Hepatotoxicity has been noted to occur in up to 20% of renal transplant recipients receiving the drug.[1-4] The exact nature of this hepatotoxicity, however, has not been defined, although it has been manifested principally, if not exclusively, as elevated serum bilirubin levels. We have observed a similar elevation of serum bilirubin levels in cardiac transplant recipients receiving cyclosporine-A and prednisone for immunosuppression. We report a more detailed description of the hepatic dysfunction occurring in these patients receiving cyclosporine than has been reported previously.

MATERIALS AND METHODS

Patients. Patients who had undergone cardiac or heart-lung transplantation at Presbyterian-University Hospital between January 1981 and April 1983 were considered as candidates for inclusion into our study. In addition, to be studied, patients had to survive at least two weeks after surgery and they had to be receiving cyclosporine and prednisone for immunosuppression.

Data collection. Charts were reviewed retrospectively for determinations of the serum values of total and direct bilirubin, transaminases, and alkaline phosphatase, both before and after transplantation. The peak bilirubin posttransplantation was recorded, as well as the corresponding enzyme levels. In addition, cardiac catheterization data, which were available in some of these same patients, were reviewed. Finally, a prospective study of serum bilirubin and bile salt levels and blood cyclosporine levels was performed in a smaller group of patients.

Chemical determinations. Total and direct serum bilirubin levels were determined spectrophotometrically by the method of Jendrassik and Grof.[5] Serum enzyme activity was determined spectrophotometrically using standard techniques.[5] Serum cholylglycine and sulfolithocholylglycine levels were determined by radioimmunoassay (Abbott Laboratories, North Chicago, IL). Blood cyclosporine levels were measured using high-pressure liquid chromatography.[6]

Data analysis. Values are reported as a mean ± SEM. Statistical comparisons were made using the Student's t test for unpaired data and a single-tail design.

RESULTS

Thirty transplant recipients had records suitable for review. The mean age of these 30 patients was 40.9 ± 1.8 years, and there were 26 males and four females.

As shown in Fig. 1, there was no significant increase in transaminase levels or biliary canalicular (alkaline phosphatase) enzyme levels after cardiac transplantation. However, the more hepato-specific of the two transaminase enzymes, serum glutamic pyruvic transaminase (SGPT), was arithmetically increased after successful transplantation.

In contrast, serum bilirubin values reached a peak elevation 2.5 times the upper limits of normal about two weeks (16.6 ± 2.1 days) posttransplantation and were markedly increased compared to the values observed pretransplantation (Fig. 2). Moreover, the serum bilirubin level remained elevated (2.2 ± 0.4 mg/dl, $n = 22, p < 0.05$ compared to pretransplant) when the patient was discharged from the hospital. In no patient was the increase in total bilirubin due to an increase in the indirect reacting bilirubin fraction. Significant increases in bilirubin levels in heart transplant patients were seen in both the total and direct reacting bilirubin, but not for the indirect fraction.

From the University of Pittsburgh, School of Medicine, Departments of Medicine, Surgery, and Pathology, Pittsburgh, PA.

Supported in part by a grant from the Gastrointestinal Medicine Research Foundation of Southwestern Pennsylvania.

Address reprint requests to Dr. R. R. Schade, 1000J Scaife Hall, University of Pittsburgh, Pittsburgh, PA 15261.

0041-1345/83/1505-0103$01.00/0

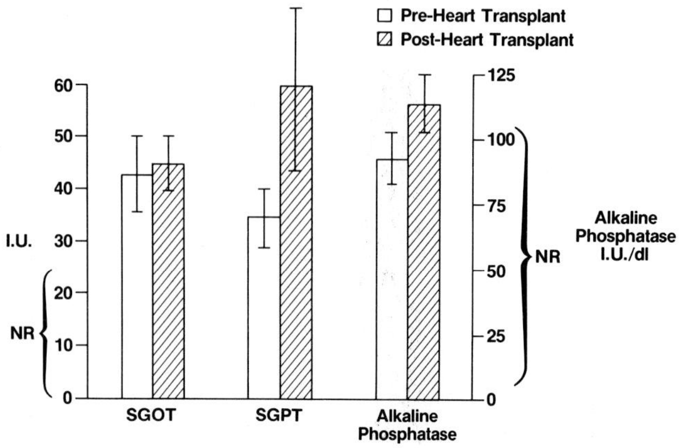

Fig. 1. Liver enzyme activity in the serum of patients before and after cardiac transplantation. There was no statistical difference between the groups, although SGPT values did increase arithmetically. NR, normal range.

Cardiac catheterization data were available in 11 patients. The mean pulmonary artery wedge pressure was 13.1 ± 1.2 mm Hg in these patients and the mean right atrial pressure was 6.9 ± 1.3 mm Hg. Despite these normal values, the mean serum bilirubin obtained at the same time as the catheterization study was elevated at 2.0 ± 0.4 mg/dl. In contrast to the increase in bilirubin, serum enzyme values were unremarkable (Table 1) at the time of catheterization.

Finally, total and direct bilirubin, serum bile salt levels, and blood cyclosporine levels were determined prospectively in 11 patients.

The mean blood cyclosporine-A level, based on 22 determinations in these 11 patients, was 474.0 ± 46.7 ng/ml. No correlation could be found between the blood cyclosporine levels and the serum bilirubin or bile salt levels obtained in these prospectively studied patients.

In normal subjects, fasting serum bile salt levels are quite low, usually less than 0.3 μM/liter. In contrast (Fig. 3), both cholylglycine and sulfolithocholylglycine levels were markedly elevated in the transplant patients studied, suggesting that pronounced cholestasis was present and was out of proportion to any abnormality present in serum hepatocellular and canalicular enzyme levels.

DISCUSSION

Cyclosporine is being used increasingly for immunosuppression in patients undergoing organ transplantation.[3,4,7,8] This drug is known to be fat soluble and to be well absorbed orally. It is also known to accumulate within the liver and to undergo biliary recirculation.[9] Several investigators have observed a "hepatotoxic" effect of the drug, which has been reported to occur in as many as 20% of renal transplant recipients.[1–4] Although elevated bilirubin levels were noted by these investigators, no descriptions of the hepatic enzyme changes present in their patients, and possibly indicative of hepatocellular injury, have been provided. In addition, in no instance was the patient's pretransplant hepatic function evaluated. Relevant to this latter issue is the fact that it is well known that renal failure patients

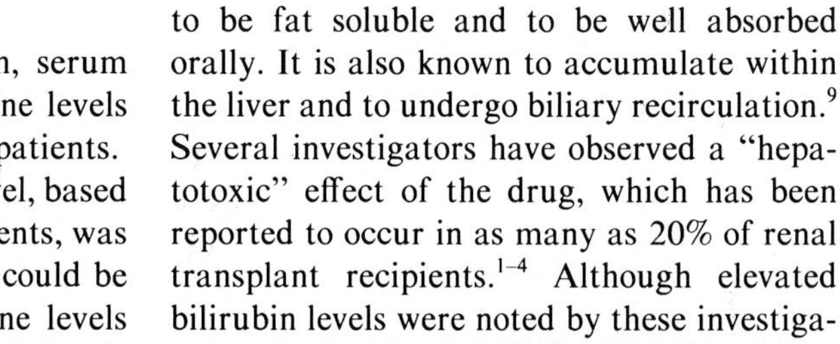

Fig. 2. Serum total bilirubin levels before heart transplantation, at their peak level following transplantation, and their level at the time of discharge from the hospital. Bilirubin levels are significantly elevated after transplantation.

Table 1. Cardiac Catheterization

	Heart Transplant	Normal Controls
RA_m	6.9 ± 1.2 mm Hg	2–8 mm Hg
PAo	13.1 ± 1.2 mm Hg	2–12 mm Hg
CO	4.9 ± 0.3 liter/min	4.4–7.2 liter/min
Bilirubin	2.0 ± 0.4 mg/dl	0.3–1.2 mg/dl
SGOT	34.8 ± 3.9 IU	<34 IU
Alkaline phosphatase	93.8 ± 17.0 IU/liter	<100 IU/liter

frequently have preexistent liver injury. Problems related to hemodialysis and transfusion, such as hepatitis-B and non-A non-B viral infections, or iron overload, frequently introduce confounding variables in the assessment of liver function in such patients. Moreover, fatty liver and hepatic necrosis are reported phenomena in diabetic patients, many of whom are included in the renal transplant recipient groups studied to date.[10]

We have noted elevations of serum bilirubin levels in patients undergoing cardiac transplants who were receiving cyclosporine-A. The bilirubin levels appeared to peak relatively early after transplantation and to remain elevated for a prolonged time. The increase in bilirubin is predominantly in the direct reacting fraction; consequently, it is not likely to be due to hemolysis or congestive heart failure. In addition, bilirubin levels were increased despite normal pulmonary artery wedge and right atrial pressures and while cardiac output was normal, thereby effectively ruling out congestive heart failure as an etiologic factor (Table 1).

Markers of liver injury (serum glutamic oxaloacetic transaminase [SGOT] and SGPT) were noted to be minimally elevated prior to transplantation. In contrast, bilirubin and alkaline phosphatase levels were consistently within the normal range pretransplant (Fig. 1). Curiously, although serum bilirubin levels were abnormal in 86% of our heart recipients, alterations in SGOT levels were not found when compared to the pretransplant values (Fig. 1). In contrast, the SGPT levels, which were increased minimally before transplant, increased further after successful transplantation, albeit not statistically. More importantly, the biliary canalicular enzyme alkaline phosphatase, which would be expected to increase during cholestasis, remained normal in the patients we studied.

Despite the absence of significant increases in enzyme levels, there was profound cholestatis. Not only were total and direct bilirubin levels increased, but so were the cholylglycine and sulfolithocholylglycine levels. This latter finding clearly indicates that a more general defect has occurred within the hepatocytes of the patients we studied and that the changes observed are not confined solely to bilirubin excretion.

The precise nature of the hepatic injury, however, remains elusive. Unfortunately, we do not have a sufficient number of cardiac transplant patients in whom azathioprine and prednisone were used instead of cyclosporine for immunosuppression to permit comparison with the cyclosporine-treated group. Regardless of the mechanisms responsible, clearly, cholestasis has developed in the patients we

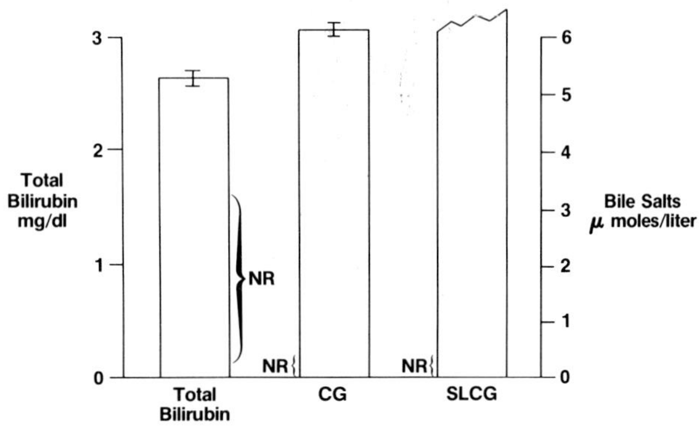

Fig. 3. Fasting serum bile salt levels in 11 heart transplantation recipients. Normal levels are low, <0.3 μM/liter. In these patients, they were strikingly elevated, indicating significant cholestasis. CG, serum cholylglycine; SLOG, serum sulfolithocholylglycine; NR, normal range.

have studied. While we may conjecture that a lipid-soluble drug that undergoes enterohepatic circulation might alter biliary canalicular function, we have no specific evidence other than cholestasis to support this contention. To define the nature of the injury, additional tests, including liver biopsy, would be required. In order to implicate cyclosporine-A as the agent responsible for its production, controlled animal investigations are needed. It is also apparent that if one hopes to monitor hepatocellular injury in transplant patients receiving cyclosporine, it would be wise to monitor the more specific SGPT and bile salt levels, than to simply follow SGOT and/or bilirubin levels.

REFERENCES

1. Goran B, Klintmalm G, Iwatsuki S, et al: Transplantation 32:488, 1981

2. Calne RY, White PJ, Thiru S, et al: Lancet 2:1323, 1978

3. Harder F, Calne RY, Pichlmayr R, et al: Lancet 2:57, 1982

4. Najarian JS, Ferguson RM, Sutherland DER, et al: Transplant Proc 15:438, 1983

5. Henry RJ, Cannon PC, Winkelman JW (eds): Clinical Chemistry: Principles and Technics. Hagerstown, MD, Harper and Row, 1974

6. Sawchuk RI, Cartier LL: Clin Chem 27:1368, 1981

7. Hakala TR, Starzl TE, Rosenthal JT: Transplant Proc 15:465, 1983

8. Starzl TE, Iwatsuki S, Van Thiel DH, et al: Hepatology 2:614, 1982

9. Kahan BD, Ried M, Newburger J: Transplant Proc 15:446, 1983

10. Cello JP, Sleisenger MH: In Zakim D, Boyer TD (eds) Hepatology—A Textbook of Liver Disease. Philadelphia, W. B. Saunders, 1982, p 1221

11. Falchuk KR, Fiske SC, Haggitt RL, et al: Gastroenterology 78:535, 1980

Cyclosporine-Associated Hepatotoxicity After Allogeneic Marrow Transplantation in Man: Differentiation From Other Causes of Posttransplant Liver Disease

K. Atkinson, J. Biggs, A. Dodds, and A. Concannon

CYCLOSPORINE (CsA) is proving to be a useful drug in bone marrow transplantation.[1,2] Although effective as an immunosuppressant in minimizing severe graft-versus-host disease[1] and associated with rapid engraftment of donor marrow,[3] it has a number of side effects. The most significant of these is nephrotoxicity,[4-6] but hepatotoxicity has also been described.[7-9] In this study, we report on the clinical features of CsA-associated hepatotoxicity after marrow transplantation and its differentiation from other causes of posttransplant liver disease.

MATERIALS AND METHODS

Twenty-one consecutive evaluable recipients of allogeneic marrow transplants immunosuppressed with CsA at St. Vincent's Hospital, Sydney, Australia, were studied. Four received histocompatibility leuckocyte antigen (HLA)–identical sibling transplants for severe aplastic anemia, 13 received HLA-identical sibling transplants for hematologic malignancy, and four received HLA-nonidentical family member transplants for acute leukemia. The conditioning regimens for marrow transplantation have been previously described.[3] The day of transplantation was designated day 0. CsA was administered at a dose of 25 mg/kg per day orally in two 12-hr divided doses, beginning on day −1 pretransplant (eight patients) or on day −7 (13 patients). The dose was reduced to 12.5 mg/kg per day on day +4 and was subsequently tapered by 5% per week starting at day +49; CsA was discontinued at 100 or 180 days posttransplant. Recipients of HLA genotypically nonidentical family member grafts received methotrexate (MTX) 15 mg/sq m intravenously on day +1 and 10 mg/sq m on day +6 in addition to CsA.

CsA serum concentration was measured by radioimmunoassay.[10] Hyperbilirubinemia was defined as a serum bilirubin concentration of greater than 20 μmol/liter on four or more consecutive days (normal range, 3–18 μmol/liter). A diagnosis of CsA-associated hepatotoxicity was made when a patient had hyperbilirubinemia associated with an increasing CsA trough serum concentration that was not explained by any other cause and that resolved on lowering or stopping the dose of CsA. A diagnosis of acute hepatic graft-versus-host disease (GVHD) was made when hyperbilirubinemia was not associated with an increasing CsA trough serum concentration, but was associated with acute GVHD of the skin or intestine, or a threefold or greater elevation of serum alkaline phosphatase (SAP) concentration,[18] or histologic documentation of hepatic GVHD.[11] A diagnosis of hyperbilirubinemia due to hemolysis was made when hyperbilirubinemia was not associated with an increasing CsA trough serum concentration, but was related to blood product transfusion and accompanied by a positive direct Coombs' test or other evidence of hemolysis (methemalbuminemia, hemoglobinuria, or a decreased serum haptoglobin value). Hepatotoxicity due to infection was diagnosed when hyperbilirubinemia was not related to a rising CsA trough serum concentration but occurred in association with overwhelming systemic infection. Hepatotoxicity due to multiple causes (conditioning regimen, bacterial sepsis, blood product transfusion) was diagnosed when hyperbilirubinemia was not associated with an increasing CsA trough serum level but occurred during or shortly after the period of conditioning and marrow infusion and was not clearly ascribable to a single etiologic factor. The criteria for the clinical and histologic diagnosis of GVHD have been previously described.[12,13] All of the patients in this study were treated on protocols approved by the Ethics and Review Committee of St. Vincent's Hospital, Sydney.

RESULTS

Of the 21 patients, 18 (86%) had one or more episodes of hyperbilirubinemia (Table 1). The 18 patients had a total of 28 episodes of hyperbilirubinemia, 10 patients having two separate episodes. Twenty-nine separate causes were identified for the 28 episodes, since two clearly distinct contributing factors were associated with one episode. CsA was the

---

From the Department of Haematology, St. Vincent's Hospital, Sydney, NSW, Australia.

Supported in part by grants from the New South Wales State Cancer Council and the National Health and Medical Research Council of Australia.

Address reprint requests to Dr. K. Atkinson, Department of Haematology, St. Vincent's Hospital, Sydney, NSW 2010, Australia.

0041-1345/83/1505-0104$01.00/0

Table 1. Patient Details

Patient No.	Age (years)	Sex	Diagnosis	Time of Episode of Hyperbilirubinemia (Days Posttransplant)	Cause of Hyperbilirubinemia
35	21	F	CML	9–129	CsA
37	16	F	AA	(i) −2– +5	Hemolysis
				(ii) 6–146	CsA
38	24	F	ALL	62–158	CsA
43	23	F	AA	4–48	CsA
55	22	F	ALL	7–116	CsA
56	52	M	ALL	(i) 5–55	CsA
				(ii) 56–95	Acute GVHD of liver
46	50	M	CML	(i) 5–15	CsA
				(ii) 16–119	Acute GBHD of liver
48	26	F	AML	(i) 4–11	Multiple factors
				(ii) 35–55	CsA
44	21	M	ALL	(i) 4–11	Multiple factors
				(ii) 21–39	CsA
52	22	F	AML	(i) 0–8	Multiple factors
				(ii) 21–59	CsA
47	16	F	ALL	10–45	Acute GVHD of liver
40	34	M	AML	(i) 1–3	Hemolysis
				(ii) 4–20	Acute GVHD of liver
49	18	M	ALL	20–35	Acute GVHD of liver
57	12	M	ALL	(i) 6–13	Multiple factors
				(ii) 32–80	Acute GVHD of liver
45	47	M	CML	46–61	Overwhelming infection
51	20	M	ALL	(i) 7–13	Hemolysis
				(ii) 28–40	Overwhelming infection
59	17	F	AA	(i) 0–12	Multiple factors
				(ii) 13–26	Overwhelming infection
60	25	M	AA	0–4	Multiple factors

GVHD, graft-versus-host disease; CML, chronic myelogenous leukemia; AML, acute myelogenous leukemia, ALL, acute lymphoblastic leukemia; and AA, aplastic anemia.

most frequent cause of hyperbilirubinemia, being responsible for 34% of such episodes.

CsA-Associated Hepatotoxicity

This occurred in 10 of 21 patients (Table 2). The mean (± 1 SD) peak serum bilirubin value in patients with CsA-associated hepatotoxicity was 222 ± 256 (range, 33–707) μmol/liter and was comparable to the hyperbilirubinemia of patients with acute GVHD of the liver or overwhelming infection (Table 3). It was higher than the hyperbilirubinemia due to hemolysis or multiple factors and was predominantly of the conjugated type. CsA-associated hepatotoxicity was characterized by a moderate increase in serum alanine transaminase (ALT) concentration (mean ± 1 SD, 109 ± 47 IU/liter), but with only a minimal elevation of SAP concentration (mean ± 1 SD, 124 ± 38 IU/liter). While patients with acute hepatic GVHD also demonstrated a moderate elevation of serum ALT concentration, they tended to have higher elevations of SAP than those with CsA-associated hepatotoxicity ($p < 0.01$). Patients with overwhelming infection had moderate elevation of both enzymes, while those with

Table 2. Causes of Hyperbilirubinemia After Allogeneic Marrow Transplantation*

Cause	Frequency as a Cause of Hyperbilirubinemia (%)	Incidence in Patients (%)
CsA	34	48
Acute GVHD of liver	21	29
Multiple factors	21	29
Hemolysis	14	19
Sepsis	10	14

*Hyperbilirubinemia due to venoocclusive disease of the liver,[18] viral hepatitis, or hepatotoxic drugs was not recognized in this series.

Table 3. Biochemical Features, Day of Onset, and Duration of Posttransplant Hepatotoxicity*

Cause of Hepatotoxicity or Hyperbilirubinemia (No. Patients)	Peak Total Serum Bilirubin Concentration† (μmol/liter) (Range)	Peak Serum Alanine Transaminase Concentration (U/Liter) (Range)	Peak Serum Alkaline Phosphatase Concentration (U/Liter) (Range)	Day of Onset Posttransplant (Range)	Duration in Days (Range)
CsA	222 ± 256	109 ± 47	124 ± 38	18.5 ± 18	72 ± 47.5
(n = 10)	(33–707)	(67–220)	(68–183)	(4–62)	(18–140)
Acute GVHD of liver	225 ± 238	220 ± 234	352 ± 222	23 ± 19	43 ± 32
(n = 6)	(40–685)	(30–660)	(92–648)	(4–56)	(15–103)
Overwhelming infection	313 ± 250	116 ± 35	217 ± 107	29 ± 17	13 ± 2
(n = 3)	(128–597)	(95–157)	(95–292)	(13–46)	(13–15)
Hemolysis	88 ± 67	68 ± 64	65 ± 14	1 ± 5	6 ± 1
(n = 4)	(37–164)	(14–139)	(50–77)	(−2–7)	(4–7)
Multiple factors	52 ± 22	186 ± 159	174 ± 158	2 ± 3	7 ± 3
(n = 6)	(29–91)	(17–440)	(55–448)	(0–6)	(4–12)

*Values represent mean ± 1SD.
†Normal range 3–18 μmol/liter.
‡Normal range 3–26 U/liter.
§Normal range 30–100 U/liter.

hyperbilirubinemia due to hemolysis had, as expected, only slight elevation of ALT values and normal values for SAP. Patients with CsA hepatotoxity or acute hepatic GVHD had a relatively lengthy hepatic illness compared to patients in the other categories (Table 3).

The weak relationship between CsA trough serum concentration and serum bilirubin concentration (correlation coefficient 0.36) is shown in Fig. 1. The relationship between serum bilirubin concentration, CsA trough serum concentration, and CsA dose before, during, and after CsA-associated hepatotoxicity is shown in Table 4.

CsA-associated hepatotoxicity occurred in one of two distinct clinical patterns. Five patients (unique patient numbers 35, 37, 43, 46, and 56) had an early, marked, and rapid increase in CsA trough serum concentration, immediately followed by an equally rapid increase in serum bilirubin concentraton (mean ± 1 SD of peak total bilirubin, 374 ± 295 μmol/liter) and serum creatinine, with acute renal failure occurring in three of the patients.[4] An example is shown in Fig. 2; all five patients at this time were clinically septic, with an infection of the Hickman right atrial catheter[14] being responsible in four. With temporary cessation or lowering of the CsA dosage, control of the sepsis, and treatment of the renal failure, the serum concentration of CsA, bilirubin, and creatinine rapidly decreased. In contrast, the other five patients with CsA-associated hepatotoxicity showed a more gradual increase in serum bilirubin concentration, temporally related to a gradual rise in CsA trough serum concentration. Their mean ± 1 SD peak total bilirubin serum concentration was 60 ± 45 μmol/liter. This hepatotoxicity was not associated with clinical symptoms.

Acute GVHD of the Liver

This occurred in six of 21 patients and was not associated with an increasing CsA trough serum concentration. Indeed, in two of the three patients with concurrent acute GVHD of the intestine, CsA trough serum concentrations were persistently low. All six patients had concurrent acute GVHD of the skin, which was severe and long-lasting in five. Three had an elevation of SAP values four or more times above the upper limit of the normal range, while the three others had acute hepatic GVHD documented histologically at autopsy.

Hepatotoxicity Associated With Overwhelming Infection

This occurred in three patients with overwhelming systemic infection. One patient had gram-negative sepsis with multiple organisms,

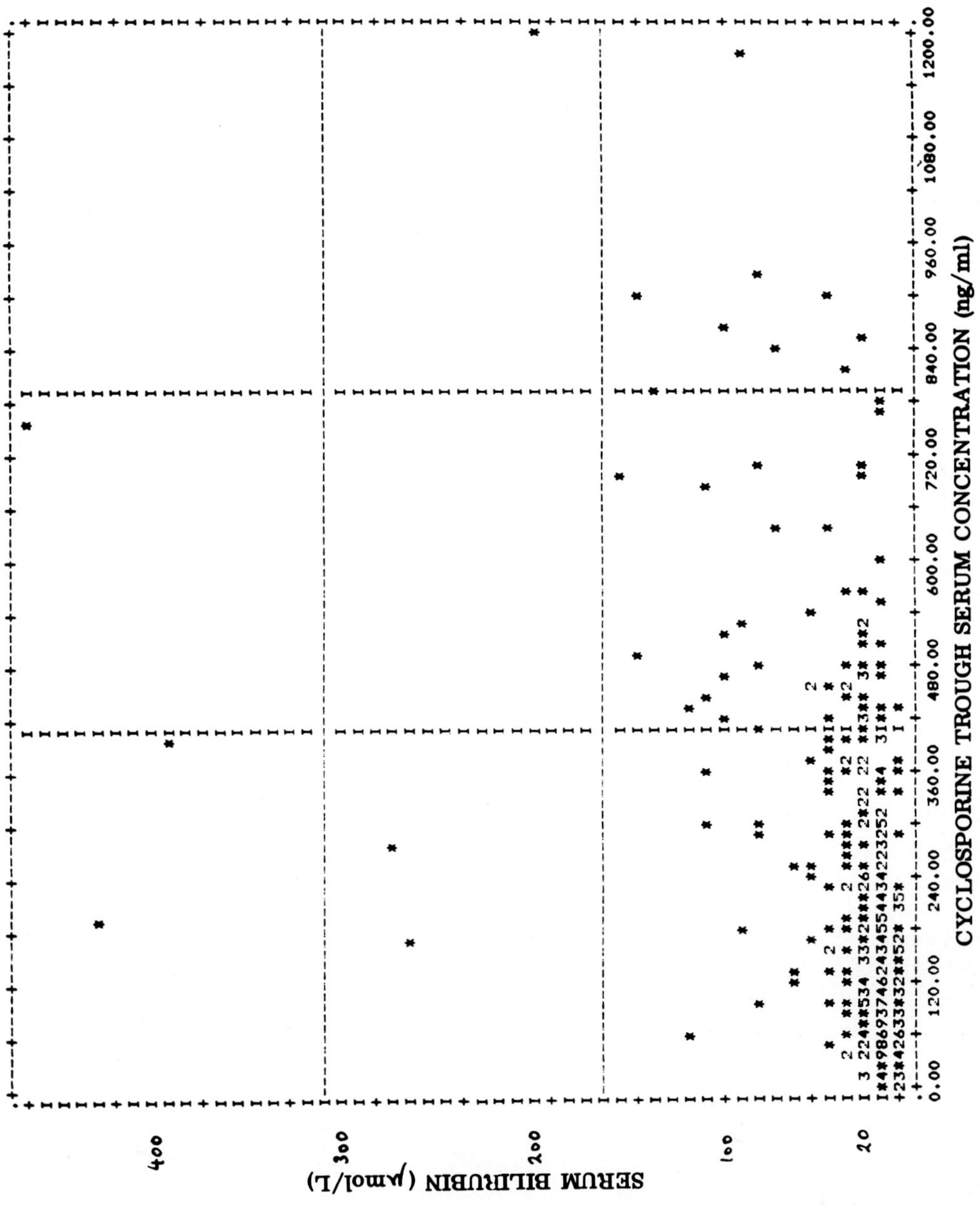

Fig. 1. Scattergram of serum bilirubin concentration and CsA trough serum concentration measured on the same blood sample in patients with CsA-associated hepatotoxicity. Numerals indicate number of samples at a particular point; 349 samples, correlation coefficient 0.36.

Table 4. Serum Bilirubin Level, CsA Dose, and CsA Trough Serum Concentration in Relationship to Episode of CsA-Associated Hepatotoxicity*

	Before	During	After
Serum bilirubin† (μmol/liter)	18 ± 7	61 ± 68‡	13 ± 5
CsA trough serum concentration (ng/ml)	248 ± 187	353 ± 252‡	140 ± 137
Daily CsA dose (mg/kg)	19.5 ± 4.0	9.8 ± 4.8	6.7 ± 3.5

*Values represent mean ± 1 SD.

†Normal range 3–18 μmol/liter.

‡Significantly different from respective "before" and "after" values, $p < 0.05–0.001$.

one had combined gram-negative and fungal sepsis, and one had disseminated cytomegalovirus infection. All three patients died from their infections. The hepatotoxicity was not associated with an increase in CsA trough serum concentration.

Hyperbilirubinemia Due to Hemolysis

This occurred in four patients, two of whom had "minor" ABO antigen differences with their donors (patient AB, donor A; patient B, donor O; respectively), and two of whom had "major" differences (patient O in each case, donor A in each case). Hyperbilirubinemia occurred much earlier than that associated with CsA or acute hepatic GVHD, with a mean onset at one day posttransplant, and had a mean duration of six days. It was related to the infusion of incompatible red cells and plasma in the marrow and subsequent platelet concentrates.

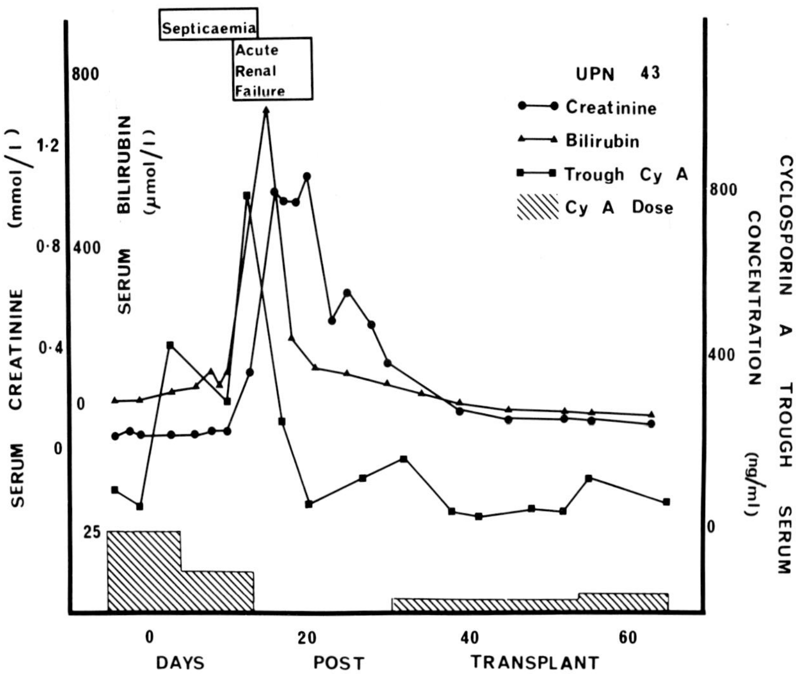

Fig. 2. Early onset type of CsA hepatotoxicity. Note rapid rise in CsA trough serum concentration, followed immediately by equally rapid rise in serum bilirubin and serum creatinine values. The clinical picture is characterized by sepsis and acute renal failure.

Hepatotoxicity Due to Multiple Causes

Six patients also demonstrated hyperbilirubinemia of early onset and short duration posttransplant unassociated with increasing CsA trough serum concentration. Moderate elevation of both serum ALT and SAP values occurred. It was felt likely that the conditioning regimen of cyclophosphamide or cyclophosphamide and total body irradiation was at least partly responsible. Additionally, all six patients had transient documented or presumed systemic bacterial infection at the time, and one of the five had a "minor" ABO difference with his donor (patient A, donor O).

DISCUSSION

Hepatotoxicity associated with CsA was common. It was characterized by conjugated hyperbilirubinemia, a moderate elevation of serum ALT concentration, and a minimal elevation of serum alkaline phosphatase concentration. Two distinct clinical patterns of CsA-associated hepatotoxicity were seen, one associated with a rapid and marked increase in CsA trough serum concentration concurrent with sepsis and renal impairment,[4] and one associated with a much more gradual and asymptomatic increase in CsA trough serum concentration. The temporal relationship between increasing CsA trough serum concentration and increasing serum bilirubin associated with both patterns of hepatotoxicity makes a causal relationship likely, as does the relationship of the dose of CsA to the onset of hyperbilirubinemia. Since CsA is predominantly excreted in the bile,[15] it is possible that the hepatotoxicity itself, as well as the sepsis and renal failure associated with the first pattern of CsA hepatotoxicity, contributed to the peak bilirubin value obtained.

As in a series of patients receiving CsA after renal transplantation,[7] CsA-associated hepatotoxicity was completely reversible upon lowering the dose of, or stopping, CsA, and in this regard, resembled the common type of CsA-associated nephrotoxicity.[4]

The first pattern of CsA-associated hepatotoxicity was easily distinguished from acute hepatic GVHD by its early onset posttransplant, the rate of climb of the serum bilirubin and CsA trough serum concentration, and the characteristic association with sepsis and renal impairment. The second pattern was distinguishable from acute hepatic GVHD by its asymptomatic nature. Both patterns were distinguishable from hepatic GVHD by absence of acute intestinal GVHD or severe acute skin GVHD, by only minimal elevation of SAP value, and by the reversibility of the hyperbilirubinemia upon lowering or stopping the dose of CsA. Although percutaneous liver biopsies were not performed in these patients, CsA does not appear to produce any consistent characteristic histologic abnormalities in the liver in humans[16] or animals,[17] with the exception of centrilobular fatty change. In contrast, bile duct atypia or proliferation appear to be characteristic histologic abnormalities of hepatic GVHD,[11,13] although sampling difficulties may occur.[16] Venoocclusive disease of the liver after marrow transplantation, although not seen in this series, is usually recognizable by an associated weight gain and ascites.[18] CsA-associated hepatotoxicity thus appears to be relatively easily distinguished from other causes of posttransplant liver disease.

ACKNOWLEDGMENT

We thank Dr. P. Isaac and Dr. R. Mrongovius of Sandoz Australia Pty. Ltd., for their help and support, and the staff of the Audio-Visual Services Department of St. Vincent's Hospital for preparation of the figures.

REFERENCES

1. Powles RL, Clink HM, Spence D, et al: Lancet 1:327, 1980

2. Hows J, Palmer S, Gordon-Smith EC: Transplantation 33:382, 1982

3. Atkinson K, Biggs JC, Ting A, et al: Br J Haematol 53:83, 1983

4. Atkinson K, Biggs JC, Hayes J, et al: Br J Haematol 54:59, 1983

5. Gluckman E, Devergie A, Lokiec F, et al: Lancet 2:144, 1981

6. Gratwohl A, Müller M, Osterwalder B, et al: Lancet 2:635, 1981

7. Klintmalm GB, Iwatsuki S, Starzl T: Transplantation 32:488, 1981

8. Laupacis, Keown PA, Ulan RA, et al: Lancet 2:1426, 1981

9. Loertscher R, Wenk M, Harder F, et al: Lancet 2:635, 1981

10. Donatsch P, Abisch E, Homberger M, et al: J Immunoassay 2:19, 1981

11. Sale GE, Storb R, Kolb H: Transplantation 26:103, 1978

12. Glucksberg H, Storb R, Fefer A, et al: Transplantation 18:295, 1974

13. Lerner K, Kao G, Storb R, et al: Transplant Proc 6:367, 1974

14. Thomas M: Br J Surg 66:673, 1979

15. Wagner O, Rietsch D: Sandoz Document 303–015, 1981

16. Sloane JP, Farthing MJG, Powles RL: J Clin Pathol 33:344, 1980

17. Farthing MJG, Clark M, Pendry A, et al: Biochem Pharmacol 30:3311, 1981

18. Shulman HM, McDonald GB, Matthews D, et al: Gastroenterology 79:1178, 1980

Infections in Kidney, Heart, and Liver Transplant Recipients on Cyclosporine

M. Ho, C. P. Wajszczuk, A. Hardy, J. S. Dummer, T. E. Starzl, T. R. Hakala, and H. T. Bahnson

OUR study involves 216 patients transplanted at the University of Pittsburgh from 1978 to 1983 (Table 1). This includes 64 kidney patients on cyclosporine (CsA), of which 21 were in a randomized trial of CsA, with 17 patients on azathioprine (AZA).[1] Since the latter was a small number, 59 renal patients on AZA from 1978 to 1980 are included for comparison. Except for the immunosuppressive drugs, all renal transplant recipients received comparable management largely from the same surgical team. In addition, from 1981 to 1983, we followed 33 heart and 43 liver transplant recipients who were all on CsA. This drug was first introduced in Pittsburgh in March 1981. A preliminary report of infections in these groups has been published.[2] This article provided additional patients, data, and follow-up material.

MATERIALS AND METHODS

All renal groups were followed for at least 6 months. Heart and liver patients were followed for a minimum of 3 months. The mean duration of follow-up for the latter 2 groups were 277 and 221 days, with a range of 90–400 and 90–594 days. Most patients received intravenous methylprednisolone 1 day prior to surgery. CsA was given according to Starzl et al.[3] On the day of surgery, 17.5 mg/kg/day was given orally, and attempts were made to reduce the dose to 3–10 mg/kg/day. Patients on AZA were begun on 5 mg/kg/day, with maintenance of 2.5 mg/kg/day. All patients on CsA and AZA also received prednisone. Patients on CsA received somewhat less cumulative prednisone than those on AZA.[4] The 3 types of transplant patients on CsA were on similar regimens, except 6 of 33 cardiac recipients also received antithymocyte globulin for rejection. They were not significantly different in terms of episodes of infection.

Infections are defined as clinically significant disease based on clinical and laboratory diagnosis, except in the case of virus infections, where the distinction between infection and symptomatic infection or disease is made.

Throat washings, urine samples, and blood buffy coats were obtained routinely for cytomegalovirus (CMV) and herpes simplex virus (HSV) cultures weekly for the first 8 postoperative weeks, biweekly during the third month, and monthly thereafter. Serum samples were obtained, when possible, from recipients and donors prior to transplantation and from recipients at monthly intervals after transplantation. CMV and Epstein-Barr virus (EBV) serology were performed as previously described.[2]

RESULTS

Table 2 is a summary of infections in all the 1981–1983 groups. Consider first the renal groups. The percent of patients who had at least one infection, as well as mean episodes of infection per patient, was significantly higher in the randomized azathioprine group (88% and 2.18) than in the CsA group (61% and 0.98). None of the infections in the renal groups was associated with deaths, of which there was only one.

The cardiac and liver transplant groups on CsA had more infection than the renal group on CsA immunosuppression. The sites of infections in the kidney, heart, and liver groups varied (Table 3). Most frequent infections for the 3 groups, respectively, were urinary tract, pulmonary and intrathoracic, and abdominal and gastrointestinal infections. Kidney recipients had the lowest frequency of bacteremias. Only the liver group had fungemia. Perhaps more important is the fact that mortality associated with severe infections was significant in the heart and liver groups. Many of the liver group died acutely with many infections. This is reflected in the fact that 50% of all episodes of infection was acquired 1 month after liver transplantation. To reach the same proportion, cardiac patients took 3 months.

From the Department of Infectious Diseases and Microbiology, Graduate School of Public Health and the Department of Medicine and Surgery, School of Medicine, University of Pittsburgh, Pittsburgh, PA.

Supported in part by NIH Grant 1-RO1-AI-19377.

Address reprint requests to Dr. Ho, Crabtree A-427, University of Pittsburgh, Pittsburgh, PA 15261.

0041-1345/83/1505-0105$01.00/0

Table 1. Transplant Groups at PUH* Followed for Infections

Time of Transplant	Type Transplant	No. of Patients	Mean Age	Immunosuppression	Duration of Follow-up
1981–1982	Kidney†	64	36	CsA	6 months–1 year
1981–1982	Kidney‡	21	41	CsA	6 months–1 year
1981–1982	Kidney‡	17	41	AZA	6 months–1 year
1978–1980	Kidney	59	33	AZA	6 months–1 year
1981–1983	Heart	33	40	CsA	3 months–1 year
1981–1983	Liver	43	36	CsA	4 months–1 year

*Presbyterian-University Hospital, University of Pittsburgh.
†All kidney patients on CsA.
‡Patients on randomized CsA, AZA trial.

Table 2. Infections and Fatalities in 1981–1983 Transplant Recipients

	Renal Transplant Groups				
Patient Characteristic	Random AZA ($n = 17$)	Random CsA ($n = 21$)	All CsA Renal ($n = 64$)	Cardiac Transpl. ($n = 33$)	Liver Transpl. ($n = 43$)
All infections					
Percent Infected*	88%	71%	61%	76%	81%
Total episodes	37	24	63	52	98
Mean episodes†	2.18	1.14	0.98	1.58	2.28
Nonviral infections					
Percent infected	82%	43%	41%	58%	65%
Total episodes	28	13	39	30	70
Mean episodes	1.65	0.62	0.61	0.91	1.63
Infection-associated deaths/total deaths	0/0	0/0	0/1	9/14	17/20

*Percent patients developing one or more infections.
†Total number of episodes divided by number of patients.

Table 3. Site of Infections According to Type of Transplant Patient on Cyclosporine

	Frequent Sites of Infection				
Type of Transplant	Site	Percent of All Infections	Bacteremias	Fungemia	Infection-Associated Deaths
Kidney	Urinary tract	41%	5%	0%	0%
Heart	Pulmonary and intrathoracic	38%	24%	0%	27%
Liver	Abdominal and gastrointestinal	35%	30%	16%	40%

Table 4. Organisms Causing Infections in 1981–1983 Transplant Recipients

	Renal Transplant Groups				
Organism	Random AZA ($n = 17$)	Random CsA ($n = 21$)	All CsA Renal ($n = 64$)	Cardiac Transpl. ($n = 33$)	Liver Transpl. ($n = 43$)
Gram-negative aerobes	18 (53)*	10 (39)	37 (34)	13 (33)	36 (49)
All gram-positive	11 (53)	7 (29)	13 (17)	10 (24)	29 (58)
Staphylococcus	7 (41)	1 (5)	4 (6)	4 (12)	12 (23)
Fungus	0 (0)	1 (5)	1 (2)	1 (3)	22 (44)
Other	12 (71)	13 (48)	30 (36)	27 (58)	23 (47)
Total	46 (88%)	13 (86%)	81 (67%)	51 (79%)	110 (88%)

*Number of isolates (percent patients infected by isolate).

Table 5. Effect of Azathioprine and Cyclosporine on Infections in Renal Transplant Recipients

Group	Bacteremias	Staph Bacteremia	Lung Infection	Lung Staph	Pneumocystis
Random AZA	5/17 (29%)	2/17 (12%)	5/17 (29%)	3/17 (18%)	
1978–1980 AZA	11/59 (19%)	5/59 (9%)	23/59 (39%)	5/59 (8%)	6/179 (3%)*
CsA	3/64 (5%)	0/64 (0%)	5/64 (8%)	0/64 (0%)	14/156 (9%)*

*Based on data for all renal transplantation 1978–1982.

Table 4 presents organisms responsible for infections in the 1981–1983 transplant groups. The following are notable. (1) Gram-negative aerobes were significant pathogens in all groups. (2) Gram-positive infections, particularly staphylococcal infections, were more common in the randomized AZA group than all other groups on CsA. (3) Severe fungus infections were a serious problem only in the liver transplant patients. Forty-four percent of liver patients had serious fungal infections and 16% were fungemic. The most common agent was Candida, which caused serious infections in 15 patients. Of these, 3 had disseminated disease, 6 had fungemia, 7 had abdominal, and 3 had lung and chest infections. Four patients had aspergillosis, in whom one produced dissemination and 3 produced pneumonia or chest infections. There was one severe Mucor wound infection and one cryptococcal meningitis. (4) Symptomatic viral infections, included here under "other," were a problem in cardiac transplant patients and are discussed below.

Renal patients on AZA had more infections that were more severe and were predominately Staphylococcal (Table 5). This statement is substantiated by including data from the 1978–1980 AZA group, whose incidence of infection was similar to the small randomized AZA group of 1981–1983.[2] The two AZA groups had 29% and 39% pneumonias, as opposed to 8% for the CsA group. Staphylococcal penumonias and bacteremias were also more common in patients on AZA. In contrast, the incidence of non-life-threatening urinary tract infections were almost identical: 41%, 39%, and 42% (not shown in table). Pneumocystis pneumonia, however, may be a special problem in renal patients on CsA. Our total Pittsburgh incidence rates for the AZA and CsA groups prior to the institution of trimethoprim-sulfa prophylaxis in September 1982 were 3.4% and 9.0%, respectively, which are significantly different. This problem is discussed by Hardy et al. elsewhere in this issue.

Virus infections, particularly of the herpesvirus group (CMV, HSV, VZV, and EBV) are frequent occurrences after organ transplantation.[5] In previous experience, the degree and type of immunosuppression has been critical in determining the morbidity. In renal transplant recipients, antithymocyte globulin has been associated with more symptomatic infection.[6] Primary infections, i.e., those

Table 6. Herpesvirus Infections in 1981–1983 Transplant Recipients

	Renal Transplant Groups														
	Random AZA (n = 17)			Random CsA (n = 20)			All CsA Renal (n = 60)			Cardiac Transpl. (n = 29)			Liver Transpl. (n = 27)		
Virus	No.	(%)	Symptomatic	No.	(%)	Symptomatic	No.	(%)	Symptomatic	No.	(%)	Symptomatic	No.	(%)	Symptomatic
All CMV	13	(76)	1	15	(75)	1	46	(77)	5	27	(93)	10*	21	(57)	12
CMV viremia	5	(26)	1	8	(40)	1	20	(33)	5	18	(62)	10*	15	(41)	10
Herpes simplex	9	(53)	6	8	(40)	6	26	(43)	14	16	(55)	8	19	(51)	9
Herpes zoster	0	(0)	0	1	(5)	1	2	(3)	2	3	(10)	3	2	(5)	2
Total symptomatic			7(41)†			7(35)			19(32)			17(59)*			18(49)

*Significantly different from other CsA groups (χ^2 test), $p < 0.05$.

†Number patients symptomatic (% of group).

Table 7. Primary and Reactivation CMV Infections in 1981–1983 Transplant Recipients

Pretransplant Serologic Status	Renal Transplant Groups: Random AZA ($n = 17$)			Random CsA ($n = 20$)			All CsA Renal ($n = 60$)			Cardiac Transpl. ($n = 25$)			Liver Transpl. ($n = 18$)		
	I/T	(%)*	Sy†	I/T	(%)	Sy	I/T	(%)	Sy	I/T	(%)	Sy	I/T	(%)	Sy
Positive	10/13	(77)	1	15/17	(88)	1	42/51	(82)	4	15/15	(100)	5	7/10	(70)	2
Negative	3/4	(75)	0	0/3	(0)		4/9	(44)	1	9/10	(90)	5	5/8	(62)	2
Total Infected	13/17	(76)	1	15/20	(75)	1	46/60	(77)	5	24/25	(96)	10	12/18	(66)	4

*I/T (%), infected/total evaluable (%).

†Sy, symptomatic patients.

occurring in seronegative recipients, have been found to be more symptomatic.[7]

Herpesvirus infections in our transplant groups are presented in Table 6. The first row describes all CMV infections diagnosed by isolating the virus from routine throat, urine, or blood buffy coat specimens. The majority of patients became infected, and the rates are indistinguishable from results from previous series of patients, most of whom were on AZA. As a group of agents, herpesviruses and gram-negative aerobes are the most frequent causes of symptomatic infections.

The incidence of CMV viremia varied from 26% to 62%. All patients who had symptomatic CMV infection were viremic, but there were also many viremic patients who were not symptomatic. The percent of patients with symptomatic disease due to CMV and herpesviruses in general was significantly higher in the cardiac group. They also had more viremia due to CMV.

Of the patients with symptomatic CMV infection, there were three cases of CMV pneumonitis in the renal group on CsA. In a separate communication (Hardy et al., this issue), the relationships of CMV infection to Pneumocystis pneumonia is discussed. Five of the ten symptomatic cases in the cardiac group were associated with CMV in the lung. One was found in association with pneumocystis in a lung biopsy and four were found at autopsy. There were 12 symptomatic cases in the liver group, including one case of interstitial pneumonia and three instances of disseminated disease found at autopsy.

Primary and reactivation CMV infections are listed in Table 7. Except for a suggestion in the case of cardiac transplant recipients that primary infection in previously seronegative subjects resulted in more symptomatic infection than reactivation infection, the numbers are too small to incriminate primary more than reactivation infections in symptomatic disease.

Rates for EBV infection are shown in Table 8. Cardiac transplant recipients had more infection, and only they had probable symptomatic disease due to EBV (see Dummer et al., this issue). However, our total experience is still relatively small.

SUMMARY AND CONCLUSIONS

Renal patients on CsA had fewer bacteremias, pneumonias, and gram-positive staphylococcal infections than renal patients on

Table 8. Epstein-Barr Virus Infections in 1981–1983 Transplant Recipients

Pretransplant IgG-VCA	Renal Transplant Groups: Random AZA	Random CsA	All CsA Renal	Cardiac Transpl.	Liver Transpl.
Negative	0/0	0/1	1/3	3/3	0/1
Positive	2/17	3/19	5/34	8/21	1/13
Total infected	2/17	3/20	6/37	11/24*	1/14
Percent	12%	15%	16%	46%	7%

*Significantly different from all other groups on CsA, $p < 0.01$. Five were symptomatic; two had primary infections, one had EBV lymphoma.

AZA. Patients on CsA may be at risk for pneumocystis.

Severity and site of infection is largely determined by type of transplantation. Heart and liver transplant recipients had serious chest and abdominal infections.

Serious fungal infections occurred largely in liver transplant recipients.

Almost every patient was infected with CMV; 8%–34% developed symptomatic disease. This was always associated with viremia.

Heart transplant recipients developed more CMV viremia and more EBV infection. They also had more symptomatic disease from all herpesviruses.

REFERENCES

1. Klintmalm GBG, Starzl TE, Iwatsuki S, et al: Transplant Proc 14:98, 1982

2. Dummer JS, Hardy A, Ho M, et al: Transplantation (in press)

3. Starzl TE, Klintmalm GBG, Weil RW, et al: Surg Gynecol Obstet 153:486, 1981

4. Hakala TR, Starzl TE, Rosenthal JE, et al: Transplant Proc 15:465, 1983

5. Ho M: Cytomegalovirus: Biology and Infection. New York, Plenum, 1982

6. Marker SC, Howard RJ, Simmons RL, et al: Surgery 89:660, 1980

7. Ho M, Suwansirikul S, Dowling JN, et al: N Engl J Med 293:1109, 1975

Infection in Renal Transplant Recipients on Cyclosporine: Pneumocystis Pneumonia

A. M. Hardy, C. P. Wajszczuk, T. R. Hakala, J. T. Rosenthal, T. E. Starzl, and M. Ho

PNEUMOCYSTIS CARINII causes pneumonia in a variety of immunocompromised individuals, including renal transplant recipients.[1] Cases of *P. carinii* pneumonia (PCP) in renal transplant patients treated with azathioprine (AZA) and steroids are generally sporadic.[2,3] At Presbyterian-University Hospital (PUH), only 6 cases of biopsy-proven PCP have been diagnosed in 179 AZA patients since 1977. The use of cyclosporine (CsA) in renal transplant patients at PUH began in 1981. Between January and December 1982, 14 cases of biopsy-proven PCP occurred in 156 patients receiving CsA and steroids. Ten of the 14 cases occurred in the last quarter of 1982. This striking increase in PCP cases prompted an evaluation of these 14 patients.

Table 1 summarizes the patients with PCP. All were recipients of cadaver kidneys and were transplanted between September 1981 and September 1982. The cases did not differ from the rest of the CsA population with respect to age, race, or underlying disease. However, the male-to-female ratio was significantly higher in those with PCP (12 males to 2 females) than in the rest of CsA patients (75 males to 67 females) ($p < 0.05$). Two of the cases were brothers; the others were unrelated. In 12 of the patients, the onset of PCP occurred in the third or fourth month after transplant; the other cases had onset of PCP in the seventh and eleventh months. The overall mortality rate in this group was 21% (3 deaths in 14 patients).

Data on cytomegalovirus (CMV) infection in these patients is shown in Table 2. All 14 patients were infected with CMV (determined by isolation of the virus and/or by appropriate serologic change). Thirteen of the patients had CMV infection detected prior to or shortly after PCP diagnosis. One patient had a fourfold rise in CMV antibody titer about 6 weeks after his pneumonia, however, because of sporadic sampling, it is likely the onset of his CMV infection actually occurred much closer in time to his onset of PCP. Four patients of 11 tested had CMV isolated from lung biopsy material taken to diagnose PCP.

Based on pretransplant serologic testing, 5 (36%) patients had primary and 9 (64%) had reactivation CMV infections. Five of the 14 patients had symptomatic CMV infections (defined by presence of typical symptoms occurring during active infection or by isolation of CMV from infected lung tissue). Five additional patients had less pronounced symptoms, which may have been caused by CMV. The last 4 patients had no indication of a symptomatic CMV infection.

Epidemiologic investigation failed to implicate any specific source of the organism or any particular mode of disease transmission. Only limited hospital contact between cases could be documented. The cases had been transplanted in 10 different months, with no more than 3 done in any month. There was no point in time when more than 4 cases were in the hospital at the same time. In only 2 instances did cases share hospital rooms prior to onset of PCP.

Prophylaxis with trimethoprim-sulfamethoxazole (TMP-SMZ) was begun in December 1982. All new transplant recipients and patients transplanted several months prior to this were started on a 3-month course

From the Department of Infectious Diseases and Microbiology, Graduate School of Public Health and Departments of Medicine and Surgery, School of Medicine, University of Pittsburgh, Pittsburgh, PA.

Address reprint requests to Dr. M. Ho, A427 Crabtree Hall, University of Pittsburgh, Pittsburgh, PA 15261.

Supported in part by NIH Grant AI-19377.

0041-1345/83/1505-0106$01.00/0

Table 1. Summary of Patients With *P. carinii* Pneumonia

Number of cases	14
Mean age (range)	40.7 years (20–65)
Male:female	12:2
White:black	13:1
Underlying diseases	2
Chronic glomerulonephritis	
Polycystic kidney disease	3
Diabetes	2
Alport's syndrome	2
Hypertension	3
Hereditary nephritis	1
Unknown	1

of this drug. To date, no additional cases of PCP have occurred in the CsA patients.

DISCUSSION

In our renal transplant recipients treated with CsA and steroids, *P. carinii* was an important cause of infection after transplantation. The reasons for this are not entirely clear. One study has suggested that CsA increases the susceptibility of rats to Pneumocystis infection.[4] More information on Pneumocystis infection in CsA-treated patients is needed to establish if patients using this drug are at an increased risk for the development of PCP.

The incidence of CMV infection in these cases was high, and a large proportion were symptomatic. CMV is immunosuppressive and may increase the susceptibility of patients to pneumocystis infection.[5] Conversely, CMV infection may just be an indication that these patients were more effectively immunosuppressed, without playing a role in the pathogenesis of PCP.

Table 2. CMV Infection in Patients With *P. carinii* Pneumonia

	No. of Patients (%)	No. Symptomatic
All CMV infection	14 (100%)	5
Primary CMV infection	5 (36%)	1
Secondary CMV infection	9 (64%)	4

Although a definite clustering of cases occurred in the last quarter of 1982, we could find little evidence for a common source, or person to person or nosocomial spread of the infection. Other investigators of possible outbreaks have also failed to identify a specific pattern of disease transmission.[6,7] Our study and others are hindered by a lack of basic epidemiologic information about *P. carinii.* We did identify the third and fourth months after transplant as the time when PCP cases were more likely to occur. This is also the time of active CMV infection, which all of our cases had. To date, 3 months of prophylactic TMP-SMZ appears effective in preventing cases of PCP. Further follow-up is necessary to see if this measure remains effective. This is the first report of proclivity toward pneumocystis pneumonia in patients on CsA.

REFERENCES

1. Walzer PD, Perl DP, Krogstad DJ, et al: Ann Intern Med 80:83, 1974
2. Rifkind D, Faris TD, Hill RB: Ann Intern Med 65:943, 1966
3. Murphy JF, McDonald FD, Dawson M, et al: Arch Intern Med 136:670, 1976
4. Hughes WT, Smith B: J Infect Dis 145:767, 1982
5. Ho M: Cytomegalovirus, Biology and Infection. New York, Plenum, 1982
6. Perera DR, Western KA, Johnson HD, et al: JAMA 214:1074, 1970
7. Singer C, Armstrong D, Rosen PP, et al: Ann Intern Med 82:772, 1975

Cellular Immune Response and Cytomegalovirus Infection in Renal Transplant Recipients Receiving Cyclosporine

C. R. Rinaldo, Jr., W. H. Hamoudi, R. L. DeBiasio, B. Rabin, T. R. Hakala, and M. Liebert

CYTOMEGALOVIRUS (CMV) infection is quite common in renal transplant recipients. The infection occurs most often during the second-to-fourth months after transplantation in patients receiving conventional immunosuppressive regimens, such as azathioprine and prednisone (Pred).[1] The high frequency of CMV infection is due to enhanced reactivation of latent virus ("reactivated infection") or increased susceptibility to primary infection caused by the immunosuppressive therapy. Clinical manifestations of CMV infection range from mild asymptomatic illness to severe pneumonitis. CMV infection can also predispose the transplant recipient to serious, secondary infections with bacteria, fungi, and parasites.[2] The severity of primary and secondary complications of CMV infection is thought to be related to the direct immunosuppressive effects of CMV that are known to occur in excess of the immunosuppression caused by the antirejection protocols.[3]

Cyclosporine (CsA) is a new nonmyelotoxic immunosuppressive drug undergoing clinical trials at Presbyterian-University Hospital in Pittsburgh. The mode of action of the drug and its effects on viral infections are not completely understood.[4] We have examined the effects of CsA-Pred treatment and CMV infection on lymphocyte blastogenesis and lymphocyte phenotypes in the peripheral blood of renal transplant recipients.

MATERIALS AND METHODS

Patients and Control Donors

Sixteen renal allograft recipients were studied prospectively for occurrence of viral infections and cellular immune function. Blood for these studies was obtained several hours prior to transplantation and at 1–3-week intervals for approximately 6 months after transplantation. The patients received CsA (Sandoz, Basel, Switzerland) orally at a daily dose of 17.5 mg/kg beginning on the day of surgery, after the pretransplant samples were taken for the immunology/virology studies. The dose of CsA was reduced to 10–12 mg/kg during the first 2 months after transplantation. The patients were begun on 200 mg of oral Pred the first day after surgery, and if possible, reduced to 20 mg/day over the next 4 days. Controls were 20 healthy laboratory and university personnel.

Viral Cultures and Serology

Urine, throat washings, and peripheral blood leukocytes were cultured at weekly intervals after transplantation on human foreskin fibroblasts, as previously described.[5] Cultures were observed for characteristic CMV-and herpes simplex virus (HSV) mediated cytopathic effects for 5 weeks before being discarded as negative. Serum antibody to CMV was determined by anticomplement immunofluorescence, and that to HSV and mumps virus by neutralization assay.[5]

Viral Antigens

Preparations of u.v.-inactivated CMV (Davis strain), HSV (Patton strain), and mumps virus (Jeryl Lynn vaccine strain; Merck, Sharpe, Dohme) antigens were made as previously detailed.[5]

Lymphocyte Blastogenesis

Mononuclear leukocytes were separated from heparinized blood on Ficoll-Hypaque gradients. A quantity of 3×10^5 cells in 0.2 ml of medium 199 with 10% heat-inactivated, human AB+ serum (negative for CMV and HSV antibodies) was placed into flat-bottom microwells (Costar). Replicate samples were treated with concanavalin-A (Con-A) or antigens known to induce maximal blastogenesis in cells from normal donors.[5] Lympho-

---

From the Departments of Microbiology, Pathology, and Surgery, University of Pittsburgh, Graduate School of Public Health and School of Medicine, and Presbyterian-University Hospital, Pittsburgh, PA.

Supported in part by Grant AI-16212 from the National Institutes of Health, Biomedical Research Support Grant RR-05451 from the USPHS, and the Pathology Education Research Fund and Research Development Fund from the University of Pittsburgh.

Address reprint requests to Dr. C. Rinaldo, A417 Crabtree Hall, University of Pittsburgh, Pittsburgh, PA 15261.

0041-1345/83/1505-0107$01.00/0

cyte blastogenesis was assessed by uptake of ^{3}H-thymidine and expressed as Δcpm, or the difference between cpm in mitogen- or antigen-treated cells and cpm in untreated or mock-antigen-treated cells.

T-Lymphocyte Identification

T lymphocytes were enumerated by direct immunofluorescence with fluorescein-conjugated monoclonal antibodies anti-Leu-4 (total T cells), anti-Leu-3a (helper-inducer T cells), and anti-Leu-2a (suppressor-cytotoxic T cells) (Becton Dickinson) with a fluorescence-activated cell sorter (FACS IV; Becton Dickinson).[6] Results were expressed as both the absolute number of lymphocytes/cu mm of blood and the relative percentage of each subset.

Statistics

Data were analyzed for statistical significance by a comparison of the mean values among patients, and between pretransplant patients and normal donors, by Student's t test.

RESULTS AND DISCUSSION

Lymphocyte Blastogenesis

All 16 patients studied were seropositive for CMV prior to transplantation. Each patient developed reactivated CMV infection by 19–78 days after transplantation, as evidenced by isolation of virus and/or a fourfold increase in serum antibody titer to CMV.

Twelve of the patients were prospectively examined for lymphocyte blastogenesis. Response to Con-A and CMV antigen decreased in 9 of the 12 patients approximately 40%–80% within 1.5 weeks after transplantation and prior to onset of CMV viremia (Table 1). The 3 transplant recipients who did not develop viremia had a 0%–15% decrease in blastogenesis to Con-A and CMV antigen (Table 2). Lymphocyte blastogenesis to HSV antigen was not appreciably altered in HSV-seroimmune patients by 1.5 weeks after allografting (Tables 1 and 2). Immune-specific response to mumps virus antigen was relatively low before and immediately after transplantation in all patients, as compared with normal, mumps virus-seroimmune donors.

During CMV viremia, mean levels of lymphocyte blastogenesis to CMV and HSV antigens decreased 40%–50% below previremia levels (Table 1). This occurred even though the mean dose of CsA-Pred was 30%–45% lower than before viremia. Response to Con-A and mumps virus antigen remained relatively stable. Blastogenesis to all three viral antigens increased approximately threefold after cessa-

Table 1. Lymphocyte Blastogenesis in Renal Transplant Recipients Receiving Cyclosporine (CsA) and Prednisone (Pred) Who Developed CMV Viremia*

		Posttransplant				
		Previremic				
Cell Treatment	Pretransplant	1.5 Weeks	Total†	Viremic	Postviremic	Normal Donors‡
Con-A	90,371§	53,293**$	56,595**$	64,148	82,400	87,188
	(±13,546)	(±10,288)	(±8,055)	(±6,526)	(±7,979)	(±3,835)
CMV antigen	19,200	4,421$	5,097	2,880$	12,335	31,479
	(±7,858)	(±1,976)	(±1,768)	(±1,810)	(±3,266)	(±6,358)
HSV antigen	12,255	11,964	16,936	9,478$	26,718	12,785
	(±3,803)	(±8,582)	(±9,064)	(±4,811)	(±7,094)	(±1,297)
Mumps antigen	4,364	3,563	3,568	3,269	10,201	10,146
	(±2,570)	(±2,775)	(±2.017)	(±2,630)	(±3,428)	(±1,833)
CsA dosages‖	0	1,094(±84)▿$	1,071(±80)▿$	764(±60)	671(±35)	0
Pred dosages‖		36.7(±7.6)▿$	32.5(±6.0)▿$	18.3(±0.7)$	14.0(±0.6)	

*Nine CMV-seropositive patients who developed CMV viremia; mean onset of viremia, 38 days posttransplant (range 19–78 days); mean duration of viremia, 29 days (range 1–91).

†Cumulative for 5–64 days posttransplantation and prior to viremia.

‡Normal donors were seropositive for the relevant viral antigen.

§Mean Δcpm (±SE).

**Significantly different from pretransplant values ($p \leq 0.05$).

$Significantly different from postviremic values ($p \leq 0.05$).

▿Significantly different from viremic values ($p < 0.05$).

‖Mean mg/day of sampling (±SE).

Table 2. Lymphocyte Blastogenesis in Renal Transplant Recipients Receiving Cyclosporine (CsA) and Prednisone (Pred) Who Did Not Develop CMV Viremia*

Cell Treatment	Pretransplant	Posttransplant		Normal Donors‡
		1.5 Week	Total†	
Con-A	72,810 §	93,820	87,894	87,188
	(±11,297)	(±8,750)	(±7,166)	(±3,835)
CMV antigen	10,964	9,206	13,553	31,479
	(±6,392)	(±4,321)	(±2,630)	(±6,358)
HSV antigen	15,860	17,540	25,688**	12,785
	(±2,375)	(±1,720)	(±2,842)	(±1,297)
Mumps antigen	3,390$	1,228	2,815	10,146
	(±1,168)	(±829)	(±891)	(1,833)
CsA dosages‖	0	1,050(±104)	768(±55)	0
Pred dosages‖		26.7(±6.7)	23.2(±5.9)	

*Three CMV seropositive patients who did not develop detectable CMV viremia (weekly samplings); two of the three had reactivated CMV infection (CMV in throat washings) without viremia.

†Cumulative for 5–157 days posttransplantation.

‡Normal donors were seropositive for the relevant viral antigen.

§Mean Δcpm (±SE).

**Significantly different from pretransplant and 1.5 wk posttransplant values ($p < 0.05$).

$Significantly different from normal donor values ($p < 0.02$).

‖Mean mg/day of sampling (±SE).

tion of viremia. By comparison, the dose of CsA-Pred decreased only 10%–20% after viremia.

These data suggest that CsA-Pred treatment has an early selective effect in certain renal transplant recipients that correlates with subsequent occurrence of CMV viremia. Depression in lymphocyte blastogenesis to Con-A, and more importantly to CMV antigen, could be a predictor of enhanced risk of developing serious CMV infection associated with viremia. One of these nine viremic patients had overt CMV disease, i.e., biopsy-confirmed CMV pneumonitis. Alternatively, lymphocyte blastogenesis to CMV antigen could simply be a more sensitive indicator of altered cellular immunity, in general, than response to other antigens, such as HSV.[7] Finally, our results indicate that CMV viremia itself is immunosuppressive in CsA-Pred-treated patients and that cellular immune reactivity increases concurrently with cessation of viremia and further decreases in drug doses.

T-Lymphocyte Subsets

Pretransplant values of absolute and relative lymphocyte counts were within normal limits for the total group of patients. Treatment with CsA-Pred resulted in a 20% decrease in total lymphocyte numbers early after transplantation, with a relative decrease in lymphocytes of approximately 30%–40% as compared with pretransplant or normal donor values. Levels of T-cell subsets decreased during viremia, but were equal to or greater than normal after cessation of viremia (Table 3). Leu-3a/Leu-2a values of less than one ("inverted ratio") were noted almost exclusively in patients who developed viremia. However, this was not a frequent finding. Indeed, a Leu-3a/Leu-2a ratio of <1.0 was noted in only 1 of 11 previremic, 4 of 14 viremic, and 4 of 15 postviremic samples.

The five patients with reactivated CMV infection without CMV viremia had no difference in mean values of T lymphocytes after transplantation as compared with pretransplant or normal levels. Their overall Leu-3a/Leu-2a ratio was 2.5 ± 0.2. Only 1 of 34 samples tested from patients not developing viremia had a ratio of <1.0. This patient was excreting HSV (throat) but not CMV at this time.

Significant inversions of T-cell ratios are known to occur during CMV mononucleosis

Table 3. Absolute and Relative Lymphocyte Counts in Relationship to CMV Viremia in Renal Transplant Recipients Receiving Cyclosporine and Prednisone*

Lymphocytes	Pretransplant	Posttransplant			Normal Donors
		Previremic	Viremic	Postviremic	
Total/cu mm	1,867(±171)	1,517(±322)	1,009(±122)**$	1,954(±208)	1,795(±119)
Percent	28(±3)	19(±4)	14(±2)	29(±3)	33(±2)
Leu-4/cu mm	1,434(±154)	954(±205)	736(±136)**$	1,324(±157)	1,194(±84)
Percent	70(±4)	59(±7)	61(±5)	80(±4)	68(±2)
Leu-3a/cu mm	902(±136)	588(±155)	403(±71)**$	885(±119)	809(±54)
Percent	44(±5)	38(±5)	38(±4)	46(±3)	47(±2)
Leu-2a/cu mm	443(±63)	346(±73)$	304(±54)$	620(±83)	387(±50)
Percent	23(±5)	24(±3)	29(±3)	32(±3)	22(±1)
Leu-3a / Leu-2a	2.4(±0.5)	1.8(±0.3)	1.7(±0.2)	1.7(±0.2)	2.4(±0.2)

*Eleven seropositive patients who developed CMV viremia; mean onset of viremia, 38 days posttransplant (range 19–78 days); mean duration of viremia, 29 days (range 1–91).

**Significantly different from pretransplant values ($p < 0.01$).

$Significantly different from postviremic values ($p < 0.02$).

in normal adults[6,8] and during reactivated CMV infection (viremic and nonviremic) and other herpesvirus infections in renal transplant recipients receiving conventional immunosuppressants.[9] Helper T-cell/suppressor T-cell ratios in these patients average 0.5 and can persist at levels <1.0 for many weeks during and after viremia.

Such persistently inverted ratios do not occur in renal transplant recipients treated with CsA-Pred and undergoing reactivated CMV infection. Preliminary studies indicate that primary CMV infection and illness also do not result in frequent or prolonged inversion of Leu-3a/Leu-2a ratios. Apparently, CsA-Pred effectively inhibits CMV infection from enhancing levels of Leu-2a-positive lymphocytes in renal transplant recipients. This could relate to the reported ability of CsA to prevent activation of T cells.[4,10] Such an immunosuppressive mechanism could be of significance in host–virus and host–allograft interactions.

ACKNOWLEDGMENT

We thank J. Toth, the Renal Transplant Unit and Clinic, and Drs. M. Ho, J. Dowling, S. Dummer, and A. Hardy for aid in these studies. We thank E. Merrall and the Division of Immunopathology for assistance in analysis of T cells, and L. Youngblood and M. Lassak for virus isolation.

REFERENCES

1. Armstrong JA, Evans AS, Rao N, et al: Infect Immun 14:970, 1976

2. Rubin RH, Cosimi AB, Tolkoff-Rubin NE, et al: Transplantation 24:458, 1977

3. Linnemann CC Jr, Kauffman CA, First MR, et al: Infect Immun 22:176, 1978

4. Britton S, Palacios R: Immunol Rev 65:222, 1982

5. Rinaldo CR Jr, DeBiasio RL: Clin Immunol Immunopathol 28:46, 1983

6. Rinaldo CR Jr, Ho M, Hamoudi WH, et al: Infect Immun 40:472, 1983

7. Gehrz RC, Christianson WR, Linner KM, et al: Am J Obstet Gynecol 140:665, 1981

8. Carney WP, Rubin RH, Hoffman RA, et al: J Immunol 126:2114, 1981

9. Schooley RT, Hirsch MS, Colvin RB, et al: N Engl J Med 308:307, 1983

10. Leapman SB, Strong DM, Filo RS, et al: Transplantation 34:94, 1982

Infections in Patients on Cyclosporine and Prednisone Following Cardiac Transplantation

J. S. Dummer, H. T. Bahnson, B. P. Griffith, R. L. Hardesty, M. E. Thompson, and M. Ho

PAST reports have documented infection as the single most important complication of cardiac transplantation, especially during the first 2 posttransplant years.[1-5] Virtually all of these reports have come out of a single institution employing a consistent regimen of immunosuppression, which included azathioprine, corticosteroids, and antithymocyte globulin. Shortly after the introduction of cyclosporine in Pittsburgh, and the initiation of regular cardiac transplantation at Presbyterian-University Hospital, our division began routine monitoring of infections in these patients in the hope of providing practical information to aid in their management, as well as insight into the clinical biology of this intriguing new agent.

MATERIALS AND METHODS

Thirty-five consecutive adult cardiac transplant patients were followed for infection. Two patients did not survive 48 hr after surgery and are excluded from the analysis. All living patients were followed for a minimum of 3 months. The mean age of the patients was 40 years, and the mean follow-up was 277 days. Patients with idiopathic cardiomyopathy, who made up 61% of the total group, did not differ from patients with coronary artery or valvular disease in age, but their follow-up was shorter.

Infections were determined by clinical and laboratory diagnoses. Minor afebrile upper respiratory tract infections, thrush, and catheter-associated bacteruria and candiduria were excluded. Major infections are those that required hospitalization for diagnosis or treatment. Surveillance cultures were routinely performed on urine, throat washes, and buffy coats of blood to ascertain the presence of herpesvirus infections. Pre- and posttransplant serum specimens for IgG to Epstein-Barr virus (EBV) viral capsid antigen, and anticomplement immunofluorescent (ACIF) antibody to cytomegalovirus (CMV) were obtained.[6]

Immunosuppressive medications included cyclosporine (CsA), 17.5 mg/kg, and prednisone, 200 mg at time of surgery with tapering after operation in accord with clinical criteria. Rejection episodes were initially treated with serial 1-g doses of intravenous hydrocortisone. Over the 9 months before May 1983, 6 patients also received courses of antithymocyte globulin for the treatment of severe rejection.

Observed proportions were compared using the chi-square test or Fisher's exact test when the numbers were small. Calculated means were compared using Student's t test.

RESULTS

Symptomatic Infections

Twenty-six patients, or 76% of the total group, had at least one symptomatic infection, and a total of 52 infections occurred for a total of 1.6 infections per patient. Major infections occurred in two-thirds of all patients and accounted for 38 episodes or 1.2 episodes per patient. Thus, three-quarters of all infections were major. Minor infections consisted of urinary tract infections and orocutaneous herpesvirus infections. Bacteremia occurred in 8 patients for a total of 10 episodes, 7 of which were caused by gram-negative rods and 3 of which were caused by gram-positive bacteria. Six of the patients with bacteremia died, 4 within a few days of the bacteremia. No patient had fungemia.

There were 14 deaths; of these, 9 were associated with infection, but only 4 were uniquely caused by infection. The other fatal infections occurred against a background of posttransplant problems, including, in 4 cases, severe acute or chronic rejection of the allograft. Three patients died with CMV pneumonitis, and one patient died while under treatment for EBV-associated lymphoma.

Risk Factors for Infection

Patients younger and older than the mean age had an almost identical incidence of infec-

---

From the Departments of Medicine and Surgery, School of Medicine, and the Department of Infectious Diseases and Microbiology, Graduate School of Public Health, University of Pittsburgh, Pittsburgh, PA.

Supported in part by NIH Grant 1-RO1-AI-19377.

Address reprint requests to Dr. Ho, Crabtree A-427, University of Pittsburgh, Pittsburgh, PA 15261.

0041-1345/83/1505-0108$01.00/0

tion. Patients with cardiomyopathy had more infections than patients with coronary artery or valvular disease, but the difference was not significant. Severe rejection by histologic criteria correlated with a higher incidence of infection. Twelve patients with severe rejection had a mean of 2.33 episodes per patient, while 21 patients with moderate, mild, or no rejection had 1.14 episodes per patient ($p < 0.01$). This was true despite the fact that their follow-up was shorter than the group as a whole.

Types of Infections

Table 1 summarizes the types of infections and the pathogens isolated in these patients. The majority of infections occurring in these patients were bacterial pneumonias, other intrathoracic suppurative complications, and herpesvirus infections. Intraabdominal infections were also prominent, but formed a heterogeneous group that included a case of intestinal salmonellosis, a case of *Acinetobacter* peritonitis associated with peritoneal dialysis, and intraabdominal infection associated with a ruptured sigmoid diverticulum. Another patient developed *E. coli* sepsis from a small cecal perforation, and the final patient developed two episodes of anaerobic abscess formation of obscure etiology, the second of which was associated with bowel infarction and led to his death. In addition, there was one case of

Table 1. Types of Infections and Isolates in 33 Cardiac Transplant Recipients

Types of Infection	Episodes	Patients	Associated* With Death
EBV-CMV	11	10	3
Bacterial pneumonia	10	9	2
Herpes simplex	8	8	0
Intraabdominal	6	5	3
Other intrathoracic	6	6	1
Herpes zoster	3	3	0
Urinary tract	3	3	0
CNS	1	1	0
Toxoplasmosis	1	1	1
Pneumocystosis	1	1	0
Otitis	1	1	0
Primary bacteremia	1	1	0

*One death associated with two infections.

Frequency of isolates: bacterial 51%, viral 43%, fungal 2%, protozoal 4%.

Listeria meningitis and a case of unrecognized disseminated toxoplasmosis in a young female suffering from severe rejection in the first month after transplantation.

Herpesviruses and bacteria accounted for almost 95% of all pathogens identified in symptomatic infections. Only one documented fungal infection has occurred in this group. That was mediastinitis due to *Staphylococcus aureus* and *Candida albicans* 12 days after surgery. This infection was cured by surgical debridement and antibiotic therapy. This low incidence of fungal infection contrasts with a published report from Stanford that 44 of 136 patients (32%) who received cardiac allografts from 1968 to 1978 developed fungal infection.[1] We have also not encountered Nocardia infection, which developed in 13% of Stanford's patients.

Herpesvirus Infections

The routine performance of surveillance cultures has helped us document a high rate of herpesvirus infections in these cardiac allograft recipients. Viral cultures were obtained for at least 1 month after transplantation for 29 patients. EBV serologies were done on 24 of these patients. Herpes simplex virus was recovered in 16, or 55%. Eight patients, or 28%, had lesions, usually stomatitis, with or without cold sores. On occasion, this caused prolonged symptoms. CMV infection occurred in 27, or 93%, of the patient group. Ten patients had associated clinical disease, which included pneumonitis, fever, leukopenia, and in most cases, atypical lymphocytosis. CMV was recovered from the blood in 18 patients or 62% of the total group. All patients with symptomatic CMV disease had viremia, and the presence of viremia correlated significantly with the development of symptoms ($p = 0.01$). Patients with symptoms were often viremic more than once. Seven of 9 patients with more than one positive buffy coat culture were symptomatic, while only 3 of 18 patients with one or fewer positive buffy coat cultures had symptoms ($p = 0.007$). Thus, the presence of viremia was a sensitive indicator of disease.

Pretransplant sera from 25 of the CMV-infected patients were assayed for CMV antibody. All 15 seropositive patients showed reactivation of CMV, and 9 of 10 seronegative patients seroconverted. Both groups contained 5 patients with symptoms due to CMV and 2 patients with CMV pneumonitis. The 55% rate of symptom development among primary CMV patients was not significantly different from the 33% rate among patients with reactivation.

Herpes zoster was determined clinically in 29 patients. It occurred in 3 patients and did not disseminate. All 3 patients experienced mild degrees of postherpetic neuralgia.

Serologic tests for IgG to EBV viral capsid antigen were performed on 24 patients from this group. All 3 seronegative patients seroconverted. Two developed symptoms compatible with EBV infection. One had fever, fleeting pulmonary infiltrates, and severe thrombocytopenia 4 months after transplantation. The other patient developed fevers, coryza, and rapid enlargement of a submandibular lymph node five months after transplantation, along with an 8-fold rise in antibody to EBV. Biopsy of the node showed histiocytic lymphoma, in which 50% of the cells stained by immunofluorescence for EBV nuclear antigen (EBNA). This was confirmed in Dr. Joe Pagano's laboratory by nucleic acid hybridization.

Of 21 seropositive patients, 8 showed a 4-fold or greater rise in antibody to EBV, and 5 of these patients also had symptoms of viral infection. Overall, 11, or 46%, of all 24 patients had serologic changes indicating EBV infection, and 7 of these were symptomatic. Only 2 of 13 patients without a serologic change of EBV infection developed symptomatic evidence of viral infection. This difference was statistically significant ($p < 0.05$). All symptomatic patients also had evidence of CMV infection, including positive buffy coat cultures. These data suggest that EBV infection may play an important role in the development of symptoms during CMV infection or that some of the symptomatic infections may indeed be due to EBV. Because of the clinical and biologic importance of EBV-related lymphoma, we are currently prospectively following all cardiac transplants for evidence of EBV infection.

CONCLUSIONS

Our careful monitoring of infections in cardiac transplant patients on cyclosporine and prednisone shows that infections were a common complication during the first 10–12 months after surgery, but fell off sharply in incidence after that. Most of these infections were major, but most could also be managed successfully, and when death did occur, it was often in the setting of other serious problems, such as acute rejection. The majority of infections were herpesvirus infections or intrathoracic bacterial infections. Severe rejection was associated with a higher incidence of infection. Every patient had herpesvirus infections, and over half of all patients had symptoms from them. These rates are similar to those reported for cardiac transplant patients on azathioprine and antithymocyte globulin.[7] The combination of EBV and CMV produced more symptomatic disease than CMV alone.

Note added in proof:

One patient who died during the study period was later found to have had cerebral aspergillosis.

REFERENCES

1. Baumgartner WA, Reitz BA, Oyer PE, et al: Curr Prob Surg 16:1, 1979

2. Remington JS, Gaines JD, Griepp RB, et al: Transplant Proc 4:699, 1972

3. Mason JW, Stinson EB, Hunt SA, et al: Ann Intern Med 85:69, 1976

4. Montgomery JR, Barrett FF, Williams TW: Transplant Proc 5:1239, 1973

5. Pennock JL, Oyer PE, Reitz BA, et al: J Thorac Cardiovasc Surg 83:168, 1982

6. Dummer JS, Hardy A, Ho M, et al: Transplantation (in press)

7. Pollard RB, Arvin AM, Gamsberg P, et al: Am J Med 73:679, 1982

Glomerular Thrombi and Infarction in Rabbits with Serum Sickness Following Cyclosporine Therapy

G. H. Neild, K. Ivory, and D. G. Williams

NEPHROTOXICITY is a major complication of cyclosporine (CsA) therapy. Usually CsA causes tubular damage and reversible renal failure in a dose-dependent manner.[1,2] However, recently, a second renal complication has been described in CsA-treated bone marrow recipients, who developed a hemolytic-uremic syndrome (HUS) with thrombocytopenia and fragmented red cells associated with glomerular capillary thrombosis.[3] During a series of experiments in which we examined the effect of CsA on acute serum sickness (ASS) (immune complex) nephritis in rabbits,[4] we noted that with a high dose of 25 mg/kg/day of CsA, some rabbits became oliguric. Examination of the kidneys showed that the most severely oliguric had macroscopic infarction of the cortex. This article describes the glomerular and tubular lesions found, which are very similar to those seen in bone marrow recipients.

MATERIALS AND METHODS

Animals

Female New Zealand white (NZW) rabbits weighing 1.8–2.5 kg were used.[5] Continuous 24-hr urine collections were made.

Experimental Model of ASS

Rabbits were injected i.v. with 250 mg/kg crystalized bovine serum albumin (BSA) dissolved in saline. BSA (100 mg/ml) was given either alone or together with 5 μg/kg of *E. coli* endotoxin (Difco Labs, LPS.W, *E. coli* 0111:B4, Detroit, MI). BSA was radiolabeled with $Na^{125}I$ by the chloramine-T method, and elimination was followed as previously described.[4,5] Antigen elimination was considered complete when less than 1% of the initial activity remained.

Serology

A reference pool of anti-BSA antibody was made from rabbits immunized with BSA.[4,5] Precipitating antibody was measured by radial immunodiffusion of neat serum into agarose-containing BSA. In addition, an enzyme-linked immunosorbent assay (ELISA) method was used to measure both total immunoglobulin antibody activity (Ig) to BSA and the IgM antibody fraction.[5] The amount of circulating immune complexes was measured by precipitation of serum globulin bound to BSA-^{125}I, as described.[4,5] The size of immune complexes was measured by ultracentrifugation of serum in 12%–40% sucrose gradients for 18 hr at 175,000 *g*, as described.[4] Serum C3 levels were measured by radial immunodiffusion.[4,5]

Proteinuria

Proteinuria was measured by the Lowry method after samples had been precipitated by TCA. Proteinuria in excess of 150 mg/dl in a 24-hr volume was considered abnormal. An episode of "significant proteinuria" was defined as 2 or more consecutive days of abnormal proteinuria.

Hematuria, Glycosuria, and Oliguria

Hematuria and glycosuria were measured in fresh urine samples using "Labstix" dip sticks (Ames, UK). A significant period of hematuria was defined as 2 or more days of 1+ or more hematuria. Oliguria was defined as a 2-day period (or longer) during which the mean daily urine volume was 50% less than the mean of the previous 4 days.

Histology

Rabbits were killed on day 12 after injection of BSA, or 2–3 days after immune elimination when elimination occurred after day 10. Whole sections of kidney were fixed in 10% buffered formal-saline. Sections were stained by the periodic acid-Schiff(PAS) reaction and with Martius Scarlet blue (MSB). Glomerular proliferation was scored on a scale of 0, ±, 1 to 4+ and was considered present when the score was ≥1+. Cryostat sections were examined with immunofluorescence (IF) using fluorescein-conjugated antisera to BSA, rabbit whole immunoglobulin (Ig), IgG, IgM, C3, fibrinogen, and albumen (Nordic Pharmaceuticals, U.K.). Paraffin-embedded tissue sections were dewaxed, pronase-

From the Department of Renal Medicine, Guy's Hospital, London, U.K.

G. H. N. and K. I. were supported by, and the project was financed by, the Medical Research Council.

Address reprint requests to Dr. G. H. Neild, Department of Renal Medicine, Guy's Hospital, London SE1, U.K.

0041-1345/83/1505-0109$01.00/0

digested, and examined for fibrinogen using a peroxidase–anti-peroxidase (PAP) technique. Renal tissue was processed for electron microscopy.[4]

Cyclosporine

Cyclosporine-A was dissolved in a solvent vehicle of Miglyol 812 and 100% ethanol at a concentration of 100 mg/ml and was given by deep intramuscular injection.

Experimental Protocol

Twenty-three rabbits were given BSA plus endotoxin but received no other parenteral treatment (untreated animals). Groups of rabbits receiving CsA (15 or 25 mg/kg/day) were given BSA plus endotoxin or BSA alone (see Table 1). Two groups of animals were used as controls. Twenty-one with ASS received equivalent volumes of solvent alone for the same period as the treated groups. Six normal rabbits were given CsA, 25 mg/kg, for 5 days; in addition, on day 0, 3 were given i.v. saline plus 5 μg/kg endotoxin, and 3 were given saline alone.

RESULTS

Clinical Data

CsA inhibited the proteinuria that normally occurs with ASS, but did not inhibit the hematuria.[4] In addition, rabbits became oliguric (30%) and developed glycosuria (44%), two features that do not normally occur in ASS. When rabbits were given BSA *alone,* the nephritis was usually mild, with slight proteinuria and hematuria. When such rabbits were also given CsA, the disease produced was as severe as in those that received BSA and endotoxin.

Serologic Data

CsA did not have any significant inhibitory effect on the humoral response as measured by (1) the time to BSA elimination, (2) the subsequent magnitude or character of the antibody response, (3) the amount or size of circulating immune complexes or (4) the fall in C3 at the time of immune elimination.[4]

Histology

Eighty-seven percent of rabbits given BSA and endotoxin developed glomerular proliferation. Proliferation was less common in those given BSA alone. Treatment with CsA significantly reduced glomerular proliferation.[4] However, CsA treatment was associated with a number of new histologic features. These were more diffuse and severe in rabbits receiving 25 mg/kg of CsA. These changes were not seen in untreated ASS or rabbits given CsA alone in equivalent doses.

Glomerular capillary thrombi. Capillary loops were partially or totally occluded by amorphous, eosinophilic material. Areas of capillary occlusion were often infiltrated with polymorphs (Fig. 1). In some cases, capillary thrombi were associated with focal and segmental glomerular infarction, (Fig. 2) and necrosis of the afferent arterioles was seen. The thrombi were PAS positive and stained scarlet with MSB. Immunofluorescence examination showed strongly positive staining

Table 1. Histopathologic Data of Rabbits With ASS Treated With Cyclosporine-A

Rabbits (No.)	Treatment: Dose (mg/kg/Day)	Treatment: Days	Glomerular Proliferation (% No.)	Glomerular Thrombi (% No.)	Cortical Infarction (% No.)
BSA, with endotoxin					
CA-treated					
(1) 12	15	−2 to +8	8	42	25
(2) 5	25	−2 to +3	0	20	20
Control					
(3) 32	—	—	84	0	0
BSA, no endotoxin					
CsA-treated					
(4) 5	15	−2 to +8	0	40	20
(5) 6	25	−2 to +3	0	83	67
(6) 5	25	0 to 5	0	80	40
Control					
(7) 12	—	—	42	0	0

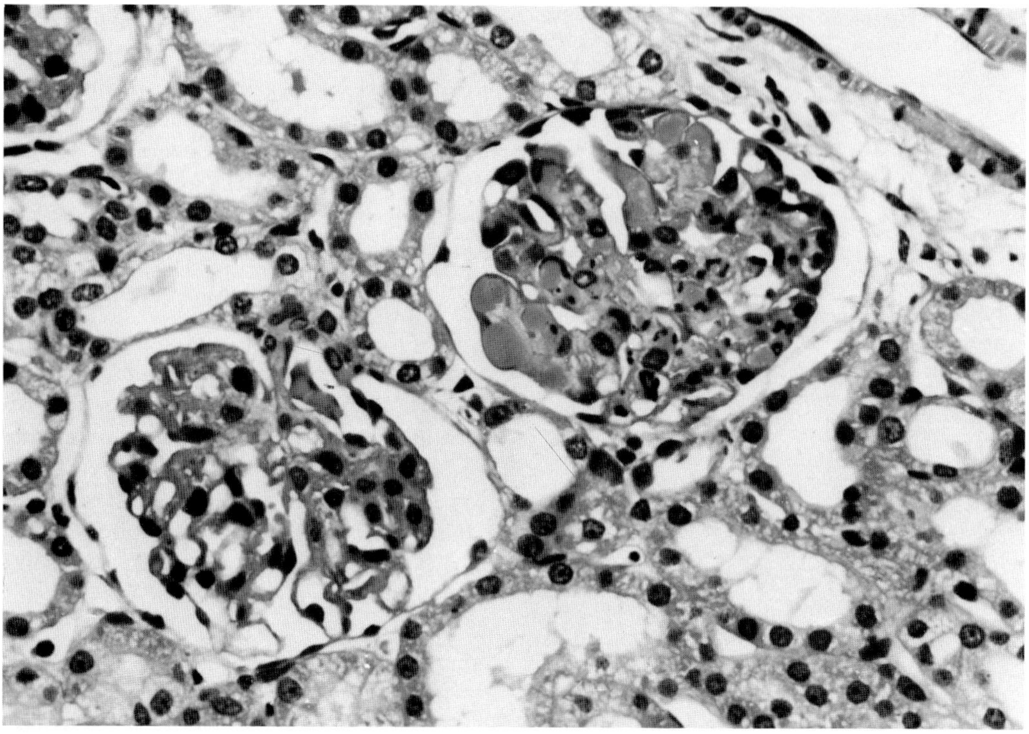

Fig. 1. Glomerulus with multiple capillary thrombi, some of which are associated with polymorph infiltration (H&E, ×25).

for BSA, but weak and equal staining for IgG, IgM, C3, and albumen. Fresh thrombi (1–2 days old) stained strongly positive for fibrinogen by both IF and immunoperoxidase.

Tubular and interstitial injury. Rabbits developed foci of dilated tubules, in which the height of the tubular epithelium was greatly reduced, or tubular cells appeared to be entirely absent. The loss in epithelium resulted in widely dilated lumina. Such tubules often contained amorphous eosinophilic casts that appeared to consist of the shed tubular epithelium. When the injury was more severe, there was total tubular necrosis. Severe, macroscopic infarction was associated with interstitial hemorrhage.

Electron Microscopy

Electron microscopy showed swelling and disruption of the endothelial cytoplasm. At times, when grossly swollen, the endothelium was indistinguishable from degranulated ("exhausted") platelets. Sometimes the endothelium was raised off the basement membrane, and the expanded subendothelial space was filled with a loose amorphous material or occasionally electron-dense material with the periodicity of fibrin. At times, capillary loops were packed with degenerating cells including platelets, polymorphs, and mononuclear cells. Strands of fibrin ran through this cellular mass. At later stages, the loops were filled with an electron-dense mass of amorphous material in which the periodicity of fibrin was not visible. Glomerular infarction was associated with accumulation of polymorphs in the capillary lumen phagocytosing chunks of this amorphous material. In areas of tubular infarction, peritubular capillaries were occluded by platelet thrombi.

DISCUSSION

In this new model of glomerular and tubular infarction, the vascular injury is initiated

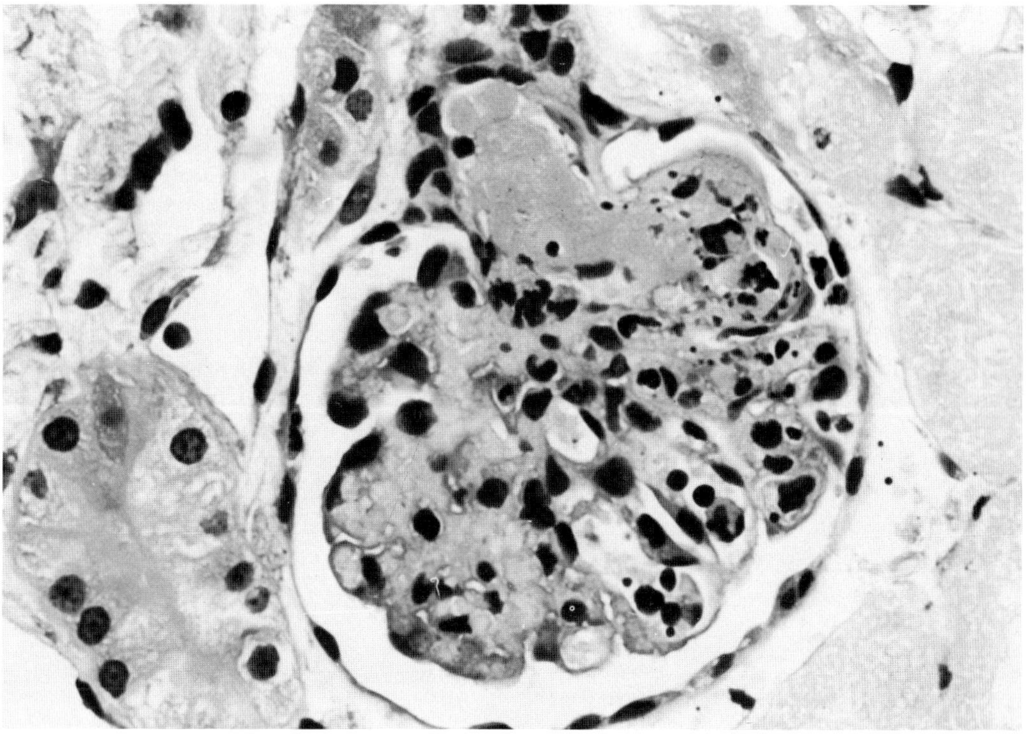

Fig. 2. Necrotic glomerulus with thrombosis of afferent arteriole. Some of the surrounding tubules are also infarcted (H&E, ×40).

during the period when immune complexes are being rapidly formed. We believe that the vascular damage and hematuria are initiated by an immune-complex-dependent mechanism. In contrast, we have suggested that the proteinuria and glomerular proliferation in unmodified ASS may be T-cell-mediated.[4] Vascular damage is a feature of acute serum sickness. Although the mechanism remains unknown, endothelial injury occurs;[6,7] there is an increase in vascular permeability and immune complexes are deposited in the vessel walls.[8] Arterial injury may progress to a proliferative and necrotic arteritis. The mediators are not known, but the fibrinoid necrosis may be inhibited by depleting the rabbits of either C3 or polymorphonuclear leukocytes[9] or by treating them with large doses of methylprednisolone.[5] However, severe endothelial injury is not a feature of ASS, and capillary thrombosis and glomerular infarction do not occur.

What is the pathogenetic mechanism of the new lesion that we have observed? There are several conditions where a similar appearance may be seen. Glomerular capillary thrombosis and cortical infarction may occur in rabbits following the Shwartzman reaction. The classic generalized Shwartzman reaction (GSR) is produced by two i.v. injections of endotoxin.[10] The first or "priming" dose prepares the animal so that the intravascular coagulation triggered by the second dose initiates widespread thombosis. Rabbits may be primed in other ways (e.g., being pregnant, pretreatment with steroids) so that a single dose of endotoxin causes a GSR. Furthermore, if rabbits are primed for a GSR, then an infusion of immune complexes can replace endotoxin and trigger off the reaction.[11] Although the pathogenesis of GSR has remained elusive, experiments suggest that the priming dose of endotoxin has a direct effect on the vascular endothelium. We propose that the priming event in the GSR is inhibition of PGI_2 production by the endothelium, with or without inhibition of fibrinolytic activity.

Secondly, it has been reported that some bone marrow recipients treated with CsA develop an HUS-like illness with glomerular and tubular infarction[3] similar to that described in our rabbits with CsA-treated ASS. HUS is an acute illness in man, which often follows a trivial viral illness. Little is known of the pathogenesis, but recently, Remuzzi et al.[12] showed that in patients with HUS, vascular synthesis of PGI_2 was reduced. Moreover, many of these patients lacked a prostacyclin-stimulating factor (PSF) in their plasma, which was necessary for synthesis of PGI_2 by vascular tissue. We have subsequently found that CsA therapy profoundly reduces PSF activity in plasma,[13] but we found no effect of CsA on platelets, or PGI_2 synthesis by aorta taken from CsA-treated animals.

A unifying hypothesis can be made from our observations, those in HUS, and those in marrow transplantation. Local production of PGI_2 by vascular endothelium limits excessive platelet aggregation and thrombus formation at sites of endothelial injury. We suggest that, in the absence of PSF, synthesis of PGI_2 is impaired, and vascular injury can progress to capillary thrombosis and necrosis of the vessel wall. We believe that ASS, graft-versus-host disease after marrow transplantation, and HUS are three examples of different mechanisms of endothelial injury which, when they occur in the absence of PSF, result in the same final vascular injury.

REFERENCES

1. Klintmalm GBG, Iwatsuki S, Starzl TE: Lancet 1:470, 1981

2. Thomson AW, Whiting PH, Blair JT, et al: Transplantation 32:271, 1981

3. Shulman H, Striker G, Deeg JH, et al: N Engl J Med 305:1392, 1981

4. Neild GH, Ivory K, Hiramatsu M, et al.: Transplant Proc (this issue)

5. Neild GH, Ivory K, Williams DG: Br J Exp Pathol 63:605, 1982

6. Kondo Y, Niwa Y, Takizawa J, et al: Lab Invest 41:119, 1979

7. Sharma HM, Geer JC: Am J Pathol 88:255, 1977

8. Kniker WT, Cochrane CG: J Exp Med 127:119, 1968

9. Kniker WT, Cochrane CG: J Exp Med 122:83, 1965

10. Thomas L, Good RA: J Exp Med 96:605, 1952

11. Lee L: J Exp Med 117:365, 1963

12. Remuzzi G, Misiani R, Marchesi D, et al: Lancet 2:871, 1978

13. Neild GH, Rocchi G, Remuzzi G, et al: Transplant Proc (this issue)

Occurrence of Hemolytic Uremic Syndrome Under Cyclosporine Treatment: Accident or Possible Side Effect Mediated by a Lack of Prostacyclin-Stimulating Plasma Factor?

C. Leithner, H. Sinzinger, E. Pohanka, M. Schwarz, G. Kretschmer, and G. Syré

IN 1980, Powles et al.[1] reported on their experience with cyclosporine-A (CsA) for prevention of graft-versus-host disease in man after allogeneic bone marrow transplantation. One of their patients had symptoms, namely thrombocytopenia, hemolytic anemia, and deterioration of renal function, which could be regarded as hemolytic uremic syndrome (HUS). Shulman et al.[2] studied the nephrotoxicity of CsA after allogeneic bone marrow transplantation, too. In a group of 16 patients, 4 subjects revealed a temporary increase of plasma creatinine to 1.4–2.5 mg/dl, probably caused by tubular injury. In 3 patients, however, a severe renal insufficiency developed, which was caused by diffuse glomerular thrombosis. These alterations were never detected in 55 patients treated without CsA. The authors concluded that CsA might cause endothelial damage resulting in microvascular thrombosis of the kidneys.

In 1978 MacIntyre et al.[3] reported on a factor present in plasma of healthy people that powerfully stimulated prostacyclin synthesis by vascular tissue. Further studies demonstrated that the activity of this plasma factor was enhanced in acute and chronic renal insufficiency.[4,5] It was therefore quite surprising when Remuzzi et al.[6] reported on a lack of plasma factor in patients who suffered from HUS or thrombotic thrombocytopenia purpura. Since the prostacyclin-stimulating plasma factor can be regarded as a kind of defense mechanism protecting endothelial integrity, these authors speculated that a lack of plasma factor would put the person at risk of microvascular thrombosis. This alteration could become more generalized, as in thrombotic thrombocytopenic purpura, or more localized to the kidneys, as in HUS. In 1982, Rocchi et al.[7] examined the influence of CsA on acute serum sickness induced by bovine serum albumen in the rabbit. Interestingly enough, the animals treated with CsA showed glomerular thrombosis and a depression of plasma factor activity. As a consequence, these authors suggested refraining from using CsA in transplant patients who had suffered from HUS as their underlying renal disease. At nearly the same time, we observed a case that seemed to support this advice.

CASE REPORT

In January 1980, a 32-year-old man was admitted to the Second Department of Internal Medicine because of hypertension (180/100 mm Hg). Since the patient presented the symptoms thrombocytopenia, hemolytic anemia, and rapidly decreasing renal function, HUS was suspected. Renal biopsy confirmed this diagnosis, showing extensive thrombosis of small arteries, arterioles, and glomerular capillaries. Rat aortic rings (4 mg wet weight) were incubated in Tris-HCl buffer (pH 7.35) and in the patient's plasma, respectively. The plasma was not able to increase prostacyclin synthesis as measured by platelet bioassay,[8] and therefore revealed a lack of prostacyclin-stimulating activity. Since all therapeutic attempts failed, chronic intermittent hemodialysis had to be started.

In April 1981, the patient was selected to receive a cadaveric renal transplant. Initial immunosuppression included prednisolone and azathioprine. The first 3 weeks passed without complications. At the end of the 4th week, the patient developed fever, a swelling of the graft demonstrable by ultrasonic scan, and an increase in plasma creatinine. The percutaneous graft biopsy confirmed the diagnosis of acute rejection, showing an interstitial infil-

From the Second Department of Internal Medicine, the First Department of Surgery, and the Department of Pathology, University of Vienna, Austria.

Supported in part by a grant of Medizinische-Wissenschaftlicher Fonds des Bürgermeisters der Bundeshauptstadt Wien.

Address reprints requests to Dr. C. Leithner, Second Department of Internal Medicine, University of Vienna, Garnisongasse 13, A-1090 Vienna, Austria.

0041-1345/83/1505-0110$01.00/0

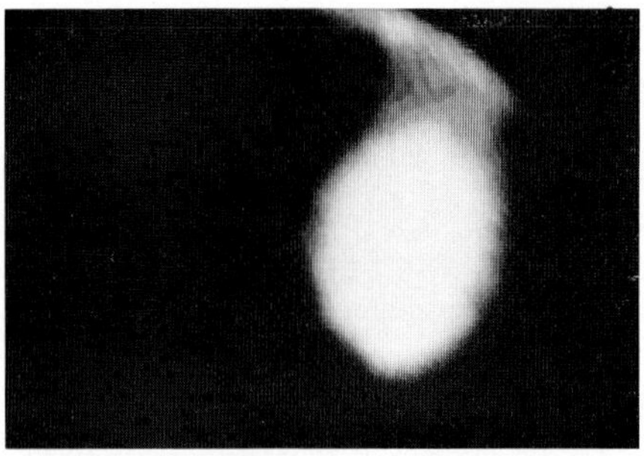

Fig. 1. Gamma camera imaging shows an intensive deposition of 111-indium-labeled autologous platelets in the graft (left iliac fossa); recurrence of hemolytic uremic syndrome after transplantation.

tration by plasma cells and lymphoblasts. Since there was no response to several grams of methylprednisolone, a transplant nephrectomy was performed. The histologic examination of this graft showed a progression of rejection with obliterative arterial lesions and parenchymal necrosis.

In March 1982, the patient underwent the second renal transplantation. Tissue typing had shown one mismatch in HLA-B and DR identity. Immunosuppression consisted of CsA (17 mg/kg body weight daily during the first 2 weeks) and prednisolone. The postoperative course was uneventful during the first 2 weeks. Plasma creatinine had decreased to 1.2 mg/dl. During the following week, the whole situation changed. The graft function deteriorated rapidly, while laboratory findings indicated the recurrence of HUS: platelet count 40,000/μl, fragmentation of red cells in peripheral blood smear, plasma bilirubin 3.8 mg/dl, lactate dehydrogenase (LDH) 1300 U/liter, fibrinogen 150 mg/dl. The labeling of autologous platelets with 111-indium-oxine was performed.[9] A massive deposition of radiolabeled platelets in the graft indicated a thrombotic process, including platelet consumption by this organ (Fig. 1). An acute rejection was rather unlikely, since fever and swelling of the graft were absent. This suspicion was confirmed by graft biopsy, which showed extensive thrombosis and glomerular capillaries and arterioles (see Fig. 2). The incubation experiments with rat aortic rings revealed that the patient plasma was not able to stimulate prostacyclin synthesis by these vascular specimens again. Since synthetic prostacyclin for treatment of platelet consumption was not available at this time, the patient received fresh plasma transfusions in an attempt to replace the missing plasma factor. However, all these treatments were in vain. The graft was removed, and the patient returned to regular hemodialysis.

DISCUSSION

We had the opportunity to observe the recurrence of HUS after renal transplantation. The question is still open as to whether HUS developed accidentally or was triggered

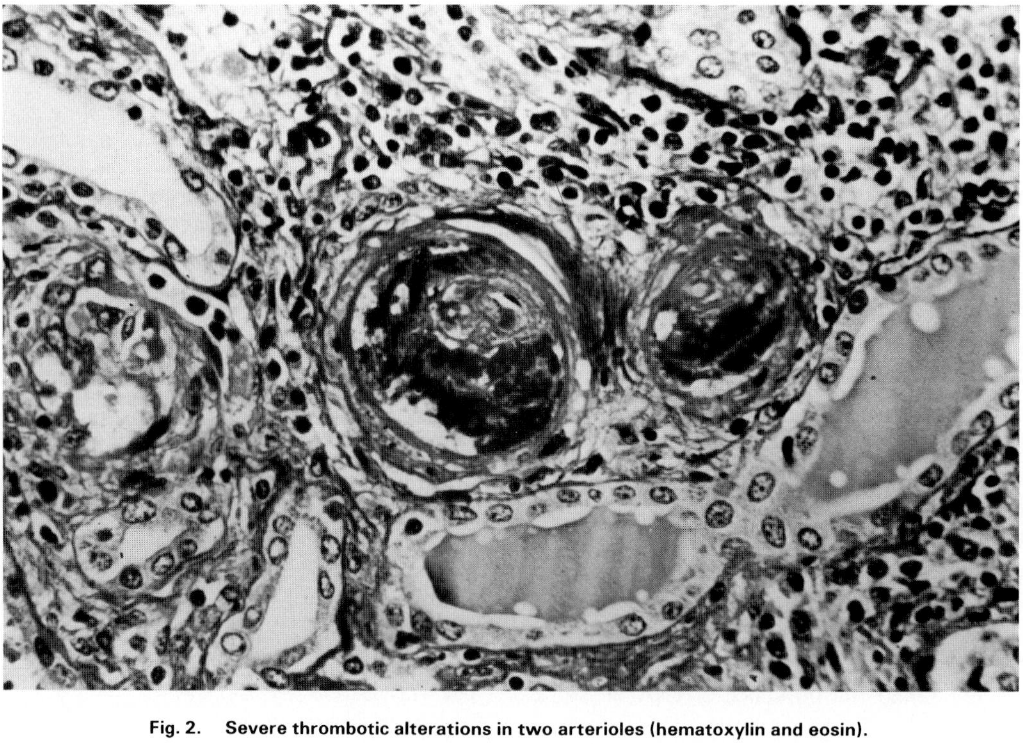

Fig. 2. Severe thrombotic alterations in two arterioles (hematoxylin and eosin).

by CsA. The arguments against a role of CsA are the following: HUS or HUS-like pictures can be encountered in acute or hyperacute transplant rejection without CsA treatment.[10] It is not always possible to discern exactly between HUS and acute transplant rejection, since both alterations of the graft are accompanied by endothelial damage, platelet deposition demonstrable with the platelet scan,[9] and a thrombotic process. There are cases in the literature, showing that the recurrence of HUS after renal transplantation may develop without CsA.[11] Recently, successful renal transplantation under CsA in a patient who had HUS as underlying renal disease has been reported.[12]

The arguments for a harmful role of CsA in our patient are as follows. In bone marrow transplant patients, HUS or related syndromes can be found under immunosuppression with CsA,[1,2] whereas conventionally treated patients are not prone to develop HUS.[2] Rocchi's finding of a depression of prostacyclin-stimulating plasma factor activity by CsA[7] seems to be conclusive. However, implications from that study are limited by the fact that a high dose of CsA (25 mg/kg) was used and that the situation in the human being could be quite different. In an attempt to solve these questions, studies on prostacyclin-stimulating plasma factor in renal transplantation are underway.

REFERENCES

1. Powles RL, Clink HM, Spence D, et al: Lancet 1:327, 1980

2. Shulman H, Striker G, Deeg HJ, et al: N Engl J Med 305:1392, 1981

3. MacIntyre DE, Pearson JD, Gordon JL: Nature 271:549, 1978

4. Leithner C, Winter M, Silberbauer KF, et al: Proc EDTA 15:418, 1978

5. Remuzzi G, Livio M, Cavenaghi AE, et al: Thromb Res 13:531, 1978

6. Remuzzi G, Marchesi D, Mecca G, et al: Lancet 1:871, 1978

7. Rocchi G, Imberti L, Fumagalli F, et al: V Int Conf Prostagland 1982, p 759 (abstr)

8. Moncada S, Higgs EA, Vane JR: Lancet 1:18, 1977

9. Leithner C, Sinzinger H, Angelberger P, et al: Lancet 2:213, 1980

10. Kohler TR, Tilney NL: Transplant Proc 14:444, 1982

11. Folman R, Arbus GS, Churchill B, et al: Clin Nephrol 10:121, 1978

12. Hamilton DV, Calne RY, Evans DB: Lancet 1:151, 1982

Lymphomas Complicating Organ Transplantation

I. Penn

THERE is an increased incidence of certain malignancies following organ transplantation and conventional immunosuppressive therapy. Mostly, these involve cancers of the skin and lips, lymphomas, in situ carcinomas of the cervix of the uterus, and carcinomas of the vulva and perineum (Table 1).[1-5] Soon after the introduction of cyclosporine-A into clinical practice, 3 lymphomas were reported among 34 transplant patients who had been treated with this agent.[6] Considerable concern arose that lymphomas might be more frequently observed after cyclosporine-A therapy than with conventional immunosuppression. To put the subject into perspective, we shall examine the problem of lymphomas that have occurred following all forms of immunosuppressive therapy, and then we shall separately consider those that arose following the use of cyclosporine-A.

LYMPHOMAS FOLLOWING ALL TYPES OF IMMUNOSUPPRESSIVE THERAPY

Incidence of Lymphomas

Up till May 1983, the Cincinnati (formerly Denver) Transplant Tumor Registry (CTTR) received data on 1767 types of tumors that arose in 1661 organ transplant recipients. Of these, 1622 patients received kidney, 33 received heart, 4 received bone marrow, and 2 received liver transplants. Lymphomas made up a disproportionately high percentage of the neoplasms seen in these patients. In the general population, they comprise 3%–4% of all malignancies. In contrast, they made up 314 of 1767 neoplasms (18%) seen in the transplant patients. However, their true incidence is higher, for if we exclude nonmelanoma skin cancers and in situ carcinomas of the cervix of the uterus, which are omitted from most cancer statistical analyses, the percentage rises to 26%, making the lymphomas the most important group of tumors seen in these patients. These findings are borne out by two epidemiologic studies done in renal transplant recipients in which the incidence of non-Hodgkin's lymphomas was increased 28-fold and 49-fold, respectively, over that observed in the age-matched population.[2]

Lymphomas are particularly prevalent in cardiac transplant recipients, making up 20 of the 34 (59%) types of malignancy noted in the 33 patients. Again, if we exclude nonmelanoma skin cancers, the incidence rises to 71%.

Age of Patients

The average age of the recipients at the time of transplantation was 39 years (range 5–70 years), much the same age as those with nonlymphomatous tumors. Of the patients with lymphomas, 54% were under 40 years of age.

Sex of Patients

Sixty-seven percent of patients were male and 33% female, similar percentages to those with nonlymphomatous tumors. These figures do not indicate that males are more prone to lymphomas than females, but merely reflect the 2:1 ratio of male-to-female patients who undergo renal transplantation.

Time of Appearance of Lymphomas

Many oncogenic stimuli in man produce their effects after a latent period lasting many years.[3,5,7] In contrast, lymphomas appear a remarkably short time after transplantation, ranging from 1 to 153.5 (average 29) months

---

From the University of Cincinnati Medical Center and Cincinnati Veterans Administration Medical Center, Cincinnati, OH.

Supported in part by Grant 6985 from the Veterans Administration.

Address reprint requests to Dr. I. Penn, University of Cinncinnati Medical Center, Cinncinnati, OH.

0041–1345/83/1505–0111$01.00/0

Table 1. De Novo Malignancies in Organ Allograft Recipients

Type of Cancer	No. of Patients*
Cancers of the skin and lips	674
Solid lymphomas	314
Reticulum cell sarcomas	155†
Kaposi's sarcomas	60†
Unclassified lymphomas	42
B-cell lymphomas	26
Hodgkin's disease	10
Lymphosarcomas	8
Plasma cell lymphomas	6
Lymphoreticular malignancies	4
Burkitt's lymphoma	1
Histiocytic medullary reticulosis	1
Mycosis fungoides	1
Carcinomas of uterus	
Cervix (111); body (12)	123
Carcinomas of the lung	86
Carcinomas of colon and rectum	66
Carcinomas of breast	55
Leukemias	45
Carcinomas of vulva and perineum (including scrotum, penis, and anus)	40
Miscellaneous	364
Total	1767

*There were 1661 patients of whom 106 had more than one type of tumor.

†One patient had Kaposi's sarcoma and a reticulum cell sarcoma.

after the operation. The interval was longer than that seen with other neoplasms that occur after transplantation, where the average interval was 58.5 months. Ten percent of lymphomas made their appearance less than 4 months after transplantation, whereas only 3% of other neoplasms appeared within this time period.

Immunosuppressive Agents Used

In the 313 patients with lymphomas, prednisone was given to 302 (96%), azathioprine in 281 (90%), antilymphocyte globulin (ALG) in 105 (34%), local radiation of the graft in 95 (30%), splenectomy in 61 (19%), actinomycin in 41 (13%), cyclophosphamide in 18 (6%), cyclosporine-A in 17 (5%), and miscellaneous other immunosuppressive treatments were used in 24 recipients.

Classification of Lymphomas

Classification of these tumors is confused by enormous differences in nomenclature. As many as 50 histologic classifications are in existence. It must be emphasized that different morphological expressions of lymphoma, which formerly were classified as separate diseases, are not absolutely distinct from one another, but frequently merge.[5] Ideally, we should classify the neoplasms according to the cell of origin, such as T cell, B cell, null cell, etc. However, only a small number of lymphomas listed in Table 1 have been studied by modern immunologic techniques. To date, all 26 cases studied have been found to be of B-cell origin.

Apart from the problem of classifying the lymphomas, pathologists have great difficulty in distinguishing certain immunoproliferative disorders from true lymphomas. The situation becomes more complicated in transplant patients, whose lymphoid tissues are exposed to a variety of foreign antigens, including those of the allograft, heterologous antilymphocyte or antithymocyte globulin, OKT_3, a broad spectrum of infectious agents, and numerous medications.[5] In one study, several posttransplant lymphomas appeared to be malignant on morphological grounds, but immunoperoxidase and cell marker techniques suggested that the lesions were polyclonal in origin.[8] They may represent a proliferative phase of poorly differentiated lymphoid cells midway in development between an Epstein-Barr virus (EBV) induced polyclonal lymphoproliferative process and a monoclonal lymphoma. A transition from polyclonal to monoclonal tumors, in association with cytogenetic transformation, has been described in three patients.[9]

Several lymphoproliferative disorders must be distinguished from lymphomas in transplant patients, including immunoblastic lymphadenopathy, lymphomatoid granulomatosis, lymphoid hyperplasia induced by antilymphocyte or antithymocyte globulin therapy, and toxoplasmosis.[5] In addition, diphenylhydantoin (Dilantin), which is used to control seizure disorders in dialysis and renal transplant patients, may cause pseudolymphomas and even lymphomas.[5]

Types of Posttransplant Lymphoma

Hodgkin's Disease

In the U.S. population, Hodgkin's disease makes up approximately 18% of lymphomas.[10] In organ transplant recipients, it was surprisingly uncommon, comprising only 10 of 314 lymphomas (3%).

In three recipients, Hodgkin's disease was localized. It involved a regional lymph node area in two patients and the liver in one recipient. The other seven patients had widespread disease, most commonly involving multiple lymph node areas.

Plasmacytoma and Multiple Myeloma

This study does not include ten patients who had multiple myeloma before transplantation or who were discovered to have the disease after transplantation, but, in retrospect, were thought to have had the malignancy before the operation was undertaken. Six recipients had myelomas that apparently developed de novo after transplantation. Three patients had plasmacytomas localized to the small intestine, large intestine, and the brain, respectively. Another three recipients had more widespread disease.

Other Non-Hodgkin's Lymphomas

Another 238 patients had other types of non-Hodgkin's lymphomas. The most frequent tumor was reticulum cell sarcoma, which occurred in 65% of patients (Table 1). This tumor is also known as a "histiocytic lymphoma," "microglioma," "immunoblastic sarcoma," "reticulo sarcoma," and "large cell lymphoma."[5]

The non-Hodgkin's lymphomas show several features that are markedly different from their behavior in the general population.[3,5] Extranodal involvement occurred in from 24% to 48% of patients in several series in the general population.[11,12] In contrast, extranodal involvement occurred in 186 of these 238 patients (78%). Most of the 52 patients with nodal involvement had widespread disease that mainly affected the liver, lungs, spleen, bone marrow, the renal allograft, and the brain. Only 3 patients had nodal disease isolated to a single area. Extranodal disease was localized to a single organ in 129 patients (69%). Of these recipients, 75 (58%) had lymphomas confined to the central nervous system (CNS). Overall, 93 of the 238 patients (39%) had CNS involvement. Patients with meningeal lesions were not included in these statistics. CNS involvement almost always affected the brain, but the spinal cord was rarely involved. Frequently, the brain tumors had a multicentric distribution. The remarkably high frequency of brain lesions contrasts with a 1% incidence of focal cerebral involvement by non-Hodgkin's lymphoma in a series of 1039 patients in the general population, in whom meningeal involvement occurred in 3.7%.[13] A possible explanation for the frequency of brain involvement is that it has poor immunologic reactions, so that lymphoma cells that arise in the brain itself or are carried there from other areas grow more readily in this relatively immunologically privileged location than in other sites.

The physician should bear in mind the possibility of a CNS lymphoma whenever a transplant patient develops neurologic symptoms.[5] A thorough workup is necessary and may include examination of the cerebrospinal fluid, computerized axial tomography, electroencephalography, radionuclide brain scan, and cerebral angiography. These tests help to exclude more common causes of neurologic symptoms in these patients, such as hypertensive encephalopathy, meningitis, brain abscess, or intracranial bleeding.

Another striking feature in the 238 recipients was frequent involvement of the allograft by lymphoma, which occurred in 31 renal transplant patients, 2 cardiac allograft recipients, and 1 hepatic transplant patient. An additional unusual manifestion was that a lymphoma presented in the soft tissues at the site of injection of antilymphocyte or antithymocyte globulin in at least 4 patients.

As lymphomas are so common in transplant patients, we might expect that leukemias, arising either from T or B lymphocytes, would also occur frequently. However, only 3 of 45 leukemias were identified as having arisen from lymphocytes. The majority arose from granulocytes and, less frequently, from monocytes.[5]

As substantial numbers of donor lymphocytes are inevitably transplanted with the allograft, questions arise as to whether the lymphomas are of donor or host origin. In animal experiments, most posttransplant lymphomas arise from host lymphocytes. In man, studies to determine donor or host origin of lymphomas have involved studies of sex chromatin, HLA specificities, and DNA restriction fragment length polymorphisms using donor and recipient lymphocytes and lymphoma cells. Of 8 lymphomas studied, 6 were of host origin and occurred in 5 renal and 1 hepatic allograft recipient, and 2 were of donor origin and occurred in bone marrow transplant patients.[5,14]

Kaposi's Sarcoma (KS)

In the general population of the U.S., KS makes up 0.02%–0.07% of all malignancies. In transplant patients, 60 of 1767 (3.3%) cancers were KS. If we exclude nonmelanoma skin cancers and in situ carcinomas of the cervix of the uterus the incidence rises to 4.9%, a remarkable figure, comparable to that seen in endemic areas of tropical Africa.

The frequent occurrence of KS in transplant patients is similar to the situation in the acquired immunodeficiency syndrome (AIDS), which afflicts male homosexuals, Haitian immigrants to the U.S., intravenous drug abusers, and hemophiliac patients. Features common to transplant and AIDS patients are marked immunosuppression; a high incidence of *Pneumocystis carinii* pneumonia, cytomegalovirus (CMV), Epstein-Barr virus (EBV) and other opportunistic infections; and the frequent development of KS. Of the transplant patients, 39 were male and 21 female, the same 2:1 ratio observed in transplant patients having other malignancies but very different from the 9:1 to 15:1 ratio seen with KS in the general population. KS appeared a remarkably short time after transplantation, an average of 17 (range 2.5–101) months. In the general population, this neoplasm occurs mainly in blacks in tropical Africa and in whites of Central and Eastern European Jewish origin or of South European ancestry. In transplant patients, the 60 cases occurred in 10 patients of Jewish background (including 9 Israelis), 8 blacks, 19 non-Israeli patients of "mediterranean" origins (Saudi Arabia, Yemen, Algeria, Italy, Greece, Spain, and Portugal), and the remainder of varying ancestries.

Six of the 60 patients (10%) had other malignancies, a figure comparable to that seen in the general population. Of the 60 patients, 42 (70%) had "benign" KS involving the skin, conjunctiva, or oropharyngolaryngeal mucosa, and 18 (30%) had the "malignant" variety with involvement of the internal organs, particularly the gastrointestinal tract and the respiratory system. Of the 42 patients with "benign" disease, 24 (57%) had complete remissions following treatment. Five of these 24 remissions (21%) occurred when the *only* treatment given consisted of a drastic reduction of immunosuppressive therapy. (This contrasts with a spontaneous remission rate of 2% in the general population.) The other remissions required surgery, radiotherapy, or chemotherapy. In the malignant group, 3 patients (17%) had complete remissions after chemotherapy or radiotherapy together with alteration of immunosuppressive therapy.

An important lesson is that we should suspect Kaposi's sarcoma whenever a transplant recipient develops reddish blue macules or plaques in the skin or oropharyngeal mucosa, or apparently infected granulomas that fail to heal. If the diagnosis is confirmed, a thorough workup is necessary to exclude any internal visceral involvement.[5]

Prognosis of Lymphomas

Modern techniques of radiotherapy or combination chemotherapy or of both have greatly improved the prognosis of patients in the general population suffering from Hodgkin's disease and non-Hodgkin's lymphomas. In contrast, lymphomas in transplant patients have a poor prognosis. Only 19% of patients with non-Kaposi's lymphomas are currently alive. Admittedly not all the deaths were from lymphomas, but the dismal outlook for these patients is borne out by a study of the mortality of renal transplant recipients with lymphoma, showing a 48-fold increase over that seen in the general population.[1]

Of the KS patients with visceral involvement, 4 of 18 (22%) are alive. Nearly all the deaths were related to the KS. Twenty-seven of 42 patients (64%) with nonvisceral KS are alive. Fatalities were generally from causes other than KS.

Treatment of Lymphomas

It is important to distinguish between polyclonal and monoclonal lymphomas. The former group may respond to treatment with antiviral agents, such as acyclovir or interferon.[8] The latter group require treatment with surgery, radiotherapy, chemotherapy, or combined modality treatment. Questions arise as to whether immunosuppressive therapy should be drastically reduced. As mentioned, this has worked well in several patients with nonvisceral KS and also in occasional patients with other lymphomas.[5]

Should the physician choose to continue with the patient's usual dose of immunosuppressive agents, there is a risk of excessive depression of the bone marrow if chemotherapeutic agents are used concomitantly to treat the lymphoma. Since many of the chemotherapeutic agents used in the treatment of lymphomas have immunosuppresive side effects, reduction or cessation of immunosuppressive therapy does not inevitably result in rejection of the organ allograft. However, if a renal allograft does undergo rejection, it should be removed and the patient maintained on dialysis.

LYMPHOMAS FOLLOWING THE USE OF CYCLOSPORINE-A

Thus far, between 2000 and 2500 patients have been treated with cyclosporine-A. To date, the CTTR has received data on 23 patients who developed malignancies following its use.[4] Fifteen were renal allograft recipients, 6 were cardiac allograft patients, and 2 received bone marrow transplants. The average age of the recipients at the time of transplantation was very similar to that of patients who developed neoplasms after conventional immunosuppressive therapy for organ transplantation. Eighteen of the recipients were male and 5 female.

The tumors that occurred were lymphomas (17), nonmelanoma skin cancers (2), carcinoma of the colon (1), carcinoma of the nasopharynx (1), carcinoma of the kidney (1), and a neuro-ectodermal tumor of the brain (1). The author is aware of several other cancers that occurred after the use of cyclosporine-A, but these have not yet been reported to the CTTR. We shall restrict our analysis only to the patients with lymphomas. If we exclude the nonmelanoma skin cancers, the lymphomas made up 81% of the neoplasms reported.

The lymphomas appeared in a remarkably short time after transplantation—between 1 and 17 months (average 6 months). This contrasts sharply with a time range of 1–153.5 months (average 30 months) for lymphomas that appeared after conventional immunosuppression given after organ transplantation. Six lymphomas were reticulum cell sarcomas, 5 were B-cell tumors, in 4 instances the type of lymphoma was not specified, and there were 2 cases of KS.

Nine of the non-Kaposi's lymphomas were widespread and six were localized to a single viscus or area of the body. In contrast with lymphomas seen in patients receiving conventional immunosuppression, in whom involvement of the CNS was common, none of the cyclosporine-A treated patients had this problem. The organs most commonly involved were the lungs (5 patients), lymph nodes (4), small bowel (3), liver (3), and the heart (3). In 2 of the 3 recipients with cardiac involvement, the lymphomas involved the cardiac allograft itself. In contrast with the lymphomas seen in cyclosporine-A-treated animals, in which at least 9 of 12 monkeys had lymph node involvement,[15] this occurred in only 4 of 15 patients. The two patients with KS had involvement of the skin only.

Seven of the patients are alive, two with KS, three with localized lymphomas, and two with widespread lymphomas. Of the ten patients who died, the malignancy caused the deaths of five patients and coronary artery disease of a sixth recipient. The cause of death of four patients is unknown. In five of the ten patients who died, the tumor was first recognized at autopsy examination.

In studies of lymphomas that developed in monkeys following the use of cyclosporine-A, it was noted that only 2 of the 12 animals were treated only with this agent. Similarly, in the patients in this series, only 1 of the 17 with lymphomas was treated only with cyclosporine-A. (Of the 6 patients with nonlymphomatous tumors, 2 had received cyclosporine-A exclusively.) Other immunosuppressive agents[15] included prednisone (16 patients), ALG (6), splenectomy (3), azathioprine (1), cytimun (1), and thoracic duct drainage (1).

POSSIBLE CAUSES OF POSTTRANSPLANT LYMPHOMAS

Multiple factors probably play a role in the etiology of the various tumors that arise de novo after transplantation.[2,3,5,7] They include disturbances of immunity; oncogenic viruses; oncogenic effects of immunosuppressive agents; possible co-oncogenic properties of these compounds; other potentially oncogenic treatments; and variations in individual susceptibility to neoplasia. Space limitations permit only a brief discussion of these possibilities, which are considered in detail elsewhere.[3,5] We shall consider those factors that account for the disproportionately high incidence of lymphomas.

One possibility is depressed natural killer (NK) cell activity.[3,5,7] Beige mice, which have a selective and marked defect in NK activity, have a high incidence of lymphomas. Patients with the Chediak-Higashi syndrome have a similar immune defect and are often afflicted by lymphoproliferative diseases. The frequent occurrence of lymphomas in transplant patients may also be related to severely depressed NK activity.

Repeated or continuous administration of foreign antigens causes a high incidence of malignant lymphomas in several experimental models.[3,5,7] Chronic stimulation of lymphoid tissues may lead to hyperplasia, which may progress to neoplasia. Chronic antigenic stimulation may also cause lymphomas through the immunologic activation of endogenous C-type oncornaviruses. The frequent occurrence of lymphomas in transplant patients may be related to the prolonged presence of the allograft with its foreign histocompatibility antigens, or to antigenic stimulation from the infections to which the recipients are so prone.

Impaired immunoregulation is another possible mechanism responsible for the development of posttransplant lymphomas.[3,5,7] Since cellular and humoral feedback mechanisms are important in controlling the extent of immune reactions, impaired control may allow the unrestrained proliferation of lymphoid cells and ultimately lead to the development of lymphomas. According to one theory, thymic suppressor function, which normally restricts lymphoid proliferation, is defective and permits unregulated growth and lymphomagenesis. Once loss of regulation occurs, the defensive ability of the immune system is impaired and other, nonlymphoid, malignancies may appear.

Another hypothesis is based on observations that immunologic reactions may activate latent oncogenic viruses and that continuous antigenic stimulation of partially immunodeficient mice may lead to the development of lymphoreticular tumors.[3,5,7] Since many transplant patients are only partially immunodeficient, it is postulated that defective antibody production fails to control lymphocyte proliferation and leads to derepression of the virogene and the activation of oncogenic viruses in an environment that favors their replication. Viruses shed from lymphoblasts infect cells in the microenvironment of the immunologic reaction and cause their malignant transformation.

Certain drugs may predispose patients to the development of lymphomas.[3,5,7] As mentioned above, the chronic administration of diphenylhydantoin (Dilantin) may cause pseudolymphomas and even lymphomas.

The short induction time of many of the lymphomas is compatible with a viral etiology.[2,3,5,7] Oncogenic viruses may be activated in transplant patients by two mechanisms: (A) as mentioned above, an immunologic reaction, such as rejection of a transplanted organ, may activate latent endogenous oncornaviruses; (B) immunosuppressed individuals are susceptible to a great variety of infectious agents, including viruses. EBV infections are common and posttransplant lymphoma cells have been found to contain EBV nuclear antigen. In addition, EBV-specific DNA sequences have been found incorporated into the human genome of these cells.[9] EBV is therefore strongly suspected as a cause of at least some posttransplant lymphomas. One question arises: If EBV causes lymphomas in organ transplant recipients, why is there no increase in the incidence in these individuals of the other human malignancy that is believed to be EBV-related, namely, nasopharyngeal carcinoma?[5]

CMV has been isolated from tissue cultures of KS in the general population. It also may be responsible for the outbreak of KS in the AIDS and for the high incidence of this disease in transplant patients.[5]

Another theory that may explain the frequent occurrence of KS in organ transplant recipients implicates a chronic immunologic reaction between antigenically altered lymphoid cells and normal lymphocytes.[5] In the course of this local graft-versus-host reaction, an angiogenesis factor is liberated and intense proliferation of mesenchymal and endothelial cells occurs. During this process, an oncogenic virus is either transferred to, or induced in, the cells responsive to the angiogenesis factor and induces their malignant transformation.

CONCLUSIONS

In reviewing the entire experience with cancers in the 1661 patients in this series, it appears that the increased incidence of cancers, and particularly of lymphomas, cannot be blamed on any single immunosuppressive agent but, rather, it is a complication of immunosuppression per se.[3,5] Concern has been expressed regarding the apparently high incidence of lymphomas following the use of cyclosporine-A. In part, this problem may be dose related.[4,16] In one study, lymphomas occurred after use of large doses of the drug, but when dosage was reduced, none was observed.[16] In addition, the length of follow-up after the use of cyclosporine-A has been short. We have mentioned that most lymphomas appear a few months after immunosuppressive therapy is started, while other malignancies manifest themselves after a longer period of time. It is therefore possible that experience with cyclosporine-A may mimic that seen with conventional immunosuppression when, early after transplantation, the most common tumors were lymphomas, but with longer follow-up, other tumor types were observed.[4] Long-term follow-up of large numbers of patients treated *exclusively* with cyclosporine-A will clarify the carcinogenic potential of this agent in man.

ACKNOWLEDGMENT

The author wishes to thank his many colleagues throughout the world who have generously contributed data concerning their patients to the CTTR.

REFERENCES

Space limitations prevent the inclusion of many references. They are listed in the references cited below.

1. Kinlen LJ, Sheil AGR, Peto J, et al: Br Med J 2:1461, 1979
2. Kinlen L: Cancer Surveys 1:565, 1982
3. Penn I: Curr Prob Cancer 6:1, 1982
4. Penn I: Cancer Surveys 1:621, 1982
5. Penn I: In Purtilo DT (ed): Immune Deficiency and Cancer: Epstein-Barr Virus and Lymphoproliferative Malignancies. New York, Plenum (in press)
6. Calne RY, White DJG, Rolles K, et al: Lancet 2:1022, 1979

7. Penn I: Cancer Surveys 1:763, 1982
8. Hanto DW, Sakamoto K, Purtilo DT, et al: Surgery 90:204, 1981
9. Hanto DW: Ann Surg (in press)
10. Silverberg E: Cancer 33:9, 1983
11. Freeman C, Berg JW, Cutler SJ: Cancer 29:252, 1972
12. Reddy S, Pellettiere E, Saxena V, et al: 46:1925, 1980
13. Herman TS, Hammond N, Jones SE, et al: Cancer 43:390, 1979
14. Schubach WH, Hackman R, Neiman PE, et al: Blood 60:180, 1982
15. Reitz BA, Bieber CP: Cancer Surveys 1:613, 1982
16. Calne RY, Rolles K, White DJG, et al: Transplant Proc 13:349, 1981

Immunoglobulin Abnormalities and Infectious Lymphoproliferative Syndrome (ILPS) in Cyclosporine-Treated Transplant Patients

J. L. Touraine, S. El Yafi, E. Bosi, C. Chapuis-Cellier, J. Ritter, N. Blanc, J. M. Dubernard, C. Pouteil-Noble, M. Chevallier, R. Creyssel, and J. Traeger

CYCLOSPORINE-A (CsA) and antilymphocyte globulins (ALG) have been administered routinely in our institution to patients with a contraindication to azathioprine and/or prednisone treatment. In a period of 5 months, 8 patients (including 1 patient not receiving CsA) developed an acute and rapidly progressing B-cell lymphoma associated with clinical symptoms of infection. This infectious lymphoproliferative syndrome (ILPS) was characterized by the presence of monoclonal or oligoclonal immunoglobulins (Ig). It was responsible for the death of six patients. Besides suggesting the possible danger of CsA and ALG association, it prompted us to investigate more thoroughly the heterogeneity of Ig in patients under CsA treatment or under conventional immunosuppression.

MATERIALS AND METHODS

Two hundred twenty-seven patients (in or out of hospital) with kidney or kidney and pancreas transplants were investigated over a 6-month period. This population included (A) 167 patients receiving azathioprine and prednisone (±ALG) for periods of time varying between 3 months and 12 years, and (B) 60 patients receiving CsA (12 mg/kg/day) and ALG (±prednisone) for 2 weeks to 2 years. Some patients were given CsA and ALG concomitantly, others sequentially with an overlap of 2 or 3 days only. Clinical characteristics of patients with acute ILPS and their immunosuppressive schedules are summarized in Table 1.

Immunoglobulin heterogeneity was investigated by isoelectric focusing on thin-layer (500 μm) acrylamide gel (T4C3) in a 3.5–9.5 pH gradient.[1]

B lymphocytes and plasma cells were studied for surface or intracytoplasmic Ig by immunofluorescence with monospecific antibodies. T-lymphocyte subsets were repeatedly determined in the peripheral blood of two patients, using monoclonal antibodies of the OKT series (Ortho Pharmaceuticals, NJ). Cytomegalovirus (CMV) was weekly searched for in the urine. CMV, Herpes simplex (HSV), Herpes zoster (HZV), parainfluenza virus, influenza virus, adenovirus, and Epstein-Barr virus (EBV) (VCA, EA, and EBNA) serologies were also routinely performed. Autopsy was performed in two patients, but permission was not granted in four other patients in whom pathology investigations were limited to biopsies.

RESULTS

Immunoglobulin Abnormalities

Among the 60 CsA-treated patients, 33 had no restriction of Ig heterogeneity (26 being totally normal, 7 being hyper- or hypoimmunoglobulinemic); 11 had a significant restriction of heterogeneity and 16 had well characterized monoclonal or oligoclonal Ig components.

Among the 167 patients under conventional immunosuppression, 131 had no restriction of Ig heterogeneity, 29 had a mild, and 2 a significant, restriction of heterogeneity; 5 patients only had well characterized monoclonal or oligoclonal Ig components.

Infectious Lymphoproliferative Syndrome

Seven of the 16 CsA-treated patients with oligoclonal Ig components and 1 of the 5 azathioprine-treated patients with oligoclonal Ig components developed the ILPS rapidly after the transplant. In most patients, CsA was given from the day of the transplant or a few weeks later to substitute for azathioprine in leukopenic patients (without demonstrated viral infection at this time). Fever occurred as

---

From the Clinic of Nephrology, INSERM U80, and the Laboratory of Biochemistry B, Hôpital Edouard Herriot, Lyon, France; and Clinica Medica VIII, San Raffaele University Hospital, Milan, Italy.

Address reprint requests to Dr. J. L. Touraine, Hôpital Edouard Herriot, Pavillon P, 69374 Lyon Cedex 08, France.

0041-1345/83/1505-0112$01.00/0

Table 1. General Characteristics of Patients With ILPS

Patients	Sex	Age (Year)	Type of Transplant	Donor	HLA Antigens (A/B)	HLA-AB Donor/Recip. Mismatches	Immunosuppression: Prior Tx	After Tx [Doses mg/kg/day × Duration (Days)]: Azathioprine	ALG	Steroids	CsA	Final Outcome
1	M	51	K + P	Cadaver	2–9/35	3	BT	2.48 × 23	9.14 × 128	0.65 × 132	10.7 × 94	Death 150 days after Tx
2	F	48	K	Related	1–9/18–35	1	TDD + BT	2.75 × 18	10 × 37	1.2 × 42	10.6 × 19	Death 42 days after Tx
3	M	46	K + P	Cadaver	1–3/15	2	BT	2.2 × 38	6.3 × 49	1.07 × 56	10.9 × 15	Death 56 days after Tx
4	M	47	K	Cadaver	2–9/12–15	4	TDD + BT	0.62 × 8	8.3 × 28	0.91 × 48	10 × 35	Death 48 days after Tx
5	M	40	K + P	Cadaver	3/15–35	3	BT	2.5 × 19	5.7 × 43	1.35 × 49	10.8 × 26	Death 49 days after Tx
6	M	33	K	Related	2–31/5–40	2	TDD + BT	1.37 × 23	6.1 × 32	2.23 × 38	0	Death 38 days after Tx
7	M	56	K	Cadaver	11–29/35–41	4	BT	*2.17 × 6	*6.5 × 39	*0.75 × 83	*6.9 × 76	Alive with functioning graft at 1 year
8	M	52	K	Cadaver	2–32/8–35	3	BT	*2.02 × 21	*7 × 31	*1.05 × 42	*11.2 × 16	Alive with functioning graft at 7 months

K, kidney; P, pancreas; TDD, thoracic duct drainage; BT, blood transfusions (random).
*Doses calculated at the time of onset of the Ig abnormality.

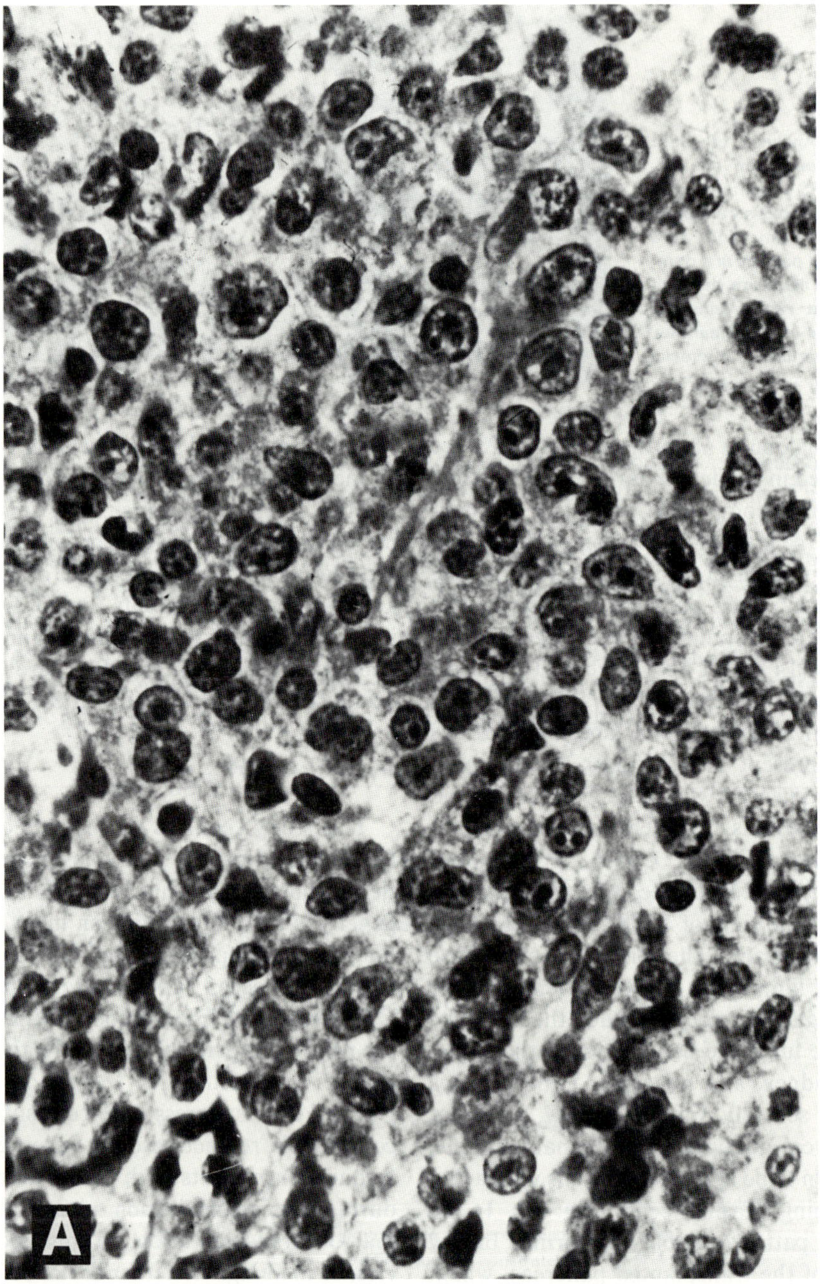

Fig. 3. Lymphomatous infiltration of the liver. Optic and immunofluorescence microscopy with anti-μ antiserum.

or in association with ATG or TLI, similarly developed a lymphoma.[8]

In our group of patients, an outbreak of lymphoma has been observed in less than 6 months, while none was detected among the 677 previous transplant patients. The development of lymphoma was not strictly dependent on CsA treatment, since one patient received azathioprine, steroids, and ALG only. However, a much higher frequency of lymphoma

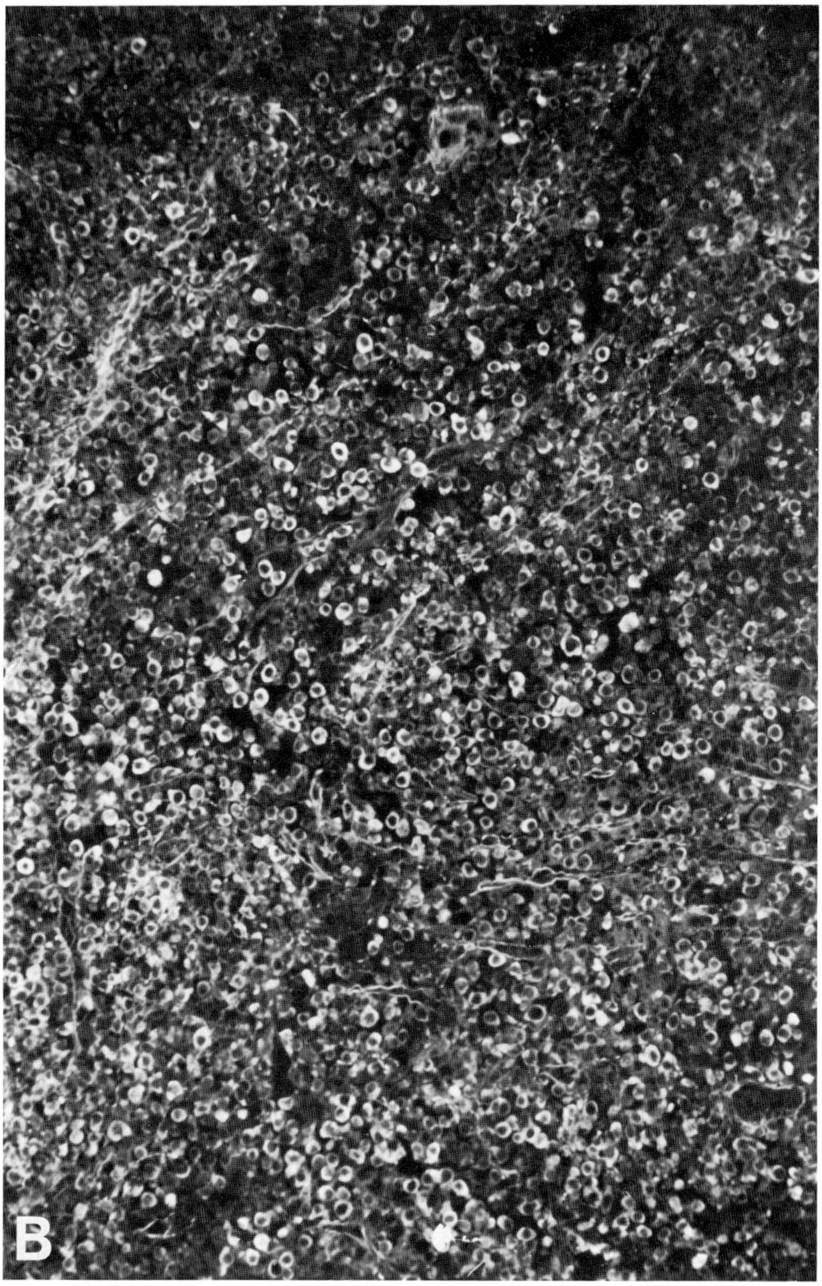

Fig. 3. Continued.

appeared to result from CsA treatment given in association with ALG. The initiation of lymphoma appeared to be very precocious after the transplant, to be rapidly progressing, and to be associated with a viral infection. The nature of the very virus responsible for this severe condition is still debatable. EBV would be a good candidate, since it activates B cells and can induce their transformation, especially in the face of insufficient T-cell "surveillance." Our results cannot, however, support the role of EBV conclusively. Several patients had no modification of EBV serology, and the alterations observed in the others may merely result from the severe immunosuppression aggravated at the time of ILPS. On the other hand, serology, in this type of patient, does not enable us to rule out a possibly important part played by EBV. Several other seroconversions for a variety of viruses have also been noted, but they may also be secondary rather than causal in ILPS. Additional investigations are currently being performed to look for human T leukemia virus (HTLV) and a number of other viruses. Whatever viral infection may be responsible for this complication, it is likely to result either from reactivation of an endogeneous virus or from transmission of a virus among patients by the means of blood transfusions.

Interestingly, an initial stage of this B-cell proliferative syndrome appears to be nonmalignant and reversible when immunosuppressive therapy is withdrawn. Production of oligoclonal Ig develops at this phase. Whether the viral infection intervenes early or after this development of restricted B-cell clones is speculative.

Finally, it may be noted that the T4+ lymphocyte subset is dramatically decreased in the peripheral blood of these patients during ILPS, to a degree comparable to findings in AIDS patients, and that correction of this abnormality is slow (over 2 months) in the surviving patients.

ACKNOWLEDGMENT

We thank Pr. P. A. Bryon and Drs. G. Lenoir, F. Touraine, S. Bosshard, and O. Gentilhomme for several of the tests performed. We are also grateful to Sandoz, Ltd., for help throughout these studies.

REFERENCES

1. Chapuis-Cellier C, Francina A, Arnaud P: In Radola BJ (ed): Electrophoresis 79. Berlin, W. De Gruyter, 1980, p 711

2. Radl J: In Adler WH, Nordin AA, Adelman RC, et al (eds): Immunological Techniques Applied to Aging Research. Boca Raton, FL, CRC Press, 1981, p 121

3. Penn I: Transplant Proc 11:1047, 1979

4. Calne RY, Rolles K, White DJG, et al: Lancet 2:1033, 1979

5. Crawford DH, Thomas JA, Janossy G, et al: Lancet 1:1355, 1980

6. Jacobs P, Gordon-Smith EC: Lancet 2:1296, 1980

7. Sandoz report on the first 1500 patients treated with CsA (personal communication)

8. Reitz BA, Bieder CP, Pennock JL: In White DJG (ed): Cyclosporin A. Amsterdam, Elsevier, 1982, p 317

Histiocytic Lymphoma in Renal Transplant Patients Receiving Cyclosporine

J. T. Rosenthal, S. Iwatsuki, T. E. Starzl, R. J. Taylor, and T. R. Hakala

THE higher incidence of cancer in immunosuppressed patients over the general population has long been recognized. A high percentage of these cancers have been called lymphomas. The first clinical trial of cyclosporine for renal transplantation reported by Calne et al.[1] included almost a 10% incidence of lymphoma (3/32). Concern was expressed for the ultimate utility of cyclosporine based on this experience. We now have experience in over 300 cases of cadaveric renal transplantation over a 3.5-year period. In this article we present the experience with lymphoma in these patients, documenting incidence, clinical presentation, treatment, and outcome following cadaveric renal transplantation.

From December 1979 to September 1980, 66 patients underwent cadaveric renal transplantation in Denver in the first trials with cyclosporine and steroid combination. The results of that trial have been reported in detail by Starzl et al.[2,3] From March 1981 to 1983 an additional 244 patients have undergone cadaveric renal transplantation in Pittsburgh, using the same immunosuppression regimen. The results of this experience have been reported.[4,5] Immunosuppression consisted of cyclosporine, 17.5 mg/kg/day, begun by mouth pretransplant and daily thereafter. Tapering occurred from 2 weeks to 6 months posttransplant. The average cyclosporine dose at 1 year posttransplant was 6 mg/kg/day. Methylprednisolone, 1 g, was given i.v. pretransplant. Prednisone was begun by mouth on day 1 posttransplant and tapered over 5 days to 20 mg/day. By 1 year, the average prednisone dose was 10 mg/day.

Six patients of the 310 (1.9%) developed "lymphoma" during the course of these trials. Two of these have been reported in detail.[2,6] Four additional cases will be discussed here in addition to these two. The clinical features of the patients are shown in Table 1. These were 5 males and 1 female; age ranged from 16 years to 57 years. Five patients developed bowel lesions, which were manifested by perforation and peritonitis. One patient developed a painless neck swelling. The time of development of the lesion was 3–6 months posttransplant. The first patient from the Denver series was receiving 16 mg/kg/day of cyclosporine at the time of development of lymphoma at 6 months posttransplant. The other 5 patients were receiving 6–11 mg/kg/day cyclosporine 3–5 months posttransplant at the time of development of lymphoma. Only one patient had been treated for rejection; this consisted of recycling of oral steroid to 200 mg/day, with a 5-day taper again to 20 mg/day. Three patients had oral herpes within 1–2 months of transplantation, while 2 patients had elevated serum creatinine indicative of cyclosporine nephrotoxicity.

The five patients with bowel lesions underwent resection of the affected segment and prompt reduction in the dose of cyclosporine. Two of these patients received small doses of cytotoxic drugs before the lesions were adequately characterized. One patient received small doses of acyclovir. The others had the cyclosporine dose reduced, but received no other treatment. The patient with the neck mass received local radiation, primarily because most of the lesion was necrotic and could not adequately be characterized. No systemic therapy was undertaken in this patient, except to lower the cyclosporine dose. Dose adjustment was in the range of 1–3 mg/kg/day cyclosporine.

From the Division of Urology, Department of Surgery, University of Pittsburgh, Pittsburgh, PA.

Address reprint requests to Dr. J. T. Rosenthal, Division of Urology, Department of Surgery, University of Pittsburgh, Pittsburgh, PA 15261.

0041-1345/83/1505-0113$01.00/0

Table 1. Clinical Features

Patient	Age/Sex	Cyclosporine Dose (mg/kg/Day)	Site	Time After Transplant
L.P.	25F	16	Bowel	6 Months
S.C.	21M	10	Bowel	5 Months
A.L.	49M	6	Neck	3 Months
P.L.	57M	8	Bowel, prostate	4 Months
E.F.	30M	10	Bowel	4 Months
L.S.	16M	8	Bowel	3 Months

All 6 patients so treated are alive and well 3 months to 4 years after treatment (Table 2). Two patients suffered irreversible rejection of the graft when immunosuppression was decreased. The other 4 patients have normal renal function.

Interpretation of the histopathology in each case was histiocytic lymphoma. Four lesions were subsequently characterized as polyclonal B-cell masses by immunoperoxidase staining. The neck mass tissue was mostly necrotic, precluding characterization. The tumor mass from one patient showed no immunoglobulin. Most of the tissue resected from the bowel was necrotic also, so that EBNA was identified in only one tumor. This also prevented DNA hybridization studies for Epstein-Barr virus (EBV) genome. Serology to EBV disclosed evidence of primary infection in one patient (L.P.) previously reported[2] and reinfection in another (E.F.), manifested by a threefold rise in antibody titer to viral capsid antigen (Table 3).

Table 2. Treatment and Outcome

Patient	Treatment	Patient Survival	Graft Survival
L.P.	Bowel resection Decrease cyclosporine	Yes	Yes
S.C.	Bowel resection Decrease cyclosporine	Yes	Yes
A.L.	Local radiation Decrease cyclosporine	Yes	Yes
P.L.	Bowel resection Decrease cyclosporine Chemo Rx	Yes	Yes
E.F.	Bowel resection Decrease cyclosporine Chemo Rx	Yes	No
L.S.	Bowel resection Decrease cyclosporine	Yes	No

DISCUSSION

Because of the high incidence of lymphoma in the early experience with cyclosporine, it was feared that the drug itself was more tumorogenic than conventional immunosuppression regimens and that its use would be severely limited by this fact. Two issues are of concern; one is the incidence, and the other is the clinical significance of these lesions. Overall incidence of lymphoma reported here is 1.9%, considerably less than the feared 10% and comparable to the 2.5% reported by Bird[7] in cyclosporine-treated cases and comparable to the incidence reported in cadaveric renal transplantation under conventional immunosuppression.[8] Evidence that the development of these lesions is related to the general level of immunosuppression comes from the higher incidence of tumors reported from cardiac transplantation,[9] where immunosuppression may be maintained at a higher level out of necessity.

The role of Epstein-Barr virus in the development of these lymphomas has been well described.[10] Epstein-Barr virus is implicated directly or indirectly in 3 of the 6 patients reported here. The majority of these lesions

Table 3. Immunologic Studies

L.P.	Polyclonal B cell	Primary EBV infection
S.C.	No immunoglobulin	EBNA positive
A.L.	—	—
P.L.	Polyclonal B cell	—
E.F.	Polyclonal B cell	Reactivation EBV infection
L.S.	Polyclonal B cell	Pending

have been found to be polyclonal, as opposed to monoclonality of killing lymphoma. Whether or not they can be distinguished by morphology is not clear.[11] All the material in our six cases was interpreted as histiocytic lymphoma prior to immunologic examination. When polyclonality is determined, the term lymphoproliferative disorder is more appropriate, or perhaps pseudolymphoma, as described by Iwatsuki.[12] The issue is of more than academic interest, since there is great enthusiasm for the use of cytotoxic drugs when the clinical diagnosis of histiocytic lymphoma appears on the chart. Previously, there was a high mortality, two of three in Calne's first group,[1] and five of six in the cases reported by Hanto.[10] If this is a virally induced B-cell proliferation, maintenance of immunosuppression and the use of cytotoxic drugs would be counterproductive. Iwatsuki treated three patients by reduction of immunosuppression only, with good outcome in all three patients.[12] In our six patients, only two received small doses of cytotoxic drugs before the exact nature of their lesions could be discerned. In all six cases, significant reductions in immune suppression were carried out immediately. Prompt resolution occurred in all patients so treated. The effectiveness of this maneuver was vividly documented in one patient who required repeat laparotomy for persistent GI bleeding. This was found to be suture line bleeding and was corrected by repeat resection. At the time of this repeat resection, 1 month following his original operation, large bowel lesions that had been seen at the first operation and left in place were entirely resolved. The question of transformation from polyclonal to monoclonal cannot be answered from the clinical data presently available. It has been suggested that monoclonal lesions in transplant patients are killing cancer and associated with development of chromosomal abnormalities in the B cells so transformed by virus.[13]

CONCLUSION

Incidence of lymphoma using cyclosporine and steroid is no different than in transplantation under conventional immunosuppression. Most of these lesions are more appropriately called lymphoproliferative disorders despite their histologic appearance. When the masses are polyclonal, prompt reduction in immunosuppression should result in excellent survival. The role for additional antiviral agents for treatment is unclear, but played no role here. Cytotoxic drugs should be avoided.

REFERENCES

1. Calne RY, Rolles K, White DJG, et al: Lancet 2:1033, 1979
2. Starzl TE, Klintmalm GBB, Wile R, et al: Surg Gynecol Obstet 153:486, 1981
3. Starzl TE, Hakala TR, Rosenthal JT, et al: Transplant Proc (this issue)
4. Hakala TR, Starzl TE, Rosenthal JT, et al: Transplant Proc 15:465, 1983
5. Rosenthal JT, Hakala TR, Starzl TE, et al: J Urol (in press)
6. Starzl TE, Hakala TR, Rosenthal JT, et al: Surg Gynecol Obstet 154:819, 1982
7. Bird AG: In White DJG (ed): Cyclosporin A. Amsterdam, Elsevier Biomedical, 1982
8. Penn I: Transplant Proc 13:736, 1981
9. Lanza RP, Cooper DKC, Cassidy MJD, et al: JAMA 249:1746, 1983
10. Hanto DW, Frizzera G, Purtilo DT, et al: Cancer Res 41:4253, 1981
11. Frizzera G, Hanto DW, Gajl-Peczalska KJ, et al: Cancer Res 41:4262, 1981
12. Iwatsuki S, Geis WP, Molnar Z, et al: J Surg Res 24:428, 1978
13. Klein G: Proc Natl Acad Sci USA 76:2442, 1979

Malignant Lymphoma in Nontransplanted Cynomolgus Monkeys Receiving Cyclosporine

N. L. Garnett, H. R. Taylor, G. J. Hoffman, R. L. Heberling, R. F. Ambinder, A. C. Huber, and B. A. Valentine

MALIGNANT lymphoma is a well documented complication of organ transplantation in both human and nonhuman primate recipients.[1–5] The relative contributions of immunosuppressive drugs, oncogenic viruses, transplantation, and other host factors in the pathogenesis of the posttransplantation lymphoma remain unresolved.[6]

The number of variables involved and the possibility of a multifactorial etiology make these lymphomas difficult to investigate in human patients. Compelling evidence has been presented to support the theory that cyclosporine-A (CsA), either as the sole drug or in combination with other immunosuppressive drugs, allows for the reactivation of Epstein-Barr virus (EBV) or other viruses, with subsequent polyclonal B-cell activation, proliferation, and eventual conversion to a monoclonal B-cell lymphoma.[1,5,7] In other studies, a chromosomal cytogenetic change has been associated with the progression from benign lymphoid hyperplasia to lymphoma.[8,9]

The extensive experience of Reitz et al.[2–4] with the use of CsA in the nonhuman primate cardiac allograft model suggests a higher risk of lymphoma in transplanted monkeys receiving CsA, either alone or in combination with conventional immunosuppressive therapy, than in those receiving conventional therapy only. This finding must be interpreted with caution, due to the greatly increased survival time, and therefore longer period at risk, for those monkeys receiving CsA.

In this article, we document the occurrence of lymphoma in two of a group of five cynomolgus monkeys (*Macaca fascicularis*) that were given CsA as part of a study on the pathogenesis of ocular infection due to *Chlamydia trachomatis*.[10] The case studies are significant due to the absence of the complicated variables of transplantation and multiple immunosuppressive drugs. The possible association of these tumors with oncogenic virus is examined. Clinical data and the results of retrospective studies conducted on the available tissues, sera, and cell cultures are presented.

MATERIALS AND METHODS

Animals

All five monkeys in this study group were received at Johns Hopkins University from Hazelton Laboratories, Alice, TX. They were all males between 18 and 19 months of age and weighed between 1.4 and 1.8 kg. Routine quarantine procedures included 3 tuberculin tests at 2-week intervals (all negative), 2 dewormings with thiabendazole via stomach tube at 2-week intervals, and collection of reference serum samples.

Experimental Infection

Chlamydial organisms were instilled bilaterally onto the conjunctivae on day 1 of the CsA protocol. Daily intramuscular injections of CsA in oil (olive oil initially, then switched to Miglyol, an oil base, on day 14) were administered for 15 weeks at a dose of 25 mg/kg. For the first 8 weeks of the study, approximately 30 mg of ketamine HCl was given daily by i.m. injection to facilitate handling. Horsfall isolation units were used for housing the animals in view of the biohazardous potential of *C. trachomatis*. The units were large enough to allow 2 compatible animals per cage. Monkeys no. 1 and no. 2 were housed together until the death of no. 1 on day 54 of

From the Division of Comparative Medicine, the Wilmer Ophthalmological Institute, the Department of Pathology, and the Oncology Center, The Johns Hopkins University School of Medicine, Baltimore, MD; and the Southwest Foundation for Research and Education, San Antonio, TX.

Supported in part by Public Health Service Grants RR00130, EY03324, RR07002, and EY01765.

Address reprint requests to Dr. N. L. Garnett, Division of Comparative Medicine, Johns Hopkins University School of Medicine, Baltimore, MD 21205.

0041–1345/83/1505–0114$01.00/0

CsA protocol. Then no. 2 was paired with no. 4 until the death of no. 2 on day 74 of CsA protocol.

Pathology

Complete systematic autopsies were performed on both monkeys. Tissue sections were fixed in 10% buffered formalin, paraffin embedded, sectioned at 6 μ, and stained with hematoxylin and eosin stain. Sections of tumor and spleen from monkey no. 1 were stored at −70°C, as was serum collected just prior to death.

Laboratory Studies on Cultured Peripheral Lymphocytes

Peripheral lymphocytes had been harvested 4 days prior to death from monkey no. 2. Approximately 10^7 frozen viable lymphocytes were cultured in RPMI 1640 medium plus 10% fetal bovine serum and 20 ng/ml cyclosporine-A until lines became established. Of 10 samples of 10^6 cells each, 8 gave rise to established lines. The time to establishment was less than 6 weeks. Smeared cells of the lines were stained for EBV antigens by indirect immunofluorescence. Subcultures were tested with a cloned EBV probe (Bam W) for EBV-like DNA sequences.

Frozen Tumor Tissue

Sections of frozen tumor tissue from monkey no. 1 were used for immunoperoxidase staining for immunoglobulins to determine the likely lymphoid cell line of origin. Directly conjugated antiisotype sera were used to examine for IgG, IgA, and IgM.

Serum

Pre- and post-CsA serum samples from all five animals were titered for antibody to the virus present in simian tumor tissue from the Reitz study,[3] and in P3JHR1K cells (human EBV-producer cell line).

Plasma Levels of Cyclosporine-A

Blood samples were taken on day 66 of the CsA protocol in order to determine plasma levels of the drug just prior to injection (24 hr after previous injection) and at 4 hr postinjection for determination of quantitative drug levels.

RESULTS

Case History: Monkey No. 1

On day 54 of the CsA protocol, a clinical call for veterinary assistance was placed by the investigator after the development of lethargy, pitting edema of the legs, and multiple soft tissue masses in the areas of the inguinal lymph nodes, injection sites on both legs, and in the periorbital region over the right eye (Fig. 1). The supraorbital mass occurred in an area that was under very close observation and had been noted only 1 week earlier. Hematology and blood chemistry analysis failed to suggest a specific diagnosis, while cytology of a chest aspirate revealed a uniform population of lymphoblastic cells with numerous mitotic figures. Due to progressive worsening of condition, the monkey was euthanized with an overdose of sodium pentobarbital and submitted for necropsy.

Case History: Monkey No. 2

On day 73 of CsA protocol, the animal was lethargic. It failed to respond to fluids and nutrients administered by stomach tube and was found dead the following day.

Case History: Monkeys No. 3, 4, and 5

Thirty-eight days after the termination of CsA, no. 3 died of undetermined causes, but with no gross or microscopic evidence of lymphoma. Monkeys no. 4 and 5 remained alive 6 months after the CsA protocol.

Gross Necropsy Findings

Monkey no. 1 was generally emaciated, with marked edema of the legs extending around the area of the penis. Extreme lymphadenopathy was evident in the inguinal, axil-

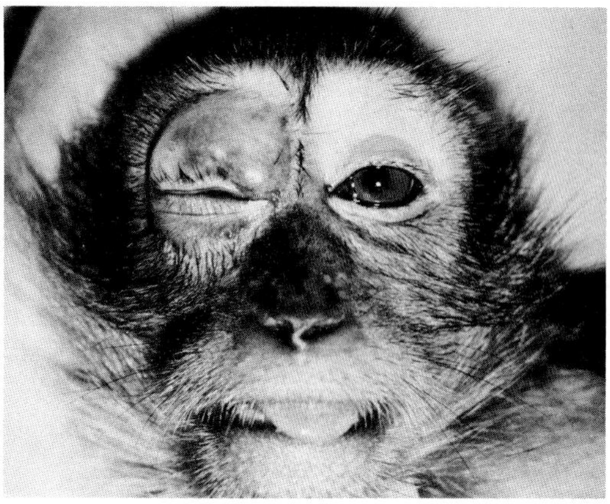

Fig. 1. Appearance of supraorbital mass 54 days after beginning administration of cyclosporine-A.

lary, and peripheral nodes, as well as within the abdominal cavity. A 1 cu cm raised soft tissue mass was present in the palpebral conjunctiva above the right eye (Fig. 1). Tumor appeared to envelope the right testis in the inguinal region, the distal abdominal aorta, and the sciatic nerve of the left leg. Other organs grossly involved by tumor included kidney (0.5 cu cm mass), adrenals, urinary bladder, and injection sites of the posterior thighs.

Monkey no. 2 was in fair general condition and had diffuse lymphadenopathy of peripheral and central lymph nodes. The mesenteric lymph nodes were from 5 mm to 8 mm in length, while periaortic and external iliac nodes ranged up to 1.5 cm × 3 cm. Hepatomegaly and splenomegaly were present, and approximately 5 ml of clear straw-colored fluid was present in the abdominal cavity. Adhesions were found between the diaphragm and the adjacent apices of lung lobes. Fibrosis was evident in the muscles of the posterior thigh injection sites.

Histopathology

Microscopically, the tumors were large cell, undifferentiated lymphomas. There was variation in nuclear size and shape, including some with cleaved nuclei and others with plasmacytoid features. In some tissues, scattered macrophages gave a characteristic "starry sky" appearance. Many of the cells had large vesicular nuclei with single prominent nucleoli. Mitotic figures were present at the rate of 6–10 per high power field. There was extensive lymphoblastoid infiltration of multiple nodal and extranodal tissues. In monkey no. 1, involved nodes, both adrenals, and portions of the kidney (Fig. 2), bladder, peripheral nerve, skeletal muscle, skin, and tonsil showed infiltration often severe enough to totally efface the normal architecture. Neoplastic aggregates were also seen in the lungs and in and around vascular structures.

Monkey no. 2 showed a more leukemic pattern, with neoplastic cells present in intravascular spaces of most tissues. There was extensive neoplastic infiltration of the spleen, liver, kidney, and bone marrow. Multiple lymph nodes, heart, skeletal muscle, diaphragm, esophagus, and choroid plexus were also involved. The thymus was identified and was not involved.

Laboratory Studies

Cultured peripheral lymphocytes. The cells showed no significant immunofluorescence staining with human sera, having specifity for Epstein Barr virus early antigen, membrane antigen, and viral capsid antigen. EB nuclear antigen was not tested for. They also failed to stain with mouse monoclonal antibodies directed against viral capsid antigen (VCA) or membrane antigen.

The cloned EBV viral DNA probes were blot-hybridized with cultured lymphocyte DNA. The probes bound strongly and showed binding consistent with approximately 100 copies of EBV genomes per cell.

Frozen tumor tissue. Immunoperoxidase staining of tumor tissue was strongly positive for IgG on the cell surface and cytoplasm.

Serum. Sera from all animals reacted positively with virus from the Reitz study[3] and with the antigens of the P3JHR1K strain of EBV. No correlation between staining and the presence or absence of tumor was demonstrated.

Plasma levels of cyclosporine-A. Plasma levels 24 hr after the last injection ranged from 120 to 127 ng/ml, while those taken at 4 hr postinjection ranged from 180 to 245 ng/ml. These levels fall within the therapeutic range discussed by Beveridge.[11]

Response to Chlamydial Infection

The chlamydial eye infection in these animals was abnormally prolonged. Although the specific antichlamydial IgM and IgG response in serum and tears was normal, the appearance of IgA was greatly delayed. In vitro testing showed that cell-mediated immunity did not develop to chlamydial antigens.[10]

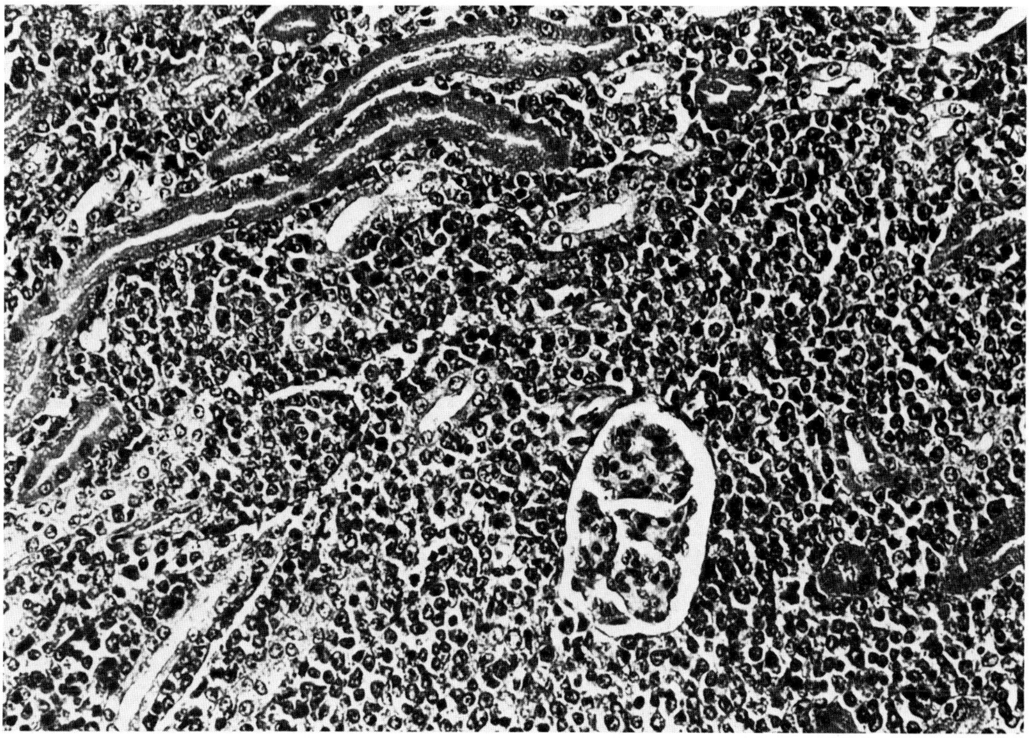

Fig. 2. Histologic section through the margin of an intrarenal tumor mass demonstrating separation of tubules and glomerulus by poorly differentiated lymphoid cells (hematoxylin and eosin, × 51).

DISCUSSION

The life-saving beneficial effects of CsA for organ and bone marrow transplant recipients are well documented.[12] The powerful, but selective, effect of CsA on T-lymphocyte subpopulations has been reported in detail.[13–15]

Previously reported experiences with posttransplantation lymphomas in human patients reveal the seriousness of this complication.[1,5,12] Numerous references exist that document or postulate the association of these lymphomas with EBV, EBV reactivation, immunosuppressive therapy, or host factors such as presenting diagnosis, age, or cytogenetic factors.[1,5,7,9,12] The questions raised by these observations are unlikely to be easily answered by retrospective human studies, due to the difficulty of controlling for multiple variables.

An animal model system is clearly needed to allow controlled, reproducible manipulation of all the factors involved in the posttransplantation lymphoma phenomenon. The nonhuman primate (especially the cynomolgus monkey) appears to be as sensitive as, or more sensitive than, the human to the development of posttransplantation lymphomas.[3]

Our work in a small sample of animals, although also retrospective, does eliminate two variables from the picture, namely, transplantation and conventional immunosuppressive drugs. Our observations do not agree with those of Borleffs et al.,[16] who reported no lymphomas in his nontransplanted animals, or those studied by Schelleken after prolonged CsA or combined CsA and conventional immunosuppressive therapy.

Our observations would suggest an association between CsA administration, EBV or EBV-like viral infection, and the development of lymphomas of B-lymphocyte origin.

Spontaneous lymphomas in nonhuman primates were considered rare prior to the publication of a review article by Manning and Griesemer (1974)[17] and the California Primate Research Center lymphoma epidemic reported by Terrell et al. (1980).[18] Considerable data have been accumulated on some simian herpes viruses, including their known oncogenicity in new world primates.[19,20] Other herpes viruses in old world primates show a remarkable similarity to EBV, both antigenically and in their behavior in vivo.[19–21]

Although toxicology studies show remarkably few deleterious side effects of CsA when compared to conventional immunosuppressive drugs,[22] and the risk–benefit ratio appears to favor widespread use of the drug, the lymphoma complication must be thoroughly investigated. Our retrospective study was greatly enhanced by the availability of cultured lymphocytes, frozen tumor tissue, and stored serum, which allowed some elements of a prospective study to be conducted. As previously stated by Conners,[6] controlled studies in nonhuman primates are required to determine the relative influence of CsA, transplantation, and oncogenic viruses. It is hoped that this report will stimulate more interest in the development of a valuable animal model system for the investigation of posttransplantation lymphomas and oncogenesis in association with immunosuppressive drug.

ACKNOWLEDGMENTS

The authors wish to express their gratitude to Shirley L. Johnson, and Drs. Elaine Young, and Judith A. Whittum of the Wilmer Eye Institute, Johns Hopkins University; Dr. Allan D. Hess of the Oncology Center, Johns Hopkins University; Drs. Gary S. Hayward and Diane S. Hayward of the Department of Pharmacology and Experimental Therapeutics, Johns Hopkins University; and to Dr. J. F. Borel of Sandoz Ltd, Basel, Switzerland, for providing the cyclosporine-A, without which this study would not have been possible.

REFERENCES

1. Penn I: Transplant Proc 11:1047, 1979

2. Reitz BA, Bieber CP, Raney AA, et al: Transplant Proc 13:393, 1981

3. Reitz BA, Bieber CP, Pennock JL: In White DJG (ed): Cyclosporin A. Amsterdam, Elsevier, 1982

4. Pennock JL, Reitz BA, Bieber CP, et al: Transplant Proc 13:390, 1981

5. Weintraub J, Warnke RA: Transplantation 33:247, 1982

6. Connors TA; In White DJG (ed): Cyclosporin A. Amsterdam, Elsevier, 1982

7. Bird AG: In White DJG (ed): Cyclosporin A. Amsterdam, Elsevier, 1982

8. Klein G: Proc Natl Acad Sci USA 76:2442, 1979

9. Dalla-Favera R, Martinotti S, Gallo RC, et al: Science 219:963, 1983

10. Taylor HR, Young E, Johnson SL, et al: Invest Ophthalmol Vis Sci 24(Suppl):196, 1983

11. Beveridge T: In White DJG (ed): Cyclosporin A. Amsterdam, Elsevier North Holland, 1982

12. Beveridge T: Transplant Proc 15:433, 1983

13. Wagner H: Transplant Proc 15:523, 1983

14. Hess AD, Tutschka PJ, Santos GW: In White DJG (ed): Cyclosporin A. Amsterdam, Elsevier North Holland, 1982

15. Hess AD, Tutschka PJ, Santos GW: Transplant Proc 15:539, 1983

16. Borleffs JCC, Neuhaus P, Marquet RL, et al: In White DJG (ed): Cyclosporin A. Amsterdam, Elsevier North Holland, 1982

17. Manning JRS, Griesemer RA: Lab Anim Sci 24:204, 1974

18. Terrell TG, Gribble DH, Osburn BI: J Natl Cancer Inst 64:561, 1980

19. Brack M: Morphological and Epidemiological Aspects of Simian Herpes Virus Infections. Berlin, Verlag Paul Parey, 1977

20. Falk LA: In Rapp F (ed): Oncogenic Herpes Viruses. Boca Raton, FL, CRC Press, 1980

21. Heberling RL, Bieber CP, Kalter SS: In Yohn DS, Blakeslee JR (eds): Advances in Comparative Leukemia Research 1981. Amsterdam, Elsevier North Holland, 1982

22. Ryffel B: In White DJG (ed): Cyclosporin A. Amsterdam, Elsevier North Holland, 1982

PROBLEMS IN DIFFERENTIAL DIAGNOSIS—DRUG TOXICITY VERSUS ALLOGRAFT REJECTION

Clinical and Laboratory Signs in Nephrotoxicity and Rejection in Cyclosporine-Treated Renal Allograft Recipients

G. Klintmalm, O. Ringdén, and C. G. Groth

WHEN THE NEW immunosuppressive drug cyclosporine A (CsA)[1] was introduced for treatment of patients requiring renal transplants by Calne et al.,[2] after extensive trials in different transplantation models, the drug was unexpectedly found to have nephrotoxic properties. However, this side effect was shown to be dose-related and reversible. By decreasing the patient's dose or changing to conventional therapy for immunosuppression, even after 8 months' use of the drug, renal function was restored.[2,3] Up to the present time, using our treatment regimen, nephrotoxicity has been found in at least half our renal transplanted patients.[4]

When a deterioration in function occurs, the clinician who is managing CsA-treated patients must be able to distinguish between the less serious condition of drug nephrotoxicity and the potentially dangerous condition of allograft rejection. The methods used to make these diagnoses have included morphological examination of the graft,[2,4,5] radionucleotide scans,[6] subcapsular pressure in the kidney,[7] determination of CsA concentrations in blood, and immunologic monitoring.[8–10] Starzl and co-workers have described how a tentative diagnosis may be made in therapeutic trials by initiating high-dose steroid therapy; if no response to the treatment is seen, the CsA dose can be lowered.[11] This has given excellent results.[12] However, unnecessary treatments with high doses of steroids are never warranted. There has been no systematic description of the clinical findings in CsA drug nephrotoxicity. The purpose of this study was to describe the clinical findings during CsA nephrotoxicity and renal graft rejection to see if some patients on clinical grounds may initially be spared invasive diagnostic procedures or high-dose steroid treatment trials.

MATERIALS AND METHODS

Patients

Since January 1980, a total of 65 renal transplant recipients have been treated with CsA and followed for a minimum of 2 months. Fifty-eight patients were treated with CsA starting at the time of operation. Thirteen patients were switched from CsA and prednisolone to azathioprine and prednisolone, 7 from conventional immunosuppression with azathioprine and prednisolone to CsA and prednisolone. Only episodes of deteriorating graft function during CsA treatment were analyzed in the present study.

The immunosuppressive routine in use calls for CsA 10 mg/kg i.v. preoperatively. After operation, CsA 15 mg/kg/day is given in divided doses twice a day. The CsA dose is lowered to 13, 11, and 9 mg/kg/day at 2, 4, and 8 weeks, respectively. Further reductions are then made, depending on the toxic side effects. Hydrocortisone 0.5 g is given i.v. during the operation at the time of revascularization. The postoperative prednisolone treatment starts with 100 mg/day on day 1 and is reduced by 20 mg/day until day 9, when 20 mg/day is given. This dose is maintained until day 30 and is then lowered to 15 mg/day. Further reductions are made at 2 months, to 12.5 mg/day, and finally at 3 months, to 10 mg/day, which is the long-term maintenance dose. Rejections are treated with methylprednisolone 0.5 g i.v. on day 1 and then for 3 more days with 0.25 g i.v. each day.

The HLA-A,B antigens were determined with the lymphocytotoxic microtechnique, using the method of Kissmeyer-Nielsen and Kjerbye.[13] HLA-DR typing was done on B cells.[14]

Thirteen recipients (6 females, 7 males) received grafts from related donors. Twelve of the donors were haploidentical, and 1 was an HLA-identical sibling. All the recipients were receiving a graft for the first time. Two of the patients had diabetes mellitus. The recipients were

From the Department of Transplantation Surgery, Karolinska Institute, Huddinge University Hospital, Huddinge, Sweden.

Reprint requests should be addressed to Dr. G. Klintmalm, Department of Transplantation Surgery, Karolinska Institute, Huddinge University Hospital, S-141 86 Huddinge, Sweden.

0041-1345/83/1505—0115$01.00/0

26 ± 12 (mean ± SD) years of age (range, 2–42 years). Two patients were not transfused. The remaining patients were given 4.8 ± 1.8 units of blood preoperatively. Fifty-two patients (19 females, 33 males) were given cadaveric grafts. Two patients had no incompatibilites for the HLA-A,B antigens. Thirty-six patients had one or two incompatibilities for HLA-A,B, and 14 patients had three or more. Twenty-three patients had no incompatibilities for HLA-DR, and 29 had one or two incompatibilities. The mean number of incompatibilities was 2.2 ± 1.1 for HLA-A,B and 0.7 ± 0.8 for HLA-DR. Eleven patients received second grafts, and 2 received third grafts. Thirteen patients had diabetes mellitus, and 31 were more than 55 years of age. The age of the group was 53 ± 11 years of age (range, 21–71 years). Three patients were not transfused. The remainder received a median of five preoperative transfusions (range, 2–95).

Methods

There were 101 episodes of deteriorating renal function in 49 patients. Deterioration in renal function was defined as an increase in serum creatinine of 30 μmol/liter or more, together with an increase in the blood urea. The baseline status was determined by calculating the mean values of the various clinical and laboratory parameters on the last 3–5 days (for inpatients or for visits of outpatients) before the day of examination (DE). The day of examination was defined as the day when a deterioration in renal function in a patient resulted in active steps to make a diagnosis of nephrotoxicity or rejection (i.e., biopsy, renogram, IVP, angiography). DE was not dependent on the day of institution of therapy: This was sometimes delayed for several days, depending on when a definite diagnosis was made.

Biopsy was performed during 81 episodes of deteriorating renal function in 38 patients. The percutaneous biopsies were performed with a Tru-cut® needle (Travenol Laboratories, Inc., Deerfield, IL), and the specimens were fixed in Stiewe's fixation fluid or Histofix (Histo-Lab, Gothenburg, Sweden) and embedded in paraffin. Light microscopic examination was carried out after staining with hematoxylin-eosin and Ladewig's modification of Mallory's trichrome stain. Eight biopsies in 6 patients were given diagnoses irrelevant to the present study and were not further analyzed (2 of the patients had pyelonephritis, 1 had an infarct, 1 an embolism with acute tubular necrosis, 1 a urinary outflow obstruction, and 3 a recurrence of the original disease). Five episodes of deterioration occurred within 5 days of transplantation, before a stable renal function had been achieved. Thus, a baseline status for comparison could not be calculated, and these episodes were consequently omitted from the study. The remaining 68 specimens form the basis of this study.

Cyclosporine A Plasma Levels

The predose morning values are reported here. A sample of 5 ml of blood was centrifuged after routine handling (>30 min at 24°C before separation). The plasma was analyzed using RIA kits provided by Sandoz Ltd.

Statistical Methods

In the statistical analysis, only the first episode to occur, nephrotoxicity or rejection, was analyzed in each patient. This results in independent samples for statistical purposes. The analyses were done by the Department of Medical Statistics at Karolinska Institute, using discriminatory analysis and Fischer's exact test.

RESULTS

Thirty-one biopsies in 25 patients showed cellular infiltrates suggestive of rejection, and the patients were subsequently given high doses of intravenous methylprednisolone. Thirty-seven specimens in 25 patients showed no significant abnormalities, and the deteriorating graft function was assumed to be due to CsA drug nephrotoxicity. The treatment for nephrotoxicity was to decrease the CsA dose or switch from CsA to azathioprine in selected cases. The correctness of treating the patients on the basis of the morphological diagnosis has already been shown.[4]

Serum Creatinine Levels

The baseline values for renal function were the same in the two groups: 196 ± 78 μmol/liter (means ± SD) for the nephrotoxic group vs. 209 ± 77 μmol/liter for the rejection group. On DE, the mean creatinine values were 252 ± 92 μmol/liter in the nephrotoxic patients and 264 ± 81 μmol/liter in the rejection patients. The number of days required for the incease to occur was 7.4 ± 7.4 in the nephrotoxic group and 3.6 ± 3.1 in the rejection group. The daily increase in serum creatinine was 19 ± 22 μmol/liter in the nephrotoxic group and 25 ± 20 μmol/liter in the rejecting group. A closer analysis reveals that late toxicity is more insidious than early toxicity. During the first postoperative month, there was no difference between the groups with regard to the daily increase in serum creatinine, which was 38 ± 30 μmol/liter and 39 ± 19 μmol/liter for the nephrotoxic and rejection groups, respectively. After the first month, the daily serum creatinine increase was 15 ± 10 μmol/liter in the nephrotoxic group and 21 ± 19 μmol/liter in the rejection group, but the difference was not significant. More than 5 months after operation the daily creatinine increase was 5 ± 5 μmol/liter at the time of nephrotoxicity and 25 ± 20 μmol/liter at the time of rejection.

Diuresis

A significant decrease in the 24-hr urine output was recorded more often with rejection. A decrease of 500–1000 ml was seen in 8% of the nephrotoxic episodes, as compared to 32% of the rejection episodes. A decrease of >1000 ml a day was noted in 4% of the nephrotoxic episodes, vs. 24% in the rejection group. In most patients in the nephrotoxic group (88%) the urinary output was essentially unchanged (±500 ml). The corresponding figure was 44% in the rejection group. The statistical analysis was not conclusive ($p = 0.062$). (See Fig. 1.)

Body Weight

A weight increase of 0.5–2.0 kg was noted in 21% of the nephrotoxic episodes and in 32% of the rejection episodes. A >2.0 kg increase occurred in 4% of the nephrotoxic episodes and in 18% of the rejection episodes. No significant increase (<0.5 kg) was seen in 75% of the nephrotoxic episodes, as compared to 50% of the rejection episodes (NS, $p > 0.05$). (See Fig. 2.)

Body Temperature

An increase in body temperature to 37.5°C or more was seen in 1 out of every 4 instances of rejection, but never during CsA drug nephrotoxicity. The highest body temperature noted during rejection was 39.2°C, compared to 37.2°C during nephrotoxicity. This difference was significant ($p < 0.05$). (See Fig. 3.)

Blood Pressure

An increase in systolic blood pressure of >20 mmHg and/or diastolic blood pressure of >10 mmHg was seen once in the nephrotoxic group and four times in the rejection group.

Combination of Clinical Findings

At least one of the following findings was seen during rejection episodes: a decrease in

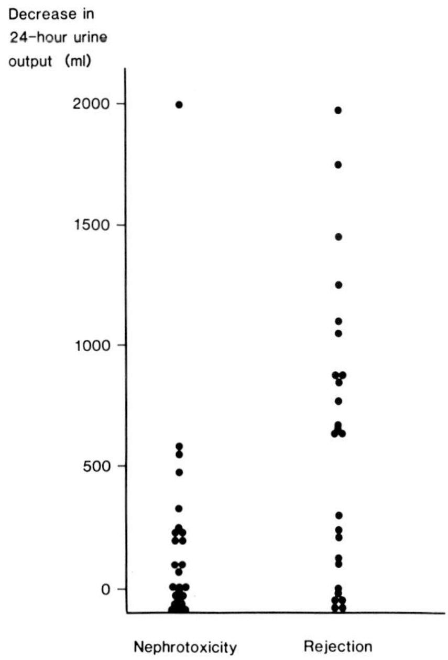

Fig. 1. Changes in 24-hr urine output during drug nephrotoxicity and graft rejection in patients treated with CsA.

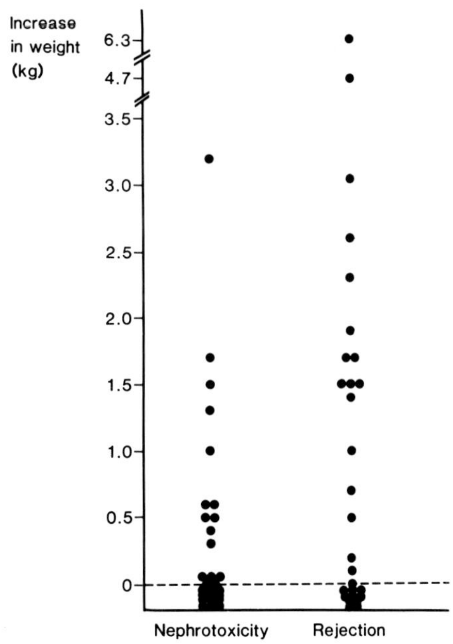

Fig. 2. Changes in body weight during drug nephrotoxicity and graft rejection in patients treated with CsA.

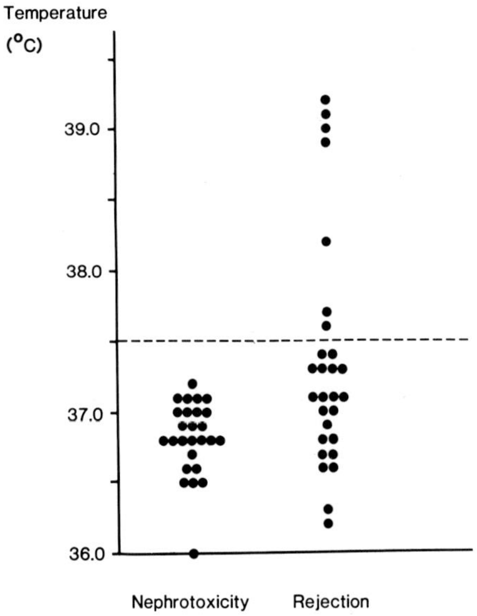

Fig. 3. Changes in body temperature during drug nephrotoxicity and graft rejection in patients treated with CsA.

diuresis of >500 ml daily, an increase in body weight of >0.5 kg, a body temperature of 37.5°C or more, or a rapidly increasing serum creatinine level (>30 μmol/liter/day). Three times, two of the findings were seen at the same time during nephrotoxicity, as compared to 11 times during rejection. Three or four findings at the same time were present only during episodes of rejection. (See Table 1.)

Nephrotoxicity and Rejection in Relation to Time After Transplantation

In the first postoperative month, rejection was as likely as nephrotoxicity to be the cause of deteriorating renal function. During the subsequent months, the incidence of rejection fell, and none was seen more than 200 days

Table 1. Number of Episodes of Deteriorating Renal Function with Zero to Four Clinical Findings During CsA Nephrotoxicity and Graft Rejection

	Number of findings		
	0	1	2–4
Nephrotoxicity ($N = 37$)	23	11	3
Rejection ($N = 31$)	10	5	16

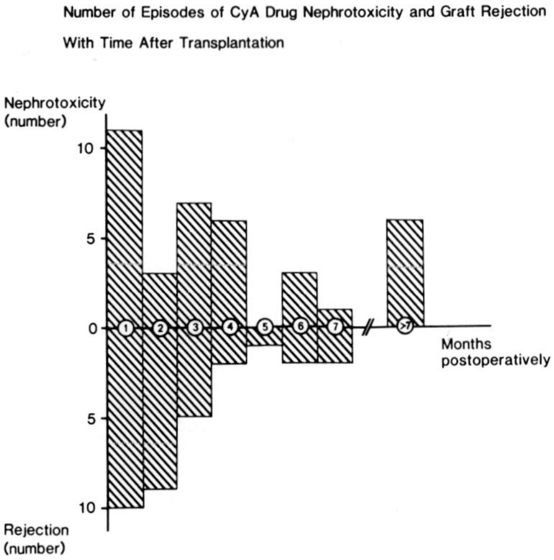

Fig. 4. Incidence of drug nephrotoxicity and graft rejection in relation to time after transplantation in patients treated with CsA.

after transplantation. Incidences of nephrotoxicity were seen during the entire follow-up period and as late as 21 months after transplantation. (See Fig. 4.)

Cyclosporine A Plasma Levels

When the CsA levels were measured, nephrotoxicity was noted with CsA levels >220 ng/ml (median, 290 ng/ml) during the first 4 months after transplantation. Late nephrotoxicity was seen with plasma levels as low as 110 ng/ml (median, 180 ng/ml). Rejections

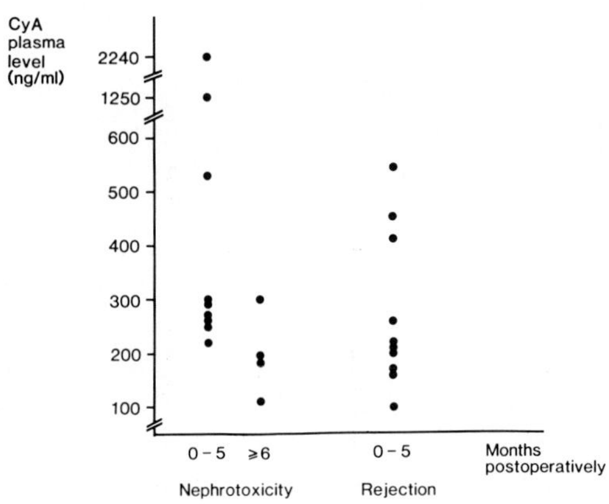

Fig. 5. CsA plasma levels during drug nephrotoxicity and graft rejection in relation to time after transplantation.

within the first 4 postoperative months were seen with CsA plasma levels with a median of 210 ng/ml, of which 7/10 times the levels were $\leq$260 ng/ml. (See Fig. 5.)

DISCUSSION

Our data suggest that when a deterioration in renal allograft function occurs, some clinical findings make the diagnosis of rejection more likely than that of CsA drug nephrotoxicity: a reduction in daily urine output, an increase in weight, an increase in body temperature, and a rapidly increasing serum creatinine. A combination of two or more of these findings occurs more frequently in subjects with allograft rejection. It was also noted that the time when the deterioration in renal function takes place after transplantation is important for the interpretation of an increase in the serum creatinine level.

The renal insufficiency seen during CsA drug nephrotoxicity is a high-output failure that tends to be associated with a slower increase in the serum creatinine level than that seen during allograft rejection. This difference between these two conditions gradually increases after transplantation. The patients with nephrotoxicity seem to be unaware of their worsening kidney function, as evidenced by an elevated serum creatinine level, possibly because their weight remains stable and diuresis is good. During rejection, changes in weight and urine output may occur, as well as an elevation of body temperature, a hallmark of inflammation. A fever was never seen during drug nephrotoxicity. This is also in accordance with the absence of signs of inflammation in the graft.[2,4,5] A comparison between CsA nephrotoxicity and rejection during conventional treatment would probably result in clear differences. The insidiousness with which rejection may occur during CsA treatment is reconfirmed by the results of this study: one-third of the rejections had none of the symptoms or signs that suggest rejection. The only sign indicating this condition is an increase in the serum creatinine level. In this study, the diagnosis of nephrotoxicity is based on the absence of morphological findings in patients with a deteriorating renal function. Subsequently, nephrotoxicity cannot initially be ruled out as occurring together with rejection. This conclusion can be reached only by using a combination of graft biopsy, CsA plasma levels, and observation of the further course of the patient's disease.

A decrease in diuresis was seen in a few patients with acute severe CsA nephrotoxicity; this occurred within a few weeks after transplantation. In these patients, sudden increases in the CsA plasma levels from previously low therapeutic levels to over 1000 ng/ml were always seen. Thus, CsA concentrations should be carried out routinely in cases with deteriorating allograft function. Nephrotoxicity was not seen with CsA plasma levels of <200 ng/ml during the first postoperative months, a finding that is in agreement with those of other authors.[8,10] However, half a year or more after transplantation, a deterioration in renal function, which could be reversed by lowering the CsA dose, was seen, with plasma levels as low as 100 ng/ml. This finding differs from those of others authors.[8,10] Commonly accepted plasma levels, 100–400 ng/ml,[8] are probably too high for patients on long-term CsA therapy if nephrotoxicity is to be avoided. Normally, these patients have CsA concentrations that were previously thought not to be therapeutic (Klintmalm, in preparation). This may be due to drug accumulation, alterations in CsA absorption or metabolism. No rejection has been seen more than 7 months after transplantation, in spite of constantly low plasma levels (<50 ng/ml). Rejections occurred earlier and with plasma levels of <250 ng/ml, but they were also seen with plasma concentrations that are usually considered to be well over therapeutic levels. The overlap between potentially nephrotoxic plasma levels and levels that are insufficient to yield adequate immunosuppression does not make monitoring of CsA concentration obsolete. We believe that with the aid of monitoring CsA plasma levels, the most obvious flaws in the management of immunosuppressive treatment can now be avoided.

In patients with increasing serum creatinine levels during CsA therapy, the serum creatinine value per se provides no guidance to the correct diagnosis. In some patients, a decrease in diuresis, an elevation in body temperature, and/or an increase in weight may be seen. If several or all of these functions are present, the diagnosis of graft rejection is more likely. CsA plasma levels may also give some guidance. However, to reach a definitive diagnosis, some other diagnostic tool, such as graft biopsy, must be resorted to, at least during the first 4–6 months after operation.

REFERENCES

1. Borel JF, Feurer C, Gubler HU, et al: Agents and Actions 6:468, 1976
2. Calne RY, White DJG, Rolles K, et al: Lancet 1:1183, 1978
3. Klintmalm GBG, Iwatsuki S, Starzl TE: Lancet 1:470, 1981
4. Klintmalm G, Bergstrand A, Ringdén O, et al: Transplant Proc 15:493, 1983
5. Ringdén O, Bergstrand A, Collste H, et al: Scand J Urol Nephrol (Suppl) 64:220, 1981
6. Klintmalm GBG, Klingensmith WC III, Iwatsuki S, et al: Radiology 142:199, 1982
7. Wagner E, Pichlmayer R, Wonigeit K, et al: Transplant Proc 15:489, 1983
8. Keown PA, Stiller CR, Ulan RA, et al: Lancet 1:686, 1981
9. Rynasiewicz JJ, Sutherland DER, Simmons RL, et al: Lancet 1:276, 1981
10. Kahan BD, Van Buren CT, Lin SN, et al: Transplantation 34:36, 1982
11. Starzl TE, Hakala TR, Rosenthal JT, et al: Surg Gynecol Obstet 154:819, 1982
12. Hakala TR, Starzl TE, Rosenthal JT, et al: Transplant Proc 15:465, 1983
13. Kissmeyer-Nielson F, Kjerbye KE: In Curtoni ES, Mattiux P, Tose RM (eds): Histocompatibility Testing. Copenhagen, Munksgaard, 1967, p 381
14. Berg B, Rindén O: Transplantation 33:291, 1982

Morphological Findings in Kidney Transplants After Treatment with Cyclosporine

M. J. Mihatsch, G. Thiel, H. P. Spichtin, M. Oberholzer, F. P. Brunner, F. Harder, V. Olivieri, R. Bremer, B. Ryffel, E. Stöcklin, J. Torhorst, F. Gudat, H. U. Zollinger, and R. Loertscher

CYCLOSPORINE A (CsA) is a new potent immunosuppressive agent[1,2] that is being increasingly used in kidney transplantation. One untoward effect of CsA is nephrotoxicity, with minor impairment of renal function up to severe acute renal failure.[3–5] Diagnostic problems therefore arise, especially in the early post-transplant period, in deciding whether impaired renal function is due either to CsA toxicity or conservation injury or rejection.[6]

Glomerular, vascular, tubular, and interstitial alterations have been described in bone marrow and kidney transplant recipients as well as in animal experiments after treatment with CsA.[7–10] The significance of these findings has yet to be determined.

The purpose of the present study, which compares a series of patients treated with CsA alone to a group of historical controls treated with azathioprine and steroids (Aza-St), is to answer two questions: (1) Does the histologic appearance of rejection differ in renal biopsies from CsA- as compared to Aza-St–treated patients? (2) Are there any characteristic morphological alterations of CsA nephrotoxicity in renal transplants?

MATERIAL AND METHODS

Patients and Clinical Data

Sixty-one renal biopsies performed in 1981 and 1982 on 32 transplant recipients undergoing basic immunosuppression with CsA alone according to the schedule of the European Multicentre Trial in 1981[11] were examined. A control group of biopsies performed between 1970 and 1982 in patients on conventional immunosuppressive therapy with Aza-St was chosen according to the time interval between transplantation and biopsy. Each biopsy of the CsA group was matched with the two most recently performed biopsies on the same day after transplantation or a day close by in patients on conventional immunosuppression. The indication for renal biopsy was always poor, clinically unexplained transplant function.

The following clinical data were considered in the CsA group: age and sex of the patients, serum creatinine, serum CsA trough level, blood pressure, thrombocyte count. In the Aza-St group, only the age and sex of the patients were considered.

Methods

The methods for light and electron microscopy and immunofluorescence have been described previously.[12] The number of cases studied by these methods in the CsA and Aza-St groups are presented in Table 1. The results are mainly based on light microscopy unless otherwise stated. Electron microscopy was used only for confirmation of light microscopic findings in both groups.

From the Pathology Institute, the Department of Internal Medicine (R. L., F. P. B., G. T.), and the Department of Surgery (F. H.), University of Basel, Switzerland, and the Department of Preclinical Research, Sandoz Ltd. (B. R.).

Reprint requests should be addressed to Dr. M. J. Mihatsch, Institut für Pathologie der Universität Basel, Schönbeinstraße 40, CH-4003 Basel, Switzerland.

0041–1345/83/1505–0116$02.00/0

Table 1. Patients and Methods

	1981–1982 Cyclosporine A	1970–1982 Azathioprine + Steroids
No. of patients	32	104
Sex ratio: Male/female	1.1/1	1.2/1
Age (mean ± SE)	42 (± 2.0) years	41 (± 1.0) years
No. of biopsies	61	138
Investigation		
Electron microscopy	59	122
Immunofluorescence	55	86

Table 2. Morphological and Clinical Data on Patients Treated with CsA

Patient No./ Biopsy No.	Clinical Data at the Time of Biopsy								Light Microscopy*							Immunofluorescence*				
									Tubules					Rejection		Vessels		Glomeruli		
	Age (years)	Sex	Biopsy (days after transplantation)	Serum CsA (ng/ml)	Serum Creatinine (μmole/liter)	Blood pressure (mmHg)	Platelets ($\times 10^3$/mm^3)	Giant Mitochondria	Vacuolization	Microcalcification	Interstitial Fibrosis	Arteriolopathy	Vascular	Interstitial	IgM	C3	IgM	C3	Follow-up†
1/1	46	F	8	626	255	155/90	231	4	1	1	2	1	1	4	1	2	1	1	
1/2	46	F	33	2860	330	185/110	214	3	1	2	2	2	1	2	2	2	1	1	
1/3	46	F	48	1760	450	180/105	315	3	4	2	2	3	1	2	3	3	1	1	Aza-St
2/1	43	M	13	630	457	135/80	286	2	1	1	1	1	1	4	1	2	1	1	
2/2	43	M	30	1180	430	120/55	145	2	1	2	1	1	1	2	1	2	1	1	
2/3	43	M	46	590	432	140/80	192	3	1	1	2	2	1	4	2	2	2	1	
2/4	43	M	104	175	407	125/80	404	3	1	1	2	2	1	4	1	2	1	2	
2/5	43	M	395	258	359	140/90	190	1	1	2	3	3	1	3	2	2	2	2	Aza-St
3/1	43	M	17	410	197	140/80	556	3	3	1	1	1	1	3	1	2	1	1	
3/2	43	M	32	190	362	190/100	434	3	3	1	2	1	3	2	2	3	2	1	Aza-St
4/1	63	M	18	950	224	140/80	428	4	2	2	2	1	1	2	1	2	1	1	Aza-St
5/1	28	F	14	1600	386	130/90	215	3	3	2	1	1	1	1	1	1	1	1	
5/2	28	F	29	3000	518	160/100	97	3	3	2	2	1	1	2	1	1	2	1	—
6/1	40	M	10	1900	920	130/90	305	2	3	2	2	2	1	2	ND	ND	ND	ND	
6/2	40	M	24	600	900	145/75	240	2	1	2	2	2	1	2	ND	ND	ND	ND	—
7/1	60	M	88	1364	306	140/90	164	3	2	2	2	2	1	2	ND	ND	ND	ND	
7/2	60	M	151	427	346	140/100	212	1	1	1	3	2	1	4	2	2	1	1	CsA
8/1	45	F	10	916	834	130/80	167	1	1	1	1	1	1	2	1	2	1	3	
8/2	45	F	66	283	594	140/100	82	1	4	2	3	2	2	1	2	2	2	2	
8/3	45	F	387	171	429	130/80	114	2	2	1	3	2	1	3	2	3	3	1	Aza-St
9/1	45	M	185	119	157	130/80	118	1	1	2	2	1	1	2	1	2	1	1	CsA
10/1	36	F	22	321	350	180/80	436	2	3	2	1	2	3	3	3	3	1	2	
10/2	36	F	42	274	660	185/70	485	1	3	1	1	1	4	1	3	3	1	2	—
11/1	46	M	21	488	420	150/100	218	1	1	1	1	1	1	3	3	3	1	2	
11/2	46	M	42	814	610	170/100	231	1	1	2	2	1	4	3	3	3	1	2	—
12/1	26	F	13	421	232	140/80	274	1	1	1	2	2	1	4	3	3	2	2	
12/2	26	F	210	121	435	120/80	297	1	1	2	4	2	1	1	1	1	2	2	Aza-St
13/1	48	F	32	626	830	150/90	156	1	1	1	2	3	1	2	4	4	1	2	

13/2	48	F	67	109	482	140/80	165	1	2	2	3	4	1	2	4	4	1	2	
13/3	48	F	172	50	158	180/130	590	1	1	1	3	2	1	4	1	2	2	2	Aza-St
14/1	34	M	12	286	793	170/100	272	2	3	2	1	1	1	1	1	2	1	2	
14/2	34	M	39	663	595	160/100	185	1	2	2	1	2	1	4	1	2	1	2	
14/3	34	M	69	78	650	120/90	130	2	4	2	2	4	1	2	4	4	1	2	Aza-St
15/1	52	M	14	654	781	135/90	323	3	2	2	1	1	1	2	2	2	1	2	CsA
17/1	28	M	25	149	192	115/70	197	2	1	2	2	2	1	3	1	2	1	1	
17/2	28	M	77	262	276	140/80	189	3	2	2	4	4	1	3	3	4	1	2	
17/3	28	M	117	256	259	165/100	249	1	1	2	4	4	1	2	4	4	1	1	Aza-St
18/1	41	M	224	332	244	120/80	283	3	1	1	3	2	1	2	1	2	2	1	CsA
19/1	20	M	12	653	408	140/80	270	1	1	2	1	2	1	3	2	2	2	1	
19/2	20	M	28	317	394	140/70	212	1	1	1	3	1	3	4	1	3	1	2	—
21/1	40	M	61	1134	253	150/90	208	4	4	1	2	1	1	1	1	1	1	1	
21/2	40	M	138	304	280	160/105	184	1	1	1	3	1	1	1	1	1	1	2	CsA
22/1	36	M	63	601	408	120/90	431	2	3	1	3	3	1	3	2	3	1	1	
22/2	36	M	135	356	267	160/100	257	1	1	2	4	3	1	4	3	3	1	1	Aza-St
25/1	56	M	129	591	223	145/100	242	3	4	1	4	4	1	2	1	2	1	2	Aza-St
26/1	38	F	13	114	905	150/90	222	ND	ND	ND	1	ND	4	1	2	2	1	1	—
27/1	55	F	10	292	168	190/90	331	1	1	2	2	1	1	3	1	2	1	1	CsA
28/1	46	F	27	200	778	120/80	411	1	3	2	1	2	2	2	2	2	1	1	
28/2	46	F	41	210	622	130/80	260	1	2	1	1	1	4	3	2	4	1	1	—
29/1	19	F	12	540	336	140/70	158	1	1	1	1	1	1	3	1	2	2	2	
29/2	19	F	30	633	280	150/80	254	1	4	2	3	4	1	4	1	2	1	1	
29/3	19	F	280	470	544	155/85	161	2	1	2	4	3	1	3	3	3	2	2	Aza-St
30/1	59	F	18	791	581	135/50	511	1	2	1	2	1	1	1	ND	ND	ND	ND	—
31/1	28	F	22	768	1601	150/100	158	ND	ND	ND	1	ND	4	1	ND	ND	ND	ND	—
32/1	60	M	40	325	168	155/100	153	1	2	2	3	3	1	3	ND	ND	ND	ND	—
33/1	42	M	179	288	267	140/30	188	1	1	2	1	1	1	1	1	3	1	3	CsA
34/1	28	F	23	207	306	140/90	330	1	1	2	2	2	3	4	1	3	3	3	—
35/1	33	F	14	408	269	150/90	296	1	1	2	1	1	1	2	2	2	2	2	
35/2	33	F	44	380	516	110/70	248	1	4	2	2	1	1	3	1	2	1	2	—
36/1	48	F	15	786	771	170/95	287	2	3	2	1	2	1	3	1	2	1	1	
36/2	48	F	36	240	849	135/60	115	1	3	2	2	2	3	2	2	2	1	1	—

*1 = 0, 4 = +++; ND = No data.

†— = Graft failure; CsA = Graft functioning, CsA treatment; Aza-St = Graft functioning, Aza-St treatment.

Table 3. Study Groups for Rejection Morphology

	Total		Time After Transplantation					
			1–28 Days		29–90 Days		>90 Days	
	CsA	Aza-St	CsA	Aza-St	CsA	Aza-St	CsA	Aza-St
No. of patients	32	95	23*	54*	18*	42*	13*	26*
No. of biopsies	61	122	23	54	18	42	13	26
Age (mean ± SE)	42 (± 2) years	41 (± 1) years	39 (± 2.5) years	42 (± 1.6) years	41 (± 2.5) years	41 (± 1.7) years	41 (± 3) years	40 (± 2) years
Sex ratio: Male/female	1.13/1	1.37/1	0.9/1	1.7/1	1/1	1.6/1	2.2/1	1.2/1
Time after transplantation (mean ± SE)	71 (± 11) days	70 (± 9) days	16 (± 1.1) days	16 (± 1) days	51 (± 4.1) days	50 (± 2.5) days	205 (± 26) days	211 (± 23) days

*No rebiopsies in the same time period.

Giant mitochondria (GM) can be identified by light microscopy using Altman's stain,[13] Gurr's stain,[14] or CAB stain.[15] The last gave the best results when the light microscopy findings were compared to those of electron microscopy. After CAB staining, GM are visible as red, sharply delineated paranuclear bodies. GM are most readily shown by electron microscopy, but unhomogeneous distribution and sampling errors make identification difficult. Tubular vacuolization is also best visualized in trichrome stains. It is easily overlooked in thin (3 μ) hematoxylin-eosin-stained sections. Kossa's stain was used for the demonstration of microcalcification.

Morphometry

An accurate GM count was obtained by calculating the number of mitochondrial profiles observed in unit cross-sectional areas of tubular epithelium (numerical area density), using the following equation:

$$N_{A(MM/EPI)} = \frac{\Sigma N_{MM}}{\Sigma P_{EPI}} \cdot \frac{m^2}{d^2} \cdot 1.155 \text{ (mm}^{-2}\text{), where}$$

N_{MM}, the number of mitochondrial profiles areas; P_{EPI}, the number of points of the test grid over tubular epithelium; m, magnification; d, distance between test points (mm); and 1.155, constant for the test grid.

Twenty consecutive microscopic fields along the longitudinal axis of the renal cortex were investigated in each CAB-stained biopsy. The overall length examined was 5 mm. The number of test points over tubular epithelium ranged from 475–831. The final magnification was 800 ×. The multipurpose grid with 100 test points (d = 11 mm) was used. Twenty consecutive biopsies of 12 patients in the CsA group biopsied in 1982 and 20 biopsies of 20 patients in the Aza-St group were analyzed. For morphometric analysis, patients with vascular rejection were not included in either of the two groups.

Mann-Whitney test (U test) and contingency tables were used in the statistical analysis.[16]

RESULTS

The following differences between CsA- and Aza-St–treated patients were found: (1) quantitative differences in the rejection pattern, (2) tubular lesions, and (3) arteriolar lesions. These findings are presented separately.

The morphological and clinical data of the individual patients of the CsA group are summarized in Table 2.

General Morphology of Rejection

The morphological features usually described in rejection[12,17] are presented in Table 3 and the quantitative differences between the treatment groups in Table 4. Qualitative differences in the morphology of rejection between CsA- and Aza-St–treated patients were not encountered. Signs of vascular rejection (endovasculitis) and associated lesions (interstitial hemorrhage, tubular dilatation) as well as IgM deposits in glomeruli were less frequently observed in the CsA group, whereas interstitial infiltrate, interstitial fibrosis, and complement (C_3) deposits in vessel walls were seen more often in the CsA group as compared to the Aza-St group.

CsA-Associated Tubular Parameters

Specificity of CsA Parameters for CsA Treatment. A comparison between CsA- and Aza-St–treated patients showed that the CsA parameters were not only found in CsA-

Table 4. Morphological Features of Rejection Different in CsA and Aza-St Treatment*

	Time After Transplantation		
	1–28 Days	29–90 Days	>90 Days
No. of patients (CsA/Aza-St)	23/54	18/42	13/26
Endovasculitis	↙ ($p < 0.05$)		↙ ($p < 0.01$)
Interstitial infiltrate, diffuse			↗ ($p < 0.025$)
Interstitial fibrosis		↗ ($p < 0.01$)	↗ ($p < 0.1$)
Interstitial hemorrhage	↙ ($p < 0.1$)	↙ ($p < 0.025$)	
Tubular dilatation	↙ ($p < 0.05$)		↙ ($p < 0.05$)
IF glomeruli (IgM)	↙ ($p < 0.05$)	↙ ($p < 0.01$)	
IF vessels (C_3)		↗ ($p < 0.05$)	↗ ($p < 0.1$)

↗ more prominent, ↙ less prominent in the CsA group

Results of U test: $p < 0.1$ (↗), $p < 0.05$ (↗, double-feathered), $p < 0.025$ (↗, triple-feathered), $p < 0.01$ (↗, solid)

*No differences were found for the following parameters: transplant glomerulitis (12), transplant glomerulopathy, glomerular necrosis and thromboses, intravascular coagulation, vascular wall necrosis, tubular necrosis, IF glomeruli (C_3), other immunoglobulins, fibrin, IF vessels (IgM), other immunoglobulins, fibrin.

treated patients but also in the Aza-St group. CsA parameters were, however, more frequent and more pronounced after CsA than after Aza-St treatment (Table 5). In the case of giant mitochondria, this was also confirmed by quantitative evaluation (Fig. 1).

Morphology of CsA Parameters. Giant mitochondria [Fig. 2 (*a, b*)], which were unhomogeneously distributed, were found in the convoluted part of the proximal tubules. They reached about half the size of a nucleus, were mostly round or oval (occasionally cigar-shaped), and lay adjacent to the nuclei. As a rule, they had very few cristae and frequently contained paracrystalline inclusions, large matrix granules, and lipid droplets.

Isometric tubular vacuolization [Fig. 2 (*c, d*)] is identical to what is known as osmotic nephrosis. To avoid any pathogenic prejudice, we use the term *isometric vacuolization.*

Table 5. Frequency of CsA Parameters and Arteriolopathy in CsA and Aza-St Treatment

	Early Biopsies (mean : 26 days)		Late Biopsies (mean : 134 days)	
	Aza-St	CsA	Aza-St	CsA
No. of patients	26	26	24	24
No. of biopsies with vascular rejection	16	3	12	6
Giant mitochondrian tubules				
0	25	12	21	15
+	1***	/	2"	3
++/+++	0	7	1	6
Tubular vacuolization				
0	14	12	15	14
+	10**	5	7*	2
++/+++	2	9	2	8
Tubular microcalcification				
0	23	11	19	10
+	3***	15	5***	14
Arteriolar lesions of any kind				
0	18	13	12	10
+	6	9	11**	7
++/+++	2	4	1	7

Contingency table:
*$p < 0.01$
**$p < 0.05$
***$p < 0.01$

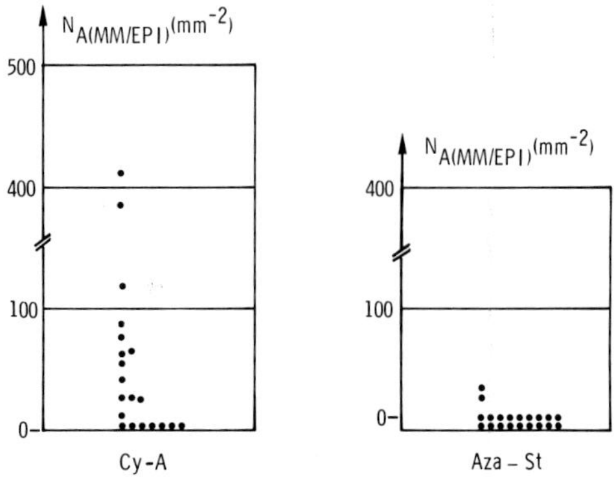

Fig. 1. Numerical area density of giant mitochondria in conventionally treated patients (Aza-St) and CsA-treated patients (CsA).

Vacuolization was unhomogeneously distributed in the kidney, primarily in the straight part of the proximal tubules. All tubular cells in one tubular cross section contained vacuoles of similar diameter [Fig. 2 (*c*)]. Both light and electron microscopy showed that the vacuoles were empty; that is, they did not contain lipids [Fig. 2 (*d*)]. Vacuolization and GM were never observed together in the same cell.

Microcalcifications [Fig. 2 (*e, f*)] were round or crescent- or polycyclic-shaped calcified structures with a diameter of either one tubular cell or a group of cells. They were detected in different parts of the nephron. The calcifications were probably the consequence of single cell necroses of tubular cells, which were sometimes observed simultaneously (dystrophic calcification). In some instances, calcium precipitates were found within intact tubular cells [Fig. 2 (*f*)].

Correlations of CsA Parameters with Other Morphological and Clinical Findings in the CsA Group. In the CsA group, GM were present in 28/59 biopsies (18/30 patients); vacuoles were observed in 29/59 biopsies (21/30 patients) and microcalcifications in 36/59 biopsies (25/30 patients) (Table 2). The combination frequencies of CsA parameters are summarized in Table 6.

A correlation between the time after transplantation and the presence of CsA parameters could not be established. CsA parameters

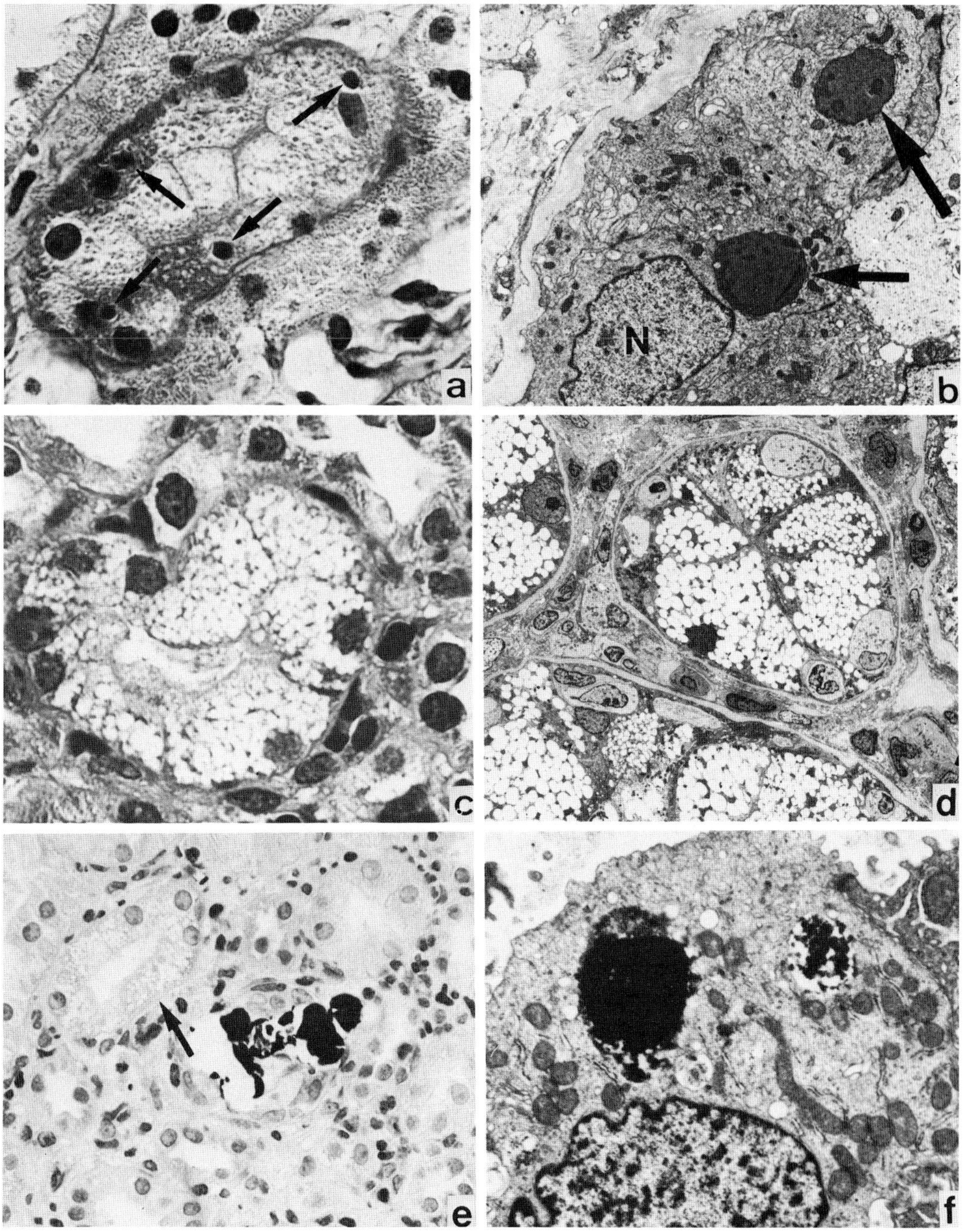

Fig. 2. Morphologic indicators of CsA nephrotoxicity in tubules (CsA parameters). (*a*) Tubular cross section with four giant mitochondria (arrow). CAB stain (×700). (*b*) Two tubular cells with giant mitochondria (arrow). N = nucleus. EM (×3500). (*c*) Isometric vacuolization of tubular epithelium. CAB stain (×875). (*d*) Isometric vacuolization as seen in the electron microscope. EM (×800). (*e*) Very large calcified bodies in a tubule. Isometric vacuolization in a neighboring tubule (arrow). Kossa stain (×350). (*f*) Intracellular calcium deposits. EM (×8500).

Table 6. Frequency and Combination of CsA Parameters in 59 Biopsies

No. of Biopsies	Parameters
9	None
5	Giant mitochondria alone
3	Vacuolization alone
11	Calcification alone
5	Giant mitochondria + calcification
6	Giant mitochondria + vacuolization
8	Vacuolization + calcification
12	Giant mitochondria + calcification + vacuolization

were found early (8–10 days after transplantation) as well as late (several months after transplantation) (Table 2). There was also no correlation between rejection, and other associated renal lesions, and the presence of CsA parameters (Table 7).

Serum CsA levels were higher in patients with GM or vacuoles than in patients without them. No such correlation was found for microcalcification (data not shown). This feature was therefore not considered further. No significant differences were present in the serum creatinine levels of patients with giant mitochondria or vacuoles (Table 8).

The serum trough CsA level did not exceed 1000 ng/ml at the time of biopsy in any of the 20 patients without GM. In contrast, the CsA level exceeded 1000 ng/ml in 2/22 patients with GM or vacuoles and in those 6/18 patients who had both GM and vacuoles in their biopsies (Table 2).

Patients with GM and/or vacuoles without associated lesions (rejection, conservation injury, and arteriolopathy) had significantly higher CsA serum levels than patients of any other group (Table 9). CsA levels in patients presenting with rejection and other symptoms, however, failed to correlate with either GM or vacuoles. Elevation of serum creatinine was most pronounced in patients with GM, vacuoles, and associated renal lesions (Table 10).

CsA-Associated Arteriolopathy (CsA-AA)

Frequency of Arteriolar Lesions in CsA and Aza-St Treatment. Arteriolar lesions of any morphology were more often found in the CsA group than in the Aza-St group, especially in late biopsies (Table 5). The medium to severe form of the arteriolopathy observed in the CsA group is here abbreviated CsA-AA.

Table 7. Association Between CsA Parameters and Different Morphological Lesions

Morphology	No. of Biopsies	None	Giant Mitochondria	Vacuolization	Calcification
Vascular rejection	10	2	2	6	6
Interstitial rejection	17	5	0	5	6
Acute tubular necrosis due to conservation injury	3	0	2	3	2
CsA arteriolopathy	13	1	6	8	10
None of the above	15	2	10	6	11

Table 8. Trough Serum CsA and Creatinine Level and CsA Parameters

	Giant Mitochondria		Vacuolization	
	Present	Absent	Present	Absent
No. of patients	18	12	21	9
Serum CsA (mean ± SE) (ng/ml)	759 (± 150)	357 (± 57)	702 (± 133)	357 (± 58)
U test	$p < 0.005$		$p < 0.025$	
Serum creatinine (mean ± SE) (μmole/liter)	447 (± 52)	373 (± 50)	463 (± 47)	312 (± 39)
U test	NS		$p < 0.1$	

Table 9. Trough Serum CsA Level, CsA Parameters, and Associated Renal Lesions

	No Giant Mitochondria or Vacuolization, with or without Calcification	Giant Mitochondria and/or Vacuolization
Rejection, conservation injury, arteriolopathy		
No. of patients	11	17*
CsA (mean ± SE)(ng/ml)	385 (± 41)	456 (± 65)
No rejection, conservation injury, arteriolopathy		
No. of patients	6	8
CsA (mean ± SE)(ng/ml)	359 (± 120)†	1421 (± 281)*†

*†U test between values with identical symbol: $p < 0.0025$.

Morphology of CsA-AA. CsA-AA was limited to the periphery of the vascular tree (arterioles and small arteries up to two layers of myocytes) without concomitant involvement of the larger arteries (except in the vicinity of the branching into arterioles). When larger arteries and arterioles were involved, this was considered as vascular rejection.

The arteriolar lesion in the CsA group was unspecific. Typically, severe arteriolar hyalinosis or necrosis [Fig. 3 (*a, b*)] was present. In some cases, a mucoid thickening of the intima was also observed [Fig. 3 (*c, d*)]. Prominent intimal proliferation or cellular infiltration of the intima was lacking.

Electron microscopy showed lumpy protein deposits in the vascular wall [Fig. 3 (*b*)], more or less extensive necroses of myocytes [Fig. 3 (*d*)], and an increased number of lysosomes and some rare GM in non-necrotic myocytes.

Glomerular lesions clearly different from those accompanying rejection were not present.

The biopsies were subdivided into two main groups for the evaluation of the immunofluorescent findings in vessels and glomeruli: (1) biopsies with vascular rejection and (2) biopsies without signs of vascular rejection, with or without arteriolopathy. In CsA-AA, the arterioles contained an increased amount of IgM and complement (C_3) in comparison with cases without or with slight arteriolopathy only (Table 11). No differences of C_3 and IgM deposits were found between biopsies with CsA-AA and those with vascular rejection (Table 11). In two biopsies with CsA-AA and in one with vascular rejection, there were slight deposits of fibrin both in and around the vessels.

Correlation Between CsA-AA and Other Clinical and Morphological Changes in the CsA Group. Of 59 biopsies, slight arteriolopathy was present in 21, and a medium to severe form in 13 performed in 9 patients (CsA-AA group) (Table 12). The severity of arteriolopathy increased with time; CsA-AA was infrequently found to occur earlier than 3 months after transplantation (Table 12).

The severity of arteriolopathy correlated to

Table 10. Serum Creatinine Level, CsA Parameters, and Associated Renal Lesions

	No Giant Mitochondria or Vacuolization, with or without Calcification	Giant Mitochondria and/or Vacuolization
Rejection, conservation injury, arteriolopathy		
No. of patients	11	17
Serum creatinine (mean ± SE)(μmole/liter)	335 (± 32)*	475 (± 47)*
No rejection, conservation injury, arteriolopathy		
No. of patients	6	8
Serum creatinine (mean ± SE)(μmole/liter)	374 (± 99)	394 (± 80)

*U test between these values: $p < 0.0025$.

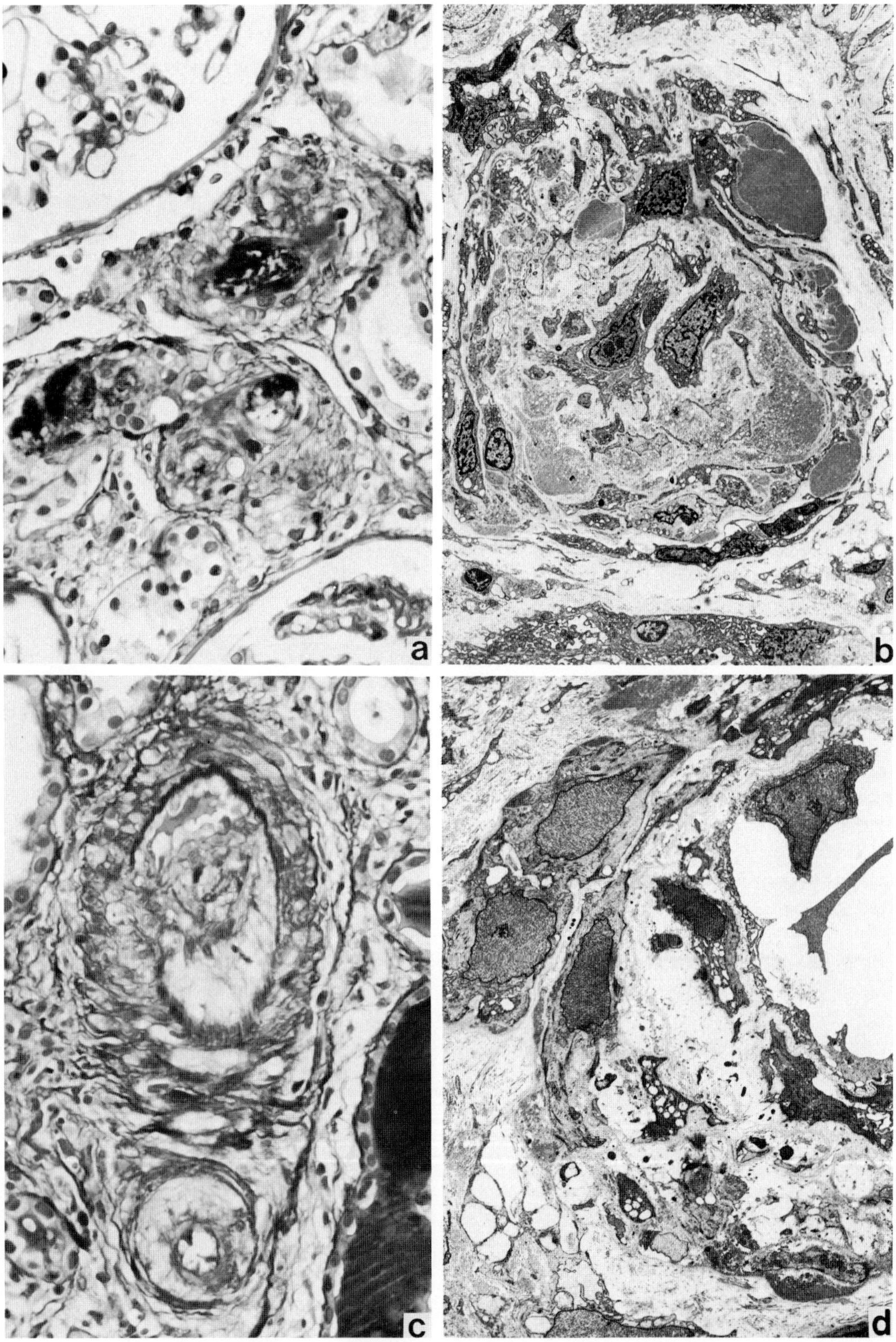

Fig. 3. Vascular lesions (CsA-AA) in CsA treatment. (*a*) Severe arteriolar necrosis with lumpy protein deposits (black) in lumens and throughout the vessel wall. AFOG[12] stain (×390). (*b*) Cross section of an arteriole with massive protein deposits throughout the vessel wall and complete occlusion of the vessel lumen. EM (×1750). (*c*) Massive mucoid thickening of the intima of an arteriole extending into the interlobular artery. AFOG[12] stain (×350). (*d*) Part of an arteriole with necrosis of myocytes and mucoid intimal thickening. EM (×2300).

Table 11. Immunofluorescence Findings in Different Forms of Vascular Lesions

	Light microscopy*			
	Arteriolopathy			
Immunofluorescence	Not Present	Slight	Medium Severe	Vascular Rejection
Arterioles				
IgM (mean ± SE)	1.2 (± 0.1)	1.5 (± 0.2)	2.8 (± 0.3)	2.1 (± 0.2)
C_3 (mean ± SE)	1.9 (± 0.1)	2.1 (± 0.1)	3.2 (± 0.3)	2.7 (± 0.2)
Glomeruli				
IgM (mean ± SE)	1.2 (± 0.1)	1.6 (± 0.2)	1.2 (± 0.1)	1.4 (± 0.2)
C_3 (mean ± SE)	1.6 (± 0.1)	1.3 (± 0.2)	1.6 (± 0.1)	1.6 (± 0.2)
No. of biopsies	19	13	12	11

*Score: 1 = 0, 4 = + + +.

Table 12. Arteriolopathy and Time After Transplantation

	Arteriolopathy		
	0	+	+ +/+ + +
No. of biopsies	25	21	13
Time (mean ± SE)(days)	41 (± 10)	81 (± 21)	114 (± 29)

the severity of interstitial fibrosis (Table 13, Fig. 4).

For comparison of the clinical findings, the 32 patients were allocated to one of the three following groups: (1) patients with CsA-AA, (2) patients without CsA-AA or vascular rejection, and (3) patients with vascular rejection (Table 14).

Mean trough serum CsA levels, maximum serum trough CsA levels, and platelet counts did not differ significantly in the three groups of patients (Table 14). There was, however, a slight but significant increase in the systolic but not the diastolic blood pressure in the CsA-AA group and in the group of patients with vascular rejection within the first 4 weeks of transplantation, as compared with the group of patients without significant vascular lesions. In the CsA-AA group, 3/9 patients received kidney irradiation (Table 14).

Table 13. Association Between Arteriolopathy and Interstitial Fibrosis

		Arteriolopathy		
		0	+	+ +/+ + +
Interstitial fibrosis	0	4	0	0
	+	8	3	2
	+ +/+ + +	2	5	6

*CC_{korr} = 64%, contingency table (3 × 3): $p < 0.05$.

In all patients in whom CsA-AA was observed, the CsA therapy was stopped. Renal function improved under subsequent Aza-St treatment (Table 2).

DISCUSSION

The reliability of the conclusions to be drawn from this study is limited for several reasons, such as the small number of patients and of biopsies per patients, the variable intervals between transplantation and biopsies, the

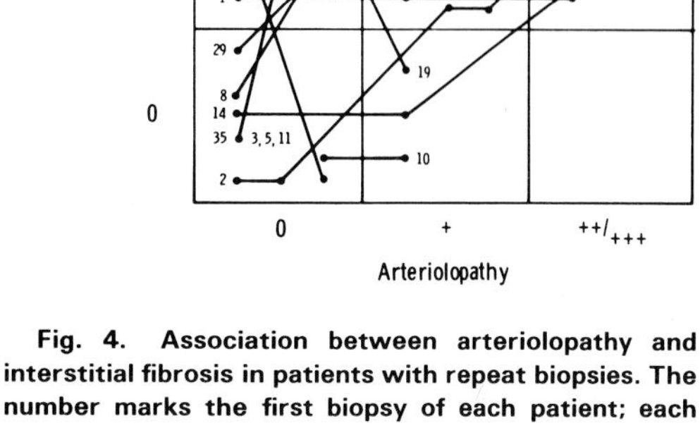

Fig. 4. Association between arteriolopathy and interstitial fibrosis in patients with repeat biopsies. The number marks the first biopsy of each patient; each point represents one biopsy.

Table 14. Clinical Findings Within 1 Month After Transplantation

	CsA-AA	No CsA-AA or Vascular Rejection	Vascular Rejection
Number of patients	9	14	9
Number of patients analyzed*	9	12	6
Serum CsA (mean ± SE)(ng/ml)	914 (± 306)	908 (± 204)	505 (± 118)
Serum creatinine (mean ± SE)(μmole/liter)	319 (± 69)	414 (± 75)	368 (± 63)
Thrombocyte count (× 10^3/mm^3 ± SE)	245 (± 21)	232 (± 21)	306 (± 48)
Blood pressure			
Systolic (mean ± SE)(mmHg)†	156 (± 4)	145 (± 2)	160 (± 6)
Diastolic (mean ± SE)(mmHg)	87 (± 3)	88 (± 3)	86 (± 2)
Kidney irradiation (3 × 150 rads)(no. of patients)	3	0	3

*Daily measurements of blood pressure and thrombocytes and weekly CsA determinations.
†U test: $p < 0.01$.

lack of a randomized control group, and the retrospective design of the study. Furthermore, other variables that may have influenced renal function of the transplanted kidneys, such as drug interaction with CsA,[18] and viral infections, were not considered.

With these reservations in mind, we dare to make the following preliminary statements.

(1) The typical morphological features of interstitial and vascular rejection that have been described previously were also observed in biopsies of poorly functioning grafts under CsA immunosuppression.[12,17] However, our CsA group appeared to display more frequently diffuse but not focal interstitial infiltrates[18] and a definitely decreased incidence of vascular rejection. Renal findings in patients receiving bone marrow transplants showed neither interstitial nephritis nor vasculitis.[5,7,19] Thus, we believe that CsA-related damage contributes little if anything to the density of interstitial infiltrates, nor does it mimic other rejection phenomena.

(2) Giant mitochondria, isometric tubular vacuolization, and microcalcifications are nonspecific tubular lesions that have been observed in kidneys of Aza-St–treated transplant recipients as well as in a variety of other nephropathies.[8,12,20–22] However, the CsA parameters were much more conspicuous in CsA-treated patients.

In the CsA group, the CsA parameters were observed in varying frequencies and combinations. This may be due to a focal distribution, sampling error, and, probably, a different biological half-life. The frequently found microcalcifications probably persisted in the kidneys for a longer time than did the GM and vacuolization. Therefore, only GM and vacuolization should be considered as indicators of actual CsA-associated renal damage.

That CsA treatment is a typical cause of isometric tubular vacuolization,[7,9,23–27] megamitochondria,[5,8,21,23,28,29] and dystrophic calcification[5,9,28] or necrosis of the tubular epithelium[5,7,9,28] has been shown both in animal experiments and in recipients of bone marrow and kidney transplants. Striking increases and polymorphism of lysosomes in the proximal tubules described by others in animal experiments and human bone marrow transplant recipients were not regularly observed in our biopsies.[7,9,27,28]

Available data are still insufficient to permit speculation on the pathogenesis of the CsA parameters and the causal relationship to impaired renal function. Mannitol or other osmotic substances as causes of isometric vacuolization can be excluded because in Basel they have neither been used in kidney transplant recipients nor been administered in animal experiments.

In patients without rejection or other associated renal lesions, the CsA levels were significantly higher when GM and/or vacuoles were present. Both lesions were absent when the serum CsA trough level was more or less within the recommended therapeutic range of 50–150 ng/ml serum, corresponding to whole blood levels of 300–900 ng/ml in our experience.

However, patients with signs of rejection showed GM and/or vacuoles to be present even at therapeutic levels of CsA. This finding might indicate a higher susceptibility to CsA-associated renal damage in the presence of contributing factors such as rejection, vasculopathy of any kind, conservation injury, or renal failure.

This interpretation has been supported by animal experiments, which showed that development of CsA parameters to be dose-dependent. Within 6 days, cytoplasmatic inclusion bodies (GM, lysosomes), tubular vacuoles, and microcalcifications developed to an increasing extent. After administration of 350 mg/day for 3 days, the tubular damage corresponded roughly to that after administration of 100 mg/day for 6 days (Table 15). Additional renal damage such as ischemia aggravated the CsA-associated tubular lesions: Within 48 hr after ischemia, GM and vacuoles were more prominent in CsA-treated animals than in the controls (Table 16).[24]

(3) The interpretation of vascular lesions in renal transplants is difficult because not only vascular rejection but also spontaneous vessel disease may occur. Vascular rejection may involve the entire vascular tree, from the renal artery up to the glomeruli. Depending on the stage of disease, intravascular coagulation and/or proliferative or even sclerosing vascular changes may ensue. In vascular rejection, however, the arterial lesions predominate, and if arteriolar changes occur, they are always associated with lesions in arteries. We have, however, never observed a vascular rejection limited to the arterioles in Aza-St–treated patients.[12] Therefore, the frequent occurrence of arteriolar lesions in CsA-treated transplant recipients was recognized as an unusual finding and termed CsA-AA. Our definition and morphological description of CsA-AA is still incomplete due to the small number of patients we have observed and the lack of objective criteria. In our preliminary definition, CsA-AA is a vascular lesion limited to the arterioles and smallest arteries (with up to two layers of myocytes). The light microscopy picture is unspecific: severe arteriolar hyalinosis, arteriolar necrosis, or mucoid thickening of the intima as seen in the hemolytic uremic syndrome.[12] The spectrum of pathogenic possibilities is wide; three possibilities in particular must be considered further: vascular rejection, hypertension, and coagulation disorder.

Vascular Rejection. Could CsA-AA be explained as vascular rejection? The following arguments speak against it: (1) The larger arteries are unaffected (see preceding discus-

Table 16. Sensitizing Effect of Ischemia on CsA-Induced Tubular Lesions

	Tubular Lesions* 20 mg - CsA - 50 mg†			
Ischemia for 90 Min.	−	+	−	+
Giant Mitochondria Lysosomes	0.0	0.9	0.4	0.9
Vacuoles	0.0	0.8	0.4	1.7

*Mean score (0–3) for 10 female rats in each group.
†Gavage feeding of CsA (mg/kg) in olive oil for 48 hr.

Table 15. Dose Dependence of Tubular Damage in the Rat

CsA (mg/kg)	Tubular* Giant Mitochondria Lysosomes	Vacuoles	Calcification	Mean Overall Damage Score*
After 6 days' i.v. administration of CsA				
7.5	0.75	0	0.5	0.40
20	0.50	0	1.0	0.50
50	1.25	1.0	1.5	1.25
100	2.50	2.25	1.5	2.08
After 3 days' i.v. administration of CsA				
350	2.25	2.0	1.0	1.75

*Mean score (0–3) for 4 female rats (200 g body weight) per group.

sion). (2) The paucicellular mucoid thickening of the intima is an unusual finding in transplant vasculopathy, which is either more proliferative or in later stages characterized by a more dense fibrous intimal thickening. (3) The strongest argument against vascular rejection is the striking improvement of renal function after substituting conventional immunosuppression for CsA. In contrast, all patients with vascular rejection experienced progressive deterioration of renal function with either CsA or conventional immunosuppression.

Hypertension. The arteriolar lesions could be attributed to hypertension. Indeed, most patients with CsA-AA were hypertensive during the first month after transplantation. However, the hypertension was usually mild, with a mean systolic blood pressure <160 mmHg and a mean diastolic blood pressure <90 mmHg. The observed arteriolar lesions in CsA-AA were developed to an extent that could not be expected in borderline hypertension.[30] Finally, severe arteriolopathy was found in one patient who received a kidney from his normotensive mother and in whom not a single increased systolic or diastolic blood pressure measurement had ever been recorded before biopsy. However, the significance of hypertension in the development of CsA-AA must not be underestimated; experimental studies with spontaneous hypertensive rats have shown that vascular lesions in the kidney develop more readily in the presence of CsA than in its absence.[31]

Coagulation Disorder. Finally, another pathogenic mechanism may have been operative. The arteriolar lesion resembled that observed in the hemolytic uremic syndrome (HUS). Despite the lack of fibrin in most cases, a pathogenic mechanism similar to a hemolytic uremic syndrome with intrarenal coagulation cannot be excluded. Fibrin deposition in HUS is time-dependent and limited to the early stages of the disease. In later phases of HUS, the immunofluorescence findings are unspecific and by light microscopy findings more similar to vascular hyalinosis or necrosis predominate.[31–33] This interpretation is further supported by the finding of glomerular thrombi and vascular hyalinosis and vascular lesions typical of HUS in bone marrow transplant recipients treated with CsA.[7,34,35] Clinically typical cases of HUS have been reported in poorly matched bone marrow transplant recipients and kidney transplant recipients treated with CsA.[7,34–36] Finally, the development of a HUS-like syndrome in rabbits treated with bovine serum albumin and CsA points in the same direction.[37]

Thus, transitory hypertension, latent disturbances of the coagulatory system, and other factors such as irradiation, drug interaction, and infections, may trigger the development of the arteriolar lesion. The common pathogenic denominator of all these factors in CsA treatment may be the suggested disturbance of prostacyclin stimulating factor synthesis.[34,38] Under experimental conditions, a vascular lesion has never been observed, even with tremendous doses of CsA, without additional damaging factors such as hypertension.[31] The development of CsA-AA is probably not dose-dependent, neither in animal experiments nor in human kidney transplants.[31]

The extent of the arteriolar lesion is correlated with the extent of interstitial fibrosis, which may be of prognostic significance. Whether interstitial fibrosis can develop independently of arteriolopathy in CsA-treated patients is still unknown.[39]

On the basis of 2 years' experience with CsA treatment in kidney transplantation we make the following suggestions regarding biopsy findings as a guide to therapy: (1) Reduce CsA dosage when GM and/or vacuolization is present. (2) Optimal blood pressure control is necessary, and if there is progressive deterioration of renal function, substitute Aza-St for CsA in case of CsA-AA. (3) Treat severe interstitial rejection with steroid pulses and low-dose oral steroids while carefully monitoring CsA dosage and blood levels. (4) The prognosis of vascular rejection is poor. Steroid pulse and oral steroid therapy should be applied, but no benefit can be expected from substituting Aza-St for CsA.

REFERENCES

1. Green JC: Diagnostic Histopath 4:157, 1981
2. Morris PG: Transplantation 32:349, 1981
3. Hamilton DV, Calne RY, Evans DB, et al: Lancet 1:1218, 1981
4. Klintmalm GBG, Iwatsuki S, Starzl TE, Lancet 1:470, 1981
5. Marbet U, Graf U, Mihatsch MJ, et al: Schweiz Med Wschr 110:2017, 1980
6. Klintmalm GBG, Bergstrand A, Ringden O, et al: Transplant Proc 15:493, 1983
7. Schulmann H, Striker G, Deeg HJ, et al: N Engl J Med 305:1392, 1981
8. Mihatsch MJ, Spichtin HP, Lörtscher A, et al: Nieren- und Hochdruckkrankheiten 11:193, 1982
9. Ryffel B: In White DJG (ed): Cyclosporin A. Amsterdam, Elsevier Biomedical, 1982, pp 45–76
10. Hamilton DV, Evans DV, Thiru S: In White DJG (ed): Cyclosporin A. Amsterdam, Elsevier Biomedical, 1982, pp 393–411
11. Report on the European Multicentre Trial: Lancet 2:57, 1982
12. Zollinger HU, Mihatsch MJ: Renal Pathology in Biopsy. Berlin, Springer Verlag, 1978
13. Bancroft JD, Stevens A: Theory and Practice of Histological Disease. Edinburgh, Churchill Livingstone, 1977, p 285
14. Gurr E: Staining. London, Leonard Hill Ltd., 1962, p 210
15. Scheuer PJ: Liver Biopsy Interpretation (3rd ed). London, Baillière Tindall, 1978
16. Sachs L: Angewandte Statistik (5th ed). Berlin, Springer Verlag, 1974
17. Olson S: In Churg J (ed): Kidney Disease. Baltimore, Williams & Wilkins, 1979, pp 327–355
18. Morgenstern GR, Powles R, Robinson B, et al: Lancet 2:1342, 1982
19. Mihatsch MJ: (unpublished data)
20. Chedid A, Jao W, Port J: Am J Gastroenterol 73:319, 1980
21. Kirwan PD, Baxter CR, Duggin GG, et al: Lancet 2:146, 1981
22. Suzuki T, Furusato M, Takasaki S, et al: Lab Invest 33:578, 1975
23. Mihatsch MJ, Olivieri V, Marbet U, et al: Lancet 1:1162, 1981
24. Thiel G, Torhorst J, Brunner FP: Proc Clin Dial Transplant Forum 10:62, 1982
25. Blair JT, Thompson AW, Whiting PH, et al: J Pathol 138:163, 1982
26. Farthing MJG, Clark ML, Pendry A, et al: Biochem Pharmacol 24:3311, 1981
27. Whiting PH, Thompson AW, Blair JT, et al: Br J Exp Pathol 63:88, 1982
28. Ryffel B, Donatsch P, Hauser R, et al: Arch Toxicol 53:107, 1983
29. Waldherr R, Horsch R, Dreikorn K: Nieren- und Hochdruckkrankheiten 11:194, 1982
30. Suwa N, Takahashi T: Morphological and Morphometrical Analysis of Circulation in Hypertension and Ischemic Kidney. Munich, Urban Schwarzenberg, 1971
31. Siegl H, Ryffel B, Petric R: Transplant Proc (this issue)
32. Fong JSC, de Chadarevian JP, Kuplan BS: Pediatric Clin No Am 29:835, 1982
33. Thoenes W, John HD: Klin Wschr 58:173, 1980
34. Powles RL, Kay HEM, Clink HM, et al: Lancet 1:612, 1983
35. Atkinson K, Biggs JC, Hayes J, et al: Br J Haematol (accepted for publication)
36. Leithner O, Sinzinger H, Pohanka E, et al: Lancet 1:1470, 1982, and Transplant Proc (this issue)
37. Neild GH, Ivory K, Hiramatsu M, et al: Transplant Proc (this issue)
38. Neild GH, Rocchi G: Transplant Proc (this issue)
39. Farnsworth A, Hall B, Bishop A, et al: Transplant Proc (this issue)

Morphology of Cyclosporine Nephrotoxicity and of Acute Rejection in Cyclosporine-Prednisone Immunosuppressed Renal Allograft Recipients

R. K. Sibley, R. M. Ferguson, D. E. R. Sutherland, R. L. Simmons, and J. S. Najarian

CYCLOSPORINE A (CsA) is an immunosuppressive agent that is a potent inhibitor of acute rejection of the renal allograft, but the incidence of nephrotoxicity (NT) caused by CsA is nearly as impressive as its potency in preventing rejection. Most reports emphasize the difficulty of separating CsA-NT from acute rejection, demonstrated by the frequency of acute rejection (9%–78%) vs. CsA-NT (50%) in various studies.[1–5] In the randomized prospective study at the University of Minnesota comparing CsA-prednisone and conventional immunosuppression, a diagnosis of acute rejection was made in 17% of patients treated with CsA-prednisone, and 66% had CsA-NT as the cause of impaired renal function.[6]

Various procedures have been used in an attempt to differentiate a patient with CsA-NT from one experiencing acute rejection. Some of these include CsA plasma or serum levels,[7–9] measurement of subcapsular hydrostatic pressure,[4] renal scintigraphy,[10] enumeration of T-cell subpopulations of the peripheral blood,[11,12] enumeration of T-cell subpopulation ratios in kidney biopsies,[13] needle aspiration cytology,[14] and renal biopsy.[2–5,7,15–19] In our initial attempt to characterize the histologic features of CsA-NT, we found that patients with acute rejection and nephrotoxicity both had a tubulointerstitial nephritis of variable severity.[19]

From the Department of Laboratory Medicine and Pathology and the Department of Surgery, University of Minnesota Medical School, Minneapolis, MN.

Supported by NIH Grant AM 13083.

Reprint requests should be addressed to Dr. Richard K. Sibley, University of Minnesota, Department of Laboratory Medicine and Pathology, Box 609, Mayo Memorial Building, 420 Delaware Street S.E., Minneapolis, MN 55455.

0041–1345/83/1505–0117$01.00/0

However, using the linear logistic regression method, it was found that the presence or absence of four histologic parameters in various combinations correctly predicted CsA nephrotoxicity and acute rejection in 94% of 116 kidney biopsies. We now report this model's usefulness in predicting nephrotoxicity and acute rejection and the results of treatment based on the histologic diagnosis in a randomized prospective study.

MATERIALS AND METHODS

Patients

The clinical charts of 44 renal allograft recipients undergoing 60 needle biopsies between August 1982 and May 1983 were reviewed. Confirmation of the renal biopsy intepretation of nephrotoxicity was based on a positive response of the serum creatinine to a lowering of the CsA dose. Chronic or nonresponsive CsA nephrotoxicity was confirmed when renal biopsy findings were incompatible with acute rejection and the serum creatinine did not improve until the cyclosporine was stopped and the patient was switched to conventional immunosuppression. An interpretation of acute rejection was confirmed when the serum creatinine decreased following therapy with increased glucocorticoids and/or antilymphocyte globulin.

Histology

Tissues obtained by percutaneous needle biopsies of the kidney were processed for light, electron microscopic, and immunofluorescent microscopy as previously described.[20] The presence or absence of four of the nine histologic parameters identified as being predictive of acute rejection or CsA nephrotoxicity as previously reported was tabulated for each biopsy.[19] The four histologic parameters found to be predictive of rejection or CsA-NT included the presence or absence of edema, vasculitis, mononuclear cell exudation within the glomerular capillaries ("glomerulitis"), and the ratio of mononuclear inflammatory cells within interstitial tissues compared to the peritubular capillaries (I/C ratio). The five histologic factors found not to be important in predicting rejection were not tabulated. These were the presence or absence of tubular necrosis, tubular ectasia, infiltration of the tubules by inflammatory cells ("tubulitis"), and the focal vs. diffuse and overall severity of the tubulointerstitial nephritis.

RESULTS

Sixty biopsies from 44 renal allograft recipients were examined. The frequency of interstitial edema, "glomerulitis," vasculitis, and the three I/C ratios are presented in Table 1. These numbers represent the frequency of each histologic parameter in acute rejection or CsA-NT. The interpretation of rejection or nephrotoxicity was derived in each biopsy by tabulating the presence or absence of the four histologic parameters and determining the probability of acute rejection or CsA-NT by the linear logistic regression method as previously reported[19] (Table 2). A diagnosis of acute rejection was made in 17 biopsies from 14 patients, and 43 biopsies from 30 patients were interpreted as CsA-NT. A highly significant difference in the occurrence of interstitial edema, the presence of a mononuclear cell exudate within the glomerular tuft, and vasculitis is evident between biopsies in patients with nephrotoxicity and acute rejection. A tubulointerstitial nephritis of minimal-mild to moderate-severe intensity was evident in all but 1 of the biopsies. In 9 (20.9%) of the CsA-NT biopsies, the majority of the mononuclear cells were found within the peritubular capillaries, while none of the acute rejection biopsies had this feature. On the other hand, a majority of the biopsies with acute rejection (70.6%) had a high IC/ratio. Nine biopsies from 5 patients with CsA-NT also had a high I/C ratio, but the infiltrate was not associated with any of the other three histologic parameters predictive of rejection. Approximately equivalent numbers of inflammatory cells in the interstitial tissues and peritubular capillaries were found in 29.4% of patients with acute rejection and 58.1% of patients with CsA-NT.

Fifty-three patients (biopsies) were initially treated with decreased cyclosporine dose (or no change in cyclosporine dose) when CsA-NT was predicted or an increase of steroid dose when acute rejection was predicted. Forty-two patients—14 with acute rejection and 28 with CsA-NT—responded to antirejection therapy in the former and reduced CsA dose in the latter. Six patients predicted as having CsA-NT received 1–3 days of increased steroids before the biopsy was performed and/or interpreted. After the diagnosis, the cyclosporine dose was decreased in each patient with return of creatinine to previous levels. Seven patients were not treated according to the acute rejection–CsA-NT probability data. One of the patients predicted to have acute rejection (98.65% probability) was treated with increased cyclosporine dose, but because of a continued elevation in the creatinine, a second biopsy was performed; this also predicted acute rejection (98.65% probability). Antirejection therapy with increased steroids was followed by return of renal function. Four patients predicted as having nephrotoxicity were initially treated with increased steroids, but because of no response or continued elevation of the creatinine, the cyclosporine dose was decreased, followed by normalization of the serum creatinine. Two further patients predicted as having nephrotoxicity were initially treated for rejec-

Table 1. Frequency of Histologic Parameters in 60 Renal Biopsies in CsA-Prednisone–Immunosuppressed Patients (Prospective Study)

Parameter	CsA Nephrotoxicity	Acute Rejection	Fisher Exact Test *p* Value
Interstitial edema	11.6%	82.4%	< 0.001
Vasculitis	2.3%	64.7%	< 0.001
Glomerulitis	20.9%	64.7%	< 0.001
I/C ratio* $\leq$ 1:3	20.9%	—	< 0.001
I/C ratio $\geq$ 3:1	20.9%	70.6%	< 0.001
I/C ratio $<$ 3:1 but $>$ 1:3	58.1%	29.4%	< 0.001

*I/C = Interstitial to intraperitubular capillary mononuclear cell infiltrate.

Table 2. Risk Factors and Probability of Acute Rejection or Cyclosporine A Nephrotoxicity* (Prospective Study)

Vasculitis	Edema	Glomerulitis	I/C Ratio†	% Probability of Rejection	Total Biopsies ($N = 60$)	Number Predicted Correctly‡ ($N = 54$)
0	0	0	1	0.004	5	5
0	0	0	2	0.24	15	14
0	0	0	3	12.59	9	7
0	0	+	1	0.056	3	3
0	+	0	1	0.086	1	1
+	0	0	1	0.42	0	—
0	0	+	2	3.23	5	4
0	+	0	2	4.86	3	3
+	0	0	2	20.04	1	1
0	0	+	3	66.56	1	0
0	+	0	3	75.28	4	3
+	0	0	3	93.82	1	1
0	+	+	1	1.17	0	—
+	0	+	1	5.57	0	—
+	+	0	1	8.17	0	—
+	+	+	1	55.48	0	—
0	+	+	2	41.39	1	1
+	0	+	2	77.60	1	1
+	+	0	2	84.29	1	1
+	+	+	2	98.65	3	3
0	+	+	3	97.68	1	1
+	0	+	3	99.52	0	—
+	+	0	3	99.69	2	2
+	+	+	3	99.98	3	3

*Linear logistic regression method.

†I/C ratio: 1 = $\leq$ 1:3, 2 = $>$ 1:3 but $<$ 3:1, 3 = $\geq$ 3:1.

‡91.6% of predictions.

tion until clinically evident viral and fungal infections were discovered and the patient was appropriately treated. Both eventually regained normal renal function following resolution of the infectious disease. Five patients did not respond to appropriate therapy as deduced from the mathematical model. Two patients predicted as acute rejection and two as CsA-NT did not respond to "appropriate" therapy but had resolution of their symptoms when treatment for acute rejection rather than nephrotoxicity or nephrotoxicity rather than acute rejection was implemented. One patient with what appeared to be CsA-NT did not respond to any type of therapy, even though the biopsy showed a minimal infiltrate and essentially normal biopsy. This patient is presently on dialysis. Thus, 55/60 (91.6%) biopsies were correctly predicted as either CsA-NT or acute rejection.

DISCUSSION

Deterioration of graft function during the first 6 months following transplantation occurs in the majority of renal allograft recipients treated with cyclosporine A.[1-6] Nephrotoxicity is a well-established side effect of CsA immunosuppression; thus, the impairment of renal function in the post-transplantation period could be related to acute rejection or due to the nephrotoxic effect of CsA or another factor such as acute tubular necrosis. Because the treatment of acute rejection requires the addition of immunosuppressive drugs and that of nephrotoxicity requires reduction in CsA dose, it is important to differentiate renal impairment secondary to nephrotoxicity from that of acute rejection.

Percutaneous renal biopsy is one procedure that has been used in an attempt to establish a diagnosis of rejection or nephrotoxicity. Nonspecific tubular changes or no significant abnormality characterize many cases of CsA-NT, while the finding of a tubulointerstitial nephritis has been thought to be characteristic of acute rejection.[1-5,7,15-18]

In our pilot study of cyclosporine A as an immunosuppressive agent at the University of Minnesota, a moderate acute tubulointerstitial nephritis was seen in renal biopsies of the first two patients with increased creatinine, and a diagnosis of acute rejection was naturally rendered. However, the patients did not respond to antirejection therapy as was expected. Because of the report of renal impairment related to CsA by Calne et al.,[1] the CsA dose in the two patients was decreased, and their serum creatinine returned to previous levels. This suggested the possibility that nephrotoxicity could simulate acute rejection not only clinically but on histologic grounds as well.

In 115/116 subsequent renal biopsies from CsA-immunosuppressed patients, a tubulointerestitial nephritis of variable severity was seen, and it appeared that CsA-NT was often associated with a significant interstitial nephritis.[19] In the retrospective analysis of the clinical symptoms, response to treatment (increase or decrease CsA or steroid doses) and the morphological features in the 116 biopsies from 51 patients, we attempted to determine whether there were any histologic parameters that would allow the differentiation of nephrotoxicity from acute rejection.[19] Using the linear logistic step-down method, we examined nine histologic parameters from the 116 biopsies and defined four histologic features, the combination of which when present or absent resulted in a probability of rejection for each biopsy. CsA-NT or acute rejection was correctly predicted in 94% of the biopsies in this retrospective analysis.[19] Our present study examined the feasability of utilizing the four histologic features in predicting the probability of CsA-NT or acute rejection on a prospective basis. Sixty biopsies from 44 recipients were studied. Acute rejection was predicted in 17 biopsies, and CsA-NT in 43. Fifteen of 17 (88.2%) patients predicted as acute rejection responded to antirejection therapy, and 40/43 (93%) patients predicted as CsA-NT responded to lowered CsA dose or a switch to conventional therapy because of chronic nephrotoxicity. Interestingly, 5 patients in whom treatment was not coordinated with the prediction of acute rejection or nephrotoxicity eventually responded when appropriate therapy was instituted. Two patients predicted as CsA-NT probably had impaired function because of viral or fungal infection. Renal function improved in the latter patients following resolution of the infectious process.

The number of biopsies interpreted correctly as acute rejection or CsA-NT was similar in both the retrospective (93.96%) and the prospective (91.8%) studies. Examination of the results from both studies (Table 3) demonstrates the importance of vasculitis in predicting acute rejection and the I/C ratio $\leq$ 1:3 in predicting CsA-NT. When the vasculitis and I/C $\leq$ 1:3 parameters are not present in a biopsy, the combination of the presence or absence of edema, "glomerulitis," and an I/C $\geq$ 3:1 and I/C $>$ 1:3 but $<$ 3:1 are highly predictive of the probability of acute rejection or CsA-NT.

These studies have not ascertained the pathophysiologic mechanism of CsA-NT, nor can the relationship of CsA-NT and the presence of an interstitial inflammatory infiltrate be explained. The finding of an interstitial mononuclear cell infiltrate in rats given toxic doses of CsA suggests that the tubulointerstitial nephritis seen in humans may in fact be an adverse response to CsA as well.[21,22] An immunofluorescent study examining the T-cell subpopulations of lymphoid cells from biopsies of kidneys diagnosed as acute rejection or CsA-NT has demonstrated that the cellular infiltrates in CsA-NT consisted of equivalent numbers of T helper and T killer-suppressor cells, whereas patients with acute rejection had increased T killer-suppressor cells as compared to the number of T helper lymphocytes.[13] It is possible that T helper cells and macrophages enter the kidney in patients

Table 3. Risk Factors and Probability of Acute Rejection or Cyclosporine A Nephrotoxicity* (Retrospective and Prospective Studies)

Vasculitis	Edema	Glomerulitis	I/C ratio†	% Probability of Rejection	Total Biopsies (N = 176)	Number Predicted Correctly‡ (N = 164)
0	0	0	1	0.004	15	15
0	0	0	2	0.24	44	43
0	0	0	3	12.59	13	11
0	0	+	1	0.056	7	7
0	+	0	1	0.086	3	3
+	0	0	1	0.42	0	—
0	0	+	2	3.23	9	8
0	+	0	2	4.86	16	15
+	0	0	2	20.04	2	2
0	0	+	3	66.56	6	4
0	+	0	3	75.28	10	8
+	0	0	3	93.82	1	1
0	+	+	1	1.17	7	7
+	0	+	1	5.57	0	—
+	+	0	1	8.17	1	1
+	+	+	1	55.48	0	—
0	+	+	2	41.39	8	5
+	0	+	2	77.60	2	2
+	+	0	2	84.29	1	1
+	+	+	2	98.65	6	6
0	+	+	3	97.68	8	7
+	0	+	3	99.52	2	2
+	+	0	3	99.69	4	4
+	+	+	3	99.98	11	11

*Linear logistic regression method.
†I/C ratio 1 = ≤ 1:3, 2 = > 1:3 but < 3:1, 3 = ≥ 3:1
‡93.2% of predictions.

immunosuppressed with CsA but the cells remain within the vasculature, as we have demonstrated by our histologic study. Perhaps presentation of antigen by the macrophages to T helper cells or some other unknown factor is hindered by CsA, thus preventing cellular immunity and acute rejection.

Our ultrastructural study in rats given various dosages of CsA revealed mitochondrial, brush border, and basilar interdigitation abnormalities, as well as increased numbers of lysosomes even at pharmacologic doses.[21] Whiting et al. have reported similar abnormalities.[22] Fine structural abnormalities were also found in 30 of our renal allograft biopsies diagnosed as CsA-NT and consisted of increased mitochondrial size, increased number of mitochondria, occasional giant matrical bodies within mitochondria, and enlarged lysosomes (unpublished data).

These immunohistochemical and ultrastructural studies suggest that CsA-NT may be the result of direct subcellular organelle injury to tubules, and the "interstitial nephritis" possibly represents an impaired type of acute rejection.

REFERENCES

1. Calne RY, White DJG, Thiru S, et al: Lancet 2:1323, 1978

2. Starzl TE, Klintmalm GBG, Weil R III, et al: Surg Gynecol Obstet 153:486, 1981

3. Klintmalm G, Bergstrand A, Ringdén O, et al: Transplant Proc 15:493, 1983

4. Wagner E, Pichlmayr R, Wonigeit K, et al: Transplant Proc 15:489, 1983

5. Wood AJ: Lancet 2:57, 1983
6. Najarian JS, Ferguson RM, Sutherland DER, et al: Transplant Proc 15:438, 1983
7. White DJG, McNaughton D, and Calne RY: Transplant Proc 15:454, 1983
8. French ME, Thompson JR, Hunnisett AGW, et al: Transplant Proc 15:485, 1983
9. Kahan BD, Ried M, Newburger J: Transplant Proc 15:446, 1983
10. Klintmalm GBC, Klingensmith WC III, Iwatsuki S, et al: Radiology 142:199, 1982
11. Van Buren CT, Kerman RH, Agostino G, et al: Transplant Proc 15:527, 1983
12. Ferguson RM, Fidelus RK, Sawchuk RJ, et al: Transplant Proc 15:535, 1983
13. Platt JL, Ferguson RM, Sibley RK, et al: Transplantation (in press)
14. Häyry P, Ahonen J, von Willebrand E, et al: Scand J Immunol 16:135, 1982
15. Fernando ON, Sweny P, Farrington K, et al: Transplant Proc 12:244, 1980
16. Thiru S, Calne RY: Lancet 2:146, 1981
17. White DJG, Calne RY: Immunol Rev 65:115, 1982
18. Morris PJ, French ME, Ting A, et al: In White DJG (ed): Cyclosporin A. New York, Elsevier Biomedical, 1982, pp 355–364
19. Sibley RK, Rynasiewicz J, Ferguson RM, et al: Surgery 94:225, 1983
20. Matas AJ, Sibley RK, Mauer SM, et al: Ann Surg 197:226, 1983
21. Simonton SC, Rynasiewicz J, Sibley RK: Lab Invest 48:78A, 1983
22. Whiting PH, Thomson AW, Blair JT, et al: Br J Exp Pathol 63:88, 1982

Effects of Cyclosporine on Human Renal Allograft Rejection: An Ad Interim Report

P. Häyry, J. Ahonen, E. von Willebrand, B. Eklund, K. Höckerstedt, K. Salmela, E. Pettersson, A. Kauste, E. Taskinen, M. Lalla, H. Sarelin, B. Kuhlbäck, M. Kääriäinen, R. Paldanius, E. Lampainen, K. Huttunen, M. Viranta, T. Vänttinen, J. Forström, V. A. Myllyniemi, L. Tarssanen, U. M. Henttula, A. Helanterä, A. Relander, H. Borgmästars, A. Linkola, E. Leijala, P. Kunelius, A. Vartia, M. Eloranta, S. Pajunen, and H. Granlund

IN A PRELIMINARY leg of this trial,[1] 20 cadaveric kidney allograft recipients were randomized for azathioprine (Aza) plus methylprednisolone (MP) or for cyclosporine A (CsA) as the only immunosuppressive agent. Both groups received intensified oral MP during rejection. All transplants were monitored by alternate-day fine needle aspiration biopsy and by transplant aspiration cytology.

This study demonstrated that some of the patients treated with CsA had a significantly decreased initial urine output associated with morphological changes in the kidney tubular component and a distinct monocytic-lymphocytic inflammation in situ. CsA-treated patients had normal levels of blood leukocytes, thrombocytes, and lymphocytes but displayed a strong initial blood eosinophilia that was absent in the control subjects. During the first 30 days after transplantation, 15 in situ episodes of inflammation were recorded in 9 patients receiving CsA, while only 6 episodes occurred in 10 patients receiving Aza + MP ($p < 0.01$). The first episode of inflammation in the CsA-treated patients occurred earlier, peaked on days 5–8, and was followed by another distinct episode on days 23–26. In the Aza + MP–treated patients, only 1 episode of inflammation occurred on the average, peaking on day 14 postoperatively. The onset of transplant function had no impact on the in situ inflammatory response of rejection in the CsA-treated patients or on the concentration of CsA in the serum. As the initial changes in the CsA-treated transplants may have been related to lack of anti-inflammatory steroids rather than to direct CsA toxicity, and as the very early inflammatory episodes under CsA could have been explained by the initial intramuscular application of this drug's resulting in very poor serum levels,[2] a second trial was designed.

In this trial, 96 new cadaveric renal transplant recipients were randomized for three treatment groups: Aza + MP, CsA, and CsA + MP. As in the previous trial, the patients were monitored—in addition to the routine clinical parameters—by alternate-day fine needle aspiration biopsy. This report contains the results when approximately 50% of the patients had passed the 6-month checkpoint. Upon completion of this trial, a separate clinical report, as well as a detailed analysis of the in situ inflammatory events in the three treatment groups, will be given.

From the Transplantation Laboratory, Fourth Department of Surgery, University of Helsinki, and the Finnish Renal Transplant Study Group, Helsinki, Finland.

Supported by Grant AM 26882-03 from the National Institutes of Health, Bethesda, MD, and grants from the Sigrid Juselius Foundation and the Association of Finnish Life Insurance Companies, Helsinki, Finland.

Reprint requests should be addressed to Dr. P. Häyry, Transplantation Laboratory, University of Helsinki, SF 00290 Helsinki 29, Finland.

0041–1345/83/1505–0118$01.00/0

MATERIALS AND METHODS

Ninety-six patients receiving first or second cadaveric renal transplants were randomized by Sandoz Pharmaceuticals, Basel, and the randomizations were distributed in 96 envelopes. An envelope was opened when the patient arrived for transplantation.

Treatment Groups

In the Aza + MP group, the patients received 2 mg/kg/day of Aza and 3.6 mg/kg/day of MP, tapered to

0.5 mg/kg/day in 15 days. In the CsA group, the patients received approximately 17 mg/kg/day CsA as i.v. infusion for the first 2–3 days, adjusted to 200–250 mg/ml plasma level after transfer to oral administration. In the CsA + MP group, the patients received CsA as above, and in addition, 3.6 mg/kg/day of MP, tapered to 0 mg/kg/day in 9 days.

All episodes of rejection were treated with 3.0 mg/kg/day of oral MP divided in four daily doses. If patients in the CsA group underwent a second episode of rejection, a small maintenance dose of steroids, consisting of ~0.3 mg/kg/day, was given to these patients thereafter.

Diagnosis of Rejection and Fine Needle Aspiration Cytology

The clinical diagnosis of rejection, and obtaining, processing, and interpreting of the aspiration biopsies, have been described in detail in previous reports.[3,4]

RESULTS

Description of the Test Groups

The three test groups were homogenous ($p > 0.05$) with respect to weight, height, weight-height ratio, total ischemic period of the transplant, total number of preoperative blood transfusions, and mismatches in HLA-A, B and HLA-DR. There were no significant differences in risk factors, including diabetes mellitus, amyloidosis, age in excess of 55 years, and a previous transplant rejected in less than 1 year, between the three groups.

Onset of Renal Function and Duration of Postoperative Hospitalization

Based on the previous trial demonstrating no differences in the inflammatory pattern or CsA serum concentration in patients with initially functioning vs. nonfunctioning grafts,[1] patients with no initial graft function were also accepted in this trial. The average onset of renal function occurred at 7.5 ± 6.6 days in the Aza + MP group, 5.9 ± 5.7 days in the CsA group, and 6.3 ± 5.6 days in the CsA + MP group. Of the patients in the Aza + MP and CsA groups, 59% required postoperative dialysis assistance, compared to 47% in the CsA + MP group. Duration of postoperative hospitalization was 30 ± 14 days in the Aza + MP group, 31 ± 12 days in the CsA group, and 33 ± 12 days in the CsA + MP group. All differences are nonsignificant.

Clinical Data and Routine Laboratory Investigations

Urine output occurred earlier and was significantly higher in the CsA + MP group, compared to patients receiving CsA only. Consequently, the highest postoperative serum creatinine levels were recorded in patients receiving only CsA. These differences were even more pronounced when only grafts with an immediate onset of function were analyzed: In this group of patients, significantly higher postoperative serum creatinine levels ($p = 0.000$) were observed in the CsA group, compared to patients receiving CsA + MP or conventional therapy.

Judged primarily on clinical signs and confirmed by aspiration biopsy cytology, 38% of patients in the Aza + MP group and 31% in the CsA + MP group, compared to only 16% in the CsA group, had no evidence of rejection during the immediate postoperative period of 30 days ($p = 0.048$). The onset of first rejection was observed significantly earlier in the CsA-treated patients (7.3 ± 4.9 days), compared to the patients receiving Aza + MP (12.3 ± 6.9 days) or CsA + MP (16.1 ± 5.5 days; $p = 0.007$ and 0.00, respectively).

Reconfirming our earlier observation,[1] a significant blood eosinophilia was recorded during the immediate postoperative period in patients receiving only CsA; this is not seen in patients receiving Aza + MP or CsA + MP. No significant differences were recorded in the incidence of thrombocytopenia among the three groups of patients; severe leukopenia ($<2.0 \times 10^9$/liter) was recorded in 13% of patients in the Aza + MP group but in no patients receiving CsA or CsA + MP.

Fine Needle Aspiration Analysis

The profiles of inflammation were distinctly different in the three groups of patients. The first episode of inflammation was recorded significantly earlier in patients receiving CsA, compared to the patients receiving Aza + MP or CsA + MP ($p = 0.021$ and 0.005, respectively) (Table 1). The intensity of the first inflammatory episode was

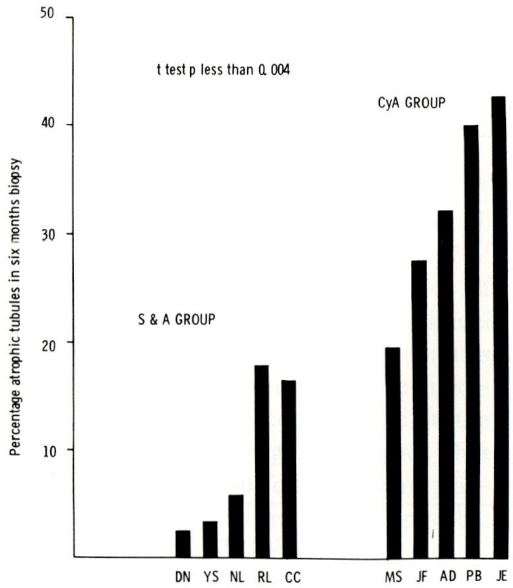

Fig. 1. Volume percentage of atrophic tubules in renal cortex of biopsy specimens.

on S+A (70.78 ± 10.1%) than those on CsA (48.08 ± 15.1%) (t test, $p < 0.02$; Wilcoxon's test, $p < 0.05$). In addition, renal function was significantly worse at 6 months in those on CsA (229.8 ± 44.4 μmole/liter) when compared to those on S+A (119.8 ± 34.5 μmole/liter). Follow-up serum creatinine and creatinine clearance values for both groups are given in Figs. 2 and 3, respectively.

The correlation between serum creatinine at time of biopsy and percentage of tubular atrophy was significant in the CsA group (Spearman's rank correlation 0.95, $p < 0.02$), but not in the S+A group. There was no significant correlation between atrophic tubules and creatinine clearance values in either group.

DISCUSSION

In early CsA toxicity, a spectrum of changes can be seen, including interstitial edema, proximal tubular epithelial cell vacuolization, and degeneration, which in severe cases can progress to frank acute tubular necrosis.[1,5] There may be intra- or extracellular microcalcification in damaged tubules. No significant glomerular or vascular changes have been reported, although recently we have noted a peculiar insudative lesion of the arterioles in some patients and are in the process of studying this lesion further. All the tubular changes described are nonspecific and can be caused by a variety of agents and conditions,

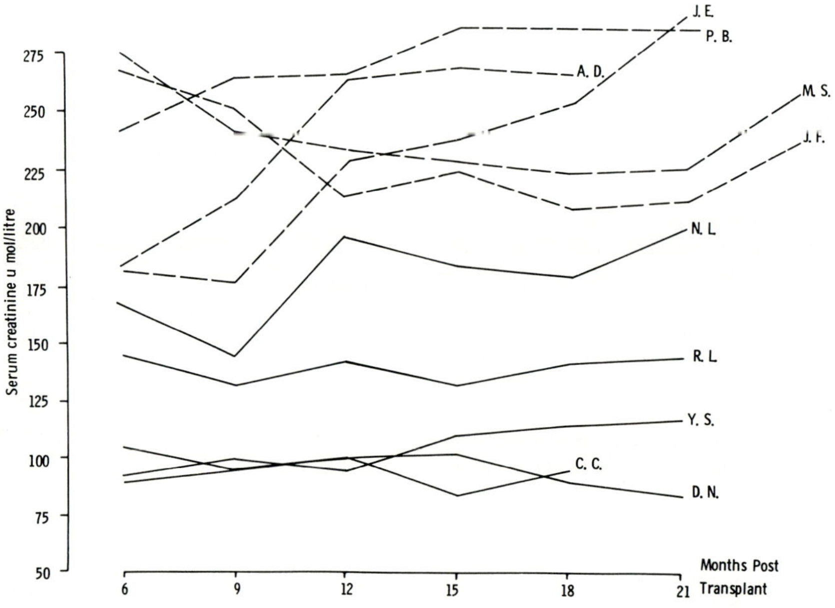

Fig. 2. Serum creatinine after transplantation (S+A patients, continuous line; CsA patients, broken line).

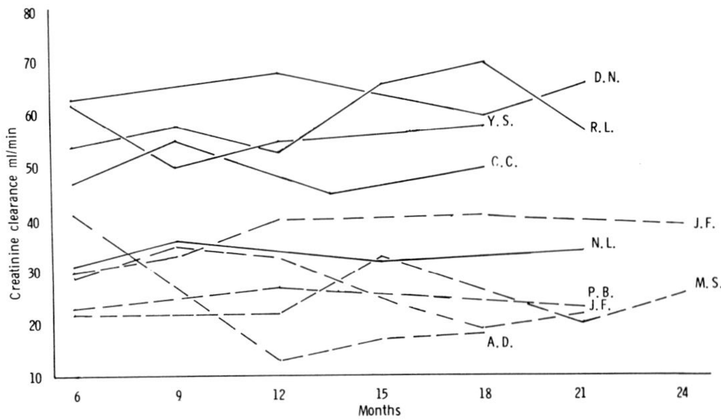

Fig. 3. Creatinine clearance after transplantation (S+A patients, continuous line; CsA patients, broken line).

including the rejection reaction itself. Acute CsA toxicity is suspected when such abnormalities are present in the absence of a significant rejection reaction in an allograft with poor function. It is well established that acute CsA toxicity is reversible in that reducing the dose or changing over to S+A is followed by improvement in function. Interpretation of the renal histology of patients on long-term CsA can be difficult, again because of the lack of specific diagnostic features. Most of these biopsies show changes of a "chronic interstitial nephritis" with tubular atrophy, vacuolization of proximal tubular cells, dystrophic calcification, interstitial fibrosis, and a mild mononuclear cell infiltration. It can be almost impossible to be certain which of these abnormalities are due to CsA and which to chronic rejection. If the biopsy includes vessels and glomeruli with typical lesions of chronic vascular rejection and allograft nephropathy, it probably means that the associated tubular and interstitial abnormalities are due chiefly to chronic rejection. The absence of such lesions, however, does not automatically exclude chronic rejection, as the biopsy may not have picked a representative sample. Perhaps in most patients both chronic low-grade rejection and CsA nephrotoxicity play some part in causing parenchymal damage.

As there has not yet been a clear documentation of abnormalities that might be present in kidneys of nonrenal transplant patients on long-term CsA, comparing the changes seen in CsA allografts with those from a comparable group of S+A allografts is an alternative way of assessing the nephrotoxic effects of CsA. In the patients studied, except for N. L., in the steroid group, none of the biopsies had the specific features of chronic rejection, yet the tubular atrophy in the CsA patients was significantly greater than that in the S+A group. These tubular changes, with simplification of the epithelial cells, basement membrane thickening, and marked atrophy, are, unlike the acute changes, quite irreversible. Superimposed on these chronic changes is probably some degree of ongoing acute damage. This may be the reason for the functional improvement that occurs when CsA patients with poor renal function have their dose of CsA reduced and/or are given supplementary steroids. It is well established that renal function is more closely related to structural changes observed in the tubules than to those in the glomeruli.[6,7] It has been postulated that there is impaired NaCl reabsorption through damaged proximal tubules, resulting in increased NaCl concentration in the tubular fluid at the macula densa; this would lead to a fall in GFR through the tubular-glomerular feedback mechanism.[8] This mechanism would explain the elevation of serum creatinine and impairment in renal function observed in CsA patients.

In a 1–4-year follow-up (to be published) of 88 patients treated with CsA at Cambridge, it appears that although renal function, as measured by serum creatinine at 6 months after transplantation, is significantly inferior to that of patients on S+A, there is no evidence of any further significant deterioration in function over the follow-up period in the CsA group as a whole. This implies that the toxic effects of CsA are most damaging in the early post-transplant period, when the graft tissue is made more vulnerable by a variety of insults, such as warm and cold ischemia and rejection; on the other hand, it can be argued that any further damage that may cause a fall in renal function is perhaps subsequently normalized at the expense of loss of a portion of the renal reserve capacity; only when the reserve capacity is exhausted will continued renal damage be reflected by functional deterioration. The length of time required for the renal reserve capacity to dissipate would presumably depend on a number of variables, including dose of CsA, supplementary steroids, antibiotics, evolution of chronic rejection, and many other unrecognized factors. Clearly, longer periods of follow-up of CsA patients are required before the argument can be settled.

Three CsA patients in this study (J. E., P. B., and A. D.) with greater than 30% atrophic tubules have a slow deterioration in function (Figs. 2 and 3). Perhaps these patients are precariously balanced, with very little functional reserve. This fine balance was recently illustrated by patient A. D. He was found to have a renal cell carcinoma of one of his kidneys and underwent a nephrectomy. Following surgery, renal function deteriorated quite dramatically but returned to preoperative levels over a period of 3 weeks (Fig. 4). An allograft biopsy done on the 10th postoperative day showed quite marked tubular atrophy (normal tubules, 40.8%; atrophic tubules, 40.4%; interstitium, 10.2%; and glomeruli, 8.5%) with superimposed acute changes. Tubules with acute degeneration and necrosis were included in the "normal" component and not in the "atrophic" component. There was no evidence of allograft nephropathy or chronic vascular rejection. Compared to the biopsy done 14 months earlier, the percentage of atrophic tubules had increased from 31.5% to 40.4%.

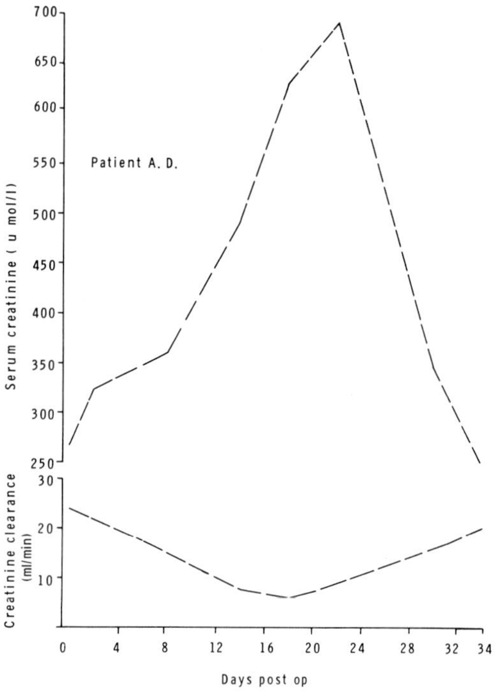

Fig. 4. **Patient A. D.: Renal function following surgery.**

The steroid patient N. L. showed glomerular and vascular evidence of chronic rejection in the 6-month biopsy. Although the tubular atrophy was not very significant at that time, the gradual deterioration in his renal function implies progressive tubular damage secondary to chronic rejection.

In conclusion, this small study has shown that transplant patients on CsA have a significant degree of tubular atrophy and a significantly lower level of renal function than patients on S+A. There is no convincing evidence, so far, of progressive deterioration in renal function in CsA patients as a group, and this implies either that CsA exerts most, or all, of its nephrotoxic effects in the early post-transplant period and/or that compensatory mechanisms are activated with utilization of the functional reserve capacity of the allograft. Sequential follow-up biopsies will help elucidate if the parenchymal damage is progressive and, by inference, give some measure of the renal functional reserve capacity.

REFERENCES

1. Calne RY, White DJG, Thiru S, et al: Lancet 2:1323, 1978

2. Whiting PH, Thomson AW, Blair JT, et al: Br J Exp Path 63:88, 1982

3. Hamilton DV, Evans DB, Henderson RG, et al: Proc EDTA 18:400, 1981

4. Aherne WA, Dunnill MS: In: Morphometry. London, Arnold Publications, 1982

5. Hamilton DV, Evans DB, Thiru S: In White DJG (ed): Cyclosporin A. Amsterdam, Elsevier Biomedical, 1982, pp 393–411

6. Risdon RA, Sloper JC, De Wardener HE: Lancet 2:363, 1968

7. Mackensen-Haen S, Bader R, Grund KE, et al: Clin Nephrol 15:167, 1981

8. Thurau K, Boylan JW: Am J Med 61:308, 1976

Pathology in Renal Transplant Patients Treated with Cyclosporine

A. Farnsworth, B. M. Hall, P. Kirwan, G. A. Bishop, G. C. Duggin, B. Goodman, J. Horvath, J. Johnson, A. Ng, A. G. R. Sheil, and D. J. Tiller

WHEN CYCLOSPORINE A (CsA) is used as an immunosuppressive in renal transplantation, episodes of deterioration of renal function may be due to rejection or CsA nephrotoxicity.[1-3] In an attempt to define the histopathology of rejection and CsA nephrotoxicity, we have examined the biopsies from renal transplant patients entered into a randomized controlled clinical trial comparing treatment with CsA alone to that of prednisone, azathioprine (Aza) and antilymphocyte globulin.

MATERIALS AND METHODS

Clinical Data

All biopsies were from patients who had consented to enter the randomized controlled clinical trial. The details of patient management have been previously reported.[4]

Biopsies were taken when clinically indicated by the physician caring for the patient. Two clinical groups of patients were identified, those with post-transplant acute renal failure who were biopsied every 7–10 days, and those with functioning grafts who had biopsies when there was deterioration in renal function suggestive of rejection. All patients gave informed consent to renal biopsy. The study was approved by the Royal Prince Alfred Hospital Ethics Committee and conformed with the statement of the NH&MRC of Australia on Human Experimentation.

Tissue Preparations

Renal biopsy specimens were divided into three pieces, one of which was fixed for light, one fixed for electron microscopy, and one frozen for immunoperoxidase stains.

Paraffin-embedded tissue cut in 4-μm sections was stained with hematoxylin and eosin, Masson's trichrome, and methanamine silver for light microscopy. Biopsies from 56 patients were examined, 32 treated with CsA and 24 treated with Aza. The sections were systematically examined by an observer unaware of the form of therapy or clinical course of the patient. A semiquantitative assessment of the degree of severity of each pathologic change was made. A comparison of the frequency and severity of each pathologic change was made between different clinical groups. The histologic changes and the score systems used have been previously reported.[5]

Fifty-seven biopsies from 22 renal transplant patients receiving CsA alone were examined by electron microscopy. Control groups were 30 transplant biopsies from 17 patients receiving Aza and 48 nontransplant biopsies from 47 patients with a variety of renal diseases on neither immunosuppressive regimen.

The indirect immunoperoxidase technique to identify the mononuclear cell subsets identified by the monoclonal antibodies T11 (E-rosette receptor), T4 (helper-inducer), and T8 (cytotoxic-suppressor) (Coulter, Inc., Hialeah, FL) has been reported.[6] Thirty-one biopsies with rejection were examined, 20 from CsA- and 11 from Aza-treated patients. Four biopsies from CsA patients with nephrotoxicity and no evidence of rejection were also examined.

RESULTS

Light Microscopic Appearances

Biopsy appearances from CsA patients and Aza patients with clinical evidence of rejection were compared. A similar frequency and degrees of severity of histologic changes were found in both groups. The changes identified were a diffuse and focal mononuclear cell infiltrate, interstitial edema, tubular cellular infiltrate, and tubular epithelial destruction. Varying degrees of vessel damage, such as intimal proliferation and medial necrosis, were also present. The histologic feature of rejection in CsA treated patients were thus found to be similar to those in patients on Aza.

Comparison of the biopsies from patients with post-transplant renal failure showed there was no difference between the two treatment groups in the frequency or degree of severity of cellular infiltrates or tubular or

From the Department of Anatomical Pathology and the Renal Unit, Royal Prince Alfred Hospital, Camperdown, N.S.W., Australia.

Reprint requests should be addressed to Dr. A. Farnsworth.

0041-1345/83/1505-0120$01.00/0

vascular changes. The only unique feature in CsA-treated patients was a diffuse interstitial fibrosis, seen in biopsies from 5 CsA patients (Fig. 1). Four of these patients showed a marked improvement in renal function after therapy was changed from CsA to Aza. One of these patients had a graft nephrectomy because of prolonged post-transplant acute renal failure. None of the biopsies from patients who had spontaneous recovery of post-transplant acute renal failure while continuing to receive CsA had this interstitial fibrosis. In the first weeks after transplantation, severe but treatable vascular rejection was seen in the biopsies from patients who developed diffuse interstitial fibrosis. This rejection was treated, and subsequent biopsies showed that the interstitial fibrosis had appeared and was not accompanied by evidence of persistent active rejection.

Since the initial analysis, a further two CsA-treated patients entered have developed interstitial fibrosis in association with impaired renal function (serum creatinine > 250 μmole/liter). They also showed a marked improvement in renal function after a change to Aza therapy. Previous biopsies from these two patients had no evidence of vascular rejection.

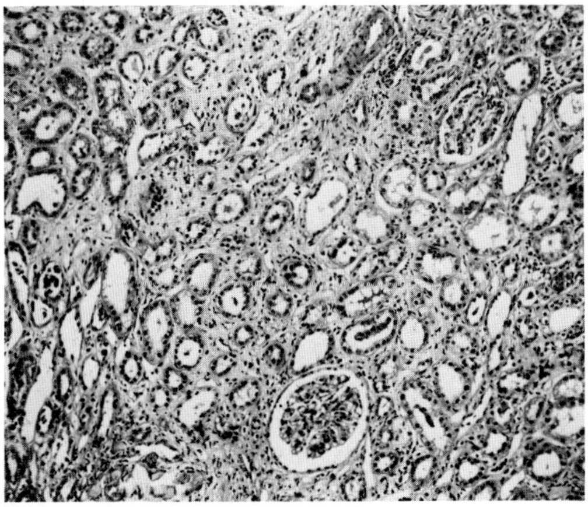

Fig. 1. Renal allograft biopsy of a patient on CsA for 80 days with no renal function. The tubules are atrophied and separated by interstitial fibrous tissue. This fibrous tissue was diffuse surrounding tubules and glomeruli. There is no evidence of chronic vascular rejection.

Immunoperoxidase Studies

The pattern of the mononuclear cell subset infiltrate was similar in both CsA and Aza-treated patients. The majority of infiltrating cells were T cells identified by T11. The helper-inducer subset (T4) predominated over or was equal in frequency to the cytotoxic-suppressor subset (T8) in all but one biopsy. The four biopsies from patients with CsA nephrotoxicity had a sparse mononuclear cell infiltrate, with an equal frequency of T4 and T8 cells.

Electron Microscopy

There was no difference in the findings associated with rejection. Of particular interest was the presence of giant mitochondria in proximal convoluted tubules. Eleven biopsies from 22 CsA and 9 from 17 Aza patients and 14 of the 47 patients with other renal disease had giant mitochondria. There appeared to be more giant mitochondria in biopsies from CsA-treated patients than in the other biopsies.

DISCUSSION

In this study, we showed that the histologic changes of rejection in CsA-treated patients are the same as those described for rejection in biopsies from patients treated with Aza.[7] Furthermore, the subsets of mononuclear cells identified by immunoperoxidase had a similar pattern in rejection in both treatment groups. Helper cells predominated over cytotoxic-suppressor cells, which is in conflict with previous reports that suggest that cytotoxic cells predominate.[8,9] The diffuse interstitial fibrosis observed in CsA-treated patients with prolonged post-transplant acute renal failure could be due to either CsA nephrotoxicity or chronic rejection. The biopsy appearances of two patients with moderate renal impairment who developed this change without any rejection episodes suggests that this change is most likely due to CsA nephrotoxicity. It is also possible that early severe rejection predisposes the kidney to the nephrotoxic effect of CsA. The presence of interstitial fibrosis appears to indicate that achievement of normal renal function is unlikely if CsA is continued.

It has been suggested that giant mitochondria are a specific feature of CsA nephrotoxicity.[10] However, we found a similar frequency of giant mitochondria in Aza-treated patients, and they were also seen in a number of other renal diseases in patients who were not receiving any immunosuppressives. Thus, giant mitochondria appear to be a relatively nonspecific finding and may be induced by a variety of pathologic processes.

In milder forms of CsA nephrotoxicity, we were unable to identify a specific pathologic marker. In particular, tubular damage was not more severe in CsA patients than in Aza patients. Other groups have suggested that focal mononuclear cell infiltrates are seen with CSA nephrotoxicity.[9] In our study, such changes were present in both treatment groups with post-transplant acute renal failure. These infiltrates could equally be due to mild, ongoing cellular rejection. Our patients with these biopsy features were treated for rejection and responded to this treatment, without reduction in the dose of CsA.

Renal biopsies will help in the management of CsA-treated renal transplant recipients, and the pathology of rejection is similar to that seen with conventional therapy. There are no specific features to identify mild CsA nephrotoxicity. The presence of diffuse interstitial fibrosis suggests severe CsA nephrotoxicity, and a change of immunosuppressive therapy is usually indicated.

ACKNOWLEDGMENTS

We wish to thank Sandoz Australia Pty. Ltd., who provided the CsA, and Shirley Davis for typing the manuscript.

REFERENCES

1. Calne RY, Rolles K, White DJG, et al: Lancet 2:1033, 1979
2. Morris PJ: Transplantation 32:349, 1981
3. Calne RY: Nephron 26:57, 1980
4. Sheil AGR, Hall BM, Tiller DJ, et al: In White DJG (ed): Cyclosporin A. Amsterdam, Elsevier Biomedical, 1982, pp 387–391
5. Farnsworth A, Hall BM, Horvath JS, et al: (submitted for publication)
6. Hall BM, Bishop GA, Farnsworth A: (submitted for publication)
7. Corson JJ: Path Ann vol. no.:251, 1972
8. Platt JL, Le Bien TW, Michael AF, J Exp Med 155:17, 1982
9. Hancock WW, Thompson NM, Atkins RC: Transplantation (in press)
10. Mihatsch MJ, Olivieri V, Marbet U, et al: Lancet 1:1162, 1981
11. Najarian JS, Ferguson RM, Rynasiewicz JJ, et al: Transplant Proc (in press)

CYCLOSPORINE CONVERSION AND USE AS ADJUNCTIVE THERAPY

Conversion Rejection Consequences by Changing the Immunosuppressive Therapy From Cyclosporine to Azathioprine After Kidney Transplantation

W. Land, L. A. Castro, G. Hillebrand, K. Günther, and J. M. Gokel

SINCE its discovery in 1976 by J. Borel, the strong immunosuppressive potency of cyclosporine has been demonstrated in both animal experiments and clinical organ transplantations.[1-5] One other remarkable advantage of its discovery represents the fact that the whole repertoire of immunosuppressive agents has extended. Thus, there is the theoretical possibility to switch from conventional immunosuppressive therapy (azathioprine) to cyclosporine and vice versa.

This article presents our own experience in changing the immunosuppressive treatment from cyclosporine to azathioprine after cadaveric renal transplantation. This type of conversion was performed in only a small percentage of our cyclosporine-treated patients (in 30 of 195 cases). The reasons for conversion trials were as follows: (1) in terms of a prospective randomized study; (2) with regard to repeated uncontrollable rejection episodes; (3) with respect to cyclosporine nephrotoxicity. The results obtained are the subject of this report.

MATERIALS AND METHODS

Patient Population

In the prospective randomized trial, 18 patients between the ages of 19 and 61 years were eligible. Conversion was started 3 months after cadaveric renal transplantation in patients with a good renal graft function [serum creatinine values (SCr) around 200 μmole/liter]. Every second patient of the 18 consecutively transplanted patients was converted from cyclosporine to azathioprine.

Conversion trials because of repeated uncontrollable rejection episodes were done in 14 patients between the ages of 25 and 51 years. All these patients had a first cadaveric renal allograft showing a severe rejection episode at the time of conversion, having had 2–3 previous rejection episodes not responding to antirejection treatment sufficiently. Conversion trials because of nephrotoxicity were done in 8 patients with either a nonfunctioning graft or a poor graft function (SCr > 4.0 mg/dl). Nephrotoxicity was assessed and scored by histologic changes (vacuolization, microcalcification, megamitochondria, segmental vascular hyalinosis). Moreover, other concomitant cyclosporine side effects were considered. Conversion in these patients was performed at least 2 months after transplantation and when previous trials of tapering the cyclosporine dose to 5–6 mg/kg body weight failed to improve graft function.

Immunosuppressive Protocol

Cyclosporine was administered intravenously prior to, and the first day after, operation in a dose of 4 mg/kg body weight and continued by oral administration in a dose of 15 mg/kg body weight for 1 month posttransplant, when it was decreased by 2 mg/kg body weight monthly to a maintenance level of 6–7 mg/kg body weight.

Methylprednisolone was begun at 8 mg daily immediately after operation and maintained at that level.

Antirejection Treatment

Antirejection treatment consisted of 3 i.v. bolus injections of 500 mg methylprednisolone during the first rejection episode. The second and the third rejection episodes were treated by administration of antilymphocyte/antithymocyte globulin (ALG/ATG) over a period of 7 days in combination with methylprednisolone in a dose of 125 mg i.v. daily until reversal.

Conversion Protocol

In all cases of conversion, we used an overlapping regimen, as shown in Table 1. Conversion because of repeated uncontrollable rejection episodes was carried out under the protection of a 7-day course of ALG/ATG treatment.

RESULTS

Prospective Randomized Trial of Conversion: Cyclosporine to Azathioprine

Actuarial graft survival of both groups (converted/nonconverted) is shown in Fig. 1.

From the Departments of Surgery and Internal Medicine I, and the Institute of Pathology, Transplantation Center, Klinikum Großhadern, University of Munich, Munich, F.R.G.

Address reprint requests to Dr. W. Land, Department of Surgery, Klinikum Großhadern, Marchioninistr.15, D-8000 München 70, F.R.G.

0041-1345/83/1505-0121$01.00/0

Table 1. Conversion Protocol: CsA → Aza

Day	CsA (mg/kg Body Weight)	Aza (mg/kg Body Weight)	MP
1	11	1.00	8 mg
2	9	1.00	8 mg
3	7	1.25	8 mg
4	—	1.50	8 mg
5	—	2.00	8 mg
6	—	2–2.50	8 mg

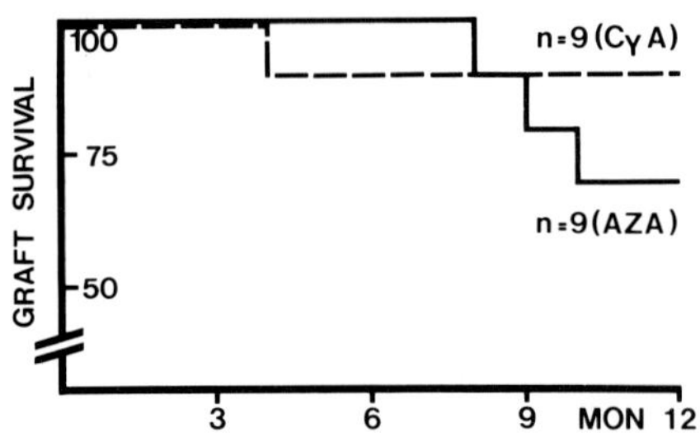

Fig. 1. Actuarial renal allograft survival rates according to the prospective conversion trial (CsA, nonconverted group; AZA, converted group).

There were three graft losses in the converted group compared to one graft loss in the control group maintained on cyclosporine. The events following conversion to azathioprine in nine patients are shown in more detail in Fig. 2. Only in two patients (G.S./H.V.) did conversion from cyclosporine to azathioprine 3 months after transplantation turn out to be without any complication. One patient (R.W.) acquired a viral infection associated with an acute rejection episode soon after conversion, requiring reconversion to cyclosporine. Interestingly enough, the same patient developed an acute rejection episode of a humoral-vascular type 4 months later. At that stage, we decided to convert him again to azathioprine and steroids. The acute rejection episode could be reversed consequently. Three patients developed acute severe rejection episodes in the second, second, and fourth weeks after conversion, respectively. All these patients received antirejection treatment; in addition, they were reconverted to cyclosporine. In all cases, the fulminant rejection could be reversed. One patient (K.E.) lost his graft following conversion due to a nonimmunologic complication during the eighth month after transplantation (complete intrarenal stenosis of the renal artery of a juvenile kidney). Two other patients (J.P., E.H.), who developed no rejection immediately after conversion, had repeated rejection episodes 6 and 8 months after transplantation that did not respond to antirejection treatment (and not to reconversion to cyclosporine in one case either). Both patients finally lost their grafts due to irre-

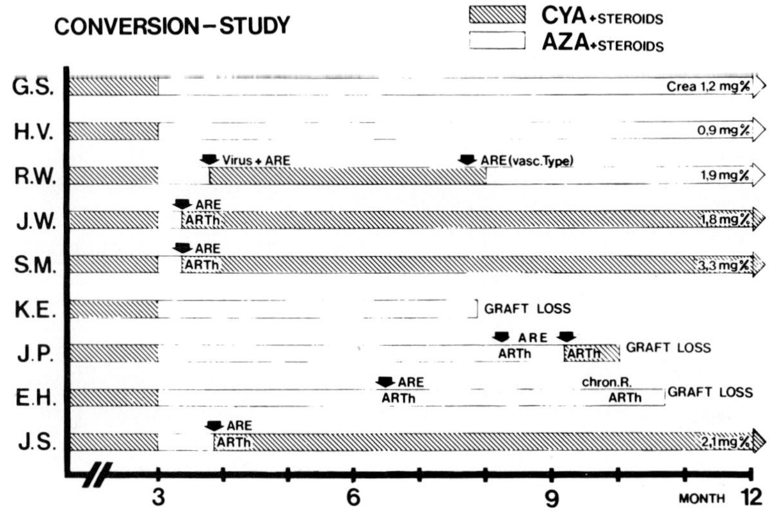

Fig. 2. Clinical course of the nine converted patients within the prospective conversion trial. (ARE, acute rejection episode; Crea, serum creatinine level; ARTh, antirejection therapy).

versible rejection in the 10th and 11th months after transplantation.

At that stage of the study, we decided to discontinue the planned prospective conversion trial with respect to these rather disappointing results.

Conversion: Cyclosporine to Azathioprine Because of Repeated Uncontrollable Rejection Episodes

Conversion from cyclosporine to azathioprine was tried in patients showing a rejection episode after having previously experienced 2–3 rejection crises not responding to antirejection treatment. Conversion was carried out under the "protection" of additional ALG/ATG therapy over a period of 7 days in most cases. The results of these attempts are shown in Table 2. Seven patients with repeated rejection episodes (histology predominantly cellular) were converted 1, 2, 2, 3, 3, 4, and 6 months following transplantation. In spite of conversion (and in 5 patients, plus administration of ALG/ATG) 4 renal allografts developed irreversible rejection; in 3 patients, reversal of rejection was achieved. Three months after conversion, these patients showed elevated but reasonable SCr levels. Five patients with repeated rejection episodes (histology predominantly cellular/chronic vascular type) were converted 1, 2, 3, 4, and 10 months after transplantation. We observed 3 irreversible rejections and 2 reversals in this type of rejection. In 2 patients with acute humoral vascular rejection episodes (which always implies a "malignant" type of rejection), conversion to azathioprine did not influence the course of rejection: both grafts were rapidly and fulminantly rejected. Thus, successful conversion from cyclosporine to azathioprine was achieved in one-third of the patients (5 of 14), whereas unsuccessful conversion to azathioprine therapy was observed in about two-thirds of the "immunologically high-responder patients."

Conversion: Cyclosporine to Azathioprine Because of Cyclosporine Nephrotoxicity

Conversion to azathioprine because of nephrotoxicity was tried in 8 patients 2–12 months after transplantation, according to our criteria described in Materials and Methods.

The results are shown in Table 3. In 3 patients (2 patients with a primarily nonfunctioning graft because of acute tubular necrosis; 1 patient with a SCr value of 7.1 mg/dl), conversion to azathioprine was followed by the occurrence of uncontrollable irreversible rejections 2–3 weeks after conversion. Two of these patients had already had rejection episodes under CsA therapy that responded to antirejection treatment at that time. Interestingly enough, in all these patients, histologic investigation revealed severe signs of cyclosporine nephrotoxicity in the renal graft.

In 5 patients, conversion to azathioprine 2, 2, 3, 6, and 12 months after transplantation was successful and led to an improvement of the impaired kidney function, as demonstrated by a fall of SCr levels by an average of about 50% 1 month after conversion. The rate of fall was most rapid during the first week

Table 2. Conversion: Uncontrollable Rejection Episodes

No. of Patients	Type of Rejection (Histology)	Time After Transplant (Months)	Additional Therapy	Outcome	SCr (mg/dl) 3 Months After Conversion
7	Cellular	1,2,2,3 3,4,5	ALG in 5 cases	4 Irrev. rej.	∅
				3 Reversal	2.9; 2.8; 4.2
5	Cellular chronic vascular	1,2,3, 4,10	ALG in 4 cases	3 Irrev. rej.	∅
				2 Reversal	3.8; 1.8
2	Acute vascular	2,2	∅	2 Irrev. rej.	∅

Total 14 patients: 5 reversals; 9 irreversible rejections.

Table 3. Results: Conversion CsA to AZA ($n = 8$) (Nephrotoxicity)

No. of Patients	SCr (mg/dl) Before	SCr (mg/dl) 1 Month After	Time After Transplant (Months)	Histologic Change, Grade I–III	Outcome
3	NF	0	2	++	Irreversible rejection
	NF		2	++	
	7.1		4	+++	
5	NF	2.0	2	+	Improvement
	4.4	2.0	12	(+)	
	4.6	2.0	2	+	
	7.9	3.1	3	+	
	6.0	1.8	6	Not done	

NF, Nonfunctioning kidney (ATN).

after conversion, with a continuing reduction in SCr in all 5 patients during the next 4 weeks. No further significant fall in SCr occurred in the following 3 months. The histologic investigation of the renal grafts after biopsy revealed only slight to moderate signs of nephrotoxicity in these patients.

DISCUSSION

Three different indications for conversion to azathioprine in cyclosporine-treated patients have been chosen by our group: conversion within a prospective randomized trial; conversion because of repeated uncontrollable rejection episodes; conversion because of cyclosporine nephrotoxicity.

The first indication was based on the fact that the supply of cyclosporine by the company was transiently limited during a short period of time at the beginning of the past year. In this situation, we decided not to treat a small number of patients over a long period of time but to treat all patients for a short period of time. For this reason, we tried a conversion to azathioprine 3 months after transplantation, which was done in terms of a prospective randomized trial.

As our results obtained show, we had a rather discouraging experience, which is in some disagreement with observations of the Oxford group.[6] These authors tried conversion to azathioprine 3 months after transplantation in 14 patients, observing 11 successful conversions and 3 irreversible rejections after conversion. Therefore, it must be investigated whether other conversion protocols at another time after transplantation (later: 6 months, 1 year?) may lead to better results than we obtained.

Conversion to azathioprine in high responders with repeated rejection episodes under cyclosporine treatment did not improve the fatal course of the graft function in two-thirds of the patients. On the other hand, in about one-third of the patients, reversal of the rejection episode could be achieved. These results may give rise to the consideration that in immunologically desperate cases, a conversion to azathioprine is a worthwhile try, although the chances of reversal are poor in the majority of patients.

Conversion to azathioprine because of nephrotoxicity is a rare indication for discontinuation of cyclosporine therapy. In our hands, only in 8 of 195 cyclosporine-treated patients (4.1%) was conversion required, which fits in very well with the observations of the Minnesota group.[7] However, the incidence of 3 irreversible rejections after conversion in 8 patients implies a warning signal. Thus, the indication for conversion because of nephrotoxicity can be mandatory, provided the diagnosis of the cyclosporine nephrotoxic episode is clear-cut, as well as a dose reduction procedure (like the alternate-day approach)[7] has been tried prior to conversion. Nevertheless, nephrotoxicity remains one of the most serious problems in cyclosporine therapy.

REFERENCES

1. Borel JF, Feurer C, Gubler HU, et al: Agents Actions 6:468, 1976
2. Calne RY, Rolles K, White DJG, et al: Transplant Proc 13:349, 1981
3. Beveridge T: Transplant Proc 15:433, 1983
4. Hakala TR, Starzl TE, Rosenthal JT, et al: Transplant Proc 15:465, 1983
5. Shumway NE: Transplant Proc 15:1221, 1983
6. French ME, Thompson JF, Hunniselt AGW, et al: Transplant Proc 15:485, 1983
7. Ferguson RM, Rynasiewicz JJ, Najarian JS: Transplant Proc 15:480, 1983

The Consequences of Conversion From Cyclosporine to Azathioprine and Prednisolone in Renal Allograft Recipients

R. F. M. Wood, J. F. Thompson, N. H. Allen, A. Ting, and P. J. Morris

CYCLOSPORINE A (CsA) represents the most significant advance in immunosuppressive therapy since the introduction of azathioprine in the 1960s. Until now, the combination of azathioprine and corticosteroids has been used universally as the standard immunosuppressive regimen and, with the possible exception of antilymphocyte globulin, additional or alternative agents have not improved graft survival rates. When CsA becomes generally available, the clinician will have a choice of effective immunosuppressive agents, and by using appropriate monitoring techniques, it may be possible to tailor therapy to the needs of the individual patient. Situations will undoubtedly arise in which conversion from one regimen to another is considered desirable. It is therefore important to achieve an understanding of the consequences of conversion.

Extensive information on the effects of conversion from CsA to conventional immunosuppression has been acquired in two randomized controlled trials of CsA that have been conducted in Oxford. These have employed a protocol of routine conversion from CsA to azathioprine and prednisolone (AP) at 3 months, and represent the only experience so far of systematic conversion from CsA to AP at a fixed time after transplantation. A small number of patients in previously published studies have been converted from CsA to AP,[1-3] but it has been difficult to assess the results of conversion in these cases because drug therapy was altered at varying times after operation and for a number of different reasons, including rejection, nephrotoxicity, and other side effects of CsA.

The decision to administer CsA for only a limited period in the Oxford trials was prompted by anxiety about the incidence of lymphomas in the first pilot study of CsA,[4] and concern that its long-term use might have other side effects, such as progressive renal impairment from nephrotoxicity. The policy of using short-term CsA was attractive, as experimental work had shown that the drug was most effective in blocking the induction phase of the immune response and inhibiting T-cell proliferation in response to alloantigen stimulation.[5] Before embarking on the clinical trials, a series of animal experiments was undertaken in Oxford. In rats, a brief course of CsA given during the first few days after renal transplantation resulted in prolonged or even indefinite survival of the grafts.[6] Further studies in dogs demonstrated that the short-term use of CsA, with subsequent conversion to AP, was not only feasible, but was associated with graft survival rates superior to those obtained by treatment with conventional immunosuppressive agents.[7]

This article considers the results of conversion from CsA to AP in cadaver allograft recipients in the two Oxford trials. In the majority of patients, conversion has been successfully accomplished and has resulted in a marked and sustained improvement in renal function. Rejection after conversion has occasionally occurred, but has, in general, responded promptly to standard antirejection therapy.

MATERIALS AND METHODS

Trial I began in January 1980, and 35 patients were entered into this initial study (CsA 21 patients, AP 14

From the Transplant Unit, Nuffield Department of Surgery, University of Oxford, John Radcliffe and Churchill Hospitals, Oxford, England.

Address reprint requests to Dr. R. F. M. Wood, Transplant Unit, Nuffield Department of Surgery, University of Oxford, John Radcliffe and Churchill Hospitals, Oxford, England.

0041-1345/83/1505-0122$01.00/0

patients). Because of the previous excellent results obtained with conventional immunosuppression in recipients of HLA-DR-compatible grafts,[8] only patients receiving HLA-DR-mismatched kidneys were included in trial I. Patients with a history of hepatic dysfunction or malignancy were excluded, as were recipients of kidneys from living-related donors. Immediate graft function was also made a prerequisite for entry because of uncertainty at the time the trial was planned about the effect of CsA nephrotoxicity on kidneys already affected by acute tubular necrosis (ATN). This restriction meant that randomization could not be performed until 6 hr postoperatively, when it was clear whether the graft was functioning or not. By November 1981, it was apparent that graft and patient survival rates in the CsA group were at least as favorable as in the control group, and entry into trial I was terminated. Trial II was then begun, with only minor modifications to the protocol, but with the removal of most of the previous restrictions to entry. In trial II, all recipients of cadaver grafts were eligible for entry, except those with liver disease or a history of cancer. Randomization was therefore possible preoperatively, and the first dose of CsA was given intravenously prior to revascularization of the graft. To date, 66 patients have entered trial II (CsA 34 patients, AP 32 patients). Patient details for both trials I and II are given in Table 1.

Drug Therapy

Cyclosporine A

In trial I, all patients received a preoperative oral dose of azathioprine (2.5 mg/kg) and intravenous hydrocortisone at the time of operation (100 mg). In the patients subsequently randomized to receive CsA, the first dose (17.5 mg/kg) was given by intramuscular injection 6 hr postoperatively. Thereafter CsA was given orally as a single daily dose (17.5 mg/kg/day on days 1–30, 15 mg/kg/day on days 31–60, and 12.5 mg/kg/day on days 61–90). In Trial II, the first dose of CsA (10 mg/kg in 1 liter of saline) was given intravenously prior to revascularization of the graft. Subsequent doses of the drug were given orally using the same dosage schedule as in trial I.

Azathioprine and Prednisolone

The immunosuppressive therapy for these conventionally treated patients was identical in the two trials. They received azathioprine 2.5 mg/kg orally before operation, with subsequent doses (2.5 mg/kg/day) given orally. Hydrocortisone (100 mg) was given intravenously at the time of operation, with prednisolone given orally thereafter. In addition, in trial I, 1 g of intravenous methylprednisolone (IVMP) was given routinely on days 6, 7, and 8 after transplantation. The prednisolone dose was 15 mg b.d. for the first 60 days, 12.5 mg b.d. on days 61–75, and 10 mg b.d. on days 76–90. From day 90 onwards, the daily dose of prednisolone was reduced by 1 mg every 2 weeks until a permanent maintenance dose of 10 mg/day was reached.

Treatment of Acute Rejection Episodes

In trial I, acute rejection episodes were treated with 1 g bolus doses of IVMP daily for 3 days. In trial II, the dose of IVMP in each bolus was reduced from 1 g to 0.5 g, and treatment was continued for 3–5 days, depending on the severity of the rejection episode. In the patients receiving CsA in trial I, the occurrence of more than two rejection episodes was considered as treatment failure, and further therapy was not specified in the trial protocol (some patients were converted to AP immediately, while others had prednisolone, 10 mg b.d., added to their CsA therapy). In trial II, the protocol specified that all patients in the CsA group having more than two rejection episodes should have prednisolone, 10 mg b.d., added to their CsA therapy.

Conversion Protocol

Patients treated with CsA in both trials were converted at 90 days to conventional immunosuppressive therapy. This was accomplished by stopping the CsA, and the following day, beginning azathioprine in a dose of 2.5 mg/kg/day and prednisolone in a dose of 10 mg b.d. The daily dose of prednisolone was then progressively reduced by 1 mg every 2 weeks until the maintenance dose of 10 mg daily was reached.

Follow-up

In both CsA and AP groups, percutaneous needle-core biopsies were performed routinely on days 7, 21, and 90 and at 1 year following transplantation. Additional biopsies were taken if clinically indicated. In the CsA group,

Table 1. Details of Patients Included in Trials I and II and of Patients Excluded From Trial I

	Trial I Patients (35)		Trial I Exclusions (44) HLA-DR-Compatible (35);	Trial II Patients (66)	
	CsA (21)	AP (14)	Oliguric (9)	CsA (34)	AP (32)
Mean age	37	37	39	42	39
HLA-A,B incompatibilities	2.1	1.6	1.6	2.1	2.5
HLA-DR incompatibilities	1.4	1.4	0.3	0.6	0.6
Not transfused before transplantation*	57%	14%	44%	39%	42%
Positive crossmatch	19%	14%	30%	15%	26%

*Nontransfused patients in both trials were given 2 U of blood during operation.

serum CsA levels were measured regularly, but the results were assessed retrospectively and were not used to regulate therapy.

RESULTS

Graft and Patient Survival

The results of trial I have now been published.[9] The minimum follow-up time is now 18 months and the 1-year graft survival rates were 71% in the CsA group and 57% in the AP group. In trial II, the mean follow-up to date is 9 months. The predicted 1-year graft survival rates in the two treatment groups are: CsA 79%, AP 70% ($p = 0.47$, log rank method of Peto). Predicted patient survival at 1 year is similar in the two groups: CsA 91%, AP 90%. In trial I, the AP-treated patients were given a mean of 3.4 courses of IVMP (10.2 g), while the patients treated with CsA received a mean of 2.7 courses (8.1 g). In trial II, the AP-treated patients have received a mean of 2.0 antirejection courses of IVMP in the first 3 months after transplantation, compared with 1.6 antirejection courses in the CsA group. The mean total dose of IVMP administered per patient in trial II has been significantly greater in the AP group (AP, 4.4 ± 3.0 g; CsA, 2.9 ± 2.4 g, $p = 0.03$, Student's t test). Of the 34 patients treated with CsA in trial II, 17 have required initial dialysis (50%) compared with 11 of the 32 patients treated with AP (34%).

Outcome of Conversion

Of the 101 patients entered into trials I and II, 55 have received CsA. Conversion to AP has so far been carried out in 36 cases. An analysis of the various aspects of conversion in these patients is presented in this section.

Conversion From Cyclosporine A Alone to Azathioprine and Prednisolone

A total of 28 patients were receiving CsA alone at the time of conversion to AP. Six of these patients were converted before 90 days because of side effects of CsA or rejection, while a further 22 patients completed the full protocol and were converted at 90 days (Table 2). Most patients treated with CsA had elevated serum creatinine (SCr) values at day 90, but following successful conversion to AP, there was a rapid and significant fall in SCr, with the mean level reaching 69% of the preconversion value 1 week after stopping CsA (see Table 2). There was a further significant fall in mean SCr to 54% of the preconversion value by 1 month after conversion, but thereafter, SCr values remained stable. By 6 months after transplantation, the mean SCr values in the CsA-treated group (126 μmole/

Table 2. Conversion From Cyclosporine A Alone to Azathioprine and Prednisolone (28 Patients)

(A) Summary of Results

No. of Patients	Day of Conversion	Reason for Conversion	Outcome of Conversion	
22	90	Completed 3 months of CsA therapy	Improved function	17
			Reversible rejection	4
			Irreversible rejection	1
2	38,55	Side effects of CsA	Improved function	2
4	15,25,25,38	Third rejection on CsA	Improved function	2
			Irreversible rejection	2

(B) Serum Creatinine Changes Following Successful Conversion

	Conversion (C)	C + 1/52	C + 1/12	C + 3/12
Mean serum creatinine (μmole/liter ± SD)	242 ± 79	167 ± 52	131 ± 34	126 ± 38
Range	141–489	104–331	72–184	67–194
Significance of fall in serum creatinine		$p = 0.001$	$p = 0.01$	$p = 0.62$
Percent fall in mean SCr		31%	46%	48%

liter) and the AP-treated group (128 μmole/liter) were not significantly different.

Conversion From Cyclosporine A Plus Prednisolone to Azathioprine and Prednisolone

A total of 8 patients on oral prednisolone (10 mg b.d.) plus CsA have been converted to AP at 90 days. In this subgroup, the SCr fell from a mean value of 168 μmole/liter preconversion to a level of 135 μmole/liter 1 week after substituting azathioprine for CsA (see Table 3). At 6 months after transplantation, the mean SCr (110 μmole/liter) was not significantly different from the value in the group converted from CsA alone to AP (126 μmole/liter).

Rejection Problems at Conversion

Of the 30 patients so far converted to AP at 90 days from either CsA alone or CsA plus prednisolone, 6 have experienced symptoms and signs of acute rejection within the first 2 weeks of conversion. In all cases, treatment with bolus doses of IVMP was instituted. Rejection was characterized by features commonly seen in a first acute rejection episode on conventional immunosuppression, namely pyrexia, malaise, oliguria, and graft tenderness. Five of the patients had an immediate response to treatment, with a rapid return to normal renal function. Three of these patients have had further rejection episodes, and in two of them, rejection has only been controlled on conversion back to CsA. Irreversible rejection has occurred in only one patient whose graft function was satisfactory prior to conversion. In this patient, symptoms and signs of rejection developed 12 days after conversion from CsA to AP. Before conversion, the SCr had been stable at a level of 119 μmole/liter. The SCr fell during the first week after conversion to reach a level of 78 μmole/liter on day 95. On day 102, there was a slight rise in SCr to 93 μmole/liter, accompanied by signs and symptoms of acute rejection. Despite treatment with IVMP, there was then a rapid and inexorable rise in SCr, with values reaching 280 μmole/liter on day 105 and 657 μmole/liter on day 107. Biopsy confirmed the presence of irreversible rejection, and a graft nephrectomy was performed 2 days later.

There were 4 patients who were converted from CsA to AP before 90 days because of continuing rejection (see Table 2). In each case, the SCr level fell for the first week after conversion. However, by 2 weeks after conversion, 2 of the patients had gone on to develop irreversible rejection.

Table 3. Changes in Serum Creatinine on Addition of Prednisolone to CsA and on Conversion from CsA Plus Prednisolone to Azathioprine Plus Prednisolone at 90 Days (8 Patients)

Patient	Pred Added (P)	Conversion (C)	C + 1/52	C + 1/12	C + 3/12
1	342	152	140	142	137
2	408	297	209	150	145
3	281	108	105	107	134
4	296	105	87	85	76
5	169	96	80	77	79
6	717	357	260	154	127
7	*	92	80	61	75
8	*	138	115	174	—
Mean serum creatinine (μmole/liter ± SD)	369 ± 188	168 ± 101	135 ± 66	119 ± 42	110 ± 32
Range	(169–717)	(92–357)	(80–260)	(61–174)	(75–145)
Percent fall in mean serum creatinine		P → C 54%	C → C + 1/52 20%	C → C + 1/12 29%	C → C + 3/12 35%

*Patients already on prednisolone at the time of transplantation.

Histology

The early graft biopsies in the CsA-treated patients show fewer of the classic features of rejection than biopsies in the AP group. They do, however, contain focal infiltrates of mononuclear cells, often concentrated around vessels. The vessels themselves rarely show rejection changes, and compared with the AP biopsies, the absence of fibrinoid necrosis is striking. By 3 months after transplantation, the focal cellular infiltrate emerges as the major difference in appearances between the two groups, with the additional development of some interstitial edema and fibrosis in the CsA-treated group. The 1-year biopsies performed so far reveal that although there is an improvement in appearances in the CsA group, there is still evidence of some underlying renal damage. The focal cellular infiltrate tends to persist and there is an increase in interstitial fibrosis compared with the patients receiving AP from the time of transplantation.

DISCUSSION

Administration of CsA for a period of 3 months after transplantation has the advantage of providing potent immunosuppression in the critical early stage of recipient exposure to graft alloantigens, while avoiding side effects of long-term treatment. It is already apparent that nephrotoxicity may be a serious problem in patients maintained on CsA, and the interstitial fibrosis seen in biopsies may indicate that the duration of useful graft function may be limited. Several lymphomas have been reported in patients treated with CsA[10] and the possibility that there will be an increased incidence of these malignancies in patients receiving prolonged CsA remains a cause for concern. In addition to these major problems, minor side effects such as hypertrichosis, gum hypertrophy, tremor, hyperaesthesia, and gastrointestinal intolerance are unacceptable in some patients. If CsA is to be used on a short-term basis, it is clearly essential to be able to convert to another form of immunosuppression without risk to the graft.

The Oxford studies have demonstrated that conversion from CsA to AP at 3 months is a feasible policy, but that occasional rejection episodes occur in the immediate postconversion period. The nephrotoxic effect of CsA appears to be fully reversible, and the majority of patients attain normal SCr levels (less than 150 μmole/liter) within 1 month of conversion (see Table 2). There has been no correlation between serum CsA levels at the time of conversion and the percentage fall in SCr.[11] Biopsies at the time of conversion have shown significant interstitial fibrosis, but this does not appear to have progressed in the patients so far biopsied at 1 year. Of the 30 patients with stable renal function converted at 90 days from either CsA alone or CsA plus prednisolone, 6 (20%) have had an acute rejection episode in the first 2 weeks after conversion. In five of these patients, rejection was easily controlled with IVMP, and only one patient has progressed to irreversible rejection. The development of these florid rejection episodes at this stage suggests that in some patients there is a rapid proliferation of cytotoxic effector cells upon withdrawal of CsA. It appears that, in the occasional case, these cells may be unresponsive to conventional immunosuppression and antirejection therapy. The one patient having irreversible rejection had previously lost a first cadaver graft at 10 days from fulminant acute rejection. Her clinical course during her 90 days on CsA was stable, with SCr levels consistently below 130 μmole/liter. In trial II, it has been our policy not to convert patients who have lost a previous graft from aggressive early rejection.

Four patients in trial I were converted to AP early because they had a third rejection episode while receiving CsA alone. Two of these patients rejected their grafts irreversibly shortly after conversion, and in retrospect, the other two patients may have had nephrotoxicity rather than rejection. The impression that conversion may have caused an acceleration in the rejection process in the two patients who lost their grafts led to the policy in trial II of adding oral prednisolone to CsA therapy in patients requiring more than two antirejection courses of IVMP. The outcome in one such patient illustrates the benefit of this policy (Fig. 1). In trial I, he was randomized to receive CsA. During the first month he had three clear-cut acute rejection episodes and was converted to AP at 25 days. He suffered progressive rejection, and a graft nephrectomy was performed on day 39. For his second cadaver transplant in trial II, he was again randomized to receive CsA. An almost identical postoperative course developed, with three acute rejection episodes in rapid succession. Following the trial II protocol, oral prednisolone was added to CsA, and this resulted in resolution of the rejection process. Conversion to AP was not undertaken at 90 days for the reasons outlined above.

The combination of CsA and prednisolone has been suggested as the optimal form of immunosuppression for all renal allograft recipients.[12] In our experience, the addition of prednisolone to CsA has consistently resulted in a marked fall in SCr (from a mean of 369 μmole/liter at the time of adding prednisolone to a mean of 168 μmole/liter at 90 days). There has then been a further fall in SCr following conversion, with mean values reaching 135 μmole/liter at 1 week postconversion and 119 μmole/liter at 1 month postconversion. Despite these apparently encouraging results, it is perhaps significant that 3 of the 4 deaths in the CsA patients have occurred in the 13 individuals on CsA plus prednisolone. Each of these 3 deaths was due to infection. CsA plus prednisolone may therefore cause excessive suppression, and a policy of adding oral prednisolone only in selected cases seems justified.

The improvement in renal function following conversion appears to be due to abolition of CsA nephrotoxicity rather than control of a low-grade rejection process. This is mirrored by the deterioration in renal function, which we have observed in 7 patients with long-standing grafts converted from AP to CsA because of steroid side effects or azathioprine intolerance.[13] In none of these 7 patients has there been any evidence of rejection. The lack

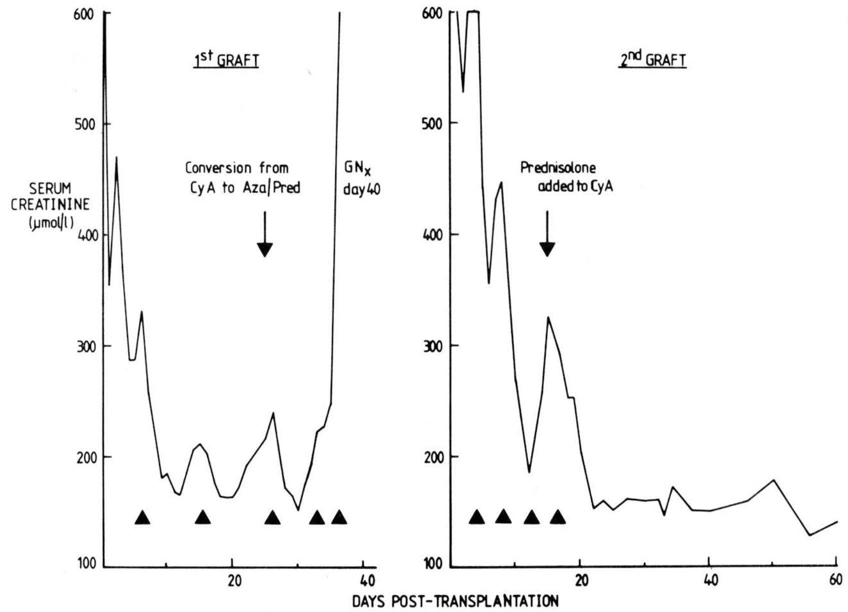

Fig. 1. Renal function in a patient treated with CsA for both first and second cadaver grafts. The first graft rejected irreversibly following conversion from CsA to AP. Rejection of the second graft was successfully controlled by the addition of prednisolone to CsA therapy.

of rejection may reflect the immunologically quiescent situation due to the development of immunoregulatory mechanisms involving circulating antibody and suppressor cells. The 20% incidence of acute rejection after conversion from CsA to AP suggests that a longer period of CsA administration may be desirable. In conventionally treated transplant patients, acute rejection is rare after 6 months, and if the initial CsA therapy had been continued until day 180 the problem of postconversion rejection might have been avoided. The abrupt substitution of AP for CsA at the time of conversion may also not be the ideal form of management, although we have found that CsA is detectable in the serum for up to 2 weeks after stopping the drug. It might nevertheless be better to start patients on steroids a week before conversion and then gradually reduce the dose of CsA while slowly increasing the dose of azathioprine.

The second Oxford trial is continuing to establish whether there is a significant increase in graft survival in the group treated initially with CsA. The basic strategy of using short-term CsA appears to be effective despite the problems with postconversion rejection. In the light of experience, some modifications to the protocol may be required, but a brief course of CsA at the time of transplantation with subsequent conversion to conventional agents may, in the long term, prove to be the most successful way of employing this powerful immunosuppressive drug.

REFERENCES

1. European Multicentre Trial: Lancet 2:57, 1982
2. Canadian Multicentre Transplant Study Group: N Engl J Med (in press)
3. Margreiter R, Spielberger M, Konig P, et al: Dial Transplant 12:108, 1983
4. Calne RY, Rolles K, White DJG, et al: Lancet 2:1033, 1979
5. Morris PJ: Transplantation 32:349, 1981
6. Homan WP, Fabre JW, Williams KA, et al: Transplantation 29:361, 1981
7. Homan WP, French ME, Millard PJ, et al: Transplant Proc 13:397, 1980
8. Morris PJ, Ting A: Immunol Rev 66:190, 1982
9. Morris PJ, French ME, Dunnill MS, et al: Transplantation (in press)
10. Beveridge T: Transplant Proc 15:433, 1983
11. French ME, Thompson JF, Hunnisett AGW, et al: Transplant Proc 15:485, 1983
12. Hakala TR, Starzl TE, Rosenthal JT, et al: Transplant Proc 15:465, 1983
13. Thompson JF, Chalmers DHK, Carter NP, et al: Transplant Proc (in press)

The Effect of Conversion From Cyclosporine to Azathioprine Immunosuppression for Intractable Nephrotoxicity

S. M. Flechner, C. T. Van Buren, R. Kerman, and B. D. Kahan

CYCLOSPORINE (CsA) and prednisone, in combination, represent a potent immunosuppressive regimen for human renal transplantation. Several centers reporting in this volume have demonstrated improved allograft survival in both cadaveric (CAD) and living-related (LRD) transplant recipients using these agents. The use of CsA, however, has been complicated by nephrotoxicity, which is experienced to a varying degree by each recipient. In most instances, nephrotoxicity is dose related and responds to a reduction in the administered daily dose of CsA by 50–100 mg.

As previously reported, the frequency of CsA-induced nephrotoxic events can be minimized by keeping 24-hr serum trough levels of drug under 200 ng/ml.[1] However, a few patients have experienced a form of intractable CsA nephrotoxicity that is not responsive to dose reduction and occurs with low CsA trough levels (<100 ng/ml).[2] We have attempted to improve renal function in these patients by conversion from CsA to azathioprine (Aza), while maintaining the same dose of steroids. This report details the results of conversion in such recipients.

MATERIALS AND METHODS

Patient Population

Between January 1981 and April 1983, 150 renal transplants (100 CAD, 50 LRD) were performed at the University of Texas Medical School at Houston using CsA and prednisone immunosuppression. No other agent was used in combination with CsA. Recipients initially received 14 mg/kg CsA orally either 48 hr (LRD) or 6–12 hr (CAD) prior to transplantation. Postoperatively, CsA was administered in tapering doses: 14 mg/kg week 1; 12 mg/kg weeks 2–3; and 10 mg/kg weeks 4–12. Tapering continued based on the determination of 24-hr serum trough levels as measured by a radioimmunoassay (reagents supplied by Sandoz, Ltd., Basel, Switzerland).[1] Dosing was adjusted in an effort to keep trough levels in a range of 100–200 ng/ml. Most recipients are receiving 7–8 mg/kg at 6 months and 5–6 mg/kg at 1 year posttransplant.

Table 1. Criteria for Conversion From Cyclosporine to Azathioprine to Improve Renal Function

(1)	Progressive renal dysfunction over several weeks
(2)	CsA trough levels <100 ng/ml
(3)	No clinical signs of rejection
(4)	Renal biopsy with no evidence of rejection
(5)	Absence of active infection
(6)	WBC >4,000, platelets >100,000

In this population, 55 patients experienced episodes of renal dysfunction in which serum creatinine elevations >25% of baseline occurred.[2] There were 17 patients in whom rejection was diagnosed, and they were treated with steroid pulse therapy. In the other 38 patients, CsA nephrotoxicity was suspected, and they were treated by continued CsA dose reduction. This was successful in 28 of the 38 patients. The remaining 10 patients (10/150, 6.7%) were felt to have intractable CsA nephrotoxicity and were subjected to a protocol of conversion to Aza to improve renal function.

These 10 patients included 5 males and 5 females with an age range of 8–55 years. Seven were recipients of cadaveric allografts and three had received living-related renal transplants. Six recipients had received prior steroid pulse therapy for presumed rejection (none within 60 days prior to conversion) without significant response.

Criteria for Conversion

Candidates for conversion to Aza to improve renal function had persistent elevations in serum creatinine (Table 1). These were demonstrated over several weeks and were >4 mg/dl in each case. During the previous weeks, the CsA dose was continually reduced until serum trough levels were <100 ng/ml. These recipients had no clinical signs of rejection, and in each instance, a percutaneous renal biopsy was performed prior to conversion.

From the Division of Immunology and Organ Transplantation, Department of Surgery, University of Texas Medical School at Houston, Houston, Tx.

Address reprint requests to Dr. S. M. Flechner, Division of Immunology and Organ Transplantation, Department of Surgery, University of Texas Medical School, Houston, TX 77030.

0041-1345/83/1505-0123$01.00/0

Table 2. Laboratory Data on 10 Patients Converted From Cyclosporine to Azathioprine for Intractable Nephrotoxicity

Patient	Posttransplant (Day)	Kidney Source	Creatinine (mg/dl)	BUN (mg/dl)	WBC (per cu cm)	Platelets (cu cm × 10^3)	CsA Dose (mg/kg)	CsA Level (ng/ml)	Prednisone (mg)
1	525	CAD	5.8	67	14,500	314	4.0	41	15
2	375	CAD	4.2	83	8,500	241	5.5	67	20
3	333	CAD	5.1	88	12,500	301	9.4	<10	20
4	231	LRD	9.1 D	85	19,000	441	6.1	83	15
5	150	LRD	3.4	53	6,800	174	5.3	37	20
6	110	CAD	5.8	120	15,600	250	5.6	76	20
7	93	LRD	4.4	121	11,600	424	6.4	112	25
8	90	CAD	4.1	74	12,200	387	4.2	43	10
9	54	CAD	4.2	139	5,300	156	8.4	39	20
10	42	CAD	7.2 D	89	5,100	212	6.3	108	25
Totals	200 ± 161	7:3	5.33 ± 1.72	91.9 ± 26.7	10,800 ± 4,400	290 ± 101	6.12 ± 1.68	57.5 ± 37.5	19 ± 4.5

D, dialysis required.

Biopsies revealed maintained renal architecture without diffuse cellular infiltrates, necrosis, or vascular thrombosis. No recipient had fever or clinical signs of infection. Laboratory criteria required prior to Aza conversion included normal liver function tests and white blood cell and platelet counts of 4,000 and 100,000, respectively (Table 2). Two recipients required supportive hemodialysis at the time of conversion. One recipient had been treated for *Escherichia coli* transplant pyelonephritis 6 weeks previously (with an aminoglycoside and ampicillin), and was producing 1000 ml of urine per day. The second had initial nonfunction 6 weeks posttransplant and was oliguric (<200 cc urine/day).

Method of Conversion

During conversion, patients were hospitalized and had complete blood count, electrolytes, blood urea nitrogen, and creatinine monitored daily. Aza was administered over 5–7 days in increasing doses, until 2 mg/kg was reached and tolerated. CsA was tapered and withdrawn by 100 mg/day only after adequate immunosuppressive doses of Aza were given. This was done in an effort to prevent breakthrough rejection episodes due to subtherapeutic doses of either CsA or Aza.

RESULTS

Each recipient completed the conversion protocol and tolerated full doses of Aza (2 mg/kg). The mean dose of Aza for these patients was 154 ± 36 mg by 2 weeks postconversion, and there were no episodes of severe leukopenia requiring withholding of the drug. No patient experienced a significant infection during conversion that required reduction in immunosuppressive drug doses. The maintenance dose of prednisone was unchanged during conversion. By the first week after CsA withdrawal, 9 of the 10 recipients demonstrated improved renal function, and the 2 patients with inadequate renal function were removed from dialysis (Table 3). With a mean follow-up of 208 ± 79 days postconversion, 8 patients retain functioning grafts and have a mean creatinine of 2.78 ± 1.07 mg/dl and blood urea nitrogen of 42.5 ± 11.6 mg/dl.

Two grafts were lost after conversion to Aza. One occurred in an 8-year-old female who was retransplanted with a cadaveric organ. Her first graft was lost due to oxalosis. After initial good function, her creatinine continued to rise to 4.1 mg/dl. Biopsy revealed oxalate deposition in her renal tubules and parenchyma. She underwent conversion on day 90, and by the first week her creatinine fell to 3.1 mg/dl. However, renal dysfunction progressed. Transplant nephrectomy on day 118 revealed extensive oxalate deposition in the allograft without chronic rejection. The second graft loss occurred in a 51-year-old diabetic male who received a cadaveric allograft. After initial acute tubular necrosis, renal function improved to a creatinine of 1.8 mg/dl. He suffered a viral infection, which resolved, but experienced progressive renal dysfunction. He underwent conversion on day 110. After some improvement in function 1 week postconversion, renal function deteriorated. Transplant nephrec-

Table 3. Results of Conversion From Cyclosporine to Azathioprine to Improve Renal Function

	Before Conversion		1 Week Postconversion		Present		Follow-up
	Cr (mg/dl)	BUN (mg/dl)	Cr	BUN	Cr	BUN	(Days)
1	5.8	67	3.5	46	3.5	44	180
2	4.2	83	3.8	76	2.1	38	139
3	5.1	88	4.5	61	2.9	40	108
4	9.1 D	85	7.0	90	3.8	58	220
5	3.4	53	3.4	59	4.5	62	160
6	5.8	120	5.0	110	Graft loss		—
7	4.4	121	3.2	145	1.6	30	298
8	4.1	74	3.1	51	Graft loss		—
9	4.2	139	3.3	77	2.1	36	290
10	7.2 D	89	5.5	71	1.7	32	275
Totals	5.33 ± 1.72	91.9 ± 26.7	4.23 ± 1.27	78.6 ± 30.1	2.78 ± 1.07	42.5 ± 11.6	208.8 ± 78.9

D, dialysis required.

tomy on day 145 revealed chronic allograft rejection and fibrosis.

DISCUSSION

CsA-induced renal dysfunction has been observed since the initial clinical trials of the drug in human transplant recipients.[3] This has created an obstacle to a simplified dosing regimen for all patients receiving CsA. In ideal circumstances, an initial loading dose of the drug should be given to saturate all tissue receptors. Thereafter, adequate maintenance doses would be given to achieve the desired immunosuppressive effect. The minimum dose required to achieve adequate immunosuppression in humans is presently not known and may differ from patient to patient. Therefore, dosing has been empiric, and is limited by the magnitude of renal dysfunction induced by the drug.

Three distinct patterns of nonimmunologic renal dysfunction in CsA-treated recipients have been observed. The first occurs in the majority of CsA-treated recipients, who experience small incremental elevations in serum creatinine (<25% baseline values) that respond promptly to a reduction in the administered daily dose. The second pattern is more severe and causes creatinine elevations >25% of baseline values, which can be difficult to differentiate from allograft rejection. CsA levels are helpful when elevated (>200 ng/ml), but this pattern can be observed with levels in a desired range (100–200 ng/ml).[2] Most of these patients do respond to a reduction in the administered dose, but about two-thirds are left with permanently impaired function. The third pattern, which represents the recipients in this report, is a progressive renal deterioration observed during continued CsA dose reduction.

This third intractable form of CsA-induced nephrotoxicity can be observed during the initial posttransplant period as persistent oligoanuria, not due to rejection. It can also occur as late as 500 days posttransplant as a progressive decline in renal function. The 10 recipients described with intractable CsA nephrotoxicity all had low CsA trough levels, mean 57 ± 37 ng/ml. The approach to improve renal function in these patients was to convert them to Aza while maintaining the same dose of steroids. The results of conversion were satisfactory, in that 8 of 10 recipients experienced improvement or stabilization in renal function with a mean change in creatinine from 5.33 to 2.78 mg/dl. No recipient suffered infections or other complications during or immediately after conversion. It is important to note that patients were first loaded with Aza (2 mg/kg) prior to discontinuing CsA in an effort to minimize breakthrough rejections, which have previously been reported.[4] Patients were also screened for active infections and leukopenia that could limit the amount of Aza tolerated, and therefore, lead to abandonment of the graft.

One graft was lost due to recurrent oxalosis after conversion and may not have represented CsA-induced nephrotoxicity. The results of transplantation in recipients with oxalosis have been variable,[5] but the use of CsA may exacerbate renal tubular injury in these recipients. The other graft loss occurred 1 month after conversion due to breakthrough rejection and illustrates that Aza is not as potent an immunosuppressive agent as CsA. The patients in this series were converted from CsA to Aza to improve renal function when intractable CsA-induced nephrotoxicity was diagnosed. Clinical, laboratory, and pathologic studies were performed to rule out acute allograft rejection in these recipients. If patients are converted during acute rejection episodes because of a poor response to antirejection therapy, a higher rate of graft loss may be predicted.

It is concluded that conversion to Aza can improve renal function in carefully selected nephrotoxic CsA-treated recipients. Breakthrough rejection episodes can be minimized by adequate preloading with Aza prior to CsA withdrawal. The long-term stability of Aza-converted patients requires longer follow-up to establish the true salvage of these impaired grafts.

REFERENCES

1. Kahan BD, Van Buren CT, Lin S, et al: Transplantation 34:36, 1982

2. Flechner SM, Van Buren CT, Kerman R, et al: Transplant Proc (this issue)

3. Calne RY, Thiru S, McMaster P, et al: Lancet 2:1323, 1978

4. Starzl TE, Klintmalm GB, Weil R, et al: Surg Gynecol Obstet 153:486, 1981

5. Alison DV, Luke RG, Curtis J, et al: Transplantation 35:161, 1983

Cyclosporine Nephrotoxicity in Renal Allograft Recipients: Conversion to Azathioprine to Improve Renal Function

D. M. Canafax, D. E. R. Sutherland, N. L. Ascher, R. L. Simmons, and J. S. Najarian

CYCLOSPORINE (CsA) has successfully prevented renal allograft rejection but occasionally produces a dose-related decrease in renal function.[1-4] In most patients, improved function is obtained by decreases in CsA dose, but when dosage reduction fails to improve renal function or concurrent nephrotoxins must be administered, patients often must be converted to another form of antirejection therapy. We have converted 28 CsA-treated patients to azathioprine (Aza) for persistently elevated serum creatinine levels (Cr). All but one patient (96%) had a subsequent decrease in Cr after conversion. Conversion is not without its problems, however: the present retrospective study details the successes and complications associated with conversion from cyclosporine to Aza immunotherapy.

MATERIALS AND METHODS

From April 1, 1980 through April 1, 1983, 159 HLA-mismatched renal transplant recipients were treated with CsA and prednisone antirejection therapy. Patients given CsA were either part of a randomized trial comparing CsA and low-dose prednisone with Aza, antilymphocyte globulin (ALG) and prednisone (57%) or an open protocol for second and third transplant recipients and older patients (43%). Only two recipients of HLA-identical sibling donor kidneys were treated with CsA—both were secondary grafts. All patients were treated with CsA, 14 mg/kg/day for 7 days and 12 mg/kd/day as maintenance. Dosage reduction was carried out in 50-mg increments to maintain optimal renal function. Prednisone was given in a tapering schedule to all patients, starting at 2 mg/kg/day and decreasing by 0.5 mg/kg/day every third day for 9 days. The dose was then more slowly decreased to a maintenance dose of 0.3 mg/kg/day by postop day 61 and 0.2 mg/kg/day at 1 year after transplantation.

The decision to convert a patient from CsA to Aza was always in response to persistently elevated Cr in the absence of obstruction, renal arterial stenosis, or rejection. In almost all cases, percutaneous biopsy confirmed the diagnosis of cyclosporine nephrotoxicity. Aza was started at 5 mg/kg/day and tapered to 2.5 mg/kg/day over 9 days in all patients. CsA was stopped 5–7 days after starting Aza. ALG was given to 7 (25%) patients for 10 days at 20 mg/kg/day. All patients were followed with frequent white blood cell (WBC) counts and Cr. Leukopenia was defined as a WBC below 3000 cells/cu mm, which required Aza dosage to be temporarily stopped. Acute tubular necrosis (ATN) was defined as poor post-transplant renal function requiring hemodialysis.

RESULTS

Twenty-eight (17%) of the 159 renal allograft recipients begun on CsA have been converted to Aza for elevated Cr. The mean time to conversion was 154 ± 111 (18–370) days after transplantation. This group of patients was 34 ± 10 (20–55) years of age, 71% male, and 50% diabetic, which is typical of our renal transplant population. More cadaver transplant recipients (82%) were converted than living-related donor recipients, even though 63% of our CsA-treated renal transplant recipients were from cadaver donors, suggesting cadaver recipients are a high-risk group of patients. Nine patients were recipients of second or third transplants (32%).

Twenty-seven of 28 (96%) patients had a decrease in Cr after conversion to Aza (Fig. 1). The mean Cr at conversion was 4.8 ± 1.8 (2.6–8.1) mg/dl, with 7 additional patients on hemodialysis. The mean Cr improved to 2.4 ± 1.1 (0.8–6.1) mg/dl. At present, the mean Cr is 2.9 ± 1.3 (1.1–4.0) mg/dl after a mean follow-up period of 654 (45–985) days post-transplant. However, five patients have died

From the Departments of Pharmacy and Surgery, University of Minnesota Hospitals, Minneapolis, MN.

Supported in part by the National Institutes of Health Grant AM 13083.

Address reprint requests to Dr. D. M. Canafax, Box 611, Mayo Memorial Building, University of Minnesota, Minneapolis, MN 55455.

0041–1345/83/1505–0124$01.00/0

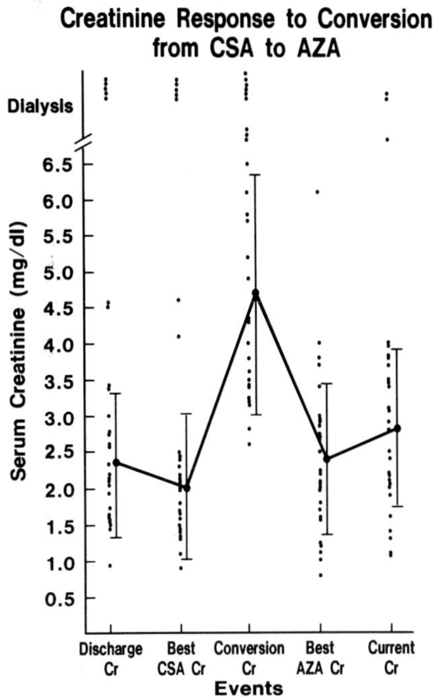

Fig. 1. Each patient's creatinine responses after transplantation are shown at discharge from the hospital, best level on CsA, at conversion to Aza, best level on Aza, and current level. Means ± SD are shown. Patients requiring dialysis are represented at the top for each event.

and two now require hemodialysis due to amphotericin B toxicity and recurrent membranoproliferative glomerulonephritis.

Seven (25%) patients were given ALG at the time of conversion. Six (86%) of the ALG-treated patients developed serious infections: three disseminated cytomegalovirus (CMV), one pneumonia, one enterococcal sepsis, and one Candida sepsis, as shown in Table 1. Three of these patients died from their infection: two CMV and one Candida sepsis. Two of the five deaths were unrelated to conversion; one patient died of a myocardial infarction and one was a suicide.

A total of 10 (36%) patients developed leukopenia, with their mean WBC counts decreasing to 2500 ± 1000 (500–3000) cells/cu mm at 14.6 ± 14.9 (1–50) days after conversion. Tables 1 and 2 show that 2 of the 6 patients not given ALG and 4 of 6 patients given ALG, developed a serious infection after a period of leukopenia. The leukopenic episodes required 9 ± 8 (1–30) days without Aza for the patients to recover their WBC.

All but three of the converted patients had a pretransplant splenectomy. The three patients with spleens left in situ all developed leukopenia and infectious complications.

A comparison of 10 (36%) patients converted in the first 3 months [mean 40 ± 16 (18–75) days] and 18 (64%) patients converted late [mean 215 ± 84 (120–340) days] is displayed in Table 2. Both groups had equally good improvement in Cr after conversion. Patients converted early had Cr decreases from 5.3 ± 2.0 to 2.5 ± 1.1 mg/dl and patients converted late had Cr decreases from 4.6 ± 1.8 to 2.5 ± 1.2 mg/dl. A comparison of the CsA doses at the time of conversion showed the late patients to be receiving less CsA. Late patients had had reductions in CsA dose to 4.9 ± 2.9 (1.2–9.6) mg/kg/day prior to conversion, while the early patients were receiving doses of 10.9 ± 2.2 (6.3–13) mg/kg/day. Five of the late patients were receiving every other day CsA and two were receiving doses every third day.

Four (14%) patients had rejection episodes after conversion to Aza. Two of these rejections were in patients given ALG during early conversion, while the other two had been converted to Aza alone. All four rejection episodes were reversible with increased prednisone doses. Of the 21 patients converted to Aza without ALG, there has been 1 death from a myocardial infarction and 2 graft losses from amphotericin-B toxicity and recurrent membranoproliferative glomerulonephritis.

Three patients developed infections on CsA that required amphotericin-B therapy and conversion to Aza for increasing creatinine levels. All three patients had a decrease in Cr and all three are currently well with functioning grafts.

DISCUSSION

The management of elevated Cr is a difficult, time-consuming, and expensive problem

Table 1. Risk Factors for the Development of Infectious Complications After Conversion From CsA to AZA and Patient Outcome

		Risk Factors				Outcome	
Patient	Organism(s)	ALG	Leukopenia	Diabetes	2nd or 3rd Graft	Graft	Patient
Patients with infections 9/28 (32%)							
R.A.	Cryptococcal meningitis, CMV, VZV and Candida esophagitis	No	Yes	Yes	2nd	Lost	Survived
A.D.	CMV	Yes	Yes	Yes	1st	Lost	Survived
D.A.	Enterococcal sepsis	Yes	Yes	Yes	2nd	Functioning	Survived
M.S.	CMV, cryptococcal meningitis	No	Yes	Yes	3rd	Functioning	Survived
R.B.	Candida esophagitis	No	No	Yes	1st	Functioning	Died (MI)
R.L.	Pneumonia, unknown etiology	Yes	Yes	Yes	2nd	Functioning	Died (suicide)
E.N.	CMV	Yes	No	No	2nd	Functioning	Died
T.M.	CMV	Yes	Yes	Yes	1st	Functioning	Died
M.P.	Candida sepsis	Yes	No	Yes	2nd	Functioning	Died
Subtotal		6/9 (67%)	6/9 (67%)	8/9 (89%)	6/9 (67%)	2/9 (22%)	5/9 (56%)
Patients without infections 19/28 (68%)		1/19 (5%)	4/19 (21%)	6/19 (32%)	3/19 (16%)	0/19 (0%)	0/19 (0%)
Total		7/28 (25%)	10/28 (36%)	14/28 (50%)	9/28 (32%)	2/28 (7%)	5/28 (18%)

Table 2. Clinical Course of Patients According to Reason for Conversion From CsA to AZA

		Discharge		Best CsA		At conversion		Best AZA		Current					
	No. of Patients	Mean Cr	Dialysis	Mean Cr	Dialysis	Mean Cr	Dialysis	Mean Cr	Dialysis	Mean Cr	Dialysis	Leukopenia	Infections	Rejections (After Conversion)	Deaths
Early prolonged ATN															
ALG	6	3.0	2/6	2.4	3/6	3.9	4/6	2.4	0/6	3.4	0/3	3/6	5/6	2/6	3/6
No ALG	4	4.6	3/4	4.4	2/4	5.8	2/4	2.6	0/4	3.0	0/4	2/4	1/4	0/4	0/4
Late persistently elevated Cr															
ALG	1	1.6	0/1	1.6	0/1	6.0	0/1	2.9	0/1	—	—	1/1	1/1	0/1	1/1
No ALG	17	2.1	0/17	1.7	0/17	4.4	1/17	2.4	0/17	2.7	2/17	4/17	2/17	2/17	1/17
Total	28	2.4	5/28	2.0	5/28	4.7	7/28	2.4	0/28	2.8	2/23	10/28	9/28	4/28	5/28

in CsA-treated renal allograft recipients. In most cases, an elevated Cr in CsA-treated patients will fall as the CsA dose decreases,[5] but a few patients will continue to have decreased renal function even after dosage reductions to less than 5 mg/kg/day. This group of patients usually will have improved renal function when converted from CsA to Aza, but normal values are seldom achieved. Interstitial fibrosis is a common renal biopsy finding.

A second group of patients that may benefit by conversion from CsA to Aza are those with poor renal function during the early posttransplant period. Such patients may even have prolonged acute tubular necrosis requiring prolonged dialysis. In addition, patients that require potent nephrotoxins, such as amphotericin B, are likely to improve their renal function when converted from CsA and Aza.

We have converted 28 patients for these indications and found that all three patient groups responded to conversion with decreased Cr. This improved renal function appears to persist for the majority of patients, even though a few (29%) show gradual increases in Cr (0.3–1.0 mg/dl) levels. Whether this represents chronic rejection or the residual of cyclosporine toxicity is not yet clear.

Four risk factors were identified that predispose patients to complications after conversion. These included cadaver allografts, ALG therapy during conversion, diabetes, and multiple grafts. Cadaver allograft recipients dominated the group of patients converted. This was possibly the result of pretransplant ischemic and preservation injury. Patients with decreased renal reserve after transplantation appear to be more sensitive to the nephrotoxic effects of CsA. The use of ALG to prevent rejection at the time of conversion resulted in a high incidence of serious infections and infection-related deaths. These infections were likely the result of overimmunosuppression at the time of conversion. In addition, the development of Aza-induced leukopenia coincided with an increased incidence of infection in these patients. Those few patients without pretransplant splenectomy were at the greatest risk of developing leukopenia and infections. This is a potentially serious problem, since splenectomy will probably not improve the transplant results with cyclosporine, but the need to convert a large proportion of cadaver recipients to azathioprine may be associated with troublesome leukopenia.

The fear that acute rejection will follow conversion from CsA to Aza appears unwarranted. Acute rejection episodes occurred less commonly after conversion than was expected, and all were easily reversed with increased prednisone doses. Leukopenia at the time of conversion and the resulting decrease in Aza doses may have played a role in causing rejection in these patients.

SUMMARY

Of 159 mismatched renal transplant recipients, 28 (17%) were converted from cyclosporine to azathioprine, primarily to reverse persistent or progressive renal dysfunction. Recipients of cadaver transplants predominated. The transition was complicated by serious infection in six of seven patients who received ALG during the conversion and three of these patients died. In 21 patients who were not given ALG, no kidneys were lost to rejection and 3 serious infections resulted. Improvement in renal function was generally seen, but return to normal values was not common.

REFERENCES

1. Calne RY, Thiru S, McMaster P, et al: Lancet 2:1323, 1978

2. Ferguson RM, Rynasiewicz JJ, Sutherland DER, et al: Surgery 92:175, 1982

3. Klintmalm GBG, Iwatsuki S, Starzl TE: Lancet 1:470, 1981

4. Hows JM, Palmer S, Gordon-Smith EC: Transplantation 33:382, 1982

5. Ferguson RM, Rynasiewicz JJ, Najarian JS: Transplant Proc 15:480, 1983

Conversion Problem—Azathioprine to Cyclosporine

K. Rolles, R. Merion, and R. Y. Calne

THE Cambridge experience with cyclosporine-A in clinical organ grafting now spans 5 years and was preceded by a 2-year extensive use of the compound in a wide range of animal models.[1-4] Nevertheless, at this point in time, the use of this unique immunosuppressant confronts us with more questions than answers to its efficient long-term clinical use.

Excellent short-term results in terms of kidney graft and patient survival have been reported by Calne, using cyclosporine-A alone,[5-7] and by Starzl,[8,9] using it in conjunction with long-term steroids. Morris,[10] in a small short-term controlled trial, found cyclosporine-A at least as good as azathioprine and steroids and demonstrated that conversion of cyclosporine-A-treated patients to azathioprine and steroids at 3 months could be achieved with ease, as long as the grafts were not rejecting on cyclosporine-A at the time of the changeover. The recent European Multicentre Trial has further confirmed the short-term efficacy of cyclosporine-A.[11]

The problems of early nephrotoxicity have, to a large extent, receded, being essentially dose related in the majority of patients, but the observation by Hamilton that functional improvement did not occur in some cases treated with cyclosporine-A for more than 1 year has been accompanied by biopsy evidence of structural changes, including tubular atrophy, interstitial fibrosis, and mild interstitial inflammation.[12,13] Morris[10] reported interstitial fibrosis as early as 3 and 6 months and suggested the lesions were progressive. With these points in mind, long-term results of cyclosporine-A immunosuppression are anxiously awaited to establish its proper place in the immunosuppressant armamentarium. If it transpires that the short-term excellence of cyclosporine-A is not maintained in the long term, then detailed information on conversion of patients to and from other immunosuppressive agents will become important.

All clinicians using cyclosporine-A in renal transplantation will have some experience of converting patients from cyclosporine-A to azathioprine and steroids and vice versa.

We report our experience of interchanging cyclosporine-A with azathioprine and prednisone in our renal allograft and liver allograft recipients.

RENAL ALLOGRAFTS

Between July 1978 and December 1982, 101 patients receiving renal allografts on an ABO-compatible and best HLA-A and B antigen match were treated with cyclosporine-A as the sole initial immunosuppressant. The first 15 patients were started on cyclosporine-A, 25 mg/kg/day, intramuscularly for the first 2 days and orally thereafter. The remaining 86 patients were begun on 17 mg/kg/day, reducing by 2 mg/kg/day every 2 weeks to a maintenance dose of 6–8 mg/kg/day.

Biopsy-proven acute rejection episodes were treated with three 1.0-g doses of intravenous methylprednisolone on consecutive days, which was repeated after an interval of a further 3 days if no biochemical improvement in renal function was seen. In those cases where no response was seen after 2 courses of methylprednisolone, cyclosporine-A was stopped abruptly and replaced by prednisone, 2 mg/kg/day, and azathioprine, 1–2 mg/kg/day.

In 16 patients, the immunosuppressive regimen was changed from cyclosporine-A to azathioprine and prednisone because of uncontrolled allograft rejection between 2 weeks and 34 months posttransplant (mean 5.6

From the Department of Surgery, University of Cambridge, Addenbrooke's Hospital, Cambridge, U.K.

Address reprint requests to Dr. K. Rolles, Department of Surgery, University of Cambridge, Addenbrooke's Hospital, Hills Road, Cambridge, CB2 2QQ, U.K.

0041-1345/83/1505-0125$01.00/0

months). Monitoring of cyclosporine-A blood levels was not available at this time. Eight of these grafts were subsequently rejected and two recipients died. Mean serum creatinine in the functioning grafts remains elevated at 270 μmole/liter. Actuarial survival of grafts and patients at 3 years is 60% and 78%, respectively.

A further 14 kidney graft recipients initially treated with azathioprine and prednisone were changed to cyclosporine-A for a variety of indications between 2 weeks and 4 months postoperatively. Ten patients were converted because of the side effects of prednisone, two patients due to pulmonary sepsis, one patient because of bone marrow suppression, and one because of continuing rejection. All ten patients changed on account of steroid side effects have survived with functioning grafts. Mean creatinine in this group is 208 μmole/liter. All four of the remaining patients died, three with functioning grafts. In the fourth patient, rejection of the allograft was not prevented by conversion to cyclosporine-A. Actuarial survival of grafts and patients at 3 years is 71%.

Actuarial survival of grafts and patients whose immunosuppression has been converted to or from cyclosporine-A is comparable to patients treated with cyclosporine-A alone (73% for grafts, 88% for patients) and to those maintained on azathioprine and prednisone alone (50% for grafts, 78% for patients) at 3 years.

Conversion of patients from cyclosporine-A to azathioprine and prednisone has been generally successful. One-half of the kidneys continuing to reject on cyclosporine-A immunosuppression were salvaged by converting to azathioprine and prednisone. The efficacy of cyclosporine-A as a steroid-sparing immunosuppressant is clearly demonstrated in those patients converted to cyclosporine-A because of steroid side effects.

LIVER ALLOGRAFTS

We have cautiously introduced cyclosporine to our liver allograft recipients since 1980. Forty-one patients have received cyclosporine-A since that time, by one of three different regimens.

Six patients initially treated with prednisone, 1 mg/kg/day, and azathioprine, 2 mg/kg/day, were converted to cyclosporine-A, 10 mg/kg/day orally, between 1.5 and 4 years posttransplant, all because of severe steroid side effects.

Two of these patients, known to suffer from severe osteoporosis preoperatively, lost several centimeters in height postoperatively due to vertebral collapse, progressively made worse by long-term steroids. In addition, two patients had chronically deteriorating graft function.

Following conversion, two patients died, one of a myocardial infarct at 4.75 years and the other of graft failure, also at 4.75 years. Four patients remain well between 3 years and 7.5 years postoperatively on maintenance doses of 5–8 mg/kg/day of oral cyclosporine-A.

Twenty-three patients were changed from azathioprine and prednisone to cyclosporine-A, 10 mg/kg/day, electively, posttransplantation, when liver function was felt to be stable. All patients were changed between 3 days and 4 months postoperatively. Two patients died within the first month of transplantation, one of septicemia and one of a preservation-related injury to the liver graft. The perioperative mortality in this group of patients appeared considerably less than anticipated from earlier experience. Five more patients died within the first 6 months, three of graft rejection, one of an intracerebral hemorrhage, and one of graft infarction. Three further patients subsequently have died, one following a fracture of an osteoporotic cervical spine at 10 months and two of tumor recurrence between 1 and 2 years.

Thirteen patients remain alive and well between 1 and 3 years postoperatively on maintenance doses of cyclosporine-A between 5 and 8 mg/kg/day.

However, in the last year, concurrent with a further change in the immunosuppressive regimen, these promising results have not been maintained. Twelve patients have received an intravenous infusion of cyclosporine-A, 4 mg/kg/day, starting within 12 hr postoperatively. Oral cyclosporine-A has usually replaced the intravenous infusion within 1 week. No azathioprine or prednisone was initially given to these patients. Three patients only remain alive and well between 5 and 9 months. One patient died of influenza at home at 4 months. Eight patients have died within 6 weeks of transplant, usually with good liver function. Pulmonary complications have been the most common, with severe pulmonary edema leading to hypoxia and terminal pneumonia. Renal failure, often requiring dialysis, and severe hypoalbuminemia have been other features in all these patients. There has been no correlation between blood levels of cyclosporine-A and toxic effects in these patients.

Intravenous infusions of cyclosporine-A at similar dosage have been used in our kidney and pancreas transplant patients without the development of major pulmonary complications, as seen in the liver recipients. This picture is similar to that described by Powles et al. (1983)[14] in bone marrow graft recipients treated with oral cyclosporine-A. At present, we feel that the circumstantial evidence against the intravenous preparation of cyclosporine-A should not be ignored. We have recently returned to our former regimen of azathioprine and prednisone in the early post-transplant period, converting to oral cyclosporine-A when liver function is stable.

REFERENCES

1. Kostakis AJ, White DJG, Calne RY: J Med Sci 5:280, 1977
2. Calne RY, White DJG, Rolles K, et al: Lancet 1:1183, 1978
3. Calne RY, White DJG, Pentlow BD, et al: Transplant Proc 11:860, 1979
4. McMaster P, Procyshyn A, Calne RY, et al: Br Med J 1:444, 1980
5. Calne RY, White DJG, Thiru S, et al: Lancet 2:1323, 1978
6. Calne RY, Rolles K, White DJG, et al: Lancet 2:1033, 1979
7. Calne RY, White DJG, Evans DB, et al: Br Med J 282:934, 1981
8. Starzl TE, Iwatsuki G, Klintmalm G, et al: Transplant Proc 13:281, 1981
9. Starzl TE, Hakala TR, Iwatsuki S, et al: In White DJG (ed): Cyclosporin A. Amsterdam, Elsevier Biomedical, 1982, p 365
10. Morris PJ, French ME, Ting A, et al: In White DJG (ed): Cyclosporin A. Amsterdam, Elsevier Biomedical, 1982, p 355
11. European Multicentre Trial: Lancet 1:57, 1982
12. Hamilton DV, Calne RY, Evans DB, et al: Lancet 1:1218, 1981
13. Keown PA, Stiller CR, Ulan RA, et al: Lancet 1:686, 1981
14. Powles RL, Morgenstern GR, McElwain TJ, et al: Lancet 1:612, 1983

Total Lymphoid Irradiation and Cyclosporine

D. E. R. Sutherland, R. M. Ferguson, M. I. Aeder, W. I. Lewis, F. R. Bentley, N. L. Ascher, R. L. Simmons, and J. S. Najarian

IN THE late 1970s, two new approaches for immunosuppression excited attention: total lymphoid irradiation[1] and cyclosporine.[2] The two regimens can be compared for their ability to prevent rejection in both experimental and clinical transplantation. Total lymphoid irradiation (TLI) and cyclosporine (CsA) can also be used together as a combination immunotherapy regimen, under the assumption that the synergistic effect of low doses will be greater for the therapeutic than for the toxic effects of either regimen alone.

Attempts to use TLI and CsA together have not been reported for clinical transplantation, but several such experiments have been performed in animals.[3–7] So far, a comparison of TLI versus CsA in clinical practice is possible only in the unique situation of retransplantation after rapid rejection of previous grafts, because it is only in such patients that TLI has had any extensive application.[8] TLI and bone marrow transplantation can result in chimerism in rodents, with permanent acceptance of organ allografts,[9] but graft-versus-host disease is not always obviated,[10–12] and tolerance has not been achieved in large animals[13] or humans.[8]

TLI alone is immunosuppressive, but the effect dissipates with time, and TLI must be combined with other immunosuppressants for long-term maintenance. In the clinical trial of TLI for retransplantation at Minnesota, TLI was administered with azathioprine and prednisone.[8,14] The current status of the patients so treated is updated in this article, and a comparison is made to a similar group of patients treated with CsA for retransplantation after rapid rejection of previous allografts. The possibility of using TLI in combination with CsA is then reviewed by summarizing the results of various experiments with this combination in animal models.

COMPARISON OF TLI-AZATHIOPRINE-PREDNISONE AND CSA-PREDNISONE FOR TREATMENT OF PATIENTS UNDERGOING RETRANSPLANTATION AFTER RAPID REJECTION OF PREVIOUS ALLOGRAFTS

From January 1970 to March 1983, 98 patients who had rejected at least one renal allograft in less than 1 year underwent retransplantation at the University of Minnesota. Since January 1979, all such patients have been treated with either TLI-azathioprine-prednisone or CsA-prednisone after retransplantation. The demographic features of the 20 patients who were treated with TLI and transplanted between February 17, 1979 and August 25, 1981 and of the 33 patients treated with CsA between June 9, 1980 and March 21, 1983 are summarized in Table 1. Actuarial patient and graft survival rates in both groups of patients were calculated on May 1, 1983.

The details of the immunosuppressive treatments have been described previously.[8,14] Briefly, the TLI patients received 1600–4150 rad (150 R per fraction) over a 24–124-day period between 1 and 330 days pretransplant. Posttransplant, azathioprine, 1.5 g/kg/day, was administered and adjusted according to white blood count. The prednisone dose was variable, ranging from 0.4 to 2.0 mg/kg initially, followed by a taper. Rejection was treated with an increase in prednisone only,

From the Department of Surgery, University of Minnesota, Minneapolis, MN.

Supported in part by NIH Grant AM13083.

Address reprint requests to Dr. D. E. R. Sutherland, Box 280, University of Minnesota Hospitals, Minneapolis, MN 55455.

0041–1345/83/1505–0126$01.00/0

Table 1. Demographic Features of Patients who Rapidly Rejected Previous Renal Allografts According to Immunosuppressive Regimen Used for Retransplantation

	TLI (n = 20)	Cyclosporine (n = 33)
Age		
Range	4–51 years	6–58 years
Mean	27 ± 13	35 ± 11
Mean time of rejection of previous allografts	5.8 ± 5.5 months	2.6 ± 2.1 months
Interval between loss of previous allograft and retransplantation	2–49 months (15.6 ± 12.8 months)	2–57 months (22.9 ± 15.8 months)
No. males/females (%)	15 M/5 F (25%)	2 M/12 F (36%)
No. 2nd/3rd transplants (%)	13/7 (35%)	25/8 (24%)
No. rel/unrel donors (%)	1/19 (95%)	8/25 (76%)
Percent diabetic	30%	24%
Follow-up		
Range	22–52 months	1–36 months
Median	38.5 months	17 months
Mean	38.8 ± 7.8 months	14.3 ± 9.0 months

except for one patient who also received antilymphocyte globulin.

In the other group, CsA, 14 mg/kg/day, was given for 1 week and then reduced to ≤12 mg/kg/day, with the dose adjusted according to clinical course and whole blood levels. Prednisone was given in a dose of 2.0 mg/kg/day and tapered to 0.2 mg/kg/day by 1 year. Six patients were switched to azathioprine between 3 and 6 weeks posttransplant.

The patient and graft survival rates in all recipients are depicted in Fig. 1. At 1 year, the graft survival rates were 80% in the TLI and 75% in the CsA group, and the corresponding figures at 2 years were 60% and 58%.

Of the 20 TLI-treated patients, 12 are

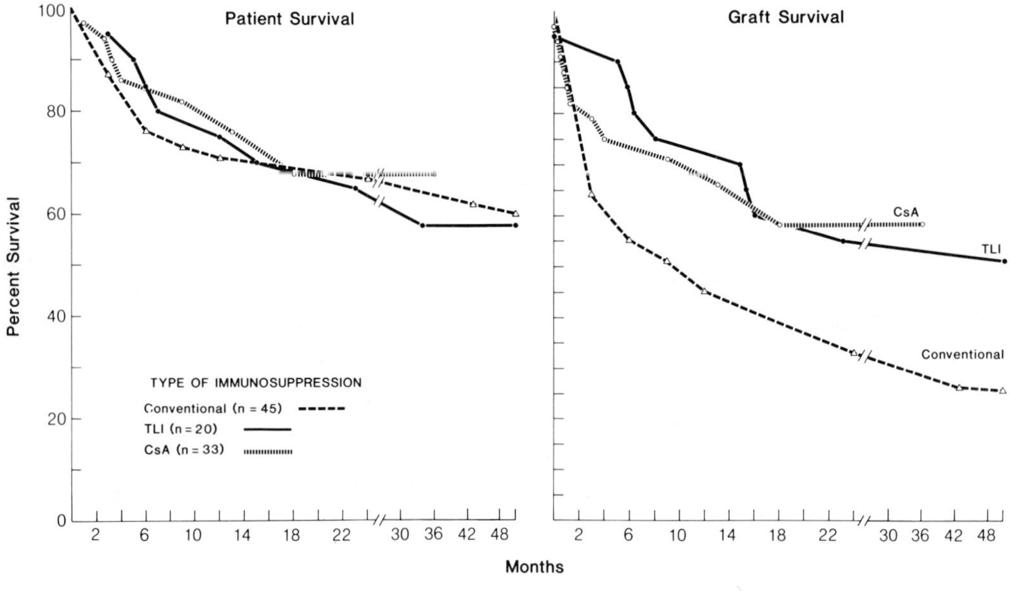

Fig. 1. Actuarial patient and renal allograft survival rates according to immunosuppressive regimen after retransplantation in University of Minnesota patients who rejected previous allografts in less than 12 months. All patients in whom treatments were initiated are included in the calculations.

currently alive and 11 have functioning grafts with a mean creatinine of 1.7 ± 0.5 mg/dl at 25–51 months posttransplant. One patient who rejected the graft at 15 months is alive at 31 months posttransplant, while four patients died after loss of graft function; 1 of a perforated gastric ulcer two months posttransplant after rejection at one month, 1 of diabetic complications at 12 months after rejection at 8 months, 1 of sepsis at 34 months after rejection at 6 months, and 1 of diabetic complications at 3 months after loss of the graft for technical reasons. Four patients died with functioning grafts, 1 at 5 months with CMV, 2 from lymphoma at 5 and 11 months, and 1 at 12 months of pneumococcal sepsis.

A previous detailed analysis of the TLI trial showed that the results were best in patients who received approximately 2500 rad.[8] Also, a short interval between TLI and transplantation was associated with fewer rejection episodes and the best long-term graft survival rates. A long interval between TLI and transplantation, or an initial low dose of prednisone, was associated with a high incidence of rejection episodes. The optimal protocol appeared to be transplantation within 3 weeks of TLI and initial administration of a high dose of prednisone, followed by a rapid taper.

Twenty-six of the 33 CsA-treated patients are currently alive and 22 have functioning grafts, with a mean serum creatinine of 2.1 ± 0.8 mg/dl, between 1 and 36 months posttransplant. Three patients with functioning grafts were switched to azathioprine between 2 and 3 months after transplantation. Four patients are alive between 2 and 13 months after loss of graft function, 1 for technical reasons and 3 from early rejections; while 2 patients died of infections at 1 and 3 months after technical losses. Five patients died with functioning grafts, 1 at 4 months of herpes viremia, 1 at 13 months of a myocardial infarct, 1 at 3 months of cytomegalvirus infection, 1 at 10 months from suicide, and 1 at 18 months of sepsis; the latter 3 patients had been switched to azathioprine in the early posttransplant period.

Since six of the CsA-treated patients were switched to azathioprine early, a comparison of TLI versus CsA was also made with these patients eliminated from the analysis, along with those in both groups whose grafts failed for technical reasons. The results of this analysis, summarized in Table 2, show that patient survival was 10% better at 12 months and 22% better at 24 months in the CsA than in the TLI group. The graft survival rates in both groups were similar at 12 months, but there was an 18% better graft survival in the CsA group at 24 months. The incidence of graft losses due to rejection was nearly the same in the TLI and CsA groups, 4 of 19 (21%) in the TLI and 3 of 21 (14%) in the CsA group (technical failures and switches to Aza excluded).

Complications occurred in both groups of patients. TLI was associated with leukopenia (WBC < 2500/cm) in 5 patients, and gastrointestinal symptoms occurred in 7 patients. Two patients in the TLI group developed lymphoma; one of them received ALG for treatment of rejection episodes; both were associated with Epstein Barr virus infections.[16] The main complication in the CsA-treated patients was an elevated creatinine from presumed nephrotoxicity. Of the 19

Table 2. Actuarial Patient and Graft Survival Rates According to Immunosuppressive Regimen Used for Retransplantation in Patients Who Rejected Previous Renal Allografts in <12 Months While on Conventional Immunosuppression. Technical Failures (1 TLI and 3 CsA) and Patients Switched From CsA to Conventional Immunosuppression (n = 9) are Excluded*

	Patient Survival (%)		Graft Survival (%)	
Time Post-Tx	TLI (n = 19)	CsA (n = 21)	TLI (n = 19)	CsA (n = 21)
1 Months	100	100	100	86
3 Months	100	100	100	86
6 Months	89	95	84	81
12 Months	79	95	79	81
18 Months	74	90	63	76
24 Months	68	90	58	76
36 Months	63	90	58	76
48 Months	63		58	

*See text for fate of excluded patients. They are included in survival rate curves of Fig. 1.

which the recipient is not dependent for survival in the one model, and recurrence of hyperglycemia in the other), the differences in graft survival times may partially be explained by differences in sensitivity in detecting rejection, but for practical purposes, and in this model, this regimen is inadequate to prevent rejection of pancreas allografts; however, multiple other regimens tested were also ineffective.[19]

Posttransplant TLI Combined With CsA in Lewis Rat Recipients of Heterotopic Heart Allografts From ACI Donors

One of the most serious drawbacks to the use of preoperative TLI for clinical renal allotransplantation was the inability to precisely time the transplant in relation to the completion of the prescribed course of TLI. It would be logistically advantageous if TLI could be given in the immediate pre- or postoperative period. In the initial attempts at application of posttransplant TLI by Rynasiewicz et al.,[3,4] the dose fraction schedules that were effective in prolonging graft survival when administered preoperatively had only a minimal effect when given postoperatively. Rejection would occur before the dose necessary to blunt the immune response had been delivered. However, if early rejection was prevented by a low dose of CsA (a dose unable to prevent rejection by itself), posttransplant TLI was effective in prolonging graft survival or preventing rejection (Table 3).

In subsequent experiments, Bentley et al.[20] devised a posttransplant TLI dose-fraction schedule that by itself significantly prolonged graft survival. For example, 300 rad/day for the first 5 posttransplant days resulted in a median graft survival time of 16.8 days (n = 4), and a schedule of 300 rad × 3 days, followed by 2 days of rest, and then an additional 5 doses of 200 rad/day (n = 4), gave a median graft survival time of 25 days. Bentley et al.[6] went on to combine posttransplant TLI in combination with a very short course of either ALG or CsA, and a synergistic effect on prolonging graft survival times was demonstrated (Table 3). The results of these experiments illustrate the long-term effect of TLI, since in the ACI to Lewis rat heart allograft model, a short course of CsA is unable to induce tolerance,[3,4,19] unlike the situation in other rat donor–recipient strain combinations.[21]

Pretransplant TLI Combined With Posttransplant CsA in Canine Renal Allograft Recipients

TLI protocols that promote organ allograft survival in rodents are less effective in dogs, and a total TLI dose of >2500 rad is poorly tolerated.[22] Thus, we have tested a variety of protocols in which TLI was combined with other immunosuppressants, including azathioprine, prednisone, and ALG.[23] Although some of the protocols were quite effective in delaying or preventing rejection, the therapeutic ratio was relatively low, since many dogs died with functioning grafts. We have also combined CsA with azathioprine, prednisone, or ALG with moderate success.[24,25] In a further search for an effective combination immunotherapy regimen, pretransplant TLI has been combined with posttransplant low-dose CsA in splenectomized and nonsplenectomized, outbred, bilaterally nephrectomized, beagle dog recipients of renal allografts from DLA-mismatched donors. The results of the pilot experiments, summarized in Table 4, show a mild synergism of CsA and TLI in delaying or preventing graft rejection, but the therapeutic ratio was relatively poor (especially compared to the results in the rat heart allograft model), and further experiments with TLI and CsA as a method to prevent or delay allograft rejection have not been done, because CsA combined with other pharmacologic agents appeared to provide a better therapeutic ratio than the CsA-TLI combination in dogs.

Comments

The combination of low-dose TLI and CsA is very effective at preventing rejection in rat heart allograft recipients, even when TLI is

Table 4. Functional Survival of Renal Allograft in Outbred, DLA-Mismatch Beagle Dogs

Treatment*	Day of Rejection (Cr >7 mg/dl)	Died With Functioning Graft	Median Days Graft Fxn
Splenectomized			
None	5,6,6,7,7,7,11,12	—	7
CSA 5	7,7,8,8,13	—	8
TLI(1,800)	8,8,8,9	—	8
TLI(2,100)	10,12,30,30,50	—	30
TLI(2,400)	25,30	15(1.1)†, 43(1.4)‡	27.5
TLI(1,800) + CSA 5	9,38,39,41,42,50	20(2.4)§	39
Nonsplenectomized			
None	6,8,12,13,15,19	—	12.5
CSA 5	7,10,37	11(4.9)‡, 15(6.7)‡ 62(2.3)†	12.5
TLI(1,000–1,400)	8,8,9,9,12	—	8.5
TLI(1,800)	9,10,32,36	22(3.9)‡, 29(2.4)‡	25.5
TLI(1,000) + CSA 5	91	33(3.5)†	62
TLI(1,200) + CSA 5	29,35	152(0.5)‖	35
TLI(1,500) + CSA 5	13,44	3(0.9)‖	29.5
TLI(1,800) + CSA 5	32	48(4.9)‡	40

*Treatment refers to total dose (rad) of TLI (given in fraction of 150 R) pretransplant and mg/kg/day of cyclosporine given posttransplant.

†From pneumonia.

‡Cause unknown.

§From peritonitis.

‖From malnutrition and dehydration.

given posttransplant.[4,6] Sadeghi et al.[7] found both pre- and posttransplant fractionated TLI (200 rad/fraction) to be synergistic when combined with CsA for prevention or delay of rejection of cardiac allografts in rats, using as little as 600 rad preoperatively and up to 1000 rad postoperatively. The most effective protocol out of 11 tried was a 600-rad course of TLI completed 14 days preoperatively, followed by postoperative CsA 2 mg/kg/day, and 1000 rad of TLI begun 6 days postoperatively (4 of 6 grafts functioned >50 days). The beneficial effect of TLI on graft survival was progressively less as the interval between initiation of TLI and transplantation lengthened.[7] A similar dissipation of the effect of TLI with time had been noted by Rynasiewicz et al.[3,4] in earlier experiments.

The TLI-CsA combinations we tested were much less effective in prolonging graft survival in the rat pancreas and dog kidney models compared to the rat heart allograft model. The only other report of the use of TLI-CsA in a large animal model is that of Pennock et al.[5] They combined fractionated TLI (100 rad/fraction) with CsA (17 mg/kg/day i.m.) to treat monkey recipients of orthotopic cardiac allografts and observed mean allograft survival times with CsA alone of 59 days, and with CsA plus TLI (600 or 800 rad) of 89 and 160 days, respectively,[5] only a slight additive effect.

There are multiple dose-fraction–time combinations of TLI and CsA that could be tested in the various allograft models, and ones more effective than those studied so far might be found. The fact that some regimens are highly effective in the rat heart allograft model is an impetus to continue to study new combination immunotherapy regimens that might be clinically applicable in the large animal allograft models.

SUMMARY AND CONCLUSIONS

Patients who rapidly reject previous renal allografts in less than 1 year continue to be a high-risk group for retransplantation, but the outlook has improved since the introduction of TLI and CsA into clinical practice. Before we began to use these modalities, the 1- and 2-year graft survival rates after retransplantation in this particular subgroup of patients were 55% and 38%, respectively. In our TLI trial, the 1- and 2-year graft survival rates were 80% and 60%; the corresponding figures in the CsA group were 75% and 58%. Nevertheless, both the 1- and 2-year graft survival rates in the retransplant group continue to be less than what we currently achieve either in CsA-prednisone-treated (1- and 2-year graft survival rates of 83% and 79%) or azathioprine-ALG-treated (1- and 2-year graft survival rates of 76% and 76%) recipients of primary cadaveric renal allografts.[26] Thus, there remains an impetus to develop more effective immunosuppressive regimens for retransplantation.

We and others have tested alternative combination immunotherapy regimens in aninal allograft models.[3–7,14,22–25] Pre- or posttransplant TLI combined with posttransplant chemical immunosuppressants had either a synergistic or additive effect on prolongation of graft survival, depending on the particular protocol and choice of allograft model. However, TLI and CsA together do not appear to be more effective than other combination immunotherapy regimens, except in the rat heart allograft model, where low-dose TLI and CsA can result in indefinite graft function, even in a donor–recipient strain combination in which a limited course of CsA does not induce a tolerant state.

It remains to be seen whether the TLI-CsA combination can be exploited for clinical organ allotransplantation. It is also uncertain what the role of TLI will now be in clinical organ transplantation, with the demonstrated effectiveness of CsA in also preventing rejection following retransplantation. TLI might allow CsA to be used without the addition of steroids, the latter being an integral part of CsA immunotherapy regimens, particularly in North America. However, further studies are needed to determine whether TLI provides a better therapeutic ratio than other agents in combination with CsA.

REFERENCES

1. Slavin S, Strober S, Fuks Z, et al: Transplant Proc 9:1001, 1977
2. Calne RY, White DJG, Pentlow BD, et al: Transplant Proc 11:860, 1979
3. Rynasiewicz JJ, Sutherland DER, Kawahara K, et al: Transplant Proc 13:452, 1981
4. Rynasiewicz JJ, Sutherland DER, Kawahara K, et al: J Surg Res 30:365, 1981
5. Pennock JL, Reitz BA, Bieber CP, et al: Transplantation 32:467, 1981
6. Bentley FR, Sutherland DER, Rynasiewicz JJ, et al: Transplant Proc 15:671, 1983
7. Sadeghi AM, Downing PP, Bieber CP, et al: Heart Transplant 2:209, 1983
8. Najarian JS, Ferguson RM, Sutherland DER, et al: Ann Surg 196:442, 1982
9. Slavin S, Strober S, Fuks Z, et al: J Exp Med 46:34, 1977
10. Ascher NL, Sullivan W, Simmons RL: Surg Forum 31:366, 1980
11. Kersey JH, Kruger J, Song C, et al: Transplantation 29:388, 1980
12. Pierce GE, Wahs LM, Kinnaman ML, et al: J Surg Res 30:398, 1981
13. Koretz SH, Strober S, Gottlieb MS, et al: Transplant Proc 13:443, 1981
14. Ferguson RM, Rynasiewicz JJ, Sutherland DER, et al: Surgery 92:176, 1982
15. Hanto DW, Frizzera G, Gajl-Peczalska KJ, et al: N Engl J Med 306:913, 1982
16. Ferguson RM, Sutherland DER, Kim T: Transplant Proc 13:1673, 1981
17. Ferguson RM, Fidelus RK, Sawchuk RJ: Transplant Proc 15:535, 1983
18. Sutherland DER, Ferguson RM, Simmons RL, et al: Urol Clin North Am 10:277, 1983
19. Rynasiewicz JJ, Sutherland DER, Ferguson RM: Diabetes 31(Suppl 4):92, 1982
20. Bentley FR, Sutherland DER, Najarian JS: J Surg Res 32:360, 1982
21. Fabre JW: Transplantation 34:223, 1982
22. Lewis WI, Sutherland DER, Najarian JS: Surg Forum 32:365, 1981
23. Lewis WI, Aeder MI, Sutherland DER, et al: Surg Forum (in press)
24. Aeder MI, Sutherland DER, Lewis WI, et al: Transplant Proc (this issue)
25. Aeder MI, Sutherland DER, Najarian JS: Surg Forum (in press)
26. Najarian JS, Strand M, Fryd DS, et al: Transplant Proc (this issue)

Use of Cyclosporine and Monoclonal Antibodies in Clinical Renal Transplantation

N. L. Tilney, R. L. Kirkman, J. L. Araujo, C. B. Carpenter, E. L. Milford, E. L. Reinherz, S. F. Schlossman, and T. B. Strom

THE renal transplant group at the Brigham and Women's Hospital treated its first recipient of a cadaver allograft with cyclosporine (CsA) in 1979, using protocols that had evolved through the early experience of Calne et al.[1,2] Because of rigid inclusion criteria, accumulation of initial patient data was slow.[3] However, with gradually increasing understanding of the clinical effects of this drug, our results in kidney transplantation using CsA as primary immunosuppression have improved markedly; thus, at present, the majority of all patients receiving both cadaver and living-related allografts are treated with the agent. In addition, during the past year, a pan-post-thymic T-cell monoclonal antibody, anti-T12, has become available to treat acute rejection episodes.[4] This report summarizes our preliminary experience with CsA, emphasizing both early discouragement with its use as the sole immunosuppressive agent and later enthusiasm with the addition of low-dose corticosteroids to our protocols. The adjunctive utilization of anti-T12 as an antirejection treatment is also described.

MATERIALS AND METHODS

The first patient in the series at the Brigham and Women's Hospital treated with CsA received a renal transplant on November 6, 1979. The course of each recipient of an allograft performed subsequently through March 1, 1983 has been reviewed. Complete follow-up on all patients was obtained through personal examination and review of hospital and clinic records. During the period of study, 137 patients received kidney grafts, 84 from cadavers, 53 from living-related sources. Forty-five recipients of cadaver allografts received CsA; 39 individuals treated with standard immunosuppressive therapy (azathioprine and steroids, A+S) received cadaver allografts during the same time and will be considered as nonrandomized but concurrent controls. Fifty-three patients received kidneys from living-related sources during this period; of those treated with standard A+S, 33 were HLA-nonidentical with high mixed lymphocyte reactions (MLR) between donor and recipient, 12 were HLA-identical with low MLR. Routine use of CsA as primary treatment for non-HLA-identical high MLC recipients of living-related grafts was initiated in July 1982; the results of 8 patients receiving this treatment are reported.

The overall population of graft recipients included 61 females and 76 males; average age was 38 years (range 20–69 years). Four patients in this series received two kidneys during the period under study; they are counted as new patients with each successive transplant. Of these, 3 received CsA during the Initial Pilot Study and later were treated with A+S for their second kidney. One individual received CsA for both kidney grafts. All recipients of cadaver grafts received at least 5 blood transfusions before transplantation. There were no differences in types of original renal disease afflicting those in the series, regardless of treatment protocols. Two CsA-treated recipients had a history of alcohol-induced liver disease; however, liver enzymes were normal in the months preceding transplantation. Donor and recipient HLA tissue typing of A, B, C, and DR locus antigens was carried out in all patients. Only individuals with negative past and current donor-specific T-cell crossmatches were accepted for cadaver transplantation. MLR was performed between recipients and their living-related donors; stimulation index of >5% was considered a high MLR.

Clinical Protocols

Our initial clinical experience using CsA as the sole immunosuppressive agent was modest in scope, with the agent administered conservatively because of the potential for lymphoma and other complications, as initially reported by Calne et al.[1,2] With increasing experience, however, our clinical protocols have evolved through three distinct phases of patient management: the Initial Pilot Study, an Interim Protocol, and a Current Protocol. All protocols were passed by the Human Subjects Committee and detailed informed consent obtained from all patients.

In the Initial Pilot Study, all patients received a single

From the Departments of Surgery and Medicine, Brigham and Women's Hospital, and the Division of Tumor Immunology, Sidney Farber Cancer Institute, Boston, Mass.

Address reprint requests to Dr. N. L. Tilney, Department of Surgery, Brigham and Women's Hospital, Boston, MA 02115.

0041-1345/83/1505-0127$01.00/0

dose of azathioprine (4 mg/kg) upon admission. If the cadaver kidney did not function immediately, CsA was not used and standard A+S given indefinitely as maintenance therapy. If the graft functioned during the first 6 hr after revascularization, azathioprine was discontinued and CsA was begun in a dose of 17 mg/kg/day. If allograft function diminished or urine volume decreased below 500 ml/24 hr, the dose of CsA was halved to 8.5 mg/kg/day. For the first rejection episode, a steroid pulse (1 g Solumedral i.v. each day for 3 days) was started. For a second rejection episode, a second pulse was administered, CsA was discontinued, and maintenance A+S begun. Because of insecurity regarding the long-term effects of CsA, all patients were switched to maintenance A+S 3 months after transplantation. Needle biopsies were performed routinely at 7 and 14 days.

In December 1980, an Interim Protocol was initiated to include for study the relatively large proportion of patients whose cadaver allografts failed to function initially. No individual received azathioprine preoperatively. CsA (17 mg/kg/day) was started the day of surgery and tapered slowly after the first 2 weeks to 10 mg/kg/day at 2 months. As in the Initial Protocol, all patients were switched to A+S at 3 months. If the individual became oliguric in the early postoperative period, CsA dose was decreased to 12.5 mg/kg/day, 3/4 dose. First and second rejection episodes were treated with i.v. pulses of Solumedrol (100 mg/day for 3 days); if a third rejection occurred, the patient was switched to A+S and treated again with a steroid pulse. In addition, 4 individuals from this group were given maintenance prednisone (30 mg/day) following their first rejection episode.

The Current Protocol, in use since November 1981, involves administration of CsA plus low-dose maintenance steroids (30 mg/day) from the time of transplantation. CsA dose is tapered as described above; steroid dose is reduced slowly after 2 months to approximately 5–10 mg/day. Rejection episodes were treated initially with Solumedrol pulses; however, during the past 6 months, with the availability of anti-T12, rejections have been treated predominantly with this material. Since July 1982, non-HLA-identical recipients of grafts from living-related donors with a high MLR between donor and recipient have also been treated with this protocol.

All control patients received a standard regimen of A+S. Azathioprine was administered in a dose of 3 mg/kg/day if renal function was satisfactory. If function declined, the dose was cut to 2 mg/kg/day. Prednisone was given in a dose of 50 mg/day beginning the day of transplantation, tapering after 2 months. Rejection episodes were treated with intravenous boluses of Solumedrol, 1 g/day for 3 days, with no more than 3 such pulses being given in the first 3 months.

Ten patients with acute renal allograft rejection occurring within 3 months of transplant while receiving primary immunosuppression with CsA and prednisone have been treated with the monoclonal anti-T12 antibody. This antibody is a mouse IgM directed against a 120K-dalton glycoprotein determinant present on all post-thymic T cells. Details of the preparation and specificity of this antibody have been presented elsewhere.[4] Rejection was confirmed by needle biopsy in all cases. The antibody was given intravenously daily for 10 days at a dose of 200 μg/kg, with adjustment of the dose to achieve free antibody level. Treatment was discontinued after 5 days if no response occurred. Baseline immunosuppression with CsA and prednisone was continued unchanged.

RESULTS

In this series, there were no significant differences in tissue matching or presensitization between CsA-treated recipients and those treated with standard A+S immunosuppression. Cold ischemic time of the perfused kidneys was also relatively similar between the two treatment groups. Anuria secondary to acute renal failure occurs relatively commonly in cadaver transplantation in our unit. As noted, the Initial Protocol precluded use of CsA in patients who became anuric or oliguric in the postoperative period. Thus, nine of the first ten recipients treated with CsA had immediately functioning kidneys. Once the inclusion criteria were broadened in the Interim and Current Protocols, 18 of 35 subsequent patients (51%) had early function. In the control group of recipients treated with A+S, 19 of 39 (49%) kidneys functioned immediately. There were 8 grafts among the 45 CsA cadaver recipients (18%) that never functioned, 8 among the 39 patients (20.5%) receiving A+S; these invariably showed changes of severe humoral rejection and cortical necrosis on biopsy or later nephrectomy. The remainder of the cadaver kidneys in both groups that were initially oliguric regained function 7–42 days later.

Patient Survival

There were 4 deaths among 137 patients in this series (3%). Three of 53 (6%) receiving CsA died within 1 year of transplantation; there have been no subsequent deaths. The first of the deceased individuals received a cadaver renal allograft that never functioned and required nephrectomy at 2 weeks. CsA was administered only during this 14-day period. At 1 week, he developed transient acute pancreatitis, and at 3 months, a left colectomy was performed for a perforation of a solitary sigmoid diverticulum. At 1 year, carcinoma of the pancreas was discovered, which rapidly proved fatal. The second patient remained anuric for 6 weeks before graft function. At 3 months, he developed transient cytomegalovirus infection with persistent fevers and malaise. At 8 months, fulminating *Pneumocystis carinii* pneumonia ultimately proved fatal. Maintenance CsA dose had been 8 mg/kg/day during this period; kidney function had been normal. The third patient experienced anuria for 2 weeks following transplantation, for which CsA was reduced to half dose (8.5 mg/kg/day) after 4 days. Subsequently, his allograft recovered and functioned normally. A spree-type alcoholic, he had had a history of elevated liver enzymes in the months prior to transplantation, although these were normal at the time of operation. Subsequently, his bilirubin rose to 2.5 mg/dl, but declined with reduced drug dosage. At 3 months, he vomited and aspirated during an alcoholic binge and was admitted with pneumonia. Multiple system failure ensued, which caused his death. The single fatality among those treated with A+S occurred in a patient with severe chronic hepatitis and general debility. She received a cadaver transplant as an emergency, and died a few weeks later of liver failure.

Allograft Function

Our primary experience with CsA included its use in 16 patients, 10 receiving the Initial Protocol and 6 receiving the Interim Protocol. Neither of these early protocols were effective. Of the 10 individuals receiving the Initial Protocol, CsA alone without adjunctive steroids, 7 kidneys were functioning at 3 months, at which time the agent was discontinued and A+S initiated. By 1 year, however, only 4 of these grafts continued to function. Only 3 grafts placed in 6 individuals receiving the Interim Protocol were functioning at 3 months when CsA was replaced by A+S. Two more of these had failed by 6 months. It is interesting that the only grafts that functioned in this group were in patients who received full-dose CsA throughout the first 3-month period.

The Current Protocol includes 29 recipients of cadaver allografts who received full-dose CsA throughout their course, regardless of initial graft function, plus low-dose maintenance steroids initiated at operation. Although follow-up is short, with the first patient entering this phase of the study in November 1981, the results have been gratifying. At 3 and 6 months following operation, 89% and 79% of allografts were functioning, respectively (actuarial figures). As described, two individuals in this group died at 3 and 6 months with well functioning grafts. The results of the control group were less impressive, with 69% functioning at 3 months and 60% at 6 months. Of the recipients of grafts from living-related sources, 100% of grafts in hosts of HLA-identical and CsA-treated recipients are functioning at 6 months; 66% of those from HLA nonidentical sources.

Rejection

It can be extremely difficult to differentiate between episodes of acute rejection or drug-induced nephrotoxicity in CsA-treated recipients. Acute rejection in patients receiving standard immunosuppression with A+S usually becomes manifest by high fevers and an enlarging, tender graft, exhibiting declining function. In contrast, rejection in those receiving CsA with or without steroids is more subtle. Rarely does fever rise over 100°F. The kidney often remains nontender, firm, and compact; no changes in size or character are noted in serial ultrasound examinations. Thus, graft dysfunction may be the only clue of rejection in these patients.

The pattern, frequency, and severity of rejection episodes have varied in this study, depending on which CsA protocol was used. Nine of 10 patients receiving the Initial Protocol experienced 17 rejections 4 days to 3 months following surgery. However, only two individuals in this group had remained on full-dose CsA (17 mg/kg/day) throughout the entire 3-month period. Similarly, 5 of 6 patients receiving the Interim Protocol experienced 7 rejection episodes 5–21 days postoperatively. Only 2 had remained on full-dose CsA during the initial 3 months. This situation changed dramatically when we adopted the Current Protocol, with initiation of relatively low-dose maintenance steroids in addition to full-dose CsA beginning the day of transplantation. Twenty of 29 individuals (69%) in this group never experienced identifiable rejection crises.

Treatment of Acute Rejection With Anti-T12 Monoclonal Antibody

Ten CsA patients were treated with the monoclonal antibody anti-T12 for acute rejection episodes occurring 3 days to 3 months posttransplant, with each confirmed by needle biopsy. Response to the anti-T12 therapy followed several different patterns. Three patients had rapid and complete resolution of rejection, with return of serum creatinine to prerejection levels. Posttreatment biopsies showed clearing of the interstitial mononuclear cell infiltrate in two cases; the third patient refused repeat biopsy. Two additional patients showed resolution of cellular infiltrate by biopsy, although serum creatinine did not change. While graft function improved in 2 patients following anti-T12 therapy, interpretation of the contribution of anti-T12 was difficult because of use of additional steroid therapy. In one, a standard steroid pulse was given when the creatinine failed to fall after 5 days of therapy; this lack of improvement in renal function may have been secondary to acute tubular necrosis (ATN), demonstrated on the pretreatment biopsy. In the other, serum creatinine fell significantly following the initiation of anti-T12, but rose again on the fifth treatment day, leading to initiation of a steroid pulse by protocol. In both cases, rejection resolved clinically and histologically after the combined treatment. Finally, no response to the anti-T12 therapy could be documented in three patients: two had humoral rejection with vascular damage, causing eventual graft loss; the third had a severe cellular rejection that responded to a subsequent steroid pulse. The only episode of acute rejection following anti-T12 therapy occurred in an individual with ATN plus rejection. Posttreatment biopsy showed the cellular infiltrate to have cleared. However, persistent low urine output led to a second biopsy 12 days later, which again demonstrated cellular rejection and ATN. A steroid pulse was administered, but renal function never improved. This patient also developed anti-mouse antibodies.

Of the 10 patients treated with anti-T12 therapy, 7 have functioning kidneys in follow-up ranging from 1 to 8 months. No significant complications have occurred from the combined use of CsA and monoclonal antibodies.

Nephrotoxicity

Nephrotoxicity secondary to CsA may occur both in the first few days after transplantation and after several weeks or months of function. It is difficult, if not impossible, to differentiate early nephrotoxicity superimposed upon ATN. Early nephrotoxicity became manifest in initially well functioning grafts in 5 patients in our series by a diminishing rate of glomerular filtration occurring 1–7 days following transplantation and lasting 1–6 weeks before normal function returned. Although CsA dosage (17 mg/kg/day) was cut by 50%–75% (8.5–12.5 mg/kg/day) in individuals given the Initial and Interim Protocols, such early dose reduction did not obviously reverse the process and may have contributed to rejection, with ultimate graft loss by undersuppression. As a result, CsA dosage has not been decreased during the first 2–3 weeks in the Current Protocol, regardless of early graft function.

Thirteen of the 53 patients, however, were considered to have developed nephrotoxicity 2 weeks to 3 months after transplantation, as manifested by elevated levels of serum creatinine to 3–4 mg/dl from baseline values of 1.5–2.0 mg/dl. Biopsies showed little cellular infiltrate. The dosage of CsA was reduced to

50%–75% dose for 2–4 days before improvement in renal function was noted. In each case, elevated levels of serum creatinine returned to normal.

Other Complications

We have noted few other complications potentially attributable to CsA.[5,6] One individual developed a fine tremor postoperatively, which decreased with reduced drug dosage, and nine females have developed hirsutism. Infections, either pneumonia or urinary tract infections, have only occurred in six patients, despite the use of maintenance steroids. Nine patients developed transient elevation in bilirubin (1.5–3.0 mg/dl direct) 1–4 weeks after surgery, reversed by reducing CsA dosage. As noted, two individuals taking maintenance CsA plus low-dose steroids died of pneumonia and multiple system failure, primarily liver failure, 3 and 8 months after transplantation, respectively. Organisms in the lungs of these individuals were *Pneumocystis carinii* and *Pseudomonas,* respectively.

Conversion from CsA to A+S

Discontinuation of CsA has occasionally produced important sequelae. The agent was discontinued for three main reasons in our study: conversion to A+S at 3 months to conform to early protocols, conversion at other times because of uncontrollable rejection, or complete cessation of immunosuppression following allograft failure. For instance, two patients with failed but completely asymptomatic allografts who had already returned to hemodialysis experienced episodes of acute rejection with fever and enlarged tender grafts within 24 hr of discontinuation of CsA. These patients required graft nephrectomy. An additional patient sustained fulminating irreversible rejection of a previously well functioning graft when CsA was discontinued in preparation for starting azathioprine.

DISCUSSION

The learning period necessary to use CsA effectively as a primary immunosuppressive agent in recipients of renal allografts has been long; it is interesting that the majority of transplant groups involved in testing the material have ultimately arrived at relatively comparable protocols by various and disparate routes using CsA, as described by Calne,[1,2] plus concomitant low doses of maintenance steroids, as suggested by Starzl.[7,8] In addition, the recent availability of an intravenous preparation of CsA may be of aid in producing therapeutic levels in the first few days following transplantation. Several variations in treatment protocols have undeniably improved our clinical results. It seems clear that the unsatisfactory experience accrued in the early phases of the study were ameliorated by several changes in drug use, including: (1) continuation of full CsA dosage regardless of graft function in the early postoperative period; (2) continuation of CsA treatment indefinitely rather than conversation to azathioprine because of the potential for severe rejection after its cessation; and (3) the addition of maintenance steroids in relatively low doses beginning at the time of transplantation. In retrospect, it seems clear that many of our initial patients were ineffectually immunosuppressed; rejection episodes were common and incidence of graft loss relatively high. Because of ignorance about drug toxicity in these early patients, the doses were reduced markedly if signs of declining function appeared. It may also be a tribute to the effectiveness of CsA that, despite low doses, seven of the ten patients receiving the Initial Protocol had functioning allografts at 3 months, at which time they were converted to A+S. However, three patients developed acute rejection crises upon discontinuation of CsA, a phenomenon that has encouraged us to continue indefinite treatment with the agent. This occurrence has also been reported by Morris et al.[9]

The addition of maintenance steroids to CsA beginning at the time of transplantation has been critical in improving our results. Acute rejection has become a relatively uncommon event with this drug combination; if it occurs, it has usually been successfully treated either with a steroid pulse, or increasingly with anti-T-lymphocyte monoclonal antibodies. In comparison to standard protocols of A+S, which include treatment of more frequent and fulminant early rejection crises with high-dose steroids, it is apparent that the use of CsA reduces markedly the overall need for steroids in the first weeks or months following engraftment. Such dose reduction is of obvious benefit in diabetic or prediabetic patients, as well as in decreasing the incidence of infections, cataracts, bone disease, and other all-too-common sequelae of these agents. In contradistinction to our experience and that of others in the United States,[10] it is intriguing that Calne et al.[2,11] have not found steroids to be necessary in their patients, nor have the participating centers in the European Multicentre Trial used steroids in conjunction with CsA.[12] The results of the Canadian Multicenter Trial, which includes maintenance steroids for the first 3 months after transplantation, however, have also shown improved results.[13]

Therapy with the monoclonal antibody, anti-T12, has been a useful adjunct in patients with rejection episodes occurring despite CsA and prednisone immunosuppression. This treatment reversed rejection completely in three of ten patients and contributed to improvement in four others. The antibody produced no significant complications and did not require changes in baseline immunosuppression. Moreover, the combined steroid-sparing effects of monoclonal antibody therapy and cyclosporine A resulted in a significant lowering of the overall steroid requirements. This is of particular benefit to the diabetic and older transplant recipient.

The potential nephrotoxicity of CsA not infrequently poses an important clinical conundrum, which may be difficult to resolve. Differentiating, in the early postoperative period, between acute tubular necrosis, acute rejection with its subtle manifestations, and nephrotoxicity may be difficult. As noted, it has become our practice increasingly to administer full CsA dose despite early acute renal failure in expectation of resumption of urine output. Serial ultrasound examination and needle biopsies have been of some aid in determining the cause, extent, and prognosis of anuria. Nephrotoxicity secondary to drug effect was noted in the original clinical experience and still remains a problem in patient management.[1] Cadaver allografts, functioning well initially, may become oliguric or anuric after relatively short periods of treatment, a circumstance corroborated by subtle tubular changes noted on light microscopy of renal biopsies. As the postoperative period of oliguria is usually self-limiting and reversible, standard doses of CsA should generally be continued. Renal function will also improve toward normal in the early period after transplantation, although many allograft recipients may run levels of serum creatinine that are slightly higher than those usually occurring in individuals treated with A+S.[2] Thus, creatinine levels of 2.0–2.5 mg/dl are not uncommon in patients receiving CsA; glomerular filtration usually improves with slight reduction of drug usage, especially in patients exhibiting late nephrotoxicity. Increased serum creatinine levels have been noted when trough serum levels of CsA are as high as 400 ng/ml or plasma levels measure over 400 ng/ml, as determined by radioimmunoassay.[14,15] Other sequelae of drug use have been noted,[5,6] including hepatoxicity, hirsutism, and tremor; these have been relatively inconsequential in one series and are usually dose-related.

Although CsA has been a difficult agent to learn to use effectively, gradual improvements in understanding its actions and toxicities with increasing experience in its administration, are beginning to suggest its real usefulness. It now seems fair to assume that CsA, probably in conjunction with relatively low-dose maintenance steroids, may represent an incremental improvement over previously available immunosuppression modalities.[2,7–10,12,13] This improvement in results of grafting without sacrificing safety for the recipient himself, will allow increasing latitude in transplantation, with larger numbers of difficult or older individuals with organ failure now becoming acceptable as recipients.

REFERENCES

1. Calne RY, White DJG, Thorin S, et al: Lancet 2:1321, 1978
2. Calne RY, Rolles K, White DJG, et al: Lancet 2:1033, 1979
3. Carpenter BJ, Tilney NL, Strom TB, et al: Kid Int 19:265, 1981
4. Reinherz EL, Meuers S, Fitzgerald KA, et al: Cell 30:735, 1982
5. Morris PJ: Transplantation 32:349, 1981
6. Bordes-Aznar J, Tilney NL: J Clin Surg 1:53, 1982
7. Starzl TE, Weil R III, Iwatsuki S, et al: Surg Gynecol Obstet 151:17, 1980
8. Starzl TE, Hakala TR, Rosenthal JT, et al: Surg Gynecol Obstet 154:819, 1982
9. Morris PJ, French ME, Ting A, et al: In White DGJ (ed): Cyclosporin A. Amsterdam, Elsevier Biomedical, 1982, p 355
10. Ferguson RM, Rynasiewicz JJ, Sutherland DER, et al: Surgery 92:171, 1982
11. Calne RY, White DJG: Ann Surg 196:330, 1982
12. European Multicentre Trial: Lancet 2:57, 1982
13. A Randomized Trial of Cyclosporin in Cadaveric Renal Transplantation from the Multicenter Transplant Study Group: N Engl J Med (in press)
14. Stiller CR, Keown PA, Sinclair NR, Ulan RA: In White DJG (ed): Cyclosporin A. Amsterdam, Elsevier Biomedical, 1982, p 379
15. Kahan BD, Van Buren CT, Lin SN, et al: In White DJG (ed): Cyclosporin A. Amsterdam, Elsevier Biomedical, 1982, p 413

EFFECTS IN AUTOIMMUNITY, VIRAL AND FUNGAL INFECTIONS

Effect of Cyclosporine on Antigen Presentation: Relationship to Lupus

M. Fischbach and N. Talal

AUTOIMMUNE DISEASES can be viewed as complex problems of disordered immunologic regulation.[1,2] Abnormalities involving B cells, T cells, and macrophages have been described.[3–5] Much valuable information has been gained by the study of murine strains that spontaneously develop autoimmunity.

For over 20 years the NZB mouse and its variants were the only murine models for systemic lupus erythematosus (SLE) available for examination. In recent years, a second model has been introduced called MRL/*lpr*, which differs from the NZB in developing a very fulminant form of disease, with early death.[6,7] A cardinal feature in this disease is the marked proliferation of an unusual T lymphocyte that is weakly expressive of the Lyt-1^+23^- phenotype.[8] Disease in this strain is related to the presence of the *lpr* gene, since a congeneic MRL mouse lacking this gene, MRL/+ +, develops only very mild disease. The *lpr* gene has also been introduced into C57B1/6, C3H, and AKR mice. Although the time of disease onset may vary, all of these *lpr* mice develop hypergammaglobulinemia, autoantibodies, immune complex glomerulonephritis, and massive lymphoproliferation.

We undertook a study of immunoregulatory factors that might be qualitatively or quantitatively abnormal in autoimmune states and found that a deficiency in the T-cell growth factor interleukin 2 (IL-2) is a common feature of autoimmune mice.[9,10] This defect arises within the first 2 months of life in the MRL/*lpr* and C57B1/6/*lpr* strains, before major autoimmune manifestations have developed.

Murine IL-2 is a 30,000-mol wt protein produced by Lyt-1^+23^- T cells in response to antigen or mitogen stimulation.[11,12] IL-2 has diverse effects on lymphocytes in vitro, including augmentation of antibody synthesis by splenocytes from nude mice,[9,13,14] long-term maintenance of specific alloreactive cytotoxic and helper T cells,[9,13,15–19] and enhancement of thymocyte proliferation after mitogen stimulation.[20–23] Receptors for IL-2 are present on activated T cells,[24,25] which are then stimulated to undergo clonal expansion. IL-2 is also active in vivo[24,25] and is an important mediator of immune function and regulation.

Deficiency of an immune-regulatory factor such as IL-2 might contribute significantly to the immunoregulatory disorder of *lpr* mice. Similar problems involving IL-2 are also present in patients with systemic lupus erythematosus[26] and rheumatoid arthritis.[27] In this respect, there is a parallel between the human disease and the animal model.

Cyclosporine A (CsA) is an immunosuppressant with a high degree of specificity for T cells.[28] While the action of CsA is not completely understood, it does inhibit the proliferation of T cells induced by mitogens and antigens by both suppressing the synthesis of IL-2 and rendering T cells unresponsive to IL-2.[28] We were interested in studying the extent to which CsA could mimic the *lpr* defect.

MATERIALS AND METHODS

Mice

MRL/Mp-*lpr*/*lpr* (MRL-*lpr*), MRL/Mp-+/+, C57B1/6J-*lpr*/*lpr* (C57B1/*lpr*), C3H/HeJ-*lpr*/*lpr*

From the University of Texas Health Science Center at San Antonio, Department of Medicine, Division of Clinical Immunology, and the Audie L. Murphy Memorial Veterans Administration Hospital, San Antonio, TX.

Supported by the Research Service of the Veterans Administration.

Reprint requests should be addressed to Dr. Michael Fischbach, Department of Medicine, UTHSC, 7703 Floyd Curl Dr., San Antonio, TX 78284.

0041–1345/83/1505–0128$01.00/0

(C3H/*lpr*) mice were obtained from our breeding colonies at The University of Texas Health Science Center at San Antonio. The normal cogenic partners, C57Bl/6J and C3H/HeJ, were obtained from Jackson Laboratory, Bar Harbor, ME.

Antigen Presentation

Antigen presentation was studied by using the method of Alkan.[29] Mice were immunized at the base of the tail with 10 μg $TNP_{25}KLH$ emulsified in complete Freund's adjuvant. Seven days later, draining lymph nodes were removed and the T cells purified by nylon-wool chromatography. Nonimmune spleen cells, 1×10^7, were incubated with TNP-KLH in the presence of mitomycin C for 1 hr at 37°C. After extensive washing, 2×10^5 antigen-pulsed spleen cells were incubated with 4×10^5 immune T cells for 5 days in culture. The incorporation of tritiated thymidine was used to measure the degree of antigen stimulation.

IL-2 Production

The number of interacting cells in the antigen-presentation assay was tripled in order to measure the IL-2 produced during the reaction. Supernatants were collected and stored at −20°C until use.

IL-2 Assay

Supernatants from antigen-presentation assays were serially diluted and added to 5×10^3 IL-2–dependent cytotoxic T cells. This IL-2–dependent cell line was a gift of Dr. Steven Gillis. Cultures were incubated for 24 hr and pulsed with tritiated thymidine during the final 6 hr of culture. The amount of IL-2 present was proportional to the amount of cellular proliferation.

RESULTS

The better to define and elucidate the cellular nature of the IL-2 defect, we studied the interaction between macrophages and T cells during the important activity of presenting antigen.

Not surprising, all murine strains possessing the *lpr* gene did not respond normally to antigen. A representative study using C57/*lpr* and its normal C57/B6 partner is shown in Table 1. The *lpr* mouse failed to respond, whereas the normal cogenic mouse gave a brisk response. To determine the cell responsible for this defect, normal antigen-presenting cells were mixed with *lpr* T cells, and vice versa. As can be seen in Table 1, the *lpr* spleen cells can present antigen to normal T cells.

Table 1. Antigen Presentation, TPN-KLH in C57B6/J and C57B6/1pr

Cells	Incorporation Tritiated Thymidine (Δcpm ± SEM)
Normal antigen presenting cells + normal T cells.	41,300 ± 4,322
1pr antigen presenting cells + 1pr T cells.	322 ± 165
Normal antigen presenting cells + 1pr T cells.	1,402 ± 629
1pr antigen presenting cells + normal T cells.	38,039 ± 4,147

Controls: Primed T cells, antigen presenting cells, unprimed T cells, or antigen presenting cell alone or in any combination gave <900 cpm.

However, *lpr* T cells are unable to respond to antigen when presented by normal spleen cells.

This finding held true for three strains possessing the *lpr* gene and demonstrates that the *lpr* macrophage can perform normally in this assay. These results imply that there is enough IL-1 produced by *lpr* macrophages to initiate a normal proliferative response.

To rule out the presence of suppressor cells, *lpr* T cells were mixed with an equal number of normal T cells, and only a dilutional effect was seen (Table 2). Likewise, adding supernatants from *lpr* cultures to antigen-presentation cultures of normal mice ruled out the presence of inhibitory factors.

$Lyt\text{-}1^+$ and $Lyt\text{-}2^+$ cells were removed by panning techniques using monoclonal antibodies. The results (Table 3) demonstrate that normal responding and proliferating T cells possess the $Lyt\text{-}1^+$ phenotype. Cells from *lpr* mice remained unresponsive, suggesting that the *lpr* defect in antigen presentation is

Table 2. Antigen Presentation TNP-KLH: Mixing 1pr and Normal T Cells

Cells	cpm
Normal antigen presenting cells + normal T cells.	36,422 ± 3,100
Normal antigen presenting cells + 1pr T cell.	425 ± 150
Normal antigen presenting cells + 50% 1pr T cells and 50% normal T cells.	15,878 ± 1,780

Table 3. Antigen Presentation, TNP-KLH by Isolated T Cells

Cells	cpm
Normal antigen presenting cell + normal Lyt 1$^+$ T cells.	25,144 ± 3,160
Normal antigen presenting cell + Lyt 2$^+$ T cells.	1,293 ± 386
Normal antigen presenting cells + 1pr Lyt 1$^+$ T cells.	800 ± 276
Normal antigen presenting cells + 1pr Lyt 2$^+$ T cells.	375 ± 150

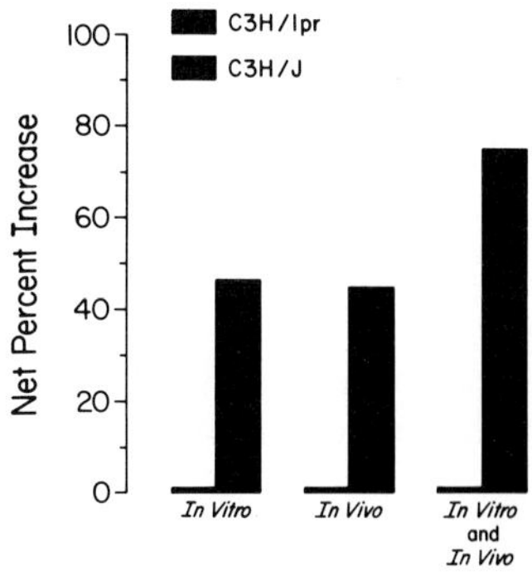

Fig. 1. Delectinated IL-2 was given daily at the base of the tail or added in vitro during antigen-presentation assay. The percentage increase above normal antigen-presentation assay values is given.

intrinsic to the Lyt-1$^+$ cell. In neither case did Lyt-2$^+$ cells respond.

Since IL-2 is necessary for T-cell proliferation, the generation of IL-2 during antigen presentation was studied. Normal T cells were able to produce IL-2, whereas *lpr* T cells could not (Table 4).

A pharmacologic attempt to simulate the defective *lpr* T cell was undertaken (Fig. 1). Purified IL-2 was added in vitro to the antigen-presentation cultures. Cells from normal mice increased their antigen-induced proliferation by 45%. The *lpr* cells did not change. IL-2 was given in vivo at the time of initial immunization, and daily therafter. Again in the normal mouse, antigen-induced proliferation increased by the same amount, 45%, but *lpr* mice remained unresponsive. Finally, IL-2 was administered both in vivo and in vitro. Normal mice increased by ~75%, but *lpr* mice could not be stimulated.

CsA was added in vitro to antigen-presentation cultures from normal mice to see whether this drug-induced IL-2–deficient state would mimic the *lpr* defect. Table 5 demonstrates abrogation of T-cell proliferation by CsA at a standard dose of 100 ng/ml. However, the addition of IL-2 restored T-cell proliferation, unlike the results obtained with the *lpr* mice. IL-2 added to control cultures of immune T cell and nonantigen-pulsed presenting cells gave only 1/3 the stimulation observed when IL-2 was added to CsA-treated cultures, demonstrating a requirement for antigen and ruling out a nonspecific augmentation by IL-2.

DISCUSSION

These studies have identified an important defect common to mice bearing the *lpr* gene. These mice possess T cells that are only weakly expressive of the Lyt-1$^+$23$^-$ phenotype[8] and are also incapable of normal proliferation when presented with antigen by H2-compatible macrophages. The mechanism responsible for this lack of normal activation is currently under study in our laboratory.

One important consequence of this failure of activation is the inability of these cells to

Table 4. IL-2 Production During Antigen Presentation*

Culture Supernatants	Dilutions			
	0	1:4	1:8	1:16
			(cpm)	
1pr	474 ± 41	394 ± 36	481 ± 50	449 ± 39
Normal	474 ± 41	7,846 ± 804	2,290 ± 266	1,144 ± 118
Control (no antigen)	474 ± 41	482 ± 45	134 ± 9	125 ± 18

*Assayed on IL-2 dependent cell line.

Table 5. Effect of Cyclosporine A on Antigen Presentation in Normal C57B6 Mice

Treatment in vitro	CPM
None*	20,144 ± 3,740
IL-2	75,435 ± 6,674
Cyclosporine A	746 ± 98
Cyclosporine A & IL-2	15,432 ± 1,870

Control: Mixtures of T cells and antigen presenting cells (with and without antigen pulse) gave <1000 cpm.

synthesize IL-2. However, the response to IL-2 is also defective in addition to the impaired production. Thus, at least two T-cell subpopulations are implicated (IL-2 producers as well as IL-2 responders), presumably the Lyt-$1^{+}23^{-}$ and Lyt-123^{+} subsets.

This inability to respond to IL-2 explains the relative ineffectiveness of IL-2 added in vivo or in vitro. Exogenous IL-2 is unable to augment the proliferative response to antigen.

At first glance, CsA appeared to mimic the action of the *lpr* gene. The presence of CsA prevented normal T cells from proliferating. However, the addition of purified IL-2 reversed this T-cell hyporesponsiveness, in contrast to the effect of exogenous IL-2 on *lpr* T cells.

This suggests that the primary action of CsA was to inhibit IL-2 production but not interfere with IL-2 response. One indication of normal T-cell priming and activation is the acquisition of IL-2 receptors,[30] which then allows a response to IL-2. This latter phase of the T-cell response can still occur in normal mice given CsA. This difference between CsA-treated normal mice and autoimmune *lpr* mice could be useful in working out both mechanisms of CsA action and the lesion in the autoimmune mice. Our results are compatible with an earlier report that CsA could not inhibit primed or memory T cells from responding to IL-2.[31] Successful antigen presentation requires the initial priming of T cells in vivo. This does not occur in *lpr* mice, as their T cells appear incapable of normal activation.

The defective production of IL-2 in patients with SLE and rheumatoid arthritis demonstrate that the animal model can provide information relevant to human disease. The diseases of immunologic dysregulation, which include SLE, may be susceptible to specific treatment with immunoregulatory molecules. Much progress has been made recently due to our understanding of the immunobiology of the interleukins and interferon. Hopefully, better definition of immunoregulatory abnormalities in animal models and patients will one day yield appropriate drugs or biologicals that can restore immune control in these diseases.

REFERENCES

1. Talal N: Autoimmunity: Genetic, Immunologic, Virologic, and Clinical Aspects. New York, Academic Press, 1977
2. Talal N: Arthritis Rheum 21:853, 1978
3. Steinberg AD, Huston DP, Taurog JD, et al: Immunol Rev 55:14, 1981
4. Theofilopoulos AN, Dixon FJ: Immunol Rev 55:179, 1981
5. McCoombs C, Hom J, Talal N, et al: J Immunol 115:1695, 1975
6. Andrews BS, Eisenberg RA, Theofilopoulos AN, et al: J Exp Med 148:1198, 1978
7. Murphy ED, Roths JB: In Genetic Control of Autoimmune Disease. Rose NR, Bigazzi PE, and Warner NL (eds): New York, Elsevier-North Holland, 1978, 207
8. Morse HC, Davidson WF, Yetter RA, et al: J Immunol 129:2612, 1982
9. Wofsy D, Murphy ED, Roths JB, et al: J Exp Med 154:1671, 1981
10. Dauphinee MJ, Kipper SB, Wofsy D, et al: J Immunol 127:2483, 1981
11. Watson J, Mochizuki D: Immunol Rev 51:257, 1980
12. Smith KA: Immunol Rev 51:337, 1980
13. Farrar JJ, Simon PL, Koopman WJ, et al: Immunology 121:1353, 1978
14. Stotter H, Rude E, Wagner H: Eur J Immunol 10:719, 1980
15. Gillis S, Smith KA: Nature 268:154, 1977
16. Rosenberg SA, Spiess PJ, Schwartz S: J Immunol 121:1946, 1978
17. Rosenberg SA, Schwartz S, Spiess PJ: J Immunol 121:1951, 1978
18. Ruscetti FA, Morgan DA, Gallo RC: J Immunol 119:131, 1977

19. Gillis S, Balcer PE, Ruscetti RW, et al: J Exp Med 148:1093, 1978

20. Shaw J, Monticone V, Mills G, et al: J Immunol 120:1974, 1978

21. Koopman WJ, Farrar JJ, Oppenheim JJ, et al: J Immunol 119:55, 1977

22. Draber P, Kisielow P: Eur J Immunol 11:1, 1981

23. Wagner H, Röllinghoff M: J Exp Med 148:1523, 1978

24. Larsson E, Coutinho A, Martinez C: Immunol Rev 51:61, 1980

25. Smith KA, Gillis S, Ruscetti FW, et al: Ann NY Acad Sci 332: p. no., 1979

26. Alcocer-Varela J, Alarcon-Segovia D: J Clin Invest 69:1388, 1982

27. Talal N, Dauphinee M, Christadoss P, et al: Adv in Nephrol (in press)

28. Britton S, Palacios R: Immunol Rev 65:5, 1982

29. Alkan S: Eur J Immunol 8:112, 1978

30. Oppenheim JJ, Gery J: Immunol Today 3:113, 1982

31. Bunges D, Hardt C, Röllinghoff M: Eur J Immunol 11:657, 1981

Response of Murine Autoimmune Disease to Cyclosporine and Thiols

M. G. Jones, G. Harris, and G. Cowing

NZB/W (F_1) HYBRID mice (NZB/W) develop a spontaneous immunoproliferative syndrome, multifactorial in origin and analogous to human systemic lupus erythematosus (SLE).[1] Female NZB/W mice are much shorter lived than males, owing to the earlier onset and more rapidly progressive glomerulonephritis. While this murine disease is under the control of multiple gene loci,[2] with environmental factors involved as triggering mechanisms, the etiology remains obscure, rendering any form of treatment difficult.

Preliminary studies showed that pyritinol, a thiol compound, and cyclosporine A (CsA), a selective immunosuppressive agent, significantly prolonged the life span of female NZB/W mice. We therefore compared the effects of pyritinol and CsA in these mice, examining various parameters to elucidate further the modes of action of these two compounds.

MATERIALS AND METHODS

NZB/W (F_1) hybrid mice reared at the Kennedy Institute were used. The mice were fed on a high-protein diet, P.M.D. (Labshore).

Pyritinol hydrochlorate (Pyrithioxine), dihydroxy 3,3′ dimethyl-2,2′-dithiodimethylene-5,5′-(Pyridyl-4-methanol) (E. Merck, Darmstadt) was dissolved in distilled water and immediately given daily by gavage to mice at a dose of 200 mg/kg^{-1}, five times a week, using a blunt-ended curved needle and syringe.

CsA (Dr. J. Borel, Sandoz, Basel) was dissolved in olive oil by stirring for 30 min and given immediately at 100 mg/kg^{-1} daily to mice in the same manner as pyritinol.

RESULTS

As shown in Fig. 1, oral administration of both pyritinol and CsA prolonged the life span of female NZB/W mice, although CsA appeared more effective.

Treatment had no adverse effect on the body weight of female NZB/W mice and did not prevent the typical progressive splenomegaly and hyperplasia of peripheral lymphoid tissue, indicated by increased mesenteric lymph node weights. Untreated mice developed thymic atrophy by the age of 10 months, the 50% mortality period. Untreated mice surviving beyond this time showed relatively good retention of thymic tissue. Treatment with CsA in particular resulted in some degree of preservation of thymic tissue, confirmed by histologic examination (Table 1).

Using the Cunningham chamber method to detect direct plaque-forming cells,[3] no significant difference was found in the response of female NZB/W mice (age < 30 weeks, 12 mice in each group) to sheep red blood cells between the untreated and pyritinol-treated NZB/W mice; however, there was a significant inhibition in the formation of plaque-forming cells in the CsA-treated mice when compared with untreated female NZB/W mice (Student's t test: $p < 0.001$; data not shown).

Hematology

Erythrocyte autoantibodies were present on the red cells of untreated and treated mice older than 40 weeks (Table 1). The development of antiglobulin positivity followed by anemia and reticulocytosis in the peripheral blood completed the typical picture of autoimmune hemolytic anemia in these mice. It can be seen that neither treatment influenced the development of this anemia.

From the Kennedy Institute of Rheumatology, Division of Experimental Pathology, Bute Gardens, London, England.

Supported by a grant from the Arthritis and Rheumatism Council, London.

Reprint requests should be addressed to Dr. M. G. Jones, Division of Experimental Pathology, Kennedy Institute of Rheumatology, Bute Gardens, London W6 7DW, England.

0041-1345/83/1505-0129$01.00/0

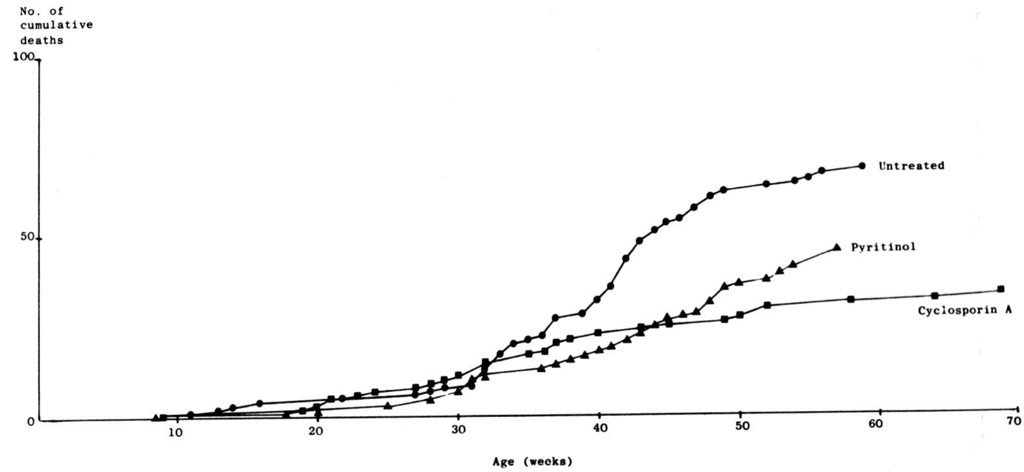

Fig. 1. **Cumulative deaths in 87 untreated, 78 pyritinol-treated, and 77 CsA-treated female NZB/W (F_1) hybrid mice.**

Total Ig Level

Serum IgM and IgG levels were determined using the radial immunodiffusion method[4] (rabbit anti-mouse IgM and IgG antiserum were obtained from Nordic). No difference was observed in the IgM levels of both untreated and treated mice, and, furthermore, the level of IgM did not change with age. In contrast, the IgG levels increased with age, but treatment of the mice did not have a significant effect on the IgG levels as compared with the untreated mice.

Anti-ds DNA Antibody

An enzyme-linked immunosorbent assay was used to detect IgG anti-ds DNA antibodies. There was a progressive increase with age in the level of anti-ds DNA antibody in both

Table 1. The Effect of Treatment on Body and Tissue Weights and on Blood Profile

Age (months)	Treatment	Body weight (g)	Thymus (mg)	Spleen (mg)	Mesenteric Lymph Node (mg)	Hemoglobin (g/dl)	Reticulocytes (%)	Antiglobulin (% positive)
4	Control	28.5 (0.9)*	61.3 (14.0)	89.0 (11.2)	89.5 (35.2)	13.0 (0.2)	1.3 (0.6)	NT
	Pyritinol	29.4 (1.7)	62.1 (9.8)	103.9 (20.5)	71.4 (14.7)	14.2 (1.4)	1.4 (0.8)	50
	CsA	31.3 (2.0)	69.3 (14.5)	112.5 (25.8)	84.4 (18.7)	13.8 (1.0)	2.0 (0.7)	90
6	Control	35.8 (4.4)	48.6 (18.1)	147.8 (55.6)	76.1 (42.4)	13.0 (1.7)	3.4 (3.0)	48
	Pyritinol	31.0 (2.6)	60.5 (17.3)	163.3 (76.3)	77.6 (18.0)	12.4 (2.0)	2.1 (1.1)	80
	CsA	33.6 (3.8)	80.3 (12.4)	179.8 (86.4)	108.0 (13.2)	12.2 (1.6)	1.4 (1.5)	59
7	Control	32.3 (5.2)	39.6 (13.8)	188.7 (50.9)	73.7 (33.5)	12.6 (1.9)	4.5 (9.7)	100
	Pyritinol	31.7 (4.4)	54.7 (12.0)	138.6 (51.1)	66.3 (31.7)	13.5 (1.3)	2.0 (1.1)	80
	CsA	34.4 (3.0)	55.8 (12.8)	174.9 (51.3)	81.7 (19.5)	13.4 (1.1)	2.7 (1.5)	55
8	Control	33.2 (0.6)	13.5 (19.0)	253.0	46.0 (25.0)	10.3 (2.3)	5.6 (4.7)	91
	Pyritinol	30.8 (1.3)	35.0 (8.5)	169.0 (38.4)	97.3 (23.2)	12.5 (1.1)	4.2 (4.8)	81
	CsA	NT	NT	NT	NT	11.7 (1.6)	3.0 (2.4)	86
9	Control	34.4	30.0	308.0	85.0	10.6 (1.8)	8.3 (7.1)	100
	Pyritinol	29.0 (1.4)	36.0 (8.6)	115.0	48.3 (7.8)	13.9 (0.9)	8.6 (7.1)	100
	CsA	33.6 (1.9)	52.6 (17.8)	390.0	82.0 (17.6)	12.3 (1.7)	3.6 (2.9)	82
10	Control	34.0 (3.3)	35.6 (38.0)	323.5 (88.5)	79.8 (45.9)	8.3 (7.1)	28.6 (23.0)	100
	Pyritinol	33.7 (3.9)	52.8 (26.5)	347.0 (116.0)	91.6 (35.2)	8.6 (7.1)	4.2 (1.5)	83
	CsA	35.9 (2.9)	41.9 (20.6)	410.1 (119.4)	105.6 (59.4)	3.6 (2.9)	13.3 (7.2)	100
11	Control	34.7 (1.5)	53.2 (31.5)	499.5 (152.1)	112.0 (27.7)	11.1 (1.3)	8.2 (5.6)	100
	Pyritinol	32.0 (0.3)	48.0 (3.6)	282.0 (84.4)	116.0 (39.9)	NT	NT	NT
	CsA	34.0 (1.0)	62.0 (9.9)	415.0 (172.4)	120.4 (29.7)	11.3 (1.1)	2.9 (0.3)	100

*Number in parentheses represents the standard deviation.

NT = Not tested.

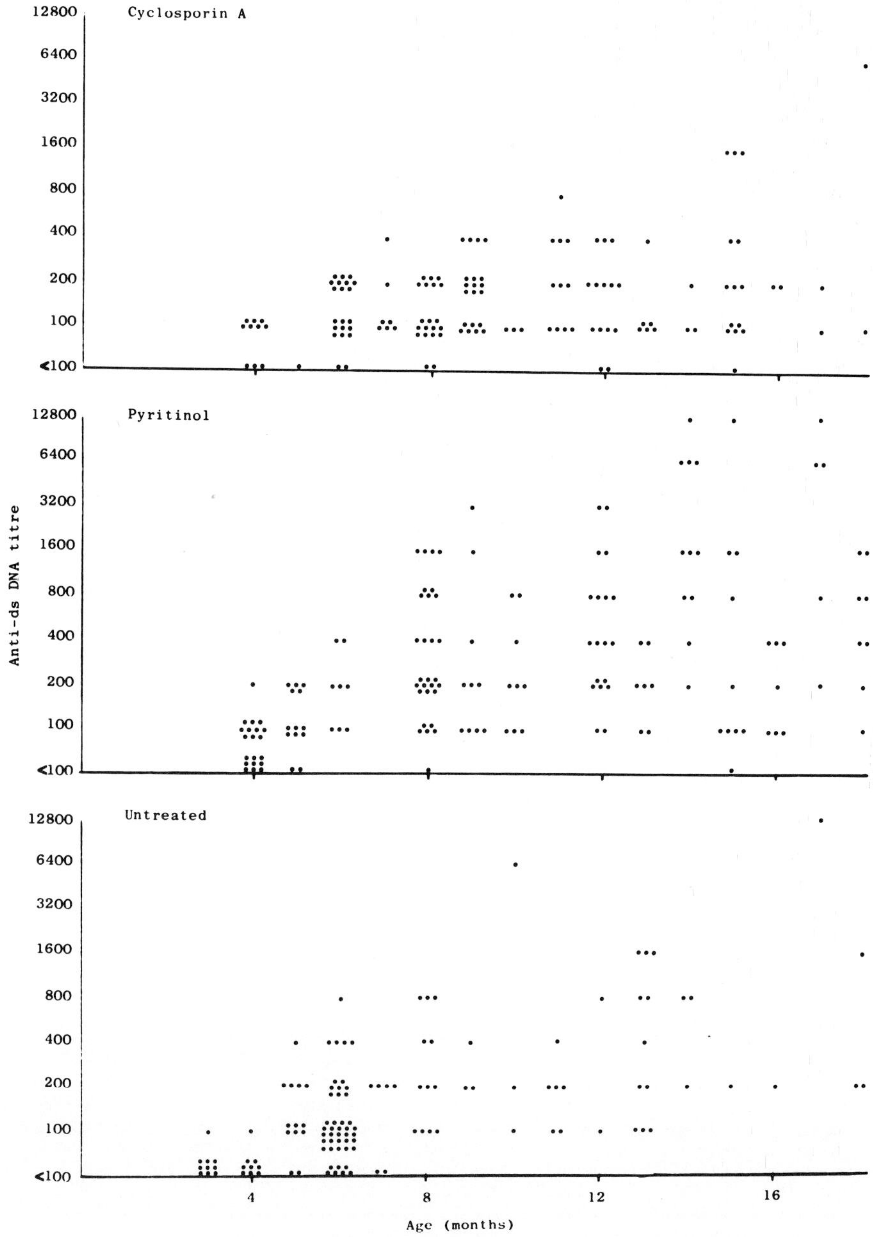

Fig. 2. Levels of anti-ds DNA antibody in treated and untreated female NZB/W (F_1) hybrid mice.

untreated and treated mice (Fig. 2). Pyritinol treatment might have actually stimulated increased levels of this antibody as compared with untreated mice. Comparisons in older animals must be cautious due to the high mortality rate in the controls. CsA treatment did, however, result in reduced levels of anti-ds DNA as compared to both the control and pyritinol-treated animals, although there was still a progressive increase with age in the CsA-treated group.

Histologic Studies of the Kidney

The perivascular infiltration with lymphoid and plasma cells so typical of murine immunoproliferative disease was similar in the kidneys, lungs, and livers from both treated and untreated mice. Treatment, however, protected the glomeruli, but immunofluorescence showed a heavy deposition of IgM, IgG, and C_3 in the glomeruli, indicating similar immune-complex deposition in both untreated and treated mice.

DISCUSSION

Previous findings that daily treatment of female NZB/W mice with pyritinol extended their longevity[5] have been confirmed, and CsA had similar efficacy. The most prominent feature of this study was that treatment prevented glomerular damage and renal failure, the main cause of death in the NZB/W mouse. Protection of the kidneys occurred despite the same degree of cellular infiltration and immunoglobulin and complement deposition in the glomeruli.

In contrast to pyritinol, CsA treatment reduced the response of NZB/W mice to T-dependent sheep red cells, and the level of anti-ds DNA autoantibody, considered to be an important disease marker, was also reduced.

CsA is an immunosuppressant that has a highly selective action on lymphocytes; in noncytotoxic doses, it leaves other nucleated cells relatively intact. It has been found to decrease antibody production to T cell–dependent antigens, prolong allograft survival, inhibit cytotoxic activity generated in the allogeneic mixed lymphocyte reaction, and abrogate concanavalin A–induced suppressor T cells.[6] CsA may act by blocking early processes in responding T cells. Proliferation of T cells in culture is maintained by interleukin 2 (IL-2), but CsA inhibits the expression of IL-2 receptors.[7]

The mode of action of pyritinol remains debatable, although it seems likely to differ from that of CsA. D-penicillamine is an effective agent in the treatment of rheumatoid arthritis.[8] In vitro studies have found D-penicillamine to depress[9] and stimulate lymphocyte function.[10,11] The most likely mode of action of pyritinol may be related to its possible action as a free radical scavenger, thus maintaining the stability of lysosomal and other cell membranes.[12] Evidence for cellular damage in autoimmune disease by free radicals was suggested by the finding of clastogenic factors[13] (CF)—chromosome breaking agents—in the serum of patients with rheumatoid arthritis and in NZB mice, where chromosomal damage is a feature. Thus, protection from damage mediated by endogenous free radicals might explain the mode of action of pyritinol in NZB/W mice. CsA is known to act at the T-cell level and may directly inhibit a T cell–mediated response directed on the kidney, or it may block the T-helper activity and thus indirectly affect the humoral immune response. The thymus may also be another level at which CsA has its effect. It is also conceivable that CsA acts like pyritinol as a free radical scavenger.

This study is now currently investigating other parameters, to elucidate the mode of action of pyritinol and CsA, and also in the hope of furthering our understanding of this autoimmune strain of mice.

REFERENCES

1. Dixon FJ, Theofilopoulos AN, Izui S, et al: In Fougereau M, Dausset J (eds): Progress in Immunology (4th ed). New York, Academic Press, 1980, pp 959–995

2. Knight JG, Adams DD, Purves HD: Clin Exp Immunol 28:352, 1977

3. Cunningham AJ, Smith JB, Mercer EH: J Exp Med 124:701, 1966

4. Mancini G, Carbonara AO, Heremans JF: Immunochemistry 2:235, 1965

5. Harris G, Chandler P: In Maini RN, Berry H (eds): Modulation of Autoimmunity and Disease: The Penicillamine Experience. New York, Praeger, 1981, pp 122–133

6. Morris PJ: Transplantation 32:349, 1981

7. Palacios R, Möller G: Nature 290:792, 1981

8. Report on the European Multicentre Trial: Lancet 1:275, 1973

9. Lipsky PE: In Maini RN, Berry H (eds): Modulation of Autoimmunity and Disease: The Penicillamine Experience. New York, Praeger, 1981, pp 79–88

10. Harris G, Hutchins D: In Turk JL, Parker D (eds):

Drugs and Immune Responsiveness. London and Basingstoke, Macmillan, 1979, pp 41–61

11. Toohey JI: Proc Natl Acad Sci USA 72:73, 1975

12. Munthe E, Kåss E, Jellum E: In Maini RN, Berry H (eds): Modulation of Autoimmunity and Disease: The Penicillamine Experience. New York, Praeger, 1981, pp 134–142

13. Emerit I: In Natarajan et al (eds): Progress in Mutation Research (vol 4). New York, Elsevier Biomedical, 1982

The Effect of Cyclosporine on Lymphocyte Subsets in Experimental Allergic Encephalomyelitis: Functional Loss of Disease-Suppressing Cells In Vivo

L. M. Fredane, G. A. Hashim, and R. E. McCabe

EXPERIMENTAL allergic encephalomyelitis (EAE) is a T cell–mediated, demyelinating autoimmune disease of the central nervous system (CNS).[1] It can be induced in a number of species by immunization using the appropriate CNS antigen. Myelin basic protein (MBP) is a native protein of CNS myelin which is extracted and used to induce EAE. For each of the species thus far examined, there is a species-specific sequence within MBP that is capable of inducing disease such that any enzymatic digest peptides containing this encephalitogenic determinant are also able to induce EAE.[2] The sequence for the guinea pig[3] is: H-Phe-Ser-Trp-Gly-Ala-Glu-Gly-Gln-Lys-OH. S3, a synthetic peptide that consists of this sequence coupled to a glycine, can itself induce EAE.[4] By deleting the four central amino acids (Gly-Ala-Glu-Gly) of the encephalitogenic determinant, tetramerizing the remaining sequence to increase its biological half-life, and synthesizing this new peptide coupled to glycine, S42, is created:[5] H-(Phe-Ser-Trp-Gln-Lys)4-Gly-OH, which is not encephalitogenic, is cross-reactive with MBP and encephalitogenic sequence-containing peptides in delayed-type hypersensitivity (DTH) reactions,[5] and, when used as the primary immunogen in guinea pigs, suppresses clinical disease induction upon later immunization with MBP.[6] Lymph node cells from protected donors can be used to passively transfer the ability to suppress disease induction.[6]

Using this unique inducer-antigen, suppressor-antigen system, we examined the in vivo effect of cyclosporine A (CsA) on lymphocyte subsets responsible for disease induction, disease suppression, and DTH reactions to MBP and S42.

MATERIALS AND METHODS

MBP was isolated from bovine spinal cord,[7] and S42 was synthesized by the Merrifield solid-phase method, as previously described.[5] Immunizations were made by hind footpad injection of 100 μg antigen in 0.05 ml saline emulsified with 50 μg *M. butyricum* in 0.05 ml of complete Freund's adjuvant (CFA). CsA was dissolved in corn oil (40 mg/kg) and given i.p. at a dose of 17 mg/kg/day.

Male Hartley guinea pigs weighing 400–500 g were divided into six groups: group 1 (disease control) received MBP alone on day 0; group 2 received MBP on day 0 and CsA on days 0–4; group 3 received MBP on day 0 and CsA on days 8–17; group 4 (suppression control) received S42 on day 0 and MBP on day 60; group 5 received S42 on day 0, CsA on days 0–4, and MBP on day 60; group 6 received S42 on day 0, CsA on day 15, and MBP on day 60. The animals were observed and weighed daily. DTH testing was performed on all groups on day 5, 9, 12, 16, and 19 by injecting 0.1 ml of saline containing 15 μg of the appropriate antigen intradermally on the animal's shaven flank. At 24 and 48 hr, the erythema at the site was measured at its maximum diameter and at right angles to that diameter. Animals either died, were sacrificed at the end of the experiment (day 25 after MBP challenge), or were sacrificed when they became premortal. Brains and spinal cords were removed for histology.

RESULTS

DTH

The results (Figs. 1 and 2) for the disease control and the suppression control groups

---

From the Jane Forbes Clark Surgical Research Laboratories, St. Luke's–Roosevelt Hospital Center, and the Department of Microbiology, Columbia University, New York, NY.

L. M. F. is a Postdoctoral Fellow of the National Multiple Sclerosis Society in the Department of Pathology (Immunology), Yale University School of Medicine.

Reprint requests should be addressed to Dr. George A. Hashim, Jane Forbes Clark Surgical Research Laboratories (S&R 10), St. Luke's–Roosevelt Hospital Center, Amsterdam Avenue at 114th Street, New York, NY 10025.

0041–1345/83/1505–0130$01.00/0

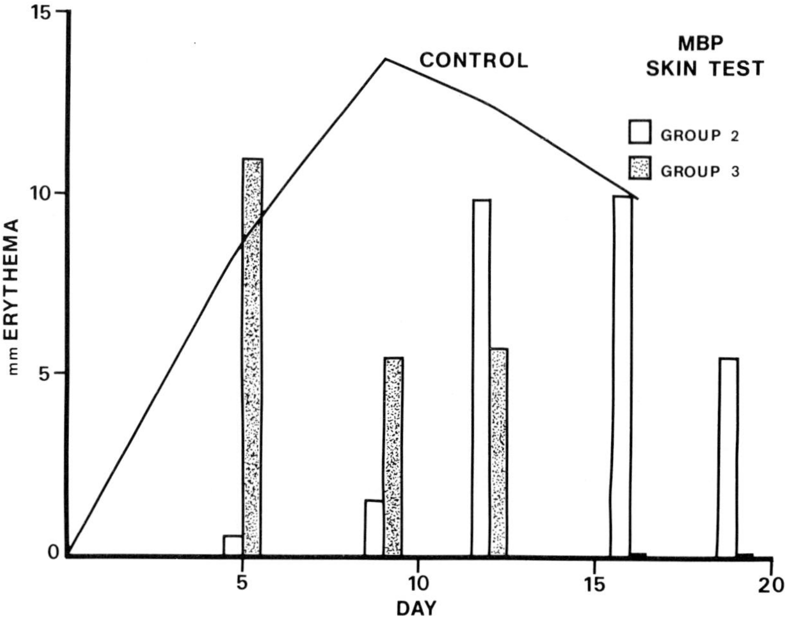

Fig. 1. Mean DTH skin-test response to MBP for Groups 2 and 3 compared with control (Group 1).

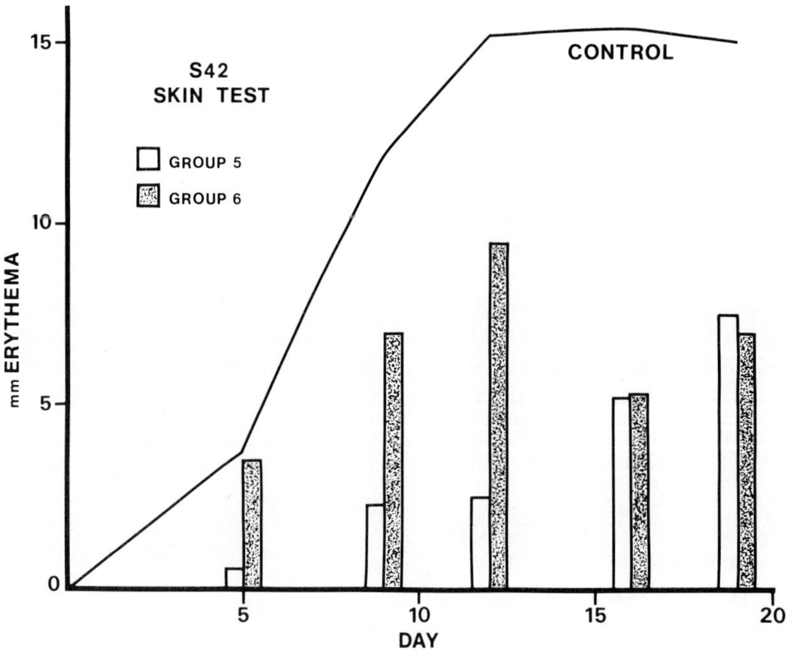

Fig. 2. Mean DTH skin-test response to S42 for Groups 5 and 6 compared with control (Group 4).

(Groups 1 and 4, respectively) are the same as they have been since DTH was first compared between the two.[5,8] Animals immunized with MBP alone reached a peak DTH response around day 10 that declined with the onset of disease, while those immunized with S42 only also reached a peak response around day 10 that remained plateaued (for > 90 days; unpublished data). Group 2 did not achieve any significant level of response until a week after the CsA is stopped, and it too declined as the animals became sick. Group 3, which appeared to have the same initial development of DTH as the control, had a significant but incomplete suppression of DTH by CsA when it was first given and required several days before DTH was completely suppressed. As with group 2, group 5, which also received CsA on days 0–4, had delayed onset and slower development of its DTH response. The animals in group 6 had a significant but incomplete suppression of DTH after a single dose of CsA on day 15, which appeared to be recovering by day 19.

Survival

As with the DTH results, the survival of the two control groups (Table 1) is consistent with previous experiments.[6] Disease control animals (group 1) all succumbed to disease by day 17 (mean survival, 15.5 days), while suppression control animals (group 4) all survived to day 25 of the experiment. In fact S42-immunized and MBP-challenged guinea pigs failed to develop any signs of disease, even when observed for extended periods of time (unpublished data). Both group 2 and group 3 animals had prolonged survival to a mean of 21 days, all of the group 2 animals developing clinical EAE. However, of the three group 3 animals that died during the course of the experiment, none showed any signs of clinical disease despite being histologically positive. Comparing the two groups histologically, group 2 is 3–4+ (on a scale of 0–4+), while group 3 is only 1+, the one surviving member of that group being histologically negative. In group 5, one animal did develop EAE, but the others remained healthy, gained weight, and survived without clinical disease to the end of the experiment. In group 6, 3/4 animals developed EAE and either died or were sacrificed before the end of the experiment, giving a mean survival of 17.5 days.

DISCUSSION

In his early work with CsA, Borel showed that its immunosuppressive effect was T cell–specific, reversible,[9] and protective of EAE.[10] Others demonstrated in histocompatibility antigen systems that its T-cell specificity went so far as to spare suppressor cells,[11] even allowing their specific induction.[12] It was our goal to examine in a nonhistocompatibility antigen system (EAE) the effect of CsA on the induction and function of antigen-specific disease-inducing and disease-suppressing T cells while monitoring its effect on DTH responses to the particular antigens. Most of our results are in agreement with previous reports about CsA in EAE;[13,14] others are new and require further evaluation.

CsA delayed the induction of DTH in the

Table 1. Survival Data for Individuals and Means of Groups

Group	Treatment	Survival (days)*	Mean
1	MBP only (disease control)	12, 16, 17, 17	15.5
2	MBP, CsA days 0–4	19, 19, 21, 25	21.0
3	MBP, CsA days 8–17	19,† 20,† 20,† > 25	21.0
4	S42, MBP, no CsA (suppression control)	> 25, > 25, > 25, > 25	> 25.0
5	S42, CsA days 0–4, MBP	19, > 25, > 25, > 25	> 23.5
6	S42, CsA day 15, MBP	13, 13, 19, > 25	17.5

*Following MBP challenge.

†Sudden death without signs of disease.

two groups in which it was given during the induction period (days 0–4), but induction did eventually take place (probably due to the continued presence of antigen at the injection site or within macrophages). In animals with developed DTH responses, at this dose level a single injection could only inhibit DTH partially and was readily reversed, while continued administration for a period of several days was necessary to completely inhibit DTH. The induction of disease-inducing cells was only delayed by approximately the period of time during which the CsA was given; the EAE produced was the same as the control except for the time interval from immunization to termination. Although one of the guinea pigs in group 5 escaped protection, CsA also had little long-term effect on the induction of disease-suppressing cells. Those animals treated during the disease period (days 8–17) were protected from disease while they received the drug, but at its cessation, with the reversal of its effect, they died suddenly without clinical signs of disease. The most devastating effect of CsA appears to have been on developed or developing disease-suppressing cells, where in 3/4 of the animals their protected state was abolished despite the fact that they received only one dose of CsA, which only partially inhibited DTH and seemed to have been reversed.

The development of cellular immunity in vivo is a complex, dynamic process involving many lymphocyte subsets in a host of interactions. The findings of Ortiz-Ortiz and Weigle[15] that the cellular events required for the development of EAE are IL-2–dependent and those of Larsson[16] that CsA inhibits the acquisition of IL-2 responsiveness when taken together leave little room for surprise at the powerful effect CsA has on all subsets in our model. Any subset of T cells that must pass through a stage that requires IL-2 for its manifestation in vivo will be affected by CsA if it is given at a time before it has acquired its IL-2 receptors. Therefore, it would appear that it is the timing of the CsA that is important to its overall effect and not the nature of the subsets involved. This issue of timing of CsA has been clearly demonstrated with regard to the passive transfer of EAE.[14]

What remains disturbing is that not all cells affected by CsA were affected reversibly, that despite recovery of the DTH response, our putative suppressor cell was functionally deleted after it had been induced and developed (group 6). Perhaps this mechanism of functional deletion was also responsible for the sudden death of those animals treated during the disease period (group 3). With the functional loss of those disease-suppressing cells induced by MBP itself and the reversal of the CsA effect on the disease-inducing cells, these effector cells would be allowed to act unopposed and could under such conditions produce a hyperacute disease without concomitant clinical signs.

Although EAE is the animal model for multiple sclerosis (MS), the implications of this study go beyond EAE and MS. All autoimmune diseases, whether experimental or natural, are dynamic in the nature of their cellular events, and without certainty in the timing, CsA therapy could have undesirable effects, especially upon cessation of therapy. Without more effective methods for immunologic monitoring of autoimmune diseases, patients placed on CsA may be forced to remain on it for life for fear of the consequences of its withdrawal. Further studies are necessary in this and other animal models of autoimmune disease before patient treatment should be undertaken with CsA for those diseases thought to be of autoimmune origin.

REFERENCES

1. Paterson PY: In Talal N (ed): Autoimmunity. New York, Academic Press, 1977, p 643

2. Hashim GA: Immunol Rev 39:60, 1978

3. Eylar EH, Hashim GA: PNAS 61:644, 1968

4. Hashim GA, Hwang F, Schilling, FJ: Arch Biochem Biophys 156:298, 1973

5. Hashim GA, Sharpe RD, Carvalho EF, et al: J Immunol 116:126, 1976

6. Hashim GA: J Immunol 126:419, 1981

7. Eylar EH, Salk J, Beveridge GC, et al: Arch Biochem Biophys 132:34, 1969

8. Lee DH, Hashim GA, Pierce JC: Neurochem Res 2:293, 1977

9. Borel JF, Feuer C, Magnee C, et al: Immunology 32:1017, 1977

10. Borel JF, Feuer C, Gubler HU, et al: Agents and Actions 6:468, 1976

11. Leapman SB, Filo RS, Smith EJ, et al: Transplantation 30:404, 1980

12. Hess AD, Tutschka PJ: J Immunol 124:2601, 1980

13. Bolton C, Allsopp G, Cuzner ML: Clin Exp Immunol 47:127, 1982

14. Hinrichs DJ, Wegman KW, Peters BA: Cell Immunol 77:202, 1983

15. Ortiz-Ortiz L, Weigle WO: J Immunol 128:154, 1982

16. Larsson EL: J Immunol 124:2828, 1980

Cyclosporine Therapy in the Treatment of Uveitis

R. B. Nussenblatt, A. G. Palestine, C. C. Chan, W. C. Leake, A. H. Rook, I. Scher, and I. Gery

UVEITIS IS A TERM used to denote any intraocular inflammatory disease, whether caused by exogenous "infectious" or putative autoimmune factors and whether the primary site of ocular inflammation is in the uvea or not. Ten percent of visual handicap in the United States is due to this disease,[1] and less severe ocular inflammatory disease is very commonly seen by the ophthalmologist, frequently secondary to other factors, such as ocular surgery. Systemic corticosteroids have been the mainstay in the treatment of severe endogenous uveitis since their use by Gordon in 1952, with cytotoxic agents the only recourse if steroids are not tolerated or ineffective.[2]

The large number of uveitic syndromes are generally classified as to their clinical appearance. The discovery and purification of the retinal S antigen by Wacker and co-workers[3] and Faure and colleagues[4] provided investigators with a highly uveitogenic ocular antigen that could be utilized in vitro in order to identify those patients with retinal autoimmunity as a possible component to their disease. Further, experimental autoimmune uveitis induced by the S antigen is a dependable animal model for human uveitis,[5] and we have reported that a subgroup of uveitis patients, with clinical evidence of retinal disease, have in vitro cell-mediated responses to this material.[5,6]

The remarkably effective prevention of experimental autoimmune uveitis by cyclosporine (CsA)[7,8] led to a pilot study in which patients with posterior uveitis were treated with CsA. We report here our experience with CsA in a group of uveitis patients and the successful outcome of this therapeutic approach.

MATERIALS AND METHODS

Sixteen adults with bilateral sight-threatening ocular inflammatory disease of noninfectious etiology were evaluated. The diagnoses of these patients included Behcet's disease, idiopathic vitritis, pars planitis, birdshot retinochoroidopathy, ocular sarcoidosis, sympathetic ophthalmia, and Vogt-Koyanagi-Harada's syndrome. These patients had had an unsuccessful therapeutic trial with either systemic corticosteroids or cytotoxic agents, or side effects rendered continued use intolerable. All patients had active intraocular inflammatory disease when therapy began, and their ocular inflammatory disease was graded. Patients were evaluated for evidence of hepatic or renal disease before the commencement of therapy. This included 24-hr urine collections with the calculation of creatinine clearance.

Baseline natural killer cell (NKC) assays were performed on six patients as detailed elsewhere.[9] In vitro lymphocyte responses to the retinal S antigen and circulating T-cell subgroups were also determined on all patients before the initiation of cyclosporine therapy as described in detail elsewhere.[6]

Patients were treated with 10 mg/kg/day of the oral preparation of cyclosporine. No other immunosuppressive medication was given systemically, but three patients used steroid drops.

RESULTS

The 16 patients treated with CsA ranged in age from 20–67 years. Of these, 8 were previously treated with systemic corticosteroids and 8 with a combination of systemic corticosteroids and cytotoxic agents (chlorambucil or methotrexate). Patient follow-up on CsA was on the average 6.4 months (range 2–16 months).

Clinical Response

Fifteen of the 16 patients treated with CsA had a positive therapeutic response as measured by an improvement in visual acuity accompanied by a diminution in ocular

From the Clinical Branch and Laboratory for Vision Research, National Eye Institute, National Institutes of Health; Division of Virology, Office of Biologics, National Center for Drugs and Biologics; Naval Medical Research Institute, Bethesda, MD.

Reprint requests should be addressed to Dr. Robert B. Nussenblatt, Clinical Ophthalmic Immunology Section, National Eye Institute, National Institutes of Health, Bldg. 10, Rm. 10 D 19, Bethesda, MD 20205.

0041-1345/83/1505-0131$01.00/0

inflammatory activity. An increase in visual acuity and diminution of the anterior-segment inflammation could be noted rapidly in the majority of patients treated, while vitreal haze and debris were slower to dissipate.

The nonocular manifestations of Behcet's disease appeared to respond particularly well to CsA therapy. One patient with severe mouth ulcers noted disappearance of the ulcers within 1 week. Additionally, the patient with Vogt-Kayanagi-Harada's syndrome noted a dramatic improvement in her hearing once on the medication.

Natural Killer Cell Activity

Natural killer cell activity was determined in six patients prior to the initiation of CsA therapy. All had normal levels of activity when compared to control levels. CsA therapy did not lower natural killer cell responses in these patients (Fig. 1).

Circulating Lymphocyte Subsets

The total number of circulating T cells did not change in a statistically different fashion with CsA administration when compared to controls. Patients, however, did demonstrate changes in their OKT4/OKT8 ratios. One group demonstrated an increase in their OKT8 fraction and therefore a drop in the OKT4/OKT8 ratio by 10 days after CsA therapy. The second demonstrated an ultimate drop in their OKT4/OKT8 fraction, but this was seen only after several weeks on CsA therapy. It should be noted that the one patient that was not a therapeutic success demonstrated a late change in his OKT4/OKT8 ratio, which returned to the pre-CsA level during an exacerbation.

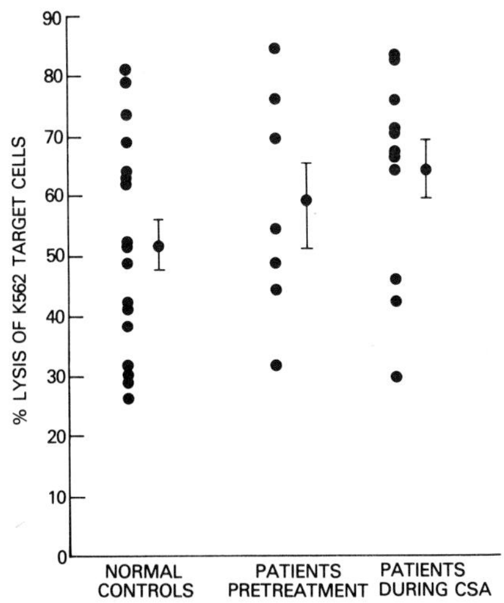

Fig. 1. Natural killer cell activity of uveitis patients before and after cyclosporine therapy, as compared to normal controls.

S-Antigen Responses

Twelve of the 16 patients treated with CsA demonstrated in vitro cell-mediated responses to the retinal S antigen. All of these individuals have to date had a positive therapeutic response to CsA. Three of the remaining 4 patients also demonstrated a good response to the medication.

CsA Toxicity

Three of the 16 patients have been noted to develop an increase in serum creatinine with a concomitant drop in creatinine clearance while on CsA therapy. Elevated serum creatinines as high as 2.3 mg/dl were seen at CsA dosages of 10 mg/kg/day. A return to a serum creatinine within normal limits could be effected by dropping the CsA level to 3–6 mg/kg/day. This dosage to date has been sufficient to control the patients' ocular inflammatory disease. In addition, minimal elevations of liver function tests, particularly the SGOT and SGPT, have been noted but have not posed any problem to date. A slight increase in the alkaline phosphatase has also been seen. An increase in the ESR has been consistently noted in the patients we have treated with CsA. Patients with clinically inactive disease have been noted to have a two- and threefold increase in their ESR. None of the patients treated has manifested lymphomatous alterations or tumors of the gastrointestinal tract.

DISCUSSION

The etiology of a large proportion of intraocular inflammatory syndromes would appear to be autoimmune. The successful prevention of S antigen–induced uveitis demonstrated the mandatory role of the T cell in this animal model that has human relevance.[5] CsA's effective control of intraocular inflammatory disease in humans further supports the important and probable mandatory role of the T cell.

The effects of any immunosuppressive agent on the immune system demands special attention. Natural killer cell alterations ascribed to CsA have been reported.[10] We found that our patients had normal natural killer cell activity prior to CsA initiation, and these levels remain within the normal range on therapy. Further, no increased incidence of infection was noted in this unique group of patients receiving this medication. However, basic clinical tests such as the ESR are altered and cannot be utilized to follow the activity of the inflammatory disease. It is because of this that other parameters must be developed. It may be that screening for changes in T-cell subsets or prior evidence of immune reactivity to a retinal antigen may be helpful.

SUMMARY

Severe intraocular inflammatory disease is an important cause of visual handicap in the United States.[1] Until now, the usual therapeutic approach has been systemic corticosteroids or cytotoxic agents, with the resultant side effects. Cyclosporine would appear to show promise as a possible alternative to these systemic medications in selected cases of severe noninfectious bilateral intraocular inflammatory disease.

REFERENCES

1. U.S. DHEW: DHS, NIH: Interim Report of the National Advisory Eye Council, Support for Vision Research. Washington, DC, U.S. Govt. Printing Office, 1976, pp 20–22

2. Nussenblatt RB: In Lichtenstein LM, Fauci AS (eds): Current Therapy in Allergy and Immunology 1983–1984. Philadelphia, Decker, 1983, pp 224–227

3. Wacker WB, Donoso LA: Invest Ophthalmol Vis Sci (Suppl) 94, 1975

4. Faure JP, de Kozak Y, Dorey C, et al: Invest Ophthalmol Vis Sci (Suppl) 94, 1975

5. Nussenblatt RB, Gery I, Kuwabara T, et al: In Helmsen RJ, Suran AA, Gery I, et al (eds): Immunology of the Eye Workshop II (A special supplement to Immunol Abst). Bethesda, MD, 1981, pp 49–66

6. Nussenblatt RB, Mittal KK, Ryan S, et al: Am J Ophthalmol 94:147, 1982

7. Nussenblatt RB, Rodrigues MM, Wacker WB, et al: J Clin Invest 67:1228, 1981

8. Nussenblatt RB, Salinas-Carmona M, Waksman BH, et al: Int Archs Allergy Appl Immunol 70:289, 1983

9. Quinnan GV Jr, Kirmani N, Rook AH, et al: N Engl. J Med 307:7, 1982

10. Ho M, Hardy AM, Gui XE, et al: 22nd Interscience Conference on Antimicrobial Agents and Chemotherapy: 124 (abst), 1982

The Effects of Cyclosporine on Viruses

X. E. Gui, R. W. Atchison, and M. Ho

THE FUNGAL METABOLITE cyclosporine (CsA) is a hydrophobic, cyclic polypeptide consisting of 11 amino acids with a molecular weight of 1203. It is insoluble in water but soluble in olive oil or alcohol. The compound is a potent immunosuppressant that has a selective action against T lymphocytes, particularly those involved in allograft rejection.[1,2] CsA is more effective than other conventional immunosuppressive agents in maintaining a heterotransplant.[3]

Surprisingly, we found that CsA at a dose of 100 mg/kg inhibited replication of murine cytomegalovirus in the lung, liver, and spleen of mice infected intraperitoneally.[4] This finding led to the present study to determine the effect of CsA on the replication of a number of viruses.

MATERIALS AND METHODS

Cell Cultures

The mouse embryo cell cultures (MECC) were prepared from the embryos of pregnant ICR mice and grown in medium 199 supplemented with 10% or 5% heat-inactivated newborn calf serum and antibiotic as previously described.[4] The Vero line of continuous African green monkey kidney cells was cultured in Eagle's minimum essential medium supplemented with newborn calf serum, antibiotics, and $NaHCO_3$ (MEM).

Human foreskin cells, originated from primary tissue obtained from Magee-Women's Hospital, Pittsburgh, PA. Passage 9 to 30 was grown in MEM.

Viruses

The Indiana strain of vesicular stomatitis virus (VSV) was grown by infecting monolayers of chick embryo cells in MEM supplemented with 10% newborn gammaglobulin-free bovine serum and stored at −70°C. The titer of the pool of virus used for these studies assayed by plaque titrations on Vero cells was 2.7×10^8 PFU/ml.

The Smith strain of murine cytomegalovirus (MCMV) was obtained from J. Osborn, University of Wisconsin, Madison, WI. Virus stocks were prepared from the salivary glands of ICR mice 3 weeks after infection and titered 2.5×10^7 PFU/ml on mouse embryo cell cultures.

The wild strain of poliovirus type 2 used in this study was originally obtained from W. M. Hammon of this department. The virus was grown in rhesus monkey kidney cell culture and titered 4×10^7 PFU/ml by plaque titration on Vero cells.

Cyclosporine

CsA, manufactured by Sandoz Inc. (East Hanover, NJ), was a gift from Dr. T. E. Starzl. CsA, 98 mg, was dissolved in 3.5 ml 95% ethanol and 1.4 ml Tween-80. Physiologic saline was added to a total volume of 49 ml, giving a final concentration of CsA of 2 mg/ml. It was refrigerated at 4°C, in darkness, and was used within 2 weeks of preparation.

Virus Titrations and the Effect of CsA

In general, the effect of CsA was tested two ways: preinfection treatment of cells and postinfection treatment of cells. For "preinfection treatment," cell cultures were overlaid with medium containing various dilutions of CsA for 24 hr before infection with virus. The drug was then washed off, virus was serially diluted, and 0.1 ml of each dilution was inoculated onto duplicate wells and adsorbed for 1 hr (VSV, poliovirus) or 1.5 hr (MCMV) at 37°C under 5% CO_2. Then 1 ml of medium was added to each well. For "postinfection treatment" with CsA, 1 ml of medium containing different concentrations of CsA was added to wells after the virus had been adsorbed. Cultures overlaid with medium without CsA, and with the diluent used to prepare CsA, served as controls. Supernatant fluids were collected 24 hr after infection with VSV and poliovirus and 5 days after infection with MCMV. To measure intracellular virus, the infected cell sheets were detached at proper times with a rubber policeman and washed two times with 5 ml of medium. The cells were resuspended in 2 ml of medium and sonicated for 5 min (Sonic Oscillator, Raytheon Manufacturing Co., Waltham, MA) before titration. The virus titers from supernatants with infected cell sheets after sonification represented the total virus.

For titration of VSV, 0.1 ml of serial 10-fold dilutions was inoculated onto duplicate wells of Vero cells in 12-well plates. One hr after inoculation, 1.5 ml of 1%

From the Department of Infectious Diseases and Microbiology, Graduate School of Public Health and Department of Medicine, School of Medicine, University of Pittsburgh, Pittsburgh, PA.

Supported in part by NIH Grant 1 RO1 AI 19377.

Reprint requests should be addressed to Dr. Monto Ho, Crabtree Hall A427, University of Pittsburgh, Pittsburgh, PA 15261.

0041–1345/83/1505–0132$01.00/0

methyl cellulose overlay medium was added to each well, and cultures were incubated for 2 days. The cell sheets were stained with gentian violet for plaque counting. For poliovirus titration, a similar procedure was followed, except 0.2 ml was used for inoculating each well of a 6-well culture of Vero cells, and 2 ml of 1% methyl cellulose overlay medium was used. For MCMV titration, MECC in 12-well plates were overlaid with 0.8% tragacanth gum medium and incubated for 6 days with plaque development.

All virus titers were expressed in $\log_{10}$ PFU/1 ml of inoculum. Where indicated, standard error of geometric mean titers are included. In all experiments with VSV and MCMV, the samples were tested on the day of harvest without prior freezing because we found that VSV became sensitive to inactivation by solutions of CsA and to a lesser extent by the solvent used to suspend CsA after storage at −70°C. Poliovirus was not affected.

Electron Microscopy

For electron microscopy studies, the viruses in the supernatant fluids from CsA-treated and untreated cell cultures were examined by the drop method of negative staining as previously described.[5] Rabbit antiserum against VSV with a neutralization titer of 1:60,000 was a gift of Dr. J. S. Youngner. It was used at a dilution of 1:100.

RESULTS

Effect of CsA on Poliovirus

Replicate Vero cell cultures were inoculated with poliovirus at a multiplicity of infection (MOI) of 0.001 and incubated with different concentrations of CsA at 37°C for 24 hr either "preinfection" or "postinfection." After preinfection treatment, when cells were only exposed to CsA for 24 hr prior to virus inoculation, or after postinfection treatment, when CsA was present during 24 hr, extracellular poliovirus was increased in a dose-responsive manner. A dose of 5 μg/ml was not effective, but yield from cells treated with 20 μg/ml CsA was almost 10 times higher than controls. The constant presence of CsA was not essential (Table 1).

To determine whether CsA affected the release of poliovirus, extracellular, intracellular, and total virus titers were separately compared (Table 1). Vero cells were infected with the virus at a MOI of 0.001 and incubated with MEM containing 20 μg/ml of CsA or MEM alone for 24 hr. In a complete experiment, 20 μg/ml CsA increased the extracellular virus titer as expected, but it had no effect on intracellular or total virus titers. To determine whether the solvent diluent used to suspend CsA had any effect on poliovirus titers in Vero cell cultures inoculated at an input MOI of 0.001, the amount of diluent equivalent to that in 10 or 20 μg/ml CsA was used to pretreat Vero cell cultures or was incorporated in the medium after infection. The difference between the log titers of virus from untreated and solvent-treated cultures in four separate experiments was 0.2 ± 0.04 and 0.4 ± 0.1. The solvent effect was inadequate to explain the above differences observed between controls and CsA-treated cultures. Taken together, these results suggest that CsA facilitated the release of poliovirus from the cells.

Table 1. Effect of Cyclosporine on Poliovirus*

Treatment with CsA	Extracellular Virus (CsA in μg/ml)				Intracellular Virus (CsA in μg/ml)		Total Virus (CsA in μg/ml)	
	0	5	10	20	0	20	0	20
Preinfection (−24 to 0 hr)	5.6	5.9	6.1	6.4	—	—	—	—
Postinfection† (0–24 hr)	5.7‡ ± 0.3	—	6.4 ± 0.3	6.7 ± 0.4	—	—	—	—
Postinfection (0–24 hr)	6.6	—	—	7.5	7.1	7.1	7.7	7.8

*Extracellular virus = virus in culture supernate; intracellular virus = virus in washed, sonicated cell monolayers; total virus = virus in supernate and cell monolayer.

†Repeated three times.

‡Virus titer in mean $\log_{10}$ PFU/ml ± SE.

Effect of Preinfection Treatment with CsA on VSV

MECC were treated with various concentrations of CsA "preinfection" and then infected with VSV at input MOI of 0.001. Controls were incubated with solvent equivalent to 40 μg/ml CsA or medium. After 24 hr of incubation, the supernatant fluids were harvested and titrated in Vero cells. The titers of replicate samples from cultures containing 40 μg/ml of CsA or diluent or medium controls were 7.9 ± 0.1, 7.2 ± 0.1, and 7.0 ± 0.2 $\log_{10}$ PFU/ml (two separate experiments). These results suggest that preinfection treatment with CsA enhanced the titers of VSV in mouse cells. A similar experiment was done in human foreskin cells. The titers of VSV from cultures pretreated with 40 μg/ml, 20 μg/ml of CsA and the solvent used to suspend 40 μg/ml of CsA, and medium controls were 8.0, 7.9, 7.1, and 6.9 $\log_{10}$ PFU/ml, respectively. The results indicated that the enhanced effect occurred not only in mouse cells but also in human cells infected with VSV.

Next we compared the effect of preinfection treatment with CsA on the intracellular as well as extracellular VSV titers. MECC were incubated with 40 μg/ml of CsA, equivalent solvent, or medium for 24 hr and washed before inoculation of VSV at a MOI of 0.001. At 24 hr after infection, in treated and control cultures, the intracellular virus titers were 6.2, 6.0, and 6.0 $\log_{10}$ PFU/ml, respectively, while the extracellular virus titers were 7.8, 7.1, and 6.8 $\log_{10}$ PFU/ml, respectively. The intracellular virus titers were not significantly changed, while the extracellular titers were enhanced. This suggests that preinfection treatment with CsA may facilitate the release of VSV from the cells, as in the case of poliovirus.

Effect of Postinfection Treatment with CsA on VSV

Figure 1 summarizes five experiments in which media containing various concentrations of CsA were added to infected MECC (postinfection treatment). The supernatant fluids were titrated after 24 hr of incubation. Contrary to results of preinfection treatment, CsA inhibited the titer of VSV in a dose-responsive manner. Controls for the amount of ethanol–Tween-80 solvent present in 10 or 20 μg/ml of CsA showed no significant effect. Inhibition was not demonstrable in human foreskin cells.

Mechanism of the Inhibitory Effect of CsA on VSV

One possible explanation for the effect of CsA on VSV was that CsA might affect the adsorption of VSV. To test this, Vero cells were inoculated with approximately 100 PFU of VSV per well and incubated for 1 hr at 37°C in the presence of 20 μg/ml of CsA. The cells were washed three times, overlay medium was added, and the cells were incubated for 2 days. The cell sheets were then stained for plaque counting. The mean number of plaques from CsA-treated and control cultures were 72 and 61, respectively. We concluded from this experiment that CsA did not inhibit adsorption of VSV.

Another possible mechanism for the inhibitory effect of CsA on VSV might be that CsA inactivated the virus directly. To determine this, VSV was incubated with medium con-

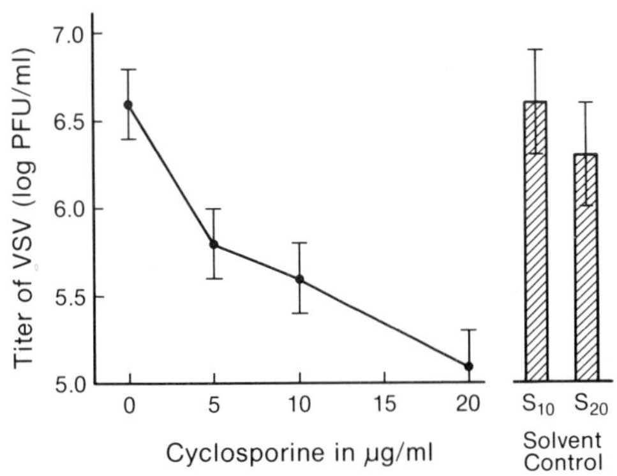

Fig. 1. Effect of CsA on the replication of VSV in MECC. Each point represents the mean and standard error of results from five experiments. S_{10} and S_{20} represent virus titers of samples from cultures treated with the amount of ethanol–Tween-80 present in 10 and 20 μg/ml of CsA suspension.

taining 20 μg/ml of CsA at 37°C for 10 hr and then titrated in Vero cells. The titers from CsA-treated and untreated samples were the same, 8.1 $\log_{10}$ PFU/ml. This indicated that the inhibitory effect of CsA was not due to inactivation of VSV.

To determine whether CsA inhibits VSV intracellularly, MECC were infected with the virus at a MOI of 0.001 for 1 hr and treated with 20 μg/ml of CsA "postinfection." Extracellular and intracellular virus was titrated from duplicate cultures of treated and control groups. The intracellular virus titers from CsA-treated and control cell cultures were 5.0 ± 0.1 and 6.4 ± 0.3 $\log_{10}$ PFU/ml, respectively, and the titers of extracellular virus were 5.7 ± 0.3 and 7.4 ± 0.2 $\log_{10}$ PFU/ml. The fact that CsA inhibited both intracellular and extracellular virus titers suggests that CsA inhibited the replication or assembly of VSV.

Similar results were obtained when Vero cells were used instead of mouse cells. However, this inhibitory effect of CsA was not observed in the human foreskin cells.

For electron-microscopic studies, harvests were obtained from MECC 24 hr after infection with VSV at a MOI of 0.001 and treated "postinfection" with 20 μg/ml CsA. An aliquot of treated and control fluids was mixed with an equal volume of rabbit antiserum against VSV and incubated for 30 min at 25°C. Grids were prepared and stained with 2% phosphotungstic acid at pH 4.5. Figure 2 shows enveloped complete particles from control fluids, a few of which are broken (*a*). These enveloped particles are better penetrated after they had been clumped with antibody (*b*). On the other hand, CsA treatment yielded particles whose outer envelopes were stripped or detached (c), irrespective of whether they were clumped with antiserum (*d*).

Effect of Postinfection Treatment with CsA on MCMV

In two separate experiments, MECC were infected with MCMV at a MOI of 0.001 and treated "postinfection" with 0, 5, 10, and 20 μg/ml CsA or solvent used to suspend 20 μg/ml of CsA. After 5 days of incubation, the respective extracellular mean log, PFU virus titers were 4.7 ± 0.2, 4.1 ± 0.2, 3.6 ± 0.1, 2.3 ± 0.4, and 4.4 ± 0.2. It is clear that at higher CsA concentrations, CsA decreased virus production of MCMV, as it did VSV.

Since CsA inhibited VSV (an enveloped RNA virus) and MCMV (an enveloped DNA virus), experiments were done to see if CsA inhibits herpes simplex virus in human foreskin cells. The results showed that, as in the case of VSV, CsA had no significant inhibitory effect on HSV-1 in human cell cultures (data not shown).

DISCUSSION AND SUMMARY

We found that infections by cytomegalovirus, herpes simplex, Epstein-Barr, and varicella-zoster viruses continue to be a problem in renal, heart, and liver transplant patients on CsA.[6] One would assume that this is because CsA is a potent inhibitor of certain T-lymphocyte functions.[1,2] However, virus infections may be facilitated by other actions of CsA. It suppresses NK cell function[7] as well as the ability of interferon to enhance NK activity.[4] CsA may also depress the generation of specific cytotoxic T cells against CMV in humans, although we could not demonstrate such an effect in mice (Breinig, Camp, and Ho, unpublished).

The present report adds to mechanisms by which CsA might facilitate viral infections. It enhances the release of poliovirus, a nonenveloped RNA enterovirus. It also enhances release of VSV, an enveloped virus, in mouse cell cultures pretreated with CsA. Whether these effects are significant factors in transplant patients is unknown. The effect described is not great; relatively large doses must be used, and the specific viruses studied are not significant pathogens in transplant patients.[8]

The enhancing effect of VSV may also be offset by an opposite effect. When cells were treated with CsA after infection and it

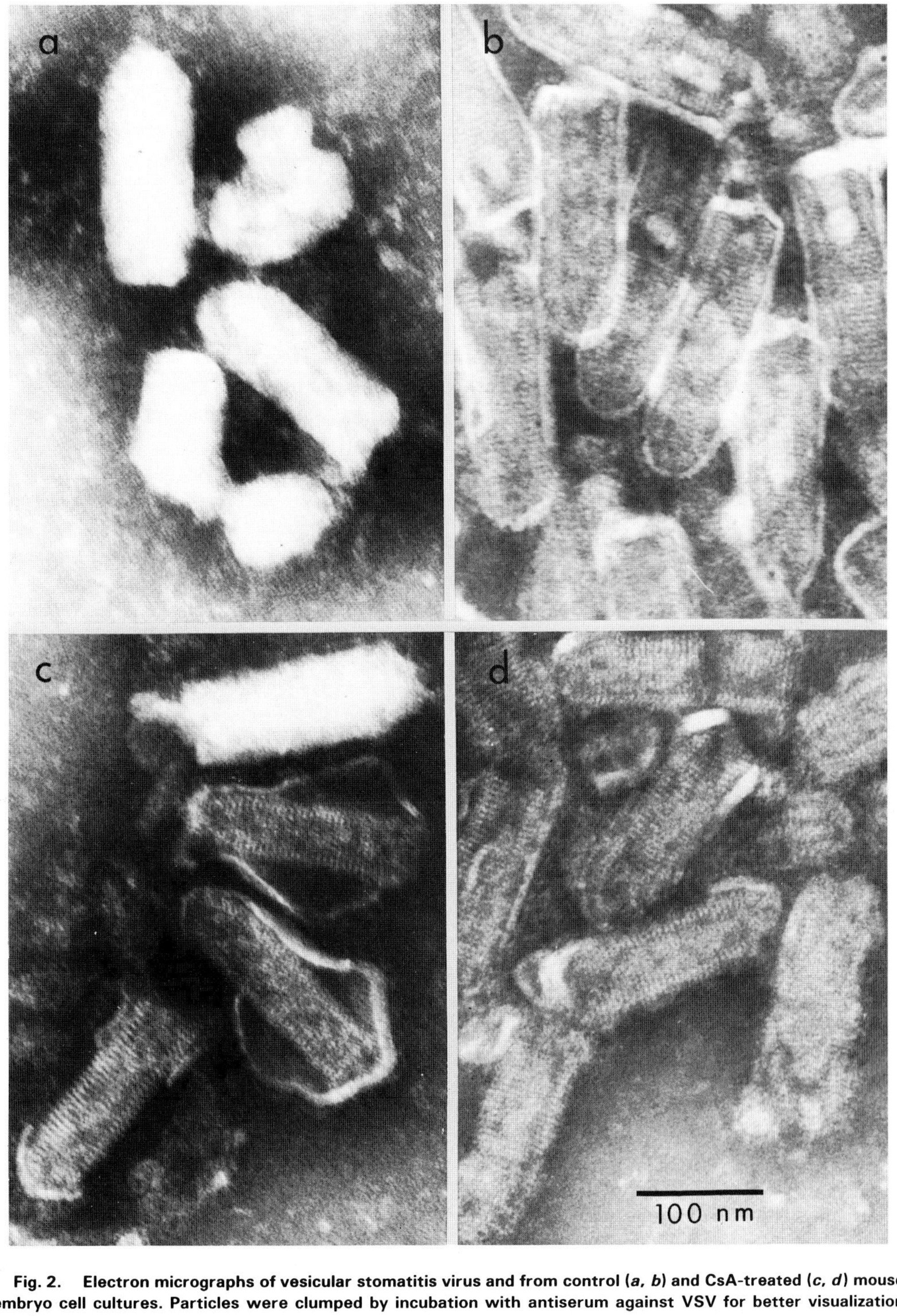

Fig. 2. Electron micrographs of vesicular stomatitis virus and from control (*a, b*) and CsA-treated (*c, d*) mouse embryo cell cultures. Particles were clumped by incubation with antiserum against VSV for better visualization (*b, d*).

remained constantly in infected cell cultures, VSV replication was actually suppressed. This suppressive effect of CsA on viral replication of both VSV and MCMV was shown only in mouse cells, as we failed to demonstrate it in human foreskin cells. Herpes simplex virus was also not affected.

It is not clear whether the difference of effect of CsA in human fibroblasts and in MECC is related to the virus or the cell. Quite possibly, there may be species variation in response to CsA. After a short period of treatment with CsA, renal allografts in rabbits and heart allografts in pigs may survive for more than 5 months.[9,10] In contrast, rejection occurred in dogs and in humans with renal allografts when administration of CsA was stopped.[11,12]

Other reports support the thesis that CsA may act on various biological agents, apart from its action on lymphocytes. Nickell reported the antimalarial activity of CsA both in vitro and in the rodent.[13]

The mechanisms by which CsA treatment enhances cellular release of enveloped and nonenveloped viruses is unclear. CsA is thought to act on the cell membrane; Palacios reports that it acts on the same receptors as OKT3 monoclonal antibody.[14] What we observed is not easily explained by such action. Cell cultures treated postinfection with CsA also produced less VSV. This may be explained by our demonstrating of stripped envelopes. It is, however, unclear whether this stripping represents a direct action of CsA or its indirect effect on cell membranes or on viral synthesis and assembly.

ACKNOWLEDGMENTS

We thank Dr. J. A. Armstrong and Dr. P. Whitaker-Dowling for valuable assistance and criticisms.

REFERENCES

1. Borel JF, Feurer C, Gubler HU, et al: Agents and Actions 6:468, 1976

2. Bunjes D, Hardt C, Röllinghoff M, et al: Eur J Immunol 11:657, 1981

3. Klintmalm GBG, Starzl TE, Iwatsuki S, et al: Transplant Proc 14:98, 1982

4. Gui XE, Ho M, Camp PE: Infect Immunol 36:1123, 1982

5. Atchison RW: Virology 42:155, 1970

6. Dummer JS, Hardy A, Ho M, et al: Transplantation (in press)

7. Introna M, Allavena P, Spreafico F, et al. Transplantation 31:113, 1981

8. Ho M: Arch Virol 55:1, 1977

9. Green CJ, Allison AC: Lancet 1:1182, 1978

10. Calne RY, White DJG, Rolles K: Lancet 1:1183, 1978

11. Dutoit DF, Homan WP, Morris PJ: In White DJG (ed): Cyclosporin A. Amsterdam, Elsevier Biomedical, 1982, p 101

12. Calne RY, Rolles K, White DJG, et al: Transplant Proc 13:349, 1981

13. Nickell SP, Schiebel LW, Cole GA: Infect Immunol 37:1093, 1982

14. Palacios R: J Clin Immunol 2:155, 1982

In Vitro Effects of Cyclosporine on Lymphocyte Responses to Cytomegalovirus

P. J. Converse, A. D. Hess, P. J. Tutschka, and G. W. Santos

ANIMAL MODELS have shown the effectiveness of cyclosporine (CsA) in the prophylaxis of graft-vs.-host disease (GVHD) and prevention of graft rejection.[1-3] Based on these studies, the drug came into clinical use in 1979. In vitro studies have demonstrated that the drug inhibits the activation of cytotoxic T lymphocytes, the cells presumably responsible for GVHD and graft rejection.[4] However, cytotoxic cells are also important in the control of viral infections such as cytomegalovirus (CMV)[5,6] that often compromise the survival of transplant recipients. To probe this potential dilemma, an in vitro model was devised to assess the effects of cyclosporine on the immune response to CMV.

MATERIALS AND METHODS

Mononuclear Cell and Lymphocyte Isolation

Blood from healthy volunteers was tested for complement fixation antibody to CMV and for the ability of cells separated over Ficoll-Hypaque to proliferate (as measured by ^{3}H-thymidine incorporation) to cytomegalovirus (Towne strain)-infected fibroblasts fixed in glutaraldehyde and irradiated (CMF$_x$). Those who responded to the stimulating cells ("responders") but not to fixed uninfected irradiated fibroblasts (UF$_x$) were used in subsequent suppressor and cytotoxic cell experiments. Responder cells (2×10^6/ml) were cocultured with fibroblast stimulator cells (2×10^4/ml) in CMV antibody-negative complete medium.[4]

Cyclosporine

CsA in powdered form was generously provided by Sandoz, Ltd. (Basel) and was dissolved in 95% ethanol and diluted to various concentrations (as indicated in the text) in complete medium.

Suppressor Cell Assays

The suppressive effects of lymphocytes primed by CMF$_x$ in vitro in the presence or absence of CsA were assessed. Bulk cultures were harvested on day 7, incubated for 1 hr at 37°C in complete medium, and further washed two times in complete medium. The cells were resuspended at 2×10^6/ml, 4×10^5/ml, and 2×10^5/ml; 0.1-ml aliquots were set up in triplicate flat-bottom microtiter wells with equal-volume aliquots of fresh responder cells at a constant concentration of 2×10^6/ml and with CMF$_x$ at 2×10^4/ml or irradiated allogeneic lymphocytes (B$_x$) at 2×10^6/ml. Control cultures consisted of autologously primed lymphocytes irradiated and added to fresh lymphocytes and CMF$_x$. After 7 days of incubation, the cultures were pulsed with ^{3}H-thymidine to measure proliferation and suppression by the following formula:

$$\%\ \text{suppression} = 1 - \frac{\text{cpm of test culture}}{\text{cpm control culture}} \times 100.$$

Cytotoxic Cell Experiments

Cells cultured for 8 days with CMF$_x$ in the presence or absence of CsA were tested after washing for their ability to lyse unfixed CMV-infected (CMVF) or noninfected (NF) fibroblast targets in round-bottomed microtiter plates. Primed cells were resuspended at a concentration of 5×10^6/ml, and 0.1-ml aliquots were set up in triplicate at a ratio of 50:1 against 1×10^5/ml of ^{51}Cr-labeled target cells for a final volume of 0.2 ml. After 4–5 hr incubation at 37°C, plates were centrifuged, and 100 μl of supernatant was harvested and counted for released ^{51}Cr. Spontaneous and maximum release were measured by harvesting supernatants in wells to which 0.1 ml of medium or 0.1 ml of 1 N HCl, respectively, had been added to target cells. Percent specific ^{51}Cr release was calculated by the following formula:

$$\%\ \text{specific}\ ^{51}\text{Cr release} = \frac{\text{cpm test} - \text{cpm spontaneous}}{\text{cpm maximum} - \text{cpm spontaneous}} \times 100.$$

Statistical Analysis

Results were analyzed for statistical significance by Student's t test.

From the Bone Marrow Transplant Program, Oncology Center, The Johns Hopkins University, School of Medicine, Baltimore, MD.

Supported by NIH-NCI Grants CA 15396 and NIH-NIADD 1RO1 AM 25602. A.D.H. is a scholar of the Leukemia Society of America.

Reprint requests should be addressed to Dr. P. J. Converse, Oncology Center, Room 3-127, Johns Hopkins Hospital, 600 N. Wolfe Street, Baltimore, MD 21205.

0041-1345/83/1505-0133$01.00/0

Table 1. The Effect of Cyclosporine on Proliferative Responses to CMF_x and Control Antigens Measured by ^{3}H-Thymidine Uptake After 6 Days in Culture

Antigen	cpm + SEM	No. of Individuals
CMF_x	38,899 ± 5,674	11
CMF_x (CsA 1.0 μg/ml)	1,288 ± 429	6
CMF_x (CsA 2.5 μg/ml)	810 ± 183	5
UF_x	3,281 ± 941	9
B_x	40,752 ± 4,101	11

RESULTS

Eleven of 28 individuals (39%) responded to CMF_x as measured by lymphocyte incorporation of ^{3}H-thymidine (38,899 ± 5,674). Responses to UF_x or irradiated autologous lymphocytes (A_x) were 10-fold less ($p < 0.001$). Lymphocyte transformation responses by the remaining 16 seronegative individuals were similarly 10-fold less for CMF_x, UF_x, or A_x. All individuals tested responded to allogeneic cells (B_x).

When cyclosporine at 2.5 μg/ml or 1.0 μg/ml was added to responder lymphocyte CMV_x cultures of five individuals, the proliferative responses were significantly reduced by 30-fold, as shown in Table 1. Kinetic studies demonstrated a peak response on day 5 or 6 and only a diminution and not an alteration or delay of the proliferative response in the presence of CsA.

The ability of CMF_x to stimulate the development of suppressor cells and the effect of CsA on this activity were also assessed. Cells primed for 7 days in vitro by CMF_x suppressed the response of an equal number of fresh autologous responder cells to CMF_x by 70%. The suppressive effect was dependent on the ratio of primed cells to fresh responder cells, as shown in Table 2. Cyclosporine added at the initiation of culture did not allow proliferation in response to CMF_x, but after thorough washing these day-7 lymphocytes were capable of suppressing the response of fresh responder cells to CMF_x to the same degree as control primed cells.

The CMF_x-induced suppressor cells were not capable of suppressing responses of fresh lymphocytes to alloantigens. However, alloantigen-primed lymphocytes not only suppressed the response to the original stimulating alloantigen but also suppressed the response to CMF_x.

Stimulation of mononuclear cells by CMF_x also induced the activation of cytotoxic cells. Mean lysis of CMV-infected fibroblasts (CMVF) by cells stimulated for 8 days in vitro by CMF_x was 35%. The CMF_x-primed cells also mediated substantial, if significantly ($p < 0.001$) less, lysis of noninfected fibroblasts (NF); the mean value was 15%. CsA added at the initiation of culture significantly ($p < 0.01$) inhibited the generation of cells

Table 2. Suppressor Cell Activity After Stimulation In Vitro*

Primed Cell Population	Fresh Micro Lymphocyte Culture	% Suppression of Fresh Micro Lymphocyte Culture: Primed Cell–to–Fresh Responder Ratio 1:1	1:5	1:10
(A × CMF_x)′	A × CMF_x	70 ± 11	47 ± 13	34 ± 9
(A × CMF_x CsA 1.0 μg/ml)′	A × CMF_x	63 ± 4	49 ± 5	39 + 6
(A × CMF_x CsA 2.5 μg/ml)′	A × CMF_x	71 ± 2	45 ± 8	36 ± 6
(A × CMF_x)′	A × B_x	29 ± 12	NT†	NT
(A × CMF_x CsA 1.0 μg/ml)′	A × B_x	24 ± 2	NT	NT
(A × B_x)′	A × B_x	96 ± 2	NT	77 ± 6
(A × B_x CsA 1.0 μg/ml)′	A × B_x	83 ± 5	NT	71 ± 5
(A × B_x)′	A × CMF_x	48 ± 7	NT	NT
(A × B_x CsA 1.0 μg/ml)′	A × CMF_x	59 ± 8	NT	NT

*Cells were stimulated in vitro for 7 days by allogeneic cells or by CMV-infected fibroblasts (CMF_x) and then added to fresh micro lymphocyte cultures for a further 7 days. Control primed cell cultures were irradiated autologously stimulated cells.

†NT = Not tested.

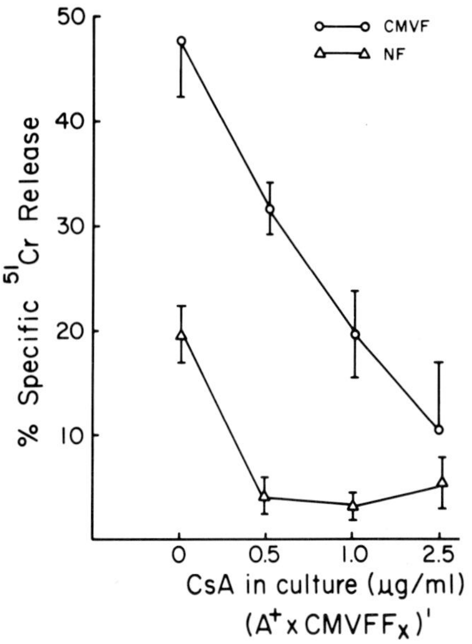

Fig. 1. The effect of CsA on the generation of cytotoxic cells to CMV-infected fibroblasts (CMVF) and noninfected fibroblasts (NF).

capable of mediating lysis of CMVF. However, this level of cytotoxicity was significantly ($p < 0.01$) above background levels. The results of an illustrative experiment are shown in Fig. 1. There was also a significant reduction of lysis of NF with the addition of CsA at ≥ 0.5 μg/ml at the initiation of culture. CsA also significantly ($p < 0.0001$) reduced the cytotoxicity to noninfected cells to levels not significantly ($p > 0.1$) different from background. Further studies indicate that the cells responsible for lysis of CMVF are a mixture of T cells and, predominantly, NK cells (data not shown).

DISCUSSION

The present studies demonstrate the effect of cyclosporine on in vitro proliferative as well as functional immune responses by cells primed in vivo to viral antigens that are highly relevant in clinical transplantation.

Previous studies have shown that CsA blocks primary proliferative in vitro responses to alloantigens and mitogens.[4] The drug was found to block the formation of cytotoxic T lymphocytes at levels as low as 0.1 μg/ml, yet the induction of suppressor cells was not impaired. In the current studies, both CMV seropositive and seronegative individuals were tested. Only those who were seropositive possessed memory lymphocytes that were capable of proliferating when presented with CMVF. This proliferation of memory cells was abrogated by the presence of CsA in culture. Experiments studying functional immune responses found that CsA did not hamper CMF_x-induced suppressor-cell activity, findings which are in agreement with the results from the mixed lymphocyte response (MLR) systems.[4] Although the presence of CsA at the initiation of culture did reduce cytotoxicity to infected fibroblasts, this function was not completely abrogated as was found in primary MLR. Furthermore, the doses of CsA necessary for impairing cytotoxicity were at least 5- to 10-fold higher than those that blocked alloreactive cytotoxic cell activation. The presence of the drug only eliminated killing of normal fibroblasts.

Cell-mediated cytotoxicity to CMV-infected cells has been correlated with protection both in murine systems and in bone marrow transplant patients.[5] The present studies may indicate that the presence or persistence of cells recognizing CMV antigens in transplant patients should be protective despite CsA treatment. The results of these studies offer some experimental support to findings reporting the use of cyclosporine—a nonlymphotoxic immunosuppressive agent—and observing a markedly reduced incidence of CMV disease in renal transplant recipients.[7,8] In our experiments, CsA did not totally eliminate immune defense function of sensitized individuals against a viral agent known to cause considerable morbidity in transplant recipients. Furthermore, our studies would also imply that effective immunosuppression preventing graft rejection and/or GVHD could be achieved with CsA without severely compromising antiviral immunity of sensitized hosts.

ACKNOWLEDGMENT

I would like to thank Mrs. Constance Rutter for her expert secretarial assistance in the preparation of this manuscript.

REFERENCES

1. Tutschka PJ, Beschorner WE, Hess AD: In Thierfelder S, et al (eds): Immunobiology of Bone Marrow Transplantation. New York, Springer, 1980, p 241

2. Deeg HJ, Storb R: In White DJG (ed): Cyclosporin A. New York, Elsevier Biomedical, 1982, p 121

3. Tutschka PJ, Hess AD, Beschorner WE, et al: In White DJG (ed): Cyclosporin A. New York, Elsevier Biomedical, 1982, p 519

4. Hess AD, Tutschka PJ: J Immunol 124:2601, 1980

5. Quinnan GV, Kirman N, Rook AH, et al: New Engl J Med 307:7, 1982

6. Elfenbein GJ, Saral R: In Allen JD (ed): Infection and the Compromised Host (2d ed). Baltimore, Williams and Wilkins, 1982, p 157

7. Najarian JS, Ferguson RM, Sutherland DER, et al: Transplant Proc 15:438, 1983

8. Peterson PK, Rynasiewicz JJ, Simmons RL, et al: Transplant Proc 15:437, 1983

In Vitro and In Vivo Antifungal Activity of Cyclosporine

M. S. Osato, T. J. Roussel, K. R. Wilhelmus, and D. B. Jones

CYCLOSPORINE A (CsA) was first isolated from fermentation broth cultures of two soil fungi, *Trichoderma polysporum* (Rifai) and *Cylindrocarpon lucidum* (Booth).[1] This agent initially generated interest as a new antifungal antibiotic but was found to have a rather limited antifungal spectrum and systemic toxicity. In contrast, topical application of 1%–5% CsA in studies of corneal transplantation[2] demonstrated that this route of therapy was nontoxic to external ocular tissues. Therefore, the antifungal activity of topical 5% CsA in a rat model of *Candida albicans* keratitis (unpublished data) was compared to the results observed with conventional antifungal therapies.[3]

MATERIALS AND METHODS

Determination of In Vitro Antifungal Activity of Cyclosporine

Fungal Cultures. Yeast cultures (*S. cereviseae, C. albicans* ST16, and *C. albicans* EP) were grown on potato dextrose agar (BBL) for 24 hr at 35°C, harvested in sterile phosphate-buffered saline (PBS, pH 7.0), and adjusted to 5–8 × 10^5 blastospores/ml. Cultures of *A. candidus* were maintained on Czapek solution agar (Difco) at 35°C for 3 weeks under 8% CO_2 tension. The conidia were harvested by washing the plates with sterile PBS containing 0.005% dioctylsuccinate (Eastman Organics) and resuspended to 5 × 10^5 conidia/ml.

Cyclosporine. CsA (donated by Sandoz Ltd., Basel) was dissolved in Tween-80 (Nutritional Biochemicals). CsA agar plates were prepared by slowly adding the diluted CsA solutions to antibiotic medium 3 (Difco) to produce final concentrations of 1.25%, 2.5%, and 5% (w/v). The inoculated plates were incubated for 48 hr at 30°C.

Preparation of Disc Sensitivities. The disc sensitivity assay was a modification of that described by Boyer.[4] Briefly, CsA dissolved in creamophor EL (Sigma) was placed in 0.02-ml aliquots onto sterile filter paper discs (Schleicher and Schuell). Drug-impregnated discs were placed in wells of a cluster dish (Corning) containing antibiotic assay medium 3 (M-3). Diffusion of the CsA was facilitated by overnight exposure to M-3 medium, at which time 0.05 ml of blastospore or conidial inocula were added to each well of the cluster dish. The inoculated dishes were incubated at 30°C for 48 hr. Both medium and carrier-vehicle control wells were included in each assay.

Determination of In Vivo Activity of Cyclosporine

Fungal Culture. *C. albicans* EP, isolated from a human infection, was used. Fresh cultures were prepared by re-isolating the yeast from discs stored at −70°C. The cultures were passed three times in brain-heart infusion (BHI) broth (Difco Laboratories, Detroit, MI) prior to intracorneal injection.

Preparation of Inoculum. Eighteen-hour broth cultures of *C. albicans* EP were harvested, washed in PBS, and adjusted to ~10^4 blastospores/10 μl. Viable counts were prepared by plating the inoculum in duplicate on BHI agar containing 50 μg/ml gentamicin. All plates were incubated at 35°C for 48 hr.

Rat Model of Candida Keratitis. Male Sprague-Dawley rats were anesthetized with 12 mg ketamine and 3 mg xylazine. The eyes were proptosed, and a micropipette containing the inoculum was inserted to a midstromal depth of the central cornea. For the early

---

From the Cullen Eye Institute, Baylor College of Medicine, Houston, TX.

Supported in part by grants from the Sid W. Richardson Foundation and Research to Prevent Blindness, Inc.

Reprint requests should be addressed to Dr. Michael S. Osato.

0041-1345/83/1505-0134$01.00/0

therapy studies, treatment was initiated at 8 hr after injection; in the late therapy studies, treatment was begun at 24 hr after injection.

Antifungal Agents. CsA was dissolved in sterile olive oil (Sigma Chemical Co., St. Louis, MO), flucytosine (donated by Hoffman-LaRoche, Nutley, NJ) in sterile PBS, and amphotericin B (E. R. Squibb and Sons, Princeton, NJ) in sterile distilled water. Natamycin (Alcon) and miconazole (donated by Janssen Pharmaceuticals) were used as supplied.

Therapeutic Trials. At 8 and 24 hr after injection, rats were randomly separated into control and treatment groups. The rats were administered one drop of a topical drug preparation per hour for 12 consecutive hours. The treatment groups included the following: control (saline), amphotericin B (0.1% or 0.5%), natamycin (5%), miconazole (1%), flucytosine (1%), cyclosporine (5%), and combined amphotericin B (0.5%)–flucytosine (1%). Amphotericin B (0.1%) was used only during the early (8-hr postinjection) treatment studies. At the termination of therapy, the rats were sacrificed by intracardiac Nembutal, and their corneas were excised and processed for quantitative fungal cultures.

Quantitative Fungal Cultures. Excised corneas were washed twice in 50 ml quantities of sterile PBS, blot-dried, and homogenized. The corneal tissue homogenates were plated in duplicate on BHI agar containing 50 μg/ml gentamicin. All plates were incubated at 35°C for 48 hr, and the growth was expressed as the number of colony-forming units (cfu) per gram of wet corneal tissue.

Statistical Analysis. All data were analyzed by CLINFO using the nonparametric, two-sample, signed ranks test of Wilcoxon.[5]

RESULTS

In Vitro Sensitivity

The determination of in vitro activity of cyclosporine was hampered by its extreme hydrophobicity. Carrier solvents used in this study included Tween-80, creamophor EL, dimethylsulfoxide (DMSO), and olive oil; all produced similar effects when added to aqueous media. Diffusion of the CsA from the drug-impregnated discs and from the compartmentalized drug-agar interfaces in the plate assays was probably inhibited due to precipitation in these media. Nevertheless, a qualitative stratification of sensitivities was demonstrated with the different fungal isolates. The data indicated that *S. cereviseae* was the most sensitive to CsA suppression, while the *Candida* species were the most resistant. *A. candidus* demonstrated an intermediate reactivity (Table 1).

In Vivo Activity

The rat model of *C. albicans* keratitis results in a gradually progressive disease that reaches it maximal response 20 hr after injection. The infection slowly subsides over the next 72 hr and is clinically resolved at 7 days (Osato, unpublished data). In these experiments, topical CsA was as effective as other commonly used antifungal agents in inhibiting the replication of the *Candida* when administered during the early phase of infection (8 hr after injection), as compared to saline-treated controls ($p \leq 0.01$). In established infection (24 hr after injection), only amphotericin B (0.5%), natamycin (5%), and combined 0.5 amphotericin B–1% flucytosine therapy effectively suppressed the growth of the injected *Candida* ($p \leq 0.05$) (Table 2). Miconazole (1%) was ineffective in both the early and late treatment phases and may reflect the in vitro antifungal sensitivity pattern of this organism.

DISCUSSION

Fungal keratitis presents a substantial therapeutic dilemma for clinicians despite advances in antifungal chemotherapy. Anecdotal reports of clinical efficacy have been difficult to interpret without a suitable animal model of fungal keratitis for objective determination of antifungal antibiotic efficacy. The rat model of *Candida albicans* keratitis (Osato, unpublished data) is highly reproduc-

Table 1. In Vitro Antifungal Activity of Cyclosporine

	Concentration of Cyclosporine*						
	Agar Plate Assay			Disc Diffusion Assay			
Fungal Isolate	5%	2.5%	1.25%	40 mg	30 mg	20 mg	10 mg
Saccharomyces cereviseae	NG†	NG	NG	2+	2+	3+	3+
Candida albicans ST 16	NG	2+	2+	2+	3+	3+	3+
Candida albicans EP	NG	2+	2+	2+	3+	3+	3+
Aspergillus candidus	NG	NG	2+	2+	3+	3+	3+

*Grading scale as compared to controls at 48 hr: 1+ = light growth, 2+ = moderate growth, 3+ = heavy growth.
†NG = No growth.

ible, especially during the first 36 hr of infection, and is susceptible to modulation by topical antifungal therapy.

Experimental *Candida* keratitis was treated with topical cyclosporine, amphotericin B, natamycin, fluctysine, and combined amphotericin B–flucytosine therapy (Table 2). During the early phase of infection, antifungal agents significantly reduced the number of viable *Candida* in corneal homogenates of treated rats when compared to matched controls ($p \leq 0.01$).

In established disease, only the polyene antibiotic–treated groups (natamycin and amphotericin B) significantly reduced the number of organisms in homogenates of corneal tissue, as compared to saline-treated controls ($p \leq 0.05$). These contrasting responses demonstrated in early and late treatments may reflect the antifungal sensitivity pattern of the microorganism.

The systemic effects of other fungus-derived antibiotics resemble CsA. For example, the imidazoles can induce renal dysfunction by a direct action on tubular cell transport systems. These agents can also produce marked immunomodulatory reactions.[6] Miconazole, a phenylethyl imidazole, inhibits mitogen-induced lymphocyte blastogenesis and mixed lymphocyte responses (MLR) in vitro.[7] Miconazole has also been shown to prolong significantly the survival of skin allografts in mice and rats, as compared to untreated companion animals.[8,9] In addition, systemic metronidazole (a benzylimidazole) can induce lung tumors and malignant lymphomas in mice,[10] similar to the effect documented with systemic cyclosporine.[11]

Considering the close pharmacologic relatedness of CsA and the imidazoles, especially miconazole, the dichotomy of therapeutic efficacy between the individual responses elicited in the *Candida* keratitis model presents an interesting paradox that may relate to differences in drug bioavailability, mechanisms of action, cellular permeability, or intracellular transport mechanisms.

Most available antifungal agents demonstrate inherent toxicity to external ocular tissues when applied topically. This has restricted their use in these infections. Ocular toxicity of 5% CsA has not been demonstrated

Table 2. Comparison of Early and Late Therapy of Experimental *Candida albicans* Keratitis*

Treatment Group	Early Therapy	*p* Value	Late Therapy	*p* Value
Control (saline)	5.31×10^5	—	5.24×10^5	—
Amphotericin B (0.1%)	2.66×10^5	0.025	—	—
Amphotericin B (0.5%)	1.01×10^5	0.001	3.22×10^5	0.037
Combined (AB + 5-FC)	1.00×10^5	0.001	2.96×10^5	0.033
Cyclosporine (5%)	1.78×10^5	0.009	3.70×10^5	0.111
Flucytosine (1%)	2.10×10^5	0.017	4.19×10^5	0.387
Miconazole (1%)	4.24×10^5	0.057	4.08×10^5	0.387
Natamycin (5%)	2.23×10^5	0.006	2.32×10^5	0.037

*Average log of colony-forming units per gram of corneal tissue (20 eyes per group).

histopathologically by Roussel et al,[2] nor were any discordant reactions observed in this study.

Because of extreme hydrophobicity, determination of in vitro sensitivities for CsA are problematic and require further investigation. Possible use of the galenic form may facilitate application in aqueous media. The in vivo efficacy of CsA in the treatment of *Candida* keratitis is promising. Further investigations into its in vivo antifungal effects are contingent upon development of more applicable carrier vehicles.

ACKNOWLEDGMENTS

The authors thank Nettie M. Robinson, M.S., for her excellent technical assistance and Frank L. Kretzer, Ph.D., for his thoughtful review of the manuscript.

REFERENCES

1. Dreyfuss M, Harri E, Hofmann H, et al: Eur J Appl Microbiol 3:125, 1976

2. Roussel TJ, Osato MS, Wilhelmus KR: Transplant Proc (in press)

3. Jones DB: In Srinivasan D (ed): Ocular Therapeutics. New York, Masson, 1980

4. Boyer JM: Antimicrob Ag Chemother 9:1070, 1976

5. Snedecor GW, Cochran WG: *Statistical Methods* (6th ed). Ames, IA, Iowa State University Press, 1979

6. Miller JJ: Transplant Proc 12:300, 1980

7. Thong YH, Ronan-Kelly B: Br Med J 1:149, 1978

8. Thong YH, Ferrante A: Clin Exp Immunol 35:10, 1979

9. Miller JJ, Salaman JR: In Salaman J (ed): Immunosuppressive Therapy. New York, JB Lippincot, 1981, p 111

10. Rustra M, Shubik P: J Natl Cancer Inst 48:721, 1972

11. Calne RY, Rolles K, White DJG, et al: Lancet 2:1033, 1979

EXPERIMENTAL TRANSPLANTATION

KIDNEY

Combination Immunotherapy With Low-Dose Cyclosporine and Azathioprine in Splenectomized Canine Recipients of Renal Allografts

M. I. Aeder, D. E. R. Sutherland, W. I. Lewis, and J. S. Najarian

ALTHOUGH cyclosporine (CsA) by itself is immunosuppressive and as a single agent can prolong allograft survival in some animal models and in humans, the doses needed to consistently prevent rejection result in renal and hepatic toxicity in humans.[1,2] Combination immunotherapy has been used clinically in transplantation for over 20 years, based on the rationale that nontoxic doses will have a synergistic therapeutic effect. Although some transplant units try to administer CsA alone, at least initially, others have combined CsA with prednisone as a standard or investigative immunosuppressive regimen in kidney,[3,4] pancreas,[5] liver,[6] and heart[7] transplantation. Although CsA and low-dose prednisone is effective and free of immediate toxicities, the long-term use of steroids, even at low doses, can result in significant side effects, apart from those related to immunosuppression.[8] For this reason, we have investigated the use of CsA in combination with nonsteroidal immunosuppressive treatments in an attempt to further reduce the potential for chronic immunosuppressive toxicity.[9–11] CsA combined with nonsteroidal antiinflammatory drugs had a small effect on graft survival.[12] Low-dose CsA in combination with azathioprine (Aza) was completely effective in preventing rejection of rat heart allografts transplanted across a major histocompatibility barrier in doses that, by themselves, could not prevent rejection.[10] Further work was performed in the mongrel dog renal allograft model, and the combination of CsA and Aza was found to significantly enhance graft survival.[13] However, the doses used were associated with leukopenia, leading to late deaths. In the experiments reported here, we have examined a wider range of doses in a beagle renal allograft model. In addition, the animals were splenectomized in an attempt to compensate for the tendency of Aza to induce leukopenia.[10] Again, the synergistic effects of CsA and Aza were apparent, and dose combinations that resulted in very prolonged graft and dog survival in most of the recipients were identified.

MATERIALS AND METHODS

Dogs

All animals were outbred beagles weighing 10–20 kg and were obtained from Laboratory Research Enterprises, Kalamazoo, MI.

From the Department of Surgery, University of Minnesota Health Sciences Center, Minneapolis, MN.

Supported in part by NIH Grants AM 27540 and 13803. M.I.A. is the recipient of the Lee McBride Fellowship at Case Western Reserve University, Cleveland, Ohio.

Address reprint requests to Dr. D. E. R. Sutherland, Department of Surgery, University of Minnesota Hospitals, Box 280 Mayo, 516 Delaware Street SE, Minneapolis, MN 55455.

0041-1345/83/1505-0135$01.00/0

Experimental Groups

Group I: Control, no immunosuppression (n = 8); group II: azathioprine 1.5 mg/kg/day (n = 6); group III: azathioprine 2.5 mg/kg/day (n = 7); group IV: cyclosporine 5 mg/kg/day (n = 5); group V: cyclosporine 10 mg/kg/day (n = 11); group VI: cyclosporine 5 mg/kg/day plus azathioprine 2.5 mg/kg/day (n = 7); group VII: cyclosporine 7.5 mg/kg/day plus azathioprine 1.5 mg/kg/day (n = 6); group VIII: cyclosporine 10 mg/kg/day plus azathioprine 1.5 mg/kg/day (n = 6); group IX: cyclosporine 10 mg/kg/day plus azathioprine 2.5 mg/kg/day (n = 8).

The first dose of drugs was given 3 hr prior to operation. The drugs were administered orally, and the doses of immunosuppressive agents remained constant until the death of the dog.

Operative Procedure

All animals undergoing transplantation were splenectomized at least 2 weeks prior to receiving a renal allograft. A two-team approach was utilized and the kidneys exchanged between pairs of dogs. The remaining kidney was excised and discarded. Kidneys were then heterotopically transplanted to the iliac fossa, utilizing an end-to-side anastomosis of the renal vein and an end-to-end anastomosis of the renal artery to the iliac vessels. A ureteroneocystostomy was created by a bladder wall tunnel and anastomosis of the spatulated ureter to the bladder mucosa.

Daily measurements of serum creatinine were obtained, as well as a weekly complete blood count. A graft was considered to be functional if the serum creatinine was <7 mg/dl and to have failed when the serum creatinine rose to >7 mg/dl. A complete postmortem examination was performed on all animals. Histologic samples of the renal graft were stained with hematoxylin and eosin and examined blindly.

Blood CsA measurements were performed on whole blood samples by high-pressure liquid chromatography (HPLC). The capabilities for measurement became available late in the course of experimentation, and therefore, only the long-term survivors (>200 days) were analyzed.

Median graft survival times were calculated and a life table analysis performed on our data.

RESULTS

A total of 64 dogs were transplanted and placed into one of 9 treatment groups. Eight animals (12.5%) died due to technical complications before the sixth postoperative day and were not included in the statistical analysis. The data obtained on the remaining 56 dogs are summarized in Table 1.

No Immunosuppression (Group I)

All 8 dogs in this group lost graft function within 12 postoperative days (median of 7 days). The mean WBC prior to death was 19,600 cells/cu mm.

Azathioprine Alone (Groups II and III)

There was one technical failure (no graft function) in each group. All grafts were rejected in animals of group II receiving Aza 1.5 mg/kg/day (median of 10 days). In group III (Aza 2.5 mg/kg/day), graft survival was seen in 4 of 6 dogs; one rejected at 44 days, and until that time, had had good renal function. The 3 dogs in group III who died with a functioning allograft all had respiratory infections, and on autopsy, gross purulence was present in one or more lung lobes. The mean WBC prior to death in those dogs surviving at least 25 days was 3400 cells/cu mm.

Table 1. Comparison of Kidney Graft Survival, Median Days of Graft Function, and Long-Term Graft Function According to Immunotherapy Regimen of Renal Allografts in 56 Splenectomized Outbred Beagles

Group	Treatment (mg/kg/Day)	Day of Rejection	Died With Functioning Graft (Days)	Currently Alive Days (Cr)	Median Days Graft Function	Graft Function >60 Days (%)
I	None	5,6,6,7,7,7,11,12	—	—	7	0/8 (0%)
II	Aza 1.5	8,9,10,11,15	—	—	10	0/5 (0%)
III	Aza 2.5	6,7,44	21,29,48	—	25	0/6 (0%)
IV	CsA 5	7,7,8,8,13	—	—	8	0/5 (0%)
V	CsA 10	7,8,8,10,12,37,46,71,75	—	240 (1.0)†	24.5	3/10 (30%)
VI	CsA 5 + AZA 2.5	8,9,10,35	43,48	—	22.5	0/6 (0%)
VII	CsA 7.5 + AZA 1.5	11	226*	226(0.2),*322(1.6)*	226	3/4 (75%)
VIII	CsA 10 + AZA 1.5	22	64,76	225(1.4),†303(0.7),†337(1.0)†	165.5	5/6 (83%)
IX	CsA 10 + AZA 2.5	10,36	71	222(0.2),†233(0.8),†242(0.8)†	146.5	4/6 (67%)

*Cyclosporine levels at >200 days range from 152 to 927 ng/ml (mean 475 ± 135) in dogs on CsA 7.5 mg/kg/day.

†Cyclosporine levels at >200 days range from 110 to 1371 ng/ml (mean 406 ± 65) in dogs on CsA 10 mg/kg/day.

Cyclosporine Alone (Groups IV and V)

Five and 11 dogs were immunosuppressed with CsA 5 or 10 mg/kg/day, respectively. One dog receiving CSA 10/mg/kg/day (group V) died due to intussusception on the fifth postoperative day and was not included in the analysis. All dogs receiving CsA 5 mg/kg/day (group IV) promptly underwent acute rejection of their allografts (median of 8 days). Nine of the 10 dogs treated with the higher dose of CsA rejected their graft, but median survival was 24.5 days. One dog (group V) is presently alive 240 days following transplantation. The mean WBC in the animals surviving >25 days was 7300 cells/cu mm.

Cyclosporine Plus Azathioprine Combination (Groups VI–IX)

Seven dogs were transplanted in group VI (CsA 5 mg/kg/day plus Aza 2.5 mg/kg/day). One animal died on the third postoperative day from a large urine leak at the ureteroneocystostomy site. Of the 6 remaining dogs, 3 rejected in the first 10 days following transplant, while 1 dog rejected its allograft 5 weeks after the procedure. Two animals died with functioning allografts, one due to pneumonia and the other with severe anemia and leukopenia. The median graft survival in this group was 22.5 days and the mean WBC of those dogs alive at 25 days was 2500 cells/cu mm.

Six dogs were allografted and immunosuppressed with CsA 7.5 mg/kg/day plus Aza 1.5 mg/kg/day (group VII). Two dogs died on the fourth postoperative day from severe vascular compromise of the graft due to an arterial thrombosis. Only 1 of the remaining 4 animals rejected its allograft and died on the 11th postoperative day. A second dog died with a functioning kidney as a complication of phlebotomy 226 days following transplant. The other two dogs are currently alive with functioning grafts. In this group, the median graft survival time is 226 days and the mean WBC is 9200 cells/cu mm.

Six dogs were immunosuppressed with CsA 10 mg/kg/day plus Aza 1.5 mg/kg/day (group VIII). Three of these dogs are still alive with functioning allografts. Only 1 animal in this group rejected its kidney, while 2 dogs died with functioning grafts, at 64 and 76 days, from pneumonia. The median graft survival in this group is 165.5 days and the mean WBC of the 5 long-term dogs is 4800 cells/cu mm.

In group IX (CsA 10 mg/kg/day plus Aza 2.5 mg/kg/day), 8 dogs were transplanted. Two dogs died on posttransplant days 2 and 3 due to an arterial thrombosis of the graft and intussusception with peritonitis, respectively. Of the remaining 6 dogs, 2 rejected their allograft at 10 and 36 days. One animal died 71 days following transplant with a normal serum creatinine (0.8 mg/dl) from pneumonia. The other 3 animals are presently alive with functioning grafts. This group has a median graft survival of 146.5 days and the mean WBC of the 5 long-term dogs is 4700 cells/cu mm.

Assessing groups VII–IX as a single group with combination immunosuppression, 8 of 16 dogs are presently alive with functioning grafts. Only 4 animals (25%) rejected their transplanted kidneys, while the other 4 had maintained good renal function at the time of death.

Histologic examination of renal tissue revealed a marked monocellular infiltrate in all animals rejecting their allograft. Additionally, large numbers of plasma cells were seen in the renal cortex of some of the animals receiving long-term treatment with CsA. Dogs dying with functioning allografts had no acute cellular infiltrate.

The capability of measuring dog CsA levels was not attained until late in the course of the experiment. Only dogs alive at >200 days had levels measured. Mean trough whole blood CsA measurements according to the doses are shown in Table 1.

DISCUSSION

Cyclosporine, used as a single immunosuppressive agent, can prevent allograft rejection, but the doses required and the drug blood levels necessary to accomplish this may result in toxicity to the kidney and liver.[1,2] Therefore, the clinical use of CsA, combined with prednisone, allows moderate, less toxic doses of each drug to be utilized. This combination has been effective when used to prevent rejection of renal allografts[3,4] and is being utilized as an immunosuppressive regimen for the transplantation of other organs as well.[5–7] Earlier work in our laboratory showed that the combination of CsA and Aza had shown a synergistic effect in 3 of 4 animal models, and the use of CsA 5 mg/kg/day in combination with Aza 2.5 mg/kg/day in a mongrel renal allograft population prolonged graft survival between 3 and 4 times that of either drug alone.[11,13] The primary side effect noted in this model was leukopenia. We have substantiated the synergistic effect of this immunosuppression combination in our study, as well as confirming that infection, secondary to leukopenia, is the major cause of animal loss with a functioning graft.

We have shown previously that splenectomy is a beneficial adjunct in human renal allograft recipients treated with an immunosuppression regimen of antilymphocyte globulin, Aza, and prednisone.[14] It has also been shown to increase tolerance to the myelosuppressive effects of Aza and increase the efficacy of CsA in prolonging graft survival in rat transplant models.[9,15]

There was little difference whether the animals received low doses of CsA (5 mg/kg/day) or Aza (1.5 mg/kg/day) when compared with no immunosuppression at all (Fig. 1). Median graft survival was 1 week, and no graft functioned for more than 15 days. When the dose of CsA was doubled (10 mg/kg/day) or the dose of Aza increased to 2.5 mg/kg/day, median graft survival exceeded 3 weeks. Two of the CsA-treated dogs rejected after 70 days, while 1 of 10 dogs is still alive 8 months following transplant. Of the Aza-treated dogs, none survived more than 50 days. The 3 animals who died with functioning allografts all had respiratory infections, a complication of the leukopenia seen with long-term myelosuppression by Aza. The combina-

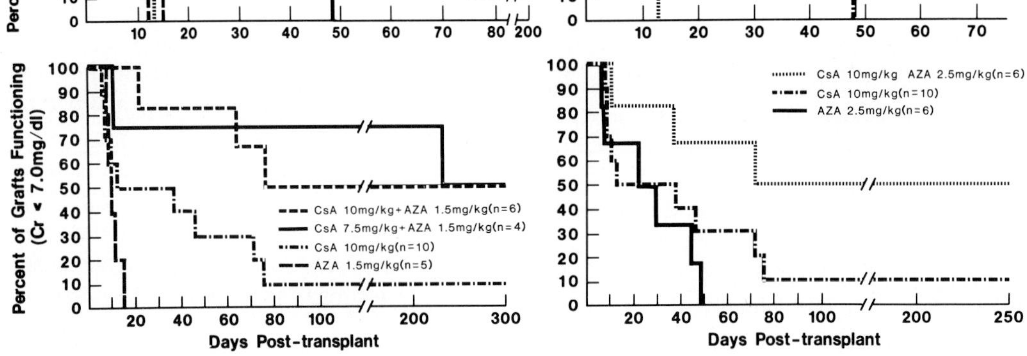

Fig. 1. Functional survival of renal allografts according to treatment groups. (Upper left) Control groups—no immunotherapy, low- and medium-dose CsA, low- and medium-dose Aza. (Upper right) Low-dose CsA and medium-dose Aza, alone and in combination. (Lower left) Medium-dose CsA and low-dose Aza, alone and in combination. (Lower right) Medium-dose CsA and medium-dose Aza, alone and in combination.

tion of CsA 5 mg/kg/day with Aza 2.5 mg/kg/day, as had been used in our earlier study, showed no difference in median graft survival versus Aza at that dose alone (22.5 days versus 24.5 days, $p > 0.1$) (Fig. 1). Four of the 6 dogs in this group rejected their allograft between 1 and 5 weeks following transplant. Once again, myelosuppression was the major factor leading to the deaths of 2 animals with long-term graft function.

Increasing the dose of CsA to 7.5 or 10 mg/kg/day in combination with low- or high-dose Aza markedly prolonged graft survival (Fig. 1). Only 2 of 16 animals (12.5%) acutely (within 2 weeks) rejected their allograft. Two others rejected their kidneys at 3 and 5 weeks. Three of 4 dogs who died with functioning grafts survived at least 2 months and succumbed from respiratory infections and anemia. The other dog died 226 days postoperatively following a technical complication. Eight of the 16 dogs receiving these combinations are presently alive with good graft function at least 7 months following transplant. The median graft survival for each of these three higher CsA dose groups is significantly greater than for either drug used alone or the combination of lower dose CsA plus Aza (group VI) ($p < 0.05$). Taken as a group, the median graft survival of these 16 dogs (groups VII–IX) is 221 days, significantly greater than each of the other groups (groups I–VI) ($p < 0.05$).

Trough whole blood CsA levels were not able to be obtained until late in the course of experimentation, and therefore, were only obtained for dogs who had survived >200 days. The range of the values was between 110 and 1371 ng/ml with 7 of 10 between 110 and 345 ng/ml. The higher results, when obtained in a human, would almost certainly be associated with nephrotoxicity or hepatotoxicity. However, we have been unable to show functional kidney or liver toxicity due to CsA in this dog model. We have studied other dogs with renal allografts and found, on similar immunosuppressive regimens, that animals with trough whole blood CsA levels <100 ng/ml rejected their grafts, a process not always seen when blood concentrations were above that level.

We are uncertain what the plasma cell cytosis in the long-term CsA-treated dogs represents. It may possibly be a CsA-induced nephrotoxicity or may be just part of the rejection morphology, and we are currently exploring this area.

We have shown that combination of CsA and Aza is synergistic as an immunosuppressive regimen in allograft transplantation. This combination would eliminate the long-term use of corticosteroids, with their debilitating side effects. The major problem with our dosages is the myelosuppression seen with the Aza. This could be remedied in the clinical population with proper dosage adjustments according to the patient's response. The therapeutic ratio in any drug combination must be individualized to the patient's own metabolism, and as such, the use of fixed doses, as we have done here, is not clinically consistent. This study has substantiated our earlier work, and we are presently employing other drug combinations in various dose schedules in a mongrel renal allograft model.

ACKNOWLEDGMENT

We would like to thank Kathryn Combs and Frances Rabe for their technical assistance.

REFERENCES

1. White DJG, Calne RY: Immunol Rev 65:115, 1982

2. European Multicentre Trial: Lancet 8289:57, 1982

3. Ferguson RM, Rynasiewicz JJ, Sutherland DER, et al: Surgery 92:175, 1982

4. Starzl TE, Weil R, Iwatsuki S, et al: Surg Gynecol Obstet 151:17, 1980

5. Sutherland DER, Goetz FC, Rynasiewicz JJ, et al: Surgery 90:159, 1981

6. Starzl TE, Klintmalm GBG, Porter KA, et al: N Engl J Med 305:266, 1981

7. Rertz BA, Wallwork MB, Hunt SA, et al: N Engl J Med 306:557, 1982

8. Kjellstrand CM: Transplant Proc 7:123, 1975

9. Rynasiewicz JJ, Sutherland DER, Kawahara K, et al: J Surg Res 30:365, 1981

10. Rynasiewicz JJ, Sutherland DER, Ferguson RM, et al: Diabetes 31 (Suppl 4):92, 1982

11. Squifflet JP, Sutherland DER, Rynasiewicz JJ, et al: Transplantation 34:315, 1982

12. Rynasiewicz JJ, Squifflet JP, Sutherland DER, et al: Surg Forum 33:344, 1982

13. Squifflet JP, Sutherland DER, Field J, et al: Transplant Proc 15:520, 1983

14. Fryd DS, Sutherland DER, Simmons RL, et al: Transplant Proc 13:48, 1981

15. Downing TP, Reitz BA, Aziz S, et al: Transplantation 32:76, 1981

Cyclosporine Enhances an Effect of Donor-Specific Blood Transfusion in Canine Renal Transplantation

T. Ochiai, M. Gunji, M. Nagata, T. Suzuki, K. Enomoto, T. Asano, N. Yamada, H. Sato, and M. Ohtsuka

A BENEFICIAL effect of pretransplant blood transfusion (BT) on graft survival time has been widely observed in humans,[1] rats,[2] mice,[3] monkeys,[4] and dogs.[5,6]

The factors responsible for a beneficial effect of BT on graft survival time are not yet fully understood. However, antigenic stimulations induced by transfused blood must be the first requirement for the following immunologic process. Our previous experiments and those others in the rat[7,8] have shown that cyclosporine (CsA) has the ability to induce donor-specific suppressor cells upon antigenic stimulation of an allograft. These observations have led us to the idea that pretransplant antigenic stimulation by means of donor-specific blood transfusion (DST) or donor splenic tissue extracts, combined with a simultaneous administration of CsA, could induce suppressor cells against a prospective donor graft and result in prolonged graft survival in canine renal transplantation.

In most of the canine experimental models, a beneficial effect was obtained by using third-party BT followed by postoperative administration of immunosuppressants to the recipient.[9] An effect of DST on graft survival time was a matter of debate in the dog. Halatz et al. reported that 2 ml of DST, 10 and 5 days prior to transplantation, prolonged graft survival time as compared with the control dog;[10] however, the result was not repeated by Obertop et al. in DLA-typed dogs.[11] Recently, Iwaki et al. reported that a beneficial effect of DST was seen only when postoperative immunosuppressants were given.[12] In the present experiment, DST and donor splenic tissue extracts were used as stimulating antigens, and the effect of combined treatment of donor antigens and CsA on graft survival time was evaluated. Postoperative immunosuppressants were avoided in order to elucidate the mechanisms of pretransplant antigenic stimulation. The article deals with the experimental result.

MATERIALS AND METHODS

Adult mongrel dogs weighing 15–20 kg were used without tissue typing. The prospective recipient was given 50 ml and 30 ml of DST 10 and 7 days prior to kidney transplantation, respectively. Splenic tissue extracts were prepared by a modification of the method of Shimada and Nathenson.[13] The procedure is outlined in Fig. 1. The extract from one spleen contained 500–1000 mg of protein. It contained the substances with molecular weights of the order of 67,000, 43,000, 20,000, and 10,000, estimated by acrylamide gel electrophoresis. Whole extract from one donor spleen was given i.v. to the prospective recipient 10 days before transplantation.

Cyclosporine, 20 mg/kg/day, was given p.o. to the recipient for 6 days from the day of the first DST or the day of administration of the donor splenic extract until 5 days prior to transplantation; it was discontinued thereafter.

Crossmatch testing was done at 37°C using the one-stage microlymphocytotoxicity test. Kidney transplantation was performed with bilateral nephrectomy. No immunosuppressants were given after kidney transplantation. The day of uremic death was treated as an end-point of the study. Complete histopathologic examination of all the grafts was done routinely. Any dog that died without histologic signs of rejection was excluded from data analysis.

RESULTS

The mean survival of the control dogs was 9.3 ± 3.4 (SD) days. Pretreatment of the recipient with CsA or DST slightly prolonged the mean survival, which was 11.3 ± 4.2 and

From the Department of Surgery, School of Medicine, Chiba University, Chiba, Japan.

Supported in part by a grant from the Department of Health and Welfare, Japan.

Address reprint requests to Dr. T. Ochiai, Department of Surgery, School of Medicine, Chiba University, 1-8-1 Inohana, Chiba, 280, Japan.

0041-1345/83/1505-0136$01.00/0

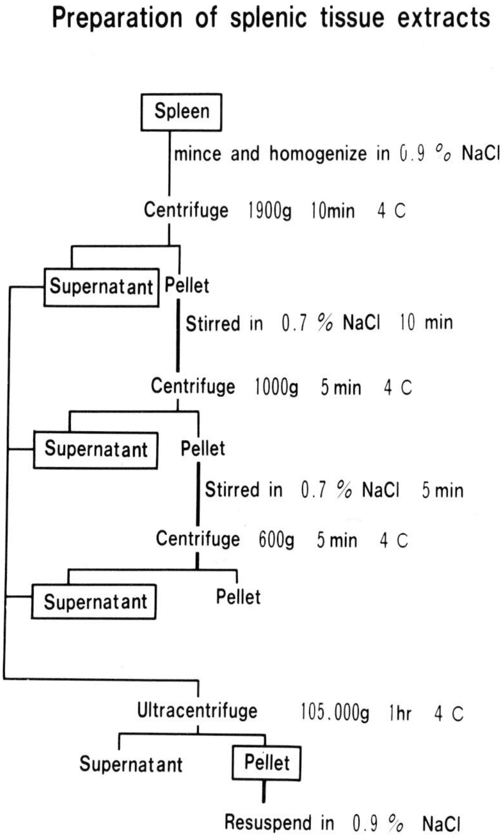

Fig. 1. Schema for preparation of tissue extracts from the spleen of the dog.

13.8 ± 4.3 days, respectively; however, there was no statistical difference compared to the control group (Table 1). The mean survival of the recipient receiving pretreatment with DST and CsA was 25.0 ± 8.7 days. Prolongation of graft survival time by pretransplant DST along with CsA was statistically significant ($p < 0.01$). On the other hand, pretreatment with donor splenic extracts and CsA did not prolong graft survival time statistically.

None of the dogs receiving DST with or without CsA developed cytotoxic antibodies against donor lymphocytes in our experiment. The dog receiving splenic extracts of the donor did not develop positive crossmatch, either.

DISCUSSION

The results obtained in the present experiment indicate that CsA enhanced a DST effect on canine renal transplantation and that it did not help splenic tissue extracts prolong graft survival time. A beneficial effect of BT has been widely accepted in human and experimental animals.[1–6] The mechanisms involved in the phenomenon have not been fully understood. Admitting that a DST effect is brought about by either selection or generation of suppressor cells, antigenic stimulations of BT must be the first trigger in the following process. Combined with CsA, antigenic stimulation of BT has induced some immunologic factors prolonging graft survival time. Even though it is not obvious how antigenic stimulations by BT and suppression of immune response by CsA resulted in prolonged graft survival, our data suggest that selection is not the sole factor for better graft survival, as Iwaki reported previously.[12]

With regard to alloantigens inducing a beneficial effect of BT, our results suggested that antigenic stimulation of splenic tissue extracts was not sufficient for initiation of the process of prolonged graft survival. The question may be raised as to whether our tissue extracts

Table 1. Survival (Days) After Kidney Transplantation and Bilateral Nephrectomy

Pretreatment	No. of Animals	No. of Positive Crossmatches	Survival (Days, Mean ± SD)	Statistical Significance
Nil	10	—	9.3 ± 3.4	
CsA	4	—	11.3 ± 4.2	NS
DST	4	0	13.8 ± 4.3	NS
DST + CsA	8	0	25.0 ± 8.7	$p < 0.01$
Donor tissue extract + CsA	4	0	11.8 ± 4.2	NS

CsA: 20 mg/kg p.o. from day −10 to −5.
DST: 50 ml on day −10 and 30 ml on day −7.
Tissue extracts: 500–1000 mg protein i.v. on day −10.
NS, not significant.

contained transplantation antigens. The methods we used for preparation of tissue extracts were described by Shimada and Natheson.[13] They reported successful solubilization of H-2 alloantigens by this method in the mouse. We did not test the functional characteristics of our tissue extracts; however, the molecular weights of the substances contained in our extracts were similar to their alloantigens.

Several investigators tried to induce prolongation of kidney graft survival by pretreatment with soluble antigens in the dog. Calne et al. reported a negative result,[14] but Wilson et al. succeeded in inducing prolonged graft survival when postoperative immunosuppression was used.[15] Recently, Iwaki et al. transfused a donor-specific spleen membrane instead of BT.[12] The graft survival time of the dog receiving spleen membrane transfusion was not statistically different from the control dog, and their results were consistent with ours.

These results suggest that alloantigens obtained by preparation of the tissue is not enough, but cells or cellular components of blood may play a role for a beneficial effect of BT.

REFERENCES

1. Opelz G, Terasaki PI: Transportation 29:153, 1960

2. Fabre JW, Morris PJ: Transplantation 14:608, 1972

3. Okazaki H, Maki T, Wood ML, et al: Transplantation 29:341, 1980

4. van Es AA, Marquet RL, van Rood JJ, et al: Transplantation 26:325, 1978

5. Fabre JW, Bishop M, Sen T, et al: Transplantation 26:94, 1978

6. Obertop H, Bijnen AB, Vriesendorp HM, et al: Transplantation 26:255, 1978

7. Sakamoto K, Ochiai T, Shinohara N, et al: Transplant Proc (this issue)

8. Hutchinson IF, Shadur CA, Duarte JSA, et al: Transplantation 32:210, 1981

9. Niessen GJCM, Obertop H, Bijnen AB, et al: Transplant Proc 14:400, 1982

10. Halatz NA, Orloff MJ, Hirose F: Transplantation 2:453, 1964

11. Obertop H, Bijnen AB, Vriesendorp HM, et al: Transplantation 26:255, 1978

12. Iwaki Y, Kinukawa T, Terasaki P, et al: Transplant Proc 15:979, 1983

13. Shimada A, Nathenson SG: Biochemistry 8:4048, 1969

14. Calne RY, Davis DR, Medawar SP, et al: Transplantation 4:742, 1966

15. Wilson RE, Rippin A, Dagher TK, et al: Transplantation 7:360, 1969

Immunosuppression of Renal Allograft Rejection by Perioperative Administration of the Combination of Histocompatibility Antigen in the Form of 3M KCl Extract or Blood Transfusion and Cyclosporine

T. Yasumura and B. D. Kahan

THE immunosuppressive effects of cyclosporine (CsA) on organ allograft rejection has been demonstrated in man[1,2] and in animal models.[3-11] Borel[9] suggested that CsA inhibits helper T-cell function, while sparing suppressor T-cell activation. This finding suggested the hypothesis that an agent that acts by specifically stimulating suppressor T cells might function synergistically with CsA to induce unresponsiveness. One possible advantage of the combined therapy would be the induction of a specific endogenous unresponsive state, wherein suppressor T cells would abort T-helper-cell differentiation without the need for continuing CsA chemical suppression. In order to test this hypothesis, CsA was combined with donor 3*M* KCl antigen, since this preparation is known to stimulate both T-helper and T-suppressor arms of the immune response. It was presumed that CsA would dampen the activation of helper cells, while permitting these antigenic preparations to stimulate suppressor cells. In addition, whole blood transfusion was tested as a source of donor histocompatibility antigen.

Because of the present restrictions of cadaveric graft preservation, the regimen was tailored to the peri-transplant period. Preliminary studies, employing 3 *M* KCl extracted donor antigen given 1 day prior to transplantation in combination with a 5-day course of 15 mg/kg/day CsA, achieved specific synergistic prolongation of graft survival in 40% of recipients.[11] Due to the significant degree of immunosuppression achieved by five CsA doses alone, the median graft survival of the entire group was not synergistically prolonged. Therefore, the studies presented herein reduced both the amount of CsA from 15 to 10 mg/kg and the length of treatment from 5 to 3 doses. Moreover, a synergistic effect of donor blood transfusions with CsA was sought, based on evidence suggesting that they induce suppressor cells.[12,13]

From the Division of Immunology and Organ Transplantation, Department of Surgery, University of Texas Medical School, Houston, TX.

Address reprint requests to Dr. T. Yasumura, Division of Immunology and Organ Transplantation, Department of Surgery, University of Texas Medical School, Houston, TX 77030.

0041-1345/83/1505-0137$01.00/0

MATERIALS AND METHODS

Animals

Inbred male rats, weighing 150–300 g, were maintained by ad libitum feedings of laboratory chow. Wistar-Furth (WFu, RT1^u) and Buffalo (Buf, RT1^b) animals were obtained from Microbiological Associates (Bethesda, MD); Brown-Norway (BN, RT1^n) animals were obtained from Charles-River (Boston, MA). Buf kidney allografts were transplanted to WFu rats; BN rats were used as the third-party control.

Renal Transplantation

Allogeneic renal transplantation was performed using a modification of the method of Lee.[14] Briefly, under light ether anesthesia, the donor renal artery attached to the aorta and the donor renal vein were anastomosed end-to-side to the recipient abdominal aorta and inferior vena cava, respectively, using microsurgical technique. A ureteroureterostomy was constructed over a fine 5-mm length polyethylene internal stent. The average total ischemic time was less than 30 min. All recipients were bilaterally nephrectomized. Graft function was assessed by recipient survival and confirmed by histopathologic examination. Statistical evaluation was performed using the Wilcoxon two-sample rank sum test.

3 M KCl Extracted Soluble Antigen

Donor and third-party antigens were prepared from Buf and BN spleen cells by the 3 *M* KCl method, previously described in detail.[15] Rats were injected intravenously (i.v.) with doses of 1.0, 2.5, 5.0, and 10.0 mg protein antigen (Ag) 1 day prior to transplantation.

Blood Transfusions

Blood was obtained from a group of three or more Buf or BN rats via cardiac puncture. Fresh, pooled, whole heparinized blood was injected i.v. into WFu recipients at doses of 0.5, 1.0, 2.0, and 5.0 ml 1 day prior to transplantation.

Cyclosporine

The CsA, donated by Sandoz (Basel, Switzerland) as a white powder, was dissolved in olive oil at a concentration of 20 mg/ml. Rats were administered 10 mg/kg by gavage on the day prior to, on the day of, and 1 day after kidney transplantation.

Mixed Lymphocyte Culture (MLC) and Suppressor Cell Assay

Recipient rats receiving CsA, 10 mg/kg/day for 3 days combined with one 5-mg dose of donor soluble antigen were sacrificed 10 days after transplantation. Peripheral blood lymphocytes (PBL), spleen cells, and lymph node cells were harvested for one-way MLC reactions performed as previously described.[11] For the suppressor cell assay, recipient PBL, spleen cells, and lymph node cells were added as a third cell to MLC reactions containing virgin WFu cells (responder:additional cell ration, 2:1) at the initiation of the reaction. Percent suppression was calculated using the formula:

Percent suppression =

$$\left[\left\{1-\frac{\text{cpm (virgin WFu} + \text{putative suppressor} + \text{stimulator cells)}}{\text{cpm virgin WFu} + \text{cpm (virgin WFu} + \text{stimulator cells)}}\right\}\right] \times 100$$

The statistical significance of the results was assessed by the Student's t test.

Adoptive Transfer of Lymphoid Cells and Serum

In order to detect suppressor cell function in vivo, PBL, spleen cells, lymph node cells, and serum harvested 10 days after transplantation from 3–5 recipients treated with CsA and 5 mg of donor soluble antigen were transferred into secondary recipients. Serial doses 2×10^8, 5×10^8, or 1×10^9 pooled cells, consisting of 2%–4% PBL and 40%–60% spleen and lymph node cells, were administered intravenously to syngeneic secondary recipients 2 days prior to Buf kidney transplantation. The significance of differences in graft survival was assessed by the Wilcoxon rank sum test.

Local Graft Versus Host Reaction (GVHR) Assay

The local GVHR assay was performed by the method of Ford et al.[16] Buf or BN rats that had been treated with 1000 rad of total body irradiation served as inert stimulators of in vivo MLC responses by lymphoid cells inoculated into the right hind footpad. Five groups of 2.5×10^6 responder cells were tested: (1) syngeneic cells, (2) allogeneic virgin WFu cells and allogeneic WFu cells from hosts, (3) 5 days after Buf kidney transplantation without immunosuppression or (4) with CsA treatment or (5) Ag-CsA treatment. Seven days after inoculation, the popliteal nodes were removed from the treated right limb, and the saline-injected left limb. The data were expressed as the ratio of the weights of right versus left popliteal nodes. The significance of differences between weight ratios was assessed by Student's t test.

RESULTS

The Effect of 3M KCl Antigen–CsA Therapy

Renal allograft survival in recipients treated with CsA combined with donor or third-party antigen is shown in Fig. 1. Untreated WFu hosts rejected Buf grafts at 7.1 ± 0.54 days. Administration of Buf or of BN antigen alone did not alter graft survival. CsA given alone at a dose of 10 mg/kg/day for 3 days prolonged graft survival slightly, but significantly, to 11.8 ± 1.82 days ($p < 0.001$). Administration of CsA combined with 2.5 mg donor antigen further prolonged graft survival to 19.3 ± 8.76 days ($p < 0.001$). On the other hand, the group receiving CsA and 2.5 mg of third-party BN antigen displayed the same survival time as the group receiving only CsA. Therefore, donor antigen produced a significant, specific, and synergistic prolongation of graft survival in CsA-treated hosts.

In order to determine the optimal dose of donor antigen, groups of WFu recipients receiving the CsA regimen were treated with various doses of donor antigen, namely 1.0, 2.5, 5, or 10 mg i.v. 1 day prior to Buf kidney transplantation (Fig. 2). Combined therapy with CsA and donor 3*M* KCl antigen at doses

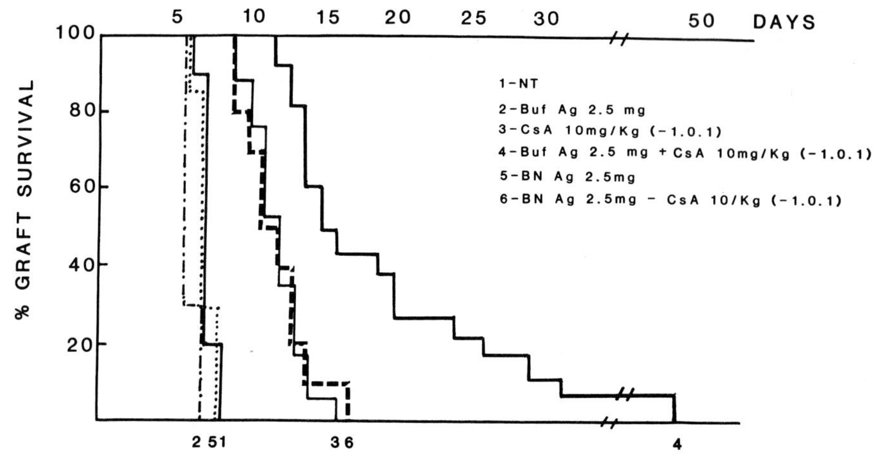

Fig. 1. **The fate of Buffalo (Buf) renal allografts in Wistar-Furth (WFu) hosts that were: (group 1) not treated, (group 2) Buf antigen 2.5 mg alone, (group 3) CsA 10 mg/kg alone, (group 4) Buf antigen and CsA, (group 5) Brown-Norway (BN) antigen only, and (group 6) BN antigen and CsA.**

of 1.0, 2.5, or 5.0 mg yielded mean survival times of 13.4 ± 2.09, 19.3 ± 8.76, and 26.5 ± 13.37 days, respectively. On the other hand, 10 mg antigen produced significantly less prolongation than 5.0 mg ($p < 0.004$); the graft survival after treatment with 10 mg was similar to that observed after 2.5 mg. Therefore, prolongation of graft survival was dependent on 3*M* KCl antigen dose.

The Effect of Donor Blood Transfusions Combined With CsA

The survival time of Buf grafts into WFu recipients pretreated with donor Buf blood transfusion is shown in Fig. 3. While 0.5 ml blood transfusion did not prolong graft survival beyond the time achieved with CsA alone, the 1.0-ml dose achieved the maximal

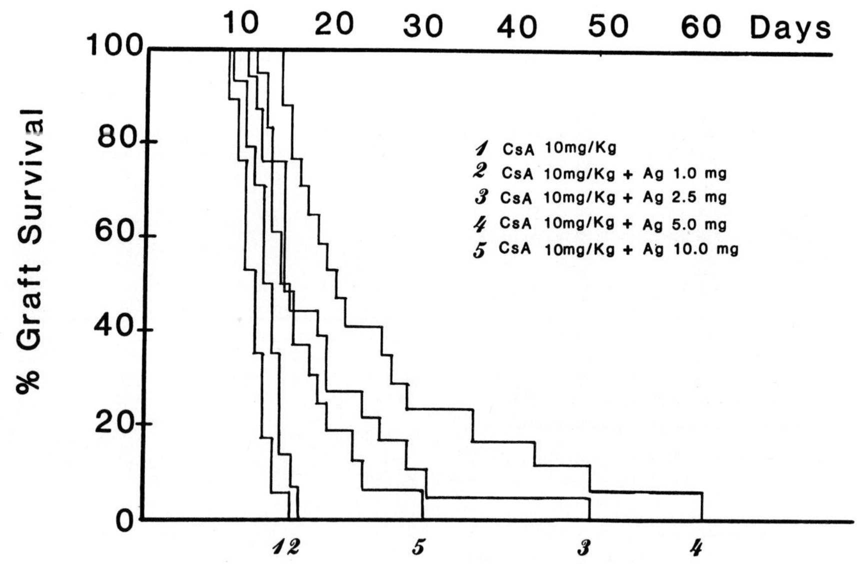

Fig. 2. **The effect of various dose of Buf antigen (Ag) in combination with CsA on graft survival: (group 1) CsA alone, (group 2) added 1.0 mg Ag, (group 3) 2.5 mg Ag, (group 4) 5.0 mg Ag, and (group 5) 10.0 mg Ag.**

8. White DJG, Timmerman W, Davies HHS, et al: Transplant Proc 13:379, 1981

9. Borel JF: Transplant Proc 13:344, 1981

10. Homan WP, Williams KA, Millard PR, et al: Transplantation 31:423, 1981

11. Tsuda T, Kahan BD: Transplantation 55:483, 1983

12. Okazaki H, Maki T, Wood ML, et al: Transplantation 32:111, 1981

13. Kerman RH, Van Buren CT, Payne W, et al: Transplantation 36:50, 1983

14. Lee S: Surgery 61:771, 1967

15. Reisfeld RA, Kahan BD: Fed Proc 29:2034, 1970

16. Ford WL, Burr W, Simonsen M: Transplant Proc 10:258, 1970

17. Green CJ, Allison AC, Precious S: Lancet 2:123, 1979

18. Nagao T, White DJG, Calne RY: Transplantation 33:31, 1982

19. Hutchinson IF, Shadur CA, Duarte A, et al: Transplant Proc 13:412, 1981

Reversal of Kidney and Prevention of Pancreas Transplant Rejection With Cyclosporine in Beagles

G. K. Kyriakides, L. Olson, C. Flaa, and J. Miller

CYCLOSPORINE is a potent immunosuppressive agent that has been shown to prevent rejection in many animal models, as well as in humans.[1,2] Its role in reversing ongoing rejection, however, has not yet been established.

In a previous study of simultaneous kidney and pancreas transplants between littermate beagles with low mixed lymphocyte culture (MLC) reactivity without immunosuppression, we demonstrated that kidney rejection (serum creatinine elevation) occurred between 4 and 26 days after transplantation, with pancreatic rejection (hyperglycemia) occurring 6–22 days (mean 10 days) later. Furthermore, institution of azathioprine and steroid therapy at the time of the onset of elevated creatinine was successful in preventing the manifestation of pancreatic rejection in 4 of 9 animals,[3] which otherwise occurred inexorably.

The purpose of the present study was to evaluate the effectiveness of cyclosporine in reversing ongoing kidney rejection and in preventing pancreatic rejection in this simultaneous kidney-pancreas allotransplant model.

MATERIALS AND METHODS

The animals used were DLA-identical littermate beagles with low MLC reactivity (stimulation index <2). Tissue typing and in vitro methods have been previously described.[4] Recipient animals underwent bilateral nephrectomy and total pancreatectomy, followed immediately by simultaneous renal and free-draining segmental pancreas transplants (FDPS) from the same donor. The surgical techniques were previously described in detail.[5,6] The serum creatinine and fasting blood sugar were determined daily. Kidney rejection was ascertained by an elevation of serum creatinine by >1.0 mg/dl from baseline and open biopsy at that time. Pancreatic rejection was determined by a rise of fasting blood sugar to >250 mg/dl. In the immediate postoperative period, no immunosuppression was used. Cyclosporine intervention (25 mg/kg/day) was started at the time of serum creatinine elevation. No steroids were used.

Open biopsies of both kidney and pancreatic allografts were performed both at the time of creatinine elevation and again two weeks after initiation of cyclosporine therapy.

Immunologic monitoring consisted of serial pre- and postoperative MLC assays, as well as cell-mediated lympholysis (CML) and antibody-dependent cellular cytotoxicity (ADCC) assays.

RESULTS

There was no operative mortality, and survival ranged from 20 to 140 days following transplantation (Table 1). Deaths were due to pneumonia. Kidney rejection occurred between 12 and 43 days posttransplantation (mean 26 ± 5 days). Seven of 8 never developed hyperglycemia. The serum creatinine elevation was reversed within 7 days of institution of cyclosporine. The course of one such animal is illustrated in Fig. 1. One animal died of terminal hyperglycemia on day 59 posttransplant, with a serum creatinine elevation at this time. Renal histology at the time of rejection showed extensive diffuse mononuclear cell infiltration. Pancreatic histology also revealed extensive mononuclear cell infiltration, but the islets appeared to be spared, as previously described.[3] The repeat biopsies 2 weeks later demonstrated moderate clearing of mononuclear cells from both renal and pancreatic grafts, with islets still spared. However, there were still some residual cellular infiltrates around perivascular areas (markedly more pronounced than in the previous study using azathioprine and steroid intervention rather than cyclosporine[3]).

From the Department of Surgery, University of Miami School of Medicine, Miami, FL.

Supported in part by National Institutes of Health Grant R01 AM 25243 and by VA research support.

Address reprint requests to Dr. G. K. Kyriakides, Department of Surgery, University of Miami School of Medicine, P.O. Box 016310, Miami, FL 33101.

0041-1345/83/1505-0138$01.00/0

Table 1. Survival of Simultaneous Kidney-Pancreas Transplants Treated With Cyclosporine Versus Azathioprine and Steroids at Onset of Rejection

Animals	Rejection (Days) Kidney	Rejection (Days) Pancreas	Survival (Days)
Cyclosporine intervention			
58453	39	0	74
58588	26	0	60
77119	14	0	140
77151	38	0	58
77178	16	0	100
79235	22	0	40
73521	12	0	20
73547	43	59	59
Azathioprine and steroid intervention*			
53696	16,21,36†	0	37
53693	45	55	56
33691	19	0	260+
58545	19,29†	0	58
53528	27,33†	40	40
52892	19	23	71
58550	23,29†	30	33
58590	19	0	73+
58594	17	46	80

*Data previously reported.

†Creatinine elevations occurred at those times at which Solu-Medrol treatment was reinstituted.

Table 2. CML Monitoring*

Animal	Preop	Prerejection	1-2 Weeks Postrejection	>3 Weeks Postrejection
58453	0	0	6	0
58588	0	0	7	0
77119	0	1	1	0
77151	0	4	13	—
77178	0	0	4	0
79235	0	44	0	0
73521	0	0	4	—
73547	0	5	—†	1

*All values expressed as percent specific ^{51}Cr release; >5% considered positive.

†Data not obtained.

The MLC remained low following transplantation. The CML was negative preoperatively in all animals (Table 2). Reactions remained negative until just prior to rejection in all but one animal (No. 79235), and then turned positive in three animals within 2 weeks following the onset of rejection. After reversal of rejection with cyclosporine, the CML reactions became negative again in all animals tested. A similar, but more pronounced, pattern was observed with the ADCC test (Table 3).

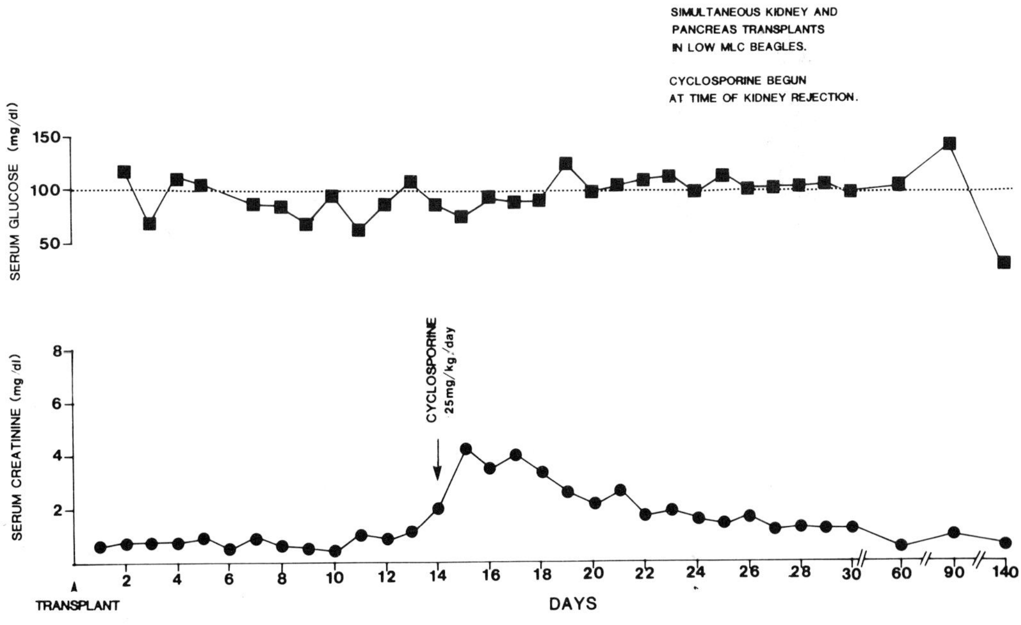

Fig. 1. Serum creatinine and fasting blood sugar in animal no. 77119. Institution of cyclosporine at the time of rise in serum creatinine reversed kidney rejection and prevented hyperglycemia.

Table 3. ADCC Monitoring*

Animal	Preop	Prerejection	1–2 Weeks Postrejection	>3 Weeks Postrejection
58453	0	0	22	—
58588	0	0	17	0
77119	0	0	42	0
77151	0	0	7	0
77178	0	11	0	0
79235	—†	—	—	—
73521	—	—	—	—
73547	0	15	—	0

*All values expressed as percent specific ^{51}Cr release; >5% considered positive.

†Data not obtained.

DISCUSSION

In a previous report of combined kidney-pancreas transplants in low MLC reactive donor–recipient pairs, we concluded that the serum creatine elevation was a sensitive indicator of the rejection process occurring in both the kidney and the pancreas allografts, and this preceded the onset of hyperglycemia by 6–22 days (mean 10.6 ± 4.6 days). Institution of immunosuppression with azathioprine and prednisone at the time of creatinine elevation reserved the rejection of the kidney and prevented hyperglycemia in slightly less than half of the animals. This recovery was accompanied by significant clearing of cellular infiltrates from both renal and pancreatic grafts within 2 weeks of the institution of therapy.

In the present study using animals with similarly good histocompatibility, it has appeared that cyclosporine alone is even more effective than the azathioprine-steroid combination in reversing ongoing acute rejection, although deaths due to immunosuppression (bacterial pneumonia) occurred. This property of cyclosporine has not been extensively described, although MacDonald et al. recently reported similar findings in humans.[7] This effect of cyclosporine may be of clinical relevance in patients who undergo repeated rejections unresponsive to other antirejection medications. We have treated 12 kidney transplant patients in this manner, with gratifying results.

The immune monitoring findings in this study are consistent with an effect of the agent on both cellular and antibody-mediated immunity.

The nature of the residual cellular infiltrate observed in both the kidney and pancreas following treatment with cyclosporine is not clear. We suspect that these cells may be suppressor in function. Studies are now in progress to characterize them after enzymatic extraction from the grafts.

REFERENCES

1. Calne RY, Rolles K, White DJG, et al: Lancet 1:1183, 1978

2. Calne RY, Rolles K, Thiru S, et al: Lancet 2:1033, 1979

3. Severyn W, Olson L, Miller J, et al: Transplantation 33:606, 1982

4. Kyriakides GK, Rabinovitch A, Mintz D, et al: J Clin Invest 67:292, 1981

5. Kyriakides GK, Sutherland D, Olson L, et al: Transplant Proc 11:530, 1979

6. Miller J, Pierce J, Varco RL: Surgery 119:811, 1964

7. MacDonald AS, Belitsky P, Cohen AD, et al: Transplant Proc (this issue)

Inhibition of Chronic Kidney Allograft Rejection by Cyclosporine

R. L. Marquet, W. Weimar, E. Heineman, and J. Jeekel

IT IS well established that cyclosporine A (CsA) is most effective in preventing organ allograft rejection when given during the induction phase of the immune response. In some models (graft-versus-host reaction and autoimmune diseases), it has been found that CsA can also suppress the effector phase.[1] However, for organ grafts, the interference of CsA with an ongoing rejection process has, thus far, not clearly been demonstrated. The present study was undertaken to investigate whether, in rats, treatment with CsA would inhibit the progression of chronic kidney graft rejection.

MATERIALS AND METHODS

Animals. Male rats of the inbred WAG ($RT1^u$) and BN ($RT1^n$) strains were used. The animals were bred under specific pathogen-free conditions, were 12–16 weeks old, and weighed 200–250 g.

Transplantation. Kidney transplantation in the BN to WAG combination was performed as described earlier.[2] Bilateral nephrectomy was performed at the time of transplantation.

Blood transfusions. Recipients were injected i.v. with 1 ml of fresh whole BN blood 7–14 days before kidney transplantation.

Immunosuppression. CsA (generously supplied by Sandoz Inc., Basel, Switzerland) was dissolved in olive oil at 70°C by constant stirring for 2 hr and administered i.m. in a volume of 0.1 ml.

Induction of chronic kidney graft rejection. Two different methods were applied to induce chronic graft rejection. The first method was pretreatment of WAG recipients with 1 ml of donor-specific BN blood 7–14 days before kidney transplantation. This procedure leads to prolonged acceptance of kidney allografts.[3] About 40% of the kidneys are rejected in 4 weeks, whereas 60% of the grafts are rejected chronically, leading to survival times that range from 60 to >200 days. A major feature of the rejection process is the occurrence of obliterative arteritis. The second method to evoke chronic rejection was treatment of WAG recipients with a single dose of 15 mg/kg CsA on the day of kidney transplantation. In the BN to WAG combination, this treatment leads to prolonged, but not indefinite, organ graft survival.[4]

Experimental procedure. WAG recipients were either conditioned with a single injection of BN blood (18 animals) or were treated on the day of grafting with 15 mg/kg CsA (25 animals). At 30 days after transplantation, the surviving animals with a serum creatinine (SCr) level below 300 μ mole/liter were divided into two groups. One group was treated with 15 mg/kg CsA on alternate days for 3 weeks; the other group received no treatment. SCr levels were determined regularly.

RESULTS

Chronic Rejection After Blood Transfusions

At 30 days after grafting, 6 of 18 animals had rejected their kidney in an acute fashion. The remaining animals were divided into two groups; 6 recipients were treated with CsA; the second group remained untreated. The mean SCr levels of the two groups was 106 ± 19 and 110 ± 21 μmole/liter, respectively. All 6 animals in the CsA-treated group survived for more than 100 days, whereas only 2 animals in the control group survived that period. The other 4 animals died at 46, 65, 78, and 93 days after transplantation, with SCr levels of >450 (Table 1). During the period of treatment with CsA, the SCr level of the experimental animals increased from 106 ± 19 to 155 ± 46, which decreased to 121 ± 31 after discontinuation of CsA (Table 2). The mean SCr after 110 days was 102 ± 44. At that time, the SCrs of the two surviving animals from the control group were 148 and 112.

Chronic Rejection After CsA Treatment

Thirty days after kidney transplantation, 18 of 25 animals treated with a single injection of CsA were still alive. None of the kidneys had been acutely rejected, and graft

From the Department of Surgery and Internal Medicine, Erasmus University, Rotterdam, The Netherlands.

Address reprint requests to Dr. R. L. Marquet, Laboratory for Experimental Surgery, Erasmus University, P.O. Box 1738, 3000 DR Rotterdam, The Netherlands.

0041-1345/83/1505-0139$01.00/0

Table 1. Kidney Allograft Survival Times in Blood-Conditioned Recipients Treated After 30 Days With CsA

Treatment	Survival Times (Days)
—	46, 65, 78, 93, >100 (2×)
CsA	>100 (6×)

CsA treatment started 30 days after kidney transplantation and was given at a dose of 15 mg/kg, on alternate days, for 3 weeks.

loss was due to technical complications only. The 18 recipients were divided into two groups; one group was treated with CsA for 3 weeks; the second group was not treated. The SCr levels in the first group ranged from 82 to 220 μmole/liter, in the second group, they ranged from 72 to 240. Five of 9 animals in the CsA-treated group survived for more than 100 days; in the control group, 4 of 9 recipients became long-term survivors (Table 3). The SCr levels during CsA administration increased from 149 ± 55 to 171 ± 46 μmole/liter. This increase was mainly the result of temporary rises in animals with relatively high preexisting SCr levels (>125 μmole/liter). The SCr in the control group remained stable (Table 4).

DISCUSSION

The present results indicate that CsA, apart from being a potent immunosuppressant in naive and sensitized recipients,[5] can, under certain circumstances, inhibit the progression of a chronic rejection process. The effect of CsA apparently was dependent on the impact of preceding therapy. In blood-conditioned animals that received no immediate postoperative immunosuppression, the effect of CsA

Table 3. Kidney Allograft Survival Times in Recipients Treated With CsA on the Day of Grafting and From Day 30 Onwards

Treatment	Survival Times (Days)
—	53, 76, 87, 89, 93, >100 (4×)
CsA	62, 67, 72, 78, >100 (5×)

See legend Table 1.

treatment was of some benefit. However, in the group that was treated with a single dose of CsA, additional CsA administration at a later stage had no effect. The reason for this discrepancy is not clear, but it is likely to be related to differences in the mechanisms of the ongoing processes. The predominant feature of rejection after a donor-specific blood transfusion in the BN to WAG combination is the occurrence of obliterative arteritis. This phenomenon is assumed to be caused by antibody-mediated rejection. In animals treated with a single dose of CsA, rejection seemed to be postponed and retarded rather than modified, as both abundant cellular infiltration and vascular lesions could be noticed in rejecting kidneys. It is a remarkable and unexpected finding that, especially in the first situation, which is known to be drug-insensitive, CsA could inhibit the progression of the rejection process. It is conceivable that a higher dose of CsA would have been effective also in the second experimental setting.

In summary, the results of this pilot study suggest that CsA may inhibit the occurrence of chronic kidney graft rejection and warrant a further exploration of this subject. The impaired function during CsA treatment apparently was due to a nephrotoxic effect of the drug. However, this nephrotoxicity was mild and readily reversible.

Table 2. SCr Levels in Recipients Conditioned With Donor-Type Blood and Treated After 30 Days With CsA

Treatment	SCr Day 30	SCr Day 45	SCr Day 60
—	110 ± 21	164 ± 62	215 ± 78
CsA	106 ± 19	155 ± 46	121 ± 31

See legend Table 1.

Table 4. SCr Levels in Kidney Allograft Recipients Treated With CsA on the Day of Grafting and From Day 30 Onwards

Treatment	SCr Day 30	SCr Day 45	SCr Day 60
—	145 ± 65	142 ± 50	150 ± 58
CsA	149 ± 55	171 ± 46	168 ± 57

See legend Table 1.

REFERENCES

1. Morris PJ: Transplantation 32:349, 1981
2. Tinbergen WJ: Transplantation 6:203, 1968
3. Marquet RL, Heystek GA, Tinbergen WJ: Transplant Proc 3:708, 1971
4. Heineman E, Marquet RL, Jeekel J: Transplantation 36, 1983
5. Marquet RL, Heystek GA, Cobussen A, et al: Transplant Proc 15:518, 1983

HEART AND LUNG

Orthotopic Cardiac Transplantation in the Cyclosporine-Treated Neonate

L. Bailey, Z. Li, F. Lacour-Gayet, P. Perier, D. Killeen, J. Perry, C. Schmidt, H. Roost, and W. Jolley

EFFICACY of orthotopic cardiac transplantation (OCT) during infancy and childhood has yet to be established. Kantrowitz and Cooley ventured into infant cardiac and cardiopulmonary transplantation without success.[1,2] Supportive research data in this age group did not exist then and remains noticeably absent today. During the past 6 years, well over 100 neonatal OCTs have been accomplished in the Surgical Research Laboratories at Loma Linda University.[3] Newborn goats have been recipients, and donors have included neonatal goats, lambs, and piglets. This report summarizes our initial experience using cyclosporine A (CsA) (Sandoz, Ltd., Basel, Switzerland) as the only immunosuppressive agent for treating 13 of 21 neonatal goat recipients surviving OCT in 1982.

MATERIALS AND METHODS

Twenty-one neonatal (<7 days of age) goat recipients underwent OCT during the spring of 1982. Animals weighed between 3 and 4 kg at the time of surgery. Donor cardiac grafts were obtained from 13 nonrelated newborn goats of differing subspecies (ALLO) and from 8 newborn lambs (HETERO). Operations were accomplished utilizing hypothermic circulatory arrest and limited extracorporeal circulation. All blood for transfusion was irradiated with 2000 rad prior to use. Donor grafts were obtained by inflow occlusion, preserved with cold cardioplegic infusion, and stored in saline at 4°C. Graft cold ischemic time varied from 60 to 90 min. Host circulatory arrest for implantation varied between 35 and 50 min. Graft implantation was accomplished with running 7–0 monofilament suture for all anastomoses. Study hosts are those who survived the first 4 postoperative (P-OP) days, i.e., survived surgery.

Each host received CsA 48 and 24 hr prior to transplantation (25 mg/kg i.m. for ALLO and 50 mg/kg i.m. for HETERO). Recipients were injected with 125 mg of methylprednisolone (Upjohn, Kalamazoo, MI) on the day of surgery. Cefamandole (Eli Lilly, Indianapolis, IN) in divided doses was administered on the day of surgery and for 48 hr P-OP. Each donor animal was injected with 200 mg of azathioprine 48 hr prior to surgery, then given 3 mg/kg of heparin (Upjohn), 125 mg of methylprednisolone, and 250 mg cefamandole at the time of anesthesia for removal of the cardiac graft. Postoperatively, each surviving recipient was administered CsA by rigid protocol on a gradually reduced schedule. Dosage protocol for administration of CsA for both ALLO and HETERO hosts is summarized in Fig. 1. CsA dissolved in Miglyol (Kay-Fries Chemical, Montvale, NJ) was administered by intramuscular injection throughout the course of these experiments. All surviving animals were bottle fed with pooled nonpasteurized goat's milk. Chronic survivors were weaned to alfalfa and feed pellets at approximately 3 months of age.

RESULTS

Eight of 13 ALLO recipients and 5 of 8 HETERO recipients survived operation Fig.

From the Cardiovascular Surgical Research Laboratory, Loma Linda University, Loma Linda, CA.

Supported entirely by the Faculty of the Department of Surgery, Loma Linda University School of Medicine.

Address reprint requests to Dr. L. L. Bailey, Department of Surgery, Director, Pediatric Cardiac Surgery, Loma Linda University Medical Center, Loma Linda, CA 92350.

0041–1345/83/1505–0140$01.00/0

POSTOPERATIVE IMMUNE SUPPRESSION

Cyclosporin-A

ALLOGRAFTED Hosts		HETEROGRAFTED Hosts	
Days	Dosage (mg/kg)	Days	Dosage (mg/kg)
1-21	25 daily	1-14	50 daily
22-60	25 QOD	15-60	Alternate 50 & 25 daily
61-120	10 QOD	61-90	25 daily
121-365	5 QOD	91-120	23 QOD
>365	None	121-365	10 QOD

Fig. 1. Dosage regimen of Cyclosporine A used for postoperative immunosuppression of newborn recipients having orthotopic cardiac transplantation.

2). Immediate perioperative mortality resulted from a variety of lethal mechanisms, including hypovolemic shock (1), cerebral vascular accident (1), respiratory insufficiency (2), acute ileo-ileal intussusception (2), low cardiac output syndrome (1), and venacaval thrombosis (1).

Six ALLO recipients survived 177, 75, 43, 23, 8, and 6 days. One female recipient remains alive and well at 350 days P-OP. One male recipient was alive and well at 365 P-OP days, at which time CsA was discontinued. During the ensuing 45 days, he began to show evidence of chronic graft rejection, including loss of coat lustre, listlessness, poor appetite, dyspnea on exertion, and cardiomegaly and perihilar infiltrates on chest roentgenography. CsA was reinstituted at 50 mg/kg for 1 week and then reduced to 5 mg/kg every other day. Although still alive, this animal continues to have evidence of reduced cardiac output. His exercise tolerance remains poor, and he has chronic ascites and persistent cardiomegaly.

Autopsy examination and microscopic analysis of cardiac grafts revealed chronic graft rejection for those ALLO recipients surviving 177 and 75 days. Graft rejection was not identified in those animals surviving 43, 23, 8, and 6 days. The animal surviving 43 days was anemic. Two packets of washed red blood cells were obtained from previously irradiated whole blood. Although laboratory crossmatching with the recipient animal showed compatibility for the first packet of washed red blood cells, there was some question about compatibility with the second packet. The animal became severely dyspneic and died during administration of the second packet of washed red blood cells. His cardiac graft showed no evidence of graft rejection on day 43 P-OP. The remaining 3 animals died of severe relapsing gastroenteritis, the etiology of

NEONATAL HOST SURVIVAL

ALLOGRAFTED Hosts		HETEROGRAFTED Hosts	
Days	Cause of Death	Days	Cause of Death
445	Alive	72	Gastroenteritis
350	Alive	34	Gastroenteritis
177	Chronic Rejection	27	Chronic Rejection
75	Chronic Rejection	15	Gastroenteritis
43	Transfusion Reaction	13	Gastroenteritis
23, 8, 6	Gastroenteritis		

Fig. 2. Survival data among newborn allografted and heterografted hosts subjected to orthotopic cardiac transplantation. Note graft rejection was infrequent cause of death.

which remains obscure. Three chronically surviving ALLO recipients had mixed lymphocyte reactions accomplished. These data were interpreted as suggesting suppression of T cytotoxic cell formation and augmentation of suppressor T-cell activity.

Five HETERO recipients survived 72, 34, 27, 15, and 13 days (mean 32 days). Only one of these recipients died of graft rejection at 27 days. HETERO hosts surviving 34 and 72 days showed minimal chronic graft rejection, virtually limited to the epicardial surface of the myocardial wall. HETERO recipients surviving 13 and 15 days showed no graft rejection. Four of the 5 HETERO recipients died of chronic relapsing severe gastroenteritis, similar to that responsible for deaths of 3 ALLO recipients. Cultures for bacterial, viral, and fungal pathogens were persistently negative. Autopsy examination of the animals dying of gastroenteritis revealed severe inflammation of both large and small bowel and one animal had acute necrotizing gastritis. Most animals dying of this complication showed prominent mesenteric lymphadenitis.

Infection among survivors was limited to 1 ALLO host that developed a purulent wound abscess during the second P-OP week. The wound was widely opened, drained, and allowed to heal by secondary intention. This recipient is presently alive at 445 days. Neoplasm has not been identified in any host, despite careful autopsy examination.

Growth and development of long-term ALLO survivors has been excellent to date, including graft and anastomotic growth. No cardiac inflow or outflow tract obstructions have been identified among chronically surviving animals.

DISCUSSION

Survival among animals in these two experimental groups is compared to survival among similar control ALLO and HETERO recipients previously reported.[3] Nine of 16 control hosts survived OCT as newborns, including 7 ALLO and 2 HETERO recipients. Control recipients received no immunosuppression. Control ALLO hosts survival was 167, 62, 45, 25, 21, and 9 days (mean 53 days). All control ALLO hosts died of subacute or chronic graft rejection. Two control HETERO recipients survived 5 and 7 days, dying of acute graft rejection. There was no statistically significant difference in survival between ALLO control hosts and ALLO recipients treated with CsA. There were significantly fewer cardiac deaths among the CsA treated group ($p < 0.002$). CsA significantly improved survival among HETERO hosts ($p < 0.04$). Minimal chronic graft rejection limited to the epicardial surface of the HETERO recipient surviving 72 days was particularly impressive.

These data tend to confirm the notion that neonates have relatively immature, albeit competent, immune systems. This immaturity is expressed as delayed graft rejection in nonimmunosuppressed hosts in the form of chronic graft rejection among ALLO recipients and acute rejection responses in HETERO recipients. Hyperacute rejections were not observed among either control or experimental groups. Neonates are, therefore, unique models for OCT. In some instances, long-term survival and growth is observed with a minimum of chronic immunosuppression. Complications other than gastrointestinal (among experimental animals) were notably absent from both control and experimental groups. Prolonged survival among several HETERO recipients is genuinely exciting.

Additional new information observed in this experimental setting is the virtually normal growth and development of ALLO recipients grafted in early infancy. It is clear from this series of experiments that newborn animals subjected to OCT by simple, well established techniques demonstrate adequate growth and function as they mature. There is no suggestion in our yearling survivors that anastomatic modifications will be necessary.

The hope for permanent graft tolerance has not been realized in this series of experiments. The ALLO host surviving 445 days developed clear evidence of graft rejection following discontinuation of CsA at the end of 1 P-OP year. This animal maintained a relative state of graft tolerance during his second 6 months of survival, while receiving remarkably small doses of CsA (5 mg/kg every other day). The female ALLO recipient, now at 350 days, shows no clinical or radiographic evidence of graft rejection. She has grown well and has excellent exercise tolerance. She has received only 5 mg/kg of CsA every other day since November 1982. She will be maintained on CsA at this level throughout the second year. There can only be speculation regarding the fate of both her graft and her fetus when she is bred in the fall of this year while still receiving CsA in reduced dosage.

SUMMARY

CsA given by rigid protocol in reduced dosages as the sole immunosuppressive agent did not statistically improve host survival among neonatal goats undergoing ALLO OCT as compared to control animals.

Administration of CsA by rigid protocol in reduced dosages significantly improved survival among neonatal HETERO OCT hosts as compared to control animals.

CsA significantly reduced death from cardiac graft rejection among neonatal recipients following both ALLO and HETERO OCT.

Long-term growth and development of both host and graft is feasible following OCT during neonatal life.

Serious infection was negligible and neoplasm absent among CsA-treated neonatal hosts undergoing OCT.

Immune tolerance following discontinuation of CsA was not observed at 12 postoperative months.

ACKNOWLEDGMENT

The authors wish to express their admiration and appreciation to the technical staff of the Loma Linda University Surgical Research Laboratories, including: Geoffrey Visbal, Joyce Ivy, Frank Rincon, Jan Smallwood, and Cindy Ghareaghadji for virtually thousands of hours of devoted effort to see these experiments to fruition. Dr. F. Rene Modglin, pathologist, has been particularly helpful in providing microscopic tissue analysis.

REFERENCES

1. Kantowitz A, Haller JD, Joos H, et al: Am J Cardiol 22:782, 1968

2. Cooley DA, Bloodwell RD, Hallman GL, et al: Ann Thorac Surg 8:30, 1969

3. Bailey LL, Lacuour-Gayet F, Perier P, et al: Proceedings of Beijing Symposium on Cardiothoracic Surgery. Copublished by China Academic and Wiley, New York, 1982, pp 342–350

Benefit From Circadian Timing of Cyclosporine Revealed by Delay of Rejection of Murine Heart Allograft

M. Cavallini, G. Magnus, F. Halberg, L. Tao, M. Y. Field, R. Sibley, J. S. Najarian, and D. E. R. Sutherland

CYCLOSPORINE (CsA) is a hydrophobic 11 amino acid cyclic polypeptide,[1] produced by two soil fungi, soluble in lipids or organic solvents, that was found to have immunosuppressive properties by Borel et al.[2,3] at Sandoz, Ltd. (Basel, Switzerland). Studies in experimental animals by Calne et al.[4] and other investigators[5] showed that CsA could prevent or greatly delay the onset of organ allograft rejection.

The mechanism of action of CsA is not well understood. The drug depresses humoral and cellular immunity, with a preferential and reversible action against T lymphocytes.[6,7] These effects are not accompanied by the bone marrow depression that is frequent during treatment with azathioprine. Among its side effects, recent clinical trials have shown nephrotoxicity and hepatotoxicity at the usual therapeutic doses in transplanted patients.[8–10] The aim of this study is to improve the toxic:therapeutic ratio of CsA by exploiting any dependence of outcome on the stage of the patient's renal, hepatic, and other circadian subsystems at treatment time.[11]

Predictably rhythmic changes of an organism can serve to enhance the desired effect and/or reduce the undesired effect, thereby improving the toxic:therapeutic ratio.[11] Time-dependent tolerance and efficacy has been documented for the toxic:therapeutic ratio of doxorubicin and the LD_{50} of whole body irradiation.[11–13] The approach by timing also relates to the clinical utilization of CsA, not only in order to reduce its toxicity, but also to improve the therapeutic effect in a murine heart allograft model.

From the Departments of Surgery and Laboratory Medicine and Pathology, University of Minnesota, Minneapolis, MN.

Supported in part by U.S. National Institutes of General Medical Sciences (GM-13981), Cancer (CA-14445) and Arthritis, Diabetes, Digestive and Kidney Diseases (AM13083). M.C. is a recipient of a fellowship from Istituto Pasteur, Fondazione Cenci-Bolognetti.

Address reprint requests to Dr. F. Halberg, 5-187 Lyon Laboratories, University of Minnesota Health Sciences Center, Minneapolis, MN 55455.

0041-1345/83/1505-0141$01.00/0

MATERIALS AND METHODS

Toxicity Study

Eighteen male inbred Lewis rats (RT1[l]), 8–11 months of age, were singly housed in cages measuring 26 × 16 × 17 cm. These cages were placed in sound-dampened environmental chambers maintained at 24 ± 1°C temperature and 50% ± 3% relative humidity. Light alternated with darkness every 12 hr (LD 12:12). Water and Purina Rat Chow were freely available. In 12 rats, CsA, in a 90% Intralipid and 10% ethanol solution (4 mg/ml), was injected daily in a single interperitoneal dose of 20 mg/kg body weight at 1 of 6 time points, 4 hr apart (2 animals per time point). These time points are expressed as hours after light on (HALO) (02, 06, 10, 14, 18, or 22). At the same time points, 6 control rats (1 rat per time point) received the same amount of vehicle (V) used for CsA injection (90% Intralipid–ethanol solution) (5 ml/kg/day, i.p.). Injections started on May 9, 1982. Intraperitoneal temperature was telemetered every 10 min from implanted transensors.[14] Hourly averages of these data were analyzed by the single cosinor method.[15]

CsA injections were continued until the animal died. Body weight and blood urea nitrogen (BUN) were checked every day and every other day, respectively.

On the day of the death of the animal, a biopsy of kidney, liver, and lung was performed for a histologic evaluation of tissue damage.

Immunosuppression—Study I

In July 1982, 18 male Lewis inbred rats (RT1[l]), 2–2.5 months of age, maintained under the experimental conditions comparable to those described for the toxicity study, received a heterotopic intraabdominal heart allograft from ACI (RT1[a]) rats. Transplantation was performed by anastomosing end-to-side the aorta and pulmonary artery of the graft to the aorta and vena cava of the recipient, respectively.[16] Revascularization of the graft was followed by satisfactory contraction of the heart. In a previous study, such a heart isograft was functioning after 200 days. Beginning on the day of transplantation, 12 animals were treated with CsA (1.25 mg/kg/day, i.p.) at 1 of 6 4-hr time points (2 animals per time point) (02, 06, 10, 14, 18, 22 HALO). Six placebo-treated rats were given the same amount of V i.p. (0.31 ml/kg/day) at the same time points (1 animal per time point). As for the toxicity study, intraperitoneal temperature was automatically recorded every 10 min by means of telemetry from implanted transensors. Rejection time was defined as the first day of cessation of palpable graft heart beat and was confirmed by laparotomy and graft histology.

Immunosuppression—Study II

In November 1982, study 1 was replicated on 18 male inbred Lewis rats, 2–2.5 months of age, with all the experimental conditions similar to those described above, except for the season.

RESULTS

Toxicity Study

Mean survival times were 27.5 ± 10.6 and 43.4 ± 11.4 days for the rats treated with CsA during the dark span (14–22 HALO) and during the light span (02–10 HALO), respectively ($p < 0.05$). As compared to the pretreatment value, after 2 weeks of treatment (2 days before the first animal died), the circadian mesor (rhythm-adjusted mean) of core temperature for placebo-treated animals had not changed. The difference in mesor was 0.03 ± 0.09°C. For CsA-treated rats, the difference, on the average, was a decrease of −1.04 ± 0.85°C ($p < 0.01$). The particular test time to check on the hypothermic effects of CsA (2 days prior to the death of the first rat) was picked in view of the hypothermia noted in rodents for several days preceding death (Table 1).

Animals treated with CsA during the dark span showed a larger temperature drop (−1.64 ± 0.66°C) than did those treated during the light span (−0.44 ± 0.55°C) ($p < 0.01$). The fit of a 24-hr cosine function to the changes in temperature mesor (after 14 days of treatment) allows the rejection of the zero-amplitude assumption, suggesting a nonrandom circadian stage-dependent response ($p < 0.02$). This finding shows that the hypothermia induced by CsA can be reduced or avoided by timing.[17]

After 2 weeks of treatment with CsA mean body weight loss (as percent of pretreatment value) was much greater in the animals injected during the dark span (−20.3% ± 4.7%) than in the group treated during the light span (−10.1% ± 5.3%) ($p < 0.01$). BUN concentrations before the treatment were 14.1 ± 3.0 mg/dl for the placebo group of animals, 15.2 ± 4.3 mg/dl for the animals that were to be injected with CsA in the light span and 16.3% ± 0.3 mg/dl for those that were to be treated in darkness. After 14 days of treatment, BUN in placebo-treated animals was 14.4 ± 2.7 mg/dl; in animals treated with CsA during the light span it was 28.3 ± 4.5 mg/dl, and it was 26.2 ± 8.6 mg/dl in those animals treated during the dark span. At this time, a statistically significant difference was found between the BUN values of the CsA-treated group and the value of the

Table 1. Body Weight (%) and Rhythm-Adjusted Mean (Mesor) of Core Temperature (°C) Changes After 14 Days From Treatment Onset, and Survival of 18 Adult Male Lewis Rats Carrying an Intraperitoneal Temperature Transsensor and Treated in Light (L) or Dark (D) Span With Cyclosporine (CsA) (20 mg/kg/day, i.p.) or Placebo (P) (90% Intralipid-Ethanol Solution) (5 ml/kg/day, i.p.), and Kept in LD12:12

			14 Days From Treatment Onset				Survival	
					*Change $p < 0.05$			
Group	No. of Rats	Rx	Change in Body Weight (%)*	$p < 0.05$ Versus†	Mesor (°C)*	Versus†	Days*	$p = 0.05$ Versus
L	6	CS	−10.1 ± 5.3	D, P	−0.44 ± 0.5	D	43.4 ± 11.4	D, P
			(−4.5 − −15.6)		(+0.3 − −1.2)		(35 − 60)	
D	6	CS	−20.3 ± 3.7	L, P	−1.64 ± 0.6 −	L, P	27.5 ± 10.6	L, P
			(−23.8 ± −14.8)		(−0.9 − −2.7)		(16 − 40)	
P	6	P	−2.3 ± 3.3	D, L	0.03 ± 0.1	D	>100	L, D
(L + D)			(+1.6 ± −6.5)		(+0.1 − −0.1)			

*Mean values ± SD (range).

†Comparisons carried out with other groups at same time.

Table 2. Blood Urea Nitrogen (BUN)* as an Index of Nephrotoxicity for Cyclosporine (CsA) Treatment (Rx) (20 mg/kg/day, i.p.) and Placebo (P) (90% Intralipid-Ethanol) (5 ml/kg/day, i.p.) given in the Light (L) or Dark (D) Span to Adult Male Lewis Rats Carrying an Intraperitoneal Temperature Transensor and Kept in LD12:12

			1†	2†		3†	
Group	No. of Rats	Rx	Before Rx Onset	14 Days From Rx Onset	$p < 0.05$‡ Versus Group Noted	2 Days Before Rat Death	$p < 0.05$‡ Versus Group Noted
L	6	CS	15.2 ± 4.3	28.3 ± 4.5	L-1	59.9 ± 30.3	L-1
			(11.8–22.3)	(25.1–36.1)	P-2	(31.1–94.4)	P-3
D	6	CS	16.3 ± 3.0	26.2 ± 8.6	D-1	40.9 ± 14.7	D-1
			(13.0–20.6)	(16.2–38.8)	P-2	(21.5–62.0)	P-3
P	6	P	14.1 ± 3.0	15.5 ± 2.7	L-2	16.6 ± 2.5§	L-3
(L + D)			(9.9 ± 18.6)	(11.3 ± 18.5)	D-2	(11.7–18.6)	D-3

*Reference range in rats is 5–29 mg/dl with a mean value of 14.5 mg/dl.
†Mean value (mg/dl) ± SD (range).
‡Comparison carried out with same group at previous times and with other groups at same time.
§35 days from Rx onset.

placebo-treated control group ($p < 0.05$) and also in a comparison with the pretreatment values of each group ($p < 0.05$). In the CsA-treated groups the BUN concentrations (at 2 days before the death of the first animal) were 59.9 ± 30.3 mg/dl for the animals treated in the light span and 40.9 ± 14.7 mg/dl for those treated in the dark span (NS) (Table 2).

The histologic abnormalities found in the liver, kidney, and lungs of 11 animals (5 treated during the light span, 6 treated in the dark span) are summarized in Table 3. Extensive pulmonary abscess formation was encountered in 2 of 5 of the "light-group" animals and 2 of 6 of the "dark-group" animals. A patchy to diffuse interstitial pneumonitis was evident in the remaining animals. These infiltrates, consisting of lymphoid cells and occasional polymorphonuclear leukocytes, were more extensive in the animals treated during darkness. Five animals had seemingly intact livers, but a mild fatty change was present in 3 of the animals treated during darkness. A patchy to mild mononuclear interstitial infiltrate was present at the cortical medullary junction in 8 of the animals. Minor degrees of tubular dilation with thinning of the epithelium was noted in 5 animals.

Immunosuppression—Study I

Delay of rejection by CsA was statistically significant:mean (±SD) rejection times for V

Table 3. Histopathologic Findings in Rats Given Cyclosporine 20 mg/kg/day

Hours After Light On	No. of Animals	Lung	Liver	Kidney
02	2		Infarction	
		Abscesses		
06	2	+IP		+ATI
		+IP		+ATI
10	1	Abscesses		++ATI
14	2	+IP		++ATI
		Abscesses	++Fatty Change	+ATI
18	2	Abscesses	++Fatty Change	
		++IP		++ATI
22	2	+IP		++ATI
		++IP	++Fatty Change	+ATI

IP, interstitial pneumonitis; ATI, acute interstitial nephritis.
(+) Minimal; (++) Mild.

and CsA-treated animals were 6.3 ± 0.8 and 12.83 ± 5.30 days, respectively ($p < 0.05$). In CsA-treated animals, no difference in delay of rejection was observed between the rats treated according to the homeostatic schedule and those treated with the sinusoidal schedule. The difference in rejection time as a function of circadian stage at treatment time was significant ($p < 0.05$); the mean (±SD) times were 9.1 ± 1.1 and 16.5 ± 5.3 days for the animals treated during the light span and dark span, respectively.

Immunosuppression—Study II

Delay of rejection by CsA was statistically significant: mean rejection times for V and CsA-treated rats were 6.5 ± 1.04 and >55.41 ± 41.84 days, respectively ($p < 0.01$). After 75 days of treatment, CsA injections were stopped in 1 animal treated during the light span (at 10 HALO) and 4 animals treated during the dark span (2 animals at 22 HALO and 1 each at 14 and 18 HALO). All the animals had a graft beating well after 100 days. The difference in rejection times as a function of circadian stage at treatment time was significant ($p < 0.05$); the mean times were ≥30.66 ± 34.15 and ≥80.16 ± 34.99 days for the rats treated during the light span and dark span, respectively. When the rejection times of CsA-treated animals in the first study (12.83 ± 5.30 days) are compared with those in the second study (≥55.41 ± 41.84 days) a $p < 0.005$ is obtained.

DISCUSSION

A mild acute interstitial nephritis has been reported in the kidneys of intact rats receiving various dosages of CsA,[31,32] but these histologic abnormalities were not correlated with renal functional studies. It appears unlikely that the interstitial nephritis alone is the cause of the renal dysfunction in the rats of the present study. Fine structural examination has revealed cytologic abnormalities even at very low doses of CsA,[31] and these changes in combination with the light microscopic abnormalities may account for renal dysfunction. Fatty change is a nonspecific finding that has an etiology involving multiple factors and could be related to sepsis and bronchopneumonia found in these rats, yet hepatoxocity is a common finding in human organ transplantation using CsA as the immunosuppressant drug. Evidence of pulmonary infection—extensive abscess formation or a minimal to mild interstitial pneumonia—was evident in most of the animals examined and appears to be the cause of death.

The toxic effect of several drugs has been reduced by timing exploiting a spectrum of susceptibility–resistance cycles.[18] Such optimization by circadian timing has been documented for nephrotoxicity.[19] Treatment timing is particularly promising in immunopharmacology, since it has been documented to account for the difference between immunosuppression and immunostimulation.[11,20] Research on experimental animals[21–24] and humans beings[25–28] has shown a spectrum of rhythms with different frequencies coordinating the immune response and/or donor antige-

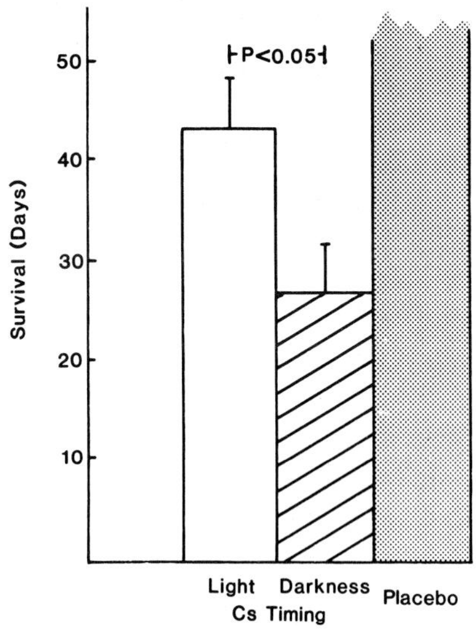

Fig. 1. Difference in mean (±SE) duration of survival of intact Lewis rats treated with cyclosporine (20 mg/kg/day, i.p. in ~5 ml/kg) during the daily light (L) ($n = 6$) or dark (D) ($n = 6$) span in LD 12:12 (with the long-term survival of 6 placebo-treated animals also indicated).

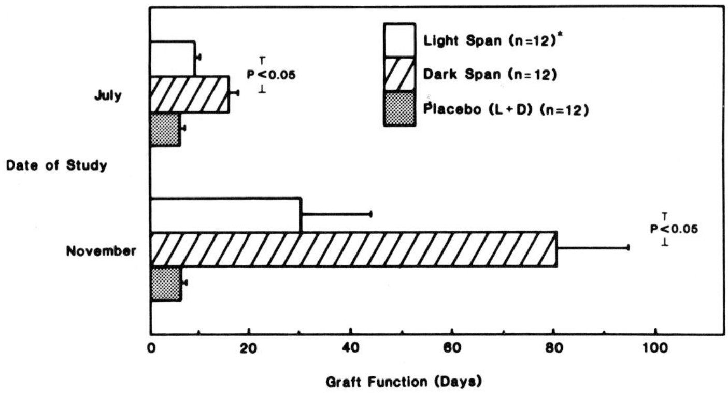

Fig. 2. Toward optimization of cyclosporine (CsA) effects by timing according to multiple frequencies; possibly converting otherwise confusing variability into useful new end-points. Circadian and circannual variation in CsA effect on mean (±SE) duration of function of ACI hearts transplanted across a major histocompatibility barrier into male Lewis rats kept in LD 12:12, and treated with CsA (1.25 mg/kg/day, i.p.) or placebo (Intralipid-ethanol solution 0.31 ml/kg/day, i.p.) during the daily L or D spans, respectively.

nicity. Among other variables, a circadian bioperiodicity has been shown for T- and B-cell counts in human peripheral blood, phagocytic activity, and natural killer cell activity.

Further transplantation studies in experimental animals with skin[29] and kidney allografts[30] have shown a circadian variation of rejection according to the time of surgery. Both experiments report a longer delay of rejection in the animals transplanted at the time when adrenal cortical hormone concentrations are spontaneously higher.

The results obtained in our studies show that both toxic and immunosuppressive effects of CsA are likely subject to the intermodulation of rhythms with several frequencies and that treatment can be optimized by timing (Figs. 1 and 2, Tables 4 and 5). In particular, the toxicity study demonstrates a reduced toxic effect when the drug is injected during the light span. The mean survival times (43.5 in the light versus 27.5 days in the dark, $p < 0.05$) and a lesser decrease in body weight (−10.1% in light versus −20.3% in darkness, $p < 0.01$) after 14 days of treatment and a lesser decrease in core temperature means (−0.4°C in light versus −1.6°C in darkness, $p < 0.01$) all support this conclusion.

At 14 days of treatment, BUN concentrations as an index of CsA nephrotoxicity are elevated in CsA-treated animals as compared to those in the placebo-treated control group ($p < 0.05$). At that time point, at 2 days before the death of the first animal, the slightly higher concentrations of BUN in the rats injected during the light span (28.3 versus 26.2 mg/dl, 59.9 versus 40.9 mg/dl) were not statistically significantly different from those of the rats injected during the dark span. Until

Table 4. Delay of Rejection (Days) of Heterotopic Intraabdominal ACI Rat Heart Allograft in 18 Male Lewis Rats Treated in July in the Light or Dark Span, 12 With Cyclosporine (CsA, 1.25 mg/kg/day, i.p.) and 6 With CsA Vehicle (Intralipid-Ethanol Solution, 0.3 ml/kg/day, i.p.)

Treatment Timing	Vehicle	Cyclosporine		
Light	8, 6, 6	7, 9, 9, 10, 10, 10	9.1 ± 1.1*	$p < 0.05$ (Light vs. Dark)
Dark	6, 6, 6	11, 13, 14, 17, 18, 26	16.5 ± 5.3	
	6.3 ± 0.8*	12.8 ± 5.3		
	$p < 0.05$ (Vehicle vs. Cyclosporine)			

*Mean (days) ± SD.

Table 5. Delay of Rejection (Days) of Heterotopic Intraabdominal ACI Rat Heart Allograft in 18 Male Lewis Rats Treated in November in the Light or Dark Span, 12 With Cyclosporine (CsA, 1.25 mg/kg/day, i.p.) and 6 With CsA Vehicle (Intralipid-Ethanol Solution, 0.3 ml/kg/day, i.p.)

Treatment Timing	Vehicle	Cyclosporine		
Light	6, 7, 6	11, 16, 17, 18, 22, >100	≥30.6 ± 34.1*	$p < 0.05$
Dark	6, 6, 7	14, 67, >100, >100, >100 >100	≥80.1 ± 34.9	
	6.3 ± 0.5*	<55.4 ± 41.8		
	$p < 0.05$			

*Mean (days) ± SD.

proof is offered to the contrary, these findings and the histologic analyses indicate that the enhanced toxic effect of CsA injected during the dark span is not necessarily the result of a difference in CsA nephrotoxicity.

On the other hand, the immunosuppressive studies show an enhanced desired effect of low doses of CsA (1.25 mg/kg/day) when the drug is injected during the dark span. In both experiments, a longer delay of rejection was statistically significant in the rats treated during the dark span: in July, 16.5 days for rats treated during darkness versus 9.1 days for those treated during light ($p < 0.05$), and in November, 80.1 days for those treated during darkness versus 30.6 days for those treated during light ($p < 0.05$). The results obtained in the studies of toxicity and immunosuppression may be two different aspects of the same effect.

Since, in the first study, the nephrotoxity of CsA is not enhanced or reduced by timing, the enhanced effect of immunosuppression by CsA during the dark span, documented by a longer delay of rejection, could be the explanation also of the greater toxic effect observed in the animals treated during darkness. In the toxicity study, the animals treated during the dark span, being more immunosuppressed, may have died earlier of infection. In any case, the results indicate that an improvement of the immunosuppressive/nephrotoxic ratio can be achieved by CsA timing.

A circannual variation in immunosuppressive CsA effect is suggested, but not proved, by the results of the allograft studies. A strikingly longer delay of rejection was obtained in the study performed in November, as compared to the results obtained in the study performed in July (55.4 in November versus 12.8 days in July, $p < 0.005$).

CsA effects are likely subject to the intermodulation of rhythms with several other frequencies, beyond any circadian and circannual changes described here. These intermodulations may account for differences in results of various laboratories and even in those of the same laboratory on the same experimental model when timing differs, e.g., as a function of season. More important, however, are the clinical implications. Information on timing should be gathered to improve the therapeutic ratio of drugs. Our data show that, in rats, the injection of CsA during the dark span (their active span) enhances the desired antirejection effect. Since rats are nocturnal, the optimal time for administration might differ from the optimal time for diurnally active human beings, but certainly the effect of time of day of dosing and, eventually, the relation of dosing to host marker rhythms awaits clinical testing.

In conclusion, it is emphasized that, in the test of the undesired effect, a lethal CsA dose was used, whereas, to the contrary, for the desired effect (of prolonging graft survival), an actually subtherapeutic dose was used. Thus, any differences as a function of timing may have come more rapidly and more markedly to the fore. A test of graded doses will be essential, of course, in the continuation of such work, if not in medium-sized animals, then eventually in the clinic. Only the principle is documented here, namely, the fact that for an efficient CsA therapy, timing must be related to dosing.

REFERENCES

1. Dreyfus M, Hyerri E, Hotman H, et al: Eur J Appl Microbiol 3:125, 1976

2. Borel JF, Feurer C, Gubler HV, et al: Agent Actions 6:468, 1976

3. Borel JF, Feurer C, Magnee C, et al: Immunology 32:1017, 1977

4. Calne RY, White DJG: IRCS J Med Sci 5:595, 1977

5. Morris PJ: Transplantation 32:349, 1981

6. Hess AD, Tutschka PJ: J Immunol 124:2601, 1980

7. Kunkl A, Klaus GGB: J Immunol 125:2526, 1980

8. Calne RY, Rolles K, White DJG, et al: Lancet 2:1033, 1979

9. Klintmalm GBG, Iwatsuki S, Starzl TE: Lancet 1:470, 1981

10. Ferguson RM, Rynasiewicz JJ, Sutherland DER, et al: Surgery 92:175, 1982

11. Halberg F: In Carpenter DO (ed): Cellular Pacemakers. New York, Wiley, 1982, p 261

12. Halberg F, Haus E, Cardso SS, et al: Experientia 29:909, 1973

13. Halberg F: Cold Spring Harbor Symp 25:289, 1960

14. Halberg F, Nelson W, Runge WJ, et al: Space Life Sci 2:437, 1981

15. Halberg F, Johnson EA, Nelson W, et al: Physiol Tchr 1:1, 1972

16. Ono K, Lindsey ES: J Thorac Cardiovasc Surg 57:225, 1969

17. Magnus G, Cavallini M, Halberg F, et al: (submitted for publication)

18. Halberg F: Chronobiologia 1(Suppl 1):27, 1974

19. Hrushesky WJM, Levi FA, Halberg F, et al: Cancer Res 42:945, 1982

20. Halberg F, Sanchez de la Pena S, Fernandes G: In Hadden J, Chedid L, Dukor P, et al (eds): Advances in Immunopharmacology. Oxford, Pergamon, 1983, p. 463

21. Halberg F: In Carpenter DO (ed): Cellular Pacemakers. New York, John Wiley, 1982, p 146

22. Fernandes G, Carandente F, Halberg F, et al: J Immunol 123:622, 1979

23. Fernandes G, Halberg F, Good RA: In Smolensky M, Reinberg A, McGovern JP (eds): Recent Advances in the Chronobiology of Allergy and Immunology. New York, Pergamon, 1980, p 289

24. Kawahara K, Levi F, Halberg F, et al: In Takahashi R, Halburg F, Walker C (eds): Toward Chronopharmacology, Proceedings of the 8th IUPHAR Congress, and Sat Symposia, Nagasaki, Japan, July 1981. Oxford, Pergamon, 1982, p 273

25. Simpson H, Tavadia HB, Fleming K, et al: In: Workshop 2 on Chronobiology and Allergy, Proceedings of an International Conference on Allergy, Tokyo, 1973, abstr 314

26. Halberg F, Dufert D, Mayersbach H: Chronobiologia 4:114, 1977

27. De Vecchi A, Halberg F, Sothern RB, et al: In Walker CA, Winget CM, Soliman KFA (eds): Chronopharmacology and Chronotherapeutics. Tallahassee, Florida A & M University Foundation, 1981, p 339

28. Knapp MS, Blaney RW, Cove-Smith HR, et al: In Reinberg A, Halberg F (eds): Chronopharmacology. New York, Pergamon, 1979

29. Halberg J, Halberg E, Runge W, et al: In Scheving LE, Halberg F, Pauly JE (eds): Chronobiology. Tokyo, Igaku Shoin, 1974, p 320

30. Ratte J, Halberg F, Kuhl JFW, et al: Surgery 73:102, 1973

31. Simonton SC, Rynasiewicz J, Sibley RK: Lab Invest 48:78A, 1983

32. Whiting PH, Thomson AW, Blair JT, et al: Br J Exp Pathol 63:88, 1982

Synergistic Effect of a Nucleotide-Free Diet and Cyclosporine on Allograft Survival

C. T. Van Buren, A. Kulkarni, and F. Rudolph

ELECTIVE dietary manipulation in allograft recipients has been a heretofore neglected instrument of the immunosuppressive armamentarium. Protein caloric malnutrition,[1] zinc deficiency[2] and essential fatty acid deprivation[3] each lead to suppression of immune responsiveness, but the associated problems with suboptimal nutrition have precluded clinical applicability of these regimens. Previous investigations in this laboratory have demonstrated that dietary nucleotide deprivation leads to depression of cellular immunity both in vivo and in vitro.[4–6] The term nucleotide refers to purine and pyrmidine bases and not to specific polynucleotides.

The current experiment addresses the role of the nucleotide-free diet (NFD) as an adjuvant to the potent suppressor of T-lymphocyte immunity, cyclosporine (CsA), in the murine heart allograft model. Preconditioning with a NFD appears to potentiate the effect of an abbreviated course of CsA.

MATERIALS AND METHODS

Eight-week-old BALB/c female mice were randomized to one of three dietary groups: chow (Purina diet no. 5008), nucleotide-free diet (NFD, Purina diet no. 5755), or nucleotide-free diet supplemented with 0.25% yeast RNA (NF-RNA specially pelleted by Purina). NFD leads to normal maturation, development, and reproduction in generations of mice. All diets are isocaloric and isonitrogenous and maintain equivalent weight gain in each of the groups.

Following 4 weeks of dietary equilibration, all animals received cardiac allografts from newborn C57BL/6 mice, employing the method of Fulmer et al.[7] Allografts were placed in subcutaneous ear pouches in the recipients. Successful engraftment was documented under the dissecting microscope by observation of vigorous contractile activity of the cardiac allograft. Cessation of pulsation of the graft was used to designate loss of function secondary to rejection.

Immediately following engraftment, mice in each dietary group were randomly assigned to receive either CsA (15 mg/kg day) dissolved in olive oil (0.1 ml) or olive oil (0.1 ml) by gavage feeding. Mice received CsA or olive oil (OO) on day 0 through day 3 following transplantation.

Difference in survival data for each group was analyzed by Wilcoxon rank sum for statistical significance.

RESULTS

Figure 1 represents the survival curves for all groups. CsA with chow or NF-RNA did not lead to prolonged allograft survival compared to chow-OO or NF-RNA-OO control groups. Thus, in this model, 4 days of oral CsA did not lead to significant immunosuppression. In contrast, NFD-OO leads to prolonged cardiac allograft survival compared to chow-OO ($p < 0.005$), chow-CsA ($p < 0.005$), NF-RNA-OO ($p < 0.005$), and NF-RNA-CsA ($p < 0.009$) control groups (see Table 1). NFD, when combined with CsA, lead to further prolongation of allograft survival compared with NFD-OO; this difference

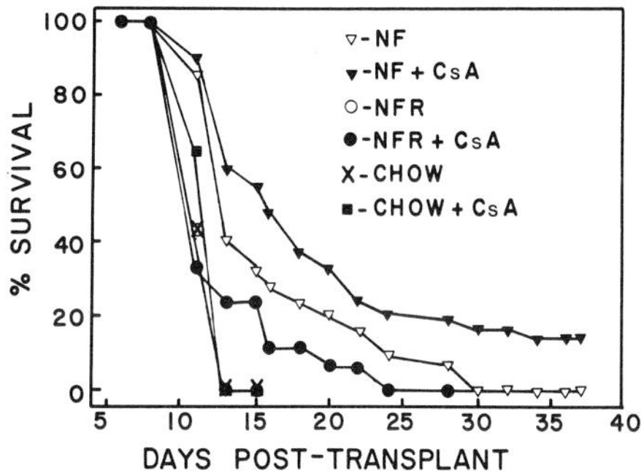

Fig. 1. Survival of C57BL/6 cardiac allografts in BALB/c mice on various diets.

From the Division of Immunology and Organ Transplantation, Department of Surgery, University of Texas Medical School, Houston, TX.

Address reprint requests to Dr. C. T. van Buren, Division of Immunology and Organ Transplantation, Department of Surgery, University of Texas Medical School, Houston, TX 77030.

0041-1345/83/1505-0142$01.00/0

Table 1. Statistical Analysis of Cardiac Allograft Survivals in Various Diet and Treatment Groups by Wilcoxon Two-Tail Test

NF + CsA	NF + OO	NFR + CsA	NFR + OO	Chow + CsA	Chow + OO
├	$p < 0.04$				
├	—	$p < 0.003$			
	├	$p < 0.009$			
		├	$p < .32$		
		├	—	$p < .22$	
	├	—	—	—	$p < .005$
	├	—	—	$p < 0.005$	
├	—	—	—	$p < 0.002$	

proved to be statistically significant ($p < 0.04$) (Fig. 2, Table 1).

DISCUSSION

Previous studies in this laboratory have demonstrated that dietary nucleotide deprivation leads to suppression of both cardiac and tumor allograft rejection.[4,8] Mice feed a nucleotide-free diet demonstrate decreased in vivo response to alloantigen using the popliteal lymph node assay. In vitro lymphocyte response to phytohemagglutinin and alloantigen in one-way MLC is depressed in NFD mice compared to chow or NF-RNA-fed controls. Primary sensitization of mice to subcutaneously injected microbial or xenoantigens is depressed on a nucleotide-free diet.[9,10] Since the demonstrated effects of dietary nucleotide deprivation have been on T-cell immunity, this diet was tested in combination with CsA, a promising agent that prevents allograft rejection. Surprisingly, dietary nucleotide deprivation led to greater immunosuppression than a short course of CsA in mice maintained on control diets. The prolongation of allograft survival by NFD was comparable to that previously reported. While CsA did not prolong cardiac allograft survival in chow or NF-RNA-fed mice, NFD and CsA increased graft survival compared with NFD alone, suggesting that the diet and CsA were synergistic in action. Thus, dietary nucleotide deprivation appears to potentiate the efficacy of CsA and may prove to be a useful adjunctive measure in the clinical management of allograft recipients.

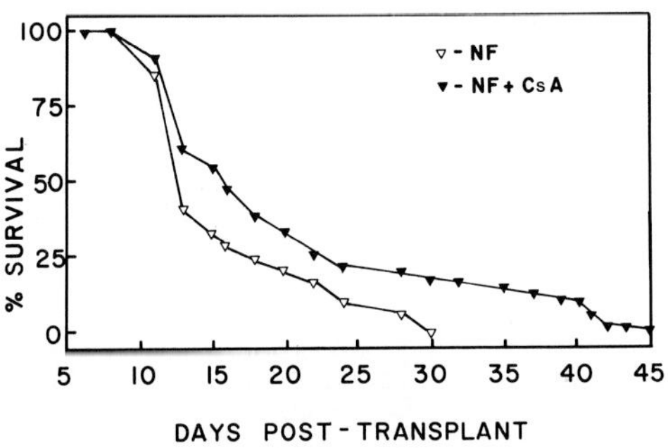

Fig. 2. Survival of C57BL/6 cardiac allografts in BALB/c mice.

REFERENCES

1. Chandra RK: Br Med J 3:608, 1974
2. Axelrod AE: In Goodhart RS, Shils ME (eds): Modern Nutrition in Health and Disease. Philadelphia, Lea and Febiger, 1976, p 493
3. Jose DG, Good RA: J Exp Med 137:1, 1973
4. Rudolph FB, Kulkarni AD, Schandle VB, et al: Adv Exp Med, Biochemical, 175–178, 1983
5. Kulkarni AD, Schandle VB, Rudolph FB, et al: Fed Proc 41:589, 1982
6. Van Buren CT, Kulkarni AD, Schandle VB, et al: Transplantation 36:350, 1983
7. Fulmer RI, Cramer AT, Liebelt RA, et al: Am J Anat 113:273, 1963
8. Van Buren D, Rudolph F, Kahan BD, et al: J Parent Ent Nutr 4:590, 1980
9. Van Buren CT, Kulkarni AD, Rudolph FB: J Parent Ent Nutr 6:582, 1982
10. Kulkarni AD, Schandle VB, Rudolph FB, et al: Fed Proc 41:589, 1982

Prolonged Heart Allograft Survival in Cyclosporine-Treated Presensitized Rats

J. A. Schulak, J. Shelby, E. Wakely, and R. J. Corry

ADMINISTRATION of cyclosporine A (CsA) at the time of initial antigen exposure usually prevents immunization, as evidenced by numerous reports of delayed or prevented rejection in experimental as well as clinical first transplants.[1] It is unclear, however, whether CsA would be as effective in the face of presensitization. While recent clinical reports have described a graft survival advantage in CsA-treated retransplanted individuals,[2,3] the efficacy of this agent in preventing rejection in experimental second-set models has been less spectacular.[4] This may be explained by the presumption that such clinical recipients were T-cell crossmatch negative with their donors, and thus, while being highly sensitized to a random population, were not presensitized specifically to their donors and therefore not truly representative of the second-set phenomenon. The purpose of this study was to evaluate the efficacy of CsA as an immunosuppressant in recipients that are clearly sensitized to their donors. In order to accomplish this goal, both graft survival and antibody response were monitored in a rat heart allograft model of second-set rejection.

MATERIALS AND METHODS

Animals

Male Lewis rats were used as graft hosts in all experiments and (Lewis × Brown, Norway) F_1 (LBN) males served as the source of both primary and secondary allografts.

Sensitization

Sensitization was achieved using a modification of a technique originally described in mice.[5] Five 1–2 cu mm fragments of LBN myocardium were grafted into the subcutaneous space of each recipient ear. Survival time for these grafts was not determined. However, immunization by this technique was verified by measurement of a donor-specific humoral response. As illustrated by the examples in Fig. 1, peak Lewis–anti-LBN antibody titers of between 1:64 and 1:256 occurred between 10 and 15 days after heart fragment engraftment in all cases and returned to negligible levels by the 35th day. We have previously demonstrated that this technique is comparable to skin graft sensitization with regard to second graft survival time.[6]

Secondary Challenge

Secondary transplantation, performed 4–6 weeks after primary grafting, consisted of standard intraabdominal heterotopic LBN heart grafts anastomosed to the infrarenal aorta and vena cava. Graft viability was monitored by daily palpation of myocardial contractions. Complete cessation of heart beat was used as an end-point in determining survival time. Group mean survival times (MSTs) were calculated, and statistical significance of the differences between group means was determined with the Student's t test.

Immunosuppression

The only immunosuppressive agent used in these studies was cyclosporine A, which was kindly supplied as a gift from Sandoz Ltd, Basel, Switzerland. CsA was mixed with a 10% fat emulsion (Liposyn, Abbott Laboratories, North Chicago, IL) and 96% ethanol to achieve a final concentration of 3 mg/ml, which was administered daily via an intraperitoneal injection. A 10 mg/kg dose was used in all short-term experiments, while a tapering schedule was employed in long-term recipients. In these latter experiments, CsA was tapered to either 2.5 mg/kg or 5 mg/kg at 6 weeks and then maintained until either 60 or 130 days.

Antibody Titers

Lewis–anti-LBN antibody titers were measured using a standard compliment-dependent microlymphocytotoxicity assay, using LBN lymphocytes as targets. After collection, serum samples were frozen at −20°C and stored until a large number of samples could be assayed simultaneously. All assays were run in duplicate.

RESULTS

Second-set rejection was observed in all Lewis recipients of vascularized LBN hearts

---

From the Department of Surgery, University of Iowa College of Medicine, Iowa City, IA.

Address reprint requests to Dr. J. A. Schulak, Department of Surgery, University of Iowa College of Medicine, Iowa City, IA 52242.

0041–1345/83/1505–0143$01.00/0

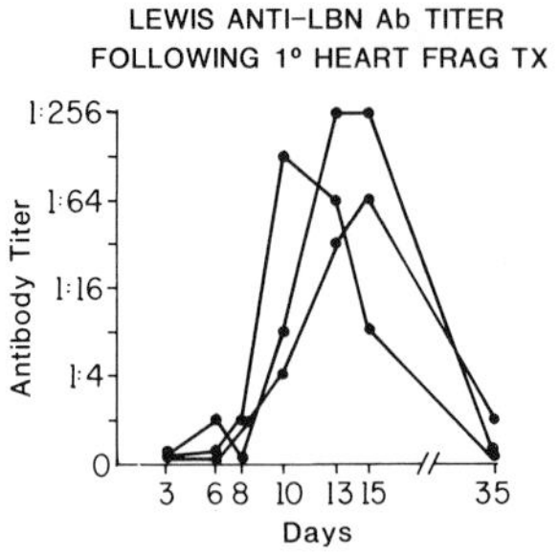

Fig. 1. Lewis rat anti-LBN humoral immune response to LBN heart fragment implantation demonstrating a brisk antibody synthesis, peaking between days 10 and 15.

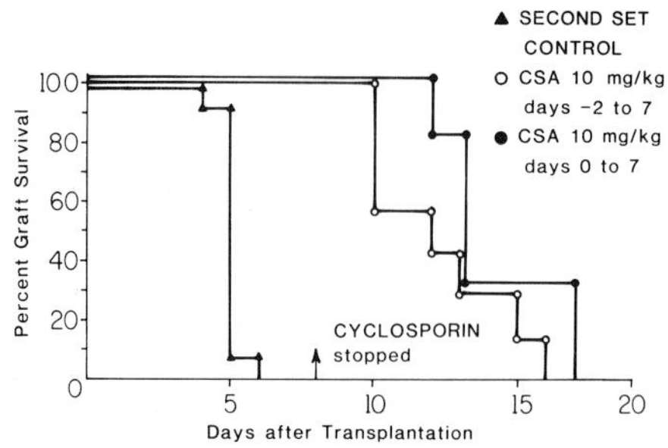

Fig. 2. The effect of CsA on secondary heart allograft survival in presensitized hosts.

when previously sensitized by heart fragment implantation. The MST of 5.0 ± 0.4 days for these recipients was significantly ($p < 0.01$) shorter than primary heart allograft survival of 9.5 ± 3.0 days. A short course of CsA, started either 2 days prior to secondary challenge or on the day of transplantation and carried on in both cases for 1 week, significantly ($p < 0.01$) prolonged graft survival, with MSTs of 12.3 ± 2.5 and 14.2 ± 2.2 days, respectively (Fig. 2).

The outcomes for two groups of similarly sensitized and transplanted animals that were maintained on long-term CsA are summarized in Table 1. The first group received a tapering dose of CsA from 10 mg/kg/day to 2.5 mg/kg/day over 6 weeks. Five of 10 recipients in this group died within the first 40 days due to either infection or anesthesia accident suffered during serum collection, all with functioning nonrejected allografts. Three of the remaining 5 had CsA stopped after 60 days and subsequently rejected their grafts at 77, 78, and 96 days, respectively. One rat experienced a cellular rejection at 93 days while on 2.5 mg/kg/day of CsA. Lewis–anti-LBN antibody was not detectable in the serum of this animal at the time of allograft rejection. The remaining rat, also still receiving 2.5 mg/kg/day of CsA, was sacrificed at 105 days, revealing a completely normal allograft with no evidence of rejection.[6]

A second group of five sensitized rats had CsA tapered to 5 mg/kg/day at 6 weeks and then was maintained on that dose until 130 days after transplantation. All of these animals had well functioning allografts while they were receiving CsA. After cessation of CsA, one graft rejected on day 142, while the remaining rats have continued graft function for >175 days. Again, no measurable donor-

Table 1. Effect of Long-Term Cyclosporine Administration on Secondary Heart Allograft Survival in Presensitized Hosts

Groups	*n*	CsA Regimen	Survival Times (Days)	Comments
Group 1		Tapering regimen*		
a	5		2, 14, 33, 37, 39	Graft losses due to recipient death
b	3		77, 78, 96	CsA stopped at day 60
c	2		93†, 105†	CsA stopped at day 100
Group 2	5	Tapering regimen‡	142, >175 × 3	CsA stopped at day 130; 1 rat died from anesthetic accident at 100 days

*CsA tapered from 10 mg/kg/day to 2.5 mg/kg/day at 6 weeks.

†One rat rejected graft on day 93 while on CsA; the other was sacrificed on day 105, revealing a normal allograft without histologic evidence for rejection.

‡CsA tapered from 10 mg/kg/day to 5 mg/kg/day at 6 weeks.

specific antibody was detected in these animals while they were receiving maintenance cyclosporine.

In contrast to the above-described long-term CsA recipients, second-set rejection was accompanied by a brisk humoral response in the control, nonimmunosuppressed group. In these animals, Lewis–anti-LBN titers routinely reached values as high as 1:8192 on the day of rejection. Eight of 11 such rats had titers of 1:128 or greater at the time of rejection (Table 2). Use of CsA markedly diminished the host humoral response in the group treated with 10 mg/kg/day for days −2 to 7. In only 1 of 6 of these rats did the Lewis–anti-LBN titer reach as high as 1:16 at rejection. In contrast, 3 recipients had either no detectable antibody present or nearly none (titer of 1:2) when the heart allograft stopped beating.

DISCUSSION

The ability of cyclosporine to inhibit the onset of rejection in presensitized hosts is clearly established in these experiments. Using a dose range of CsA easily within the limits necessary for safe clinical application, we have demonstrated that an 8–10-day course of the drug will significantly delay the onset of rejection in a model of the second-set immune response. However, in contrast to the experience with short course CsA in primary heart allotransplantation in this strain combination,[7] tolerance did not develop in these sensitized recipients, as all lost their grafts shortly after administration of CsA was stopped.

Similar data have been presented recently by others regarding a limited duration of CsA administration in sensitized animals, however, long-term studies have not been reported.[8] In our present experiments, we demonstrate that a maintenance regimen of 5 mg/kg/day will prolong graft survival significantly in recipients sensitized to their donor. One recipient did reject his graft at day 93 while on only 2.5 mg/kg/day of CsA, suggesting that that dose may have been too low to be effective in the face of presensitization.

The mechanism of prolonged graft survival observed in these experiments is not yet clear. It has been suggested that CsA favors the development of suppressor cells, which protect the allograft even after the drug is withdrawn.[7] Data from our study suggest that a suppressor cell mechanism may not be operative in the presence of presensitization, as it appears that some of our sensitized rats eventually reject their secondary hearts after CsA is stopped. On the other hand, these experiments demonstrate a marked influence of CsA on the humoral immune response in this model. CsA has been shown by others to inhibit antibody synthesis if administered during initial antigen exposure; however, to date, it has been thought that secondary humoral activity was resistant to CsA.[9] The use of CsA in this model clearly blunted the host humoral response in our sensitized recipients. Whether or not the decreased antibody synthesis was coincidental with or responsible for graft prolongation is not clear. However, it has been demonstrated histologically that CsA administration appears to eliminate an antibody-mediated component to rejection in sensitized rats.[4] Nevertheless, caution must be exercised in interpreting these data in this manner, since it remains uncertain whether humoral immunity plays an important role in murine allograft rejection.

Table 2. Effect of Cyclosporine in Blunting the Humoral Response in This Model of Second-Set Rejection

Experimental Group	MST*	Host Anti-Donor Antibody Titer† at Time of Rejection
Controls—no CsA	5.0 ± 0.4	16, 32, 32, 128, 160, 1024, 1024, 1600, 4096, 8192, 8192
CsA 10 mg/kg/days −2 to 7	12.3 ± 2.5	0, 0, 2, 8, 8, 16

*Mean survival time ± standard deviation.

†Reciprocal value.

In conclusion, we have demonstrated that CsA can prevent rejection of heart allografts in rats presensitized to their donor. A maintenance regimen of the drug results in what appears to be indefinite graft survival. Lastly, donor-specific antibody synthesis is inhibited by use of CsA, suggesting that the use of this drug in species such as man, where humoral immunity is known to be associated with the accelerated rejection observed in sensitized individuals, may be appropriate.

REFERENCES

1. Morris PJ: Transplantation 32:349, 1981
2. Starzl TE, Hakala TR, Rosenthal JT, et al: Surg Gynecol Obstet 154:819, 1982
3. Ferguson RM, Rynasiewicz JJ, Sutherland DER, et al: Surgery 92:175, 1982
4. Homan WP, Fabre JW, Millard IR, et al: Transplantation 30:354, 1980
5. Jirsch V, Kraft N, Diener E: Cardiovasc Res 8:145, 1974
6. Schulak JA, Monson D, Shelby J, et al: Transplantation 36:289, 1983
7. Hutchinson IF, Shadur CA, Duarte A, et al: Transplantation 32:210, 1981
8. Marquet RL, Heystek GA, Cobussen AC, et al: Transplant Proc 15:518, 1983
9. Borel JF, Feurer C, Magnic C, et al: Immunology 32:1017, 1977

Effect of Cyclosporine on Lymphocyte Migration in Rat Cardiac Transplantation

N. Kuromoto, C. Iga, R. Fawwaz, R. Nowygrod, K. Reemtsma, and M. A. Hardy

CYCLOSPORINE A (CsA) has been repeatedly demonstrated to be a potent immunosuppressive agent, following its introduction in 1976 by Borel et al.[1] Numerous studies, many of which are described in this issue of *Transplantation Proceedings*, have shown CsA to lead to significant prolongation of allografts in many experimental animals, as well as in human clinical trials. Despite the demonstration of its efficacy, the mechanism of action of CsA remains uncertain. Many experimental studies suggest that CsA acts by an inhibitory effect on in vitro proliferation of lymphocytes,[2–5] selective sparing of suppressor T cells,[6,7] blocking of lymphocyte surface receptors leading to inactivation of T helper cells and cytotoxic T cells,[8–10] and by production of an inhibitory substance or suppressor factor.[11] Little is known about the in vivo effect of CsA on the homing pattern of effector cells in recipients of vascularized organ allografts, and this may be important, since antigenic stimulation of the host leads to changes in lymphocyte recirculation to peripheral lymphoid organs and allografts.[12,13] In order to further define the in vivo mechanism responsible for graft prolongation in CsA-treated recipients, the present study was designed to evaluate the changes in homing patterns of indium-111 (^{111}In) labeled lymphocytes (untreated or in vivo CsA-treated) in untreated and CsA-treated rat recipients of cardiac allografts. Based on our previous studies using ^{111}In-labeled cells,[14,15] we postulated that CsA will delay the early lymphocyte infiltration of the cardiac allograft in rats, as well as change the previously described specific homing patterns of host lymphocytes to the peripheral lymphoid organs during acute allograft rejection.

MATERIALS AND METHODS

Animals

Adult male Lewis ($RT1^l$) and ACI ($RT1^a$) rats, weighing 200–250 g, were purchased from Harlan Sprague Dawley Inc., Walkersville, MD.

Heart Transplantation

Cardiac allografts from ACI rats or syngeneic grafts from Lewis rats were heterotopically transplanted into the abdomen of either untreated or CsA-treated Lewis recipients by the method of Ono and Lindsey.[16] Cardiac graft survival was determined by daily palpation, and rejection was considered complete with the cessation of palpable cardiac beat.

The Preparation of ^{111}In-Labeled Lymphocytes

Lymphocytes were isolated from lymph nodes of either untreated or CsA-treated Lewis rats.[14] ^{111}In-oxine solution was purchased from Diagnostic Isotope Inc., Bloomfield, NJ. ^{111}In has a half-life of 67 hr and gamma photon emission at 173 KeV (89%) and 247 KeV (93%). The isolated lymphocytes were washed twice at 200 *g* for 10 min with phosphate-buffered saline (PBS), and the resulting pellet was suspended in normal saline and incubated with 2–3 mCi of ^{111}In-oxine for 15 min at room temperature, as described by Thakur et al.[17] The cells were washed twice before counting and resuspended at a concentration of 2×10^7 cells/ml for infusion. Labeling efficiency was more than 80%, and the viability of the cells after labeling was greater than 95%, as determined by trypan blue exclusion.

From the Departments of Surgery and Nuclear Medicine, Columbia College of Physicians & Surgeons, New York, NY, and the Medical College of Osaka, Department of Surgery, Osaka, Japan.

Supported in part by NIH Grant HL 14799-10.

Address reprint requests to Mark A. Hardy, M.D., Columbia College of Physicians and Surgeons, 630 West 168 Street, New York, NY 10032.

0041–1345/83/1505–0144$01.00/0

Experimental Design

Since the purpose of this study was to evaluate the effect of CsA in vivo on the lymphocyte migration patterns in Lewis recipients of ACI hearts, the following schema was adopted. Group I consisted of Lewis recipients of heterotopic abdominal cardiac allografts from ACI donors or syngeneic grafts from Lewis donors (controls). Four recipients (from each subgroup, syngeneic or allogeneic grafts) were sacrificed daily, 24 hr after being intravenously infused with 2×10^7 ^{111}In-labeled untreated Lewis lymph node lymphocytes. This procedure was repeated daily for 7 days (time of complete rejection of ACI hearts in untreated Lewis recipients). Radioactivity of native and transplanted hearts, spleen, mesenteric lymph nodes (MLN), cervical lymph nodes (CLN), liver, lung, kidney, bone marrow (BM), thymus, and blood was determined per gram of isolated tissue by scintillation counting. Group II consisted of Lewis recipients of allogeneic (ACI) or syngeneic grafts who were immunosuppressed with daily intramuscular injections of CsA (8 mg/kg/day) from the day of transplantation until the day of sacrifice (day 7). CsA (OL27-400; Sandoz Ltd., Basel, Switzerland), which was provided in powder form, was initially dissolved in anhydrous ethynol (10% formulation), then in Miglyol 812 (Dynamit Nobel Chemicals, Witten/Ruhr, Germany). All animals were infused daily with 2×10^7 ^{111}In-labeled Lewis untreated lymph node lymphocytes and were sacrificed 24 hr after infusion of the cells, in an identical manner to that described in group I. Group III consisted of Lewis recipients of ACI or syngeneic heart grafts and were not immunosuppressed, analogous to group I. The Lewis rats that served as donors of daily infusion of 2×10^7 ^{111}In-labeled lymph node lymphocytes were injected i.m. with 20 mg/kg/day of CsA for 2 days prior to lymphocyte isolation. Thus, this group differed from group I only in that the labeled lymph node lymphocytes were obtained from Lewis rats treated with CsA and are referred to as "CsA-treated lymphocytes." Twenty-four hours after infusion of the labeled cells, four recipients of allogeneic or syngeneic cardiac grafts were sacrificed on a daily basis for 7 days after transplantation, and the various organs were excised for direct scintillation counting as described previously. Group IV consisted of Lewis recipients of allogeneic or syngeneic cardiac grafts and were all treated with 8 mg/kg/day of CsA from day of transplantation until day of sacrifice. All animals were infused daily with 2×10^7 ^{111}In-labeled lymphocytes obtained from CsA-treated donors (same as group III), and 24 hr following infusion of labeled cells, four animals from each subgroup were sacrificed to determine the radioactivity in the various organs, as described previously.

RESULTS

Cardiac Allograft Survival

The mean survival time (MST) of ACI cardiac allografts in untreated Lewis recipients is 6.6 ± 0.5 days. Immunosuppression with CsA resulted in survival of all ACI cardiac allografts for the duration of the experiment, i.e., 7 days. All syngeneic grafts survived for the duration of the experiment in both the CsA-treated and untreated animals.

Migration of Host ^{111}In-Labeled Lymphocytes

Most of the adoptively transferred, radiolabeled lymphocytes were recovered in the spleens and mesenteric or cervical lymph nodes in all transplanted animals. The uptake of radioactivity by bone marrow, thymus, and

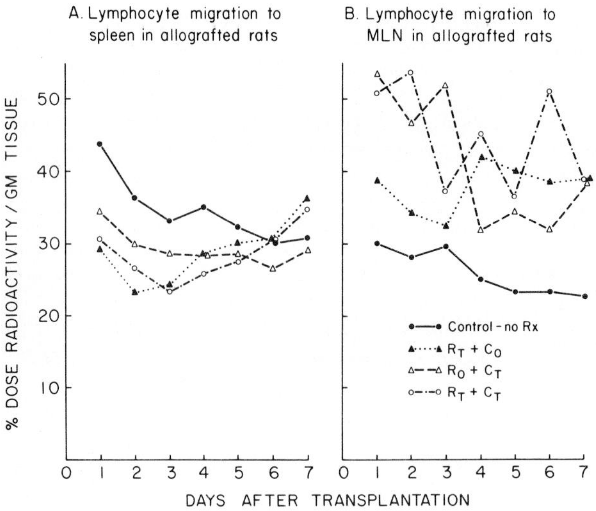

Fig. 1. Accumulation of ^{111}In-labeled syngeneic (Lewis) lymphocytes in spleen (A) and mesenteric lymph nodes (B) of ACI cardiac allografted Lewis rats. Each point represents results obtained in 4 animals in each group on a daily basis after allografting. The decrease in splenic accumulation on days 1–4 is contrasted with increased lymph node accumulation in recipients treated with CsA and/or CsA-treated lymphocytes.

other nonlymphoid organs was relatively very small throughout the study. In syngeneic transplantation, there was little change observed in adoptively transferred lymphocyte migration between untreated controls and experimental groups where either recipients and/or lymphocyte donors were treated with CsA.

Spleen

As shown in Fig. 1A, there was a significant decrease in the accumulation of ^{111}In-labeled lymphocytes in the spleens of allografted animals treated in vivo with CsA and/or infused with CsA-treated cells, as compared to the levels of radioactivity recovered in the spleen of the untreated controls. This difference was significant from day 1 to day 4 after transplantation, but subsequently became insignificant due to the decrease in splenic accumulation in the controls and the gradual rise in splenic accumulation in the experimental groups. No statistically significant difference in lymphocyte accumulation patterns was observed in the spleens of recipients of syngeneic cardiac grafts, regardless of whether they were treated with CsA or not.

Cervical and Mesenteric Lymph Nodes

In contrast to the splenic lymphocyte accumulation, recipients of allografts receiving CsA-treated cells and/or treated in vivo with CsA (groups III and IV) showed a high accumulation of radiolabeled lymphocytes on day 1 after transplantation, and this continued throughout the experimental period. This was also true, to a lesser extent, in group II (CsA treatment in vivo only) and was most apparent from day 4 after transplantation until day 7, as compared to the results obtained in untreated recipients of allografts. Recipients of syngeneic cardiac grafts demonstrated no significant increase in lymphocyte accumulation in mesenteric lymph nodes (MLN). Recipients of allografts treated in vivo with CsA and/or infused with CsA-treated lymphocytes had a significantly higher daily accumulation of lymphocytes in the cervical lymph nodes than did the untreated control recipients of allografts, and the results were similar to those seen in MLN. CsA treatment had no apparent effect on lymphocyte migration in isografted animals. The accumulation of adoptively transferred radiolabeled lymphocytes in the thymus of allografted animals was very small in all experimental groups, and no significant differences were observed from the results obtained in untreated allografted animals. CsA treatment of recipients and/or lymphocyte donors did not alter the migration pattern of host cells to the liver, bone marrow, lung,

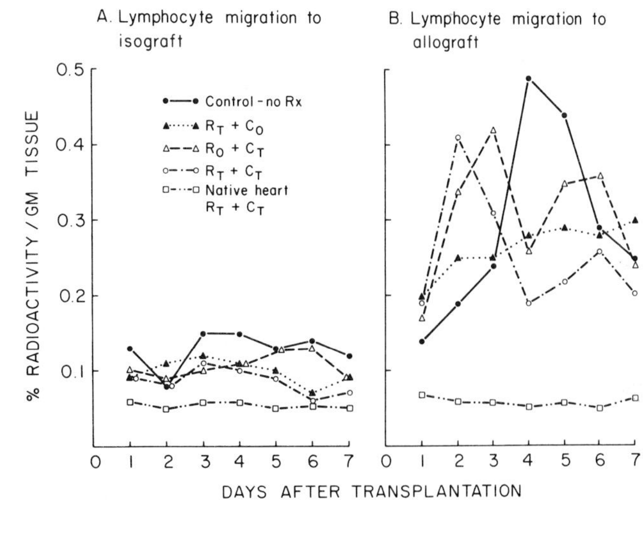

Fig. 2. Accumulation of ^{111}In-labeled syngeneic (Lewis) lymphocytes in Lewis cardiac isografts (A) and ACI cardiac allografts (B) compared to accumulation in recipients' native hearts (A and B). CsA does not alter lymphocyte accumulation in cardiac isografts or native hearts, but alters significantly lymphocyte migration to cardiac allografts as compared to controls.

kidney, or blood as compared to the very low levels of accumulation of radiolabeled cells in these organs in the control groups.

Accumulation of Cells in Transplanted Hearts

As shown in Fig. 2 (A and B), there was a significant difference in accumulation of radiolabeled host lymphocytes in the transplanted hearts between the isografted controls (treated and untreated) and the allografted groups. Accumulation of ^{111}In-labeled lymphocytes in syngeneic heart grafts was stable and very low throughout the experimental period, regardless of CsA treatment. In the untreated recipients of cardiac allografts, there was a marked increase in lymphocyte accumulation by day 4 after transplantation and this gradually decreased by day 7 (time of rejection). In contrast, recipients of in vivo CsA-treated lymphocytes (groups III and IV) showed an initial (day 2 posttransplantation) increase in accumulation of radiolabeled cells in the allograft, which gradually decreased by day 4 after transplantation. Group II, where the recipients were treated in vivo with CsA, had a relatively steady daily uptake of radiolabeled untreated syngeneic cells and showed no significant changes in uptake throughout the experimental period, while those that were both treated with CsA and received CsA-treated cells showed a precipitate decrease in radioactivity by day 4, which remained low. Simultaneous measurement of radioactivity in native hearts was low and stable both in the allografted and isografted animals.

DISCUSSION

Many experimental and clinical studies have demonstrated that CsA is a unique and powerful immunosuppressive agent. Heart and kidney allografts have functioned indefinitely in rat and rabbit recipients treated with a short course of CsA.[18-20] Prolonged graft survival has also been reported in CsA-treated dogs,[21] pigs,[22] and primates.[23] The initial report by Calne[24] that CsA can prevent kidney rejection in man has been followed by many recent clinical trials that indicate that this drug alone, or in combination with prednisone, is a very effective immunosuppressive agent in man.[25-28] It has been suggested that CsA acts by its inhibitory action on Interleukin-2, which prevents activation of both helper and cytotoxic T cells.[10] Leapman et al.[7] showed that the drug reduces Ia-like antigens on lymphocytes, while Hess et al.[6] showed that CsA preferentially inhibits induction of such toxic effector cells, while allowing the expression of alloantigen-activated suppressor cells.

Other postulated mechanisms on the immunosuppressive activity of CsA include alteration of the antigen recognition process and modification of the early differentiation of T lymphocytes.[29]

In the present study, we hypothesized that CsA acts by altering the antigen recognition process in the afferent limb of immune response as a result of its blocking effect on the surface receptors on T lymphocytes,[8-10] and therefore, in vivo treatment with CsA of recipients of allografts or of adoptively transferred lymphocytes would alter the homing patterns of effector cells to the peripheral lymphoid organs in cardiac allografts. We have previously reported[30] that unsensitized syngeneic cells localize preferentially in the lymph nodes, while sensitized syngeneic and allogeneic cells localize preferentially in the spleen of the ungrafted and cardiac allografted hosts. The localization of unreactive (syngeneic) cells in lymph nodes relative to the spleen has been attributed to the affinity of the cells for the specialized endothelium and the postcapillary venules in the lymph node cortex[31-34] and positive recognition of HLA identity.[35] Since the spleen appears to be the prominent site for antigen localization and processing during immune responses,[36,38] it is not surprising that the preferential accumulation of alloreactive cells is in the spleen. The present study demonstrates that there is preferential homing of adoptively transferred radiolabeled lymphocytes to the lymph nodes, with concomitant splenic lymphocyte depletion in recipients of cardiac allografts treated with CsA and/or infused with in vivo CsA-treated cells. It appears that the localization of such adoptively transferred CsA-treated lymphocytes in the lymph nodes in untreated or CsA-treated recipients of cardiac allografts depends on failure of sensitization of the cells by the graft alloantigens. This can only be true if CsA blocks the surface receptors of the adoptively transferred lymphocytes. Previous reports by Palacios and Möller[8] and Leapman et al.[9] complement such interpretation of our results.

The early accumulation of CsA-treated cells in the rat cardiac allografts may result from nonspecific immune response to the graft histocompatibility antigens. An interesting major difference in the accumulation of radiolabeled cells in the allograft was noted when there was a significant decrease of radioactivity on days 4 and 5 after transplantation in CsA-treated recipients, as compared to the controls that showed peak cardiac allograft radioactivity on day 4 (Fig. 2, A and B), Parallel with these observations, the accumulation of radiolabeled lymphocytes in the lymph nodes of control animals showed a sharp decline on day 3 after transplantation, while it rose significantly in the lymph nodes on day 3 in the CsA-treated groups. These findings suggest that CsA treatment of the recipient and/or of the lymphocytes (in vivo) leads to the inactivation of the lymphocyte cells' surface receptors, thereby preventing the graft histocompatibility antigens from sensitizing circulating cells that pass through the cardiac allograft. The preferential appearance of such cells in the lymph nodes after their apparent disappearance out of the graft is probably due to their joining the lymphocyte recirculating pool, as would be expected from unsensitized lymphocytes.

The results of this study, by showing that CsA treatment of cardiac allograft recipients and/or of host lymphocytes (in vivo) alters syngeneic lymphocyte migration patterns to the peripheral lymphoid organs and cardiac allografts, confirms, in a different experimental model, a previous observation[8–10] that CsA exerts its major immunosuppressive action probably by blocking surface receptors on lymphocytes, thereby abolishing the recognition phenomenon in allografting. This study further suggests an approach to evaluate other immunosuppressive agents or methods that may be synergistic or additive to the immunosuppressive action of CsA.

REFERENCES

1. Borel JF, Feurer C, Gubler HV, et al: Agents Actions 6:468, 1976
2. Borel JF, Feurer C, Mangee C, et al: Immunology 32:1017, 1977
3. White DJG, Plumbo AM, Pawelee G, et al: Transplantation 27:55, 1979
4. Leapman SB, Filo RS, Smith EJ, et al: Transplant Proc 13:405, 1981
5. Gordon D, Nouri AME: Clin Exp Immunol 44:287, 1981
6. Hess AD, Tutschka PJ: J Immunol 124:2601, 1980
7. Leapman SB, Filo RS, Smith EJ, et al: Transplantation 30:404, 1980
8. Palacios R, Möller G: Nature 290:792, 1981
9. Leapman SB, Strong DM, Filo RS, et al: Transplantation 34:94, 1982
10. Britton S, Palacios R: Immunol Rev 65:5, 1982
11. Ferguson RM: (personal communication)
12. Kupiec-Weglinski JW, Tilney NL: Transplantation 32:121, 1981
13. Baldwin WM, Hutchinson IF, Meijer CJLM, et al: Transplantation 31:117, 1981
14. Oluwole S, Wang T, Fawwaz R, et al: Transplantation 31:51, 1981
15. Satake K, Kuromoto N, Oluwole S, et al: Heart Transplant 1:208, 1982
16. Ono K, Lindsey BS: J Thorac Cardiovasc Surg 57:225, 1969
17. Thakur ML, Coleman RE, Welch MJ: J Lab Clin Med 89:217, 1977
18. Kostakis AJ, White DJG, Calne RY: IRCS Med Sci 5:280, 1977
19. Green CJ, Allison AC, Precious S: Lancet 2:123, 1979
20. Homan WP, Fabre JW, Williams KA, et al: Transplantation 29:361, 1980
21. Calne RY, White DJG: IRCS Med Sci 5:595, 1977
22. Calne RY, White DJG, Rolles K, et al: Lancet 2:1181, 1978
23. Pennock JL, Reitz BA, Bieber CP, et al: Transplant Proc 13:390, 1981
24. Calne RY, Rolles K, White DJG, et al: Lancet 2:1323, 1978

25. Calne RY, Rolles K, White DJG, et al: Transplant Proc 13:349, 1981

26. Rynasiewicz JJ, Sutherland DER, Ferguson RM, et al: Diabetes 31(Suppl 4):92, 1982

27. Starzl TE, Klintmalm GBG, Porter KA, et al: N Engl J Med 305:266, 1981

28. Oyer PE, Stinson EB, Jamieson SW, et al: Heart Transplant 1:285, 1982

29. Borel JF, Wiesinger F: In Lucas DO (ed): Regulatory Mechanisms in Lymphocyte Activation. New York, Academic Press, 1982, p 716

30. Oluwole S, Satake K, Kuromoto N, et al: Transplantation (in press)

31. Gowans JL, Knight EJ: Proc R Soc Biol 159:257, 1964

32. Nieuwenhuis P, Ford WL: Cell Immunol 23:254, 1976

33. Carey GD, Chin Y, Woodruff JJ: J Immunol 127:976, 1981

34. Ford WL: Prog Allergy 19:1, 1975

35. Degos L, Pla M, Colombani JM: Eur J Immunol 9:808, 1979

36. Ford WL, Simmonds SJ: Cell Tissue Kinet 5:175, 1972

37. Gowans JL: Ann NY Acad Sci 99:432, 1962

38. Atkins RC, Ford WL: J Exp Med 141:664, 1975

Studies With T Cells From Long-Term Surviving Canine Lung Allograft Recipients: Reduced Lymphocyte-Mediated Cytotoxicity But Not Reduced Mixed Lymphocyte Reactivity

A. J. Norin, E. E. Emeson, K. L. Pinsker, S. L. Kamholz, and F. J. Veith

UNTIL recently, immunosuppressive techniques for lung transplantation in outbred species were relatively unsuccessful as compared to other organs. The use of cyclosporine (CsA), in combination with other drugs, has resulted in a significant improvement in the survival of lung allografts in dogs, rats, monkeys, and man.[1-6] Furthermore, a number of studies with different organ transplant models have indicated that CsA therapy could be terminated without the subsequent rejection of the graft.[3,7-12] These findings raise the possibility that CsA therapy may, under certain circumstances, be effective in inducing a state of tolerance to allografts in man.

Effects of CsA on cytolytic T-cell (CTC) activity may be important to the suppression of rejection and/or the induction of unresponsiveness. This is a preliminary report of our investigations of mixed lymphocyte reactivity (MLR) and CTC activity of lymphocytes obtained from long-term surviving lung allograft recipients that have received CsA therapy. These experiments suggest that CTC and their precursors are depleted from the blood but are present in the allografted lungs. In contrast to CTC precursors, other T lymphocytes are present in the blood that proliferate in response to irradiated donor lymphocytes (i.e., a donor-specific MLR).

MATERIALS AND METHODS

Left lung allotransplantation was performed in male mongrel dogs (Biomedical Associates, Inc., Friedensberg, PA) as previously described.[2,13] CsA (Sandoz Ltd., Basel, Switzerland) was administered alone or in combination with azathioprine (2 mg/kg for 14 days) and/or steroids, as detailed elsewhere.[3] Lung allografts were evaluated by previously reported techniques.[2,3] The diagnostic procedures included: chest roentgenograms, radionuclide ventilation-perfusion lung scans, analysis of cells in bronchoalveolar lavage (BAL), and open lung biopsies or necropsies.

CTC activity was measured as previously reported.[14] The washed cell preparations from BAL were enriched for T lymphocytes by the nylon column technique and incubated in RPMI 1640 medium with 15% fetal bovine serum, penicillin (100 IU/ml), streptomycin (100 μg/ml), and glutamine (2 mM) (RPMI-complete). One hundred microliters of T cells was added to 100 μl of ^{51}Cr-labeled Raji cells (lectin-dependent cytotoxicity, LDC) incubated with 10 μg/ml concanavalin-A (Con-A) in 96-well round-bottom microtiter plates (Nunc, Roskilde, Denmark). Specific cytotoxicity assays were performed with ^{51}Cr-labeled Con-A-stimulated lymphocytes from the donor or third-party dogs. Two-to-four-day-old blast cells were washed with methyl-α-D-mannoside–RPMI-complete to remove Con-A. Effector-to-target cell ratios were varied from 100:1 to 6.25:1, with the number of target cells kept constant. After 3–4 hr at 37°C, 100 μl of supernatant from triplicate samples were harvested and the ^{51}Cr radioactivity determined in a gamma spectrophotometer (Model 1185, Searle Analytic, Inc., Des Plaines, IL). The percent cytotoxicity was calculated by the formula: (cpm experimental − cpm spontaneous) ÷ (cpm maximum − cpm spontaneous) × 100.

One-way mixed lymphocyte cultures (MLC) were initiated by incubating Ficoll-Hypaque, nylon column purified peripheral blood T cells with ^{60}Co-irradiated (2000 rad) stimulator cells at a concentration of 10^6 responders/ml and 10^6 stimulators/ml for 7 days at 37°C. At the end of the culture period, quadruplicate 200-μl samples were incubated in microtiter wells with ^{3}H-thymidine, 1 μCi/ml, 3 Ci/mM (Schwarz Mann, Orangeburg, NY) to determine proliferation.[15] The remainder of the cells were washed twice and resuspended at an appropriate concen-

---

From the Departments of Microbiology and Immunology, Surgery, Pathology, and Medicine, Montefiore Medical Center, Albert Einstein College of Medicine, New York, NY.

Supported in part by NIH Grant HL17417 and the Manning Foundation.

Address reprint requests to Dr. A. J. Norin, C416, Montefiore Medical Center, Albert Einstein College of Medicine, 111 East 210th Street, New York, NY 10467.

0041-1345/83/1505-0145$01.00/0

tration for cytotoxicity determinations on specific and third-party Con-A-stimulated ^{51}Cr-labeled blasts.

RESULTS

We have previously demonstrated that MLC of canine peripheral blood T cells not only generate cytolytic activity to the specific target cells, but also to Raji target cells in the presence of Con-A, i.e., LDC.[14] The data presented in Table 1 indicate that T cells obtained from an allografted lung also have the ability to kill specific donor-type target cells, as well as the ability to kill nonspecific lectin-coated target cells. Significantly less cytotoxic activity was detected in the T-cell population obtained from the recipient's own right lung or the blood.[14,16]

Seven lung transplant recipients with long-term graft survival are listed in Table 2. These dogs may be separated into two groups based on lung survival, the level of LDC, and other signs of rejection. The allografted lungs of the first group of four recipients were eventually rejected despite high-dose methylprednisolone therapy.[3] These dogs had high levels of LDC (>20%) and moderate to severe evidence of rejection as judged by chest films, perfusion scans, and histologic sections of open lung biopsies. In contrast, the lung allografts of the second group of recipients survived with good function until completion of this study. Dogs 15 and 19 had LDC levels that were ≤15%, and dog 1 had LDC ≤5%. Other evidence of rejection was slight in dogs 15 and 19 and could not be detected in dog 1. Despite prednisone therapy, LDC in serial BAL in both groups remained relatively constant when compared to the initial study of each dog at 3 weeks after transplantation. However, the steroid therapy did reduce the total number of lymphocytes that were recovered by BAL.

Table 1. In Vivo Generation of Lectin-Dependent and Specific Cytolytic T-Cell Activity

Source of T Cells*	E:T	Percent Cytotoxicity Target Cells: Raji	Donor 27
BAL, left lung	100	21.2 ± 2.1	13.6 ± 2.8
BAL, right lung	100	5.3 ± 0.7	0.3 ± 0.1

*Nylon-column-purified lymphocytes from recipient 27 at 121 days after transplantation.

E:T, effector-to-target cell ratios.

The ability of peripheral blood T cells from lung allograft recipients to proliferate in response to donor alloantigens and to generate donor-specific cytotoxicity was examined. Recipient T cells had a normal MLR to donor stimulator cells as compared to the response of normal dog T cells to the same stimulators (Fig. 1 and Table 3). The MLR of recipient T cells in response to donor cell stimulation was also similar to the MLR of recipient T cells induced by third-party lymphocytes (Table 3). Donor stimulators generated high cytolytic activity after MLC with third-party lymphocytes (Fig. 1 and Table 3). Furthermore, third-party stimulators generated high cytolytic activity after MLC with recipient T lymphocytes (Table 3). In contrast, MLCs of recipient T cells and irradiated donor lymphocytes generated poor cytolytic activity to ^{51}Cr-labeled donor target cells (Fig. 1 and Table 3).

DISCUSSION

We have previously demonstrated the generation of specific cytolytic T cells and LDC in MLCs of canine peripheral blood lympho-

Table 2. Cytolytic T-Cell Activity and Other Evidence of Rejection in Cyclosporine-Treated Canine Lung Allograft Recipients With Long-Term Survival

Dog No.	Lung Survival (Days)	Percent Cytotoxicity*	Index of Rejection†
4, 8, 17, 23	352, 282, 175, 189	54, 54, 28, 26	4+, 3+, 3+, 2+
1, 15, 19	>1053, >415,‡ >460	4, 13, 15	0, 1+, 1+

*Lectin-dependent cytotoxicity, E:T, 100:1.

†Based on periodic chest films, lung ^{99}Tc perfusion scans, and histologic sections of open lung biopsies or necropsies.

‡Dogs 1 and 15 were killed at 1053 and 415 days, respectively.

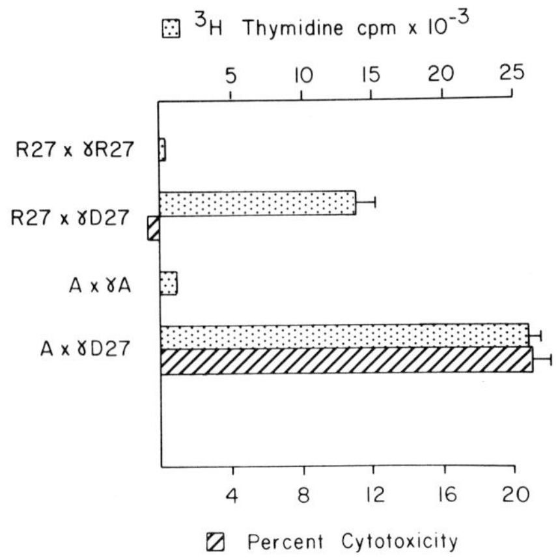

Fig. 1. Peripheral blood T cells of recipient 27 (R27, at 121 days after transplantation) and a normal dog (A) were analyzed for MLR and specific cytotoxicity as described in Materials and Methods.

cytes.[14] In the present report, we show that LDC and specific cytotoxicity are mediated by T cells obtained from the BAL of lung allografts. Both types of cytotoxic activity are reduced, or are not present, in the cell populations from the normal right lung and blood. These findings are a further indication that LDC can be used in the absence of specific target cells to identify the in vivo generation of T-cell-mediated cytolytic activity against an allografted lung.

Our initial results suggest that the LDC at 3 weeks after transplantation correlates with other manifestations of rejection and graft survival. T cells from BAL of normal dogs had LDC of less than 5% at an E:T ratio of 100:1.[14] In 4 lung allograft recipients that survived less than 6 months, LDC was greater than 25% (E:T, 100:1) and all had rejection.[16] Another recipient died of a wound infection at 68 days with no evidence of rejection and LDC of 2.0% (E:T, 20:1). In this report, we show that lung allograft recipients that survived greater than 6 months and had low LDC also had better graft survival with less clinical evidence of rejection than long-surviving recipients with high LDC. Interestingly, the lungs of recipients that had low levels of LDC survived indefinitely after CsA therapy was stopped, whereas the lung allograft of one recipient (dog 23) with a higher level of LDC was rejected at 100 days after termination of CsA therapy.[3,7] This preliminary finding suggests that the level of LDC may be useful in predicting those recipients in which CsA therapy may be discontinued without rejection.

In several experiments, we found that the peripheral blood T cells of lung allograft recipients (with >25% LDC) proliferated in a one-way MLR to irradiated donor lymphocytes. However, cells from these responding cultures had reduced ability to kill donor target cells. Since a high level of CTC was found in the BAL of their allografted lungs, we postulate that CTC precursors also accumulate in the graft and thus account for their relative depletion from the blood.

The role of CTC in rejection is not firmly established, though a number of studies have suggested their importance.[16,17] In CsA-treated lung allografts, it is clear that CTC are associated with the presence of focal peri-

Table 3. In Vitro Mixed Lymphocyte Reactivity and Specific Cytotoxicity of Lymphocytes From a Long-Term Surviving Canine Lung Allograft Recipient

MLC	MLR (^{3}HTdR cpm/Culture)	Target	Percent Cytotoxicity at E:T 100	50	25	12
(R23 × γD23)	13,302 ± 1,556	D23	7.4	4.2	2.6	2.6
		3rd	0.9	−0.2	0.2	0.3
(R23 × γ3rd)	10,160 ± 2,633	D23	0.4	0.2	0.8	1.0
		3rd	46	29	20	14
(3rd × γD23)	19,674 ± 2,366	D23	51	44	33	25
		3rd	−0.3	0.6	1.0	1.7

R23, Lymphocytes from lung allograft recipient 23 (cells obtained 85 days after termination of CsA therapy); D23, lymphocytes from lung allograft donor for recipient 23; 3rd, lymphocytes from a third-party dog. ^{3}HTdR, ^{3}H-thymidine.

The MLR of (R23 × γR23) = 745 ± 58, and the MLR of (3rd × γ3rd) = 1,443 ± 388.

vascular and interstitial mononuclear cell infiltrates and reduced lung blood flow.[1,3,16] Maintenance prednisone therapy begun after initial methylprednisolone treatment was beneficial in inhibiting these reactions.[3] Recent evidence suggests that a subset of inducer/helper T cells (those that mediate delayed hypersensitivity) play an even more pivotal role in mediating the rejection of organ grafts than CTC.[18–20] The same class of T cells is a major responding cell type in mixed lymphocyte reactions.[21] Future studies will be required to elucidate the effects of CsA on the activity of these cells. It is important to determine the relative level of MLR of T cells from blood as compared to T cells from the BAL of lung allografts. Also of interest is an examination of the suppressive effect of T cells from BAL on inducer/helper T-cell activity after CsA therapy is terminated.

REFERENCES

1. Norin AJ, Veith FJ, Emeson EE, et al: Transplantation 32:259, 1981
2. Veith FJ, Norin AJ, Montefusco CM, et al: Transplantation 32:474, 1981
3. Norin AJ, Emeson EE, Kamholz SL, et al: Transplantation 34:372, 1982
4. Prop J, Bartels HL, Petersen AH, et al: Transplant Proc 15:511, 1983
5. Reitz BA, Beiber CP, Raney AA, et al: Transplant Proc 13:393, 1981
6. Reitz BA, Wallwork JL, Hunt SA, et al: N Engl J Med 306:557, 1982
7. Norin AJ, Emeson EE, Veith FJ: Transplant Proc 15:508, 1983
8. Homan WP, Fabre JW, Morris PJ: Transplantation 28:439, 1979
9. Nagao T, White DJG, Calne RY: Transplantation 33:31, 1982
10. Green CJ, Allison AC: Lancet 1:1182, 1978
11. Dunn DC, White DJG, Herbertson BM, et al: Transplantation 27:359, 1979
12. Calne RY, White DJG, Rolles K, et al: Lancet 1:1183, 1978
13. Veith FJ, Richards K: Ann Surg 171:553, 1970
14. Emeson EE, Norin AJ, Veith FJ: Transplantation 33:365, 1982
15. Norin AJ, Short MK: J Immunol 129:2377, 1982
16. Emeson EE, Norin AJ, Kamholz SL, et al: Transplant Proc 15:550, 1983
17. Loveland BE, McKenzie IFC: Transplantation 33:217, 1982
18. Loveland BE, Hogarth PM, Caredig RH, et al: J Exp Med 153:1044, 1981
19. Loveland BE, McKenzie IFC: Transplantation 33:174, 1982
20. Dallman MJ, Mason DW: Transplantation 33:221, 1982
21. Reinherz EL, Kung PC, Goldstein G, et al: Proc Natl Acad Sci USA 76:4061, 1979

LIVER, PANCREAS, INTESTINE

Histologic Evidence of Modification of Liver Allograft Rejection in Inbred Miniature Swine by Cyclosporine

M. W. Flye

PREVIOUSLY, we have demonstrated[1] that there will be long-term survivors among unimmunosuppressed domestic farm pigs or SLA-matched inbred miniature swine receiving orthotopically placed liver transplants. However, if the donor and recipient are mismatched for the major histocompatibility complex (MHC), death results within 14.6 ± 3.6 days from massive liver rejection. This fatal immune response can be modified by the administration of a short course of cyclosporine (CsA).[1]

Battersby et al.[2] showed by serial biopsies that although a progressive round cell infiltration, consistent with rejection, occurred in all outbred pig liver allografts, this usually spontaneously resolved within a month in long-term survivors. Similarly, in the rat, the liver graft has been found to be under immune attack with a profuse cellular infiltrate between 5 and 15 days, during the establishment of donor-specific unresponsiveness.[3,4]

However, the histologic pattern in the liver has not been examined during and following treatment with CsA. The use of miniature swine inbred for the MHC allows comparison of animals of similar genetic disparity treated with or without CsA.

MATERIALS AND METHODS

Miniature Swine

Animals of the NIH colony of well characterized miniature swine were a generous gift from Dr. David Sachs.[5] Three herds, differing at the MHC and designated a, c, or d, were used to insure SLA-matched or mismatched donor–recipient combinations. The offspring of controlled breeding were SLA-typed by trypan blue exclusion and mixed lymphocyte culture (MLC) reactivity.

Liver Allografts

The recipient's liver was orthotopically replaced by a liver of the appropriate SLA type during extracorporeal shunting of the portal and inferior caval blood to the internal jugular vein. No homologous blood transfusions were given. Immediately postoperatively, cyclosporine was begun in a dose of 10 or 20 mg/kg/day for 25–50 days. Initially given intramuscularly, this was changed to oral administration when the animal was eating.

Histologic Examination

Serial percutaneous needle biopsies were examined by light microscopy after staining with hematoxylin and eosin. At the time of death or sacrifice, a complete autopsy was performed and grafts examined histologically.

Renal and Skin Grafts

One to three months after completion of CsA treatment, a renal graft of the liver donor SLA was trans-

---

From the Department of Surgery, Yale University School of Medicine, New Haven, CT.

Supported in part by the Zelda Zinn Casper Foundation.

Address reprint requests to Dr. M. W. Flye, Department of Surgery, Yale University School of Medicine, New Haven, CT 06510.

0041–1345/83/1505–0146$01.00/0

planted to the liver recipient. A cutaneous ureterostomy allowed monitoring of urine output. Rejection, as defined by cessation of urine output, was confirmed by renal biopsy. The liver allograft was simultaneously biopsied. Cryopreserved skin grafts from the liver donor and from other SLA matched or mismatched animals were placed on the liver recipient 1–2 months following renal graft rejection.

RESULTS

SLA-Mismatched Liver Recipients

Two or more liver biopsies were taken from 10 SLA-mismatched recipients. Biopsies taken 1 hr after transplantation appeared normal. A rise in serum bilirubin 4–7 days following transplantation correlated well with the onset of histologic evidence of rejection. Initially, there was infiltration and widening of the portal tracts by lymphocytes, mononuclear cells, and eosinophils. This infiltrate spread into the parenchyma as rejection progressed. There was resulting necrosis of hepatocytes, with disruption of the lobular architecture as early as 8 days. At the time of death from progressive liver failure after 14.6 ± 3.6 days, there usually were few viable hepatocytes remaining within the dense cellular infiltrate.

SLA-Matched Liver Recipients

The biochemical, clinical, and histologic course varied greatly between animals receiving SLA-matched liver allografts. In 2 of 8 animals serially biopsied, there was a minimal portal cellular infiltrate and widening of the portal tracts without hepatocyte involvement over the 2 years prior to sacrifice. Two animals died from marked rejection after 79 and 95 days. The remaining animals demonstrated lesser degrees of rejection. This ongoing chronic rejection allowed the development of fibrosis and intrahepatic scarring. The resulting portal hypertension was manifested by dilated abdominal veins. In the more severe cases, there was collapse and fibrosis of the hepatic lobule. Occasionally, regenerating hepatocytes were present. Cholestasis was present when sloughing bile duct cells resulted in intrahepatic biliary obstruction.

Cyclosporine-Treated SLA-Mismatched Liver Recipients

The survival of SLA-mismatched animals was increased to greater than 170 days after receiving 20 mg/kg/day CsA for 25–50 days. Serial biopsies showed minimal to absent cellular infiltration in the portal areas, with good preservation of the hepatocyte cords. After 4–6 months, some animals had widening of the interlobular septae consistent with fibrosis. This histologic picture was strikingly different than for the non-CsA-treated SLA-mismatched recipients and similar to several of the SLA-matched animals without rejection.

When 10 mg/kg/day of CsA was used to treat these liver recipients, survival was not prolonged and death resulted in 16.0 ± 4.0 days with a histologic pattern of severe rejection.

Renal Grafts Following Cyclosporine Treatment

Three liver recipients received renal transplants of the liver SLA type 1–3 months after CsA was stopped. Urine output from the transplant cutaneous ureterostomy stopped after 8–12 days. Renal biopsy at that time demonstrated severe cellular infiltration, while a simultaneous liver biopsy showed minimal signs of rejection. Subsequent biopsies demonstrated progressive fibrosis. A second renal transplant of the same SLA resulted in hyperacute rejection without urine production. While no cytotoxic antibody was detectable in the liver recipient prior to renal grafting, within 3–5 days of the renal transplant, antibodies cytotoxic to both T and B cells were present.

Skin Grafts Following Cyclosporine Treatment

Following renal grafting, cryopreserved liver donor and SLA matched and mismatched skin grafts were placed on the liver recipient. Liver donor skin survival was prolonged 5–8 days, while third-party SLA matched or mismatched skin was rejected in normal first-set time. A second set of the same skin grafts was rejected in an accelerated fashion. Throughout the rejection of renal and skin grafts, there was no change in the histology of the liver transplant.

DISCUSSION

Unlike the SLA-matched miniature swine and some domestic farm pigs, the degree of genetic disparity in the SLA-mismatched miniature pig induces violent rejection from which the nonimmunosuppressed liver cannot recover. However, a short course of CsA, 20 mg/kg/day, allows long-term engraftment of an SLA-mismatched liver. This is associated with minimal histologic signs of rejection. Even in the presence of rejection of kidney and skin of the same SLA type and the development of cytotoxic antibodies, rejection of the transplanted liver does not occur. We do not yet know whether a liver graft would be more readily rejected if it followed a renal graft and a course of CsA. This phenomenon of continued acceptance of the liver, while kidney and skin grafts are being rejected, is different from the acceptance of a second renal allograft from a third-party donor[6] by CsA-treated rabbits bearing a long-surviving renal allograft.

In farm pigs not genetically characterized, Degen et al.[7] have found MLC suppression by lymphocytes from kidney-transplanted animals but not from liver-bearing pigs. On the other hand, they found that MLC blocking antibodies were always present in liver-transplanted pigs and caused 85% MLC suppression compared to 15% inhibition by kidney transplanted sera. We have been unable to demonstrate significant MLC suppression.

Davies et al.[3] have shown that PVG rats bearing DA long-term liver grafts are specifically depleted of clones effecting graft rejection, and suppression was not detected. Lymphocytes from liver-grafted rats showed normal GVH reactivity and proliferation in MLC, but had a specific deficiency in the ability to generate cytotoxic cells. However, the mechanism of the induction of unresponsiveness in this rat strain is not yet known.

Some investigators have suggested that CsA may lead to clonal depletion of antigen-reactive T cells.[8] This does not seem to be the case in the present studies, since in these partially inbred miniature pigs, SLA skin and kidney were rejected, while Davies et al.[3] found that DA liver-grafted PVG rats were specifically depleted of clones capable of effecting DA skin graft rejection.

CONCLUSION

A state of unresponsiveness to SLA-mismatched liver grafts is induced in inbred miniature swine by a short course of CsA. The lack of significant cellular rejection is demonstrated on histologic examination. This persists despite rejection of the liver donor SLA type kidney and skin with the production of MHC cytotoxic antibodies.

REFERENCES

1. Flye MW, Rodgers G, Kacy S, et al: Transplant Proc 15:1269, 1983
2. Battersby C, Egerton WS, Bilderson G, et al: Surgery 76:617, 1974
3. Davies HffS, Kamada N, Rosen BJ: Transplant Proc 15:831, 1983
4. Zimmerman FA, Knoll PP, Davies HffS, et al: Transplant Proc 15:1272, 1983
5. Sachs DH, Leight G, Cone J, et al: Transplantation 22:559, 1976
6. Dunn DC, White DJG, Herbertson BM: Transplantation 29:349, 1980
7. Degen H, Bachhorn H, Baron DP, et al: Transplant Proc 15:737, 1983
8. Leoni P, Garcia RC, Allison AC: J Clin Lab Immunol 1:67, 1978

Induction of Liver Graft Tolerance in a Primarily Nontolerant Rat Strain Combination with Temporary Treatment of Cyclosporine

R. Engemann, K. Ulrichs, A. Thiede, W. Müller-Ruchholtz, and H. Hamelmann

IN LIVER transplantation, especially in some inbred rat strain combinations, the phenomenon of spontaneous long-term survival of animals with fully MHC allogeneic liver grafts has been described.[1,2] As recently observed,[3] such findings may be also dependent on methodological parameters. Following orthotopic rat liver transplantation (ORLT), syngeneic recipients exhibited improvement of graft survival, liver morphology, and cell-mediated lymphocytotoxicity (disappearance of nonspecific cytotoxicity) only after rearterialization of the hepatic artery. Furthermore, in the fully allogeneic strain combination BN ($RT1^n$) → LEW ($RT1^l$), spontaneous long-term survival occurred. To study further possibilities for manipulation of the liver allograft rejection, a donor–recipient combination was found in which, in spite of rearterialization, all animals died of graft rejection. Manipulation of rejection was performed with cyclosporine A (CsA), a nonsteroidal fungal metabolite that was first used for an immunosuppressive regimen by Calne[4] and has proved to be a powerful immunosuppressive agent in various species.[5] Though the drug has been used in clinical liver transplantation with promising results,[6] analytical data on CsA in rat liver transplantation are not yet available. Therefore, the aim of the present study was to investigate survival, liver morphology, and cell-mediated lymphocytotoxicity in the DA ($RT1^{avl}$) → LEW ($RT1^l$) combination after CsA therapy.

MATERIALS AND METHODS

Male LEW rats ($RT1^l$), weighing 250–300 g, were used as recipients. Male BDV ($RT1^d$), F344 ($RT1^{lvl}$), BN ($RT1^n$), or DA ($RT1^{avl}$) were used as liver donors and DA as skin and F344 as third party skin donors. Using microsurgical techniques, ORLT was performed with reanastomosis of the hepatic artery, as described in detail elsewhere.[3] For immunosuppression, CsA (Sandoz AG, Basel, Switzerland) was suspended in olive oil at 50 mg/ml and given orally in a concentration of 15 mg/kg body weight/day from the day of operation to the 13th postoperative day only. For in vivo studies, survival times were evaluated, and in long-term survivors, tolerance was tested by grafting donor-specific and third party skin at day 100 postoperation. For in vitro monitoring of graft recipients, cell-mediated reactivity was tested in the microcytotoxicity assay (MCA)[7] according to the procedure of Bröcker et al.[8] Reactivity of the recipients' lymphocytes of the various lymphatic compartments (blood, B; spleen, S; peripheral lymph nodes, PLN; mesenteric lymph nodes, MLN; Peyer's patches, PP) was tested against donor and third party strain fibroblasts in Terasaki microtest plates for 48 hr. The result was read microscopically and is indicated in the figures as integral of cell-mediated lysis. In vitro reactivity of the allogeneic graft recipients was always compared to background reactivity of the syngeneic control animals. Liver histology was performed with biopsies, usually taken at days 14, 20, 40, at the day of death, or at the day of in vitro testing. Stainings were done with hematoxylin and eosin.

To study the pattern of liver rejection followed by the death of the animals, various strain combinations were investigated: BDV → LEW ($n = 5$), F344 → LEW ($n = 5$), BN → LEW ($n = 12$), DA → LEW ($n = 10$), and LEW → LEW ($n = 17$) as syngeneic control group. Of all groups tested, only the DA → LEW combination was selected for experiments, since none of the graft recipients survived beyond day 14, while in all other combinations, long-term survivors could be observed. According to these pilot studies, the following experimental groups were chosen: group I, DA → LEW (without CsA treatment) with a total number of 17 animals, and group II, DA → LEW (with CsA treatment) with a total number of 32 liver-grafted animals up to now.

From the Department of General Surgery and the Department of Immunology, University of Kiel, Kiel, F.R.G.

Supported in part by the Deutsche Forschungsgemeinschaft, SFB 111, Projekt B 9. Cyclosporine A was generously supplied by Sandoz, AG., Basel, Switzerland.

Address reprint requests to Dr. R. Engemann, Department of General Surgery, University of Kiel, Hospitalstr. 40, 2300 Kiel 1, F.R.G.

0041-1345/83/1505-0147$01.00/0

Table 1. DA → LEW Combination with CsA Treatment: Of the 7 Animals Retained for the Long-Term Surviving Group, the Day and Cause of Death, as well as Liver Histology at the Day of Death, are Indicated

	Animal No.						
	3	4	1	2	6	5	7
Day of death	14	38	40	53	149	150	153
Cause of death	LI	LI	LI	LI	Test	Test	Test
Test							
Liver histology at the day of death	Ø	+	F	+	+F	Ø	+F

LI, Lung infections; Ø, no periportal mononuclear cell infiltrates, no fibrosis; +, slight periportal mononuclear cell infiltrates; F, slight fibrosis, restricted to the periportal field; Test, cell-mediated in vitro reactivity.

RESULTS

Survival and Tolerance

In the syngeneic LEW → LEW control group, 80% of the animals survived more than 100 days ($n = 17$). In group I without CsA treatment, none of the LEW rats bearing a DA liver allograft survived beyond day 14 (MST = 10.5 ± 2.3) in a survival study ($n = 10$). In contrast to this finding, in the CsA-treated group II, long-term survivors beyond day 100 could be obtained (survival study: see Table 1). Long-term survivors, who received donor-specific (DA) and third party (F344) skin grafts on the 100th day postoperation, showed specific nonresponsiveness, since the DA skin was accepted indefinitely, while F344 skin was rejected in a normal way ($n = 5$).

Cell-mediated In Vitro Reactivity

From previous observations,[9] one had to expect that cell-mediated in vitro reactivity of the recipients' lymphocytes against the allograft is suppressed in CsA-treated rats compared to nonimmunosuppressed rats. Four liver graft recipients in each experimental group were tested for cell-mediated in vitro reactivity at day 10; additionally, 3 tolerant rats of the CsA-treated group were tested at days 149, 150, and 153. The results are shown in Figs. 1 and 2. The analysis yields the following findings. (A) Group I vs. group II at day 10: in all 5 lymphatic compartments investigated, reactivity of the recipients' lymphocytes against donor antigen as well as against third party antigen is remarkably stronger in nonimmunosuppressed individuals of group I than in CsA-treated individuals of group II. (B) Group II at day 10 vs. day 150 (B.1): reactivity in the lymphatic transport compartment (blood) is clearly stronger at day 10 than at day 150, where it is almost zero. (B.2): in contrast, reactivity in the lym-

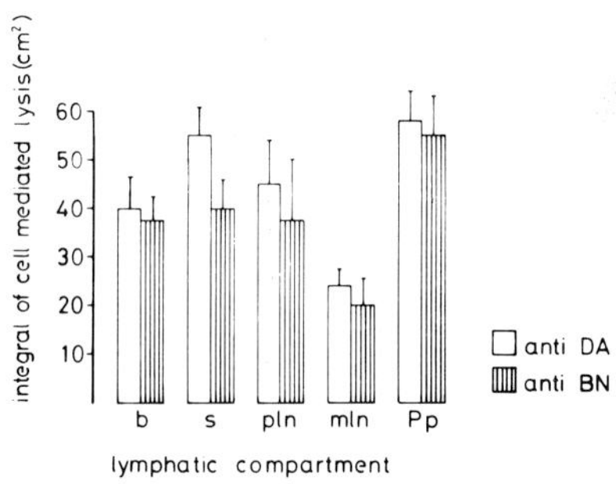

Fig. 1. Cell-mediated in vitro reactivity of liver graft recipients (group I, DA → LEW) in various lymphatic compartments at day 10 p.o., $n = 4$. b, Blood; s, spleen; pln, peripheral lymph nodes; mln, mesenteric lymph nodes; Pp, Peyer's patches.

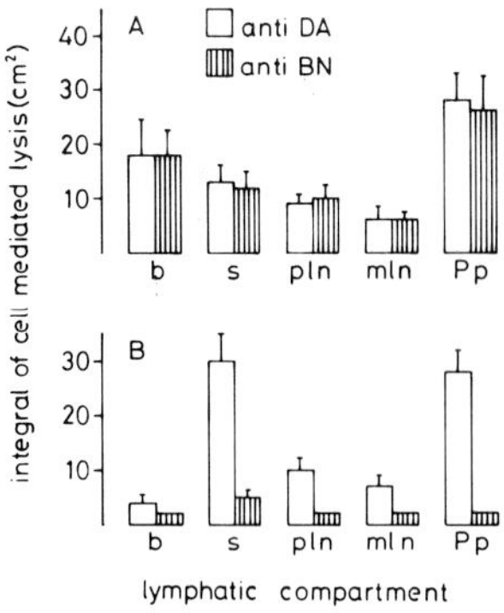

Fig. 2. Cell-mediated in vitro reactivity of liver graft recipients (group II, DA → LEW, CsA treatment) in various lymphatic compartments. (A) At day 10 p.o., $n = 4$, (B) at approximately day 150 p.o., $n = 3$.

phatic tissue compartment (spleen) is clearly lower at day 10 than at day 150. (B.3): reactivity in the 3 other lymphatic tissue compartments, i.e. peripheral and mesenteric lymph nodes and Peyer's patches is similar at both test times. (C) Specificity of cell-mediated in vitro reactivity: it was alloantigen specific in the long-term survivors, since reactivity against a third party strain (BN) was not elevated above the background reactivity of the syngeneic control animals; however, it was alloantigen nonspecific in the early p.o. phase, since third party reactivity (BN) was elevated above background reactivity.

Liver Macroscopy and Histology

(A) LEW → LEW: at all stages of their postoperative life (days 20, 50, 150, or 270), the syngeneic graft recipients showed a normal appearance of the liver ($n = 17$). The liver lobes had sharp edges and possessed few connective tissue adhesions. Histologically, in this syngeneic control group, evidence of liver alterations could not be found. (B) DA → LEW without CsA treatment: in contrast to the above findings, the DA livers of the non-immunosuppressed, nonsurviving LEW rats looked spotted and were swollen with round-edged lobes. Histology of these livers revealed severe periportal as well as intrahepatic mononuclear cell infiltrates, which finally lead to the destruction of the organ (Fig. 3). (C) DA → LEW with CsA treatment: the livers of the CsA-treated LEW rats bearing a DA graft, including some long-term survivors, were only slightly swollen and possessed round-edged liver lobes. Four of the 7 rats listed in Table 1 died of lung infections (histologically documented) at days 14, 38, 40, and 53. No death occurred due to graft rejection. Investigation of animal no. 1 at the time of death showed slight fibrosis restricted to the periportal field. Animals 2 and 4 had slight periportal mononuclear cell infiltrates, and animal 3 possessed a totally unaltered liver morphology. In the 3 long-term survivors, periportal mononuclear cell infiltrates could not be detected at day 14, only a few were

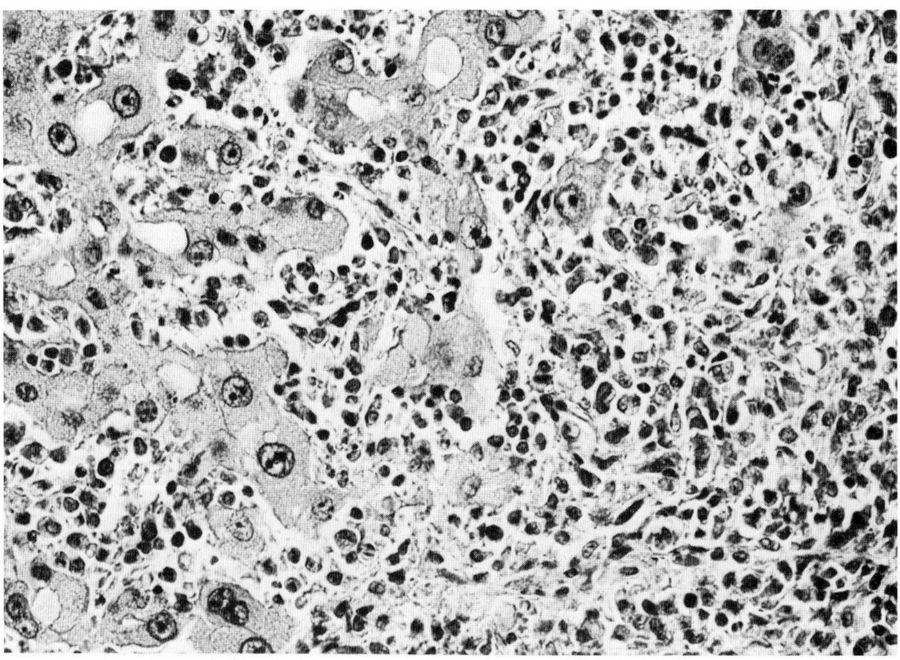

Fig. 3. Histology of an allogeneic untreated DA → LEW liver transplant at day 9 p.o.: severe allograft rejection, as documented by periportal and intrahepatic mononuclear cell infiltrates (hematoxylin and eosin, × 100).

present at day 20, and at day 40, round cell infiltrates appeared to be restricted to the periportal area. Histological examination of these rats at days 149, 150, and 153 revealed only very slight liver fibrosis and a few mononuclear cell infiltrates (see Table 1, animals 6 and 7), similar to those found at earlier stages. Absolutely no liver alteration could be detected in rat 5 (Fig. 4); the DA graft having functioned in a CsA-treated LEW recipient for 150 days had the appearance of a normal liver.

DISCUSSION

Experimental and human liver transplantation still yield heterogeneous and partly conflicting results. At present, some parameters causing this heterogeneity are becoming more apparent and may have to be carefully considered if liver transplantation is to be consistently successful in the future. In liver transplantation in several fully MHC allogeneic rat strain combinations (e.g. DA → PVG or DA → LEW), long-term graft survival occurs,[1,10] as well as rapid genetically determined graft rejection. So far, very little is known about the nature of this genetic determination in the experimental rat system, and even less about its equivalent in humans. A second important parameter is the microsurgical technique; orthotopic rat liver transplantation is usually performed without reanastomosis of the hepatic artery.[1,10] The striking differences in long-term graft survival, e.g. in the DA → PVG combination, ranging from 10%[10,11] to approximately 100%,[2] may indicate the influence of surgical skill and the value of the chosen technique on the transplantation result. In our own experiments, long-term graft survival in the BN → LEW combination was achieved with the improved orthotopic technique, whereas without it, all graft recipients died within 3 weeks.[3] In strain combinations with genetically determined graft rejection (rejection in spite of the optimized technique with reanastomosis of the hepatic

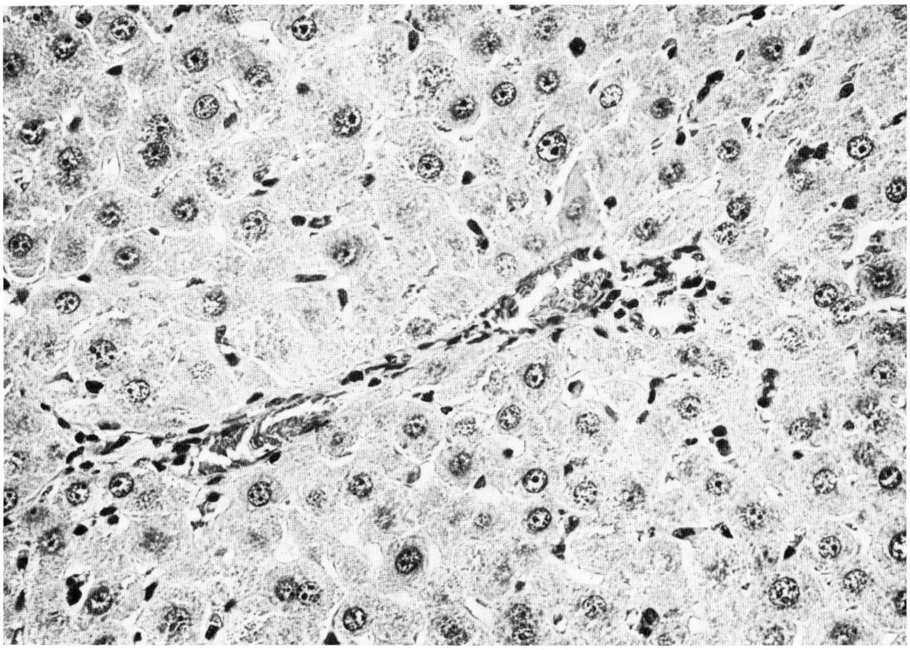

Fig. 4. Histology of an allogeneic CsA-treated DA → LEW liver transplant at day 150 p.o.: compared to the syngeneic control, there is normal structure of the periportal field and liver parenchyma (hematoxylin and eosin, × 100).

artery), it is obvious that the transplantation barrier can be overcome by treating the recipient with an immunosuppressive drug such as CsA. So far, promising results have been achieved with this drug in other transplantation models, including rats bearing kidney[12] or heart[13] allografts, and also in human liver transplantation.[6] In the clinical situation, a systematic analysis of these parameters is extremely difficult to achieve. Therefore, it seemed desirable to investigate them further in our experimental model.

In the survival study of group II, 4 of 7 rats died from lung infections rather than from graft rejection. Therefore, it cannot be excluded that the dosage, based on the standard regimen for successful graft survival in the rat, was too high and that a less immunosuppressive dosage would improve the results. We now use only 10 mg/kg/body weight and have less infection mortality.

Histological data of organ-grafted animals with CsA treatment are rarely documented in the literature. In our experiments, all rats who did not die from lung infections lived in very good health until the day of testing. Nonoccurrence or, alternatively, the occurrence and precise site of the (almost negligible) morphological expression of immunological reactions to the target organ liver could only be documented adequately by histological examination. In the CsA-treated liver recipients, in vitro cell-mediated reactivity was clearly reduced compared to the nontreated animals. The nearly complete lack of reactivity in the blood, combined with reactivity in the four tissue compartments at day 150, may represent a "locking-in phenomenon" of graft-damaging cytotoxic effector lymphocytes. This is supported by the observation that the decrease of reactivity in the blood is accompanied by an increase of reactivity in the spleen (Fig. 2).

Two similar "locking-in phenomena" (nonreactivity in the blood vs. positive reactivity in the splenic compartment) have been observed in fully allogeneic, cyclophosphamide-treated, and crosstransfused rats, specifically tolerant to skin allografts[14] and in F_1-hydrid rats that had survived a GVHR crisis after receiving a small intestine graft.[15] Further analysis of this most interesting finding is in progress.

Specific nonresponsiveness in organ-transplanted rats, induced by a short course of CsA, is already known for heart[13] and kidney[12] and has been confirmed with regard to another organ, namely liver, according to the results presented in this article. One major aspect of nonresponsiveness, its kinetics, has become a matter of growing interest.[5] Kinetic studies have recently been carried out in CsA-treated and heart-allografted rats,[13] with the result that there appears to be a stable nonspecific suppression in the early postoperative stage, which further develops into a weak specific and finally into a strong long-lasting donor-specific suppression. From the data presented here, it may be concluded that a similar time course of nonresponsiveness also develops in liver-grafted, CsA-treated rats. The strong nonspecific cell-mediated in vitro reactivity of group I may be correlated with the lethal rejection crisis of these animals. The relatively lower nonspecific in vitro reactivity in group II at the early stage may be explained by the fact that CsA is still administered at day 10 p.o.. However, skin grafts, donor type and third party (F344), transplanted at the 20th p.o. day were rejected in a slightly delayed fashion (unpublished data). When these animals were tested at about day 40 p.o., 4/5 showed nonspecific cell-mediated in vitro reactivity and 1/5 specific cell-mediated in vitro reactivity. A similar phenomenon was observed in mixed lymphocyte culture experiments (unpublished data) where the spleen cells of these liver graft recipients were tested for suppressor cell activity: in 4/5 there was indication of nonspecific suppressor cells and in 1/5 specifically acting suppressor cells could be found. This has been reported after rat heart transplantation by others too.[16,17] Though our long-term survivors have not yet been tested for suppressor cell activity, there are other parameters (skin grafts and cell-mediated in vitro reactivity) that indicate the occurrence of specific nonresponsiveness in the late p.o. stage. This is in good concordance with our previous data,[18] showing that in the BN → LEW combination, in which long-term survival occurs without immunosuppressive regimen, specific nonresponsiveness develops after an early nonspecific phase. So it may be possible that this time course of nonresponsiveness is a general mechanism in rat liver transplantation.

ACKNOWLEDGMENT

The excellent technical assistance of Frauke Blunck and Linda Hoffmann is gratefully acknowledged.

REFERENCES

1. Kamada N, Brons G, Davies HffS: Transplantation 29:429, 1980

2. Kamada N, Davies HffS, Roser B: Nature 292:840, 1981

3. Engemann R, Ulrichs K, Thiede A, et al: Transplantation 33:566, 1982

4. Calne RY, White DJG: IRCS J Med Sci 5:595, 1977

5. Morris PJ: Transplantation 32:349, 1981

6. Starzl TE, Klintmalm GBG, Porter KA, et al: N Engl J Med 305:266, 1981

7. Takasugi M, Klein E: Transplantation 9:219, 1970

8. Bröcker EB, Kuhlencordt KM, Müller-Ruchholtz W: Int Archs Allergy Appl Immunol 53:234, 1977

9. Leapman SB, Filo RS, Smith EJ, et al: Transplant Proc 13:405, 1981

10. Zimmermann F, Butcher GW, Davies HffS, et al: Transplantation Proc 11:571, 1979

11. Limmer J, Herbertson BM, Calne RY: Eur Surg Res 12:343, 1980

12. Homan WP, Fabre JW, Williams KA, et al: Transplantation 29:361, 1980

13. Nagao R, White DJG, Calne RY: Transplantation 33:31, 1982

14. Schienle W, Bröcker EB, Müller-Ruchholtz W: Z Immun Forsch 150:235, 1975

15. Ulrichs K, Deltz E, Thiede A, et al: In Nieuwenhuis P (ed): In Vivo Immunology. Histophysiology 9th Lymphoid System. New York, Plenum, 1982, p 591

16. Hutchinson IF, Shadur CA, Duarte A, et al: Transplant Proc 13:412, 1981

17. Bordes-Aznar J, Lear PA, Strom TB, et al: Transplant Proc 15:500, 1983

18. Engemann R, Ulrichs K, Thiede A, et al: Transplant Proc 15:729, 1983

The Effect of Cyclosporine Alone and in Combination With Steroids on Experimental Segmental Pancreatic Allografts in the Baboon

D. F. Du Toit, J. J. Heydenrych, G. Louw, T. Zuurmond, L. Laker, D. Els, and S. Woolfe-Coote

SUCCESSFUL long-term immunosuppression of immediately vascularized segmental pancreatic allografts with conventional immunosuppression (steroids and azathioprine) in large outbred animals has been difficult.[1,2] Apart from technical failures experienced and the limitations imposed by models used, corticosteroids have been shown to be diabetogenic and to have an adverse effect on the function of pancreas and islet grafts.

Cyclosporine A (CsA), a new and potent immunosuppressive agent, has recently been shown to be highly effective in prolonging segmental pancreatic allograft survival in pancreatectomized dogs, but in doses much higher than used in humans.[2,3]

The present study was undertaken to evaluate the efficacy of CsA alone and in combination with steroids in suppressing segmental pancreas allograft rejection in totally pancreatectomized outbred baboons.

MATERIALS AND METHODS

Unrelated, outbred, conditioned, and disease-free Chacma baboons of both sexes, weighing between 15 and 25 kg, were used. All animals were anesthetized with ketamine hydrochloride, sodium pentobarbitone for induction and ethrane for maintenance. An endotracheal tube was utilized for continuous delivery of oxygen during anesthesia. Ringers lactate solution was administered during surgery at a rate of 100 ml/hr, and at 500 ml/day intravenously postoperatively for 4 days. Parenteral penicillin and streptomycin were given for 5 days. Thereafter, a standard primate pellet diet was given daily with the addition of pancreatic extract (Cotazyme-Organon) to the diet to compensate for the lack of pancreatic enzymes produced by the pancreatectomy.

Recipient baboons underwent meticulous total surgical pancreatectomy, followed by segmental (tail) pancreatic autotransplantation with free duct drainage as a two-stage procedure or allotransplantation at the same operation. The technique of segmental pancreatic transplantation with unligated ducts has previously been described.[4]

Following allotransplantation, plasma amylase, electrolytes, fasting plasma glucose, and creatinine were determined daily for 1 month and on alternate days, thereafter, until rejection of the graft was diagnosed. These parameters were repeated more often if the recipient appeared sick. Liver function tests were performed weekly. Intravenous glucose tolerance tests (IVGTT) were performed under general anesthesia on all baboons before and after transplantation, using 0.5 g of a 50% glucose solution/kg body weight after an overnight fast. K values (percentage disappearance of glucose per minute) were calculated from the 10, 15, 20, 25, 30, 35, 40, 45, 50, 55, and 60 min samples, as previously reported.[5] Insulin was measured by a solid-phase ^{125}I radioimmunoassay using human insulin standard technique (Coat-A-Count). The low-end sensitivity of the assay was taken as 10 μU/ml. Cyclosporine serum levels were determined using the method described by Donatsch and coworkers.[6]

Graft failure was recognized when the fasting venous plasma glucose rose above 8.0 mmole/liter for 2 consecutive days or the day on which the recipient died.

Biopsy material of autografts and allografts were stained with hematoxylin and eosin and aldehyde-fuchsin and examined by light microscopy. Ultrathin sections were prepared from the transplant for transmission electron microscopy after preservation in cacodylate-buffered gluteraldehyde.

The Mann-Whitney U test was used for statistical comparison between groups, and the difference was considered statistically significant at $p < 0.05$. All data shown here are expressed as SEM.

Cyclosporine A administration began on the day of transplantation (Table 1).

Experimental Groups

One hundred and sixty-two baboons were divided into 9 groups.

Group I. Normal baboons (n = 100) provided the

From the Departments of Surgery and Pediatric Surgery, University of Stellenbosch Medical School, Tygerberg, Republic of South Africa.

Supported in part by grants from the Harry Crossley Fund, Medical Research Council, University of Stellenbosch, and The Cape Provincial Administration.

Address reprint requests to Dr. D. F. du Toit, Department of Surgery, University of Stellenbosch, P. O. Box 63, Tygerberg, 7505, Republic of South Africa.

0041–1345/83/1505–0148$01.00/0

Table 1. Effect of Cyclosporine-A Alone and in Combination With Steroids on Survival of Segmental Pancreatic Allografts in Pancreatectomized Outbred Baboons

Group	Treatment	No Baboons	Duration of Normoglycemia (Days)	IVGTT *K* Values
I	Normal baboons	100	—	2.4% ± 0.09%
II	Pancreatectomy alone	6	<1 × 6	0.3% ± 0.1% (3 days)
III	Segmental autografts	10	42 × 10	1.0% ± 0.1% (6 weeks)
IV	Segmental allograft, no immunosuppression	11	2,4,†5,6,7,10,12,14,14,14,14	0.5% ± 0.2% (7 animals at 7 days)
V	Segmental allograft, CsA 25 mg/kg/day (orallly) (indefinitely)	8	1,*3,*14,19,20,27,28,60	0.5% ± 0.03% (6 animals at 7 days)
VI	Segmental allograft, CsA 50 mg/kg/day (orally) (indefinitely)	10	6,7,11,21,23,§25,26,33,42,§50	0.69% ± 0.06% (9 animals at 7 days)
VII	Segmental allograft, CsA 85 mg/kg/day (orally) (indefinitely)	5	5,7,9,21,26	0.5% ± 0.2% (4 animals at 7 days)
VIII	Segmental allograft, CsA 25 mg/kg/day (orally) a.m. and 10 mg/kg/day (i.m.) p.m.	5	15,20,21,60,60	0.65% ± 0.07% (5 animals at 7 days)
IX	Segmental allograft, CsA 25 mg/kg/day (orally), prednisolone 2 mg/kg/day i.m. indefinitely	7	5,7,7,22,25,28,30	0.6% ± 0.02% (4 animals at 7 days)

Rejection was considered to have occurred on the first 2 consecutive days on which the plasma glucose was above 8 mmole/liter. CsA was administered on the day of transplantation.

*Arterial thrombosis.

†Died of pancreatitis.

‡Intentionally sacrificed.

§Developed pancreatic ascites and pseudocyst.

normal range of electrolytes, creatinine, liver function tests, blood glucose levels, plasma amylase, plasma insulin, glucose tolerance, and glucose degradation values (*K* values).

Group II. Total surgical pancreatectomy as a one-stage procedure ($n = 6$). These animals received neither transplants nor exogenous insulin.

Group III. Total surgical pancreatectomy and segmental heterotopic autotransplantation of the pancreatic tail with the duct unligated ($n = 10$).

Group IV. Total surgical pancreatectomy and simultaneous segmental, heterotopic allotransplantation of the tail of the pancreas with unligated duct and no immunosuppression ($n = 11$).

Group V. Total surgical pancreatectomy and simultaneous segmental pancreatic allotransplantation; CsA 25 mg/kg/day (oral solution) indefinitely ($n = 8$).

Group VI. Total surgical pancreatectomy and simultaneous segmental pancreatic allotransplantation; CsA 50 mg/kg/day (oral solution) indefinitely ($n = 10$).

Group VII. Total surgical pancreatectomy and simultaneous segmental pancreatic allotransplantation; CsA 85 mg/kg/day (oral solution) indefinitely ($n = 5$).

Group VIII. Total surgical pancreatectomy and simultaneous segmental pancreatic allotransplantation; CsA 25 mg/kg/day (orally) 8:00 a.m. and CsA 10 mg/kg/day (intramuscularly) 3:00 p.m., indefinitely ($n = 5$).

Group IX. Total surgical pancreatectomy and segmental pancreatic allotransplantation; CsA 25 mg/kg/day (orally) indefinitely plus methylprednisolone, 125 mg, given intravenously at transplantation and for 3 consecutive days; thereafter, prednisolone 2 mg/kg i.m. daily indefinitely ($n = 7$).

RESULTS

The overall survival and metabolic results are given in Table 1.

Group I: Normal Baboons ($n = 100$)

The mean fasting PLG level was 5.66 ± 0.13 mmole/liter (range 1.6–9.5 mmole/liter) and the mean plasma amylase level was 845 ± 147 Street-Close units (range 689–992 Street-Close units). The mean *K* value was 2.44% ± 0.09% (range 0.52%–4.66%). Serum insulin values increased from 134.58 ± 35.43 μU/ml to 360.26 ± 72.27 μU/ml during IVGTT.

Group II: Totally Pancreatectomized Baboons ($n = 6$)

The 6 apancreatic control animals died between 3 and 12 days after pancreatectomy (median survival 5 days). The fasting PLG levels rose immediately after pancreatectomy and remained elevated until death occurred. The PLG at death was 18.0 ± 1.37 mmole/liter and the mean K value 3 days after pancreatectomy was 0.36% ± 0.02%. Plasma insulin levels before and after stimulation with glucose during IVGTT were below the lowest level of insulin assay sensitivity (10 μU/ml).

Group III: Segmental Autografts With Unligated Ducts (n = 10)

Amylase levels were transiently elevated in all animals 2–4-fold (>1000 Street-Close units) after transplantation. The peak occurred at 48 hr, but in all recipients, there was a return to normal within 7 days. Transient hyperamylasemia was observed in allograft recipients (groups IV–IX). K values were 1.03% ± 0.01% at 6 weeks and differed significantly from control animals in group I ($p < 0.05$). Serum insulin levels increased from 20.0 ± 2.31 μU/ml to 53.5 ± 6.14 μU/ml.

Histologic evaluation of the grafts at 6 weeks revealed total obliteration of the pancreatic duct by fibrosis. Evidence of widespread pancreatic fibrosis, dilatation of the pancreatic ducts, and atrophy of the exocrine parenchyma associated with a cellular infiltrate was present at 6 weeks. Ultrastructurally, the islets appeared normal, but graft evaluation at 6 months (2 animals) revealed extensive fibrosis in association with marked ultrastructural changes of nuclear and cytocavitary components of the islets. Both these animals were normoglycemic.

Pancreatic ascites and steatorrhea were not observed in this group.

Group IV: Untreated Segmental Pancreatic Allografts (n = 11)

All animals showed evidence of rapid rejection of the pancreas between 2 and 14 days (median 10 days) after transplantation. K values were reduced to 0.5% ± 0.2% (7 animals). Serum insulin levels increased from 36.25 ± 11.66 μU/ml to 92.5 ± 14.88 μU/ml. One animal died of graft pancreatitis and another was sacrificed because of paraplegia. Postmortem examination demonstrated a thrombus of the lower end of the aorta in the latter animal.

Histologically, the grafts showed necrosis and hemorrhage and were heavily infiltrated with large numbers of polymorphs and mononuclear cells.

Group V: Segmental Pancreatic Allograft and Cyclosporine-A 25 mg/kg/Day (n = 8)

CsA-treated allograft recipients showed a modest but significant prolongation of graft survival (median 20 days) when compared to untreated allografts in group IV ($p < 0.05$). K values were reduced to 0.57% ± 0.03% (6 animals at 7 days). Serum insulin levels increased from 12.1 ± 1.11 μU/ml to 46.0 ± 12.63 μU/ml. Rejection of the pancreas was characterized by an abrupt and unremitting rise in plasma glucose levels, findings consistent with other allograft groups (VI–IX). Plasma amylase levels were within normal limits before and at the time of rejection.

Free duct drainage into the peritoneal cavity resulted in severe pancreatic ascites in 2 baboons, which necessitated paracentesis within the first 14 postoperative days, and 2 grafts were lost due to arterial thrombosis.

Histology of the rejected grafts showed hemorrhagic necrosis in all animals, findings similar to those seen in group IV.

Group VI: Segmental Pancreatic Allografts and Cyclosporine A 50 mg/kg/day (n = 10)

Allograft recipients sustained normoglycemia for a period of 23 days (median) (range 6–50 days). Compared to animals in group V, there was no difference in graft survival ($p > 0.05$).

K values were 0.69% ± 0.06%, and serum insulin values increased from 23.33 ± 3.78 μU/ml to 65.55 ± 8.45 μU/ml during IVGTT.

One animal had abdominal paracentesis for pancreatic ascites and two developed pseudocysts adjacent to the grafts. Intraabdominal sepsis was not observed in this group. Two animals developed a severe intention tremor. Loss of appetite was apparent in most animals in this group.

In one normoglycemic animal, the graft was intentionally sectioned at 50 days for histologic examination. Microscopically, the exocrine parenchyma was replaced by dense fibrous tissue, as in the autografts, in which islets of Langerhans were observed. Aldehyde-fuchsin staining confirmed the presence of poorly granulated beta cells. A mild mononuclear round cell infiltrate was present within the pancreas and around the islets.

Plasma creatinine levels and liver function tests in animals of groups IV–VI remained within normal limits. Histologic examination of the liver and kidneys obtained (autopsy) from recipients in these groups showed no abnormalities that could be ascribed to cyclosporine A toxicity.

Group VII: Segmental Pancreatic Allografts and Cyclosporine A 85 mg/kg/day (n = 5)

Allografts survived between 5 and 26 days, with a median of 9 days. Despite exocrine supplementation of the diet, all animals developed severe diarrhea, which was attributed to the large volume of CsA administered. Renal failure was not observed.

Group VIII: Segmental Pancreatic Allografts and Cyclosporine A 25 mg/kg/day (Orally) 8 a.m. and 10 mg/kg/day (Intramuscularly) 3 p.m. (n = 5)

Allograft recipients rejected their grafts between 15 and 60 days, with a median of 21 days—values not significantly different from animals in groups V and VI. *K* values were 0.65% ± 0.07% (5 animals at 7 days), and serum insulin levels increased from 12.2 ± 1.11 μU/ml to 46.0 ± 12.63 μU/ml during IVGTT. Two animals died of acute renal failure on days 15 and 20, and another had paracentesis for severe pancreatic ascites on day 21.

Group IX: Segmental Allograft Cyclosporine Immunosuppression Combined With Steroids (n = 7)

Allograft recipients immunosuppressed with CsA and steroids showed a modest prolongation of graft survival (median 20 days) that did not differ significantly from animals treated with CsA alone. *K* values (in 5 animals at 7 days) were 0.58% ± 0.1%. Autopsy revealed diffuse purulent peritonitis in one animal at 7 days.

Serum Cyclosporine A Levels in Immunosuppressed Pancreatic Allografts (Groups V–IX)

Radioimmunoassay of CsA serum levels in allograft recipients in groups V–IX showed levels that varied widely from animal to animal and in course of time. Cyclosporine A levels ranged from 100 to 600 ng/ml postoperatively, and although the results are preliminary, there was no correlation between the absolute level of serum CsA and nephrotoxicity.

DISCUSSION

The dose–response studies confirm the immunosuppressive activity of CsA, which was used to suppress segmental pancreatic allograft rejection in the outbred baboon. The results show that the administration of CsA in doses ranging from 25 to 50 mg/kg/day to pancreatectomized allograft recipients produced a modest prolongation of graft survival, there being no significant difference in survival between treated groups. Similar results were reported by Du Toit et al. in a comparable dog model[3] in which it was possible to obtain considerable segmental pancreatic allograft survival with a dose of 40 mg/kg/day, doses much higher than used in man or necessary to obtain long-term survival of renal allografts in dogs.[9] The need for the unusually high doses of oral CsA to ensure prolonged graft survival might be explained by poor CsA absorption in the pancreatectomized animal; Calne et al. have recently shown that frequent dose adjustments of oral CsA are necessary in the first few days after renal transplantation in man so as to ensure adequate immunosuppression.[7]

Our data show that the combination of CsA and prednisolone in a low dose had no synergistic immunosuppressive effect in prolonging pancreatic allograft survival in the baboon,

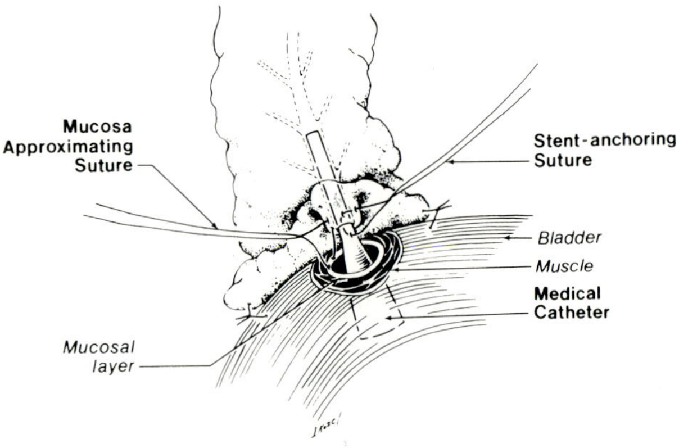

Fig. 1. Techniques of pancreaticocystostomy. The pancreatic duct is sutured to the bladder mucosa. A no. 18 angiocatheter is used as a shunt.

RESULTS AND DISCUSSION

Of the 36 animals transplanted, 6 had to be excluded because of postoperative complications not specifically related to the pancreas transplant. Two animals were sacrificed because of intususception, 2 animals died from infection, and 2 animals had early graft thrombosis. There were no technical complications related to the pancreaticocystostomy. All animals had good graft function, with fasting blood glucose values below 125 mg/dl 48 hr after the transplant. Graft survival in the individual groups is shown in Table 1. In group 1, without immunosuppression, mean graft survival was 7.5 days. Immunosuppression with imuran and prednisone resulted in minimal improvement in graft survival to 9.3 days (group II). Low-dose cyclosporine-A (starting dose 10 mg/kg/day i.v.) combined with prednisone resulted in significantly improved graft survival to 14.7 days, but no long-term surviving animal was observed. In the high-dose cyclosporine-A/prednisone group, all animals survived beyond 60 days. The longest surviving animal was followed for 120 days. Four animals were sacrificed with a normal functioning pancreas because a sufficient amount of cyclosporine-A was not available to continue immunosuppression. In this group, all animals had normal fasting blood glucose values, gained weight, and appeared clinically well. Intravenous administration of high-dose cyclosporine-A was extremely well tolerated. Renal function at the termination of the experiment was normal in all animals tested. Histologic examination of the pancreas, as demonstrated in 1 animal sacrificed 90 days after transplantation, showed normal-appearing exocrine and endocrine tissue with well preserved pancreatic islets (Fig. 2). The bladder mucosa was found to be macroscopically and microscopically normal. No damage secondary to exocrine pancreatic secretions was found. The pancreatic duct was noted to be patent, and usually a number 18 or 16 angiocatheter could be passed at autopsy from the bladder into the pancreatic duct. The arteriovenous fistula was patent in two animals after 60 days. In three animals, the arteriovenous fistula had ceased to function, but at autopsy, it could not be determined if this was a postmortem event. Encouraged by these results, we have now transplanted 3 patients using high-dose intravenous cyclosporine-A and low-dose prednisone. The operative technique used was identical as described in the experimental animals above. In all cases, pancreaticocystostomy was used as the drainage procedure. One patient developed early vascular thrombosis, which necessitated

Table 1. Survival of Segmental Pancreas Allografts

Group	Immunosuppression	n	Graft Survival (Days, Mean ± SD)
I	None	13	7.5 (±2.1)
II	Imuran + prednisone	5	9.3 (±3.7)
III	Low-dose cyclosporine + prednisone	7	14.7 (±1.4)
IV	High-dose cyclosporine + prednisone	5	>60, >60, >60, >60, >60

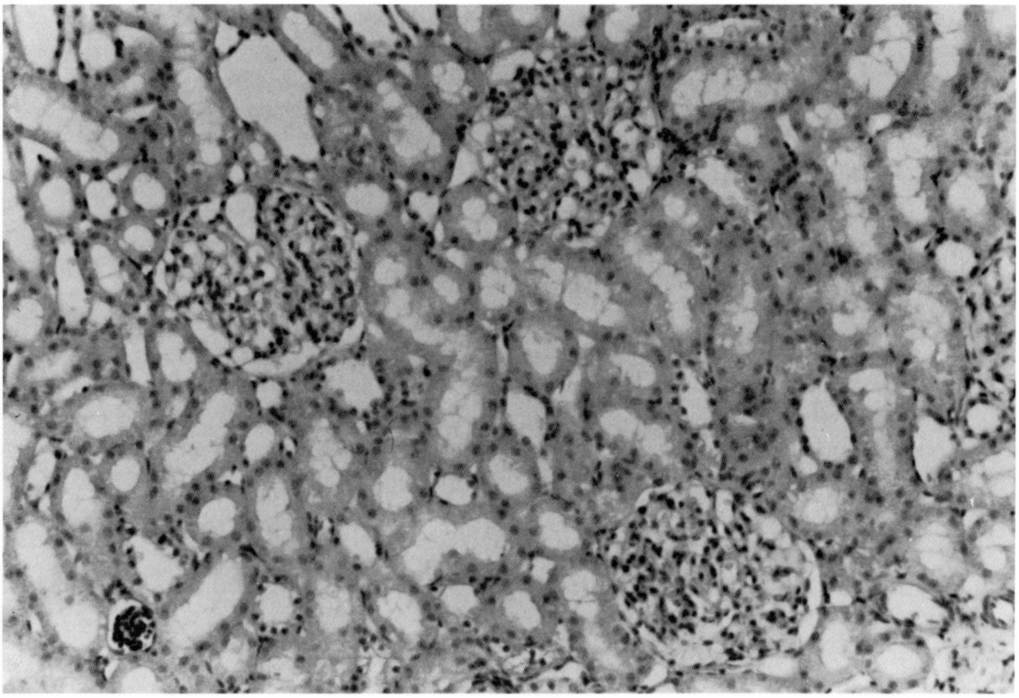

Fig. 2. Histology of an allogeneic pancreas removed 3 months after transplantation. Exocrine and endocrine tissue appear normal.

the removal of the pancreas after 24 hr. In this case, the cimino fistula was not functioning well at the time of the operation and anticoagulation was suboptimal. Two other patients have well functioning grafts, indicated by normal fasting blood glucose and normal glucose tolerance tests. The patient with the greatest graft success has now been followed for 5 months with normal pancreatic function. His clinical course and immunosuppressive

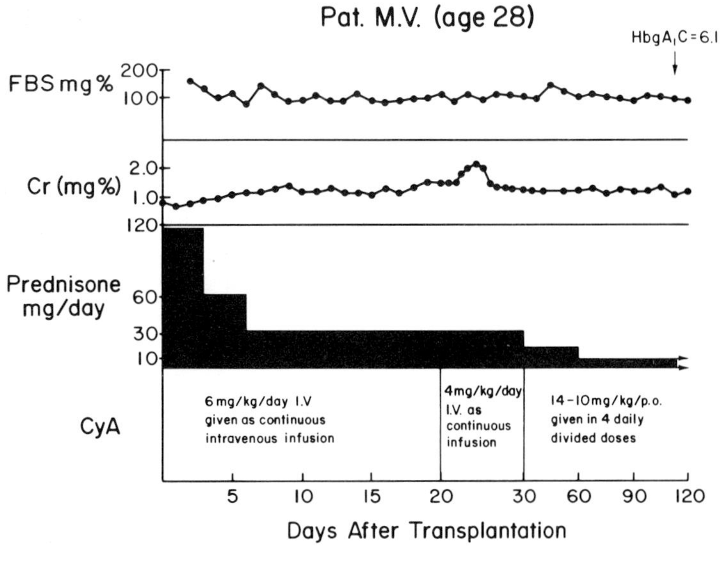

Fig. 3. Immunosuppressive regimen used in pancreas recipient M.V. Patient had received cadaveric kidney 2 years prior to pancreas transplant.

therapy is demonstrated in Fig. 3. The starting dose of prednisone was 120 mg/day for 3 days, which was rapidly tapered to 30 mg/day after 1 month, and he is now maintained on 10 mg/day p.o. Cyclosporine-A was started as a continuous intravenous infusion at a dose of 6 mg/kg/day i.v. It is our preliminary impression that continuous infusion of cyclosporine-A reduces nephrotoxicity during the period of administration of high doses. After 20 days, the dose was lowered to 4 mg/kg/day i.v. and was also given as a continuous infusion. In the transitional period, the i.v. dose was lowered, while the patient was started on oral cyclosporine-A. He was discharged 30 days posttransplant at a dose of 14 mg/kg p.o. given in 4 daily divided doses. This was tapered between day 60 and 90 to 10 mg/kg p.o., also given in 4 daily divided doses. Hemoglobulin AlC obtained 4 months after transplantation was in normal range of 6.1. At no time postoperatively did the patient have any complaints regarding his urinary tract. He is maintained on TMP sulfa, 2 tablets a day, for the prophylaxis of urinary tract infection. Urine amylase is ranging between 10,000 U and 70,000 U/dl.

In summary, our preliminary experience demonstrates that high-dose intravenous cyclosporine-A in the initial phase after transplantation effectively prevents early pancreatic rejection, and when given as an intravenous infusion, has minimal nephrotoxicity. Also, pancreaticocystostomy has been demonstrated to be a safe and simple procedure for exocrine drainage. Although long-term follow-up of these patients will be necessary to determine the usefulness of this method in pancreatic transplantation, we believe that this method will find its place as a valuable alternative method for exocrine pancreatic drainage.

ACKNOWLEDGMENT

We would like to thank Dr. J. Borel (Sandoz, Basel, Switzerland) for supplying us with cyclosporine-A.

REFERENCES

1. Klempnauer J, Kasahara K, White DJG, et al: Presented at the 17th Congress of the European Society of Surgical Research, 1982
2. Klempnauer J, Wagner E, Wonigeit K, et al: Transplant Proc (this issue)
3. Calne RY, McMaster P, Rolles K, et al: Transplant Proc 12(Suppl 2):51, 1980

Pancreas and Kidney Allograft Rejection Responds Differently to Cyclosporine Immunosuppression

J. Klempnauer, E. Wagner, B. Steiniger, K. Wonigeit, and R. Pichlmayr

CYCLOSPORINE (CsA) has led to a major improvement in the results of clinical renal allotransplantation.[1,2] In vascularized pancreas transplantation, however, the clinical outcome is still disappointing, even with the use of CsA.[3] Besides technical problems, mainly related to the management of the exocrine pancreatic secretion, this may also reflect immunologic peculiarities of pancreas transplantation. In order to investigate whether pancreas and kidney rejection responds differently to CsA, we have compared the survival of vascularized pancreas and kidney allografts in rats receiving identical CsA immunosuppression.

MATERIALS AND METHODS

Inbred rats of the strains DA ($RT1^a$) and LEW ($RT1^l$) were used in this study. These strains differ at their major histocompatibility complex (MHC) and a multitude of non-MHC alloantigens.[4]

Orthotopic left kidney transplantation was performed, using a small patch of the donor bladder for ureteric anastomosis. The recipient's left kidney was removed at the time of transplantation, and the remaining right kidney 5 days later. Rejection was defined by the death of the transplant recipient and was confirmed by histologic examination.

Pancreas whole organ transplantation was performed in streptozotocin diabetic rats. After complete pancreatectomy in the donor, the duct-ligated pancreas was transplanted heterotopically to the infrarenal aorta and vena cava of the recipient. Rejection was defined by recurrence of hyperglycemia above 14 mmole/liter on at least 2 consecutive days and was confirmed histologically.

Immunosuppression consisted of CsA, 15 mg/kg body weight, dissolved in olive oil and administered intramuscularly from days 0 to 13.

RESULTS (TABLE 1)

Isografts and Untreated Allografts

Kidney isograft recipients all survived beyond 100 days with good renal function. Diabetic recipients of vascularized pancreas isografts became normoglycemic within 6 hr after transplantation and maintained normoglycemia for the whole observation period of 100 days. Graft removal on day 100 was followed by prompt recurrence of hyperglycemia.

Untreated kidney allografts in the strain combination DA ($RT1^a$) to LEW ($RT1^l$) were rapidly rejected within 9 days. Histologically massive infiltration of lymphocytes and severe glomerulopathy and vasculopathy were demonstrated in these rejected grafts.

The rejection times of vascularized pancreas allografts did not differ from those of kidney allografts. Rejected grafts had increased in size and turned firm and fibrotic. In addition to the sequelae of duct ligation, the histologic picture of rejected grafts was dominated by a massive fibrosis and dense infiltration of lymphocytes both in the exocrine pancreas and the islets that underwent severe disintegration.

Allografts Treated With CsA

Kidney allograft recipients treated with a 14-day course of CsA, 15 mg/kg body weight, intramuscularly, all survived beyond 100 days. The creatinine levels did not differ from isografts. Macroscopically, these grafts were undistinguishable from isografts; histologically, however, distinct perivascular lymphocytic infiltrates were detected in all grafts.

From the Klinik für Abdominal- und Transplantationschirurgie, Medizinische Hochschule Hannover, Hannover, F.R.G.

Supported in part by Stiftung Volkswagenwerk, AZ I/38 510.

Address reprint requests to Dr. J. Klempnauer, Klinik für Abdominal- und Transplantationschirurgie, Medizinische Hochschule Hannover, D-3000 Hannover, F.R.G.

0041-1345/83/1505-0150$01.00/0

Table 1. Survival Times of Vascularized Rat Kidney and Pancreas Isografts (LEW) and Allografts in the Strain Combination DA (RT1[a]) to LEW (RT1[l])

	n	Kidney	Pancreas
Isografts	6	>100	>100
Allografts			
untreated	10	7.8 ± 0.8	8.6 ± 1.2
Allografts			
CsA 15 mg/kg i.m.,			
days 0–13	5	>100	47.8 ± 7.1

In the same strain combination, all vascularized pancreas allografts were rejected following cessation of CsA immunosuppression. Rejection occurred after a mean of 48 days. Without exception, the functional demonstration of rejection was confirmed histologically. The pattern of rejection did not differ from untreated pancreas allografts (Fig. 1).

DISCUSSION

In experiments using identical CsA immunosuppression in identical rat strain combinations, we could demonstrate that kidney and pancreas allografts respond differently to CsA.

A 14-day course of CsA led to a significant prolongation of both kidney and pancreas allograft survival. None of the grafts was rejected while CsA was being administered. This indicates that, when CsA is used in appropriate dosages, it is capable of suppressing kidney as well as pancreas allograft rejection in the rat. However, following cessation of CsA immunosuppression, pancreas allografts were regularly rejected, while kidney allografts survived for a very prolonged period of time. Using the same experimental protocol, we have previously demonstrated a similar phenomenon for pancreas and heart allografts. In the strain combination DA (RT1[a]) to WAG (RT1[u]), heart allografts survived permanently after short-term immunosuppression with CsA, while all pancreas allografts were rejected following cessation of CsA.[5] This indicates that pancreas and kidney or heart allografts evoke differential alloim-

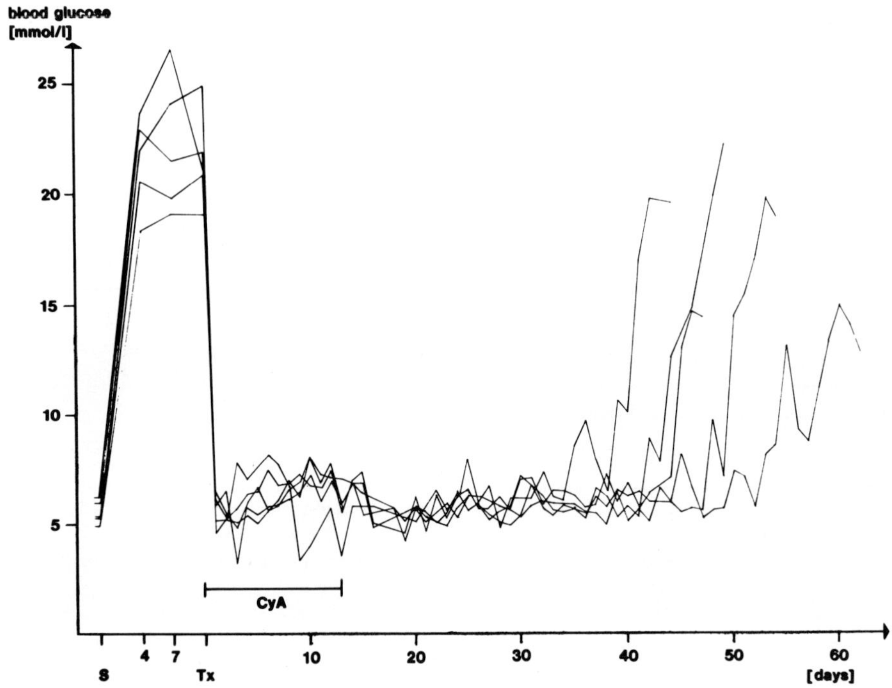

Fig. 1. Course of blood glucose in streptozotocin diabetic LEW (RT1[l]) rats that received a vascularized pancreas allograft from DA (RT1[a]) donors and short-term CsA immunosuppression. S, induction of streptozotocin diabetes; Tx, time of pancreas transplantation.

mune reactions, which respond differently to CsA immunosuppression. Since alloimmune reactions are caused by histocompatibility differences between donor and recipient tissue, it is conceivable that the differential susceptibility to CsA immunosuppression of vascularized pancreas and kidney or heart allografts is due to differences in the antigenicity of these organs.

The difference in the survival of pancreas and kidney transplants under CsA treatment may be related to the differential functional importance of MHC and non-MHC alloantigens in transplantation of these organs. Incompatibility at MHC alloantigens causes rapid rejection of pancreas as well as heart and kidney allografts.[4,6] Incompatibility exclusively at non-MHC antigens, however, causes rapid rejection of pancreas, but not of kidney or heart allografts.[7,8] Since the strain combinations DA → LEW and DA → WAG, in addition to incompatibility at their MHC, also differ at non-MHC alloantigens as well, the question arises whether the differential effect of CsA on rejection of pancreas and kidney or heart allografts is due to the strong effect of non-MHC alloantigens in pancreas transplantation.

REFERENCES

1. Calne RY, White DJG, Thiru S, et al: Lancet 2:1323, 1978

2. Beveridge T: Transplant Proc 15:433, 1983

3. Sutherland DER: Transplant Proc 15:1303, 1983

4. Günther E, Stark O: In Götze D (ed): The Major Histocompatibility System in Man and Animals. New York, Springer Verlag, 1977, pp 207–253

5. Klempnauer J, Kasahara K, White DJG, et al: Eur Surg Res 14:128, 1982

6. Klempnauer J, Wonigeit K, Steiniger B, et al: Transplant Proc 15:1308, 1983

7. Klempnauer J, Wonigeit K, Günther E, et al: Transplant Proc (in press)

8. Thoenes GH, Urban G, Doering I: Immunogenetics 3:239, 1974

Effect of Cyclosporine on Allotransplanted Pancreatic Islets in DLA-MLC-Compatible Dogs

M. D. Williams, R. Walshaw, R. W. Bull, W. D. Schall, G. A. Padgett, V. V. Gossain, and R. F. Nachreiner

THE feasibility of pancreatic islet cell transplantation has been demonstrated by numerous investigators through successful islet tissue autografts in dogs.[1-3] In these studies, dispersed pancreatic islet tissue, prepared by collagenase digestion without separation of exocrine and endocrine components, ameliorated diabetes when autotransplanted into the splenic pulp or portal vein of totally pancreatectomized dogs. This technique has also been successful in human beings who underwent near total pancreatectomy to relieve the pain of chronic pancreatitis.[4,5] In these cases, however, islet cell mass and function were often compromised prior to transplantation, and pancreatic fibrosis hampered islet tissue preparation.[6] Isogenic transplantation of isolated islets has been successful in ameliorating experimental diabetes in highly inbred strains of rodents.[7-9]

In man and large animals, islet cell allotransplantation has been less successful than iso- and autotransplantation.[10-13] Rejection has likely played a major role in this lack of success. Pancreatic islet preparations are highly immunogenic and are extremely susceptible to allograft rejection,[14-17] especially across strong histocompatibility barriers. Islets appear to be rejected more rapidly than kidney, heart, and skin following allograft transplantation.[14,18]

Cyclosporine-A (CsA) is an immunosuppressive agent that prolongs survival of various organ allografts in a number of species.[19-28] Some evidence suggests that CsA reduces the incidence of graft rejection compared with standard methods of immunosuppression.[23,29]

In this study, the efficacy of CsA was evaluated in totally pancreatectomized dogs receiving intrasplenic transplants of dispersed allogeneic pancreatic islet tissue from histocompatible donors. Related and unrelated donor–recipient pairs were used.

MATERIALS AND METHODS

Animals

Conditioned Labrador retrievers, Siberian huskies, beagles, golden retrievers, and a variety of mixed-breed dogs, weighing between 10 and 25 kg, were used. The dogs were free of intestinal parasites and heartworms and were vaccinated against distemper, leptospirosis, hepatitis, and parvovirus.

Histocompatibility Testing

Serologically defined dog lymphocyte antigens (DLA) A,B, and C were determined by the two-stage lymphocytotoxicity method.[30-32] Cell-mediated assays were performed using the mixed lymphocyte culture (MLC) technique.[33] Donor–recipient pairs were then selected on the basis of DLA identity and nonstimulation of recipient lymphocytes by donor cells in the MLC.

Immunosuppressive Therapy

Cyclosporine-A, dissolved in olive oil, was orally administered at doses of 25 mg/kg/day or 40 mg/kg/day. When the drug was used at the latter rate, it was given in divided doses. In those allograft recipients that were immunosuppressed, therapy was initiated 2 days before transplantation.

Pancreatectomy and Preparation of Dispersed Pancreatic Fragments

General anesthesia was induced with thiamylal sodium and maintained with halothane, oxygen, and nitrous oxide. The pancreas was exposed through a ventral midline incision, extending from the xiphoid process to the caudal umbilicus. The left limb and body of the pancreas were quickly removed and immediately immersed in iced

From the Colleges of Veterinary Medicine and Human Medicine, Michigan State University, East Lansing, MI.

Address reprint requests to Dr. M. D. Williams, Department of Pathology, Michigan State University, East Lansing, MI 48824.

Supported in part by NIH Grants 5 F32 AM06630-03, 3 P40 RR01173-03S1, and 5 R01 AM27876-03.

0041–1345/83/1505–0151$01.00/0

Hanks' balanced salt solution (HBSS). This segment was taken directly to the laboratory for preparation. The right limb of the pancreas was meticulously dissected in order to preserve the pancreaticoduodenal vessels and bile duct. Resection of this segment was usually completed within 30 min after removal of the initial segment. The tissue was placed in iced HBSS and promptly transported to the laboratory for preparation.

The pancreas was weighed and then distended by direct infiltration with cold (4°C) HBSS. The edematous organ was freed of major blood vessels and connective tissue and then manually minced into fragments with a maximal diameter of 2 mm. The diced tissue was washed 3 times by sedimentation in cold HBSS. The tissue was then suspended in 37°C HBSS to a total volume of 100–125 ml and digested for 20 min in a shaking water bath (37°C) with 1350 U of collagenase (Worthington, Type IV) per gram of tissue. After digestion, the tissue was washed 4 times by sedimentation in cold HBSS. The tissue was then placed into 50-ml centrifuge tubes and pelleted by centrifugation at 1000 rpm for 1 min. The digested tissue was adjusted in cold HBSS to a total volume of 35–50 ml and placed in a 50-cc syringe for implantation into the spleen of recipient animals.

Islet Tissue Implantation

In each recipient, the splenic capsule was directly punctured with a 14-gauge 5.5-inch needle catheter, which was inserted parallel to the longitudinal axis of the spleen, and the tissue was injected as the catheter was slowly withdrawn. The catheter was passed at least twice in order to achieve wide dispersal of pancreatic fragments throughout the splenic pulp. Hemostasis was achieved at each of the puncture sites by placing a 5-0 chromic gut mattress suture over an absorbable sponge.

Experimental Groups

Each dog in groups 2, 3, 4, 5, and 6 was made diabetic by total pancreatectomy and received intrasplenic transplants of autologous or allogeneic dispersed pancreatic islet tissue.

Group 1 ($n = 16$). Normal dogs were used to establish the ranges of normal fasting plasma glucose values and normal intravenous glucose tolerance test (IVGTT) curves.

Group 2 ($n = 4$). Received autologous dispersed pancreatic islet tissue.

Group 3 ($n = 3$). Received allogeneic islet tissue from DLA-MLC-compatible littermates. Immunosuppressive treatment was not administered.

Group 4 ($n = 4$). Received allogeneic islets from DLA-MLC-compatible littermates. Cyclosporine-A was administered at a dose of 25 mg/kg/day.

Group 5 ($n = 4$). Received allogeneic islet tissue from DLA-MLC-compatible littermates. Cyclosporine-A was administered at a dose of 40 mg/kg/day.

Group 6 ($n = 4$). Received allogeneic islet tissue from unrelated DLA-MLC-compatible donors. Cyclosporine-A was administered at a dose of 40 mg/kg/day.

Postoperative Care

Dogs received Ringer's lactate solution intravenously until they had returned to normal oral alimentation. All animals were treated with ampicillin (10 mg/lb, t.i.d.) subcutaneously for the first 5 postoperative days. No oral intake was allowed for the first 1–2 days following surgery. After this time, water was given in small amounts, and if no vomiting occurred, small quantities of semisolid food were offered every 4 hr. For the first 24–48 hr postoperation, plasma glucose concentrations were determined every 4 hr, and if values fell below 60 mg/dl, intravenous boluses of 50% dextrose were administered in amounts adequate to establish euglycemia. Normal oral alimentation had usually returned by 3–4 days following surgery, and dogs were then fed a standard kennel diet with pancreatic extract (Viokase, A. H. Robbins Co.) added to compensate for the exocrine deficiency produced by pancreatectomy.

Metabolic Studies

Normal carbohydrate metabolism was verified in all donors and recipients prior to surgery by multiple fasting plasma glucose determinations and one IVGTT. Intravenous glucose tolerance tests were performed using 0.5 g of 50% glucose/kg of body weight. The glucose bolus was administered as a rapid injection into the cephalic vein. Peripheral blood samples were collected before injection (0 min) and at 5, 10, 15, 30, 45, 60, 90, and 120 min thereafter. Samples were assayed for glucose and insulin concentrations. K values (percentage of decline of plasma glucose concentration per minute) were calculated from the 5, 10, 15, 30, and 45-min postinjection plasma glucose values, using the method of least squares. Plasma glucose concentrations were measured by the glucose oxidase method, using a Beckman Glucose Analyzer 2. Euglycemia was defined as a plasma glucose level of less than 150 mg/dl after a 12-hr fast. Plasma insulin was measured by radioimmunoassay using Corning's Immophase® insulin radioimmunoassay test system.

Fasting plasma glucose concentrations were determined in recipient animals daily for 2 weeks following transplantation and a minimum of 3 times weekly thereafter. In surviving animals, IVGTTs were performed at 3 and 8 weeks after transplantation.

Termination of Experimental Animals

Surviving dogs were studied for a maximum of 60 days, after which time splenectomies were performed. Multiple sections of spleen were fixed in 10% buffered formalin and Bouin's solution for histologic examination. Daily fasting plasma glucose determinations and one IVGTT were done on each splenectomized subject. Animals were sacrificed 3–5 days after splenectomy.

Other criteria for terminating study on individual animals were death and sacrifice because of debilitation with severe hyperglycemia, ketoacidosis, weight loss, and inappetence.

Histologic Studies

Necropsy examinations were performed and multiple sections of tissue from lungs, heart, kidneys, liver, lymph nodes, and spleen were fixed in 10% buffered formalin, embedded in paraffin, sectioned, and stained with hematoxylin and eosin. Sections of spleen were also fixed in Bouin's solution and stained by immunoperoxidase technique for identification of beta cells.

Data Analysis

One-way analysis of variance (ANOVA) and the Walker-Duncan Adaptive Procedure were used to analyze the data. All evaluations were conducted at a probability level of 0.05.

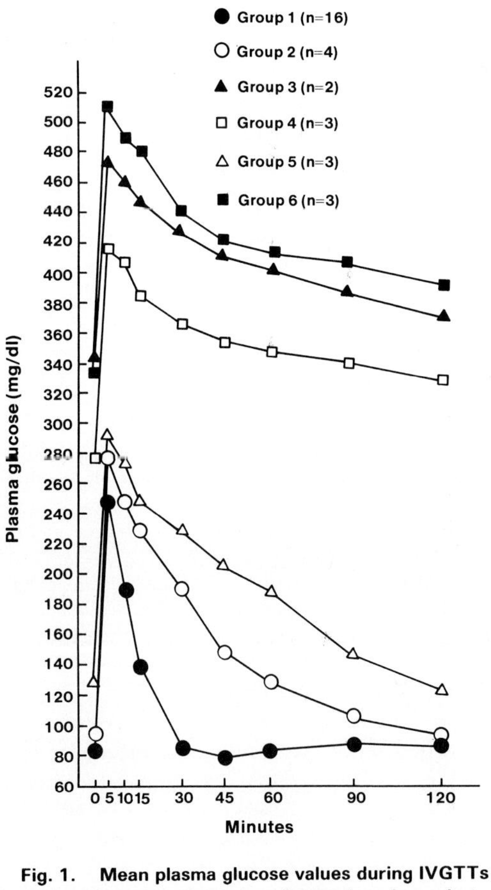

Fig. 1. Mean plasma glucose values during IVGTTs 3 weeks after transplantation. Comparison is made to normal dogs (group 1).

RESULTS

Survival and Metabolic Studies

Group 1. Normal dogs had mean (±SE) fasting plasma glucose values of 82 ± 2.42 mg/dl and mean K values of 2.9% ± 0.2%. The mean of fasting basal plasma insulin values prior to IVGTTs was 19 ± 1.6 μU/ml, and following administration of a glucose load, mean plasma insulin values peaked at 68 ± 9.0 (Figs. 1–4).

Group 2. The 4 dogs receiving autologous islet tissue became euglycemic 4.5 ± 1.5 days after transplantation. Three animals remained euglycemic until splenectomized 60 days following surgery. The dog that did not maintain normal fasting plasma glucose for 60 days developed hyperglycemia from day 35 to day 49. Daily fasting plasma glucose during this period was 202 ± 16.1 mg/dl (additional information given in Table 1). The mean K value of the 4 animals 3 weeks posttransplant was 1.5% ± 0.2%. At 8 weeks, the mean K value for the 3 dogs that were euglycemic for 60 days was 1.8% ± 0.3%, indicating a signifi-

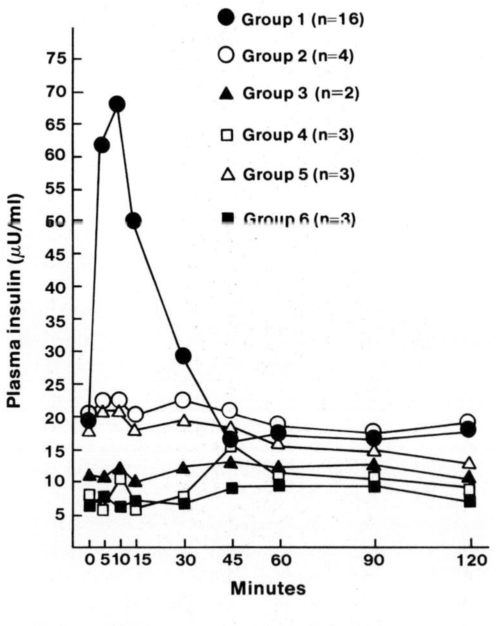

Fig. 2. Mean plasma insulin levels during IVGTTs 3 weeks after transplantation. Comparison is made to normal dogs (group 1).

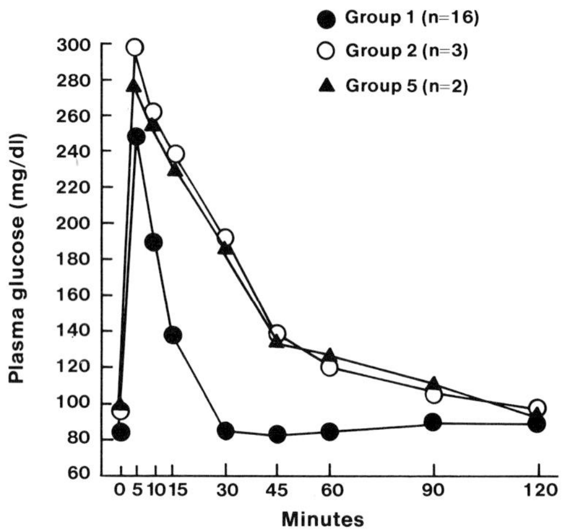

Fig. 3. **Mean plasma glucose values during IVGTTs 8 weeks after transplantation. Comparison is made to normal dogs (group 1).**

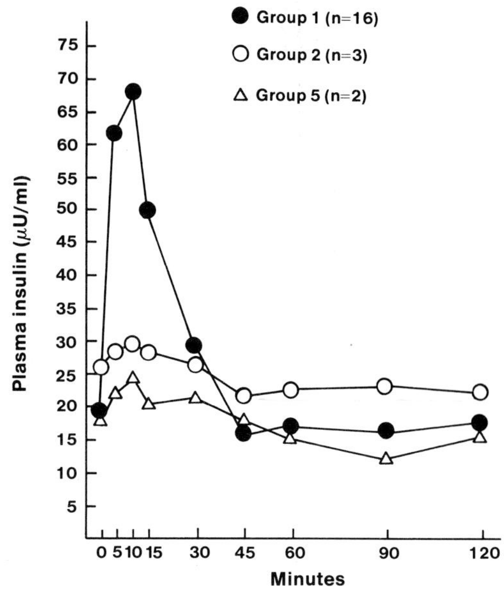

Fig. 4. **Mean plasma insulin levels during IVGTTs 8 weeks after transplantation. Comparison is made to normal dogs (group 1).**

cant impairment of glucose degradation when compared to the normal dogs ($p < 0.05$), although the animals maintained euglycemia.

During the 8-week IVGTT, plasma insulin increased from a basal concentration of 26 ± 2.2 μU/ml to a peak of 29 ± 3.2 μU/ml.

Splenectomies were performed at 60 days on the 3 dogs that maintained euglycemia for the entire posttransplant period; mean plasma glucose was 97 ± 6.5 mg/dl before splenectomy. Hyperglycemia developed in all of these animals, and the mean *K* value of IVGTTs performed 2 days later was 0.4% ± 0.03%. The dogs were sacrificed 3–5 days after splenectomy. Mean plasma glucose values prior to sacrifice were 395 ± 5.6 mg/dl (Figs. 1–4).

Group 3. Three nonimmunosuppressed dogs received allogeneic islet tissue from histocompatible littermates and 2 of them never became euglycemic; the other animal had a short duration of euglycemia from day 6 to day 10. The mean survival time was 21 ± 6.6 days. The mean *K* value of 2 surviving dogs 3 weeks posttransplant was 0.3% ± 0.0%. During IVGTT, plasma insulin increased from a basal concentration of 11 ± 1.0 μU/ml to a peak of 12 ± 0.0 μU/ml. The mean plasma glucose of this group at the time of death was 399 ± 26.6 mg/dl (Table 2, Figs. 1, 2).

Group 4. Four dogs receiving allogeneic islet tissue from histocompatible littermates were administered CsA (25 mg/kg/day) and

Table 1. Metabolic Data of Groups 2 and 5 Following Transplantation. All Subjects in These Groups Survived the Maximal 60-Day Length of the Study (Mean ± SE)

Group	Treatment	Test Subjects	Days Until Euglycemia Achieved	Maintained Euglyucemia Until Day 60	*K* Values at 3 Weeks	K Values at 8 Weeks	Final Plasma Glucose (mg/dl) Before Splenectomy (Day 60)
2	Pancreatectomy +	A, B, C	5.0 ± 2.0	Yes	1.6 ± 0.2	1.8 ± 0.3	97 ± 6.5
	autotransplant	D	3	No*	1.3	1.0	148
5	Pancreatectomy +	A, B	6.0 ± 0.0	Yes	0.9 ± 0.4	1.7 ± 0.2	97 ± 8.0
	allograft (related) + CsA	C	12	No†	0.8	0.6	214
	(40 mg/kg/day)	D	Never	—	0.8	0.3	309

*Developed hyperglycemia from days 35 to 49. Daily plasma glucose during this period was 202 ± 16.1 mg/dl.

†Became hyperglycemic on day 31 and remained so for duration of study. Daily plasma glucose during this period was 218 ± 5.1.

Table 2. Metabolic and Survival Data of Groups 3, 4, and 6 Following Transplantation (Mean ± SE)

Group	Treatment	Test Subjects	Days Until Euglycemia Achieved	Number of Days Before Sacrificed	Mean Days Before Sacrificed	*K* Values at 3 Weeks	Final Plasma Glucose (mg/dl)
3	Pancreatectomy + allograft (related) + No CsA	A, B, C	Never*	8, 26, 29	21.0 ± 6.6	0.3 ± 0.0	399 ± 26.6
4	Pancreatectomy + allograft (related) + CsA (25 mg/kg/day)	A, B, C, D	Never	20, 24, 29, 30	25.8 ± 2.3	0.4 ± 0.1	365 ± 35.6
6	Pancreatectomy + allograft (unrelated) + CsA (40 mg/kg/day)	A, B, C, D	Never	13†, 26, 29, 39	26.8 ± 5.4	0.5 ± 0.1	336 ± 31.1

*Subject B had a short period of euglycemia days 6–10.

†Subject A was sacrificed on day 13 due to development of severe acute hemorrhagic enteritis. Parvovirus infection was suspected.

none became euglycemic. The mean survival time was 25.8 ± 2.3 days. The mean *K* value of 3 surviving dogs 3 weeks posttransplant was 0.4% ± 0.1%. During IVGTT, plasma insulin increased from a basal concentration of 8 ± 0.5 μU/ml to a peak of 16 ± 8.5 μU/ml. The mean plasma glucose of this group at the time of death was 365 ± 35.6 mg/dl (Table 2, Figs. 1, 2).

Group 5. Four dogs receiving allogeneic islet tissue from histocompatible littermates were given CsA (40 mg/kg/day) and 3 animals became euglycemic 8.0 ± 2.0 days after transplantation. Two animals remained euglycemic until splenectomized 60 days following surgery. The dog that did not maintain normal fasting plasma glucose for 60 days became hyperglycemic on day 31 and remained so for the duration of the study. Daily fasting plasma glucose from day 31 to day 60 was 218 ± 5.1 mg/dl (additional information given in Table 1). At 3 weeks posttransplantation, the mean *K* value of the 3 animals that were euglycemic was 0.9% ± 0.2%. At 8 weeks, the mean *K* value for 2 dogs that were euglycemic was 1.7% ± 0.2%; this value was significantly lower than that of the normal dogs ($p < 0.05$), but not significantly different from group 2 at 8 weeks.

During the 8-week IVGTT, plasma insulin increased from a basal concentration of 18 ± 2.5 μU/ml to a peak of 24 ± 0.5 μU/ml.

Splenectomies were performed at 60 days on the 2 dogs that maintained euglycemia for the entire posttransplant period; mean plasma glucose was 97 ± 8.0 mg/dl before surgery. Hyperglycemia developed in both animals, and the mean *K* value of IVGTTs performed 2 days later was 0.4% ± 0.0%. The dogs were sacrificed 4 days after splenectomy, with final mean plasma glucose values of 356 ± 7.0 mg/dl (Figs. 1–4).

Group 6. Four dogs receiving allogeneic islet tissue from histocompatible unrelated donors were given CsA (40 mg/kg/day) and none became euglycemic. The mean survival time was 26.8 ± 5.4 days. There was no significant difference between the survival times of groups 3, 4, and 6 ($p < 0.05$). The mean *K* value of 3 surviving dogs 3 weeks posttransplant was 0.5% ± 0.1%. During IVGTT, plasma insulin increased from a basal concentration of 7 ± 1.3 μU/ml to a peak of 9 ± 3.2 μU/ml. The mean plasma glucose of this group at the time of death was 336 ± 31.1 mg/dl (Table 2, Figs. 1, 2).

DISCUSSION

The results of autologous transplants confirm that diabetes produced in dogs by total pancreatectomy can be ameliorated by intrasplenic dispersed pancreatic fragments. After glucose loading, however, glucose decay and insulin peaks are of a lesser magnitude than those observed in normal dogs. These findings are similar to those of other investigators.[3,12]

Intrasplenic dispersed pancreatic fragments obtained from histocompatible related donors were ineffective in ameliorating diabetes when no immunosuppressive agent was administered, nor when CsA was administered at a dose of 25 mg/kg/day.

Diabetes in dogs produced by pancreatectomy was ameliorated, however, by intrasplenic dispersed pancreatic fragments obtained from histocompatible related donors when CsA was administered at a dose of 40 mg/kg/day. Furthermore, glucose decay and insulin peaks after glucose loading were not different from those of dogs receiving autologous tissue (at 8 weeks).

Cyclosporine-A, administered at a dose of 40 mg/kg/day, was ineffective when administered to dogs receiving tissue from unrelated histocompatible donors. This finding emphasizes the limitations of DLA and MLC as a means of determining histocompatibility and underscores the importance of minor histoincompatibility.

The dose–response curve evident from differences between groups of related histocompatible dogs treated with the two doses of CsA raises the question as to whether CsA at a dose greater than 40 mg/kg/day would be effective and tolerated if used in dogs receiving tissue from unrelated histocompatible donors. Animals in this study tolerated the drug well, and there was no consistent histologic or biochemical evidence of hepatotoxicity or nephrotoxicity.

Because it is known that islet tissue is less immunogenic than the remainder of the pancreas,[34] another approach for further investigation is to transplant canine islets uncontaminated with collagen and exocrine pancreatic tissue. Using the improved technique for the isolation of islets from compact pancreata, described by Lacy and coworkers,[35] it may be possible to successfully transplant insulin-producing tissue between unrelated histocompatible dogs using CsA at a dose of 40 mg/kg/day or less.

ACKNOWLEDGMENT

The authors gratefully acknowledge Florence Williams, Peggy Coffman, Eileen Salmond, Janet Grace, Marc Bailie, Joanne Otto, Naomi Green, Mae Sunderlin, Frances Whipple, and the I.C.U. animal technicians for excellent technical assistance, and Janice Fuller for expertise in typing the manuscript. We thank the Sandoz Corporation for generously supplying us with cyclosporine-A.

REFERENCES

1. Mirkovitch V, Campiche M: Transplantation 21:265, 1976

2. Kretschmer GM, Sutherland DER, Matas AJ, et al: Surgery 82:74, 1977

3. Kolb E, Ruckert R, Largiader F: Eur Surg Res 9:419, 1977

4. Najarian JS, Sutherland DER, Baumgartner D, et al: Ann Surg 192:526, 1980

5. Sutherland DER, Goetz FC, Najarian JS: Transplant Proc 13:291, 1981

6. Traverso LW, Abou-Zamzam AM, Longmire WP: Ann Surg 193:191, 1981

7. Ballinger WF, Lacy PE: Surgery 72:175, 1972

8. Leonard RJ, Lazarow A, Hegre OD: Diabetes 22:413, 1973

9. Bowen KM, Andrus L, Lafferty KJ: Diabetes 29:98, 1980

10. Sutherland DER: Diabetes 31:112, 1982

11. Sutherland DER, Matas AJ, Goetz FC, et al: Diabetes 29:31, 1980

12. DuToit DF, Reece-Smith H, McShane P, et al: Transplantation 33:302, 1982

13. Sutherland DER, Kretschmer GJ, Matas AJ, et al: Trans Am Soc Artif Intern Organs 23:723, 1977

14. Reckard CR, Barker CF: Transplant Proc 5:761, 1973

15. Barker CF, Naji A, Silvers WK: Diabetes 29:86, 1980

16. Naji A, Barker CF, Silvers WK: Transplant Proc 11:506, 1979

17. Sutherland DER, Rynasiewicz JJ, Kawahara K, et al: J Surg Res 29:240, 1980

18. Nash JR, Peters M, Bell PRF: Transplantation 24:70, 1977

19. Norin AJ, Veith FJ: Transplantation 32:259, 1981

20. Deeg JH, Storb R, Gerhard-Miller L: Transplantation 29:230, 1980

21. Reitz BA, Burton NA, Jamieson SW, et al: J Thorac Cardiovasc Surg 80:360, 1980

22. Borel JF, Mesyaros J: Transplantation 29:161, 1980

23. Calne RY, Rolles K, Thiru S, et al: Lancet 2:1033, 1979

24. Green CJ, Allison AC: Lancet 1:1182, 1978

25. Dunn DC, White DJG, Herbertson BM, et al: Transplantation 27:359, 1979

26. Jamieson SW, Burton NA, Breber H, et al: Surg Forum 30:289, 1979

27. Homan WP, Fabre JW, Williams KA, et al: Transplantation 29:361, 1980

28. McMaster P, Procyshyn A, Calne RY, et al: Br Med J 280:444, 1980

29. Williams JW, Peters TG, Haggitt R, et al: J Surg Res 32:576, 1982

30. Albert ED, Storb R, Erickson VM, et al: Tissue Antigens 3:417, 1973

31. Terasaki PI, McClelland JD: Nature 204:998, 1964

32. Vriesendorp HM, Albert ED, Templeton S, et al: Transplant Proc 8:289, 1976

33. Bijnen AB, Vriesendorp HM, Grossewilde H, et al: Tissue Antigens 9:187, 1977

34. Mandel TE: Immunol Today 3:175, 1982

35. Lacy PE, Lacy ET, Finke EH, et al: Diabetes 31:109, 1982

The Effect of Cyclosporine on Simultaneous Skin and Pancreatic Islet Allografts in the Rabbit

W. B. Jolley, K. Knierim, J. Ham, and J. K. Longerbeam

THE selective immunosuppressive activity of the cyclic peptide cyclosporine-A (CsA) has generated a new surge of activity and hope for more successful tissue transplantation. From the available data, it would appear that the suppression is predominantly involved with certain T-lymphocyte-dependent mechanisms, while the B-lymphocyte activity is not impaired. It also appears that the T-suppressor cell population is not inhibited. Some data seem to indicate that there might even be some tissue differences in these responses.[1–3]

We have started a series of studies in which we are investigating the effectiveness of CsA in maintaining rabbit allografts of skin and pancreatic islets of Langerhans. The present report focuses mainly on preliminary studies on the time for rejection of simultaneously allografted skin and islets in diabetic rabbits. Particular emphasis was placed on the degree of tolerance noted after cessation of CsA treatment.

MATERIALS AND METHODS

Animals

Female California and New Zealand white rabbits (2.5–3.5 kg) were used as donors and recipients. In previous studies, it had been shown that this strain combination has histoincompatibility for skin, kidneys, heart, and pancreatic islets. These outbred animals were housed in single cages, fed a pellet diet, and water ad libitum.

Induction of Diabetes

Fasting rabbits were given two doses of alloxan, 65 mg/kg body weight, 1 hr apart to induce diabetes. The rabbits were monitored for blood glucose for a minimum of 2 weeks to assure that they were not recovering from the alloxan. A Yellow Springs Instrument glucose analyzer was used for the glucose testing. Only animals that had blood glucose levels above 300 mg/dl were used in the studies.

Transplantation

Full-thickness ear allografts of 2 sq cm were exchanged between the rabbit pairs. The animals were inspected daily and photographed to define graft rejection. Histologic sections were made at various stages to define cell infiltration.

Pancreatic islets were prepared by a method developed in our laboratories and transplanted to the liver via the portal vein by techniques previously described.[4] Viability and functioning of the islet transplants were ascertained by monitoring blood glucose. Rejection was presumed to be occurring when the glucose levels reached 200 mg/dl for 3 consecutive days and was judged complete when pretransplant levels were reached.

Immunosuppression

CsA was dissolved in olive oil and injected intramuscularly. To define the proper concentration to use in diabetic rabbits, three different concentrations were tested; 20 mg/kg body weight (BW)/day, 15 mg/kg BW/day, and 10 mg/kg BW/day. The 10 mg/kg BW/day dosage was used in all of the experiments, since skin grafts survived at this level, and the higher concentrations produced anuria within 3 days and the rabbits stopped eating. Several rabbits showed very dry compacted food in the stomach when autopsied. It appeared that gastric motility and perhaps even secretory activity had been reduced. The CsA was generously supplied by Sandoz Ltd., Basel, Switzerland.

Study Groups

Group A was the skin allograft controls and received no CsA. Group B was the islet allograft controls done on diabetic rabbits and received no CsA. Group C received skin allografts only and CsA 10 mg/kg BW/day. The CsA treatment ended after 60 days, and the grafts were inspected daily to define the time of rejection. Group D,

From the Loma Linda University School of Medicine, Department of Surgery, and the Jerry L. Pettis Veterans Administration Hospital, Loma Linda, CA.

Supported in part by the Southern California Chapter of the American Diabetic Association.

Address reprint requests to Dr. W. B. Jolley, Department of Surgery, Loma Linda University School of Medicine, Loma Linda, CA 92354.

0041–1345/83/1505–0152$01.00/0

diabetic rabbits, received islet allografts from a single donor and CsA 10 mg/kg BW/day for 60 days. Blood glucose levels were determined prior to transplantation and every third day thereafter. Group E received both skin and islet allografts to diabetic rabbits. The skin and islets came from the same donor. The CsA treatment protocol was identical to that in groups C and D. Graft rejection was also defined as above.

RESULTS AND DISCUSSION

Group A, skin allografts and no treatment (14 rabbits), survived 7.2 ± 0.8 days.

Group B, islet allografts and no treatment, showed graft function for 0, 2, 3, 3, 2, and 4 days.

Group C, CsA treatment and skin allografts (8 rabbits), survived as long as we continued the CsA. One animal showed what appeared to be a very slow rejection in which the hair on the graft was gradually reduced, with some small foci of obvious rejection and areas of necrosis.

Group D, CsA treatment and islet allografts, 4/7 rabbits survived and remained normoglycemic during the period in which the animals received the CsA.

Group E, 6 animals, received both skin and islet allografts and CsA; 6/6 rabbits had viable skin grafts, while only 3/6 had functional islet grafts. One animal rejected the skin graft within 20 days of cessation of CsA treatment. The islets continued to function for an additional 3 weeks, followed by a slow rejection, as evidenced by a steady rise in the blood glucose. The second animal rejected the skin 42 days after cessation of treatment. The rabbit remained normoglycemic for an additional 60 days, at which time the animal was sacrificed for histologic studies. The third animal rejected the skin graft 30 days after CsA was stopped, while the islets have continued to function for 120 days.

The renal and gastric toxicity observed in our early studies is in agreement with the experience of others.[5–8] Our animals showed greater sensitivity to the drug at 15 mg/kg than others using a different rabbit strain combination of donors and recipients.[9] Another explanation for a difference could be that the alloxan used to induce diabetes had caused systemic changes, making the rabbits more responsive to the CsA.

Although permanent tolerance to skin allografts did not occur after cessation of the CsA, successful skin grafts were possible during the entire period of drug administration. Hair growth was normal and very few infiltrating cells were observed.

The most intriguing observation of these studies was the continued survival and functioning of the transplanted islets after the rejection of skin grafts. This observation, if true in a greater number of animals, raises the possibility of immune cell populations having differential sensitivities and resistance to CsA when related to a specific tissue. Current studies are in progress to see if such cells can be identified.

REFERENCES

1. Norin AJ, Emeson EE, Veith FJ: Transplant Proc 15:508, 1983

2. Homan WP, Fabre JW, Morris PJ: Transplantation 28:439, 1979

3. Nagao T, White DJG, Calne RY: Transplantation 33:31, 1982

4. Hinshaw DB, Jolley WB, Knierim KH, et al: Surg Forum 32:381, 1981

5. Gratwohl A, Forster I, Speck B: Transplantation 31:136, 1981

6. Gratwohl A, Forster I, Speck B: Transplantation 33:361, 1982

7. Deeg HJ, Storb R, Gerhard-Müller L, et al: Transplantation 29:230, 1980

8. Prop JM, Bartels HL, Petersen AH, et al: Transplant Proc 15:511, 1983

9. Gratwohl A, Forster I, Speck B: Transplant Proc 15:497, 1983

Pharmacokinetics of Cyclosporine in a Canine Intestinal Transplantation Model

Z. Cohen, S. R. Nordgren, R. D. Mackenzie, A. G. Lossing, C. R. Stiller, and B. Langer

CYCLOSPORINE (CsA) is a recently developed immunosuppressant drug that interferes with early stages of the immunologic response. CsA has a predominant effect on the T cell and inhibits lymphocyte activation and cytotoxic T-lymphocyte generation following allogeneic stimulation.[1] It is effective in prolonging survival of several transplanted organ systems, both in animal and man.[2,3] CsA is also effective in inhibiting graft-versus-host disease (GVHD) in experimental bone marrow transplantation.[4] The effects against both allograft rejection and GVHD are of specific importance when considering small intestinal transplantation. We recently demonstrated that parenterally administered CsA significantly prolonged survival after total small intestinal allotransplanation (TSIA) in the dog to an average of over 100 days.[5,6]

Intestinal transplantation, however, may impede enteral absorption of nutrients and drugs. Reasons for this may be changes in the portal flow, intestinal denervation, and the disruption of intestinal lymphatics. Intestinal rejection presents a further potential challenge to absorption of orally administered nutrients and drugs.

The oral route of administration of CsA has been preferred in clinical transplantation due to the lipophilic character of the drug. However, absorption of orally administered CsA is not well studied, and oral CsA given as the only immunosuppressant following TSIA did not significantly prolong survival in our previous investigation.[5,6] The aim of the present study was to investigate absorption of orally administered CsA in dogs after transplantation of the total small intestine. Specific interest was focused on the contribution of intestinal lymphatics in the absorption of CsA.

MATERIALS AND METHODS

Determination of CsA in Plasma

Throughout the study, blood for CsA analysis was drawn in heparinized tubes (Vacutainer). Plasma was recovered and stored at −70°C until assay. The assay was performed at the Transplantation Laboratory, University of Western Ontario, London, Ontario, employing a radioimmunoassay devised by Sandoz Ltd., Basel, Switzerland. The antibody was supplied by Sandoz Ltd. Unless otherwise stated, samples were drawn at 0, 3, 6, 9, 12, and 24 hr after administration of an oral dose of CsA, 25 mg/kg dissolved in olive oil.

CsA Absorption in Normal Dogs

Five adult mongrel dogs were used. These dogs had no previous surgery and were not previously exposed to CsA. The dogs were given CsA in the morning, following an overnight fast. Free access to food was allowed after the 3-hr samples.

CsA Absorption in Autotransplanted Dogs

Small intestinal autotransplantation was performed in four dogs, according to our previously described technique.[6] The total small intestine was resected on its vascular pedicle. The vascular bed of the transplant was perfused with 1 liter of cold heparinized Ringer's lactate. Ischemic time was 60–80 min. The intestine was transplanted back into the donor in an orthotopic fashion, anastomosing the superior mesenteric artery to the abdominal aorta and the superior mesenteric vein to the inferior vena cava. Intestinal continuity was restored with

---

From the Department of Surgery, Toronto General Hospital and the University of Toronto, Toronto, Ontario, and the Department of Medicine, University of Western Ontario, London, Ontario, Canada.

Supported in part by grants from the Division of General Surgery, University of Toronto, the Toronto General Hospital Foundation, the PSI Foundation, Toronto, Canada, and the Greenmeadow Charitable Foundation.

Address reprint requests to Dr. Z. Cohen, Room Eaton 9-211, Toronto General Hospital, 101 College Street, Toronto, Ontario, Canada M5G 1L7.

0041–1345/83/1505–0153$01.00/0

a proximal and a distal end-to-end anastomosis. No attempts were made to ligate or reconnect the intestinal lymphatics. All four dogs withstood the surgery well, and three are presently alive and well 40–60 weeks posttransplant. One dog died from a volvulus of the graft at 32 weeks. CsA absorption was studied 1 and 10 weeks after transplantation.

CsA Absorption in Allotransplanted Dogs

Total small intestinal allotransplantation was performed in 13 dogs. Three of these died prior to the sixth day from surgical complications and were excluded from the study. Allotransplanted dogs were given CsA, 25 mg/kg/day p.o., starting on day 1 posttransplant. Samples for CsA assay were drawn every second or third day before and 6 hr after administration of the drug. Histologic monitoring of the allograft was performed by means of mucosal biopsies from an isolated segment of the terminal end of the graft, accessible from the skin surface, but out-of-continuity from the remaining graft.[7]

CsA Absorption After Diversion of Thoracic Duct Lymph

Thoracic duct cutaneous fistulae were created under general anesthesia in four normal mongrel dogs. Through a left paramedian neck incision, the thoracic duct terminus was exposed at the confluence of the left jugular and subclavian veins. By ligating the brachiocephalic vein proximally, the subclavian vein distally, numerous small veins close to the confluence, and the jugular vein high in the neck, a venous conduit was created for lymph (Fig. 1). Lymph was delivered to the skin via this conduit as described by Markowitz et al.[8] After completing the neck dissection, a small upper abdominal laparotomy was

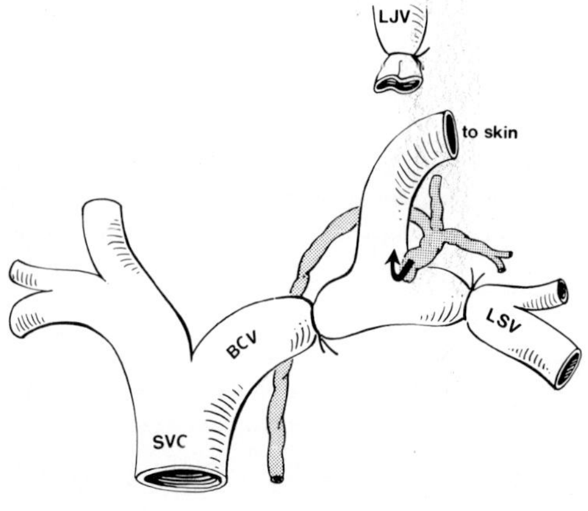

Fig. 1. Schematic representation of the technique for construction of the thoracic duct fistula. LJV, left jugular vein. LSV, left subclavian vein. BVC, brachiocephalic vein. SVC, superior vena cava.

performed, and CsA, 25 mg/kg in olive oil, was administered as a bolus injection in the upper jejunum. Anesthesia was reversed, and lymph was collected at intervals, as for the blood samples, in the recovering dogs. In four dogs, a sham operation of similar duration was performed, including minilaparotomy and jejunal instillation of CsA.

The lymph and blood samples were centrifuged, and the supernatant recovered and stored at −70°C until assay. In one of the lymph-diverted dogs, the fistula was patent more than 48 hr, and a second dose of CsA was given orally the day after surgery. Plasma and lymph samples were then collected for another 24-hr period.

CsA Absorption From the Peritoneal Cavity

CsA dissolved in alcohol, 10 mg/kg, was suspended in Intralipid (5 ml), heated to 37°C under gentle agitation, and injected intraperitoneally in 5 normal (nontransplanted) awake dogs. Blood samples were drawn as stated above.

RESULTS

CsA Absorption in Normal Dogs

A significant increase of plasma CsA was noted in the 3-hr sample. However, the peak value was consistently recorded 6 hr after the oral dose. The peak reached 1683 ± 154 ng/ml (mean ± SE). Thereafter, the plasma level tapered off in a logarithmic fashion. The 12-hr level was 543 ± 125 ng/ml, and after 24 hr, a plasma CsA level of 143 ± 34 ng/ml was recorded (Fig. 2).

CsA Absorption in Autotransplanted Dogs

At day 7 after transplantation, the animals appeared well, although their body weight was 10%–15% below that recorded preoperatively. All autotransplanted dogs had diarrhea. The appearance of CsA in plasma after an oral dose showed a time course similar to the normal dogs. However, the average peak reached at 6 hr was 678 ± 348 ng/ml or approximately 40% of the peak level reached in normal dogs (Fig. 2). The difference is statistically significant at $p < 0.05$. The 24-hr CsA level was 85 ± 24 ng/ml. At 10-weeks after autotransplantation of the total small bowel, the dogs produced formed feces and all had regained their preoperative weight. However, the administration of CsA in olive oil

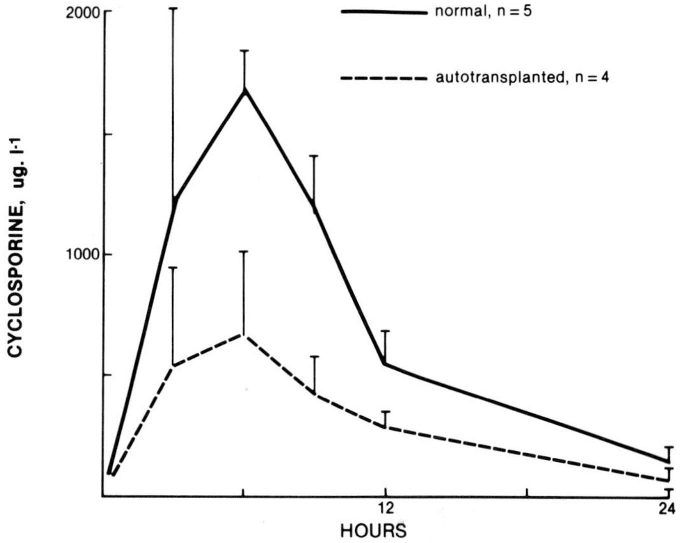

Fig. 2. Plasma levels of cyclosporine after an oral dose, 25 mg/kg in olive oil, in normal dogs and in dogs after intestinal autotransplantation.

caused short-lasting diarrhea in all four dogs. The 6-hr peak plasma level of CsA at 10 weeks was 528 ± 85 ng/ml. Twenty-four hours after the 10-week test dose, the plasma level was 88 ± 26 ng/ml.

CsA Absorption in Allotransplanted Dogs

Ten successfully allotransplanted dogs survived a mean of 34 days. At day 7 posttransplant, normal allograft histology was documented in 5 dogs. Predose plasma CsA in these dogs was 172 ± 69 ng/ml. The 6-hr peak CsA level was 1005 ± 328 ng/ml. The increase in mean plasma CsA 6 hr after oral administration of the drug amounted to 833 ng/ml, which is comparable to the increase noted in autotransplanted dogs after a single dose of oral CsA. Five dogs showed histologic signs of rejection at day 7. Predose CsA levels in these dogs were 99 ± 47 ng/ml and 6-hr peaks 368 ± 31 ng/ml. The difference between the peak CsA levels in nonrejecting and rejecting allotransplanted dogs is statistically significant at $p < 0.05$.

CsA Absorption After Diversion of Thoracic Duct Lymph

The flow rate of lymph after surgery was completed was approximately 50 ml/hr. The lymph had a clear appearance before instillation of CsA in olive oil, but turned milky 2–3 hr after CsA administration. Plasma levels of CsA remained low in lymph-diverted dogs. A peak of 147 ± 25 ng/ml was reached in plasma in lymph-diverted dogs at 6 hr after instillation of CsA (Fig. 3). The CsA content of the diverted lymph, however, increased considerably to a peak of 1759 ± 615 ng/ml (Fig. 3). In one dog, the lymph level of CsA reached 10,000 ng/ml, coinciding with the milky appearance of the lymph. At 24 hr after the intrajejunal administration of CsA, lymph levels were 114 ± 3 ng/ml and plasma levels were 30 ± 8 ng/ml.

Plasma levels of CsA after intrajejunal administration in sham-operated dogs were higher than those recorded from lymph-diverted dogs. At 6 hr, mean plasma levels in the sham-operated dogs were 229 ± 79 ng/ml. This peak was significantly higher than the peak in dogs with diversion of the thoracic duct lymph, $p = 0.05$, (Mann-Whitney U test).

In the one dog with a persisting lymphatic fistula, an oral dose of CsA was given 24 hr after the preceding dose. Lymph levels of CsA in this dog rose to over 150,000 ng/ml within 3 hr. The 6-hr level in plasma was 722 ng/ml in

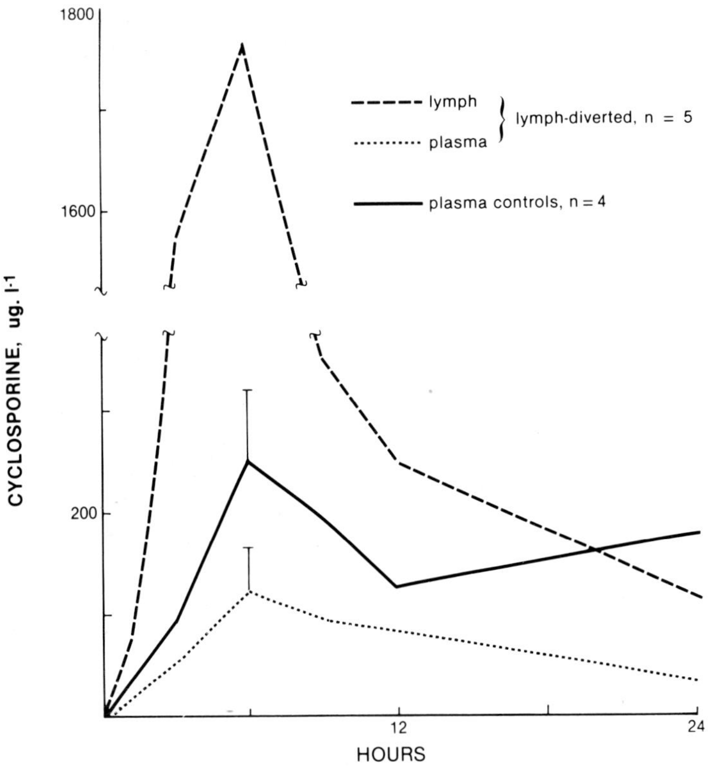

Fig. 3. Plasma and lymph levels of cyclosporine after jejunal instillation of 25 mg/kg in olive oil in dogs with a thoracic duct fistula. Sham-operated dogs served as controls.

this dog, comparable to the average obtained in autotransplanted dogs.

CsA Absorption From the Peritoneal Cavity

The appearance of CsA in peripheral plasma was noted earlier after intraperitoneal injection than after oral administration. A peak value of 200 ± 50 ng/ml was recorded at 3 hr after administration. The 6-hr level was 140 ± 27 ng/ml. The plasma levels tapered off to 67 ± 19 ng/ml at 24 hr.

DISCUSSION

Transplantation of the total small intestine presents a unique challenge to the efficient absorption of nutrients and drugs. The surgical procedure, as described above, disrupts mesenteric nerves and lymphatic channels completely and alters portal flow. All of these factors may influence the function of the transplanted intestine.[9] To elucidate some of the functional aspects of the intestinal allograft, we studied the absorption of orally administered CsA in olive oil in normal dogs and in dogs after intestinal auto- and allotransplantation. We also investigated the effects of lymphatic diversion on CsA absorption.

The results demonstrate that a peak plasma level is reached on average 6 hr after an oral dose of CsA, both in autotransplanted and in normal nonoperated dogs. This indicates that the kinetics of absorption are not changed significantly by the operative procedure. However, the absolute level of CsA at 6 hr in the autotransplanted dogs was only 40% when compared to the controls.

This reduced absorption in the autotransplanted state may be caused by trauma to the intestine from resection and cold preservation, altered venous return (systemic versus portal), the effects of severing the autonomic nerve fibers to the bowel, or the disruption of intestinal lymphatics. Ruiz et al. demonstrated that absorption of d-xylose was reduced to approximately 40% of normal after skeletonization of the small intestinal mesenteric root in dogs.[10] A similar quantitative reduction of d-xylose absorption in allotransplanted dogs was reported by Toledo-Pereyra.[11] These findings imply that division of intestinal nerves and lymphatics has a greater impact on absorption of carbohydrates than does the altered venous return.

Recovery from postoperative diarrhea to normal intestinal function in autotransplanted dogs has been reported to occur after several weeks or months.[10] The return to normal bowel function also coincides with reconnection of intestinal lymphatics, which takes place approximately 4 weeks after intestinal autotransplantation[12] and allotransplantation.[5] However, we were not able to demonstrate any improvement in absorption of CsA 10 weeks after autotransplantation. This may be explained by the explosive diarrhea that was produced in these animals after administration of oral CsA in olive oil. In animals receiving a daily dose of olive oil, a better tolerance to a fat load may have developed, allowing for a more efficient absorption of the drug.

Intestinal absorption of CsA in allotransplanted animals was studied in dogs with histologically normal graft mucosa and in dogs undergoing rejection. Absorption in nonrejecting dogs was comparable to that in autotransplanted dogs. The low values recorded from allografted dogs in rejection were not unexpected and stress the importance of functional monitoring of the intestinal allograft for maintaining adequate absorption of nutrients and drugs.

A lipophilic substance like CsA should theoretically be absorbed through intestinal lymphatics. We studied the lymphatic contribution to plasma levels of CsA after oral administration by creating a thoracic duct fistula in normal nontransplanted dogs. The peak plasma level after jejunal instillation of CsA was significantly lower in dogs with lymph fistulas when compared to sham-operated controls. This supports the hypothesis that lymphatics play a major role in the intestinal absorption of CsA in olive oil. However, it is not possible to draw quantitative conclusions from this experiment, due to the generally low absorption in these dogs recovering from a general anesthesic. The high levels of CsA documented in the diverted lymph also support the hypothesis that lymphatics play a major role in absorption of CsA. More physiologic conditions prevailed in one dog with a persisting lymph fistula. In this dog, when studied awake, plasma CsA reached only 42% of the mean in normal dogs. This represents a plasma level of CsA comparable to that found in autotransplanted dogs. This also indicates that, after an oral dose of the drug, drainage of thoracic duct lymph in this dog resulted in a plasma level of CsA similar to that seen after intestinal autotransplantation.

We have observed chylous ascites in dogs shortly after intestinal transplantation. This has made us believe that lipid compounds, having entered the intestinal lymphatics, are poured freely into the peritoneal cavity through the cut lymph channels. If true, the fraction of CsA that is transported from the intestine into the intestinal lymph channels does not leave the body but enters the abdominal cavity. We assume that a reabsorption of CsA may take place through the peritoneal membrane. To test this hypothesis, we instilled a suspension of CsA in Intralipid[13] into the peritoneal cavity in normal dogs and studied the plasma CsA levels. Appearance of CsA in the plasma was rapid, indicating that some peritoneal absorption may well occur directly into the circulation.

The immunosuppressive effect of CsA is well documented, although relatively little is known of the correlation between plasma CsA levels and optimal drug effect. Recent studies in human kidney transplantation indicate that plasma trough levels in the range of 100–300 ng/ml are adequate in the initial posttransplant period and that considerably lower levels may be sufficient at a later stage after transplantation.[14] To support this concept, we have shown that survival of orally treated dogs in this study was significantly shorter than survival in previously reported dogs receiving parenteral and then oral CsA treatment.[5] Three dogs from the previously reported parenterally treated group were maintained on oral CsA for a mean of over 200 days. Also, in this study, three of the dogs treated with oral CsA alone survived an average of 60 days. This strongly suggests that adequate plasma levels of CsA were maintained for long periods of time in these dogs, despite the oral route of drug administration. In this particular animal model, rejection presents a further challenge to the effective absorption of orally administered CsA. Therefore, during episodes of rejection, parenteral administration of the drug will be necessary to achieve both optimal plasma levels and immunosuppression.

In conclusion, the present study demonstrates that oral CsA in olive oil is absorbed from the autotransplanted and allotransplanted small intestine in dogs. The absorption occurs despite the extensive surgical procedure, including complete disruption of intestinal nerves and lymphatic channels. Therefore, the oral route of CsA administration may be used shortly after intestinal transplantation. However, we do not feel that this will provide maximal immunosuppression. Close monitoring of plasma levels of CsA will be necessary in order to provide the graft and the host with optimal immunosuppression.

ACKNOWLEDGMENT

Cyclosporine was kindly provided by Sandoz Ltd., Basel, Switzerland.

REFERENCES

1. Keown PA, Essery GL, Stiller CR, et al: Transplant Proc 13:386, 1981
2. Morris PJ: Transplantation 32:349, 1981
3. Borel JF: Transplant Proc 13:344, 1981
4. Deeg HJ, Storb R, Weiden PL, et al: Transplant Proc 13:402, 1981
5. Reznick RK, Craddock GN, Langer B, et al: Can J Surg 25:51, 1982
6. Craddock GN, Nordgren SR, Reznick RK, et al: Transplantation 35:284, 1983
7. Lossing A, Nordgren S, Cohen Z, et al: Transplant Proc 14:643, 1982
8. Markowitz J, Archibald J, Downie HG: In: Experimental Surgery (ed 5) Baltimore, Williams & Wilkins, 1965, p 425
9. Ruiz JO, Lillehei RC: Am J Proctol 23:379, 1972
10. Toledo-Pereyra LH, Simmons RL, Najarian JS: Am J Surg 129:192, 1975
11. Ruiz JO, Uchida H, Schultz LS, et al: Am J Surg 123:297, 1972
12. Kocandrle V, Houttuin E, Prohaska JV: Surg Gynecol Obstet 122:587, 1966
13. Homan P, Fabre J, Williams A: Transplantation 29:361, 1980
14. Stiller CR, et al: Transplant Proc (this issue) 1983

Successful Small Bowel Allografts in Piglets Using Cyclosporine

C. Ricour, Y. Revillon, F. Arnaud-Battandier, D. Ghnassia, P. Weyne, A. Lauffenburger, J. Jos, J. L. Fontaine, P. Gallix, and M. Vaiman

WITHOUT immunosuppressive drugs, rejection of small bowel allografts occurred within 10 days.[2-4] Various assays of immunosuppression were without success, delaying rejection for approximately 20 days.[5-8] Recent demonstration of cyclosporine-A's (CsA) immunosuppressive capacity, allowing (in animals and man) the prevention of kidney, bone marrow, heart, liver, and pancreas rejection,[9] prompted us to reconsider the possibility of an intestinal graft. This work studied the effects of CsA on the survival of piglet small intestinal allografts.

MATERIALS AND METHODS

Animals

Forty large white piglets, 20–40 kg, were used. Donor and recipient were histoincompatible for one or two haplotypes for the major histocompatibility system (SLA) and were mixed lymphocyte culture (MLC) positive.[10]

Transplantation

Transplantations were performed as previously described[11] after luminal and vascular washings using a Collin's solution at 4°C and with a vascular orthotopic mesenteric anastomosis.

Experiments were done with paired animals, each animal being donor and recipient. Two different procedures of intestinal graft were employed: (1) 200-cm small intestinal grafts were transplanted, with each extremity exteriorized as cutaneous enterostomy (n = 30), and recipient residual bowel continuity reestablished by end-to-end anastomosis; (2) 600-cm small intestinal grafts were transplanted and placed immediately in continuity with the recipient small intestine (n = 11).

CsA

CsA was used alone, beginning 48 hr before transplantation, in both donor and recipient. Treatment was given in 3 different ways: (1) every other day intramuscularly at the dose of 25 mg/kg (n = 6); (2) every day orally at the same dose (n = 27); and (3) every day intravenously, using a central venous catheter, at the dose of 8 mg/kg for 5–10 days, then orally 25 mg/kg (n = 3). The control group consisted of 4 animals receiving no CsA and no other treatment.

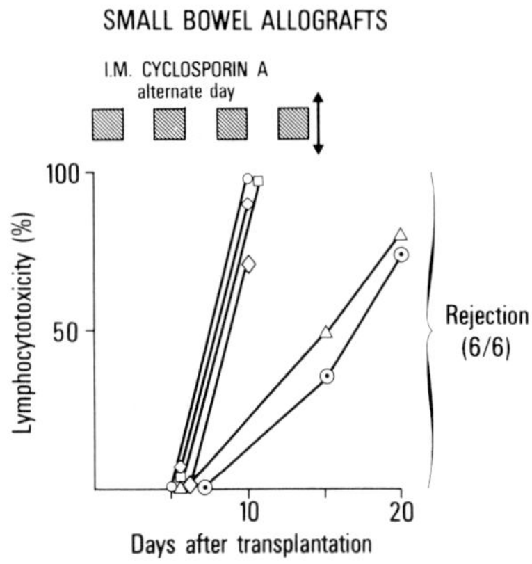

Fig. 1. Serum percent lymphocytotoxicity of the host against the donor lymphocytes in 6 cases with CsA given every other day intramuscularly.

Monitoring

Every 3 days during the first month, then once a month, the following parameters were determined: (1) histologic studies of the graft mucosa, only in the enterostomy group; (2) serum complement-dependent cytotoxicity (percent lymphocytotoxicity—%LCT) as previously described;[10] and (3) plasma CsA levels by radioimmunoassay for the last 20 experiments.

From the Service de Gastroentérologie Pédiatrique et de Nutrition et Clinique Chirurgicale Infantile, Hôpital des Enfants Malades, Paris, France, and the Commissariat à l'Energie Atomique, IPSN, Département de Protection, Laboratoire de Radiobiologie Appliquée, Jouy-en-Josas, France.

Supported in part by a grant from the Scientific Council of CHU Necker, Paris.

A preliminary communication of this work was reported at the European Society of Pediatric Gastroenterology and Nutrition, 1981.[1]

Address reprint requests to Dr. C. Ricour, Service de Gastroentérologie Pédiatrique et de Nutrition, Hôpital des Enfants Malades, 149, rue de Sèvres F, 75730 Paris Cedex 15, France.

0041-1345/83/1505-0154$01.00/0

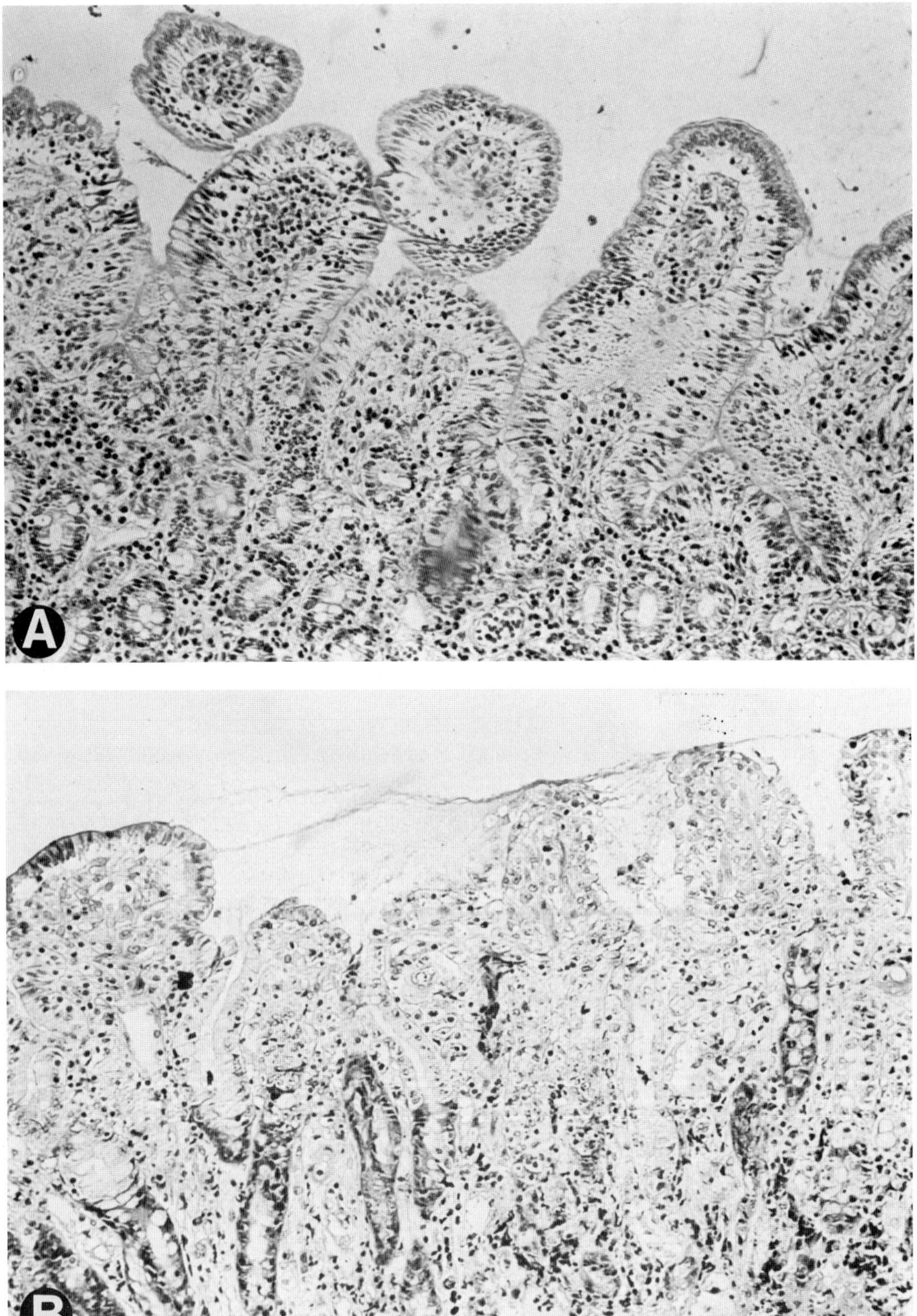

Fig. 2. Histologic aspects during subacute rejection. Normal mucosa on day 0 (A); crypt hypertrophy, decrease in villous height, low increase of the lymphoid population in the lamina propria on day 8 (B); flattening of the mucosa with cellular infiltration on day 12 (C); necrosis on day 20 (D) (hematoxylin and eosin ×100).

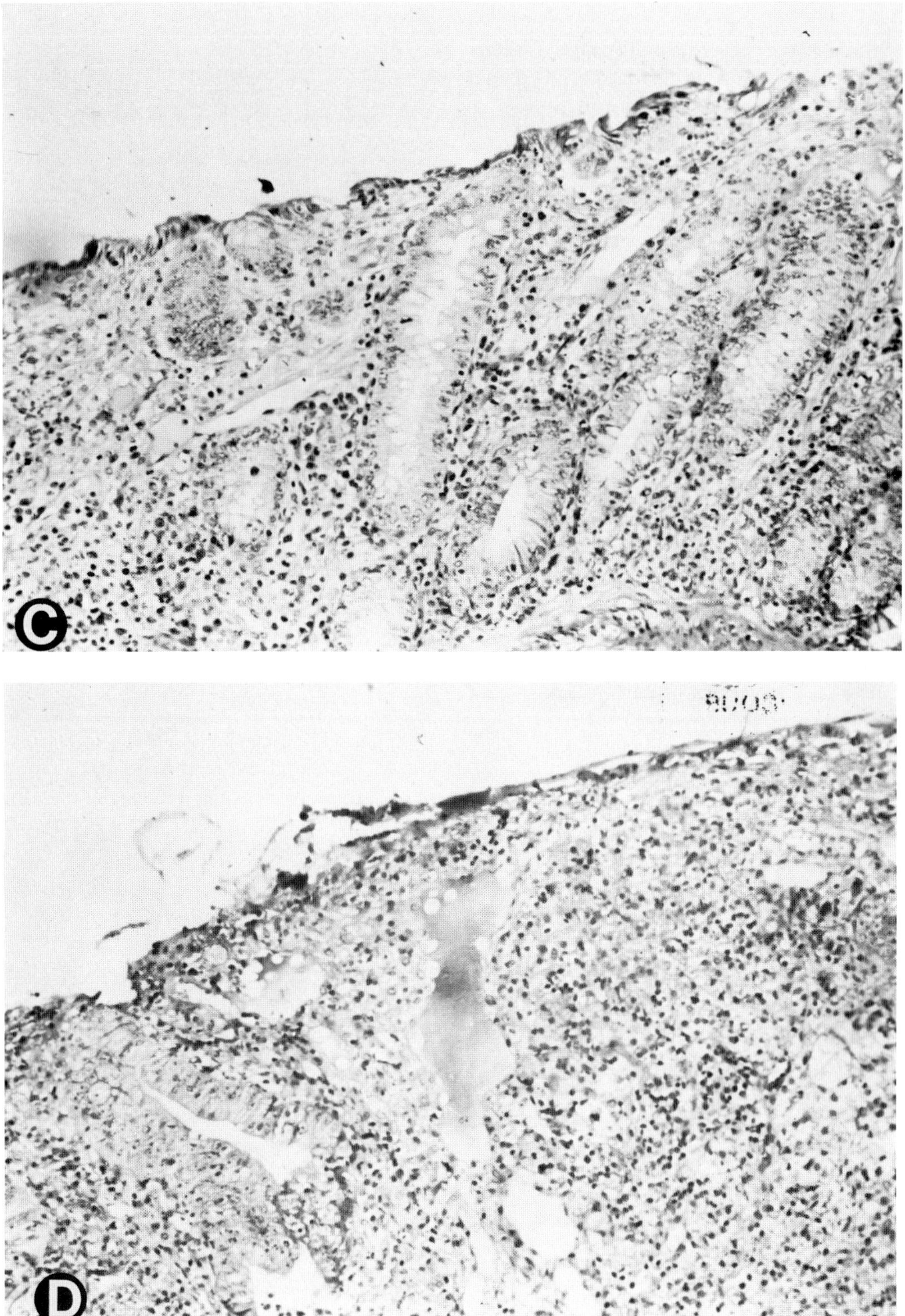

Fig. 2. continued

RESULTS

Seven experiments failed because of immediate necrosis and/or death of the animal within 5 days after surgery.

I. First Group: Double Enterostomy

(I_1) Without CsA ($n = 4$): acute rejection with graft necrosis always occurred within 8 days.

(I_2) CsA intramuscularly, every other day for 15 days ($n = 6$). In 4 cases, graft necrosis occurred on the tenth day, with a %LCT reaching 75%–90%. In 2 other cases, histologic rejection and increase in %LCT occurred on day 20 (Fig. 1).

(I_3) Oral CsA every day ($n = 13$). Four cases presented a subacute rejection; histologic examination revealed an atrophic mucosa with lymphocyte and plasmocyte infiltration on day 15, with necrosis 5–15 days later (Fig. 2); %LCT was above 50% on day 10 (Fig. 3); plasma CsA levels, measured in 2 cases, were below 150 ng/ml.

No rejections were observed in 9 cases; mucosa was normal, except in 2 cases where it was transitorily flat on day 15. Percent LCT was negative in 4 cases and below 40% on day 10 in the other cases (Fig. 3). Plasma CsA levels, measured in 7 cases, varied between 250 and 2000 ng/ml (Fig. 4). After 30 days, CsA was stopped in 5 cases, and rejection occurred 30–60 days later. In the 4 other cases, CsA was continued (12 mg/kg); intestinal continuity between the graft and the recipient small bowel was reestablished without any complication, the animal's growth being normal. The %LCT remained null, and plasma CsA levels varied between 250 and 1500 ng/ml. Animals were sacrificed on days 80, 95, 122, and 390; grafted small bowels were normal. No hepatic or kidney alterations were observed (Fig. 5), and no signs of graft-versus-host reaction were noted.

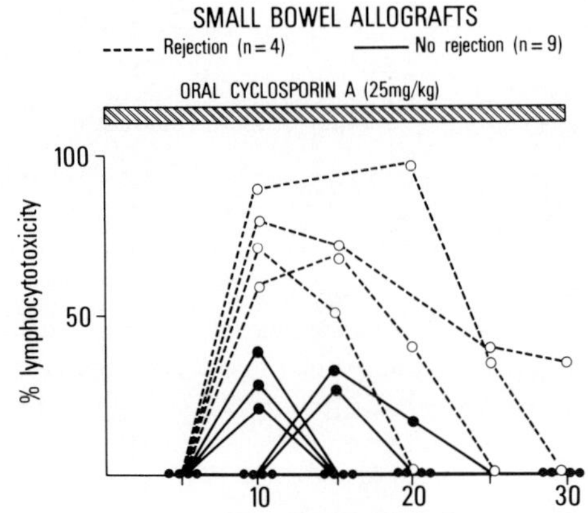

Fig. 3. Serum percent lymphocytotoxicity in 13 cases with CsA given orally every day. (●—●) No rejection; (O·····O) rejection before 30 days.

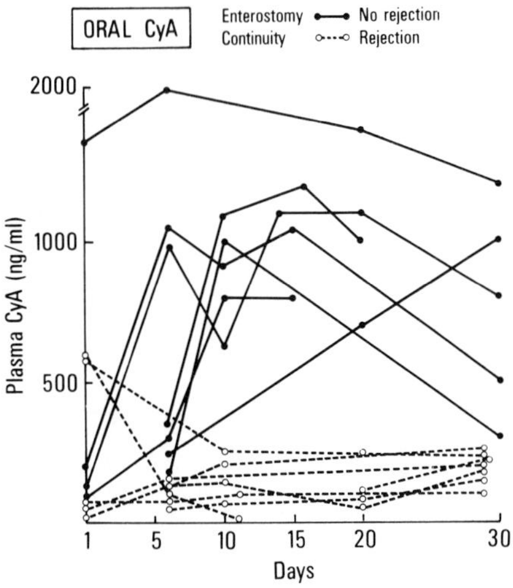

Fig. 4. Plasma CsA levels. (●—●) Double enterostomy; (O·····O) immediate end-to-end anastomosis.

II. Second Group: Immediate Small Bowel Continuity

(II_1) Oral CsA ($n = 7$). In 6 cases, an acute or delayed rejection occurred, with death of the animals on days 11, 28, 36, 49, or 71; grafts were necrosed or characterized by a complete disappearance of the mucosa. The %LCT varied between 50% and 70%, and plasma CsA levels varied from 50 to 200 ng/ml (Fig. 4). In one case, no rejection was observed (after 95 days); histologic study of the transplanted bowel was normal; %LCT was null; and plasma CsA levels varied between 150 and 300 ng/ml.

(II_2) Intravenous then oral CsA ($n = 3$). No graft rejection was observed on day 100,

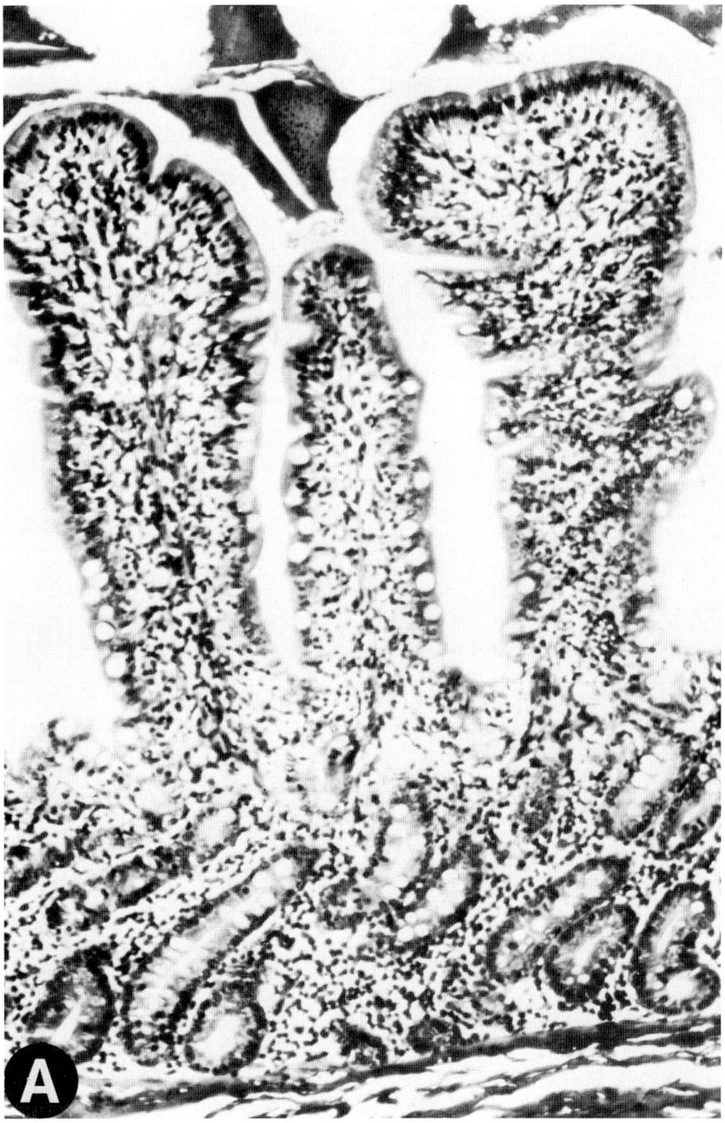

Fig. 5. Normal histology, 14 months posttransplantation, of the intestinal graft (A), the liver (B), and the kidney (C) (hematoxylin and eosin ×100).

150, and 200. Weight gain started 1 month after surgery, and there was no increase of %LCT and plasma CsA levels were above 250 ng/ml.

DISCUSSION

When donor and recipient are histoincompatible, intestinal allografts are characterized in rat,[12] dog,[2] and pig[3] by an acute rejection within a few days. Furthermore, because of the great number of lymphoid cells within the gut, the possibility of graft-versus-host reactions were raised.[8,13] These two risks and the disappointing results of most of the immunosuppressive treatments (transplant irradiation,[8] antilymphocyte serum,[14,15] prednisone and azathioprine[5–7]) led the different groups to stop any intestinal transplantation program.[15]

Our results using only CsA were thus particularly remarkable; they confirm our preliminary results,[1] as well as concomitant results obtained in dogs.[16]

In piglets, without CsA or when given every

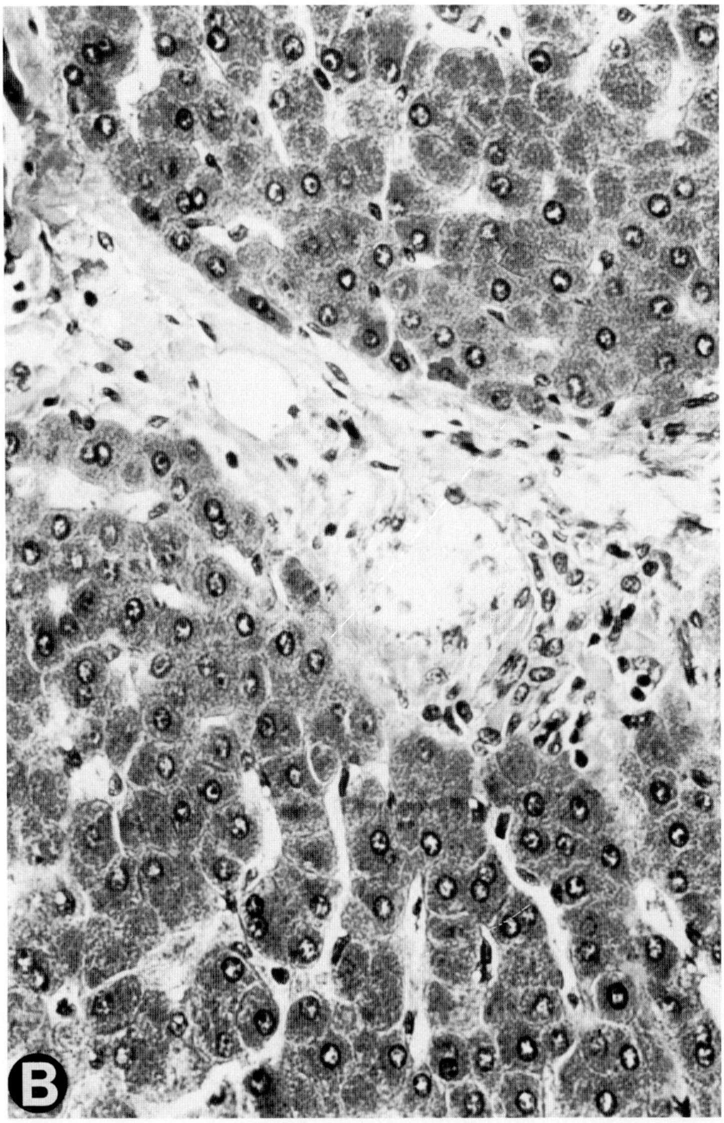

Fig. 5. *(Continued)*

other day, it was evident that rejection of the small bowel allograft occurred between 5 and 20 days. With this experimental model, two markers appeared to be discriminative and predictive of the graft rejection. As it was described in kidney graft,[17,18] an increase in the %LCT (more than 50%) 10 days after grafting was always followed by rejection. At the same time, histologic studies revealed a mucosal atrophy with lymphoid infiltration of the lamina propria, then a rapid necrosis. Similar histologic data announcing or confirming intestinal graft rejection were observed in pigs[4] and dogs.[19]

Furthermore, the survival of the intestinal grafts were dependent on the ways of CsA administration, one of the more specific and difficult problems that had to be resolved. CsA is a liposoluble drug; when ingested orally, its intestinal absorption and lymphatic transport imply functional enterocytes and lymphatic pathway. However, it was demonstrated that interruption in the lymphatic flow during transplantation reduced absorption by

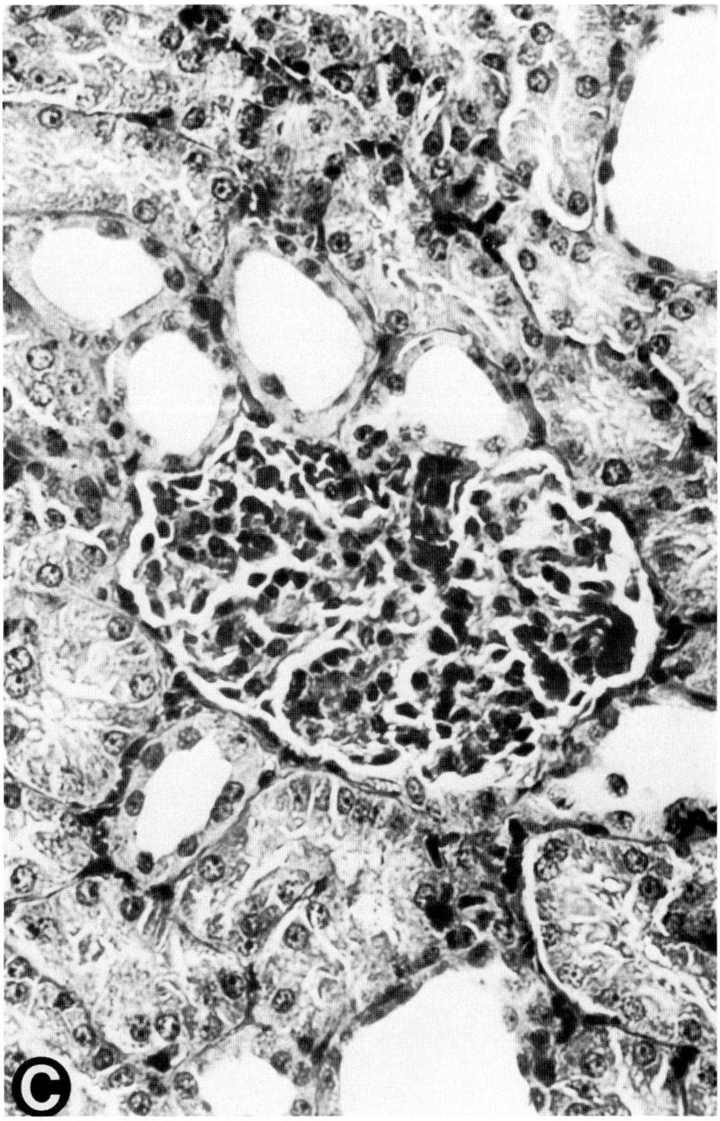

Fig. 5. (*Continued*)

nearly 60%;[20] it was only 2–8 weeks later that intestinal lipid absorption became normal, probably concomitant to veinolymphatic anastomosis.[21] These abnormalities in intestinal transport of lipids explained the difficulties we have encountered, as well as those of others,[20] when CsA was orally administered immediately after the transplantation. Subacute or delayed rejections were observed in 10 cases (4 enterostomies and 6 immediate end-to-end anastomosis) when CsA was given orally, and were probably due to its malabsorption, as demonstrated by the null or below 250 ng/ml plasma CsA levels. The other 13 cases (3 immediate end-to-end anastomosis and veinous CsA perfusion and 10 enterostomies) with perfect graft tolerance received a sufficient amount of CsA, as shown by plasma CsA levels always above 250 ng/ml.

From the results, it is clear that prevention of the "vicious circle" of malabsorption–rejection and the success of intestinal transplantation depend on the veinous path of the administration of CsA, until normalization of intestinal transport occurs. Later, when oral ingestion is substituted for parenteral administration, it is necessary to control the plasma CsA levels by adapting the dose and way of administration.

CsA tolerance, in particular renal or hepatic, was good, as shown in nine cases that received CsA over a long period of time (more than 1 year in one case). Only hisurtism appeared to be constant, beginning after 2 months of treatment. The immunosuppressive effect decreased rapidly when CsA was stopped.

In conclusion, in view of these experimental results and those obtained in man with other organ transplantations,[9,22] allotransplantation of the small bowel in patients undergoing a total intestinal resection should now be reconsidered, with CsA as an immunosuppressive treatment and parenteral feeding as a nutritional support.

REFERENCES

1. Ricour C, Revillon Y, Lauffenburger A, et al: Pediatr Res 5:356, 1981
2. Westbroeck D, Rothengatter C, Vriesendorp HM, et al: Transplant Proc 3:157, 1971
3. Hay JM, Fagniez PL, Parc R, et al: Ann Chir 28:1063, 1974
4. Stauffer UG: Prog Pediatr Surg 8:1, 1975
5. Preston FW, Macalalad F, Graber R, et al: Transplantation 3:224, 1965
6. Holmes JT: Ann R Coll Surg 52:165, 1973
7. Ruiz JO, Uchida H, Schultz LS, et al: Am J Surg 123:297, 1972
8. Cohen Z, MacGregor AB, Moore KTH, et al: Arch Surg 111:248, 1976
9. White DJG, Calne RY: Immunol Rev 65:115, 1982
10. Vaiman M, Renard C, Lafage Ph, et al: Ann Biol Anim Biochem Biophys 11:41, 1971
11. Ricour C, Revillon Y, Pletyncx M, et al: Gastroenterol Clin Biol 5:977, 1981
12. Thiede A, Deltz E: Laugenbecks Arch Chir 346:119, 1978
13. Garrido H, Lucea C, Ruiperez S, et al: Rev Eur Etudes Clin Biol 15:547, 1970
14. Hardy MA, Quint J, State D: Ann Surg 171:51, 1970
15. Telford GL, Corry RJ: Arch Surg 113:615, 1978
16. Nordgren S, Craddock GN, Lossing A, et al: Fed Proc 41:70, 1982
17. Stiller CR, Sinclair NR, Abrahams S, et al: N Engl J Med 294:978, 1976
18. Keown PA, Stiller CR, Ulan RA, et al: Lancet 1:686, 1981
19. Lossing A, Nordgren S, Cohen Z, et al: Transplant Proc 14:643, 1982
20. MacKenzie R, Nordgren S, Lossing A, et al: Transplant Proc 14:646, 1982
21. Chomette G, Cerf M, Hay JM, et al: Ann Anat Pathol (Paris) 20:343, 1975
22. Britton S, Palacios R.: Immunol Rev 65:5, 1982

Prevention of Graft-Versus-Host Reaction Following Small Bowel Transplantation by Temporary Cyclosporine Treatment

E. Deltz, K. Ulrichs, R. Engemann, T. Schack, B. Friedrichs, W. Müller-Ruchholtz, H. K. Müller-Hermelink, and A. Thiede

THE immunosuppressive properties of cyclosporine-A (CsA) have been proved in various types of clinical organ transplantation[1] and different experimental settings of animal transplantation models. Its effect lies in the impairment of interleukin release.[2] As the expression of graft-versus-host reactions (GVHR), as well as rejection reactions, depends on the grade of histoincompatibility between donor and recipient,[3] immunosuppressive agents can be assumed to influence the development of GVHR. The effectiveness of CsA for suppression of GVHR in bone marrow transplantation[4] has been shown.

Another type of transplantation in which GVHR plays an important role is the transplantation of the small intestine. As the small bowel graft contains a large amount of immunocompetent cells within the mesenteric lymph nodes and the Peyer's patches, strong GVHR after small bowel transplantation can cause death of the recipient.[5] Circumvention of GVHR, therefore, is an indispensable condition for successful small bowel transplantation.

In order to investigate the ability of CsA to prevent GVHR, small bowel transplantations in the rat have been carried out.

MATERIALS AND METHODS

Heterotopic transplantation has been carried out by grafting total small intestine accessory to recipient's small bowel. The technique is described in detail elsewhere.[6]

A semiallogeneic donor–recipient combination has been established by using BN ($RT1^n$) donors and BN × Lewis ($RT1^l$)F_1 hybrid recipients, as only in this combination can a unidirectional GVHR develop. Animals of group 1 ($n = 22$) received no additional treatment postoperatively. Rats of group 2 ($n = 26$) were given CsA orally (15 mg/kg body weight) dissolved in olive oil for 14 days following transplantation.

Cytotoxic anti-host activity of T lymphocytes in the lymphatic compartments of the graft (mesenteric lymph nodes, Peyer's patches) and the recipient (mesenteric lymph nodes, Peyer's patches, peripheral lymph nodes, spleen) as well as in recipient's blood was measured by microcytotoxicity assay (MCA)[7] using Lewis fibroblasts as target cells. MCA was performed 14 days (group 1), 20 days, and 120 days (group 2) after transplantation. Histologic examination of all above mentioned tissues was done with special regard to T-dependent areas of lymph nodes and spleen.

RESULTS

All animals of group 1 died within 22 days after transplantation with severe GVHR disease.[5] Of the animals of group 2, 71% (20/28) survived until 120 days posttransplant without clinical signs of GVHR disease. Anti-host T-cell cytotoxicity values (Fig. 1) of group 1 showed high GVHR activity in all lymphatic compartments, except Peyer's patches, of the graft and the recipients.

This pattern changed after CsA treatment (group 2) (Fig. 1). GVHR activity within mesenteric lymph nodes and Peyer's patches decreased both 20 and 120 days after transplantation. The same phenomenon could be found in the mesenteric lymph nodes and the blood of the recipients. Residual GVHR activity remained in the spleen and peripheral lymph nodes 20 days posttransplant and decreased to zero after 120 days. Only within Peyer's patches of recipients' small bowel did

From the Department of General Surgery, the Department of Immunology, and the Department of Pathology, University of Kiel, Federal Republic of Germany.

Supported in part by Deutsche Forschungsgemeinschaft, SFB 111.

Address reprint requests to Dr. E. Deltz, Department of General Surgery, University of Kiel, Hospitalstr. 40, Kiel, F.R.G.

0041-1345/83/1505-0155$01.00/0

a distinct anti-host reactivity remain 20 and 120 days postop.

Histologic examination of the lymphatic compartments of group 1 14 days after transplantation, when GVHR is at its climax, showed evidence of maximal immunologic stimulation within the T-dependent areas. Both paracortical areas of the mesenteric lymph nodes of the graft (Fig. 2), the peripheral lymph nodes of the recipients, and the periarteriolar sheaths of the spleen (Fig. 3) showed a high amount of immunoblasts and macrophages, thus expressing T-dependent immunologic stimulation. The same organs of the animals of group 2 examined 20 days after transplantation revealed a normal histologic picture (Figs. 4 and 5). The same findings could be shown 120 days posttransplant.

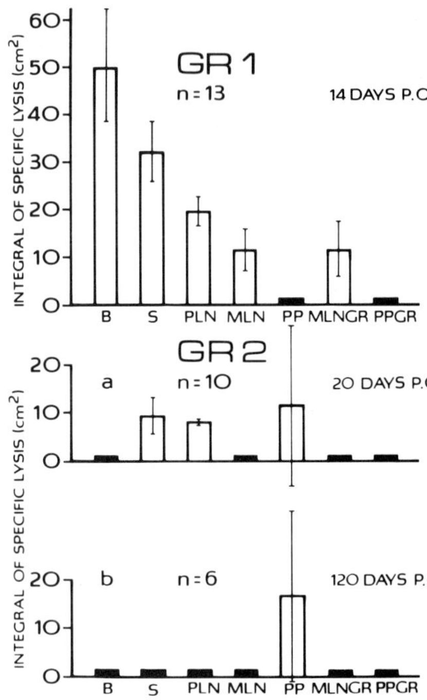

Fig. 1. Anti-host T-cell cytotoxicity within several lymphatic compartments (B, blood; S, spleen; PLN, peripheral lymph nodes; MLN, mesenteric lymph nodes; PP, Peyer's patches; GR, graft). Group 1 ($n = 13$) 14 days postop. Group 2 ($n = 10$) (A) 20 days postop, (B) 120 days postop (median ± standard error).

DISCUSSION

The considerable increase of survival rates of small bowel recipients after CsA treatment without clinical signs of GVHR disease is the most conspicuous feature of these experiments. Whereas untreated animals (group 1) die with severe GVHR disease within 22 days after small bowel transplantation, with death mainly caused by severe erosive enteritis of recipient's small bowel,[3] CsA-treated animals remain healthy more than 120 days after transplantation. Gross examination of these animals fails to show the typical damaged thin-walled small intestine of the recipients and the mesenteric lymph nodes of the graft, with the recipients' peripheral lymph nodes and spleen heavily enlarged by hyperplasia in the course of lymphatic stimulation. Histologic findings of the lymphatic compartments of both groups correspond to clinical outcome. The immunologic stimulation within the T-dependent areas by proliferation of immunoblasts and macrophages seen in the untreated animals at the time of GVHR is lacking after CsA treatment, at the GVH period as well as after 120 days.

In complete accordance with these morphological findings are the functional data representing GVHR. The most outstanding feature of the flourishing GVHR is the high anti-host cytotoxic activity in the blood of small bowel recipients, which decreases to zero with CsA treatment. Furthermore, there is an abrogation of anti-host activity in the lymphatic compartments (except the recipients' Peyer's patches) after CsA medication.

As the morphological pattern in the T-dependent areas of the graft, mesenteric lymph nodes, and the spleen of the recipients represents the immunologic stimulation of the immunocompetent cells of the graft against donor antigen and their continuing proliferation within the recipient, respectively, it can be concluded from the absence of these findings after CsA treatment that CsA is able of suppressing induction of anti-host-directed immunologic stimulation in GVHR following small bowel transplantation. Not only is the

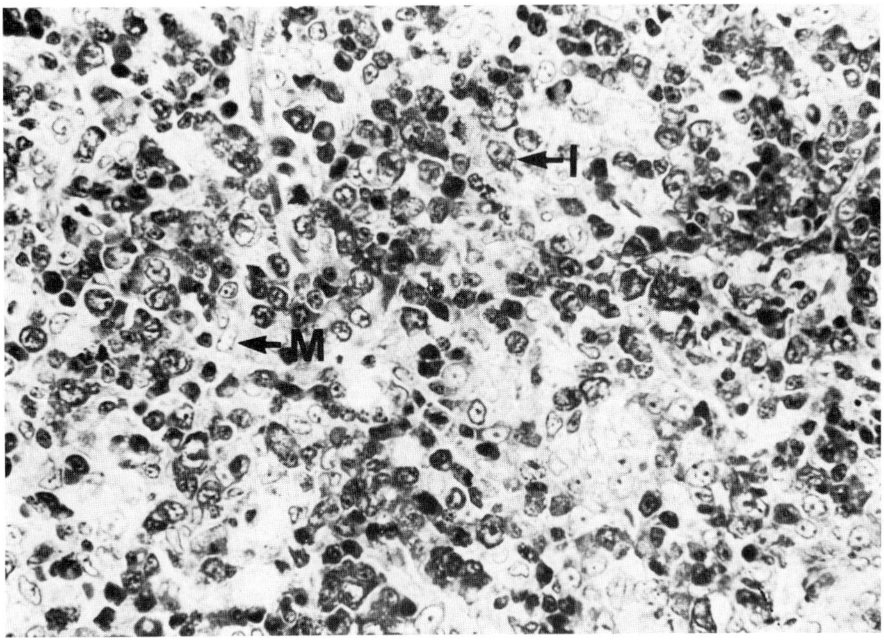

Fig. 2. Paracortical area of mesenteric lymph node (graft, group 1, 14 days postop) with immunologic stimulation by proliferation of immunoblasts (I) and macrophages (M) (400×).

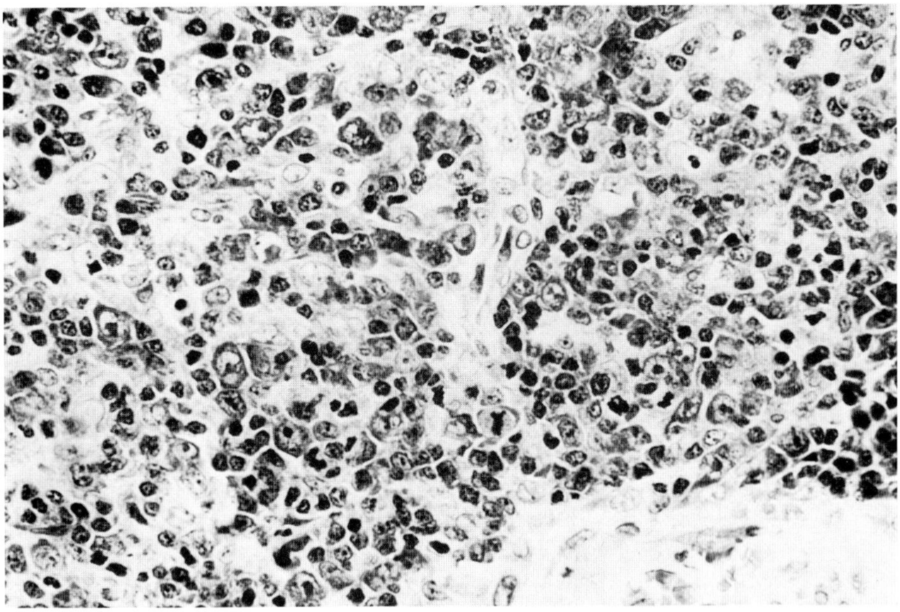

Fig. 3. Immunologic stimulation within the periarteriolar sheath of recipient's spleen (group 1, 14 days postop) (400×).

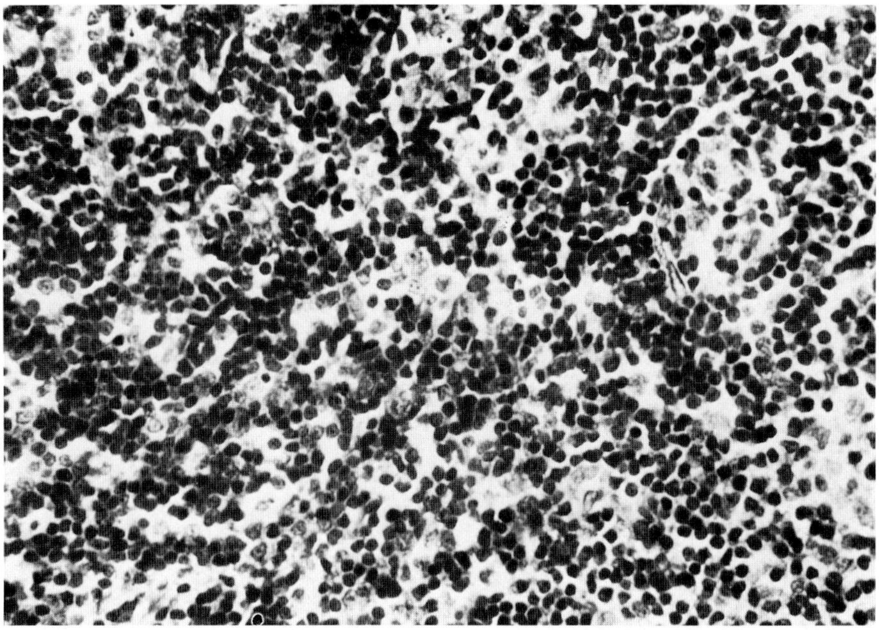

Fig. 4. Normal appearance of T-dependent areas of mesenteric lymphnodes (graft, group 2, 20 days postop) (×400).

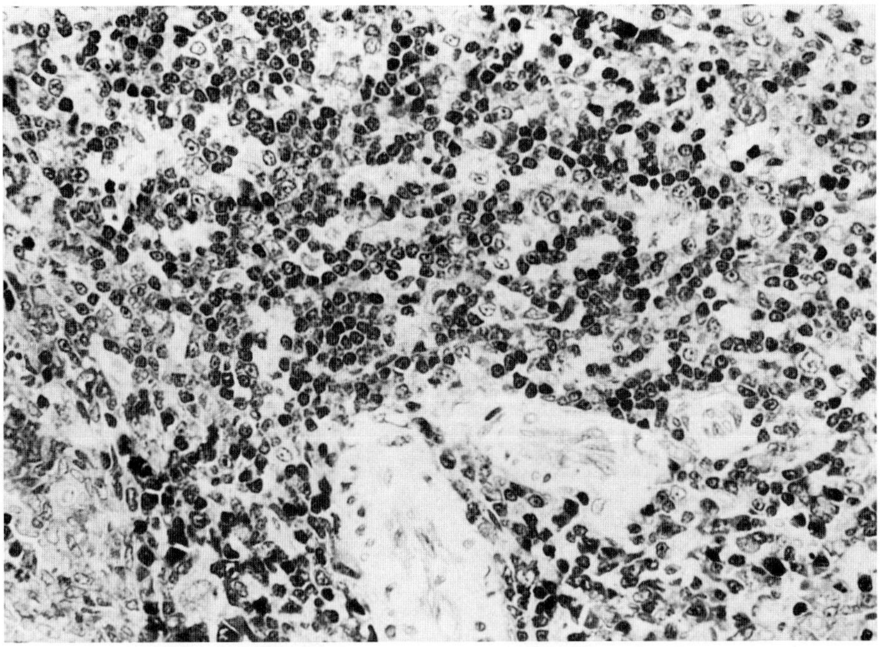

Fig. 5. Recipient's spleen (group 2, 20 days postop) (×400).

inductive phase of GVHR influenced by CsA, but so are the anti-host effector activities of T lymphocytes in the peripheral blood and the lymphatic compartments of graft and recipient, thus causing avoidance of GVHR and survival of the recipients, which show the analysis of functional parameters of MCA values after CsA treatment.

The prevention of GVHR by CsA has been demonstrated after bone marrow transplantation,[4] and there is evidence that CsA favors the early induction of cells that suppress the GVHR.[1] In our model, CsA suppresses both the inductive phase of the anti-host immune response (sensitization), as far as can be concluded from histologic pictures, and the effector phase of GVHR, which is revealed by functional investigations.

The decisive prerequisite for this GVHR suppressing effect is the administration of CsA immediately after small bowel transplantation in the sensitization period of GVHR. Once the development of GVHR has been hampered, CsA treatment can be ceased.

This temporary treatment of GVHR following small intestine transplantation makes it possible to keep the frequency of side effects, low and provides an indispensible condition for clinical small bowel transplantation.

REFERENCES

1. Borel JF: Heart Transplant 1:237, 1982

2. Bunjes D, Hardt C, Röllinghoff M, et al: Eur J Immunol 11:657, 1981

3. Deltz E: Habilitationsschrift. Kiel, FRG University of Kiel, 1981

4. Gluckman E, Arcese W, Devergie A, et al: Transplant Proc 13:368, 1981

5. Deltz E, Müller-Hermelink HK, Ulrichs K, et al: Transplant Proc 13:1215, 1981

6. Deltz E, Thiede A: Handbook of Microsurgery. Boca Raton, FL, CRC Press (in press)

7. Bröcker EB, Kuhlencordt KM, Müller-Ruchholtz W: Int Arch Allergy Appl Immunol 53:234, 1977

Uptake of ^{14}C-Glucose by the Transplanted Small Intestine

S. Nordgren, Z. Cohen, R. Mackenzie, D. Finkelstein, G. R. Greenberg, and B. Langer

WE HAVE previously reported a mean survival of 103 days after total small intestinal allotransplantation in the dog,[1] using cyclosporine (CsA) as an immunosuppressant. Allograft rejection was encountered in some of these dogs even after 200 days posttransplant and was associated with low plasma levels of CsA, which at that time was given orally to the dogs. Monitoring of the condition of the graft presents a problem in intestinal transplantation due to the relative inaccessibility of the graft. With the use of isolated pouches constructed from both ends of the transplant and sutured to the abdominal wall as mucous fistulae, we have investigated the course of histologic events in intestinal allograft rejection.[2]

The aim of the present investigation was to explore the intestinal transplant from a functional point of view, in order to develop a physiologic marker for rejection. Uptake of radiolabeled glucose from the proximal (jejunal) isolated pouch was investigated and correlated with the histologic findings in the distal (ileal) pouch in autotransplanted dogs and in allotransplanted dogs that were allowed to reject the grafts.

MATERIALS AND METHODS

Animals and Operative Technique

Outbred mongrel dogs were used. Total small intestinal transplantation was performed in 19 dogs. Autotransplantation was performed in 4 and allotransplantation in 15 dogs. The entire small intestine was resected on its vascular pedicle from the donor. The vascular bed of the graft was perfused with 1 liter of cold (+4°C) Ringer's lactate. The small intestine was resected from the recipient. Vascular anastomoses were performed between the superior mesenteric artery and the abdominal aorta, and between the superior mesenteric vein and the inferior vena cava. A 10-cm segment of the proximal end of the graft and a 5-cm segment of the distal end of the graft were isolated and closed in one end. The other end was brought through the abdominal wall and flat stomas were matured. End-to-end anastomoses were then performed between recipient duodenum and the proximal end of the graft and between the recipient terminal ileum and the distal end of the graft.

Immunosuppression

All allotransplanted dogs received cyclosporine, 7.5 mg/kg/day s.c., starting the day before transplantation for 14 days. At that time, the immunosuppression was discontinued, and the dogs were allowed to reject the allografts.

Measurement of ^{14}C-Glucose Uptake

A solution containing 2 μCi ^{14}C-glucose (13 μmole/liter) in isotonic saline was instilled into the proximal (jejunal) pouch. Blood samples were taken at 0, 5, 10, 15, 30, and 60 min after instillation of the isotope. Plasma radioactivity was determined in a liquid scintillation counter and reported as counts per minute (cpm). The test was performed at 7, 14, and 21 days after the transplantation in the autotransplants, and at 14, 21, and 28 days in surviving allotransplanted dogs.

Histologic Assessment

Biopsies were obtained from the distal (ileal) pouch when the ^{14}C-glucose uptake test was performed and daily from day 14 in allotransplanted dogs. The biopsies were mounted on filter paper, fixed in buffered formalin, and stained with hematoxylin and eosin. The diagnosis of rejection was based on the finding of blunted intestinal villi and the occurrence of an increased inflammatory infiltrate in the lamina propria and the submucosa.[2]

RESULTS

Survival

Autotransplants. All four autotransplanted dogs recovered well from the surgery

From the Departments of Surgery and Medicine, University of Toronto, Toronto, Ontario, Canada.

Supported in part by the Division of General Surgery, Toronto General Hospital, Toronto General Hospital Foundation, the PSI Foundation, Toronto, Canada, and the Greenmeadow Charitable Foundation.

Address reprint requests to Dr. Z. Cohen, Division of General Surgery, Toronto General Hospital, Eaton 9-211, 101 College Street, Toronto, Ontario, Canada, M5G 1L7.

0041-1345/83/1505-0156$01.00/0

and have remained well for 30–60 weeks. All four have exceeded their preoperative weight.

Allotransplants. Six allotransplanted dogs died at or before day 6 posttransplantation from surgical complications. Three allotransplanted dogs died at days 9–10 of an ill defined death with normal graft mucosa. These 9 dogs were not tested for ^{14}C-glucose uptake. The remaining 6 dogs all survived to day 14, when the immunosuppression was discontinued. These 6 dogs survived an additional 12 ± 4.5 days after day 14. All 6 died of rejection.

Uptake of ^{14}C-Glucose

Autotransplants. Eleven tests were performed in the autotransplanted dogs. One test was omitted for technical reasons. The graft histology was normal in all biopsies. Peak plasma radioactivity was noted after 5 min in 9 of the tests and after 10 min in 2 tests (Fig. 1). The average of the 11 individual peak values was 1304 ± 74 cpm (mean ± SE). The plasma radioactivity then decreased in a logarithmic fashion, with a half-life of approximately 45 min.

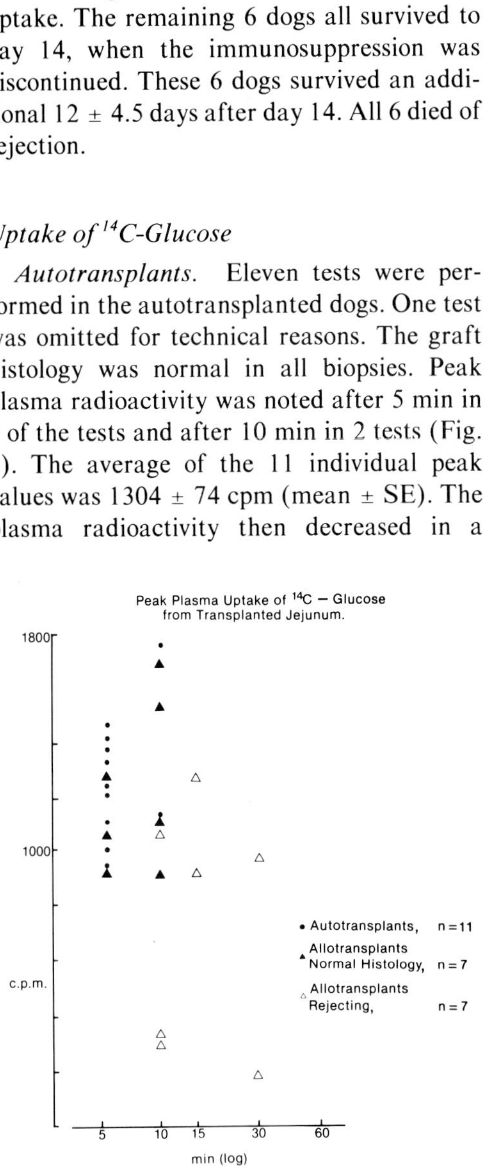

Fig. 1. Diagram showing the peak activity values in all ^{14}C-glucose uptake tests plotted against time. Note the delay in the appearance of the peak activity in allotransplanted dogs undergoing rejection.

Allotransplants. Seven tests were performed in allotransplanted dogs with normal histology in the mucosal biopsies. Peak plasma radioactivity was recorded in the 5-min sample in 3 tests and in the 10-min sample in 4 tests (Fig. 1). The average peak plasma activity was 1156 ± 101 cpm. This peak was not significantly different from the peak in the autotransplanted dogs. Seven tests were performed in allotransplanted dogs undergoing rejection as diagnosed from biopsies from the distal isolated pouch. Peak plasma activity in the dogs undergoing rejection was documented in the 10-min sample in 3 tests, in the 15-min sample in 2 tests, and in the 30-min sample in 2 tests. Mean peak plasma activity was 682 ± 175 cpm. This activity level is significantly lower than the average peak noted in the allotransplanted dogs with normal graft mucosa ($p < 0.01$).

DISCUSSION

The uptake of ^{14}C-glucose from an isolated segment of allotransplanted small intestine was investigated by Cohen et al.[3] in heterotopic cervical intestinal pouches. A good correlation to histology was documented, showing reduced uptake as rejection proceeded. Holmes et al.[4] performed a similar study on allografted small intestine transplanted as Thiry-Vella loops into the abdominal cavity. In the latter study, it was shown that the glucose uptake actually increased when the allograft was undergoing rejection, but it also increased when infection was noted in the Thiry-Vella loops. However, in the study by Holmes,[4] a high glucose concentration was used, allowing for a possible passive flux of glucose across the impaired mucosal barrier. In the present study, a low concentration of glucose was used and infection of the pouches was not seen. The use of a low glucose concentration does not rule out passive transport of glucose against the concentration gradient, but the results show a consistently low uptake of the isotope in dogs undergoing rejection. It

Table 1. ^{14}C-Glucose Uptake Index in Autotransplanted and Allotransplanted dogs

		Allotransplants	
	Autotransplants	Normal Mucosa	Rejecting
	195	186	118
	297	168	36
	214	147	6
	279	92	25
	187	246	85
	117	112	33
	288	212	60
	249		
	247		
	225		
	265		
Mean ± SD	233 ± 53	166 ± 54	51 ± 38
		$p < 0.01$	

is not known whether this decreased uptake is due to an impairment of the active mechanism for glucose absorption or a change in the regional mucosal blood flow. It is also possible that rejection causes decreased permeability for glucose through the mucosa. These aspects have not been investigated.

From the results it appears that both the uptake rate and the absolute uptake of ^{14}C-glucose is reduced in dogs undergoing rejection. We therefore suggest the use of an "uptake-index" as a mathematical expression for diagnosing rejection. This would be calculated as the ratio between the absolute uptake in cpm and the time point when the peak was recorded in minutes. This index represents the theoretical slope of the initial uptake of the isotope from the jejunal pouch. A reduced absolute uptake and a delay in the peak uptake would both reduce the numerical value of this uptake index. Uptake index was calculated for the ^{14}C-glucose uptake tests performed in this study (Table 1). From Table 1 it is found that uptake index in autotransplanted dogs and in allotransplanted dogs with normal histology was not significantly different. However, dogs undergoing rejection demonstrated a significantly lower uptake index. It is suggested that an uptake index below 100 is consistent with rejection.

In clinical intestinal transplantation, it will be useful to expose one part of the allograft to the abdominal wall for monitoring purposes.[5] As in other forms of organ transplantation, histologic monitoring of the graft integrity will probably constitute the most important means of monitoring. We propose that studying the uptake of radiolabeled glucose from the jejunal end of the transplant can be used as a physiologic test of graft integrity to help in the diagnosis of rejection.

REFERENCES

1. Craddock G, Nordgren S, Reznick R, et al: Transplantation 35:284, 1983
2. Lossing A, Nordgren S, Cohen Z, et al: Transplant Proc 4:643, 1982
3. Cohen WB, Hardy MA, Quint J, et al: Surgery 65:440, 1969
4. Holmes JT, Yeh SDJ, Winawer SJ, et al: Ann Surg 174:101, 1971
5. Fortner JG, Sichuk G, Litwin SD, et al: Transplantation 14:531, 1972

BONE MARROW

Studies on the Immunobiology of Syngeneic and Autologous Graft-Versus-Host Disease in Cyclosporine-Treated Rats

A. Glazier, P. J. Tutschka, and E. Farmer

LETHALLY irradiated rats reconstituted with allogeneic, syngeneic, or autologous bone marrow and treated with cyclosporine-A (CsA) develop clinical and pathologic lesions of graft-versus-host disease (GVHD) upon CsA withdrawal.[1,2] In this article, we describe a series of experiments designed to explore the immunobiology of this phenomenon.

MATERIALS AND METHODS

Rats

Lewis female $RT1^l$ and ACI female $RT1^a$ rats, 6–8 weeks of age, were purchased from Harlan Sprague Dawley, Inc.

Radiation

Lewis rats were irradiated on day −1 with 1020 rad at 120 rad/min from a ^{137}Cs small animal irradiator.

Marrow Transplantation

Donor marrow was suspended at 6×10^7 nucleated cells/ml in Hanks' solution supplemented with penicillin and streptomycin. On day 0, recipient rats received 1 ml i.v. via the tail vein.

Antibiotics

Rats received drinking water supplemented with Bactrim, neomycin, and polymixin-B. In addition, gentamicin, 2.5 mg/kg/day subcutaneously (s.c.), was given for 20 days. Rats that developed clinical infections were sacrificed and excluded from the study.

Assessment of GVHD

Rats were examined daily for signs of clinical GVHD, such as red ears, dermatitis, or diarrhea. Skin biopsies were taken at frequent intervals. When rats developed severe clinical GVHD characterized by weight loss, hunched appearance, and extensive dermatitis, they were sacrificed and autopsied.

RESULTS

GVHD in CsA-Treated Rats Following Allogeneic Marrow Transplantation

Lewis rats were transplanted with ACI bone marrow and treated with graded doses of CsA from day 0 to day +19. As shown in Table 1, 6/6 control rats not receiving CsA developed clinical and histologic GVHD by day 14. A CsA dose of 7.5 mg/kg/day suppressed clinical GVHD, and CsA at 15 mg/kg/day or above suppressed both clinical and histologic GVHD. By day 52, all CsA-treated rats developed clinical GVHD or had histologic changes of GVHD (Fig. 1).

GVHD in CsA-Treated Rats Following Syngeneic Transplantation

Lewis rats were lethally irradiated and transplanted with syngeneic marrow or mar-

---

From the Bone Marrow Transplantation Unit, Oncology Center, The Johns Hopkins University School of Medicine, Baltimore, MD.

Supported in part by NIH-NIADD Grant 1R01-AM 26502.

Address reprint requests to Dr. A. Glazier, Department of Pediatrics, Tufts New England Medical Center, 171 Harrison Avenue, Boston, MA 02111.

0041-1345/83/1505-0157$01.00/0

Table 1. Suppression of Acute Allogeneic Graft-Versus-Host Disease by Cyclosporine-A

CsA Dose mg/kg/Day × 20 Doses	Cumulative Fraction of Rats With Histologic GVHD Day 14	Day 30	Day 37	Day 52	Fraction Alive Day 150
0	6/6				0
2.5	6/6	6/6			0
7.5	3/6	3/6	6/6	6/6	0
15.0	0/7	2/7	7/7	7/7	2/7
25.0	0/9	0/9	8/8	8/8	5/9

Lewis rats were lethally irradiated, transplanted with ACI marrow cells, and treated with CsA from day 0 to +19.

row and spleen cells. CsA or control diluent was given for 40 days posttransplant. As shown in Table 2, GVHD did not develop in control rats not receiving CsA. In contrast, 66/70 rats treated with CsA at 7.5–25 mg/kg/day develop GVHD ($p < 0.001$). Normal Lewis spleen cells given at day 0 did not suppress the development of GVHD. Similarly normal thymic fragments (2 thymuses/rat) implanted in the peritoneal cavity on day 0 did not suppress the development of GVHD. The GVHD developed 7–40 days after CsA was stopped (Fig. 2).

Pathology of Syngeneic GVHD

Table 3 summarizes the pathologic changes observed in rats with syngeneic GVHD. The spectrum of tissue injury is strikingly similar

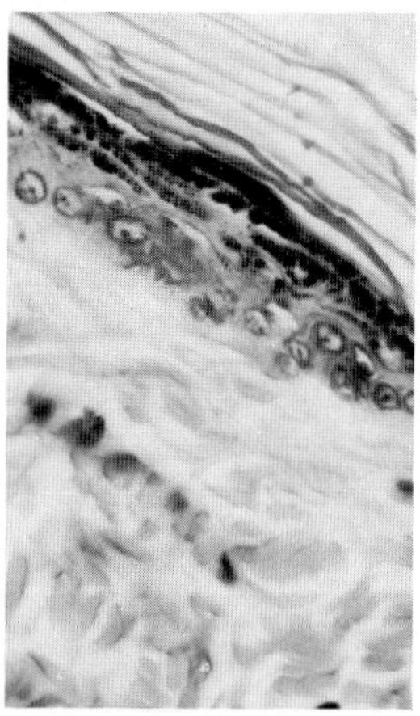

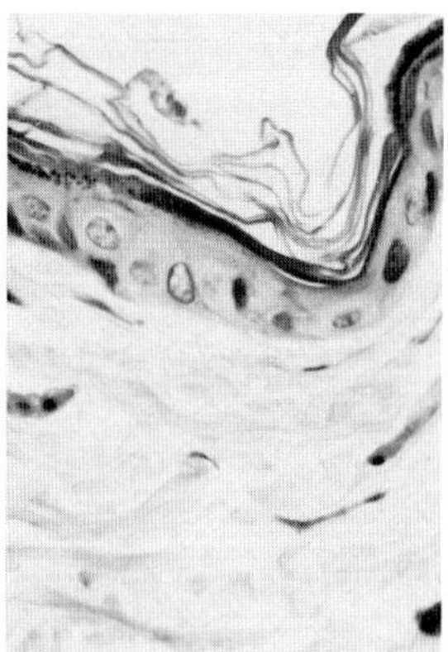

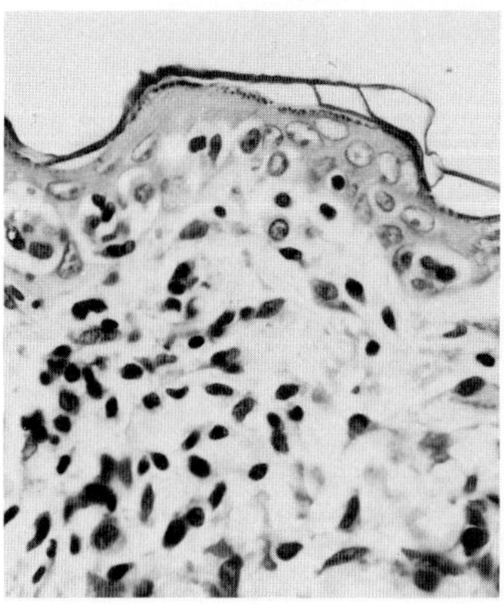

Fig. 1. Sequential skin biopsies are shown from a Lewis rat transplanted with ACI marrow and treated with 25 mg/kg/day of CsA for 20 days. No GVHD is seen at day 14 (left) or day 30 (center). At day 44 (right), contiguous grade II epidermal GVHD is present, accompanied by a mononuclear dermal infiltrate (310×).

Table 2. Syngeneic Graft-Versus-Host Disease

Cells Transplanted	CsA mg/kg/Day × 40 Days	Fraction With Grade II Histologic GVHD by Day 70
Marrow	0	0/6
Marrow + spleen	0	0/5
Marrow	7.5	15/16
Marrow + spleen	7.5	12/12
Marrow	15.0	13/16
Marrow + spleen	15.0	12/12
Marrow	25.0	8/8
Marrow + thymus	7.5	6/6

Lewis rats were lethally irradiated with 1020 rad on day −1. On day 0, the rats were transplanted with 6×10^7 syngeneic Lewis marrow cells and 10^8 syngeneic Lewis spleen cells, as indicated above. The rats received CsA or control diluent from day 0 to day 40. One group received normal Lewis thymus fragments intraperitoneally on day 0.

to that seen in allogeneic rat radiation chimeras. Dramatic histologic changes are observed in the thymuses of syngeneic chimeras treated with CsA (see Figs. 3, 4, 5). While receiving CsA, prior to the development of GVHD, distinct medullary regions are virtually absent. A near uniform cellularity, similar to normal cortex, is present throughout the entire thymus. Upon the discontinuation of CsA, a medullary configuration reappears. With the onset of syngeneic GVHD, there is a variable degree of thymic atrophy and lymphoid hypoplasia.

Autologous GVHD

Lewis rats were irradiated with 1020 rad, with the right tibia shielded with a lead donut. Four of four CsA-treated rats developed clinical and histologic GVHD. No GVHD was seen in seven untreated leg-shielded rats (Fig. 6) ($p < 0.05$).

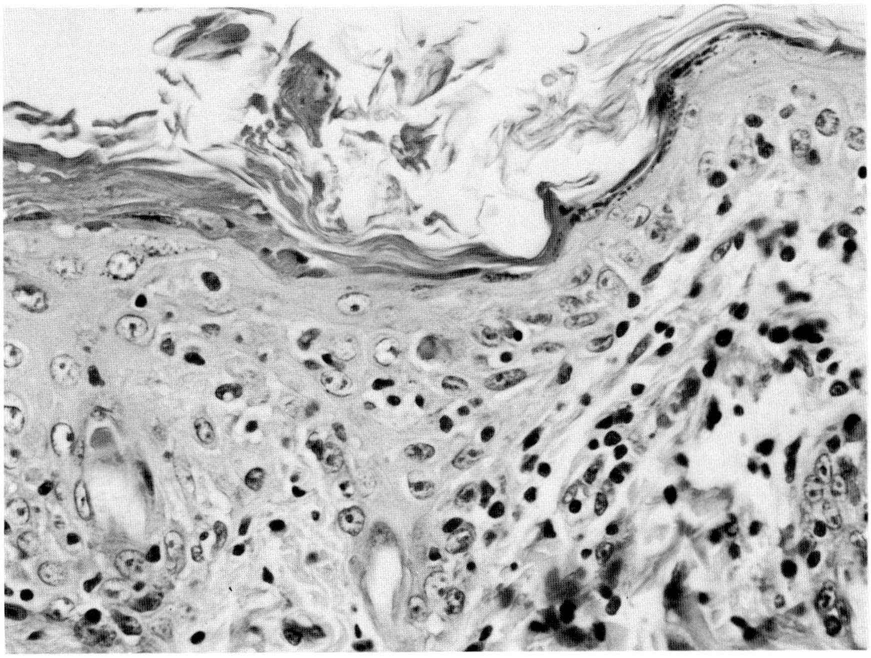

Fig. 2. Skin from syngeneic radiation chimera treated with CsA 7.5 mg/kg/day for 40 days, on day 52. Note extensive mononuclear dermal and epidermal infiltrate, with destruction of epidermal cells (240×).

Adoptive Transfer of Autologous and Syngeneic GVHD

As shown in Table 4, both syngeneic and autologous GVHD may be adoptively transferred to irradiated syngeneic recipients. Syngeneic GVHD may not be adoptively transferred to normal unirradiated recipients. Addition of 10^8 normal syngeneic spleen cells at the time of adoptive transfer did not suppress the appearance of GVHD (data not shown).

Effects of CsA in Normal Rats

Normal rats treated with CsA at doses from 7.5 mg/kg/day to 100 mg/kg/day do not develop GVHD upon CsA withdrawal. It thus appears that radiation plays an important role in the pathogenesis of autologous and syngeneic GVHD. Normal rats treated with CsA develop thymic changes similar to those described in CsA-treated syngeneic chimeras. CsA causes a rapid depletion of medullary thymocytes. With continued administration of CsA, steroid-sensitive small thymocytes repopulate the medullary region. After 2 weeks of CsA at 50 mg/kg/day, distinct medullary regions are absent in most lobules. Following the discontinuation of CsA, medullary regions rapidly reform, and normal thymic architecture is restored within 10 days.

Table 3. Pathologic Changes in Rats With Syngeneic GVHD

Organ	Pathological Changes
Tongue	Submucosal mononuclear infiltrate with lymphocytic exocytosis vacuolization and destruction of epithelium (2+ acute GVHD), myositis
Skin	Lymphocytic exocytosis into epidermis, epidermal destruction with vacuolar changes of basal layer and dyskeratotic cells (2+ acute GVHD)
	Follicular lymphocytic infiltrate and destruction
Esophagus	Lymphocytic infiltration of mucosa
Liver	Mononuclear infiltrate in portal triads
Thymus	Gross thymic atrophy with variable cortical and medullary hypocellularity
Spleen	Depletion of periarteriolar sheath
Lymph nodes	Decreased lymphoid cellularity, depletion of follicles, accumulation of lymphoblasts
Kidney	Focal mononuclear perivascular or peritubular infiltrates
Marrow	Normal cellularity, hypocellularity, myelofibrosis (rare)
Heart	No pathologic changes
Salivary glands	Mononuclear interstitial infiltrate

Absence of Syngeneic GVHD in Thymic-Shielded CsA-Treated Chimeras

Four Lewis rats were given 1020 rad of radiation with the thymus shielded, transplanted with Lewis marrow, and treated with CsA at 7.5 mg/kg/day for 40 days. Detailed autopsies failed to reveal GVHD. This result contrasts strikingly with the consistent development of GVHD seen in similarly treated rats given total body irradiation (Table 3) (Figs. 2 and 3).

DISCUSSION

The data presented demonstrate the consistent development of GVHD in lethally irradiated CsA-treated rats following allogeneic, syngeneic, and autologous bone marrow reconstitution. Normal spleen cells at doses as high as 10^8 cells/rat failed to suppress the development and adoptive transfer of syngeneic GVHD. Thymic fragments implanted in the peritoneal cavity also failed to prevent the development of syngeneic GVHD, while shielding of the thymus during pretransplant irradiation prevented GVHD in 4/4 rats.

The existence of autologous GVHD indicates that histocompatibility differences are not absolutely necessary for the development of GVHD. The mechanisms by which self-tolerance develops following bone marrow transplantation is enigmatic.

CsA is a potent inhibitor of T-cell growth factor (TCGF) production and inhibits the development of responsiveness to TCGF.[3–5]

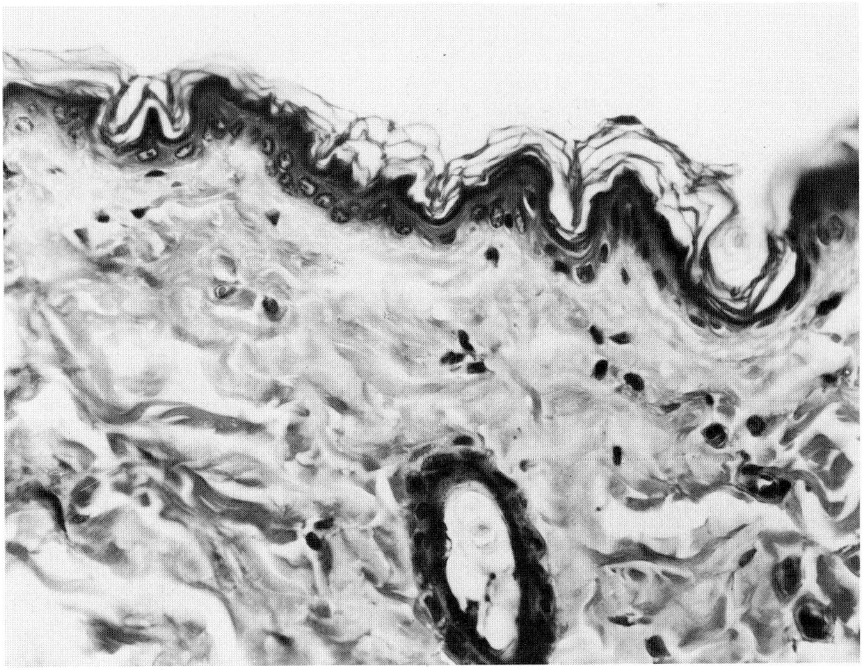

Fig. 3. Skin from thymus-shielded syngeneic chimera treated with CsA, 7.5 mg/kg/day for 40 days, on day 70. Note absence of GVHD.

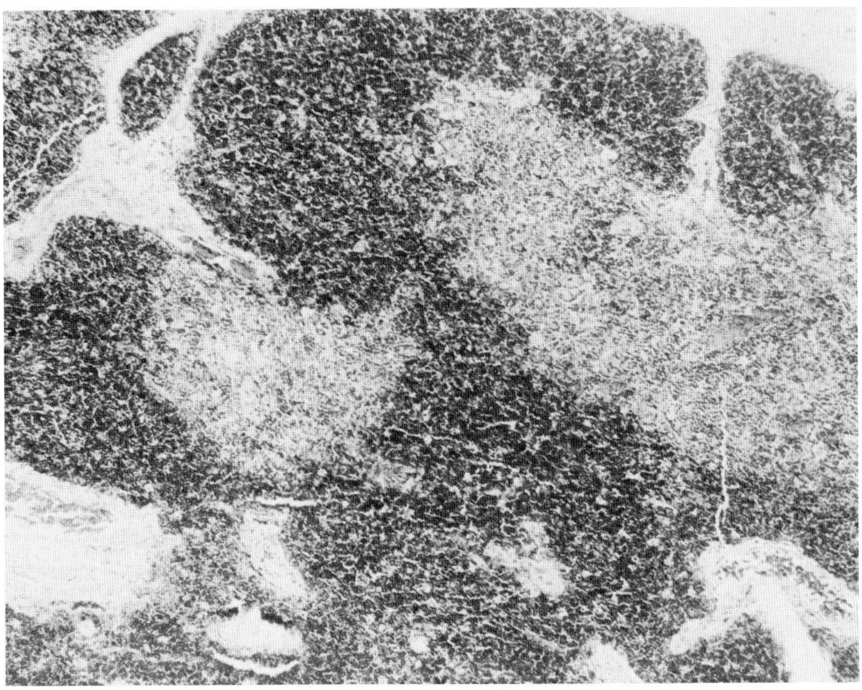

Fig. 4. Thymus from syngeneic chimera not treated with CsA. Note prominent medulla (60×).

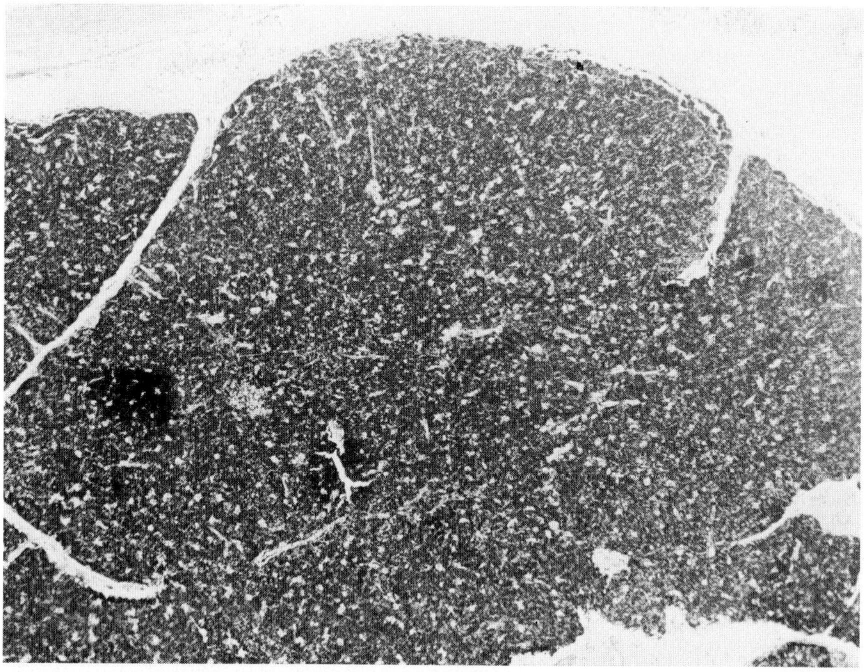

Fig. 5. Thymus from syngeneic Lewis chimera treated with CsA, 7.5 mg/kg/day for 38 days, on day 38. Note normal cortical cellularity and absence of normal medulla (×60).

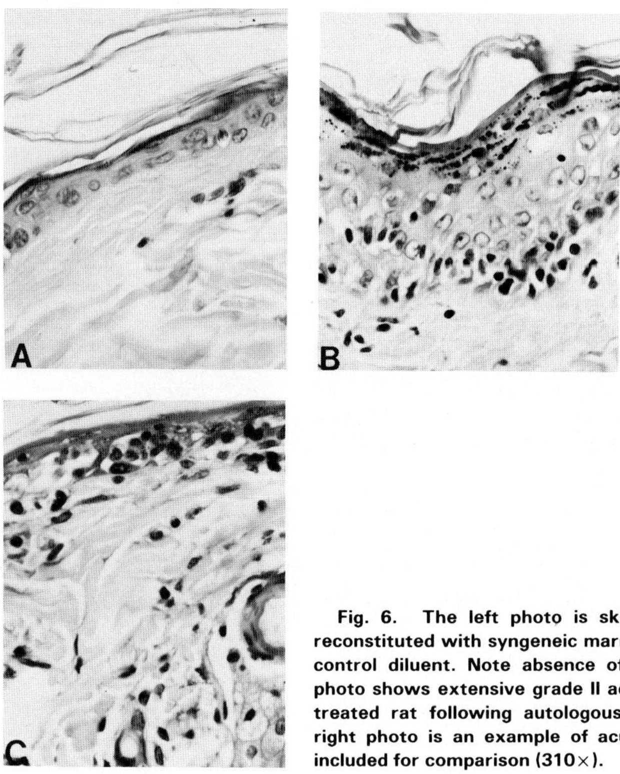

Fig. 6. The left photo is skin from a Lewis rat reconstituted with syngeneic marrow and treated with control diluent. Note absence of GVHD. The center photo shows extensive grade II acute GVHD in a CsA-treated rat following autologous reconstitution. The right photo is an example of acute allogeneic GVHD included for comparison (310×).

Table 4. The Adoptive Transfer of Syngeneic and Autologous GVHD

Pretreatment of Secondary Recipient	Fraction of Secondary Recipients With GVHD
No radiation	0/5
420 rad	2/2
1020 rad	12/13
1020 rad*	4/4

10^8 spleen cells from CsA-treated rats with syngeneic GVHD or autologous GVHD* were transferred along with 6×10^7 syngeneic Lewis marrow cells. Data pooled from four independent experiments ($p < 0.005$).

CsA does not significantly impair thymic cortical cellularity or interfere with cortical regeneration following syngeneic marrow transplantation. This suggests that the production and response to TCGF is not critical for the maturation and proliferation of most thymocytes within the thymic cortex. This is supported by the inability of cortical thymocytes to generate cytotoxic T-cell activity unless exogenous TCGF is added.[6,7] The nature of the interactions between thymic epithelium and cortical thymocytes remains unknown. It is likely that thymocytes with high affinity for thymic antigens are functionally deleted.[7] This may represent an important initial step in the development of self-tolerance. Thymocytes that survive passage through the thymic cortex, enter the thymic medulla. The marked sensitivity of medullary thymocytes to CsA suggests that the production and response to TCGF is a key event in the thymic medulla. This is supported by the localization of IA+ dendritic cells within the thymic medulla and the ability of medullary thymocytes to proliferate and generate cytotoxic T-cell activity in the absence of exogenous TCGF.[8–11] The thymic medulla may thus represent a physiologic "autologous mixed lymphocyte reaction." Both suppressor and autoreactive cytotoxic cells may arise in vitro in autologous MLRs.[12–14] The majority of thymocytes that migrate from the thymus have characteristics of medullary thymocytes.[15–16] The medullary thymic reaction may thus represent a key regulatory site in the restriction of the T-cell repertoire and the generation of self-tolerance. The mechanisms by which CsA facilitates the development of GVHD are unknown. Inhibition of the medullary thymocyte "autologous mixed lymphocyte reaction" by CsA may be important.

Regardless of the underlying mechanisms, the data presented in this article demonstrate the consistent reproducible development of classic graft-versus-host disease in CsA-treated rats following allogeneic, syngeneic, and even autologous marrow reconstitution. This necessitates a reevaluation of the biology of GVHD, its prevention, and the mechanisms of self-tolerance.

ACKNOWLEDGMENT

This paper is dedicated to the memory of Gerald Glazier, a brother, a friend, and research colleague who had contributed so much.

REFERENCES

1. Glazier A, Farmer E, Tutschka PJ, et al: J Exp Med 158:1, 1983
2. Glazier A, Tutschka PJ, Beschorner WE, et al: Exp Hematol 10:38, 1982
3. Larsson EL: J Immunol 124:2828, 1980
4. Palacior R, Moller G: Nature 290:793, 1981
5. Hess AD, Tutschka PJ, Santos GW: J Immunol 128:355, 1982
6. Wagner H, Harot C, Klaus H, et al: Immunol Rev 51:215, 1980
7. Kruisbeek AM, Hodes RJ, Singer A: J Exp Med 153:13, 1981
8. Barclay AN, Mayrhofer G: J Exp Med 153:1666, 1981
9. Wagner H, Harris AW, Feldman M: Cell Immunol 4:39, 1971
10. Kruisbeek AM, Sisistra JJ, Urose TJM: J Immunol 125:995, 1980
11. Mosier DE, Cantor H: Eur J Immunol 1:459, 1971
12. Kunkel HG, Halper JP, Weksier ME: J Exp Med 146:1809, 1977
13. Tsuyoshi S, Green I: J Immunol 123:584, 1979
14. Makoto G, Zvaifer NJ: J Exp Med 157:1309
15. Scollay R, Chen WF, Mitchell G: *In*: In Vivo Immunology. New York, Plenum, 1981, p 269
16. Scollay R, Jacobs S, Jerabek L, et al: J Immunol 124:2845, 1980

Suppressor and Cytotoxic Cells in DLA Nonidentical Canine Radiation Chimeras Given Cyclosporine and Methotrexate as Prophylaxis for Graft-Versus-Host Disease

H. J. Deeg, R. F. Raff, E. Severns, F. R. Appelbaum, E. D. Thomas, and R. Storb

GRAFT-versus-host disease (GVHD) following allogeneic marrow transplantation is due to histocompatibility differences between donor and recipient. Although the mechanisms involved may differ, dependent on whether major or minor histocompatibility differences exist, it is generally accepted that T lymphocytes of donor origin contained in the marrow inoculum recognize non-self antigens on host cells, in response to which they proliferate and attack host targets.[1,2] This graft-versus-host reaction may be self-limited or progress to the clinical manifestations of GVHD. The administration of immunosuppressive agents, such as cyclophosphamide, methotrexate (MTX), antilymphocyte globulin, or cyclosporine (CsA), can prevent or modify the course of GVHD in various models.[3] We have used extensively a canine model to examine mechanisms of GVHD and the development of tolerance.[4] In the present study we investigated in vitro functions of chimera lymphocytes (i.e., cells of donor origin) obtained from dogs given marrow grafts from DLA nonidentical unrelated or littermate donors and treated with a combination of MTX and CsA after transplantation.

From the Fred Hutchinson Cancer Research Center and the University of Washington School of Medicine, Seattle, WA.

Supported in part by Grants CA 31787, CA 28941, CA 18221, CA 18105, CA 30924, and CA 15704 awarded by the National Cancer Institute, DHHS. E.D.T. is the recipient of Research Career Award AI 02425 from the National Institute of Allergy and Infectious Diseases.

Address reprint requests to Dr. H. J. Deeg, Fred Hutchinson Cancer Research Center, 1124 Columbia Street, Seattle, WA 98104.

0041-1345/83/1505-0158$01.00/0

MATERIALS AND METHODS

Details of the procedures used have been presented elsewhere.[5,6] Briefly, dogs of various breeds were obtained from commercial kennels. They were 7–15 (median 8.5) months old at the time of transplantation. Typing for erythrocyte antigens and the antigens of the major histocompatibility complex, DLA, as determined by serologic typing, mixed leukocyte culture (MLC), and cell-mediated lympholysis (CML) assays, were carried out as described. Littermate pairs were chosen as follows. In all instances, donor and recipient shared one DLA haplotype. The donor was either homozygous for this haplotype (AA), and the recipient heterozygous (AB), or both donor (AB) and recipient (AC) were heterozygous.[7] Unrelated pairs were selected on the basis of nonidentity for DLA-A, B, and C; lymphocytes of donor and recipient were mutually reactive in MLC and generated cytotoxic effector cells against each other in CML. Before transplantation, 150–200 $\times$ 10^6 lymphocytes (host lymphocytes) from each recipient were cryopreserved for postgrafting studies. Total body irradiation (TBI) and marrow transplantation were carried out as described.[6] Recipients were given 9 Gy of TBI delivered at 7 cGy/min from 2 opposing ^{60}Co sources. Within 4 hr of TBI, recipients were given 1–13 (median 3.2) $\times$ 10^8 marrow cells/kg and, on days 1 and 2, 3–26 (median 12) $\times$ 10^8 viable buffy coat cells/kg from the donor. Postgrafting immunosuppression consisted of MTX, 0.4 mg/kg, given i.v. on days 1, 3, 6, and 11 and CsA, 15 mg/kg/day, given i.m. on days 0–7 and then orally until day 25. The CsA dose was decreased to 10 mg/kg/day on day 26 and to 5 mg/kg/day on day 51. From day 76 to day 100, CsA, 5 mg/kg, was given every other day.

Postgrafting care and methods for assessment of marrow engraftment have been described.[6] At monthly intervals, until day 100, and less frequently thereafter, MLCs with lymphocytes from donor, chimera, host, and unrelated controls were carried out.[5,7] Suppressor cell assays were carried out as described.[5] Briefly, peripheral blood mononuclear cells from the chimera were added at ratios of 1:1 to 0.2:1 to donor cells to examine their potential suppressive effect on donor cells in MLC against host or control lymphocytes. Chimera cells were either unfractionated peripheral blood mononuclear cells or nylon-wool-adherent or nonadherent cells. In some experiments, chimera cells that had been irradiated with 2000 rad were used. CML assays involving cells from donor, chimera, and control dogs as effectors, and lymphocytes from donor, chimera, host, and control as targets, were carried out at irregular intervals following transplantation, as described.

RESULTS AND DISCUSSION

DLA Haploidentical Littermate Chimeras

All 10 dogs had sustained engraftment. One dog died on day 57 from bronchopneumonia, one on day 107 with GVHD, and one on day 204 with a convulsion. Seven dogs are surviving 240–523 days after transplantation. Five are well and two have chronic GVHD. These results are superior to those obtained previously with MTX as the only postgrafting immunosuppressive agent.[8] In those studies, only 10% of the dogs became long-term survivors. All dogs with delayed GVHD died within 275 days.[7,9] The reason for prolonged survival with GVHD in the present study is unknown, but it is conceivable that a different mechanism of graft–host interaction induced by CsA is responsible.

Chimera cells obtained from dogs without GVHD were generally unresponsive in MLC to host cells, although in two dogs, there was a transient rise of the stimulation index following discontinuation of immunosuppression after day 100. In 3 dogs that developed GVHD, the proliferative response of chimera lymphocytes to stimulation by host cells increased concurrently with the clinical development of GVHD (Table 1A). These findings are in agreement with the results obtained previously in DLA haploidentical littermate chimeras treated with MTX alone after transplantation.[7]

In order to further elucidate the mechanism involved in unresponsiveness of chimera cells against host cells, we searched for the presence of suppressor cells in the chimera. Following the in vitro observation that lymphocytes primed by allogeneic stimulators in the presence of CsA could be fractionated over nylon-wool columns into adherent cells with the functional properties of suppressor cells and nonadherent cells without suppressor activity,[10] we studied nylon-wool-fractionated chimera peripheral blood lymphocytes for their suppressive effect when added to donor lymphocytes in MLC.[5] While unfractionated cells were moderately effective, nylon-wool-adherent cells caused profound suppression. During the first 100–150 days after grafting, suppression by cells from chimeras both with and without GVHD was nonspecific. Subsequently, suppression by cells from chimeras without GVHD was host specific and was most pronounced 200–300 days after transplantation, reaching peaks of suppression of 47% and 66% for unfractionated and nylon-wool-adherent cells, respectively. After day 300, chimera adherent cells were no longer suppressive. Cells from three dogs with GVHD showed slight nonspecific suppression during the entire period of observation. Suppression was not significantly affected by irradiation with 2000 rad. These results are in contrast to those obtained with cells from MTX-treated chimeras in whom we found no evidence for suppressor cells.[7] On the other hand, these results are quite similar to those obtained with spleen cells in a rat model.[11,12] After initial nonspecific suppression, a host-specific suppression was observed for about 1 year after transplantation. The subsequent disappearance of suppression was explained on the basis of clonal reduction of the suppressor cells. It is conceivable that a similar mechanism, possibly related to the use of CsA, may be operative in the present model. In the present model, however, removal of nylon-wool-adherent suppressor cells from chimera cells did not result in a nonadherent population that was able to respond to host cells. Since nonadherent cells did not have suppressor activity, it appears unlikely that unresponsiveness of these cells was due to remaining suppressor cells. Rather, it suggests that, consistent with our earlier findings, clonal deletion had taken place.[13] This might have been mediated by suppressor cells directed at the host reactive clone.

Results in CML assays were as predicted from previous studies. Chimera lymphocytes, regardless of whether or not the dog suffered from GVHD, failed to produce cytotoxic effector cells against host targets or unrelated targets from animals homozygous for one of the host's DLA haplotypes. However, chimera cells showed vigorous cytotoxicity, comparable to that of donor cells against targets from third-party donors that are histoincompatible with donor or host. These results suggest a restriction of the cytotoxic unresponsiveness by the major histocompatibility complex, presumably DLA-D.

DLA Nonidentical Unrelated Chimeras

All 9 dogs had sustained engraftment.[6] Six dogs developed GVHD 77–220 days after grafting, and 4 of these died. Two are surviving with chronic GVHD 790 and 949 days after transplantation. One dog without GVHD died on day 157 from a convulsion. Two dogs are well without GHVD 663 and 928 days after transplantation.

Although in vitro studies were carried out in parallel to those described for DLA haploidentical littermates, results were more complex. In MLC, lymphocytes not only from dogs *without,* but also from dogs *with,* clinical GVHD, were generally unresponsive to stimulation by host cells, i.e., there was no correlation of MLC reactivity and GVHD (Table 1B). It is of interest in this context that, in suppressor cell assays, the proliferative response of donor cells to host lymphocytes was suppressed by chimera cells regardless of whether the chimera did or did not have GVHD. Furthermore, in the small number of dogs that could be studied, suppression was nonspecific[14] and no clear pattern over time was apparent. Additional studies will be necessary in order to characterize the events involved.

In CML assays, cells from chimeras both with and without GVHD failed to generate cytotoxic effector cells against host targets.[15] Moreover, chimera cells were unable to generate cytotoxic effectors against histoincompatible third-party targets.[16] The mechanisms underlying this generalized unresponsiveness are unclear. Conceivably, a lack of helper cells, helper factor, or defective interaction between different functional subsets of cells might be responsible.[15–17] However, the failure to restore cytotoxicity by the addition of supernatants from primary MLCs with donor cells or small numbers of donor cells to chimera cells argues against this possibility.

In conclusion, our results are consistent with previous findings in DLA nonidentical littermate chimeras that tolerance was mediated by clonal abortion. The data in unrelated chimeras, however, are more complex. The observation of a generalized inabil-

Table 1. Reactivity of Chimera Cells in MLC*

Clinical Status	Responding Cells	Stimulating Cells (cpm)			
		Chimera x	Donor x	Host x	Control x
(A) DLA haploidentical littermate chimera (dog B869)					
Well	Chimera	609	710 (1.1)	597 (1)	15,824 (26)
(day 120)	Donor	1,724 (0.9)	1,941	11,327 (5.8)	9,826 (5.1)
GVHD	Chimera	255	500 (1.9)	1,976 (7.8)	21,516 (84)
(day 218)	Donor	140 (0.6)	235	26,678 (113)	16,717 (71)
(B) DLA nonidentical unrelated chimera (dog B778)					
Well					
(day 103)	Chimera	748	362 (0.5)	261 (0.4)	5,588 (7.5)
	Donor	582 (0.9)	644	2,936 (4.6)	5,417 (8.4)
GVHD	Chimera	375	504 (1.3)	525 (1.4)	8,530 (22)
(day 141)	Donor	549 (0.9)	597	10,370 (17)	15,790 (26)

*10^5 responder and 10^5 irradiated (2000 R) stimulator cells (peripheral blood mononuclear cells, unfractionated). Shown are median cpms (stimulation index).

ity of cells from completely allogeneic chimeras to generate cytotoxic effector cells is intriguing. This may be related to the lack of sharing one haplotype between donor and recipient. Although evidence for suppressor cells was found in all chimeras, their role in vivo remains to be determined.[18] It is possible that they might be involved, at least in haploidentical littermates, in mediating clonal abortion.

REFERENCES

1. Grebe SC, Streilein JW: Adv Immunol 22:119, 1976

2. Tsoi M-S, Storb R, Thomas ED: In RP Gale (ed): Recent Advances in Bone Marrow Transplantation, UCLA Symposia on Molecular and Cellular Biology. New York, Alan R. Liss, 1983, p 291–312

3. Storb R, Thomas ED: Immunol Rev 71:77, 1983

4. Deeg HJ, Storb R, Thomas ED: In RP Gale (ed): Recent Advances in Bone Marrow Transplantation, UCLA Symposia on Molecular and Cellular Biology. New York, Alan R. Liss, 1983, p 527–546

5. Deeg HJ, Storb R, Raff RF, et al: In Baum SJ, Ledney GD, Thierfelder S (eds): Experimental Hematology Today, Basel, Karger, 1982, pp 127–133

6. Deeg HJ, Storb R, Weiden PL, et al: Transplantation 34:30, 1982

7. Atkinson K, Storb R, Weiden PL, et al: J Immunol 124:1808, 1980

8. Storb R, Kolb HJ, Graham TC, et al: Eur J Clin Biol Res 17:680, 1972

9. Atkinson K, Shulman HM, Deeg HJ, et al: Am J Pathol 108:196, 1982

10. Hess AD, Tutschka PJ, Santos GW: J Immunol 126:961, 1981

11. Tutschka PJ, Hess AD, Beschorner WE, et al: Transplantation 32:203, 1981

12. Tutschka PJ, Ki PF, Beschorner WE, et al: Transplantation 32:321, 1981

13. Nossal GJV, Pikc BL: Proc Natl Acad Sci USA 78:3844, 1981

14. King DP, Strober S, Kaplan HS: J Immunol 126:1140, 1981

15. Waterfield JD, King ID, Dutton RW: Immunology 47:219, 1983

16. Duprez V, Hamilton B, Burakoff SJ: J Exp Med 156:844, 1982

17. Mori T, Tsoi M-S, Gillis S, et al: J Immunol 130:712, 1983

18. Hilgert I: Immunol Rev 46:27, 1979

The Effect of Cyclosporine on Host-Versus-Graft Disease in Canine Bone Marrow Transplantation

A. M. Miller, E. P. Walma, W. Klapwijk, and D. W. Van Bekkum

CYCLOSPORINE-A (CsA) is a fungal metabolite that has been shown to be a potent immunosuppressant.[1] Animal studies have shown the drug to be effective in preventing graft-versus-host disease (GVHD) following histoincompatible marrow grafts.[2] Deeg et al. have shown that CsA is capable of inducing graft–host tolerance across minor (non-DLA) histocompatible barriers, but not across major (DLA) histocompatible barriers in canines.[3]

The present studies were conducted to further explore the role of CsA in reducing the conditioning regimen necessary to allow successful bone marrow transplantation in DLA-identical canines receiving stem cell grafts. This would allow a reduction in the morbidity associated with the conditioning regimen itself. Experiments were also performed in DLA one-haplotype mismatched canines. Although successful bone marrow transplantation has been achieved with HLA one-haplotype mismatched donors, the success rate is low, and the incidence of GVHD is high. The current studies utilized CsA to determine its role in abrogating the host-versus-graft disease (HVGD) across the one-haplotype mismatched barrier. In addition, stem cell grafts were used to reduce the incidence of GVHD.

MATERIALS AND METHODS

Dogs

Recipients of bone marrow cells were beagles of either sex purchased from the Central Breeding Colony for Experimental Animals of TNO, Zeist, The Netherlands. Their weight ranged from 7.5 to 15.5 kg. The dogs ranged in age from 6 months to 5 years. They were vaccinated against hepatitis, distemper, and leptospirosis.

Bone marrow cell donors were beagles from the same source or mongrels obtained from licensed dog handlers.

Genetics

The major histocompatibility complex of the dog (DLA) was analyzed for serologically defined and lymphocyte-defined determinants, as outlined in the Joint Report on Canine Immunogenetics.[4] DLA-identical combinations were always serologically identical, as well as negative in reciprocal unilateral mixed lymphocyte cultures. DLA one-haplotype mismatched donors were related dogs obtained from the same source.

Total Body Irradiation (TBI)

Dosimetry and biologic response to the radiation protocol were as described by Vriesendorp et al.[5] Two opposing Philips-Muller x-ray machines were used. Physical parameters were 300 kV, 10 mA HVL, 3.0 mm Cu and dose rate 0.16 Gy/min. During irradiation, animals were confined via a closed fitting aerated wooden box. Anesthesia was not used. The LD_{50} for the gastrointestinal syndrome and the bone marrow syndrome for a single treatment in this radiation protocol has been previously determined to be 8.5 and 3.7 Gy, respectively.[6]

Cyclosporine-A (CsA)

The cyclosporine-A was kindly supplied by Dr. J. F. Borel, Sandoz Limited, Basel, Switzerland. The CsA was dissolved in olive oil and administered orally daily in a single dose of 15 mg · kg^{-1}. CsA levels were measured utilizing a radioimmunoassay kit supplied by Sandoz Limited, Basel, Switzerland (OL 27-400).

Preparing Dogs for TBI

Prior to irradiation, the oral cavity of each dog was inspected and dental calculus was removed. Pretreatment stool cultures were performed, and animals with parasites were treated with oral Piperazine adipate (300 mg orally) or Dichlorvos (472 mg orally). Dogs whose feces contained Pseudomonas were given a prophylactic course of oral colistin or polymyxin-B (20 mg · kg^{-1}/day × 5). Pretreatment hematologic and biochemical studies were also performed. On the day before irradiation, the sensitivity of aerobic fecal microorganisms to eight antimicrobial agents was determined.

From the Radiobiological Institute TNO, Rijswijk, The Netherlands.

Address reprint requests to Dr. A. M. Miller, Radiobiological Institute TNO, Lange Klerweg 151, 2280 HV Rijswijk, The Netherlands.

0041-1345/83/1505-0159$01.00/0

Animals were housed in individual cages and received autoclaved commercial dry food supplemented with vitamins. Acidified tap water was provided daily (pH 3 to prevent the growth of Pseudomonas). Daily input and output records were maintained. The dogs received no food for 1 day prior to and 1 day following irradiation.

Bone Marrow Transplantation

The marrow cavities of the long bones of the donors were aspirated aseptically under general anesthesia. Two to four milliliters were removed and transferred to a bottle containing 10 ml of Hanks' Balanced Salt Solution, to which 1500 IU preservative-free heparin (Thromboliquine, Organon) and a trace of DNAse I (Calbiochem) had been added. The bone marrow suspension (volume 100–250 ml) was then centrifuged for 20 min at 1000 *g*. The buffy coat was removed and filtered through a sieve consisting of 6 layers of autoclaved gauze tissue. The nucleated cell concentration was determined and adjusted by subtracting the leukocyte concentration in the peripheral blood (assuming a maximum contamination of the bone marrow cells with blood).

Discontinuous Albumin Gradient Centrifugation

Purified stem cell fractions were obtained as described by Dicke et al.[7] The cells were suspended in a 17% bovine serum albumin (BSA) solution and pipetted on top of a graduated BSA gradient (BSA concentrations of 21%, 23%, and 25% from top to bottom). The tube was centrifuged for 30 min at 10°C in an International model PR-2 centrifuge at 2000 rpm (1000 *g* at the bottom of the tube). After centrifugation, distinct cell layers were visible at the density interfaces in the gradient. Following this, each fraction was collected with a pipette, washed in HBSS, and the cell concentration determined in a hemocytometer using Türck solution. The cell fraction between 17% and 21% BSA was designated as fraction 1 + 2; the cell fraction between 21% and 23% BSA as fraction 3, etc. A tube was chosen with a diameter of 2.3 cm, allowing for fractionation of cell numbers up to 2×10^9 cells/tube.

Albumin fraction V powder (Sigma, St. Louis, MO) was dissolved to a concentration of 35% in Tris buffer (pH 7.2, 250 mosmole/liter) by diluting the 35% stock solution with increasing volumes of sodium chloride-sodium phosphate buffer. Two percent albumin solutions (25% to 17%) were prepared. The final albumin concentration was checked by refractometry.

Treatment of Dogs After TBI

Caretakers used clean overalls, shoes, gloves, and masks. These were changed daily. Before and after handling an animal, the gloved hands were washed in a 2% sapoform solution. Rectal temperatures were recorded daily. Antibiotics were administered intramuscularly if rectal temperatures rose above 39.7°C. Two antibiotics were administered based on the antibiogram of the pretreatment fecal cultures. Antifungal therapy was administered simultaneously. Antibiotic treatment was continued until 5 days after the rectal temperature returned to normal. Subcutaneous Ringer's lactate was administered on an as-needed basis, depending on the daily intake of each dog. Complete blood counts, including the leukocyte differential, were done on a daily basis until the leukocyte and platelet values had reached stable levels. Blood for transfusions was collected from dogs negative for DEA 1.1 and DEA 1.2.[4] Platelet transfusions were given if platelet levels fell below 20×10^9/liter. If the hematocrit was below 30, whole blood was given. All blood products were irradiated with 15 Gy from a Cs source before administration. Blood chemistries, including a serum protein electorphoresis, urea nitrogen, AST (aspartate aminotransferase), ALT (alanine aminotransferase), and alkaline phosphatase were determined.

RESULTS

TBI, CsA, and DLA-Identical Bone Marrow Transplantation

The results are summarized in Table 1. All five dogs had evidence of engraftment based on the leukocyte and platelet response. In three of the five dogs (801914, 801916, and 800124), confirmation of engraftment was possible via donor chromosome studies. The CsA serum levels were determined 2–3 times per week (trough level) immediately preceding the daily oral CsA administration. Figure 1 is a representative curve for the CsA serum levels throughout the period of CsA administration.

Table 1. Conditioning With 1 × 5.0 Gy TBI, DLA-Identical Stem Cell Grafts, and Cyclosporine-A

Dog	Sex	No. of Gradient Cells Transfused	Leukocytes ($\times 10^9 \cdot 1^{-1}$) 10	15	20	25	CsA ($15\ mg \cdot kg^{-1} \cdot day^{-1}$)	Take
T156	M	$3.3 \times 10^7 \cdot kg^{-1}$	0.6	1.7	1.9	2.6	+	+
801914	M	$4.0 \times 10^7 \cdot kg^{-1}$	1.3	1.3	2.5	2.1	+	+
801916	M	$4.0 \times 10^7 \cdot kg^{-1}$	1.1	3.0	4.6	1.8	+	+
800120	F	$4.0 \times 10^7 \cdot kg^{-1}$	0.6	2.1	5.6	4.4	+	+
800124	F	$4.0 \times 10^7 \cdot kg^{-1}$	2.0	2.5	3.6	3.5	+	+

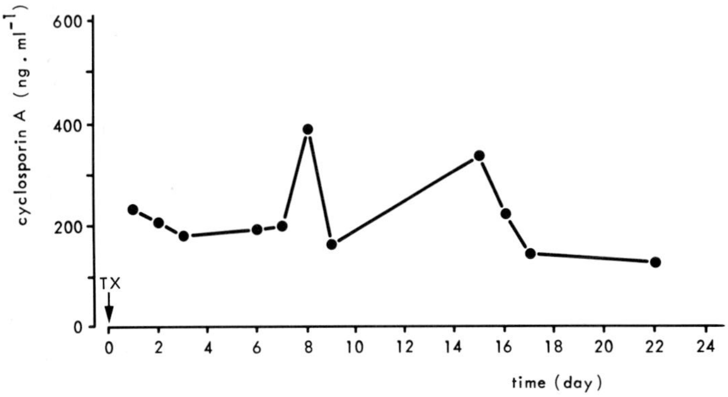

Fig. 1. Cyclosporine-A serum trough levels as determined by radioimmunoassay. A representative curve from 1 dog after bone marrow transplantation. Dose of CsA was 15 mg · kg^{-1} · day^{-1} orally.

TBI, CsA, DLA One-Haplotype Mismatch Dogs

The results are summarized in Table 2. No evidence of engraftment was observed in 5/6 dogs. One dog died early (day 9) from an intesusception. The remaining 5 dogs died of infectious complications. Marrow specimens obtained at autopsy failed to show evidence of engraftment.

DISCUSSION

CsA has been shown to be a potent immunosuppressant in preventing organ graft rejection. In an attempt to ameliorate some of the conditioning regimen toxicity, these studies were carried out using lower dose TBI (1 × 5.0 Gy), previously shown to be insufficient as a conditioning TBI dose with lymphocyte-depleted grafts,[8] engraftment with stem cell grafts, and concurrent administration of CsA from day −1 to day 27. Each of the 5 dogs were transplanted successfully. Early morbidity, as assessed by general clinical observation, number of febrile days, and episodes of overt bleeding were reduced in comparison to the morbidity observed in similar experiments utilizing the fractionated dose of TBI (2.0 × 4.5 Gy).[8] This fractionated dose is necessary to provide sustained engraftment with stem-cell-enriched grafts without the use of CsA.[8] No significant gastrointestinal, hepatic, or renal toxicity could be attributed to the CsA at the dose utilized. As can be seen from Fig. 1, trough CsA levels were consistently above 100 ng · ml^{-1}, the level believed to correlate with CsA immunosuppressive efficacy.[9]

The results in the DLA one-haplotype mismatched dogs were not as gratifying. Previous studies have shown that fractionated total body irradiation (2.0 × 4.5 Gy) and engraftment with stem cell grafts in DLA-identical

Table 2. Conditioning With 2 × 4.5 Gy TBI, DLA One-Haplotype Mismatch Stem Cell Grafts, and Cyclosporine-A

Dog	Sex	No. of Gradient Cells Transfused	CsA (15 mg · kg^{-1} · Day^{-1})	Take	Comments
801913	M	$3.1 \times 10^7 \cdot kg^{-1}$	+	−	Survival 12 days Death due to pneumonitis
801915	M	$3.5 \times 10^7 \cdot kg^{-1}$	+	−	Survival 22 days Death due to aplasia, sepsis
T167	F	$4.0 \times 10^7 \cdot kg^{-1}$	+	−	Survival 17 days Death due to aplasia, sepsis
T163	M	$4.0 \times 10^7 \cdot kg^{-1}$	+	−	Survival 9 days Death due to intesusscception
T164	M	$4.0 \times 10^7 \cdot kg^{-1}$	+	−	Survival 14 days Death due to aplasia, sepsis
T165	F	$4.0 \times 10^7 \cdot kg^{-1}$	+	−	Survival 23 days Death due to aplasia, sepsis

canines resulted in successful bone marrow transplantation in a majority of the dogs.[8] The lymphocyte-depleted grafts reduced the number of immunocompetent cells transplanted, which are presumed responsible for GVHD, while still providing equal numbers of stem cells as found in whole bone marrow grafts.[8] Five of six dogs failed to achieve engraftment with the stem cell grafts and died of infectious complications. The sixth dog died before engraftment could be expected. Again, the CsA levels were consistently above 100 ng · ml^{-1}.

In conclusion, CsA, a potent immunosuppressive agent, facilitates bone marrow transplantation and graft acceptance in DLA-identical dogs. However, CsA appears to be ineffective in abrogating the HVGD across a DLA one-haplotype mismatch barrier which would allow for successful engraftment of the bone marrow stem cell graft. Toxicity due to the CsA was not encountered.

REFERENCES

1. Borel JF, Feurer C, Gubler HU, et al: Agents Actions 6:468, 1976

2. Van Bekkum DW, Knaan S, Zurcher C: Transplant Proc 12:278, 1980

3. Deeg HJ, Storb S, Weiden PL, et al: Transplant Proc 13:402, 1981

4. Joint Report Second International Workshop on Canine Immunogenetics: Transplant Proc 8:289, 1976

5. Vriesendorp HM, Van Bekkum DW: In Shifvine M, Wilson FD (eds): B. The Canine as a Biomedical Research Model. Oak Ridge, TN, DOE Technical Information Center, 1980, p 153

6. Vriesendorp HM, Klapwijk WM, Van Kessel AMC, et al: Transplantation 31:347, 1981

7. Dicke KA, Van Bekkum DW: Transplant Proc 3:666, 1971

8. Walma EP, Vriesendorp HM, Klapwijk WM, et al: (in press)

9. Keown PA, Valn RA, Wall WJ, et al: Lancet 1:686, 1981

EFFECTS ON WOUND HEALING, COMPOSITE GRAFTS, SKIN, CORNEA, AND VEIN ALLOGRAFTS

Effects of Cyclosporine on the Healing of Vascularized and Nonvascularized Bone Allografts in Rodents

P. F. Halloran, M. Bushuk, and J. A. Stewart

BONE transplantation has considerable potential for the reconstruction of osseous defects, frequently as an alternative to limb amputation. Because syngeneic grafts are obviously limited by the size and configuration of the defect, allografts, either vascularized or nonvascularized, have been used with some success.[1] As the therapeutic index of immunosuppression improves, the possibilities for the use of bone allografts will increase. The purpose of the present studies was to examine the effect of cyclosporine (CsA) on bone graft healing in animal models. The results indicate that CsA does not improve healing in devascularized segmental bone allografts, because it directly depresses bone healing; however, in vascularized bone grafts in rats, cyclosporine improves graft survival and even permits limited growth of transplanted bone, despite strong histocompatibility differences.

MATERIALS AND METHODS

Two previously described experimental models were used: segmental nonvascularized bone allografts in mice[2] and vascularized limb grafts in rats.[3,4] In brief, the nonvascularized murine bone grafts were performed by excising a segment of the tibia of a recipient (BALB/cByJ, H-2[d]) and of a donor (C57BL/6J, or "B6," H-2[b]) under general anesthesia and replacing the recipient tibia with donor bone, which was held in place by an intramedullary pin. The skin was closed, and the mouse was immediately permitted full ambulation. Donor-specific alloantibody responses were tested in a complement-dependent microcytotoxicity assay, using sera obtained by periodic bleedings from the retroorbital plexus. Bone healing was assessed radiographically, using high resolution industrial grade film. The incidence of union at the proximal and distal fracture sites was assessed by three independent observers using coded radiographs. The principal measure of the degree of bone healing was the tensile strength, which was measured in absolute terms per unit of cross-sectional area of bone (in kg/sq mm) and expressed as well as a percentage of the strength of the contralateral, nonoperated control limb. Details of this testing will be published elsewhere (Bushuk and Halloran, in preparation).

The vascularized limb graft model in the rat was performed in two rat strain combinations: F344 (RT1[l]) recipients of ACI (RT1[a]) grafts [a strong major histocompatibility complex (MHC) difference, plus minor histocompatibility (MiHA) differences], and F344 recipients of Lewis (RT1[l]) grafts (MHC matched, but with multiple MiHA differences). Controls consisted of F344 recipients of F344 grafts. The graft consisted of the distal femur, knee joint, intact tibia, and all the intrinsic musculature of the leg, including the gastrocnemius. The foot, being denervated, was amputated to avoid complications of a flail foot. The femoral artery and vein were anastomosed by a microsurgical technique; the nerves were not repaired. The donor skin was not transplanted; skin coverage consisted exclusively of recipient skin to preserve some sensation and to avoid skin breakdown due to the high susceptibility of skin to rejection. Occasionally, due to trauma or impaired blood supply, the skin over the stump broke down and was revised immediately to prevent sepsis.

These grafts were studied by serial x-rays (using high resolution film as above), bone scans (using technetium-labeled methylene diphosphonate[5]), donor-specific antibody determinations, and histologic evaluation after sacrifice. Growth was assessed on the basis of measurements on the x-rays and was confirmed by examination of the bones at the time of sacrifice.

CsA was a generous gift of Dr. Borel of Sandoz Laboratories, Basel, Switzerland, and was administered by gastric lavage, dissolved in olive oil, in a fixed volume of 0.1 ml/10 g body weight. Mice were obtained from Jackson Laboratories, Bar Harbor, ME and were 6–12 weeks old as the experiments began; rats (200 g) were obtained from Charles River Breeding Laboratories, Boston, MA (F344) or from Laboratory Supply Co., Indianapolis, IN (ACI, Lewis).

From the Harold Tanenbaum Department of Medical Research, Mount Sinai Hospital, Toronto, Ontario, Canada.

Supported in part by grants from the Medical Research Council of Canada (MA5739) and from the Mount Sinai Research Institute.

Address reprint requests to Dr. P. F. Halloran, Mount Sinai Hospital, Suite 435, 600 University Avenue, Toronto, Ontario M5G 1X5, Canada.

0041-1345/83/1505-0160$01.00/0

RESULTS

Mice tolerated the administration of CsA in olive oil by gastric lavage well, with no pronounced excess in mortality over the 30 days of administration. Plasma CsA levels (measured by RIA) varied with the dose and with the duration of therapy, the 24-hr trough level after 10, 20, and 30 days of therapy being 25 ng/ml on 25 mg/kg/day, and 1553, 132, and 274 ng/ml on 100 mg/kg/day. The measurement of a variety of biochemical parameters failed to reveal significant differences between the CsA groups and the olive oil group, except for depression of the alkaline phosphate and a mild rise in serum creatinine. There was some hair loss in the mice given CsA, which was not observed in the control groups.

One consistent side effect of animals given CsA was failure to gain weight and grow at the expected rate. For this reason, in one experiment, we included a "food limitation" control group (4 g of food per day, compared to the normal intake of approximately 6 g). We had previously found that mice on such a diet gain weight at a rate similar to that of the CsA 100 mg/kg group. We could thus distinguish effects of caloric malnutrition from those of CsA.

Table 1. The Effect of CsA on the Healing of Nonvascularized Tibial Grafts in BALB/c Mice

	Mean Tensile Strength (± Standard Error) in kg/sq mm	
Treatment Group	Syngeneic Grafts (BALB/c Donors)	Allogeneic Grafts (B6 Donors)
No treatment	1.7 ± 0.2	1.0 + 0.1*
Olive oil control	1.8 ± 0.2	1.1 ± 0.3*
CsA 25 mg/kg	1.4 ± 0.2‡	1.1 ± 0.2
CsA 50 mg/kg	1.1 ± 0.1†‡	1.2 ± 0.4
CsA 100 mg/kg	1.2 ± 0.4†‡	1.1 ±0.2

*Significantly different from the syngeneic control.
†Significantly different from the untreated control.
‡Significantly different from the olive-oil-treated control.

When alloantibody responses were studied at 1 month, we found that CsA 25 mg/kg blunted the response, whereas CsA 100 mg/kg abolished the alloantibody response. Bone healing, as assessed by radiographs and, as shown in Table 1, by tensile testing, was abnormal in the allogeneic grafts. We and others have previously presented evidence that this impaired healing is a function of the donor-specific immune response.[6–8] However, CsA did not improve the healing of the allo-

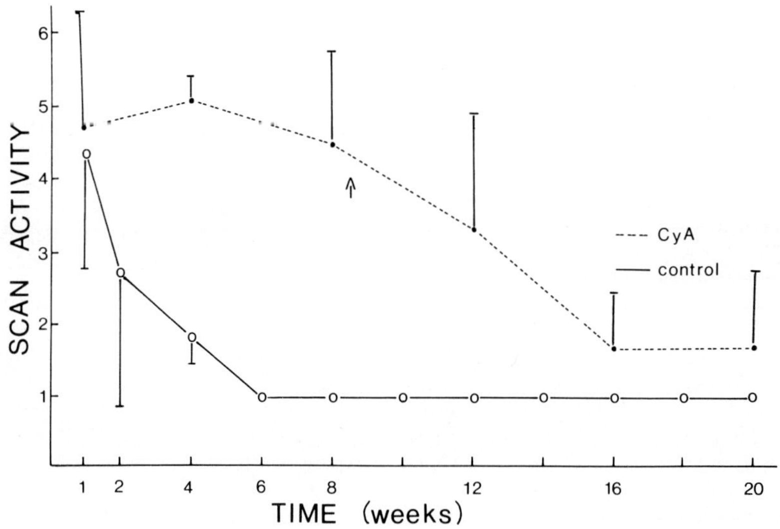

Fig. 1. Viability of bone grafts, as assessed by bone scans, across a strong MHC difference (ACI into F344) when treated with CsA 10 mg/kg/day for 8 weeks. Arrow indicates time of discontinuation of CsA therapy. Five animals per group were tested at each point.

grafts; the reason for this failure was apparently a direct CsA-dependent depression of bone healing, since the healing of the syngeneic grafts was depressed by the CsA administration. This effect was not due to the generalized decreased nutrition seen in CsA-treated animals, because it was observed in the animals treated with 25 mg/kg, which gained weight normally during this period. Moreover, CsA 100 mg/kg/day depressed healing significantly more than did food deprivation, despite a similar degree of weight loss in both groups (not shown). Thus, in the devascularized murine bone graft model, CsA depressed the immune response but did not improve allograft healing, apparently because CsA depressed the healing of these segmental bone grafts, as seen in the syngeneic controls.

In the vascularized rat limb allografts, the findings were different. CsA markedly prolonged graft survival (as demonstrated by bone scans) across the strong MHC difference, although graft viability declined when CsA was withdrawn (Fig. 1). Across the weak MiHA difference, the bones remained viable by bone scans even after the CsA therapy was discontinued (not shown). Although CsA itself did cause some impairment of growth and weight gain, the bones of the allografts grew on CsA therapy: a small but significant amount across the MHC disparity and a larger amount across the MiHA difference (Fig. 2). Thus in vascularized allografts, CsA permits prolonged viability and some growth, particularly if combined with MHC matching.

DISCUSSION

The differences between the devascularized segmental tibia graft model and the vascularized femur-knee-tibia graft model should be emphasized, because these differences probably explain the different actions of CsA in these two graft models. Species differences (mouse versus rat) could play a role in the results, but for the present, we shall ignore this factor. The healing of the segmental allograft demands maximal activity of the host osteoprogenitor elements, but also requires some recipient marrow-deprived cells for optimal healing.[7,8] The graft must be replaced by creeping substitution, a large scale operation that is probably more complex and demanding than simple fracture healing. The immune response can presumably impede such healing at many levels, including the destruction of the donor cells required for optimal healing.[8] The vascularized graft, in the absence of an immune response, remains viable, and healing is simply the repair of one fracture, not the replacement of the donor bone. Since the donor bone is vascularized, it receives a continuous supply of the hematogenous cells required for healing. This graft can thus be monitored by its viability and growth

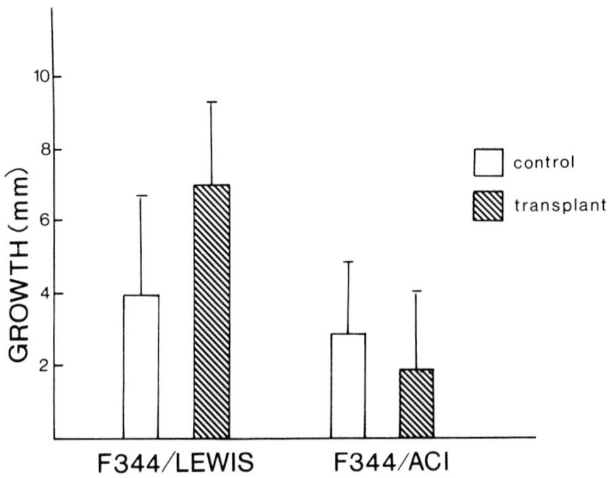

Fig. 2. Growth of bone grafts across weak (Lewis into F344) and strong (ACI into F344) histocompatibility differences, as measured at 5 months. CsA therapy was administered for the initial 2 months. Comparison of nonoperated control leg with the transplanted leg.

rather than by tensile strength. It is like a vascularized organ graft in this respect.

The mechanism by which CsA impairs healing and replacement of the devascularized grafts could be either indirect or direct. In considering indirect effects, we have excluded gross effects of CsA on nutrition as the cause, but subtle nutritional, metabolic, or hormonal effects are more difficult to exclude. Alternatively, it is possible that CsA interferes with organization, differentiation, and intercellular communication in some complex healing processes in the same manner as it arrests the immune response. Such a hypothesis would still be compatible with the concept that CsA has less direct depressive effects on healing than other immunosuppressives (e.g., corticosteroids).

The ability of a fully allogeneic tibia graft to survive and even grow on CsA should encourage further work on the potential of this approach for safe reconstitution of skeletal defects in children, as well as in adults. However, it is not established that long-term CsA therapy is safe enough to permit its use for this purpose. The present work merely demonstrates that the basic concept of transplantation of large vascularized skeletal grafts under CsA coverage, particularly with MHC matching, is feasible; the actual clinical application of such a technique and its ethics remain to be established.

REFERENCES

1. Mankin HJ: N Engl J Med 300:543, 1979

2. Halloran PF, Ziv I, Lee EH, et al: Transplantation 27:414, 1979

3. Lipson R, Kawano H, Halloran PF, et al: Transplantation 35:293, 1983

4. Lipson R, Kawano H, Halloran PF, et al: Transplantation 35:300, 1983

5. Lipson R, Dief H, Greyson N, et al: Clin Orthoped 160:279, 1981

6. Elves MW: Clin Orthoped 120:232, 1976

7. Kliman M, Halloran PF, Lee EH, et al: Transplantation 31:34, 1981

8. Esses SI, Halloran PF: Transplantation 35:169, 1983

Modification of Experimental Limb Allograft Rejection With Cyclosporine and Prednisone: A Preliminary Report

B. H. J. Press, R. K. Sibley, and A. R. Shons

THE primary obstacle to the clinical use of limb allografts has been the failure to develop pharmacologic means of immunosuppression sufficiently selective and safe to allow allotransplantation of a nonvital body part. In addition, technical limitations have prevented experiments using genetically defined strains of small laboratory animals. The recent emergence of cyclosporine as a highly effective and selective immunosuppressive agent and the refinement of microsurgical techniques in the last 10–15 years[1] led us to reexamine the limb allograft problem in inbred strains of laboratory rats. We report our preliminary experience.

MATERIALS AND METHODS

Male Fischer ($RT1^{lvl}$) rats (250–400 g) were used as donors and Lewis ($RT1^{l}$) rats as recipients. Under general anesthesia, the recipient's limb was amputated at mid-thigh level, with division of all neurovascular structures as far distally as possible. The donor limb was then amputated with proximal division of all nerves and vessels. Limb shortening was not required with this technique. Bony fixation was achieved with a 23-gauge needle as an intramedullary rod and interosseous wiring to avoid rotation. The soft tissues of the leg were reapproximated, and the femoral artery, vein, nerve, and sciatic nerve reanastomosed with standard microsurgical technique. A plastic collar was placed around the animal's neck to prevent automutilation of the anesthetic limb. Normal saline (25cc) was given intraperitoneally (i.p.) for fluid replacement, and penicillin G (100,000 U) was given i.p. 1 hr prior to operation and again on the first postoperative day. No systemic anticoagulation was used; the irrigating solution contained heparin (20 U/cc). Mean ischemic time for the cooled limb was 1.5 hr, with a mean operating time of 2.75 hr.

Immunosuppressive treatment was given as outlined in Table 1. Animals were weighed 3 times weekly to calculate immunosuppressive dosage.

Animals were sacrificed either electively at selected intervals postoperatively or as necessary because of infection or rejection. Biopsies of limb allograft skin, muscle, vessel, and nerve were fixed in Bouin's solution, embedded in paraffin, stained with hemotoxylin and eosin, and examined by light microscopy.

RESULTS

Group I animals were sacrificed at postoperative intervals of 1, 3, and 6 days to define early histologic changes, and at 11 days when rejection was grossly apparent. The elective intervals were chosen for comparison with a previous study of early histopathologic changes attendant with limb replantation.[2]

Microscopic changes in group I allografts were indistinguishable from replants at 1 and 3 days postoperatively. Edema and hemorrhage were prominent on the first postoperative day, with an inflammatory cell infiltrate appearing by day 3 and reaching maximum by day 6. Spotty muscle fiber necrosis also was prominent in these early postoperative specimens. At 6 days postoperatively, a perivascular lymphocytic infiltrate as well as increased numbers of lymphocytes in the dermis near the dermal–epidermal junction were noted (not seen in autografts). Some small vessels were involved by early vascular rejection, characterized by a subendothelial mononuclear cell infiltrate (Fig. 1). By 11 days posttransplantation, the limbs were swollen, with incipient skin breakdown. Gross examination showed firm pale muscle with good femoral arterial and venous blood flow. Microscopic sections showed severe rejection in all tissues of the limb with a marked necrotizing vasculities (Fig. 2) and many interstitial lymphocytes in muscle and skin.

From the Division of Plastic and Reconstructive Surgery, Department of Surgery, and the Department of Laboratory Medicine and Pathology, University of Minnesota, Minneapolis, MN.

Address reprint requests to Dr. B. H. J. Press, Division of Plastic and Reconstructive Surgery, Department of Surgery, University of Minnesota, Minneapolis, MN 55455.

0041–1345/83/1505–0161$01.00/0

Table 1. Experimental Design

Group	No. of Animals	Immunosuppression (mg/kg/day i.p.)*	
		Cyclosporine†	Prednisone‡
I	9	0	0
II	8	5	6
III	12	5	4
IV	6	5	0

*All immunosuppression began 1 day pretransplant and continued daily until sacrifice.

†4 mg/cc: prepared as 800 mg cyclosporine in 180 cc Intralipid-10 + 20 cc 90% ethanol.

‡Hydeltrasol (prednisolone sodium phosphate, MSD).

In group II, 2 rats were lost in the first 24 hr postoperatively due to thrombosis of the vascular anastomoses. Excluding these 2 animals, the mean survival in this group was 11 days. Of these 6 rats, 3 had overwhelming peritoneal or thoracic infection. In three animals sacrificed at 3, 6, and 16 days postoperatively, microscopic change was largely confined to muscular atrophy. There was no microscopic evidence of rejection in any of the three.

In group III, there was one perioperative death and one animal was sacrificed electively 6 days postoperatively. In the remaining 10 animals, mean survival was 10.5 days. Eight of 10 had grossly infected limb allografts at the time of sacrifice; 5 of 10 had gross lung abscesses. Microscopically, at 6 days postoperatively, a dermal infiltrate of lymphocytes was again noted. Infection rendered several limbs microscopically unevaluable because of massive leukocytic infiltration and abscess formation. The longest surviving animal (20 days) had no microscopic evidence of rejection in any tissues of the limb.

In group IV, 3 animals were sacrificed electively at 6, 7, and 20 days postoperatively. In the other 3, mean survival was 16.3 days (range 14–29 days). Four of 4 animals surviving longer than 7 days postoperatively had gross infection. This included wound and deep soft tissue infections of the transplanted limb as well as variable degrees of pulmonary involvement with abscesses and pleural effu-

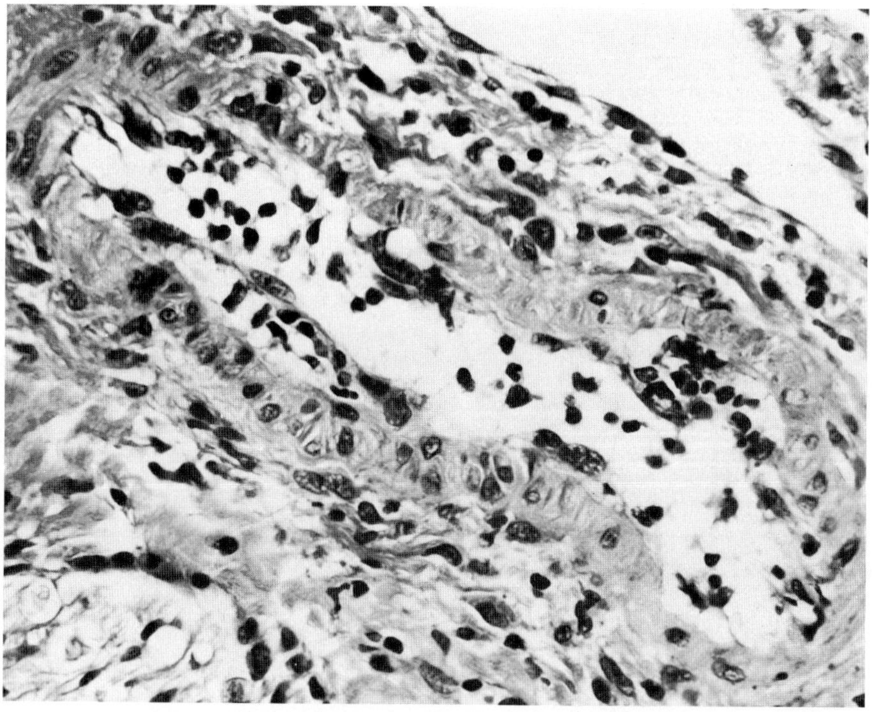

Fig. 1. Group I, postoperative day 6. A small muscular vessel. The endothelium is separated from the subintimal tissues by a mononuclear inflammatory cell infiltrate (original magnification ×480).

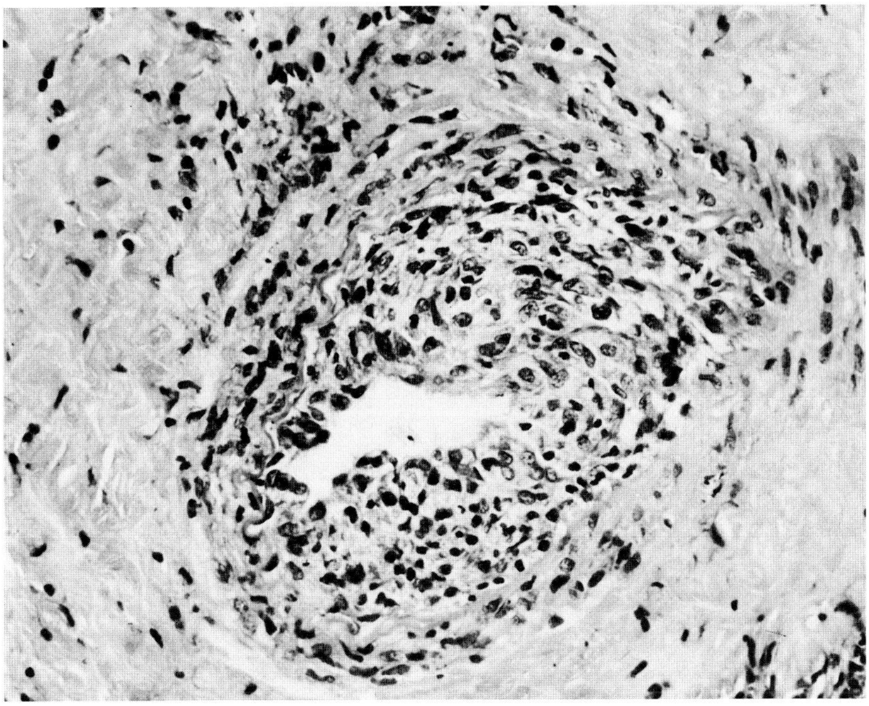

Fig. 2. Group I, postoperative day 11. Small muscular vessel. Extension of the vasculitic process with infiltration of mononuclear cells throughout the wall of the vessel (original magnification ×300).

sions. Again at 7 days postoperatively, a mild increase in lymphocytes was seen in dermis and around small muscular vessels. At 15 days postoperatively, a further increase in lymphocyte numbers was noted as well as increasing numbers of other mononuclear cells, especially mast cells and macrophages (Fig. 3). At 20 and 29 days posttransplantation (the longest survivors), mast cells and macrophages were still present; persistent collections of lymphocytes were concentrated near the dermal–epidermal junction (Fig. 4).

Postoperatively, a weight loss of greater than 20% of body weight at the time of transplantation correlated well with high mortality. As the dose of prednisone was decreased, the rate of weight loss lessened and the mean length of survival increased.

Though evidence of cyclosporine cytotoxicity was searched for, histologic examination of the heart and kidneys of randomly selected cyclosporine-treated animals showed no changes typical of cyclosporine-induced cardiac or renal toxicity.

DISCUSSION

Only a few reports of experimental limb allotransplantation exist in the literature. Schwind[3] successfully implanted limbs heterotopically onto rats in which tolerance had been induced by parabiosis and splenic grafts. In 1966, Lapchinsky[4] reported a long functioning limb allograft in a dog that had been made tolerant by cross-transfusion at 6 days of age. Goldwyn et al.,[5] in 1966, reported rejection by 7 days posttransplantation in untreated canine limb allografts. In 7 of 11 animals treated with azathioprine, limb survival was lengthened up to 28 days with a mean survival of 18 days.

In 1971, Lance et al.[6] reported allotransplantation of hind limbs at the mid-thigh level between unrelated beagle dogs. An unacceptably high rate of technical failure was reported. Dogs with technically successful grafts were treated with antilymphocyte serum alone or in combination with hydrocortisone or azathioprine. These animals were

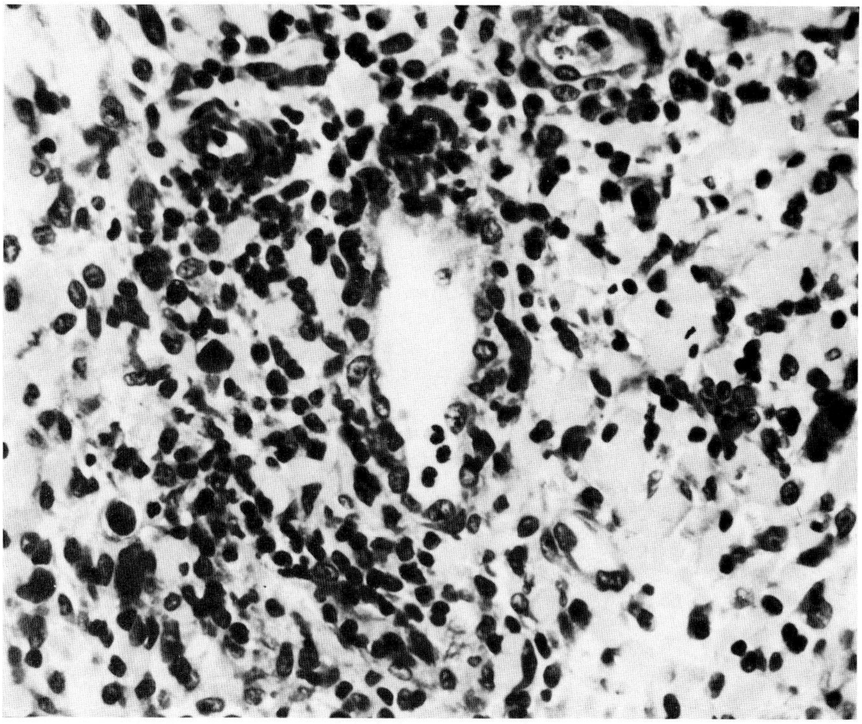

Fig. 3. Group IV, postoperative day 15. An intense mononuclear cell infiltrate is evident in the dermis. It is composed of variably sized lymphocytes and macrophages (original magnification ×495).

sacrificed at 24–112 days postoperatively because of sepsis, bone marrow depression, or automutilation of the limb. Fifty percent had no evidence of rejection. It was apparent, however, that the immunosuppressive regimen used was unable to allow graft survival without fatal complications. Somewhat better results were achieved using an immunosuppressive regimen of induced tolerance. The dogs treated in this fashion fared much better than those on continuous pharmacologic immunosuppression. Grafts were retained longer with fewer complications; two animals survived for 7 and 13 months. In all limbs, the first manifestations of rejection were noted in the skin. Those animals surviving 5 months or more had evidence of protective paw sensation and lower extremity musculature motor function.

Recently, preliminary rat experiments have been reported by Black et al.[7] in which donor limbs were taken from Lewis × Brown Norway F_1 progeny and transplanted onto Lewis recipients. Cyclosporine was administered subcutaneously (20 mg/kg/day) for 20 days and then discontinued. Untreated animals had a mean allograft survival of 18 ± 5 days, while cyclosporine-treated allografts had a mean survival of 101 ± 13 days.

Cyclosporine allows transplantation of almost all organs in all animal models tested.[8–12] It is synergistic with other immunosuppressive agents,[11] and when administered continuously, can indefinitely prevent rejection of heart allografts transplanted across a major rat histocompatibility barrier.[11] It can prolong the survival of islet allografts transplanted across a minor but not a major rat histocompatibility barrier.[11] Because of its synergism with other agents, we chose to combine cyclosporine with prednisone in an immunosuppressive regimen to maximize graft acceptance while minimizing toxic side effects.

In our experiments, rejection of untreated

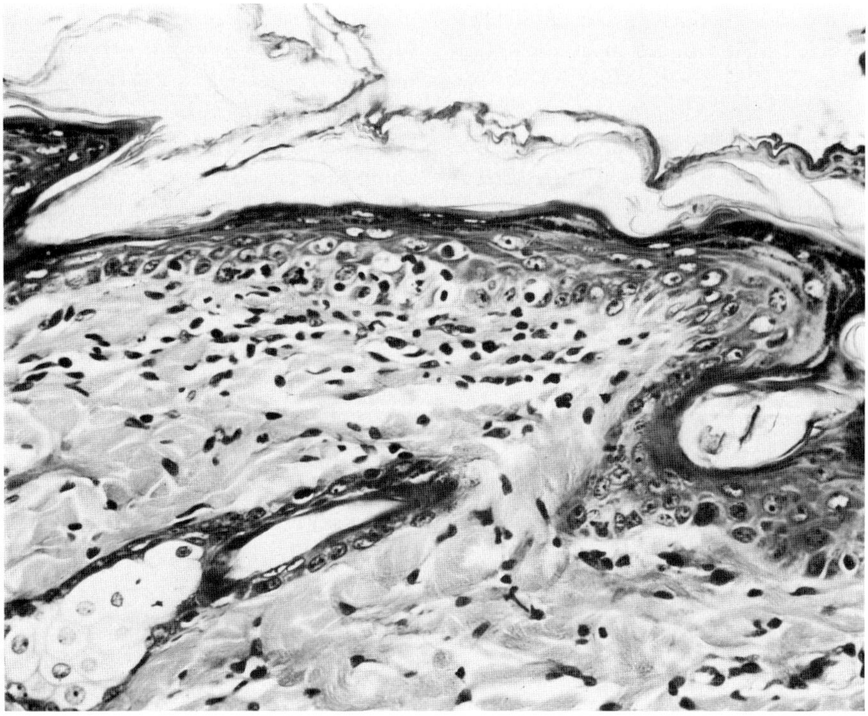

Fig. 4. Group IV, postoperative day 29. The epidermis shows acanthosis and hyperkeratosis with disruption of the basal layer and basal lamina of the skin by an infiltrate of small lymphocytes (original magnification ×300).

allografts across a minor rat histocompatibility barrier was characterized by a pattern of typical vascular rejection beginning on or about 6 days posttransplantation. This led to skin breakdown and gross rejection by 11 days posttransplantation. With the combination of 5 mg/kg/day of cyclosporine with either 6 or 4 mg/kg/day of prednisone (groups II and III), virtually no microscopic evidence of rejection was seen. However, almost all animals treated with these combinations succumbed to overwhelming infection, either in the graft or the pleural or peritoneal cavities. Infectious complications thus precluded extended survival of the limb allografts.

In group IV, a different histologic picture was noted. Although mortality from infection was still unacceptable, 4 animals (50%) survived more than 14 days. In these rats, microscopic changes were observed that were probably masked by the rejection response occurring in untreated animals prior to 14 days posttransplantation. The primary site of later cellular infiltration was dermis (near the dermal–epidermal junction), and by 15–29 days posttransplantation, the number of dermal lymphocytes had decreased from that seen at 10–15 days. A corresponding increase was also seen in the number of macrophages and mast cells infiltrating the dermis. In these longest survivors, the tissues of the limbs appeared healthy, with only mild muscular atrophy and excellent healing.

The biologic events that underlie this histologic appearance remain unclear. Similarities to the morphological appearance described here can be seen in acute and chronic graft-versus-host-disease, an analogous situation in which immunocompetent cells attack in situ skin rather than free grafts.[13] More precise characterization of the cells infiltrating the graft at various times posttransplantation and of the reason for the preferential attack on skin in the cyclosporine-treated animals will be necessary to further elucidate the mechanisms involved in the rejection of such composite tissues.

The improved results that were noted as the dosage of immunosuppression was lowered have encouraged us to proceed with further experiments using lower doses of both cyclosporine and prednisone as well as the addition of other immunosuppressive agents. The effective dosage ranges in this model are similar to those effective for other tissues transplanted across the same histocompatibility barrier.[11] With further understanding of rejection mechanisms, transplantation of composite tissue allografts may be no more difficult than allografts of heart, pancreas, or kidney.

REFERENCES

1. Shapiro RI, Cerra FB: J Surg Res 24:501, 1978

2. Press BHJ, Sibley RK, Shons AR: J Hand Surg (in press)

3. Schwind JV: Radiology 78:806, 1962

4. Lapchinsky AB, Medvedeva GV, Gadalina ID: In Kovanov BB (ed): Induction of Tolerance and Homotransplantation. Moscow, Moscow Press, 1966, p 6

5. Goldwyn RM, Beach PM, Feldman D, et al: Plast Reconstruct Surg 37:184, 1966

6. Lance EM, Inglis AE, Figarola F, et al: J Bone Joint Surg 53-A:1137, 1971

7. Black KS, Hewitt CW, Fraser LA, et al: N Engl J Med 306:368, 1982 (letter)

8. Watt DJ, Partridge TA, Sloper JC: Transplantation 31:266, 1981

9. Veith FJ, Norin AJ, Montefusco CM, et al: Transplantation 32:474, 1981

10. Reznick RK, Craddock GN, Langer B, et al: Can J Surg 25:51, 1982

11. Rynasiewicz JJ, Sutherland DER, Ferguson RM, et al: Diabetes 31:92, 1982

12. Morris PJ: Transplantation 32:349, 1981

13. Saurat JH: Int J Dermatol 20:249, 1981

Cyclosporine and Long-Term Survival of Composite Tissue Allografts (Limb Transplants) in Rats (With Historical Notes on the Role of Plastic Surgeons in Allotransplantation)

D. W. Furnas, K. S. Black, C. W. Hewitt, L. A. Fraser, and B. M. Achauer

INVESTIGATORS from the ranks of plastic surgery helped to launch the field of transplantation surgery in their quest for allografts for structural material. Through the ages, effective allografts of skin and "composite tissue" (skin, subcutaneous tissue, plus nerves and vessels, and/or muscles, and bone) have been elusive. Tagliacozzi, the "First Professor of Plastic Surgery," gained fame for skill in nasal reconstruction;[1] his work also generated some fanciful reports of allografting by imaginative writers of his day. The "Sympathetic Slave" reportedly donated a parabiotic flap from his arm to a gentleman who had lost his nose in sword-play. In exchange, the slave was freed upon detachment of the flap. The reconstructed nose was a success for three years, but then it darkened and necrosed, leaving the patient with his original defect. Inquiry revealed that the slave had died of a common ailment at exactly the same time. A philosopher, Tommaso Campanella, determined that the slave's soul remained as a whole, residing both in the slave proper and in his donated part; when the soul left the slave's body it also left the donated part, and the part was rejected.[2] Thereafter, successful allografts were reported from time to time through history, but none were substantiated.[3] Padgett carefully observed 40 patients on whom he, his associates, or his colleagues performed allografts of skin. None survived beyond 35 days, and he concluded that reports of permanent allograft survival should be "relegated to medical mythology."[4] He carried out exchange of skin grafts between two pairs of identical twins (four procedures) and saw no sign of rejection after a 2–3-month follow-up. He concluded that these skin grafts would survive indefinitely. J.B. Brown confirmed the permanence of survival of skin grafts exchanged between identical twins[5] and Brown reported further that the temporary wound closure achieved by skin allografts could be a turning point for a patient with a life-threatening problem such as a burn.[5]

Burns sustained by R.A.F. pilots in the Battle of Britain were the impetus for the Medical Research Council to form a burn unit at the Glasgow Royal Infirmary.[6] In this unit, Gibson observed accelerated rejection of a second set of pinch grafts placed from father to daughter.[6] The Medical Research Council sent a young zoologist, Medawar, to join him in investigating this phenomenon.[7] Medawar later returned to England to continue this path of investigation which led to his receipt of the Nobel Prize in 1960.

Converse resurfaced the wounds of a French soldier with skin grafts from his twin,[8] and also pursued laboratory investigations.[9] He started the biannual International Conferences on Transplantation in New York which developed into the International Transplantation Society and he followed Medawar as President in 1969.[10]

Conway investigated skin allografts in rats with an in vivo transparent chamber;[11] his organizational efforts led to the inception of the *Transplantation Bulletin* as part of the journal, *Plastic and Reconstructive Surgery.*

From the Division of Plastic Surgery, University of California, Irvine, CA.

Address reprint request to Dr. David W. Furnas, Division of Plastic Surgery, University of California, Irvine, CA 92717.

0041–1345/83/1505–0162$01.00/0

The *Transplantation Bulletin* evolved into the journal, *Transplantation.*[12]

Murray, who had worked with J. B. Brown and with Conway, began studies with skin allografts; but he then sought a more tractable model than skin grafts for the study of allograft phenomena. He succeeded in obtaining functioning kidney transplants in dogs.[13] He led the team which obtained the first clinical successes with kidney transplantation between identical twins[14] and then with kidney allografts, using azathioprine for immunosuppression.[15,16] These successes led to a dramatic surge of clinical accomplishments in organ transplants, but placed skin, composite tissue, and most plastic surgeons in the background.

Another major surgical advance occurred when Malt succeeded in replanting an arm;[17] Ch'en successfully replanted a hand soon thereafter.[18] Plastic surgeons took their cue from these two general surgeons and pursued techniques for replantation and transplantation of autologous vascularized composite tissue.

Buncke and Schulz developed microsurgical sutures and instruments that brought them success in ditigal replants on monkeys' hands.[19] Krizek et al. transplanted a free vascularized skin flap from the abdomen to the neck of a dog.[20] Buncke et al. transferred the great toe of a monkey to replace a thumb.[21] The first clinical success in microsurgical replantation came when Komatsu and Tamai replanted a thumb.[22] Snyder, et al. successfully replanted a thumb with an arterial repair only.[23] Cobbett reconstructed a thumb by microvascular transplantation of a great toe.[24] McLean and Buncke repaired a scalp-skull defect by microvascular transplantation of omentum[25] and they carried out a free groin flap to an oral defect that suddenly failed after 6 weeks of viability.[26] Daniel published the first unqualified success with a free flap of skin and subcutaneous tissue when he transferred a groin flap to a leg defect.[27] Harii and Ohmori reported a free flap of scalp.[28] During this time, to improve results in conventional tissue transfer, the principles of vascularized flaps (axial flaps, myocutaneous flaps, and island flaps) were exploited and many new flaps were developed, most of which were potential microvascular free flaps. Littler revived the neurovascular island flap of the digit,[29,30] Bakamjian developed the deltopectoral flap,[31] and McGregor developed the groin flap.[32] Furlow described the dorsalis pedis flap,[33] musculocutaneous flaps were described,[34–37] and muscle flaps that had been used to repair defects or for tendon transfer were recognized as vascularized units.[38] Buncke pushed the fields of allotransplantation and microsurgery toward a merger when he repaired a scalp defect in one twin with a pedicle of scalp from an identical twin[39] emulating Murray's first kidney transplant.

The effectiveness of CsA[40,41] in preventing rejection of organ allografts stimulated our group to try, in animal models, to bring this merger closer yet. We showed that CsA in a dosage of 25 mg/kg/day prolonged survival of allografted limbs in 4 rats to a median time of 101 days (limb temperature drop below 32°C).[42] This communication describes our further studies.

LONG TERM SURVIVAL OF COMPOSITE TISSUE ALLOGRAFTS (LIMB TRANSPLANTS) WITH CsA

In the foregoing work we endeavored to obtain indefinite survival of composite tissue allografts (limb allografts) in the presence of a strong histocompatibility barrier with a dosage level of CsA that would be free of toxic side effects.

MATERIALS AND METHODS

Experimental Model

Two regimens of CsA were studied: (A) A *20-day course only* of CsA 8 mg/kg S.C. was given without subsequent maintenance injections (one rat). (B) A *20-day course* of CsA, 8 mg/kg S.C. was given *followed by a maintenance regimen* of 8 mg/kg twice weekly (5 rats).

Animals

Six Lewis (LEW) (RT-1^{l}) rats (weight, 300 grams) each received an orthotopic transplant of a Lewis x Brown Norway (LBN) (Rt-1^{l+n}) (weight, 300 grams) hind limb.

The recipient and donor animals were anesthetized and prepared simultaneously.

Operative Technique

The transplantation was carried out by isolating the femoral vessels and the femoral and sciatic nerves of the rats. The muscles and the femur were then divided at mid-shaft level. The vessels and nerves were divided, retaining as much extra length as possible. The donor femur was joined to the recipient femur with an interosseous wire. The femoral vessels were anastomosed under the microscope with 10-0 nylon sutures. The femoral and sciatic nerves were repaired with epineural sutures, the muscles were repaired, and the skin was closed.

Preparation and Administration of CsA

CsA was dissolved using 20% Tween 80 in anhydrous alcohol (15 mg/ml). The single rat in group A was given CsA (25 mg/kg/day) for the first 20 days only with no maintenance dose (as in the 4 rats originally reported).

In experimental group B, five rats received S.C. injections of CsA (8 mg/kg/day) for the first 20 days, and then a maintenance dose of 8 mg/kg twice weekly thereafter. We deviated from this regimen several times in an effort to see if the limb would continue to survive without a maintenance dose. If rejection signs were then noted, the maintenance administration was renewed.

Signs of Rejection—Criteria

Two criteria were selected to determine the onset of rejection response: (1) the onset of erythema in the visible areas of the allografted limb, and (2) the core temperature of the limb; observation of a core temperature drop 5°F below normal was interpreted as a rejection response.

Clinical and Pathologic Evaluation

The limbs were evaluated daily for skin color, edema, eschar-necrosis, hair growth, nail growth, and reaction to painful stimuli. Weekly blood chemistry and hematology assays included blood urea nitrogen (BUN), bilirubin, complete blood count (CBC), and counts of total lymphocytes, total neutrophils, and total monocytes. Necropsy was performed after rejection of the limb. The allografted hind limb, the normal limb, kidney, liver, and spleen were examined histologically with hemotoxyln- and eosin-stained sections.

Other Examinations

Two rats in group B were tested for chimerism with Lewis anti-Bn allosera. Postmortem nerve stimulation was carried out.

RESULTS

Control Rats

Rejection signs and allograft necrosis. The first 5°F drop in core temperature was at 15.6 ± 4.3 days; the first visible sign of erythema appeared at 5.6 ± 2.9 days. Signs of frank necrosis appeared soon thereafter.

Experimental Rats

Limb survival and rejection signs. The allografted limb of the single rat in group A and the allografts of 2 of the 5 rats in group B survived indefinitely and were completely free of rejection signs. The allografted limbs of the other 3 rats in group B persisted in their survival, but they showed rejection signs (Table 1) (Fig. 1).

Variations in dosage schedule and comments. To determine if a state of induced tolerance had been achieved, we altered the maintenance schedule in several rats. In rat no. 126, the maintenance injection was discontinued at day 191 and the limb has survived without sign of rejection to day 404.

In rat no. 121, maintenance injections were discontinued at day 229; however, signs of rejection were noted on day 238, and therefore CsA was resumed, starting with 2 "3-day bursts" (days 244–246 and days 249–251), followed by the regular maintenance schedule. The hair of the leg fell out during this rejection crisis and the skin showed persistent erythema and chronic desquamation of its outer layers. All of these signs persisted to some degree even after maintenance dosage was resumed. Two rats (no. 117 and no. 125) showed persistent signs of rejection while receiving an uninterrupted maintenance regimen of CsA; in each case the allografted leg survived for the life of the rat.

These observations suggest that this regimen of CsA approximates a threshold dose for control of rejection.

Clinical examination. The wounds healed normally on all rats. The single rat in group A (no. 115), and 2 of the rats in group B (no. 122, and no. 126), which had been free of rejection signs, showed consistently normal hair and nail growth. The other 3 rats showed normal hair and nail growth until the onset of rejection signs.

The first evidence of rejection was noted on

Table 1. Summary of allograft Survival and Rejection Signs

Regimen, Rat No.	Rejection Signs: Erythema (Postop Day)	Rejection Signs: 5° Temperature Drop (Postop Day)	Indefinite Survival	Final Status (Postop Day)
A				
115	None	None	Yes	Limb alive at 504 days
B				
117	133	265	Yes*	420 (Killed)
121†	238	335	Yes*	441 (Killed)
122	None	None	Yes	84 (Died)‡
125	66	None	Yes*	95 (Died)‡
126§	None	None	Yes	404 (Killed)

NOTE. Regimen A consisted on CsA (25 mg/kg) for 20 days with no maintenance dose, and regimen B consisted of CsA (8 mg/kg) for the first 20 days and then 8 mg/kg twice weekly.

*Histologic signs of rejection were primarily noted in the skin.

†Maintenance dose of CsA was stopped on day 229 and then resumed on day 244.

‡Died from murine mycoplasma pulmonis.

§The maintenance dose of CsA was stopped on day 191.

clinical inspection of the limbs. This consisted of erythema followed by edema and desquamation of the skin, and inhibition of hair growth. Complete hair loss was noted in rat no. 121 when the maintenance dose of CsA was interrupted (see "variation in dosage schedule"). Two of the 3 legs with rejection signs showed a drop in core temperature of 5° (see table).

The allografted limbs showed purposeful muscle contraction, as well as withdrawal from painful stimuli; although the rats with rejection signs were less effective in their movements, perhaps due to the mechanical effect of edema.

Blood chemistry and hematology. The blood chemistry and hematology studies were normal throughout the period of this study.

Histologic examination. Rats which were free of signs of rejection (no. 115, no. 112, and no. 126) appeared normal histologically.

The 3 rats with signs of rejection (no. 117, no. 121, and no. 125) showed cystic hair follicles, areas devoid of hair and hair follicles,

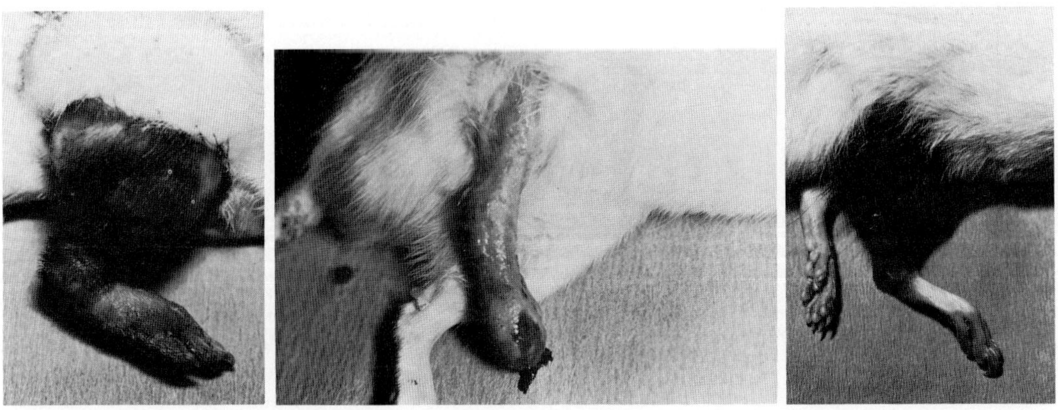

Fig. 1. (A) Control Lewis rat showing advanced rejection of hind limb of Brown Norway (F_1) at day 10. (No CsA). (B) Brown Norway (F_1) limb allograft to Lewis rat showing indefinite survival with chronic rejection signs. (CsA treated). (C) Brown Norway (F_1) limb allograft to Lewis rat with indefinite survival showing no rejection signs. (CsA treated).

and areas of dermal fibrosis; there were also some mild and scattered findings in muscle including atrophy, degeneration of muscle fibers, and areas of fatty infiltration of muscle. One rat (no. 125) showed lymphocytic infiltrates in the muscle.

Deaths. Two animals died one at day 84 (rat no. 122) and one at day 95 (rat no. 125), while still receiving CsA (8 mg/kg/day) twice weekly. They showed signs of chronic respiratory disease and the serum assay for murine mycoplasma pulmonis was strongly positive. One rat (no. 122) was free of any signs of rejection, while the second rat (no. 125) showed erythema, desquamation and edema of the allograft, but showed no temperature drop. Necropsy studies in these two rats showed normal liver, spleen, and kidneys; the lungs showed gross congestion.

Chimerism. Testing for chimerism was carried out in two rats with Lewis anti-BN allosera. In both rats tested (no. 117 and no. 121) chimerism was seen in peripheral blood, spleen, and donor and recipient bone marrow.

Postmortem nerve stimulation. At necropsy the sciatic nerve was stimulated distal (and proximal) to the nerve repair, and contraction of the soleus and gastrocnemius muscles was seen.

SUMMARY

In experimental rats treated with CsA, we have observed indefinite survival of allografted limbs in the presence of a strong histocompatibility barrier, with no obvious toxic effects.

One rat was treated with a single course of 20 days of CsA (25 mg/kg/day) and no maintenance dose. This rat has retained its allografted limb for 504 days at the time of this writing, and probably represents a state of induced tolerance.

Five rats were treated with CsA (8 mg/kg/20 days) and were maintained with CsA (8 mg/kg twice weekly); all of the allotransplanted limbs survived. Two of these limbs showed no signs of rejection response; 3 limbs showed erythema, edema, and desquamation of skin; and 2 of these showed a drop in the core temperature of the limb. The allotransplanted limbs were alive at days 404, 420, and 441 on the 3 rats which were killed, and at days 84 and 95 on the two rats which died of intervening pulmonary infection.

REFERENCES

1. Tagliacozzi G: De Curtorum Chirurgia per Insitionem. Venice, 1597
2. Gnudi MT, et al: The sympathetic slave. In: The Life and Times of Gaspare Tagliacozzi. Los Angeles, Zeitlin & Ver Brugge, 1976, pp 285–286
3. Hamilton D: in: Morris, P. (ed): "Tissue Transplantation (Clinical Surgery International no. 3). Edinburgh, Churchill, Livingstone, 1982, pp 4–5
4. Padgett EC: South Med J 25:895, 1932
5. Brown JB: Surgery 1:558, 1937
6. Gibson T: Personal Communication, 1983.
7. Gibson T, Medawar PB: J Anat 77:299, 1943
8. Converse JM, Duchet G: Plast Reconstruct Surg 2:342, 1947
9. Converse JM, Rapaport FT: Ann Surg 143:306, 1956
10. Obituary. John Marquis Converse. Plast Reconstruct Surg 68:665, 1981
11. Conway H, et al: Plast Reconstruct Surg 20:103, 1957
12. Obituary. Herbert Conway. Plast Reconstruct Surg 45:308, 1970
13. Murray JE, Lang S, Miller BF, et al: Surg Gynec Obstet 103:15, 1956
14. Murray JE, Merrill JP, Harrison JH: Surg Forum 6:432, 1956
15. Murray JE, Merrill JP, Harrison JH, et al: N Engl J Med 268:1315, 1963
16. Murray JE, Tilney NL, Wilson RE: Ann Surg 184:565, 1976
17. Malt RA, McKhann CF: JAMA 189:716, 1964
18. Ch'en CW, et al: Chinese MJ 82:633, 1963
19. Buncke HJ, Schulz WR: Plast Reconstruct Surg 36:62, 1965
20. Krizek TJ, et al: Plast Reconstruct Surg 36:538, 1965
21. Buncke HJ, et al: Br J Plast Surg 19:332, 1966
22. Komatsu S, Tamai S: Plast Reconstruct Surg 42:374, 1968
23. Snyder CC, Stevenson RM, Browne EZ: Plast Reconstruct Surg 50:553, 1972
24. Cobbett JR: J Bone Joint Surg 51:677, 1969
25. McLean D, Buncke H: Plast Reconstruct Surg 59:268, 1972

26. Kaplan EN, Buncke HJ, Murray DE: Plast Reconstruct Surg 52:301, 1973
27. Daniel RK, Taylor GI: Plast Reconstruct Surg 52:111, 1973
28. Harii K, Ohmori K, Ohmori S: Plast Reconstruct Surg 53:410, 1974
29. Littler JW: Neurovascular Skin Island Transfer in Reconstructive Hand Surgery. Edinburgh, Livingstone, 1960
30. Littler JW: J Bone Joint Surg 38A:917, 1956
31. Bakamjian VY, et al: Br J Plast Surg 24:174, 1971
32. McGregor IA, Jackson IT: Br J Plast Surg 25:3, 1972
33. Furlow LT: Plast Reconstruct Surg 55:177, 1975
34. Orticochea M: Br J Plast Surg 25:106, 1972
35. Mathes SJ, McCraw JB, Vasconez LO: Surg Clin North Am 54:1337, 1974
36. Mathes SJ, Nahai F (eds): Clinical Applications for Muscle and Musculocutaneous Flaps. St. Louis, C.V. Mosby, 1982
37. McCraw JB, Dibbell DG: Plast Reconstruct Surg 60:212, 1977
38. Ger R: Br J Plast Surg 29:199, 1976
39. Buncke HJ, Hoffman WY, Alpert BS, et al: Plast Reconstruct Surg 70:605, 1982
40. Borel JF, Meszaros J: Transplantation 29:161, 1980
41. Deeg HJ, Storb R, et al: Transplantation 29:230, 1980
42. Black KS, Hewitt CW, Fraser LA, et al: New Engl J Med 306:368, 1982

Diagnosis of Rejection and Functional Analysis of Composite Tissue (CT) and Skin Allografts Prolonged with Cyclosporine

K. S. Black, C. W. Hewitt, E. B. Howard, L. A. Fraser, B. J. Mah, J. C. Koumas, and B. M. Achauer

THE possibility of indefinitely surviving composite tissue (CT) allografts (skin, muscle, bone, vessels, nerves) opens a new realm of afflictions and disfigurements that could be effectively, functionally, and completely treated. Reconstructive surgeons have almost exclusively utilized autografts to repair peripheral tissue defects. This has severely limited their efforts due to the scarcity of donor sites and suitable tissues. Now, with the advent of cyclosporine (CsA), the concept of composite tissue allograft used in reconstructive surgery could become reality. Also, it has been previously shown that CT allografts can be sustained on rats and rabbits when the animals are treated with CsA.[1–4]

Transplantation surgeons have amassed large numbers of successful organ allografts. A key to success for these surgeries is the ability to assess the postoperative status of the newly transplanted organ. Function of the organ is the most important parameter that can be observed, and it can be impaired after rejection has developed. Therefore, any indication of rejection is important to observe.

Most previous investigations of CT allografts used their definition of the first sign of rejection of the skin as an end-point.[5–11] This assessment did not evaluate the rejection of the structures beneath the skin. Goldwyn et al. noted this problem and discussed some parameters that could elucidate the rejection process of structures other than skin in CT allografts.[12] We have examined several parameters to assess the structure and function of our peripheral composite tissue allografts (CT) and compared these to the first sign of the onset of rejection. A dose–response study was initiated to examine the effects of various CsA doses on composite tissue (limb) allograft survival. A study was also done to correlate transcutaneous oxygen and the survival of skin allografts.

MATERIALS AND METHODS

Five groups of animals were studied for correlation of the first sign of rejection to internal (muscle) temperatures, serum creatine kinase (CPK) levels, and sensory function return (Table 1). Groups 6 and 7 were studied for correlation between transcutaneous oxygen and skin allograft survival. For groups 1–5, Lewis (LEW) ($RT1^{l}$) rats (300 g) were recipients of a Lewis × Brown Norway (LBN) ($RT1^{l+n}$) (300 g) hind limb. The animals were anesthetized with acepromazine malate (1 mg/kg) and ketamine hydrochloride (100 mg/kg). The animals were prepared simultaneously. Surgery, which has been previously described,[1,3] began by isolating the femoral vessel and nerve and the sciatic nerve. The muscles and femur were then divided at mid-femur, and the vessels and nerves ligated with as much extra length on the donor and recipient as possible. The bones were then joined using 4-0 stainless steel interossure wires. The femoral vessels were anastomosed using a Zeiss (OPMI-2 operating quadrascope and 10-0 suture (70-μm needle). An epineural repair of the femoral and sciatic nerves was performed using the same equipment. The muscles were then approximated and the skin closed. CsA was mixed in a 20% Tween and 80% alcohol solution at 15 mg/ml and was injected subcutaneously.

Groups 6 and 7 used the same donor and recipient model as groups 1–5. The skin grafts were harvested with a Padgett dermatome. They were placed on (0.18-in

---

From the Reconstructive Microsurgery and Transplantation Laboratories, Division of Plastic Surgery, and Division of Urology, University of California, Irvine, and the Department of Pathology, University of Southern California School of Medicine, Los Angeles, CA.

Supported in part by the American Association of Plastic Surgeons, the Smart Family Foundation, the UCI Committee on Undergraduate Scholarships, and the American Society for Surgery of the Hand.

Address reprint requests to Dr. K. S. Black, Reconstructive Microsurgery and Transplantation Laboratories, Division of Plastic Surgery, University of California, Irvine, CA 92717.

0041-1345/83/1505-0163$01.00/0

Table 1. Experimental Groups

Group Number	Treatment
1	Limb allograft; controls
2	Limb allograft + CsA (2 mg/kg/day) daily for 20 days postop
3	Limb allograft + CsA (4 mg/kg/day) daily for 20 days postop
4	Limb allograft + CsA (8 mg/kg/day) daily for 20 days postop
5	Limb allograft + CsA (25 mg/kg/day) daily for 20 days postop
6	Skin allograft + CsA (25 mg/kg/day) daily for 20 days postop
7	Skin allograft; controls

thick) full-thickness defects (skin excised to muscle fascia) and sutured in place. CsA was mixed and injected similarly to the limbs. Temperatures were obtained on groups 1–5 every other day using a 23-gauge needle thermister probe (Yellow Springs Instruments). The needle was inserted 2 mm into the muscle of the outer thigh. The animals were bled once a week and the total CPK levels determined (Sigma Chemical Co. St. Louis, MO, Technical Bulletin #520). Transcutaneous oxygen levels (Roche Medical Electronics Model 623) were determined every other day on groups 6 and 7. Visual observations of color, edema, serous exudate, hair loss, and necrosis were performed daily on all groups. The first sign of rejection was noted as an erythema of the glabrous port of the limb or skin graft. Sensory function of the limb was mostly performed by noting withdrawal to painful stimuli. At random times a nerve stimulation set at 8 V was applied to the foot of the allograft and withdrawal was recorded.

RESULTS

There was no correlation between transcutaneous oxygen levels and skin allograft rejection. The transcutaneous oxygen levels fluctuated independently of allograft status.

Groups 1–5 showed no consistent pattern for total CPK levels. The experimental animals had elevated CPK levels compared with normal Lewis CPK levels.

The first 5°F temperature decline of the limb correlated with the first sign of rejection ($r = 0.84$) (Fig. 1). Both first sign of rejection and the first 5°F temperature drop demonstrated a logarithmic relationship when plotted against the CsA dose (Figs. 2 and 3).

Reaction to the needle stick was demonstrated as early as three weeks. None of the animals in groups 1 and 2 responded to the needle stick. The mean and standard deviation for the other groups was: 3 of 6 animals responded at 65 ± 40 days (group 3); 6 of 6 animals responded at 74.5 ± 17 days (group 4); 3 of 5 animals responded at 83 ± 20 days (group 5).

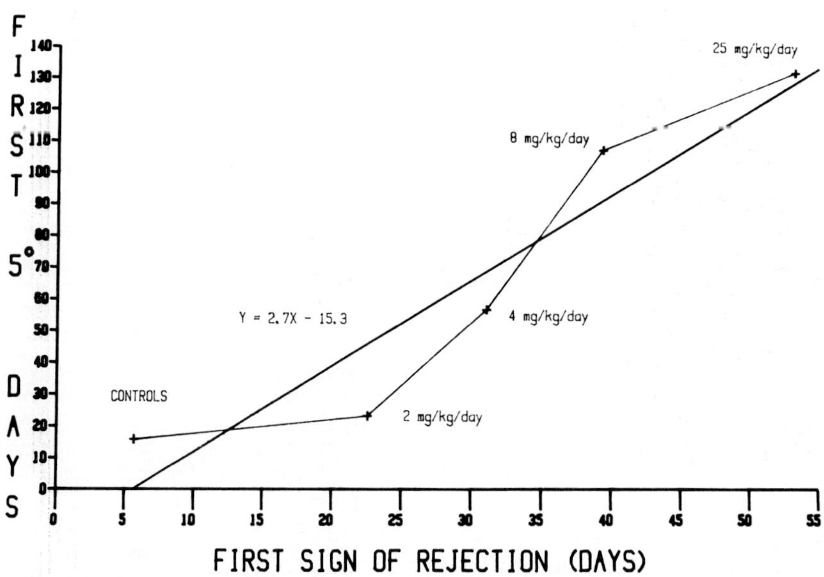

Fig. 1. Composite tissue (limb) allografts demonstrate a linear relationship when the first 5°(F) temperature drop is plotted against the first sign of rejection ($r = .84$).

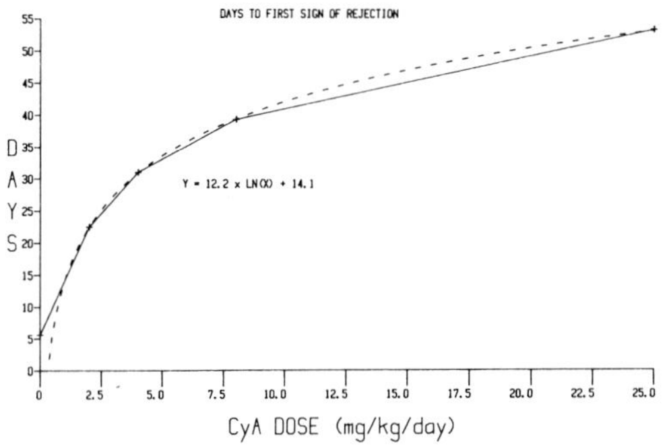

Fig. 2. A logarithmic relationship is demonstrated for a cyclosporine dose response in composite tissue allografts as determined by the first sign of rejection.

DISCUSSION

Most methods to evaluate CT allografts superficially were destined to give the same point: the time when the skin alone loses function. All other structures remain obscured by the altered or necrotic skin.

The fact that the transcutaneous oxygen did not correlate to the first visual signs of rejection might be explained by the findings that although there is no visual rejection evident in the skin there are histological signs of rejection evidenced by cellular infiltrates (13). Transcutaneous oxygen might be a more sensitive monitor of rejection of skin than visual observations, but this would have to be proven with a correlation of transcutaneous oxygen valves and histological examinations.

Many factors influence CPK levels, as well as muscle deterioration. It seems that this

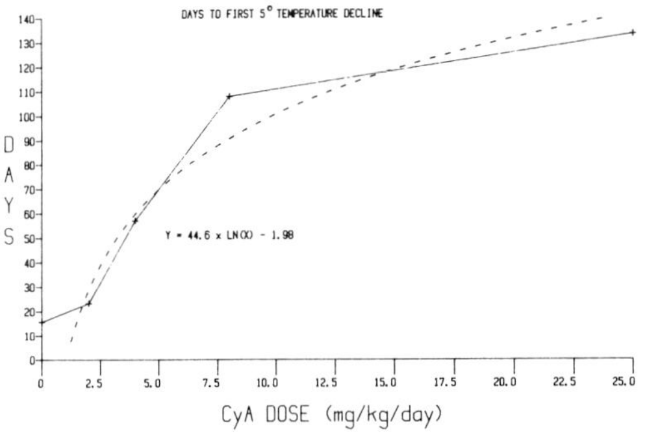

Fig. 3. A logarithmic relationship similar to Fig. 2 for a cyclosporine dose response in composite tissue allografts is demonstrated except this is determined by the first 5°(F) temperature drop of the limb.

background noise has obscured any noticeable correlation with the first sign of rejection.

The return of sensory function was noted only in the animals that had the longer surviving limbs. The rejection process, as determined by the first visual sign, had already begun in most of the animals responsive to painful stimuli. This indicated that the skin could reject and yet up to a point the nerve could continue to function.

Temperature and first sign of rejection have been shown to define a "window" of the rejection process—the first sign of rejection being the initial event and the first 5° temperature drop the later event. These two events seem to remain proportional to one another over a large dose range of CsA, as indicated by the linearity in Fig. 1 and the similarity of the logarithmic relationship demonstrated in Figs. 2 and 3.

We feel that this window might define a time when rejection has begun (first sign) and a time when the rejection process cannot be reversed (first 5° drop). If this is the case, then a rejection crisis can be defined and a necessary dose level of CsA identified that can reverse the crisis. But this will also define when the crisis is irreversible and no amount of CsA can help.

In conclusion, since we are examining a composite tissue allograft, we feel it is necessay to define survival parameters for each of these tissues (muscle, skin, nerves, vessels, bone, and connective tissue) because there is no reason to assume that if one is rejecting, then all will reject at the same time, speed, or at all. We have found the first 5°F drop of the internal temperature of the limb to be the most repeatable and reliable method we have studied to date for the objective evaluation of the rejection process in composite tissue allografts.

ACKNOWLEDGMENTS

We would like to thank Dr. David L. Winter of Sandoz Inc., for generously supplying cyclosporine. We would also like to acknowledge the expert technical assistance provided by Alexander Ingerman, Ben Philosophe, and Ana G. Bejinez, and the editorial assistance provided by Janet Inkster, Erin McLaren, and Christine Black.

REFERENCES

1. Black KS, Hewitt CW, Woodard TL, et al: J Microsurg 3:162, 1982

2. Black KS, Hewitt CW, Fraser LA, et al: N Engl J Med 300:368, 1982

3. Hewitt CW, Black KS, Fraser LA, et al: Transplant Proc 15:514, 1983

4. Siliski JM, Green CJ: N Engl J Med 310:1642, 1982

5. Schwind JV: Ann NY Acad Sci 99:933, 1962

6. Schwind JV: Radiology 78:806, 1962

7. Lance EM, Inglis AE, Figarola F, et al: J Bone Joint Surg 53A:1137, 1971

8. Doi K: Plast Reconstruct Surg 64:613, 1979

9. Porter BB, Lance EM: Clin Orthoped 104:249, 1974

10. Salyer KE, Kyger ER III: Plast Reconstruct Surg 51:672, 1973

11. Poole M, Bowen JE, Batchelor JR: Transplantation 22:108, 1976

12. Goldwyn RM, Beach PM, Feldman D, et al: Plast Reconstruct Surg 37:184, 1966

13. Gratwohl A, Forster I, Speck B: Transplantation 33:361, 1982

Cyclosporine Prolongs Skin Allografts in a Rat Burn Model

B. M. Achauer, C. W. Hewitt, K. S. Black, B. Philosophe, R. L. Linfesty, and D. W. Furnas

A MAJOR problem in massive thermal injuries is the lack of sufficient autograft (autologous skin grafts) to close the burn wound in timely fashion. Skin is a natural barrier to microbes, and its destruction may expose the patient to infection, fluid loss, and nutritional collapse.

There are many types of temporary burn wound coverings available. These include pig skin, synthetic membranes, collagen products, and allografts. Cadaver allografts were first used for burn patients in 1881,[1] but did not become common clinical practice until the 1950s. Because allograft reject 1–2 weeks after they are applied, they are used as biologic dressings and not as permanent grafts. In 1975, Burke introduced the use of allografts in conjunction with conventional immunosuppressants to postpone rejection for 30–60 days.[2] These drugs also suppressed the patient's ability to combat bacterial infections, thereby greatly complicating treatment. Cyclosporine (CsA) apparently does not affect granulocytes and monocytes and, therefore, would be more appropriate for burn patients.[3]

Natural immunosuppression has been demonstrated in both rats and humans who have sustained a severe thermal injury.[4,5] Suggested mechanisms associated with decreased immune responsiveness induced by thermal injury involve suppressor lymphocytes,[6] burn wound toxin,[7] humoral suppressor factors,[8,9] and bacterial endotoxin.[10] These factors could thus affect the dosage and use of immunosuppressive agents in prospective patients receiving skin allografts.

MATERIALS AND METHODS

In this study (Brown Norway × Lewis) F_1 (LBN, $RT1^{l+n}$) were used as skin donors to Lewis (LEW, $Rt1^{l}$) recipients.

Three groups (groups 3–5) of LEW rats underwent a 30% total body surface area (BSA) full-thickness burn by exposure to 90°C water for 10 seconds (Table 1). Groups 4 and 5 were then given partial thickness (BN × LEW) F_1 skin grafts, following primary excision of burned skin 5 days postburn. The first two groups (groups 1 and 2) received no burns and had the same percentage of skin excised surgically. They were immediately grafted with (BN × LEW) F_1 donor skin. Donor skin was harvested with the use of a Padget dermatome at a thickness setting of 0.020 in.

Table 1. Group Characteristics

Group	Number of Rats	Characteristic
1	5	Skin graft
2	7	Skin graft + CsA
3	5	Burn
4	7	Burn + skin graft
5	5	Burn + skin graft + CsA

Group 2 and group 5 received subcutaneous injections of CsA at a dose of 25 mg/kg/day for 20 days. CsA was dissolved in a solution of 20% Tween 80 and 80% ethanol.

Postthermal and surgical injury studies included segmented neutrophil (PMN) counts, white blood cell (WBC) counts, and serum blood urea nitrogen (BUN) levels. Graft survival was monitored daily by direct visual observation. Contracture of the wound and graft was monitored by mapping the graft weekly.

RESULTS

The median survival time of the skin allografts was significantly increased in both CsA groups as compared to controls. The median survival time of group 1 was 8 days; for group 2, 41 days (Table 2). Median survival time for group 4 was 6 days; for group 5, 34 days (Table 3). In both cases, a p value of <0.001 was obtained by the Mann-Whitney U test.

From the Division of Plastic Surgery, University of California, Irvine, CA.

Address reprint requests to Dr. B. M. Achauer, Division of Plastic Surgery, University of California, Irvine, CA 92717.

0041-1345/83/1505-0164$01.00/0

Table 2. LBN Allograft Survival Times in LEW Recipients Treated With Cyclosporine

Group No.	Group	n	Allograft Survival Time (Days)	Median Survival Time (Days)	p†
1	LBN skin (control)	7	6, 7, 7, 8, 8, 9, 9	8	—
2	LBN skin + cyclosporine*	7	36, 37, 40, 41, 41, 41, 42	41	0.001

*Cyclosporine was administered for 20 days at 25 mg/kg/day.
†p Values were determined by the Mann-Whitney U test.

Table 3. LBN Skin Allograft Survival Times in LEW Recipients Receiving a Thermal Injury and Cyclosporine

Group No.	Group	n	Allograft Survival Time (Days)	Median Survival Time (Days)	p†
4	LBN skin + thermal injury*	7	5, 5, 6, 6, 6, 6, 7	6	—
5	LBN skin + thermal injury + cyclosporine‡	5	28, 29, 34, 36, 38*	34	0.001

*Thermal injury consisted of a hot water scald (90°C for 10 sec) over 30% of the total body surface area.
†p Values were obtained by the Mann-Whitney U test.
‡Cyclosporine was administered for 20 days at 25 mg/kg/day.

All groups demonstrated normal WBC counts each week for 5 consecutive weeks during the course of the experiment (Fig. 1). Group 5 demonstrated a transient increase in WBC the first week, but not a significant degree ($p > 0.20$) (Fig. 1, Table 4).

Segmented neutrophil counts were taken weekly. It was observed that no significant differences existed between the groups each week for the duration of the experiment ($p > 0.05$).

Weekly monitoring of BUN levels indicated that the CsA groups were significantly different from the controls. Group 2 showed a transitory increase in BUN levels at week 3 ($p < 0.05$). Group 5 demonstrated an increase

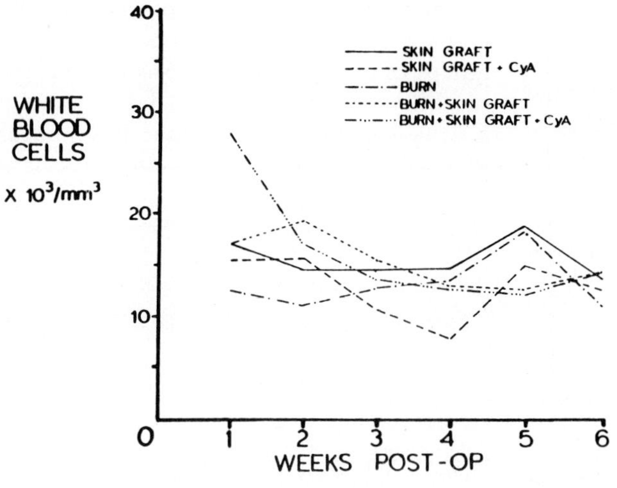

Fig. 1. Mean white blood cell counts ($\times 1000/mm^3$).

Table 4. Standard Error Limits for WBC Counts (×1000/μl)

Group	Weeks 1	2	3	4	5	6
1	3.29	1.25	0.75	3.38	5.85	1.50
2	2.65	3.11	1.15	1.36	1.30	1.47
3	1.03	2.02	1.61	3.03	4.23	2.17
4	2.09	2.03	1.05	0.66	0.54	1.24
5	7.09	1.68	1.19	1.60	4.33	2.21
*p**	<0.20	>0.20	<0.20	<0.20	<0.20	>0.20

*The *p* values were obtained by one-way analysis of variance.

at weeks 4 and 5, which dropped to normal levels by week 6 (Fig. 2; Table 5).

In addition, it was seen that thermally injured rats receiving CsA did not gain a significant amount of weight after an initial drop ($p < 0.05$). All other groups displayed normal weight recovery. The mean weight of group 5 never reached 100% of the original mean, while all others did (Fig. 3; Table 6).

DISCUSSION

CsA dramatically prolonged survival of skin allografts. Massive burns are thought to induce immunosuppression, but group 5 (burn and skin graft and CsA) did not show any additional compromise of the immune system. The experimental animals in group 2 and group 5 rejected their skin grafts at similar rates. Hence, the natural immunosuppression witnessed in other studies was not observed. Differences could be attributed to different strains of rats and to smaller total percent BSA burns.

Nephrotoxicity has been previously associated with high doses of CsA. Thermal injury may also contribute to impaired renal function, therefore BUNs were closely monitored. Both CsA groups displayed significantly ($p < 0.05$) elevated BUN levels. By week 6, the values were normal, indicating reversible toxicity with the removal of the drug. The thermally injured rats (group 5) displayed a longer lasting toxicity once the drug was removed.

The thermally injured rats receiving CsA displayed a significant decrease in weight during CsA administration. By the fifth week, all the other groups were at least at 100% of their original weights, while group 5 was at 84.8% of its original weight. Thermal injury by itself or in conjunction with skin grafts (groups 3 and 4) did not affect weight gain.

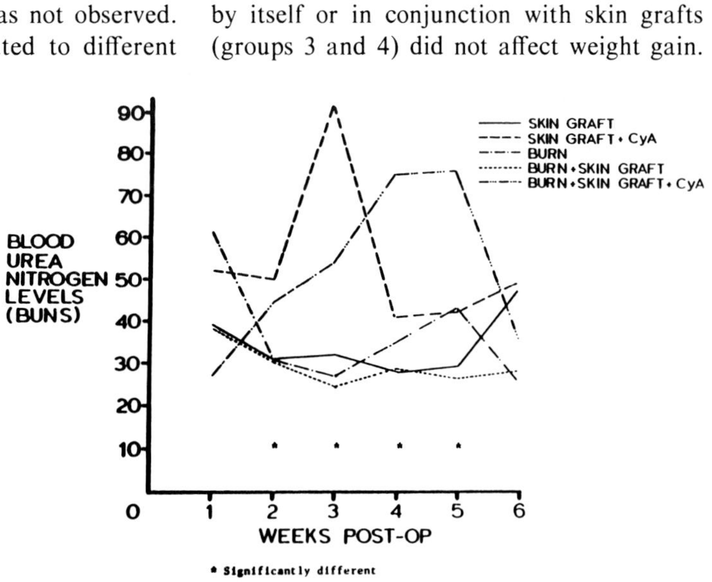

Fig. 2. Mean blood urea nitrogen levels (mg/100 ml). Asterisks represent significant differences at week indicated.

Table 5. Standard Error Limits for BUN Levels (mg/100 ml)

Group	Weeks 1	2	3	4	5	6
1	4.9	6.5	4.7	6.0	3.2	10.2
2	12.1	6.2	19.6	7.1	8.4	8.7
3	21.0	2.8	5.1	9.1	12.9	2.8
4	8.0	2.6	3.1	1.9	1.7	2.2
5	1.1	5.9	15.8	4.9	3.6	1.1
p*	>0.02	<.05	<.005	<.001	<.005	>.05

*p Values were obtained by one-way analysis of variance.

Table 6. Standard Error Limits for Weights

Group	Weeks 1	2	3	4	5	6
1	0.6	1.3	2.2	2.5	3.7	5.2
2	1.0	1.5	2.8	4.2	4.6	5.2
3	3.0	3.9	3.0	4.3	1.6	2.9
4	2.2	2.0	1.6	1.6	0.8	1.3
5	0.9	1.7	2.0	2.9	3.2	3.4
p*	>0.20	<.05	<.001	<.01	<.001	>0.10

*The p values were obtained by one-way analysis of variance.

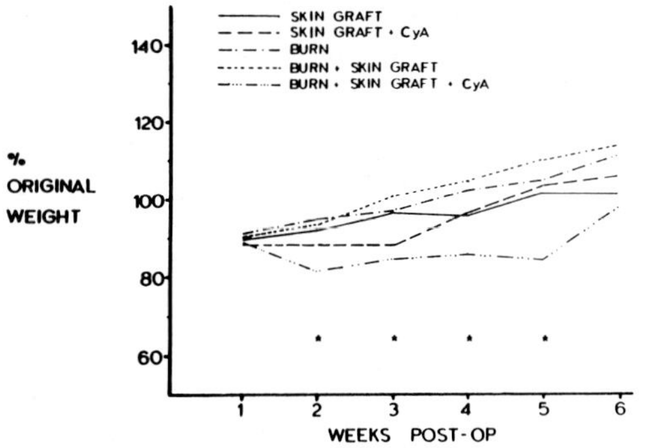

Fig. 3. Mean weight changes as determined by percent original weight. Asterisks represent significant differences at the week indicated.

Neither did skin grafts alone nor with CsA (groups 1 and 2) affect weight gain. Hence, the combination of a thermal injury and the administration of CsA at a dose of 25 mg/kg/day does adversely affect weight gain. This effect appears reversible (the mean weight of group 5 jumped to 98% of the original mean by week 6).

This study demonstrates that CsA is an effective immunosuppressant in preventing skin allograft rejection in a burn model. It did not appear that neutrophil function was affected in the CsA burn model, since neutrophil counts remained normal during the course of the investigation and the rats did not show an increased rate of bacterial infection. This area of research merits more investigation and possibly clinical application.

REFERENCES

1. Girdner JH: Med Rec 20:119, 1881
2. Burke JF, Quinby WC, Bondoe CC, et al: Ann Surg 182:183, 1975
3. Wiesinger P, Borel J: Immunobiology 156:454, 1979
4. Ninnemann JL, Fisher VC, Frank AA: Transplantation 25:69, 1978
5. Ninnemann JL: J Trauma 20:206, 1980
6. Ninnemann JL: Stein MD: J Trauma 20:959, 1978
7. Shoenenburger GA: Monogr Allergy 6:72, 1975
8. Cooperband SR, Davis RC, Mannick JA: J Immunol 109:157, 1972
9. Constantain MB: Ann Surg 188:209, 1978
10. Morrison DC, Ryan JL: Adv Immunol 28:293, 1979

Concomitant Transfusion and Cyclosporine-Induced Enhancement of Rabbit Skin Allografts: Histocompatibility Requirements

G. J. A. Clunie, L. J. Dumble, H. P. King, L. G. Bowes, P. Masendycz, and A. Mirisklavos

SIMULTANEOUS pretransplant donor-specific blood transfusion and immunosuppression have been shown to induce significant allograft enhancement in a number of animal models.[1–3] Some factors that determine the extent of graft enhancement induced by the concomitant treatment have been determined in the rabbit skin allograft model; Cyclosporine-A (CsA) is a more effective immunosuppressant than methylprednisolone with which to amplify blood transfusion-induced graft prolongation,[3] while preoperative treatment induces significantly greater graft enhancement than pretransplant treatment.[4] Although the rabbit model utilizes outbred stains, it is still suitable for investigating the histocompatibility requirements for blood transfusion/CsA-induced allograft enhancement. The experiments reported here utilize preoperative treatment with CsA and transfusion to estimate the possible relevance of histocompatibility (antigen-sharing) between the allograft and blood transfusion donors, and a comparison is made with results obtained where there is histocompatibility between the allograft recipient and the blood transfusion and allograft donor. The reduced effectiveness of third-party blood and CsA, compared with donor-specific blood and CsA, in prolonging skin graft survival indicates that transfusion-induced allograft enhancement is specificity dependent. However, results from donor-specific transfusion experiments indicate that specificities shared by the recipient and transfusion donor may be as important as those shared by the allograft and transfusion donor(s).

MATERIALS AND METHODS

CsA was provided by Sandoz Company, Basel, Switzerland. The crystalline powder was dissolved in olive oil at 50 mg/ml and injected i.m. in a dose of 20 mg/kg. Blood transfusions were collected on the day of administration in preservative-free heparin and transfused (20 ml) via the marginal ear vein to recipients in appropriate animal groups.

Outbred male rabbits (1.5–2.5 kg in weight) were obtained from three genetically distinct (Anglo-lop eared, Belgian half-lop, and New Zealand white) and geographically isolated colonies. Animals from the Belgian half-lop strain were used in a source of third-party transfusion for Anglo-lop eared recipients of a skin allograft from New Zealand white donors. This same donor–recipient strain combination was also treated with donor-specific transfusion from the New Zealand white skin donors. Donor-specific transfusions were also administered to related recipients in a series of mother to offspring (1 haplotype shared) allograft experiments.

Skin from donor animals was grafted to recipients in the manner previously described.[4] Grafts were inspected daily, and rejection time recorded as the day on which 50% necrosis occurred.

Groups of recipient animals for each of the three strain combinations were treated peroperatively with: (1) nil; (2) CsA, 20 mg/kg; (3) blood transfusion, 20 ml; and (4) CsA, 20 mg/kg and blood transfusion, 20 ml.

RESULTS

Comparisons between groups were made using a two-tailed Mann-Whitney U test. Differences at the 5% level ($p < 0.05$) were considered to be statistically significant. Skin allograft survival times in the six animal groups receiving unrelated grafts are shown in Table 1. The mean survival time in group 1 (untreated) animals was 7.1 ± 0.8 days. Peroperative CsA (group 2), donor-specific blood transfusion (group 3), and third-party blood

From the Department of Surgery, Royal Melbourne Hospital, University of Melbourne, Victoria, Australia.

Supported in part by a grant from the Australian Kidney Foundation.

Address reprint requests to Dr. G. J. A. Clunie, Department of Surgery, Royal Melbourne Hospital, University of Melbourne, 3052, Victoria, Australia.

0041–1345/83/1505–0165$01.00/0

Table 1. Effect of Peroperative CsA and/or Blood Transfusion on Unrelated Rabbit Skin Allografts

Group	Treatment	Transfusion Source	Allograft Survival (Days)	Mean Allograft Survival (Days) ± SD
1	Nil	—	6, 6, 7, 7, 7, 8, 8, 8	7.1 ± 0.8
2	CsA	—	11, 11, 11, 12, 12, 13, 13, 17	12.5 ± 2.0
3	Blood transfusion	Donor-specific	6, 7, 7, 8, 10, 16, 16, 19	11.1 ± 5.1
4	Blood transfusion	Third-party	7, 8, 9, 9, 9, 10, 12, 12	9.2 ± 2.2
5	CsA plus blood transfusion	Donor-specific	11, 12, 12, 17, 43, 45, 45, 45	28.8 ± 16.9
6	CsA plus blood transfusion	Third-party	9, 9, 10, 12, 12, 12, 13, 14	11.4 ± 1.8

Allograft prolongation with statistical significance at 5% level:
group 2 compared with group 1, $p < 0.001$ and group 4 $p < 0.02$
group 4 compared with group 1, $p < 0.008$
group 5 compared with group 1, $p < 0.001$, group 3, $p < 0.01$, group 4, $p < 0.004$, and group 6, $p < 0.05$
group 6 compared with group 1, $p < 0.001$

extended mean allograft survival times to 12.5 ± 2.0, 11.1 ± 5.1, and 9.2 ± 2.2 days, respectively. CsA treatment induced allograft prolongation that was statistically significant compared with animals who were untreated (group 1, $p < 0.001$) or who received third-party blood (group 4, $p < 0.02$). The mean survival after third-party blood transfusion (group 4) was statistically significant compared with untreated controls ($p < 0.008$), but donor-specific blood induced a wider range of results, and the mean survival time, 11.1 ± 5.1 days, was not significantly prolonged compared with any other group. Simultaneous preoperative treatment with donor-specific blood and CsA (group 5) induced significant graft enhancement compared with animal groups that were untreated ($p < 0.001$), preoperatively transfused with donor-specific blood ($p < 0.01$) or third-party blood ($p < 0.004$), or treated peroperatively with third-party blood and CsA ($p > 0.05$). The mean survival time in group 5 animals, 28.8 ± 16.9 days, was not statistically different ($p > 0.05$) from that observed in animals treated with CsA alone (group 2). Peroperative CsA and third-party transfusion (group 6) produced only modest graft prolongation, and the mean survival time (11.4 ± 1.8 days) was not statistically different from that observed in animals treated with CsA or blood transfusion alone.

The effect of CsA and/or donor-specific transfusion on skin allograft survival in recipients of related or unrelated skin grafts is shown in Table 2. The related grafts (mother to offspring) are assumed to share transplantation antigens determined by one-haplotype of the histocompatibility complex. The mean survival times (11.3 ± 9.6 and 7.1 ± 0.8 days) in untreated recipients of related (group 1) and unrelated grafts (group 2) were not significantly different from each other. Peroperative CsA treatment significantly prolonged the mean skin survival time of related (group 3) and unrelated grafts (group 4) to 16.6 ± 2.6 and 12.5 ± 2.0 days, respectively, with the treatment being more effective in the related model ($p < 0.008$). The mean graft survival times (12.3 ± 4.1 and 11.1 ± 5.1 days, $p < 0.01$) obtained in preoperatively transfused recipients of related (group 5) and unrelated grafts (group 6) were not significantly prolonged when compared with each other or the untreated control groups. Concomitant treatment with CsA and blood transfusion induced significant graft prolongation (mean > 40.9 ± 11.7 and 28.8 ± 16.9 days) in recipients of related (group 7) and unrelated grafts (group 8). The enhancement in both recipient groups was statistically significant when compared with untreated and similarly blood transfused groups. However, the result in recipients of related grafts was also signifi-

Table 2. Effect of Peroperative CsA and/or Donor-Specific Transfusion on Related and Unrelated Rabbit Skin Allografts

Group	Treatment	Donor–Recipient Relationship	Allograft Survival (Days)	Mean Allograft Survival (Days) ± SD
1	Nil	Mother-to-offspring	7, 7, 7, 8, 8, 9, 9, 35	11.3 ± 9.6
2	Nil	Unrelated	6, 6, 7, 7, 7, 8, 8, 8	7.1 ± 0.8
3	CsA	Mother-to-offspring	13, 14, 15, 17, 19, 19, 19	16.6 ± 2.6
4	CsA	Unrelated	11, 11, 11, 12, 12, 13, 13, 17	12.5 ± 2.0
5	Blood transfusion	Mother-to-offspring	6, 8, 9, 14, 14, 14, 15, 18	12.3 ± 4.1
6	Blood transfusion	Unrelated	6, 7, 7, 8, 10, 16, 16, 19	11.1 ± 5.1
7	CsA plus blood transfusion	Mother-to-offspring	12, >45, >45, >45, >45, >45, >45, >45	>40.9 ± 11.7
8	CsA plus blood transfusion	Unrelated	11, 12, 12, 17, 43, 45, 45, 45	28.8 ± 16.9

Allograft prolongation with statistical significance at 5% level:

group 3 compared with group 1, $p < 0.02$, group 2, $p < 0.002$, and group 4, $p < 0.008$

group 4 compared with group 1, $p < 0.02$, group 2, $p < 0.001$

group 7 compared with group 1, $p < 0.002$, group 2, $p < 0.0009$, group 3, $p < 0.02$, group 4, $p < 0.004$, group 5, $p < 0.005$, group 6, $p < 0.003$, and group 8, $p < 0.008$

group 8 compared with group 1, $p < 0.004$, group 2, $p < 0.001$, group 6, $p < 0.03$

cantly prolonged when compared with CsA treatment of recipients of related and unrelated grafts ($p < 0.02$ and $p < 0.004$), blood transfusion in recipients of unrelated grafts ($p < 0.003$), and CsA and blood transfusion treatment of recipients of unrelated grafts ($p < 0.008$).

DISCUSSION

Concomitant immunosuppression has proved to be a useful means of amplifying pretransplant blood transfusion-induced allograft enhancement, which is not readily demonstrated in animal models.[5] The results in recipients of unrelated skin allografts indicate that peroperative treatment with donor-specific transfusion and CsA promotes significant graft prolongation in the rabbit model. In contrast, peroperative third-party blood and CsA does not induce graft enhancement any further than that achieved by CsA alone. The absence of the transfusion/CsA synergy in the third-party transfusion model indicates that CsA-amplified transfusion-induced graft prolongation is dependent on antigen-sharing between the transfusion and allograft donors. This result implies that the transfusion effect is antigen-specific and would be consistent with the high graft survival rate achieved in one-haplotype-matched related human renal transplants following donor-specific transfusion.[6]

Further information regarding the specific requirements of the transfusate was obtained from the experiments comparing the effect of donor-specific transfusion and CsA on the survival of related and unrelated skin allografts. Results in groups that were untreated or treated with CsA or blood transfusion alone were similar in the two strain combinations, although the allografts are theoretically mismatched for one (related) and two (unrelated) haplotypes determining the histocompatibility antigens. However, the indefinite survival in 7 of 8 recipients of related grafts, peroperatively treated with donor-specific (related) transfusion, may be an indication that antigen sharing between recipient and transfusion donor has a strong influence on graft outcome. It is possible that the induction of allograft enhancement by transfusion, in addition to being antigen-specific with respect to the donor, is also affected by major histocompatibility gene restrictions operative in the recipient. Consequently, in experimental models that favor enhancement at the expense of sensitization, e.g., CsA and transfusion, histocompatibility between recipient and transfusion donor may be an important factor in determining the degree of enhancement achieved. Further experiments are in progress to determine the influence of recipient-related transfusion on unrelated allografts, which could offer wide benefits in clinical situations to prolong survival of human cadaveric transplants.

REFERENCES

1. Homan WP, Williams KA, Millard PR, et al: Transplantation 31:423, 1981

2. Miller CM, Martinelli GP, Racelis D, et al: Transplantation 33:335, 1982

3. Dumble LJ, King HP, Clunie GJA, et al: Transplant Proc 15:1000, 1983

4. King HP, Clunie GJA, Bowes LG, et al: Transplantation 34:299, 1982

5. Okazaki H, Maki T, Wood ML, et al: Transplantation 32:111, 1981

6. Salvatierra O, Iwaki Y, Vincenti F, et al: Transplantation 32:528, 1981

Cyclosporine and Experimental Corneal Transplantation

T. J. Roussel, M. S. Osato, and K. R. Wilhelmus

SINCE the advent of corneal allograft surgery in the early 19th century, progressive advances in technique and instrumentation have permitted technically successful corneal transplantation. Clear corneal grafts, however, may ultimately fail due to immune-mediated allograft rejection. Recent reports indicate that systemic,[1,2] retrobulbar,[3] and topical[4,5] administration of cyclosporine significantly prolongs corneal allograft survival in animals that are primed for rejection either by a skin graft or by eccentric placement of the corneal allograft. Our study was designed to verify that topical ocular administration of cyclosporine delays the onset of corneal allograft rejection in a rabbit model. We also wanted to determine if established rejection could be suppressed by cyclosporine and, if so, whether pretreatment with cyclosporine was a necessary requisite.

MATERIALS AND METHODS

Ten pairs of male outbred rabbits, weighing between 1.7 and 2.5 kg, underwent penetrating keratoplasty. General anesthesia was induced by subcutaneous administration of ketamine hydrochloride (150 mg) and xylazine (15 mg); 5 ml of bovine sodium heparin (1000 U/ml) were administered intravenously via the marginal ear vein to inhibit clotting of the secondary aqueous. All surgery was performed under microscopic visualization, using standard ophthalmic microsurgical instrumentation.

After placement of a lid speculum, a 6-mm trephine was used to cut a partial-thickness corneal button located eccentrically in the superonasal quadrant 1 mm from the limbus. The anterior chamber was entered with a razor blade, and the incision was completed with corneal scissors. Corneal discs were exchanged between animals and secured with a continuous 10-0 nylon suture. Following completion of the corneal surgery, a 3–4-mm midline incision was made in the scalp. The skin was undermined, and a cylindrical osmotic pump (Alza, Palo Alto, CA) with attached polypropylene tubing was inserted in a randomly coded, masked fashion. The tubing was secured to the cartilaginous portion of the nictitating membrane with 7-0 monofilament nylon suture, and the scalp incision was closed with a running 4-0 silk suture.

All animals were examined with the slit-lamp biomicroscope every other day following surgery. Any or all of the following signs were considered to represent onset of allograft rejection: (1) epithelial rejection line, (2) cellular infiltration of a portion of the corneal stroma that had previously been clear, (3) endothelial rejection line. When any of the above were noted, the graft was observed for one additional day to verify progression, at which time the initial osmotic unit was removed and replaced by the second unit containing cyclosporine. These animals were then further observed for signs of suppression or progression of the rejection reaction. Statistical comparisons were analyzed with the Wilcoxon nonparametric two-sample sign ranks test.

Topical Drug Delivery

Cyclosporine, 1% in olive oil (experimental group), or olive oil alone (control group) were delivered to the surface of the operated eye at a continuous rate of 2.5 μl/hr (25 μg/hr) for 28 days via polypropylene tubing connected to the subcutaneous osmotic pump. Following rejection, the osmotic pump was replaced with a second unit that delivered cyclosporine, 5% in olive oil, to the ocular surface at a rate of 10 μl/hr (500 μg/hr) for 7 days.

RESULTS

Three animals from the experimental group were excluded from the study; two because of malfunctioning osmotic pumps and a third because of wound dehiscence. Four of the 7 remaining cyclosporine-treated eyes remained clear at 80 days. In the other 3 eyes, rejection occurred on postoperative day 32 in two animals and day 34 in the third animal. All corneal allografts in the control group underwent rejection by the 27th day, with a mean survival time of 21 ± 1.1 (SEM) days. The onset of rejection of grafts in the experimental group was significantly delayed compared with those of the control group ($p < 0.001$) (Fig. 1).

From the Cullen Eye Institute, Baylor College of Medicine, Houston, TX.

Supported in part by grants from the Sid W. Richardson Foundation and Research to Prevent Blindness, Inc.

Address reprint requests to Ocular Microbiology Laboratory, Cullen Eye Institute, Baylor College of Medicine, Houston, TX 77030.

0041–1345/83/1505–0166$01.00/0

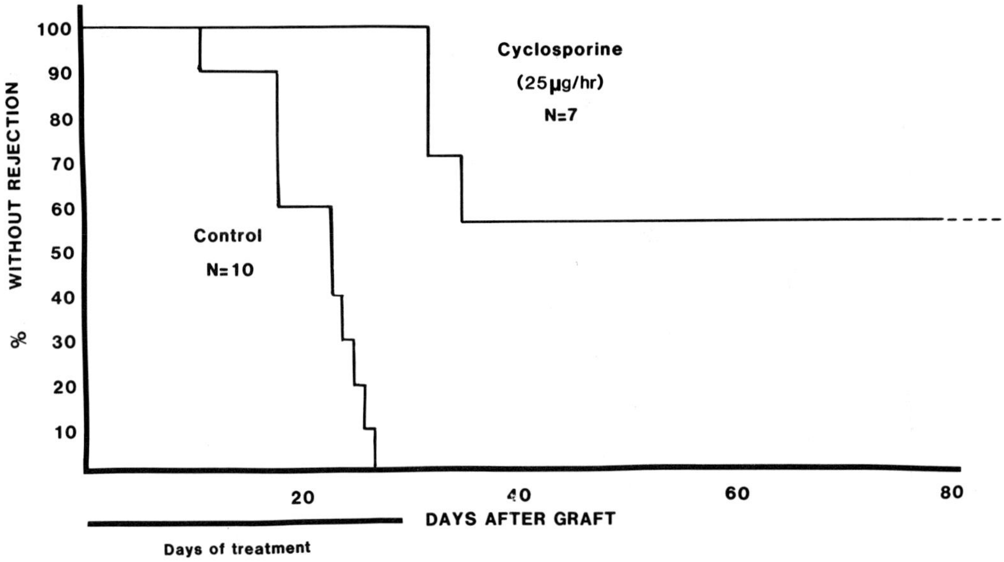

Fig. 1. Comparison of onset of corneal allograft rejection between controls and animals treated with continuous cyclosporine to the ocular surface at 25 μg/hr for 28 days. Difference between groups is statistically significant ($p < 0.001$).

Institution of cyclosporine at a delivery rate of 500 μg/hr failed to alter the course of rejection in control animals; within 5–7 days, all control grafts progressed to complete opacification and vascularization (Fig. 2A). In the cyclosporine-treated animals that subsequently rejected, the reinstitution of topical cyclosporine at 500 μg/hr suppressed the reaction; minimal progression was observed during the 7-day course of additional therapy (Table 1). Although these corneas did not clear completely, translucency improved (Fig. 2B).

DISCUSSION

The delay in rejection produced by cyclosporine following experimental corneal transplantation has been previously reported.[1–5] Our study verifies these observations in a rabbit model that does not require remote-site skin grafting to ensure corneal rejection. These findings suggest that cyclosporine may have a regional effect on antigen recognition or processing following keratoplasty. Although mucous membrane absorption of cyclosporine could produce systemic immunodulation, the average total daily dose of 0.3 mg/kg/day administered topically to our animals is far less than that utilized by other investigators to suppress corneal rejection.[1,2,4] Because 4 of 7 (57%) cyclosporine-treated animals had no signs of rejection and maintained clear grafts, we suspect that limited topical therapy may induce prolonged tolerance in some animals.

We have demonstrated for the first time that topical cyclosporine can suppress the corneal graft reaction after it begins. This effect, however, is limited to those animals who had previously received cyclosporine. These findings are consistent with those of Deeg,[6] who found that systemic cyclosporine begun on the day of surgery prevented skin allograft rejection, but discontinuation of the agent allowed rejection to occur; reinstitution of cyclosporine reversed first, second, and third rejection episodes.

Allograft rejection in control animals rapidly proceeded to complete opacification of donor tissue, despite subsequent topical cyclosporine administration. Previous reports regarding transplantation of other tissues have similarly shown that allograft reactions

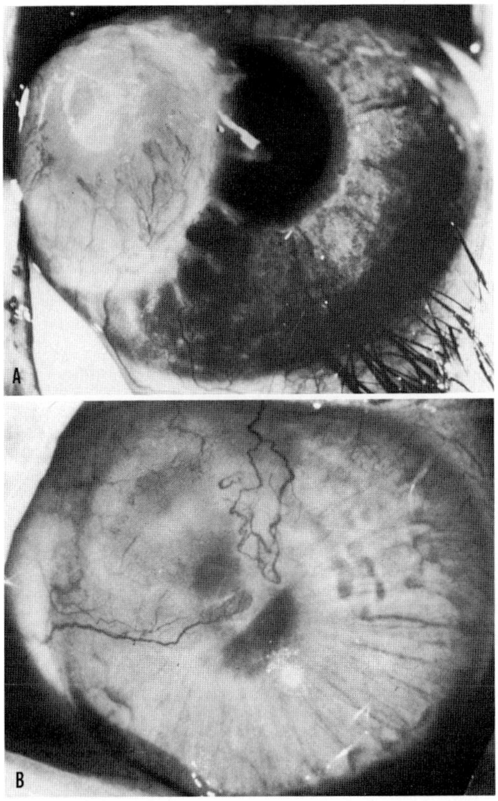

Fig. 2. Comparison of peripheral corneal allografts 10 days after onset of rejection following a 7-day course of cyclosporine to the ocular surface at 500 μg/hr, beginning at onset of rejection. Control graft (A) developed complete opacification and vascularization, while experimental eye (B), pretreated with cyclosporine, maintains central graft clarity.

Table 1. Effects of Cyclosporine on Corneal Allograft Rejection

	Control Group	Cyclosporine Group
Allograft reaction	10/10 (100%)	3/7 (43%)
Suppression of allograft reaction with CsA	0/10 (0%)	3/3 (100%)

are not generally inhibited by cyclosporine, even if the drug is begun as early as 4 days after transplantation.[7] Also, because 3 of 7 (43%) experimental corneal grafts rejected soon after discontinuation of topical cyclosporine, but prior to regression of neovascularization (usually complete by the fifth to sixth week), we suggest that cyclosporine prevents rejection in the presence of vascularization and should probably be administered until neovascularization regresses.

We conclude that, in our rabbit model, topical cyclosporine is effective in prolonging corneal allograft survival. It can also suppress an established allograft reaction in eyes that have had previous exposure to this agent during the early postoperative period. The osmotic infusion pump system could be used in further animal studies to determine the optimal drug delivery rate required to suppress corneal allograft rejection. Clinical trials are needed to verify the efficacy of this agent in human corneal transplantation.

REFERENCES

1. Coster DJ, Shepherd WFI, Chin Hook T, et al: Lancet 2:688, 1979

2. Bell TAG, Easty DL, McCullagh KG: Br J Ophthalmol 66:303, 1982

3. Salisbury JD, Gebhardt BM: Arch Ophthalmol 99:1640, 1981

4. Hunter PA, Garner A, Wilhelmus KR, et al: Br J Ophthalmol 66:292, 1982

5. Kana JS, Hoffmann F, Buchen R, et al: Invest Ophthalmol Vis Sci 22:686, 1982

6. Deeg HJ, Storb R, Gerhard-Miller L, et al: Transplantation 29:230, 1980

7. Homarn WP, Fabre JW, Williams KA, et al: Transplantation 29:361, 1980

Improved Survival of Venous Allografts in Dogs Following Graft Pretreatment With Cyclosporine

K. O. Bandlien, L. H. Toledo-Pereyra, M. I. Barnhart, S. P. Choudbury, A. Diaz-Velez, G. H. MacKenzie, and J. A. Cortez

THE venous allograft represents a fascinating alternative to the artificial prothesis for reconstruction of peripheral vessels in cases where autografts are not available secondary to previous vein stripping and/or diseased peripheral veins. An intensive search for methods of reducing the antigenicity of vein grafts was started more than 2 decades ago in an attempt to prevent the otherwise inevitable rejection and occlusion of the grafts.[1-3]

A great number of different treatment modalities has been investigated; however, lack of potency of the conventional immunosuppressive regimens and their inability to consistently prolong vascular allograft survival has been discouraging.[4,5] Cyclosporine (CsA) represents a new highly potent immunosuppressive drug, and our objective in this study has been to investigate its effect on venous allograft survival when utilized as a pretreatment modality. Recent results from our own laboratory indicate a prolongation of allograft survival following graft pretreatment with CsA in a variety of experimental models.[6-8]

MATERIALS AND METHODS

Sixty-six mongrel dogs, weighing between 12 and 25 kg, were utilized in this study. Under general anesthesia, using sodium thianyl (1.25 mg/kg) for induction and flurothane (0.5%–2%) for maintenance, the jugular vein of each donor animal was exposed, and under aseptic technique, a 5–6-cm segment was excised. The vein grafts were subsequently flushed with 100 cc of plasma protein fraction (PPF) at 4°C. The grafts then underwent various modalities of pretreatment before they were implanted into the common carotid artery of a different animal. In the recipient animal, a 4–5 cm segment of the carotid artery was excised, and the venous allograft was implanted in the artery in an end-to-end fashion, using 6–0 prolene running suture.

Postoperatively, the animals were all given i.v. penicillin (250,000 U) for 3 subsequent days. No anticoagulants were administered. Animals that died during the surgical procedure or on the day of surgery were excluded from the study.

During the follow-up period, the animals were examined weekly with a Doppler flowmeter to determine the patency of the grafts. If a graft was found to be occluded, the dog was killed and the graft was studied macroscopically and by light microscopy. If the Doppler studies were equivocal, the grafts were explored and patency determined by direct palpation.

Grafts that were patent at the time of sacrifice were also submitted for scanning electron microscopy (SEM) to determine the degree of intimal changes in the transplanted vein grafts. SEM was further utilized to examine the grafts for intimal changes caused by the various modalities of pretreatment.

Electron Microscopy Preparation

The veins were grasped at one end with forceps and repeatedly immersed in 0.06 *M* cacodylate-buffered 1% glutaraldehyde adjusted to pH 7.4 and 300 mosmole. Immersion fixation was selected because we wanted to compare the stored frozen vein, which had to be stored in the collapsed state, with the transplanted frozen-thawed veins that survived for various periods in the live dogs. Fixation by immersion in fresh glutaraldehyde continued for 18–24 hr in a refrigerator at 4°C. The fixed veins were next cut longitudinally along a midline axis using iris scissors. The half vein segments were placed for several more hours in fresh glutaraldehyde. Next, the vein segments were gently flattened while being placed between filter paper. The paper was stapled together to ensure maintenance of the flattened state through the dehydration and critical-point drying processes. Such preparations were returned to fresh glutaraldehyde for several hours. Dehydration was accomplished by sequently passing the paper-shrouded veins through 70%, 85%, 95%, 100%, and a second time in 100% ethanol solutions prior

---

From the Department of Surgery, Mount Carmel Mercy Hospital, and the Department of Physiology, Wayne State University, Detroit, MI.

Supported in part by an Institutional Grant from the Mount Carmel Research and Educational Corporation and from the Bargman Laboratory for Cell and Molecular Research.

Address reprint requests to Dr. L. H. Toledo-Pereyra, Department of Surgery, Mount Carmel Mercy Hospital, 6071 West Outer Drive, Detroit, MI 48235.

0041–1345/83/1505–0167$01.00/0

to critical-point drying in CO_2. Specimens were sputter-coated with gold after mounting on aluminum stubs which were stored in a dessicator until ready to examine in an ETEC Autoscan microscope at 10 kV and tilting to 30° for regular display by secondary electron imaging (SEI) or to 10° for backscatter electron imaging (BEI).

For backscatter electron imaging to visualize endothelial cell nuclei, methenamine silver reduction staining was used after glutaraldehyde fixation, as previously reported by Becker and Sogard[9] and Sedar, Silver, and Ingerman-Wojenski.[10] Glutaraldehyde-fixed specimens were rinsed repeatedly throughout the day in at least 6 changes of cacodylate buffer and left immersed overnight in fresh cacodylate buffer at 4°C. The veins were rinsed for 20 min in distilled water using 5 changes, then stained 5 min in methenamine silver solution: 20 ml GSM stock (5 ml of 5% silver nitrate added dropwise to 100 ml of 3% methenamine), 20 ml distilled water, and 1.5 ml of 5% sodium borate. This solution was replaced with fresh solution and placed in a 50°C water bath until the solution became gray and the specimens turned brown (about 1 hr). Specimens were next washed in 100 ml of fresh distilled water for 10 min with 5 repetitions. The staining and rinsing procedures were repeated, and the specimens next treated for 10 min with 5% sodium thiosulfate. After rising for 10 min in distilled water (5 changes), the specimens were dehydrated in ethanol. The absolute ethanol was replaced with ethanol:amyl acetate 50:50 (v:v) and then with absolute amyl acetate. The specimens were critical-point dried, using CO_2 as the intermediate fluid. The backscatter detector (G & W Electronics, Inc., Norcross, GA30092) in an ETEC scanning electron microscope was used at magnifications of 300–3000×, with inverted signal polarity and an accelerating voltage of 10 kV and 10° tilt.

Experimental Groups

Group I (n = 11) served as a control group, and the animals received fresh allografts without pretreatment or subsequent immunosuppression. Group II (n = 5) consisted of animals that received fresh allografts, as in group I, followed by mild immunosuppression with azathioprine (2.5 mg/kg/day) for the duration of the study.

Group III (n = 5) consisted of animals that received venous allografts cryopreserved in 25 cc of a 15% dimethyl sulfoxide (DMSO) solution in human plasma protein fraction (PPF) by −196°C for 22–55 days prior to implantation. (Small plastic containers containing the graft and the cryopreservative were immersed in liquid nitrogen.)

Group IV (n = 5) received venous allografts that had been flushed with 100 cc of a 15% DMSO solution in PPF containing cyclosporine (CsA) at 50 mg/liter at 4°C and subsequently cryopreserved as in group III in the same solution as was used for flushing.

Group V (n = 15) received venous allografts that had been cryopreserved as in group IV. The animals in this group subsequently received mild systemic immunosuppression with azathioprine at 2.5 mg/kg/day.

Group VI (n = 10) consisted of animals receiving venous allografts that had been stored in a PPF solution containing CsA at 50 mg/liter for 24 hr at 4°C prior to implantation. The animals then received mild immunosuppressive therapy, as in group V.

Group VII (n = 15) consisted of animals that received fresh allografts and subsequently were treated with CsA in olive oil orally for a total of 4 weeks following the vein transplantation (20 mg/kg/day for the first 2 weeks, then 15 mg/kg/day for the following 2 weeks). First oral dose was given 3 hr prior to transplantation. No further immunosuppressive therapy was administered after cessation of the CsA.

RESULTS

Graft Survival

Table 1 gives an overview of all the animals involved in the study and the patency rates of their vein grafts at different time intervals.

In the control groups (n = 11), one dog was killed at 1 week with a patent graft. At 2 weeks, 4 of the remaining 10 grafts were found to be occluded, and after 4 weeks, only 3 grafts remained open. None of the grafts in the control group were found to be open beyond 8 weeks. In group II (n = 5), 2 grafts thrombosed after one week, and at 1 month, the remaining 3 grafts were also found to be closed. In group III (n = 5), one graft occluded after 3 weeks and 2 more occluded at 7 weeks. Only one graft in this group remained open beyond 2 months. In group IV (n = 5), one dog died with a patent graft in the fifth postoperative week. At 8 weeks, 3 of 4 remaining grafts proved to be patent. In group V (n = 15), 2 dogs died on the third day after surgery with patent grafts. All the remaining 13 dogs were found to have patent grafts at 1 month. However, 7 animals died of unrelated causes between 5 and 7 weeks postoperatively. All but one of the grafts in these animals were found to be open on postmortem examination. All the remaining grafts in this group were open at 2 months. In group VI (n = 10), 2 grafts were closed at 1 week. Two dogs died of unrelated causes after 1 week, as did one other dog after 3 weeks; all 3 animals had patent grafts at time of death. After 4 weeks, one

Table 1. Experimental Results

	1 Week	2 Weeks	3 Weeks	4 Weeks	5 Weeks	6 Weeks	7 Weeks	8 Weeks
Group I (*n* = 11)	11 / 11*	6 / 10	6 / 6	3 / 6	3 / 3	3 / 3	3 / 3	0 / 3
Group II (*n* = 5)	3 / 5	3 / 3	3 / 3	0 / 3	0 / 0	0 / 0	0 / 0	0 / 0
Group III (*n* = 5)	5 / 5	5 / 5	4 / 5	4 / 4	4 / 4	4 / 4	2 / 4	1 / 2
Group IV (*n* = 5)	5 / 5	5 / 5	5 / 5	5 / 5	4 / 4	4 / 4	4 / 4	3 / 4
Group V (*n* = 15)	13 / 13	13 / 13	13 / 13	13 / 13	10 / 10	8 / 8	4 / 5	4 / 4
Group VI (*n* = 10)	8 / 10	6 / 6	5 / 5	4 / 5	4 / 4	4 / 4	4 / 4	4 / 4
Group VII (*n* = 15)	15 / 15	9 / 9	5 / 5	5 / 5	5 / 5	4 / 5	4 / 4	4 / 4

*Numbers indicate no. of patent grafts divided by no. of animals at risk at various time intervals.

graft was found to be occluded and the dog was killed. The grafts of the remaining 4 dogs were all patent at 8 weeks. In group VII (*n* = 15), all grafts were patent after 1 week; however, between 2 and 3 weeks, a total of 10 animals died of unrelated causes (distemper, intussusception, heart worms, unknown), all of which had patent grafts when explored. One graft showed thrombosis after 6 weeks and was excised. The four remaining animals in this group all had patent grafts at 8 weeks. Figure 1 shows a comparison of the effects of the different modalities of pretreatment on graft survival.

Light Microscopy Studies

The comparison of the vein grafts from various groups by light microscopy at time of death or sacrifice of the animals showed a pronounced difference of the findings between the control groups and the treatment groups. The marked cellular infiltration and the significant degenerative changes seen in group I, and to a lesser degree in groups II and III, were markedly reduced in groups IV–VII, in which CsA had been utilized.

SEM Studies

The fresh fixed veins in group I, which were studied prior to implantation, showed a lining of endothelial cells that displayed small microvilli and bulging nuclei, since fixation was in the collapsed state (Fig. 2). The nuclei were oriented in the direction of blood flow, as occurs in other normal vessels. The creases and folds of the luminal lining are artifacts due to the contraction of the muscle layers upon excising the vein and during fixation of the vein segments without the vein pinned to its in vivo length.

The endothelial lining of the veins in group III, which were stored frozen in the presence

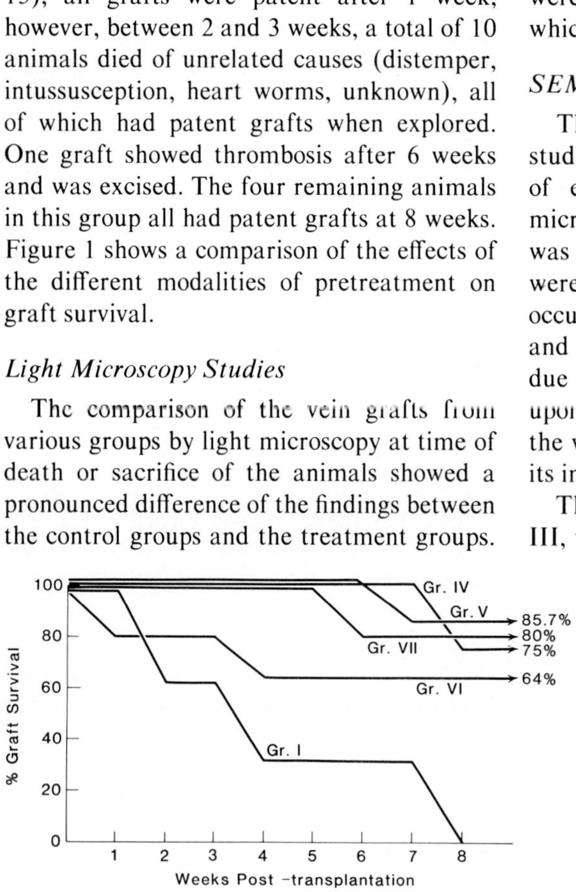

Fig. 1. Comparison of the effect of various modalities of pretreatment on graft survival.

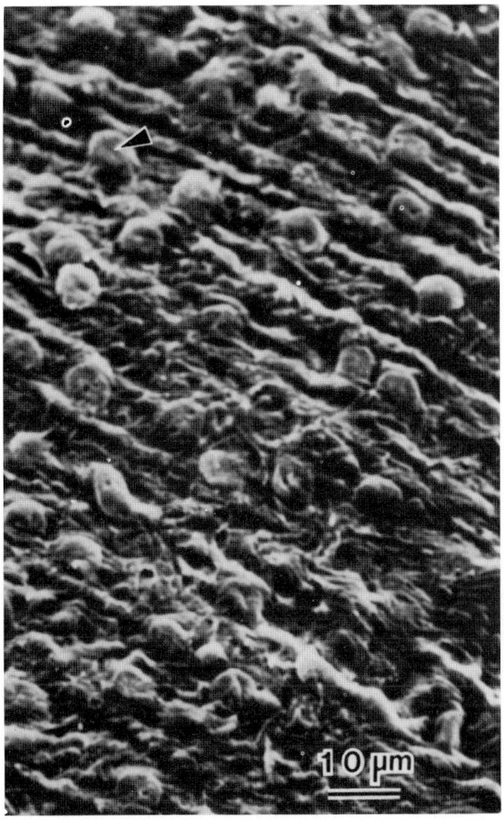

Fig. 2. Luminal surface of a glutaraldehyde-fixed, fresh, normal jugular vein. The bulges (arrowhead) overlay the endothelial cell nuclei.

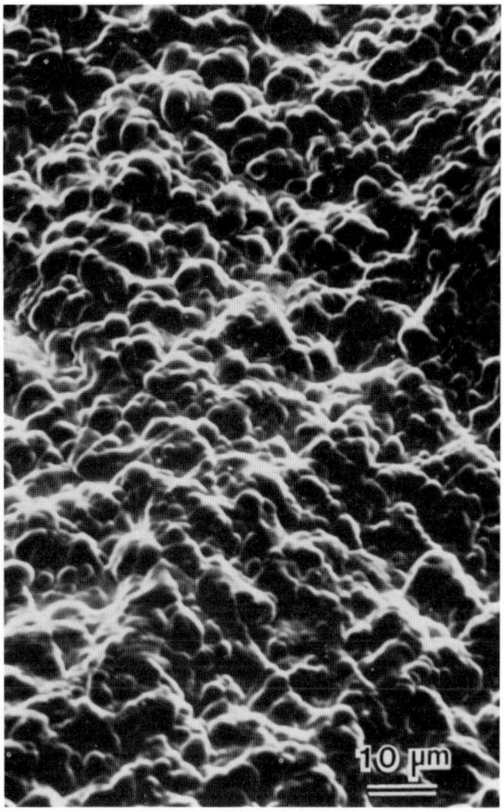

Fig. 3. Luminal surface of vein stored frozen in DMSO for 1 month (group III).

of DMSO for 1 month, remained intact according to information gained using SEM. Endothelial bulges were observed, but only some of these were over the endothelial cell nuclei (Fig. 3). Proof that the lining consisted of nucleated endothelium was gained using silver staining and BEI (Fig. 4). The only allograft that remained open in this group was examined by SEM at 2 months after implantation and revealed a lining with patches of endothelium but also fibrin deposition with adherent platelets and trapped red cells (Fig. 5).

In groups IV and V, the endothelial lining appeared relatively intact, with nuclei easily demonstrated by BEI in veins stored frozen in DMSO and CsA for 1, 2, and 3 months prior to implantation.

Two different vein allografts, from group IV in place for 2 months, were examined by SEI and BEI. The endothelium appeared intact, and endothelial cells displayed microvilli and compared favorably with normal fresh control veins (Fig. 6). Nuclei were well defined by the silver stain using BEI (Fig. 7).

The one allograft studied in group V at 2 months after implantation showed an intact endothelium with some nuclei displayed by the silver stain and BEI. An occasional red cell adhered to the vein's lining (Fig. 8). However, no significant differences were noted between the patent allografts of groups IV and V.

DISCUSSION

The findings of the SEM study should be considered as qualitative and preliminary,

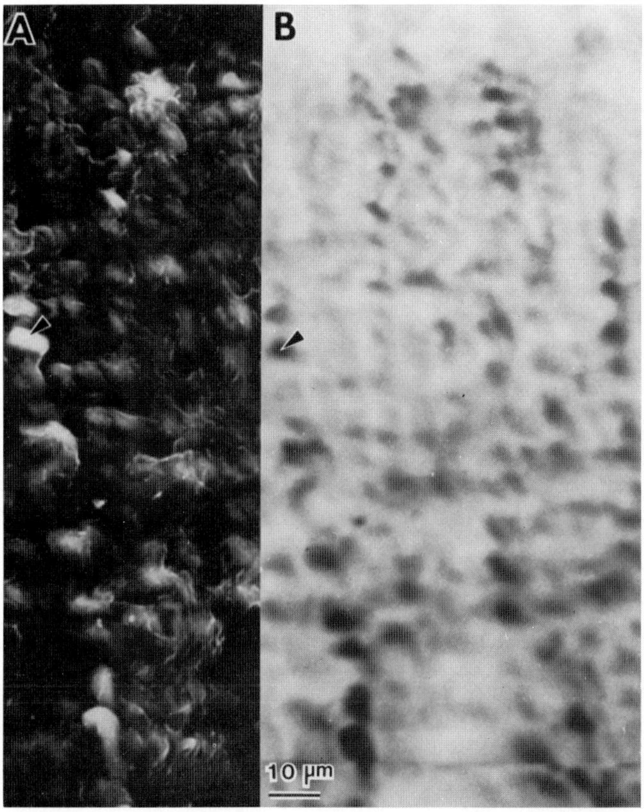

Fig. 4. Companion scanning electron micrographs (same magnification) of a silver-methenamine-stained jugular vein after DMSO storage for 1 month. (A) Secondary electron imaging of endothelial lining. Surface features and the underlying nuclei (arrowhead) are indicated by the brightest images. (B) Backscatter electron imaging of the same venous area plus the adjacent area was done with reversed polarity in order to provide an image somewhat similar to that achieved by light microscopy of histologic specimens. Match the black nuclear patterns of panel B with the bright images in panel A.

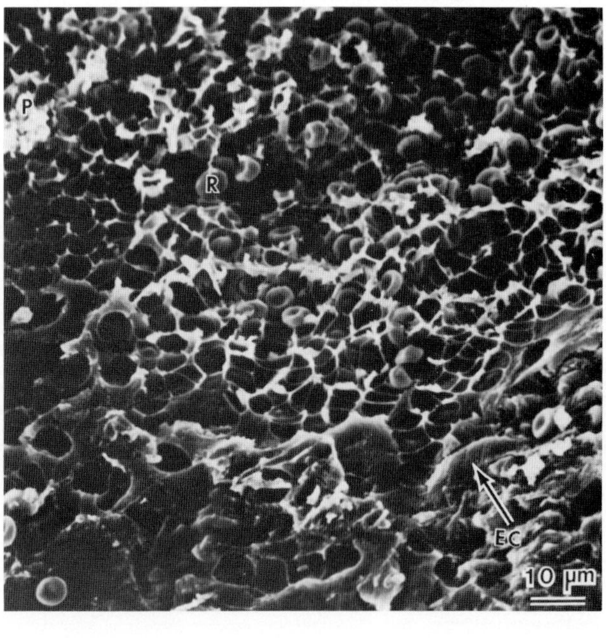

Fig. 5. Note the fibrin (bright) network spread over much of the luminal surface of this DMSO allograft in situ for over 2 months (group III). An area of endothelial cells (EC) is displayed in the lower part of the micrograph. Aggregates of platelets (P) appear in the upper left and also to the left of the arrow. Red (R) cells are caught in the fibrin thrombus.

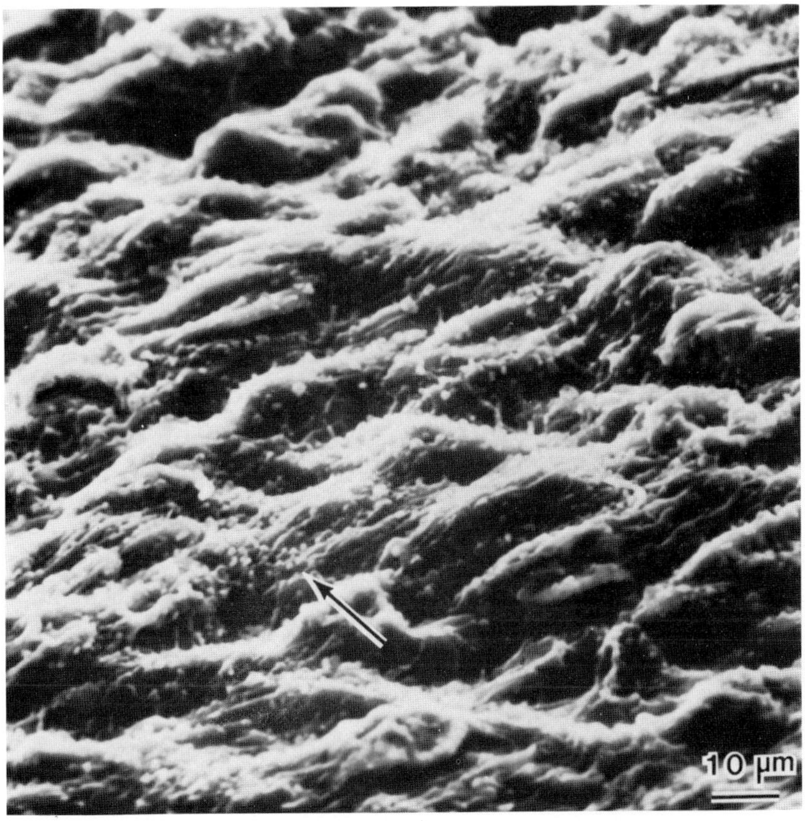

Fig. 6. Conventional scanning electron micrograph of the lining of an allograft from a group IV dog. Note the intact endothelial cell lining with prominent microvilli (arrow). This allograft was in the dog for 2 months.

since only one or two jugular vein segments before and after allografting from groups I, III, IV, and V were studied. It was demonstrated that the endothelium appears to be fairly well preserved and still in place after frozen storage in the presence of DMSO and cyclosporine for periods up to 3 months. This confirms and extends the findings of Weber, Lindenauer, and others regarding DMSO cryopreservation.[11,12] The allografted veins studied after 2 months in 5 dogs appeared to have intact endothelium, and nuclei were evident by BEI of silver-stained specimens. However, the distortions in the vein linings by the selected means of fixation prevents any quantitative judgments. Future studies will involve reexpansion of frozen stored veins using PPF and the physiologic pressure expected after the allografts are secured in vivo. Then glutaraldehyde fixation will also be done using the same perfusion pressure. Such preparations can then be evaluated quantitatively for loss of endothelial cells resulting from the frozen storage procedure. Similarly, allografts in place for various times can be fixed in situ using perfusion fixation procedure and the number of endothelial cells quantified. Certain added techniques may permit an accurate assessment to be made of the numbers of recipient endothelial cells versus retained donor endothelial cells.

The results show that CsA protects the venous allograft from early rejection and occlusion when the graft is exposed to the drug prior to implantation in the recipient animal.

The results in the control group are conclu-

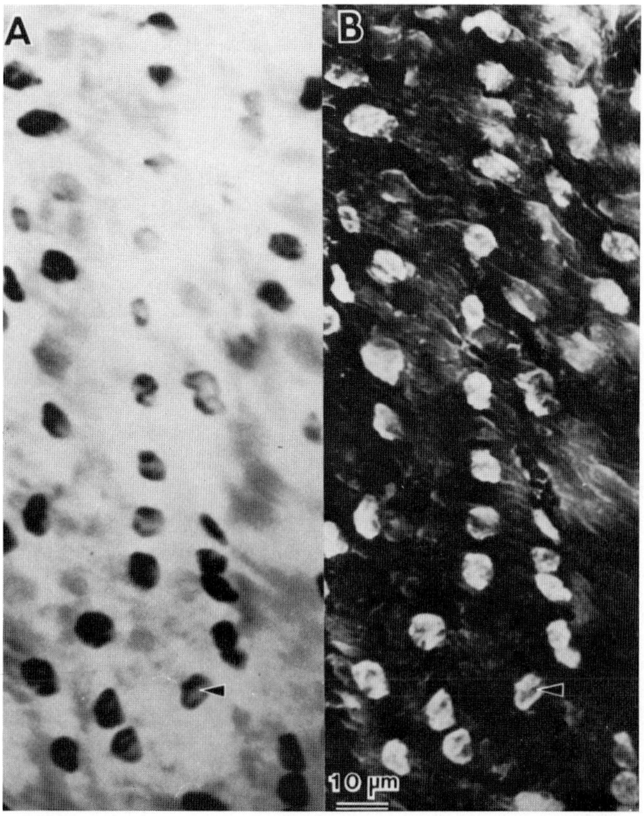

Fig. 7. Matched micrographs from another jugular vein allograft (from group IV). (A) A view by backscatter detection that reveals the internal silver-stained nuclei (arrowhead). (B) The secondary electron image of the surface of the same area. The pattern of endothelial cell nuclei is perfectly matched in panels A and B.

sive of a massive rejection of the venous allograft when introduced to a nonhistocompatible host without any immunosuppressive protection. However, mild systemic immunosuppression with azothioprine, as given in group II, is apparently not sufficient to prolong venous allograft survival significantly.

Most interesting is the relatively high early patency rate of the veins in group III, which were cryopreserved with DMSO alone prior to implantation. The patency rate at 6 weeks approaches those of the CsA-pretreated groups; however, it drops drastically between 6 and 8 weeks and subsequently shows little difference to the control group.

The early posttransplant survival of the grafts in group VI, in which the grafts were pretreated with CsA in cold storage, appears to be similar to that of group III. However, all the grafts that were open at 6 weeks remained open beyond 8 weeks. This observation might be explained by the ability of DMSO cryopreservation to preserve a smooth and intact endothelial layer with reduced suceptibility for early thrombosis, without affecting the antigencity of the graft and thus the inevitable rejection. On the other hand, it is likely that the improved results in group VI is a reflection of reduced antigenicity of the allografts with subsequent prolonged survival. This theory is supported by our light microscopy and SEM studies, which show evidence of a marked reduction in cellular infiltration and degenerative changes in the CsA-treated groups.

The most promising results with prospects for future clinical application are undoubtedly to be found in the groups IV and V. These results indicate an enhanced effect of CsA pretreatment by DMSO cryopreservation and make a future establishment of vein banks perceivable. The patency rates of the grafts pretreated with the combination of CsA and

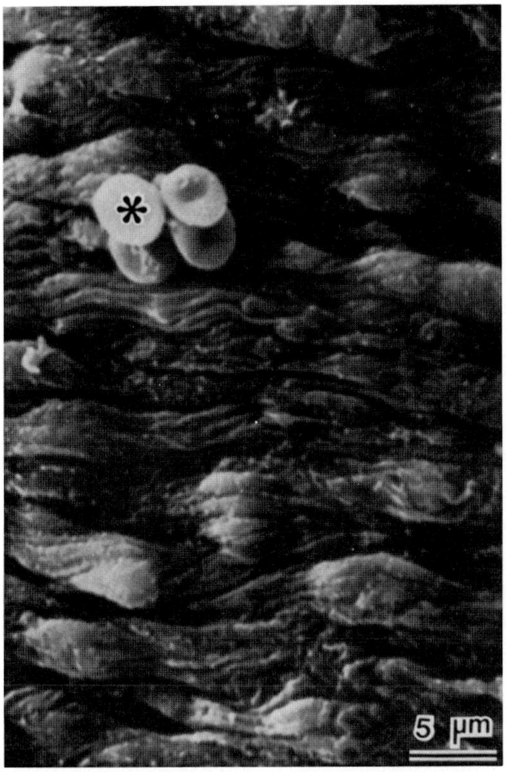

Fig. 8. Another jugular vein allograft after 2 months in the dog (group V). Again, a relatively intact luminal lining of endothelial cells is present. Microvilli appear on endothelial cells that also have bright bulges, indicating the internal silver-stained nuclei. A clump of red cells (*) are in the center of the field.

DMSO cryopreservation (groups IV and V) compare well with those that were protected by systemic CsA during the first 4 weeks of implantation (group VII).

The observation that grafts that remained open for a critical period of 6–8 weeks all showed long-term patency may be related to the process of repopulation of the intima with host-specific endothelial cells and the subsequent reduced antigenicity of the grafts.[13]

This study strongly suggests that the effect of CsA as an immunosuppressant is exhibited not only at the site of the proliferation of alloreactive cells, but also in the allograft as well. We postulate an actual binding of the CsA molecule to the surface of the endothelial cells of the graft, with possible masking of surface antigens and subsequent interference with recognition and early immune response. When considering the endothelium–host blood interface as the initial site of graft–host confrontation, we believe these results warrant further investigation of the place of the endothelial cell in the process of allograft rejection.

ACKNOWLEDGMENTS

Mr. H. L. Hill and Mrs. D. MacKinnon are acknowledged for technical assistance and aid in completion of this paper.

Cyclosporine was a gift from Sandoz, Inc.

REFERENCES

1. Perlhoff JL, Rechard CR, Rowlands DT, et al: Surgery 72:961, 1972
2. Barner HA, DeWeese JA, Schenk EA: Angiology 17:389, 1966
3. Mieny CJ: S Afr Med J 42:798, 1968
4. Ricotta JJ, Collins GF Jr, Rich HM, et al: Arch Surg 115:99, 1980
5. Calhoun AD, Bauer GM, Porter FM, et al: J Surg Res 22:687, 1977
6. Toledo-Pereyra LH, MacKenzie GH, Gordon DA, et al: Transplantation 33:329, 1982
7. Toledo-Pereyra LH, MacKenzie GH, Gordon DA, et al: Am Surg 49:261, 1983
8. Toledo-Pereyra LH, Gordon DA, MacKenzie GH, et al: Surg Gynecol Obstet (in press)
9. Becker RP, Sogard M: Scan Electron Micros 2:835, 1979
10. Sedar AW, Silver MJ, Ingerman-Wojenski CM: Scan Electron Micros (in press)
11. Weber RR, Lindenauer SM, Dent TC, et al: Ann Surg 184:706, 1976
12. L'Italien GJ, Maloney RD, Abbott WM, et al: J Surg Res 27:239, 1979
13. William GM, Krajerski CA, Dagher FJ, et al: Transplant Proc 3:869, 1971

Effect of Cyclosporine on Wound Healing

J. Ahonen, A. Nemlander, K. Wiktorowicz, E. von Willebrand, R. Hekali, M. Lalla, and P. Häyry

GLUCOCORTICOSTEROIDS delay wound healing by affecting the early inflammatory reaction. This is a potential source of complications in organ transplantation. In this study, we have compared the effects of methylprednisolone (MP) to cyclosporine (CsA) on the formation of granulation tissue in subcutaneously implanted viscose cellulose sponges, which is a commonly used model for studies on wound healing.

MATERIALS AND METHODS

Granulation tissue formation was induced by subcutaneous implantation of four viscose cellulose sponges in Spraque-Dawley rats under ether anesthesia. Postoperatively, the rats were given CsA 40, 10, or 2.5 mg/kg intraperitoneally once a day. Rats receiving MP (12 mg/kg/day) or CsA solvent were also studied, as were saline-treated controls.

The animals were killed and the sponges removed 4, 7, or 10 days after the operation. In some sponges, the infiltrating cells were released by compression and the exudate collected. After lysing red cells, smears were made with a cytocentrifuge and stained. Some of the sponges were used for chemical analysis of the relevant granulation tissue components: determination of DNA for the total amount of cells, acid phosphatase and B-glucuronidase for quantitation of macrophages, hydroxyproline for collagen accumulation, and hemoglobin for the quantitation of the development of new vascularity into the granulation tissue. The trough level of CsA was measured by radioimmunoassay.

RESULTS

The CsA concentrations obtained were quite high, ranging from 10,000 ng/ml in the group receiving 40 mg/kg/day to 3000 ng/ml in the group receiving 2.5 mg/kg/day. CsA treatment did not affect the total number of cells in granulation tissue. Instead, a clear reduction in the total cell number (DNA determination) and in the number of inflammatory cells was observed in the group receiving MP on days 4 and 7 ($p = 0.025$ and $p = 0.004$, respectively, when compared with the controls); on day 10, these differences balanced. Differential count of the inflammatory cells on day 7 revealed no major differences between the groups, except for a somewhat higher frequency of macrophages in the CsA groups when compared with the others. However, the *total* number of monocytes and macrophages was clearly lower in the MP-treated granulation tissue than in other groups, which is also reflected in the low contents of beta-glucuronidase and acid phosphatase ($p = 0.019$ and $p = 0.001$, respectively, when compared with the controls).

CsA did not reduce the accumulation of collagen, measured as hydroxyproline into the granulation tissue, as MP did. Indeed, there was a tendency, which did not reach the level of statistical significance, of higher hydroxyproline amounts in the groups receiving 10 and 2.5 mg/kg/day of CsA than in the controls. The content of hemoglobin was significantly higher in the groups receiving 10 and 2.5 mg/kg/day of CsA when compared to controls ($p = 0.047$ and $p = 0.001$, respectively). Significantly lower values of both markers were observed in the MP-treated group.

DISCUSSION

The results of this study show that cyclosporine does not affect the formation of granulation tissue in viscose cellulose sponges in the rat. Viljanto has shown that collagen accumulation in this model corraborates with the development of tensile strength in a healing skin wound.[1]

The sponge model allows a quantitative

From the Transplantation Laboratory, University of Helsinki, and the Fourth Department of Surgery, Helsinki University Central Hospital, Helsinki, Finland.

Supported by NIH Grant 1 RO1 AM 26882-03 and a grant from the Sigrid Juselius Foundation, Helsinki, Finland.

Reprint requests should be addressed to

0041-1345/83/1505-0168$01.00/0

analysis of various events in the formation of granulation tissue. Our findings deserve a few further comments. The results show that MP greatly reduced the number of macrophages in granulation tissue. This is thought to be the mechanism by which MP delays wound healing,[2] since macrophages appear to be the most important stimulators of fibroblasts.[3] On the other hand, the number of macrophages tended to be highest in the CsA-treated groups. Furthermore, especially in rats treated with lower doses of CsA, there was increased accumulation of collagen and higher content of hemoglobin, which has been shown to correlate well with the ingrowth of capillaries into the new granulation tissue.[4] Thus, at an appropriate dosage level, cyclosporine might even enhance repair.

REFERENCES

1. Viljanto J: Acta Chir Scand (Suppl) 333, 1964
2. Salmela K, Roberts PJ, Lautenschlager I, et al: Acta Chir Scand 146:541, 1980
3. Leibovich SJ, Ross R: Am J Pathol 78:71, 1975
4. Holmström H, Zederfeldt B, Ahonen J: Scand J Plast Reconstr Surg 7:97, 1973

SUMMATION

Basic Science Summation

J. F. Borel and K. J. Lafferty

ASIDE FROM its importance as a drug in clinical immunosuppression, cyclosporine (CsA) has made an impact on fundamental immunology where it is used as a tool. This summary will mainly deal with this second aspect. Based on the high quality results that were presented at this congress, we will attempt to summarize a number of important aspects of CsA and to highlight what may be presently considered the major trends and issues.

The apparent lack of congruent results, when trying to summarize some 80-odd basic science presentations, is bewildering. This might be less surprising if one considers the almost unlimited diversity of experimental protocols and varieties of techniques used. It is most difficult, to express it optimistically, to find one's way through this experimental jungle and to endeavor to construct any "Unité de doctrine." Although this may seem to be a truism to scientists, one should nevertheless keep in mind that constantly comparing apples with pears may lead to serious pitfalls. For example, spleen cells, thymocytes, peripheral blood lymphocytes, and lymphoid cell lines from many species were used; moreover several mitogens or antigens were often added in different concentrations and at various times, in order to induce different cellular functions or trigger the release of a variety of lymphokines. This applies to in vitro as well as to in vivo work. It is known that in mice and rats some experiments will only work in certain strain combinations and not in others. Among the recipient animals some were normal, others were irradiated or preconditioned by other means; transferred cells were injected at various times, in various amounts, either purified or mixed with those from normal animals. Wide concentration and dose ranges of CsA were used. Therefore, it may become irrelevant to ask such questions as: Why are certain results obtained in experimental animals not seen in man? It is obvious that in humans genetic manipulation of organ donors and recipients is not feasible and, at best, only limited tissue matching and/or negative crossmatches can be realized. We can be optimistic that once these differences are understood, it will become feasible to obtain positive effects more predictably.

The complete synthesis of CsA allows almost unlimited molecular manipulation and thus the study of structure-activity relationships.[1] Once that part of the molecule responsible for the immunological activity is known, it might be feasible to elucidate the chemical structure of the receptor on or in the lymphocyte. Furthermore, it is hoped that in the future the antiparasitic component may be separated from the immunosuppressive activity, since both effects seem to be independent from each other.[2]

Binding Studies

No one seems to have demonstrated specific receptors for CsA restricted to the lymphocytes, and no competition between this compound and mitogens for a common receptor site on these cells has yet been found (B. Ryffel, Basel, personal communication). A saturable and high cellular uptake by lymphoid cells from thymus and spleen and other tissues (especially brain and kidney) has been shown.[3] The drug concentration in the lymphocytes seems to be ~ 50-fold higher than in the surrounding medium, and ~ 75% of cell-associated drug appears located in the cytosol.[3] Apparently, CsA is not metabolized

From the Department of Preclinical Research, Sandoz, Ltd.

Address reprint requests to Dr. Borel, Preclinical Research, Sandoz, Ltd., CH-4002, Basel, Switzerland.

0004–1345/83/1505–0169$01.00/0

inside the cell (M. Merker, New Haven, personal communication).

It has been proposed that partitioning of the hydrophobic CsA molecules in the membrane bilayer perturbs the homeostatic control of membrane function[4] and the CsA may resemble the steroids that do not bind to the cell membrane, but have a receptor site inside the cytosol. This needs to be tested.

What happens at the level of molecular cell biology remains terra incognita. One group has recently suggested that the compound is inhibiting the activation of ribosomal genes in the nucleus of lymphocytes (R. Weil and J.-F. Gauchat, Geneva, personal communication). To our knowledge, however, this difficult but important area of research is not being sufficiently pursued.

Humoral Mediators of the Immune Response

Most investigators agree that the production of lymphokines is inhibited by CsA. Thus γIF (interferon), but not the virus-induced α/β IF, is suppressed.[5–7] Other lymphokines mentioned were: IL-2 (interleukin 2),[5,8] IL-3, MAF (macrophage activating factor), MIF (macrophage inhibiting factor), MPCA (macrophage procoagulant activity) and LDCF (lymphocyte-derived macrophage chemotactic factor).[9] CsA does not seem to influence the function of these factors in vitro; it was shown, e.g., that it had no effect on the antiviral activity of reference γIF itself.[6] More remarkably, the compound does not exert any direct effect on the monocyte or macrophage responses to the various lymphokines.[9] Human thymocytes in vitro absorb and consume IL-2 and this absorption was prevented by the drug, though their combined IL-2 and PMA (phorbol myristate acetate) induced proliferation after 120 hr of culture was not.[5] It was also inferred from studies using murine T-leukemia cell lines that under some, but not all conditions the effect of CsA can be overridden by the addition of exogenous IL-2.

The Effects of CsA on Lymphocytes In Vitro

It appears essential to distinguish between the subset model on the one hand and the signaling model on the other hand when considering the mechanism of action of CsA. The subset model claims that the T-cell subsets are functionally different from one another, whereas according to the signaling model, it is thought that all T cells are potentially the same, but that their receptor specificity regulates the expression of different functions.[10]

CsA inhibits the expression of helper function, i.e. the capacity of T cells to synthesize and release lymphokines. Although CsA affects the production of lymphokines, it does not interfere with their effects on target lymphocytes, e.g., IL-2 dependent T-cell proliferation,[8,10–12] or on the phagocytic or migratory activity of macrophages.[9]

The steps in the activation of resting T cells (T) to activated T cell (T′) with a receptor for IL-2, and the function of these T′ cells, such as lymphokine production, have differing sensitivities to CsA.

We can describe these different reactions as follows:[13]

Reaction A: Primary activation, $T \xrightarrow[(2)]{(1)} T'$

Reaction B: Clonal expansion, $T' \xrightarrow[(2)]{} nT'$

Reaction C: Triggering of lymphokine release, $T' \xrightarrow{(1)} l.$

Signal (1) is provided by antigen or mitogen binding to a receptor on the T-cell surface. Signal (2) is provided by costimulator activity known to be expressed by IL-1,[11] or other putative products of antigen-presenting cells. Reaction B is mediated by the T-cell product IL-2 or TCGF.

CsA interferes with reaction C in the 10–100-ng/ml concentration range, but has no effect on reaction B at concentrations below 2–4 μg/ml. The interference with reaction C is not due to an effect of the drug on binding to the T-cell receptor (B. Ryffel, Basel, and D. White, Cambridge, unpublished results). It was also reported that CsA does not alter the binding of DR antigens to the T-cell surface (S. LeGrue, Houston, unpublished results).

Reaction A, because of its multifactorial nature, is more difficult to analyze. In fact, the involvement of multiple interactions in the conversion of T to T′ may account for the varying results reported from different laboratories.[8,10,12] There is no doubt that future studies in this area will have to consider dose-response relationships and all possible interactions that may determine the effect of the drug.

The tumor promoter PMA can provide an alternate source of signal (1): PMA triggers lymphokine release from T′ cells; however, PMA triggering of T′ cells is not sensitive to CsA (R. K. Fidelus, Houston, personal communication). This finding is not in conflict with the general concept that CsA interferes with delivery of the antigen mediated signal. It was suggested that antigen may trigger a reaction sequence (A-B-C etc.) and that CsA could interfere with the A-B step but not later ones in the sequence (B-C etc.). The available evidence indicating that PMA short-circuits this process at the A-B step would explain why PMA triggering of lymphokine release is not sensitive to CsA. This model would also account for the finding that the combined IL-2 plus PMA induction of T-cell proliferation is insensitive to CsA.[5] PMA can similarly bypass CsA mediated inhibition of resting T cell activation by PHA (R. K. Fidelus, Houston, personal communication). In the process of T-cell activation by PHA, the lectin provides a source of signal (1) and also facilitates the interaction of the accessory cell, as a source of signal (2), with the T cell. CsA inhibits this process by interfering with the delivery of signal (1) by PHA.[10] In the presence of PMA, the CsA-sensitive step in the delivery of signal (1) is once again short circuited.

Although there is agreement concerning the regulation of activation, clonal proliferation and triggering of T cells expressing helper function, there is disagreement about how other T cells might respond to CsA. These differences lead to two theories of T cell biology: (*a*) All T cells are physiologically similar and have similar effector potential.[10] On the basis of this proposal, CsA affects all T cells in essentially the same way. However, different functions of the T cell have differing sensitivities to CsA. (*b*) CsA defines two T-cell subsets:[8] those sensitive to CsA (this includes helper and cytotoxic cells) and those that are insensitive to CsA (this includes suppressor cells).

Both models are viable at present until further critical experiments can be designed to distinguish between them.

Finally, there is a suggestion that CsA may be affecting B cell function in a manner similar to the way it regulates T cells, i.e., that CsA defines B cells that are either at differing stages of differentiation along the pathway to immunoglobulin synthesis, or that physiologically different B-cell subsets exist and only one is CsA sensitive.[12,14]

Tolerance Induction

Using several different transplantation models, it was shown that CsA treatment can be stopped after a short course (approximately two weeks) without compromising the subsequent survival of kidney[15] and heart[16–18] allografts in MHC-incompatible rat strains. However, indefinite allograft survival was not observed when skin allografts were examined in a rabbit model.[19] Evidence was presented that clearly demonstrated the tissue specificity of this phenomenon. A comparative study carried out in the rat with major and minor antigenic differences demonstrated that indefinite kidney survival could be achieved, but only limited prolongation of pancreas survival was observed when it was transplanted under the same conditions.[15] Thus, a short course of CsA treatment can facilitate indefinite allograft survival, even after withdrawal of the drug. However, the effect is tissue specific and different results may also be obtained when the same organ is transplanted across different strain combinations.

A special situation was encountered in mongrel dogs grafted with a jugular vein segment. It was shown that the combined cryopreservation of the allografts with CsA and DMSO prevented their rejection and occlusion.[20] It is known that CsA reduces the release of IL-1 by monocytes,[21] while at the same time the reticulo-endothelial cells of the venous tissue graft (which synthesize IL-1) are rapidly replaced by the recipient's own cells, thereby changing the antigenic composition of the allograft. In this particular in vivo model tolerance might, therefore, be induced through an early suppression of Il-1 release by donor cells lasting until their replacement by corresponding recipient cells. These interesting results need to be confirmed and analyzed in more detail.

It is unlikely that the treatment of the animal with CsA per se is responsible for tolerance induction; soon after cessation of treatment the graft can be rejected if the recipient is challenged with a donor skin graft; thus, the graft is in a metastable condition. This metastable graft-host relationship moves, with the passage of time and in the absence of continued CsA administration, to a stable form of tolerance.[16] It would appear that CsA allows engraftment and that the continued provision of graft antigen is required for the establishment of tolerance without need for the continued presence of CsA.[16]

Analysis of this stable graft-host relationship induced by grafting under the cover of CsA showed the development of graft specific tolerance in the recipient.[16] This tolerance was not due to clonal deletion because both lymph node and splenic lymphocytes responded normally to donor antigens in vitro.[22] It was further demonstrated in dogs that had become tolerant to a single lung allograft[23] that their peripheral blood lymphocytes were still able to mount a specific mixed lymphocyte reaction against donor cells, but that their ability to mount specific lymphocyte-mediated cytotoxicity against these same targets was impaired.[24]

In one study both the transfer of cells from the tolerant animal, as well as heroic efforts to transfer specific unresponsiveness to normal syngeneic recipient animals with serum failed to transfer tolerance.[16] However, in what appears to be a more sensitive test system,[17] it could be shown that the tolerant animals possessed cells that were specifically suppressive and that suppression also could be transferred with serum. T-suppressor cell function was also demonstrated in another system involving heart allografting under the short-term cover of CsA.[25]

The exact nature of the suppressive factor(s) in serum of tolerant animals has not been resolved. Possible candidates must include antibody, antigen-antibody complexes, and other as yet undefined suppressive factors. More work is also required to elucidate the mechanism underlying the cell-mediated suppression. Does it result from the inhibitory action of suppressor cells? Or, does it result from the provision of helper activity for B cells that produce the component involved in the humoral suppression?

A most intriguing phenomenon is the development of a syngeneic and autologous graft-versus-host reaction (GVHR) after discontinuation of CsA treatment of previously lethally irradiated rats reconstituted with syngeneic or autologous bone marrow.[26] A prerequisite for induction of this peculiar type of GVHR is the elimination of thymic functions. Though the mechanism by which CsA causes this phenomenon remains speculative, it was suggested that the compound possibly depletes cytotoxic T cells autoreactive to nontolerant lymphocytes, which may play a crucial role in the establishment and maintenance of self-tolerance.

Antigen-Induced Unresponsiveness

The development of donor-specific unresponsiveness was demonstrated[27] when mice were challenged with antigen at the time of CsA administration. Spleen cells from the challenged animals, when tested in vitro, showed a specific inability to produce a cytotoxic T-cell response to donor antigen. This approach to the induction of specific unresponsiveness in the adult animal was examined in kidney and skin transplantation models;[28,29] extended allograft survival was shown to result from the donor treatment in the presence of CsA. Studies in a renal allograft model showed a significant effect of antigen dose on the degree of extended allograft survival.[28]

A significant finding was that CsA treatment at the time of antigen administration eliminated the generation of graft-specific antibody as a result of donor-specific transfusion.[29,30]

Effects in Autoimmune Diseases (AID)

The papers concerned with AID were surprisingly few. One study dealt with the response of NZB/W mice to preventive, long-term CsA treatment and disclosed that this compound did not influence the histological parameters or the synthesis of autoantibodies as shown by the continuous presence of immune complexes and the positive Coombs test reactivity, but somehow protected the target tissues from damage. There was indeed no renal damage seen despite continuous deposition of immunoglobulins and complement in the glomeruli.[31] These results are surprising in view of other reports showing a clear diminution of the anti-DNA antibody titers concomitant with a significant improvement of the kidneys in affected animals.[32,33] (J. F. Bach, Paris, personal communication).

CsA has a dramatic beneficial effect on the mouse lupus model possessing the lpr-gene (G. Harris, London, personal communication). In these lpr-mice there is an intrinsic hyporesponsiveness of the Lyt 1^+ T cell and IL-2 is not produced by the lpr-lymphocytes during antigen presentation. Addition of IL-2 cannot restore T cell responsiveness. However, when CsA was added in vitro to an antigen-presentation assay of normal mouse cells, the T-cell proliferation was completely eliminated, but addition of IL-2 was able to restore the response to normal. These results suggest that CsA can interfere with a key step in macrophage/T-cell interaction and reproduce some of the immunologic deficits of lupus mice.[34]

The effect of CsA on lymphocyte-subsets in experimental allergic encephalomyelitis in the guinea pig was investigated. Depending on the timing of treatment, it was shown that the inhibitory effect of CsA on mature disease-inducing cells and those producing delayed type hypersensitivity was fully reversible, but that the inhibition of disease-suppressing cells was not; this led to sudden death when the drug was discontinued.[35]

However, in retinal autoimmunity (uveitis), it was demonstrated that the clinical symptoms regressed under CsA therapy, although the patients' lymphocytes maintained a positive cell-mediated response to the retinal S-antigen. The NK cells were not significantly altered.[36]

Finally it was reported that the generation of syngeneic cytotoxic lymphocytes (CTL) was 10- to 100-fold more sensitive to CsA than the allogeneic CTL generation, although the inhibition kinetics were identical. It was suggested that this very sensitive inhibition of syngeneic CTL may prove beneficial in AID.[37]

Nephrotoxicity

One interesting observation reported concerning the nephrotoxicity of CsA, its major side effect, may have consequences for the clinic. The drug is thought to increase the sympathetic nerve activity in spontaneous hypertensive (SH) rats as indicated by hypertension, tachycardia, and hyperglycemia. This is likely to lead to the stimulation of RAAS (renin-angiotensin-aldosterone system), as observed in CsA-treated rats and dogs.[38] An increased angiotensin II level might alter renal hemodynamics and possibly contribute to the well known nephrotoxic symptoms, thus explaining the reversibility of these effects. Similar nephrotoxic findings consisting of tubular and vascular lesions as described in the SH rat were also found in patients.[39]

Conclusions

The First International Congress on Cyclosporine has brought together an unprecedented number of investigators, who will undoubtedly contribute to an ever-increasing cooperation among those involved in this exciting area. This Congress has further fostered a vast interest in this still novel compound, which should not only provide a better understanding of its mechanism of action, but also improve its efficiency in the various clinical indications.[2]

REFERENCES

1. Wenger R: Transplant Proc (this issue)
2. Borel JF: Transplant Proc (this issue)
3. Merker M, Rice JD, Schweizer B, et al: Transplant Proc (this issue)
4. LeGrue S, Friedman A, Kahan BD: Transplant Proc (this issue)
5. Reem GH, Cook LA, Palladino MA: Transplant Proc (this issue)
6. Kalman V, Klimpel G: Transplant Proc (this issue)
7. Abb J, Abb H, Deinhardt F: Transplant Proc (this issue)
8. Hess A, Tutschka PJ, Santos GW: Transplant Proc (this issue)
9. Thomson AW, Moon DK, Geczy CL, et al: Transplant Proc (this issue)
10. Lafferty KJ, Borel JF: Transplant Proc (this issue)
11. Gery I, Benjamin WR, Jones S, et al: Transplant Proc (this issue)
12. Bouwer HGA, Hinrichs DJ: Transplant Proc (this issue)
13. Borel JF, Lafferty KJ: Transplant Proc, 15:1881, 1983
14. Klaus GGB, Dongworth DW: In D. J. G. White (ed): Cyclosporin A. Amsterdam, Elsevier Biomedical Press, 1981, pp 233–241
15. Klempnauer J, Wagner E, Wonigkeit K, et al: Transplant Proc (this issue)
16. White DJG: Transplant Proc (this issue)
17. Hall BM, Jelbart ME, Dorsch SE: Transplant Proc (this issue)
18. Ochiai T, Sakamoto K, Asano T, et al: Transplant Proc (this issue)
19. Jolley WB, Knierim K, Ham J, et al: Transplant Proc (this issue)
20. Bandlien K, Toledo-Pereyra LH, MacKenzie G, et al: Transplant Proc (this issue)
21. Andrus L, Lafferty KJ: Scand J Immunol 15:449, 1982
22. Bailey LL, Li Z, Lacour-Gayet F, et al: Transplant Proc (this issue)
23. Kambholz SL, Veith FJ, Pinsker KL, et al: Transplant Proc (this issue)
24. Norin AJ, Emeson EE, Veith FJ: Transplant Proc (this issue)
25. Kupiec-Weglinsky J, Lear PA, Bordes-Aznar J, et al: Transplant Proc (this issue)
26. Glazier A, Tutschka PJ, Farmer E, et al: J Exp Med 158:1, 1983
27. Wang BS, Heacock EH, Xue ZC, et al: J Immunol 129:1382–1385, 1982
28. Clune GJA, Dumble LJ: Transplant Proc (this issue)
29. Yasumura T, Kahan BD: Transplant Proc (this issue)
30. Ochiai T, Asano T, Gunji M, et al: Transplant Proc (this issue)
31. Jones MG, Harris G, Cowing G: Transplant Proc (this issue)
32. Gozes Y, Theofilopoulos AN, Park CM, et al: Fed Proc 41, 547 (No. 1619), 1982
33. Bowles CA, Holley KE, Handwerger BS: Am Rheum Assoc, 1983 (abstr)
34. Talal N, Fischbach M: Transplant Proc (this issue)
35. Fredane LH, Hashim GA, McCabbe RE: Transplant Proc (this issue)
36. Nussenblatt RB, Palestine AG, Chan CC, et al: Transplant Proc (this issue)
37. Ballas ZK: Transplant Proc (this issue)
38. Siegl H, Petric R, Ryffel B: Transplant Proc (this issue)
39. Mihatsch MJ: Transplant Proc (this issue)

Clinical Aspects of Cyclosporine Therapy: A Summation

T. E. Starzl

IN DESCRIBING the Australian trials, Sheil complimented those in the Sandoz Corporation for their professionalism and integrity, a remark that is germane to the Houston meeting. The program was developed not as a triumphant forum but in order to assess the problems as well as the prospects that transplantation will face in the new era which will be started this summer with the general availability of cyclosporine. A good look has been taken at this new pharmacologic emperor without its clothes, and cyclosporine has withstood the scrutiny quite well.

The reason for the excitement can be stated simply. With cyclosporine, it has been possible to transplant some of the solid organs with a success not previously possible and to carry out other kinds of solid organ transplantation that were previously beyond our grasp. Such successes provided half of the clinical story of this meeting. The other half concerned the price for these increased expectations.

The most extensive experience has been with the kidney, and certainly the most meaningful data have come from cadaveric transplantation. One-year graft survival after familial transplantation in good centers has been so high (greater than 70%) for almost two decades that statistically significant further increases with a new form of immunosuppression would be difficult to achieve. Thus, the superior results from Kyoto, Japan, with greater than 90% 1-year graft survival after parent-to-offspring transplantation under cyclosporine-steroid therapy were not considered better than those obtainable with conventional treatment in this group's historical experience. The same reservation applied to about 45% of the cases in the Minnesota randomized trial, in which the 1-year graft survival after consanguineous transplantation was better than 85% with both cyclosporine-steroid therapy and with the combined use of azathioprine, prednisone, and ALG.

Cadaveric renal transplantation under cyclosporine-steroid therapy (with a variable steroid component) versus conventional therapy were compared in multicenter trials in Europe and in Canada. Both studies showed a 20% 1-year advantage in the cyclosporine group. Adverse factors for the cyclosporine limb in the Canadian trials were said to be machine perfusion of the renal grafts for more than 24 hr or an ischemia time of more than 45 min during the construction of vascular anastomoses. It was interesting that one of the participating teams, from the Mount Sinai Hospital, Toronto, presented what amounted to a minority Canadian report. Their preexisting policy had been to treat cadaveric kidney recipients with azathioprine, prednisone, and Minnesota ALG. With this triple-drug therapy, they achieved better than 90% graft survival, compared to 74% with the proscribed cyclosporine-steroid combination; the results barely missed statistical significance. In a subset of the European trial reported from Birmingham, England, the 1-year graft survival was almost identical (70%) in the experimental and conventional groups, but the enormous advantage in the cyclosporine arm was that about half of the successfully treated recipients were not being given steroids. In a Helsinki report, the 1-year control and test groups both had 80% graft survival.

From the Department of Surgery, University of Pittsburgh, Health Center, University of Pittsburgh, Pittsburgh, PA.

Supported by research grants from the Veterans Administration, by Project Grant AM 29961 from the National Institutes of Health, and by Grant RR 00084 from the General Clinical Research Centers Program of the Division of Research Resources, National Institutes of Health.

Reprint requests should be addressed to T.E. Starzl, 3601 Fifth Avenue, Room 103 Falk Clinic, Pittsburgh, PA 15213.

0041-1345/83/1505-0170$01.00/0

The importance of giving weight to the quality of life by avoiding excessive steroid treatment was most strongly emphasized in the descriptions of the randomized Australian trials in which cyclosporine alone was compared to conventional azathioprine-prednisone treatment. Although the life survival curves of the grafts were about the same, with 70% 1-year cadaveric kidney function at 2 years, the quality of life was better in the experimental series.

In the United States, randomized trials of cadaveric transplantation in single centers were conducted by the Pittsburgh, Boston, Houston, and Minnesota teams. Because of the wide divergence of results between the experimental and conventional azathioprine-prednisone groups, the trials in Pittsburgh and Houston had to be stopped. The trials have continued at the University of Minnesota for the simple reason that there has been no difference at that institution with cyclosporine-steroid therapy versus treatment with azathioprine, prednisone, and ALG. The cadaveric graft survival has been in the 80% range, with a 1-year patient mortality of about 10% in both conventional and test groups.

Throughout their investigations of cyclosporine and in the period preceding their use of this new drug, the Houston team has made a particular effort to stratify all of their recipients on the basis of preexisting immune reactivity. By so doing, they have been able to classify their recipients over the last several years into high, intermediate, and low immunologic responders. The value of cyclosporine-steroid therapy was particularly striking in the high-responder group; in the low-responder group, the results were already so good with conventional therapy that cyclosporine was more a convenience than an overriding advantage. In discussing the Minnesota experience at one of the forum meetings, Kahan speculated that high responders may have been culled out by preoperative preparation with at least 10 transfusions; the consequence would be to convert many high responders to a nontransplantable state because of stimulation of preformed antibodies. The transfusions plus the obligatory splenectomy in the Minnesota study could have edged those patients who made it through the full preoperative preparation into the nonresponsive group. No one could really argue with this carefully thought-out "strategy" of transplantation, but what was questioned was if this kind of pretransplant preparation was really going to be necessary or desirable in the future. The ability to treat patients efficiently and effectively without extensive preparation (including a major operation) before transplantation may be especially important in patients who are at high risk because of advanced age or other adverse factors. Groth of Stockholm reported an outstanding series of cadaveric transplantations under cyclosporine-steroid therapy in a group of patients who were 55 to more than 70 years old. The results were twice as good as in historical controls.

A summary statement avoiding excessive enthusiasm as well as undue pessimism would have to note that the results with cyclosporine-steroid therapy have never been inferior to those achieved by any of the investigating groups using their own version of conventional therapy for controls and that they usually have been superior. This in itself says a lot about the quality of the immunosuppression provided by cyclosporine-steroid therapy, since its effective use has required a major intellectual adjustment by those accustomed to the use of azathioprine and prednisone (with or without ALG). Nephrotoxicity has been the most serious side effect of cyclosporine, meaning that a reduction in cyclosporine dosage is frequently the most appropriate response to a secondary decline in renal function, rather than the reflex increase in steroid doses that has been so often called for in the past.

The role of plasma or blood cyclosporine analysis in reaching a final dose under such circumstances is by no means clear. All groups are trying to use pharmacologic monitoring, but Ferguson, in a study of 70 consecutive Minnesota cases, found no correlation whatever between blood cyclosporine levels and nephrotoxicity. The Houston and London, Ontario, groups were in sharp disagreement. Yet all observers conceded that the blood-level determinations have permitted identification of specific situations in which the trough levels of cyclosporine were either much too high or surprisingly low. It is hard to believe that blood or plasma analysis will not have some value, at least in isolated cases. At the same time, it is equally clear that good clinical management can be carried out without this luxury.

It has always been comforting for clinicians to turn to the pathologist for final arbitration of disputes about the pathogenesis of complications. These roles have almost been reversed in trying to clearly distinguish cyclosporine nephrotoxicity and homograft rejection. Efforts were reported by the Minnesota group to categorize the histologic findings in subnormally functioning kidney grafts according to the clinical response to steroid therapy. Absolutely reliable guidelines for adjustment of therapy have not been delineated by this approach. K. A. Porter of London looked at a number of renal graft biopsies from our early cyclosporine experience. Rejection was common, but its features differed from those seen with conventional immunosuppression only in a somewhat greater proportion of the eosinophils in the infiltrating cells. In kidneys examined from both heart and hepatic recipients, Porter could not find specific lesions of drug nephrotoxicity. Discussion of this problem is certain to enliven clinical and pathologic conferences for years to come.

Since the beginning of clinical trials in renal transplantation, the unquestioned nephrotoxicity has explained higher average levels of serum creatinine in cyclosporine-treated kidney recipients than in successfully treated controls. Even if the creatinine is high early after transplantation (as high as the 3–4 mg/dl range), there is no urgency to reduce the cyclosporine dose if the patient feels well and if the abnormal creatinine is not rising. Our own policy has been to try to invest about 2 months of maximum cyclosporine dosage during the induction of graft acceptance. A premature pullback of dosage can lead to rejection. The coexistence of nephrotoxicity and rejection suggested by us some time ago has been supported strongly by the Houston, Stockholm, and Minnesota clinicians with evidence presented at this meeting. Personally, I believe that the extensive and beautiful Minnesota pathology studies could be interpreted as an expression of this dual problem. Anyone using cyclosporine at this time should carefully read the therapeutic strategies that have been developed by the various groups including ours to accommodate both possibilities of rejection and nephrotoxicity.

The other side effects of cyclosporine were mentioned frequently throughout the meeting. The hypertension and hyperkalemia that have been subjects of separate papers are certainly manifestations of the drug's nephrotoxicity. Hepatotoxicity, hirsutism, tremors (and even possibly seizures), and gingival hyperplasia have been reduced or relieved by dose reduction. When life-threatening infections have appeared in any large numbers under cyclosporine and steroids, the usual conclusion has been that overimmunosuppression with one or the other of the two agents has been responsible. In earlier reports from the University of Minnesota, it appeared that infections with bacteria, fungi, protozoa, and viruses were all markedly less under cyclosporine-steroid therapy than under conventional immunosuppression, but Najarian reported that this advantage in Minneapolis had been narrowed if not lost in their later experience, with the striking exception of the cytomegalovirus syndromes. The bewildering cross section of infections and how the patterns differed with different kinds of transplantations in Pittsburgh were described by Ho.

A striking observation in almost all of the renal trials has been the remarkably good results in cadaveric renal retransplantation, even including patients with widely reacting

T-warm antibodies or with a history of aggressive rejection of multiple previous organs. In the past, the justification for trying too hard to retain kidney grafts (with a resulting high mortality) has been the clouded future of recipients who rejected kidneys and then faced cadaveric retransplantation. That justification does not seem to exist anymore using cyclosporine-steroid therapy. As that new fact of life becomes broadly appreciated, the 1-year patient mortality after primary transplantation is apt to reach the 5% or lower level that will represent an irreducible minimum imposed by disease of other organ systems.

It would be easy to spend this entire summary talking about renal transplantation—and with some justification because of the broad applicability of the lessons being learned. The ripple effect certainly has been felt with liver transplantation, which (under cyclosporine) has become about twice as safe as in the past. The great improvement made possible with cyclosporine has increased the frequency and boldness with which liver replacement has been carried out, and now the prospect of escalating this advantage into other improvements (including technical) is a very bright one. Since the liver is the major site of metabolism of cyclosporine, all kinds of problems could easily be visualized about dose control. The major prediction in liver recipients could be of astronomical overdosage, but in fact the opposite has occurred, in that unreliable absorption of the drug has been the most consistent problem with consequent underdosage. Our liver recipients are now receiving double-route cyclosporine therapy, beginning with intravenous doses and continuing this intravenously for at least 2 weeks, long after the resumption of an oral diet and oral cyclosporine. The changeover from the double-route administration to an oral dose alone can be greatly aided by the systematic measurement of blood cyclosporine levels. The several groups who discussed their experience with liver transplantation under cyclosporine did not carry out randomized trials, and it is unlikely that this will ever be done.

The same lack of enthusiasm about randomized trials in cardiac transplantation was evident. The Stanford heart transplanters have achieved a 1-year survival of 80%, with a 2-year actuarial survival in excess of 70%. The fact that other groups have been able to do almost as well in Pittsburgh, Cambridge, and Houston means that pressure to expand this type of clinical service is bound to increase. At Stanford, the more complex heart-lung transplantations, which were not previously possible either in experimental animals or humans, have been successful in 8/11 patients who have been followed for 2 months to 2 years. In Pittsburgh, the survival record with heart-lung transplantation has been 3/5. Shumway has speculated that isolated lung transplantations may be infinitely more difficult than composite thoracic organ transplantation, but the merits of that argument aside, Veith has accomplished single-lung transplantation in dogs using cyclosporine, although he has not yet succeeded in human patients.

With cyclosporine, it will be surprising if major advances cannot be made in pancreas transplantation. Sutherland pointed out that this has not been achieved at the University of Minnesota. The same conclusion was reached by Dubernard of Lyon, but Groth has had successes with half of his cadaveric segmental pancreas transplantations in Stockholm during the last year. The prospect of using the pancreatico-duodenal-jejunal composite grafts now that better immunosuppression is available was raised, and two successful cases with perfect results after 1 and 3 months were presented from Pittsburgh. Parenthetically, both of these recipients are carrying about 3 ft of donor small intestine. Several groups are poised to attempt intestinal transplantation in humans, a procedure that has been successfully carried out in mongrel dogs with survival of almost 2 years.

Most of what I have summarized has come from recent trials. In chronic survivors after various kinds of transplantation, the question keeps coming up of the possible desirability of early or late conversion from cyclosporine to maintenance therapy with azathioprine. This will be necessary in some patients, but at what frequency is debatable. In our renal graft recipients treated 3 years ago, the conversion rate was about 20%, and in this subgroup, 40% subsequently rejected their grafts, as Klintmalm has reported. Our switch rate has steadily declined; it is now about 5%. The opposite trend is identifiable in the data presented from Minnesota, and, of course, all patients at Oxford have been converted at 90 days.

In the recipients of hearts and livers, the predominant conversion has been in the other direction—from conventional azathioprine-prednisone therapy to cyclosporine. Typically, a patient whose survival with one of these organs years after transplantation depends on unacceptably high steroid doses has been switched to cyclosporine and the prednisone has been discontinued. We have carried out this change in half a dozen liver recipients. The hepatic function has not deteriorated in any case, and in most it has actually improved. The advantages and dangers of this switch-over were discussed in one full session and cannot be adequately summarized here. It should be noted that there is a potential risk of mixing drugs, especially in the early postoperative period, as was exemplified by the frightening experience in Lyon, which resulted in a nearly 50% incidence of lymphoproliferative complications in a small series of patients given azathioprine, prednisone, ALG, and cyclosporine, in that general order.

Except for this experience, the incidence of de novo malignancies under cyclosporine-steroid therapy has been acceptable. It looks as if the incidence of lymphoproliferative complications is going to be less than 2%, but the implications of even that figure are relatively bland. Rosenthal reported that the simple discontinuance or reduction of immunosuppression (both cyclosporine and steroid doses) in patients with so-called lymphomas resulted in the involution and disappearance of the lesions. Most of the lymphomas seen under immunosuppression are probably associated with (or caused by) the Epstein-Barr virus.

Where cyclosporine will fit in the future of bone marrow transplantation is difficult to predict. The cross section of side effects of cyclosporine in bone marrow recipients has been very broad, and almost invariably some other potentially toxic drug was thought to have had an adverse interaction with the cyclosporine. The most common culprits were antibiotics, especially those used for their antifungal effect. It may be that cyclosporine will not influence practices in bone marrow transplantation to the extent that looks probable with solid organs, but it would be less than fair not to point out that the pioneering observations of Powles about the control of graft-versus-host reactions in humans made 4 years ago have been confirmed under a number of clinical circumstances.

So much material was presented at this conference and with such immediate clinical applicability that I find it impossible to do justice to the conference and to its participants in this summary. The conference came at a uniquely propitious moment, since cyclosporine will become available to all clinicians within the next few weeks or months. I believe that we of the transplantation community owe a unique debt to the fathers of cyclosporine, Jean Borel, David White, and Roy Calne, (who could not be here); to those highly responsible men and women in the Sandoz Corporation who have permitted and encouraged us to look at the blemishes as well as the perfections of cyclosporine; and to the masterful host of this conference, Barry Kahan, who, as I have remarked to others, is one of the great scientist-surgeons in the world today.

AUTHOR INDEX

Abb, H., 164
Abb, J., 164
Abramoff, P., 178
Achauer, B.M., 526, 847, 853, 857
Adu, D., 307, 538
Aeder, M.I., 665, 717
Ahonen, J., 626, 876
Aikawa, I., 82, 118, 285
Allen, N.H., 646
Ambinder, R.F., 592
Appelbaum, F.R., 404, 826
Aprile, M., 297
Arakawa, K., 82
Araujo, J.L., 673
Arnaud-Battandier, F., 803
Asano, T., 124, 723
Ascher, N.L., 247, 658, 665
Atchison, R.W., 701
Atkinson, K., 214, 230, 545

Bahnson, H.T., 337, 357, 490, 541, 552, 563
Bailey, L., 740
Ballas, Z.K., 107
Bandlien, K.O., 868
Barnhart, M.I., 868
Barry, E.P., 187
Baughan, A., 492
Belitsky, P., 319
Belzer, F. O., 781
Benjamin, W. R., 95
Bentley, F. R., 665
Bernstein, R. L., 490
Beschorner, W. E., 397
Bettcher, K. B., 322
Beveridge, T., 193
Biggs, J., 214, 230, 545
Billingham, M., 330
Bishop, G. A., 636
Black, K. S., 526, 847, 853, 857
Blanc, N., 582
Boake, R., 322
Boileau, M., 253
Boland, J., 214
Boldt, L., 357
Borel, J. F., 3, 26, 881
Borgmästars, H., 626
Bortin, M. M., 178
Bosi, E., 386, 460, 582
Boulas, J., 269
Bouwer, H. G. A., 90
Bowes, L. G., 861
Bremer, R., 605
Brewer, E. D., 312
Britton, K., 214, 230
Brölsch, C., 315, 370
Brookmeyer, R., 397
Brown, Z., 182
Brunner, F. P., 605
Buckels, J., 307
Buckner, C. D., 404
Bull, R. W., 788
Bunzendahl, H., 315
Burdelski, M., 370
Burke, M. D., 496
Buscetta, S., 157
Bushuk, M., 837

Calne, R. Y., 630, 662
Canadian Transplant Study Group, 263, 274, 297, 532
Canafax, D. M., 658
Cannarella, S. N., 362
Carpenter C. B., 673
Carruthers, G., 222
Castro, L. A., 301, 483, 641
Cavallini, M., 744
Chan, C. C., 698
Chapuis-Cellier, C., 582
Chevalier, M., 582
Chinn, P. L., 390
Chipping, P. M., 418
Choudbury, S. P., 868
Clift, R. A., 404
Clunie, G. J. A., 861
Cohen, A., 319
Cohen, Z., 797, 816
Cole, G. A., 55
Concannon, A., 230, 545
Conley, S. B., 312
Converse, P. J., 707
Cook, K., 781
Cook, L. A., 171
Cooley, D. A., 351
Corneo, M., 401
Cortez, J. A., 868
Corry, R. J., 753
Cory-Pearce, R., 343
Cowing, G., 688
Creyssel, R., 582
Crocker, J., 319
Crofts, M., 408
Cunningham, C., 496

Davies, H. ff. S., 62
DeBiasio, R. L., 559
Debski, R. F., 337
Deeg, H. J. 200, 404, 826
Delmonte, L., 112
Deltz, E., 811
Dereg, H. J., 826
Devergie, A., 226, 412
Devineni, R., 479
Dhein, B., 946
Diaz-Velez, A., 868
Dieperink, H., 520
Dixon, J. F. P., 160
Dodds, A., 230, 545
Donatsch, P., 503
Doney, K., 404
Donnenberg, A. D., 127
Dossetor, J. B., 322
Drath, D. B., 151
Du Toit, D. F., 776
Dubernard, J. M., 386, 460, 582
Duggin, G. G., 269, 636
Dumble, L. J., 861
Dummer, J. S., 552, 563
Duplan, J., 479

Egel, J., 490
Eklund, B., 626
El Yafi, S., 386, 582
Elick, B. A., 390
Eloranta, M., 626
Els, D., 776
Emeson, E. E., 362, 763
Engel, P., 127
Engemann, R., 770, 811
English, T. A. H., 343
Enomoto, K., 723
Evans, B., 408
Evans, D. B., 630
Ezzibdeh, M., 307

Fairhead, S. M., 418
Farmer, E. R., 397, 819
Farnsworth, A., 636
Farrell, C., 230
Fauci, A. S., 99
Fawwaz, R., 757
Fehrman, I., 291
Ferguson, R. M., 134, 247, 620, 665
Fidelus-Gort, R., 134
Field, M. Y., 744
Finkelstein, D., 816
Fischbach, M., 683
Flaa, C., 734
Flechner, S. M., 77, 86, 218, 253, 312, 473, 653
Flournoy, N., 404
Flye, M. W., 767
Foley, R. J., 570
Fontaine, J. L., 803
Forström, J., 626, 847, 853
Fraser, L. A., 526, 847, 853

Frazier, O. H., 351
Fredane, L. M., 693
Friedman, A. W., 43
Friedrichs, B., 811
Fryd, D. S., 247
Fukuda, M., 118
Fumagalli, F., 182
Furnas, D. W., 526, 847, 853, 857

Gallix, P., 803
Garnett, N. L., 592
Gartner, J. C., Jr., 366, 376
Geczy, C. L., 174
Gelet, A., 386
Gery, I., 95, 148, 698
Ghnassia, D., 803
Gibbons, S., 218
Ginchereau, E., 357
Glass, N. R., 781
Glazier, A., 819
Gliedman, M. L., 362
Gluckman, E., 226, 412
Goetz, F. C., 390
Gokel, J. M., 641
Goldsmith, J., 234, 362
Goodman, B., 636
Gordon-Smith, E. C., 206, 418, 492
Gossain, V. V., 788
Graf, A., 210
Granlund, H., 626
Gratwohl, A., 401
Greenberg, A., 490
Greenberg, G. R., 816
Griffith, B. P., 337, 357, 490, 541, 563
Groth, C. G., 291, 599
Gudat, F., 605
Guglielmi, A., 541
Gui, X. E., 701
Gunji, M., 723
Günther, K., 301, 483, 641
Gupta, R., 319
Gurland, H. J., 483

Haines, I., 538
Hakala, T. R., 243, 366, 552, 557, 561, 589
Hall, B. M., 269, 636
Hallberg, F., 744
Halloran, P. F., 297, 837
Ham, J., 795
Hamelmann, H., 770
Hamilton, D. V., 630
Hammer, C., 301
Hamner, R. W., 510, 514
Hamoudi, W. H., 559
Handschumacher, R. E., 49
Harder, F., 605
Hardesty, R. L., 337, 357, 490, 541, 563
Hardy, A. M., 552, 557
Hardy, M. A., 757
Harley, J. B., 99
Harris, G., 688
Harris, J. P., 269
Hashim, G. A., 693
Hashimoto, I., 82, 118, 285
Haynes, I. G., 307
Häyry, P., 500, 626, 876
Heberling, R. L., 592
Heineman, E., 737
Hekali, R., 876
Helanterä, A., 626
Henttula, U. M., 626
Hess, A. D., 32, 127, 397, 707
Hewitt, C. W., 526, 847, 853, 857
Heydenrych, J. J., 776
Hillebrand, C., 301
Hillebrand, G., 483, 641
Hinrichs, D. J., 90
Ho, M., 552, 557, 563, 701
Höckerstedt, K., 626
Hodgkin, P., 26
Hoffman, G. J., 592
Horvath, J. S., 269, 636
Howard, E. B., 526, 853
Hows, J. M., 206, 418, 492
Howson, W., 222
Huber, A. C., 592
Hughes, G., 408
Hunt, S. A., 330
Hutchinson, I. V., 71
Huttunen, K., 626

Iga, C., 757
Illner, W. D., 210, 301
Imberti, L., 182
Ingerman, A., 526
Ioka, J., 285
Itzkoff, J., 357
Ivory, K., 566
Iwatsuki, S., 243, 366, 376, 589

Jamieson, S. W., 330
Jeannet, M., 401
Jeekel, J., 737
Johnsen, A. M., 357
Johnson, J. R., 269, 636
Jolley, W. B., 740, 795
Jones, D. B., 711
Jones, M. G., 688
Jones, S., 95
Jos, J., 803

Kääriäinen, M., 626
Kadotani, Y., 285
Kahan, B. D., xxv, 43, 77, 86, 151, 197, 218, 253, 312, 351, 425, 433, 449, 473, 653, 726
Kaleya, R., 234, 362
Kalman, V. K., 167
Kamada, N., 62
Kamholz, S. L., 234, 362, 763
Kamps, D., 781
Kauste, A., 626
Kennedy, M. S., 200, 404
Keown, P. A., 222, 479
Kerman, R. H., 77, 86, 253, 473, 653
Killeen, D., 740
King, H. P., 861
Kirkman, R. L., 673
Kirwan, P., 636
Klapwijk, W., 830
Klaus, G. G. B., 105
Klempnauer, J., 315, 785
Klimpel, G. R., 167
Klintmalm, G., 291, 599
Knierim, K., 795
Koegler, J., 222
Kondoh, Y., 118
Koumas, J. C., 853
Kovithavongs, T., 322
Kretschmer, G., 571
Kuhlbäck, B., 626
Kulkarni, A., 757
Kunelius, P., 626
Kunkl, A., 105
Kupiec-Weglinski, J. W., 141
Kuromoto, N., 757
Kuwabara, T., 148
Kwok, D., 218
Kyriakides, G. K., 734

Lacour-Gayet, F., 740
Lafferty, K. J., 26, 881
Laker, L., 776
Lakey, W. H., 322
Lalla, M., 626, 876
Lampainen, E., 626
Land, W., 210, 301, 483, 641
Lang, W., 370
Langer, B., 797, 816
Lannon, S. G., 319
Lauffenburger, A., 803
Laupacis, A., 532
LeGrue, S. J., 43
Leake, W. C., 698
Lear, P. A., 141
Leijala, E., 626
Leithner, C., 571
Lemaire, M., 203
Lewis, W. I., 665, 717
Leyssac, P. P., 520

Li, Z., 740
Liebert, M., 559
Lien, J., 297
Linfesty, R. L., 857
Linkola, A., 626
Loertscher, R., 605
Lokiec, F., 226, 412
Longerbeam, J. K., 795
Lossing, A. G., 797
Louw, G., 776
Ludwin, D., 297

MacDonald, A. S., 319
MacKenzie, G. H., 868
Mackenzie, R. D., 797, 816
Mackintosh, P., 307
Magnus, G., 744
Mah, B. J., 853
Maher, E. R., 630
Malatack, J. J., 366, 376
Maletic-Staschak, S., 914
Marquet, R. L., 737
Martin, D. C., 526
Masendycz, P., 861
Mason, D. W., 71
Matsumura, T., 82
Maurer, G., 193, 203
McCabe, R. E., 693
McCormick, P., 322
McDonald, R., Jr., 357
McKenzie, N., 222, 479
McMaster, P., 307, 538
McMichael, J., 222
Merion, R., 662
Merker, M., 49
Michael, J., 307, 538
Mihatsch, M. J., 503, 605
Milford, E. L., 673
Miller, A. M., 830
Miller, J., 734
Mirisklavos, A., 861
Mochizuki, M., 148
Mokhtarian, F., 55
Mollenkopf, F. P., 234, 362
Montefusco, C. M., 234, 362
Moody, F. G., xxi
Moon, D. K., 174
Morris, P. J., 71, 646
Mraz, W., 210
Muller, A., 503
Müller-Hermelink, H. K., 811
Müller-Ruchholtz, W., 770, 811
Myllyniemi, V. A., 626

Nachreiner, R. F., 788
Nagao, T., 62
Nagata, M., 723
Najarian, J. S., 247, 390, 620, 658, 665, 717, 744
Nehlsen-Cannarella, S. L., 234
Neild, G. H., 182, 566
Nelson, D. S., 174
Nemlander, A., 876
Neuhaus, P., 370
Newburger, J., 197
Ng, A., 636
Nickell, S. P., 55
Niederberger, W., 193, 203
Nissen, C., 401
Nomura, H., 285
Nordgren, S. R., 797, 816
Norin, A. J., 362, 763
Nowygrod, R., 757
Nussbaumer, K., 203
Nussenblatt, R. B., 95, 148, 698

Oberholzer, M., 605
Ochiai, T., 124, 723
Ohmori, Y., 82, 118, 285
Ohtsuka, M., 723
Oka, T., 82, 118, 285
Olivieri, V., 605
Olson, L., 734
Osato, M. S., 711, 865
Öst, L., 291
Osterwalder, B., 401
Oyer, P. E., 330

Padgett, G. A., 788
Painvin, G. A., 351
Pajunen, S., 626
Paldanius, R., 626
Palestine, A. G., 698
Palladino, M. A., 171
Palmer, S., 418
Parker, J. W., 160
Paull, P., 230
Payne, W. D., 86, 253
Pedrazzini, A., 408
Penn, I., 574
Perier, P., 740
Perlroth, M., 330
Perry, J., 740
Petric, R., 503
Pettersson, E., 626
Philosophe, B., 526, 857
Pichlmayr, R., 315, 370, 785
Pinsker, K. L., 362, 763
Pohanka, E., 571
Poirier, O., 226, 412
Pollard, C., 408
Poole, C., 408
Pouteil-Noble, C., 582
Powles, R. L., 408
Pozza, G., 386
Preis, D., 210
Press, B. H. J., 841
Puschett, J. B., 490

Rabin, B., 559
Raff, R. F., 826
Reem, G. H., 171
Reemtsma, K., 757
Reeves, R., 357
Reinherz, E. L., 673
Relander, A., 626
Remuzzi, G., 182
Revillon, Y., 803
Rice, J., 49
Ricour, C., 803
Ried, M., 218
Rinaldo, C. R., Jr., 559
Ringdén O., 291, 599
Rios, A., 157
Ritter, J., 582
Robinson, W. T., 187
Rocchi, G., 182
Rodger, R. S. C., 538
Roger, S., 307
Rogers, J. R., 269
Rolles, K., 662
Rook, A. H., 698
Roost, H., 740
Rosenthal, J. T., 243, 366, 557, 589, 865
Roussel, T. J., 711, 865
Rudolph, F., 751
Ryffel, B., 503, 605

Sakamoto, K., 124
Salmela, K., 626
Sanders, J. E., 404
Sanghvi, A., 541
Santos, G. W., 32, 127, 397, 707
Saral, R., 397
Sarelin, H., 626
Sato, H., 124, 723
Schack, T., 811
Schade, R. R., 366, 541
Schall, W. D., 788
Scheibel, L. W., 55
Scher, I., 698
Schlossman, S. F., 673
Schmeller, N., 301
Schmidt, C., 740
Schmidt, E., 370
Schneider, B., 301, 483
Schran, H. F., 187
Schulak, J. A., 753
Schulte, W. E., 107
Schwarz, M., 571
Schweitzer, B., 49
Secchi, A., 386

Sells, R. A., 279
Severns, E., 826
Shapiro, A. P., 357
Shaw, B. W., Jr., 243, 366, 376
Sheil, A. G. R., 269, 636
Shelby, J., 753
Shih, C. C.-Y., 178
Shinohara, N., 124
Shoemaker, P., 503
Shons, A. R., 841
Shulman, H., 404
Shumway, N. E., 330
Sibley, R. K., 620, 744, 841
Siebert, W., 210, 301
Siegl, H., 503
Signer, E., 401
Simmons, R. L., 247, 620, 658, 665
Simpson, J. G., 486, 496
Sinclair, N. R., 222
Sinzinger, H., 571
Smith, J. M., 206, 492
Sollinger, H. W., 781
Speck, B., 401
Spichtin, H. P., 605
Starklint, H., 520
Starzl, T. E., 243, 366, 376, 552, 557, 589, 887
Stawecki, M., 222
Steiniger, B., 785
Stephen, M. S., 269
Stewart, J. A., 837
Stewart, P., 404
Stiller, C. R., 222, 263, 274, 479, 797
Stinson, E. B., 330
Stock, S., 307
Stöcklin, E., 605
Storb, R., 200, 404, 826
Strand, M., 247
Strom, T. B., 141, 673
Sullivan, K. M., 404
Sutherland, D. E. R., 247, 381, 390, 620
Suzuki, S., 285
Suzuki, T., 723
Syré, G., 571

Talal, N., 683
Tao, L., 744
Tarssanen, L., 626
Taskinen, E., 626
Taylor, H. R., 592
Taylor, R. J., 589
Thiede, A., 770, 811
Thiel, G., 605
Thiru, S., 630
Thomas, E. D., 200, 404, 826
Thompson, J. F., 646
Thompson, M. E., 357, 490, 541, 563
Thomson, A. W., 174, 486
Tillegård, A., 291
Tiller, D. J., 269, 636
Tilney, N. L., 141, 673
Ting, A., 646
Toledo-Pereyra, L. H., 157, 868
Tonnesen, A. S., 514
Torhorst, J., 605
Touraine, J. L., 386, 582
Traeger, J., 386, 582
Truitt, R. L., 178
Turney, J. H., 307, 538
Tutschka, P. J., 32, 127, 397, 707, 819

Ulrichs, K., 770, 811
Usui, T., 82
Uyemura, K., 160

Vaiman, M., 803
Valentine, B. A., 592
Van Bekkum, D. W., 830
Van Buren, C. T., 77, 86, 218, 253, 312, 462, 473, 510, 653, 751
Van Thiel, D. H., 366, 541
Vanttinen, T., 626
Vartia, A., 626
Veith, F. J., 234, 362, 763
Viranta, M., 626
Vlassis, T., 307
von Willebrand, E., 500, 626, 876

Wagner, E., 785
Wagner, O., 203
Wajszczuk, C. P., 552, 557
Wakely, E., 753
Wall, W., 222
Wallace, A., C., 479
Wallwork, J., 343
Walma, E. P., 830
Walshaw, R., 788
Warner, T., 781
Warty, V., 541
Weimar, W., 737
Weinmann, E. J., 510, 514
Wenger, R., 14
Weyne, P., 803
Wheatley, D. N., 496
White, D. J. G., 62
White, J., 319
White, N., 297
Whiting, P. H., 486, 496
Wiktorowicz, K., 876
Wilczek, H., 291
Wilhelmus, K. R., 711, 865
Williams, D. G., 182, 566
Williams, M. D., 788
Witherspoon, R. P., 404
Wonigeit, K., 315, 370, 785
Wood, A. J., 193
Wood, R. F. M., 646
Woolfe-Coote, S., 776

Yamada, N., 723
Yasumura, T., 726
Yee, G. C., 200
Yin, J. L., 418
Yoshimura, N., 82, 118

Zink, R. A., 210, 301
Zitelli, B. J., 366, 376
Zollinger, H. U., 605
Zöttlein, H., 210, 301
Zuurmond, T., 776